MW01202127

Handbook of Research on Student Engagement

Amy L. Reschly • Sandra L. Christenson
Editors

Handbook of Research on Student Engagement

Second Edition

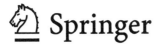 Springer

Editors
Amy L. Reschly
University of Georgia
Athens, GA, USA

Sandra L. Christenson
University of Minnesota
Minneapolis, MN, USA

ISBN 978-3-031-07852-1   ISBN 978-3-031-07853-8   (eBook)
https://doi.org/10.1007/978-3-031-07853-8

This Springer imprint is published by the registered company Springer Nature Switzerland AG
The registered company address is: Gewerbestrasse 11, 6330 Cham, Switzerland

Contents

Part IV   Measurement

About the Authors

Howard Adelman, PhD, is Professor of Psychology and co-director of the national Center for MH in Schools & Student/Learning Supports at the University of California, Los Angeles (UCLA, which operates under the auspices of the School Mental Health Project). He began his professional career as a remedial classroom teacher in 1960. In 1973, he returned to UCLA in the role of Professor of Psychology and also was the director of the Fernald School and Laboratory until 1986. Adelman and Linda Taylor have worked together for over 40 years with a constant focus on improving how schools and communities address barriers to learning and teaching, re-engage disconnected students, and promote healthy development. Over the years, they have led major projects focused on dropout prevention, enhancing the mental health facets of school-based health centers, and developing comprehensive, school-based approaches for students with learning, behavior, and emotional problems. Their work has involved them in schools and communities across the country. Their present focus is on policies, practices, and large-scale systemic transformation. This work includes facilitating the National Initiative for Transforming Student and Learning Supports.

Kelly-Ann Allen, PhD FAPS, is an educational and developmental psychologist, a senior lecturer at the Faculty of Education, Monash University, and an honorary senior fellow at the Centre for Wellbeing Science, University of Melbourne. She is also the co-director and founder of the Global Belonging Collaborative, which represents a consortium of belonging researchers and advocates from around the world. Dr. Allen is the Editor-in-Chief of *The Educational and Developmental Psychologist* and both the present and founding Co-Editor-in-Chief of the *Journal of Belonging and Human Connection*. She holds the esteemed grade of Fellow for both the Australian Psychological Society and the College of Educational and Developmental Psychologists.

Eric M. Anderman is Professor of Educational Psychology and of Quantitative Research, Evaluation, and Measurement in the College of Education and Human Ecology, Ohio State University. He received his PhD in Educational Psychology from the University of Michigan, and he also holds a Master's degree from Harvard University. Before attending graduate school, he worked as a middle school and high school teacher. His research over the past 25 years has focused on academic motivation, focusing in particular on the relations between motivation and (a) academic integrity and (b) adolescent risk-taking behavior. His research has been funded by the National Institutes of Health, the Institute of Education Sciences, and the Department of Health & Human Services Office of Population Affairs. He is a fellow of both the American Psychological Association and the American Educational Research Association. He is the editor of the journal *Theory into Practice*, and he co-edited the 3rd edition of the *Handbook of Educational Psychology*, and the *Visible Learning Guide to Student Achievement* with John Hattie. He is the co-author of three text books, as well as over 100 peer-reviewed articles and invited chapters. His research has been featured in numerous media outlets, including CBS News, NBC News (Dateline NBC), CNN, NPR, *The Huffington Post*, *The Wall Street Journal*, *New York* magazine, and numerous other outlets.

Isabelle Archambault holds the Canada Research Chair on school, youth well-being, and educational success, and is co-holder of the Myriagone McConnell-UdM (Université de Montréal) Chair in youth knowledge mobilization. Her work focuses on the differential effects of school or its practices on the engagement, well-being, and educational success of youth from vulnerable populations.

Robert W. Balfanz is a research professor at Johns Hopkins University School of Education, the director of the Everyone Graduates Center, and a co-director of the Center for Social Organization of Schools. He publishes and leads technical assistance efforts on secondary school reform, early warning systems, chronic absenteeism, social-emotional learning, and instructional improvements in high-poverty schools, and focuses on translating research findings into effective school improvement strategies and interventions.

Janine Bempechat is a clinical professor at Boston University Wheelock College of Education & Human Development. She is a developmental psychologist with a deep interest in the socialization of achievement. She studies family, cultural, and school influences in the development of student motivation and academic achievement in low-income children and youth, both nationally and cross-nationally. A former National Academic of Education Spencer Fellow, her research has been supported by the Spencer Foundation and the William T. Grant Foundation.

Joe Betts, PhD, EdS, MMIS, is the Director of Measurement and Testing at the National Council of State Boards of Nursing (NCSBN). Dr. Betts has been involved in the fields of psychology and measurement for over two decades. He has a unique view of testing and measurement as a user of psychological and educational assessments, and the test development side with respect to educational, psychological, and clinical assessments, and new product R&D. Additionally, he has worked in a managerial and directorial role for over a decade leading operational and research teams with HMH, Riverside Assessments, Pearson, and NCSBN. In addition, he has had his research published in a number of diverse areas along with over 100 professional presentations. He has contributed over a decade to service on professional journals as an associate editorial board member, editorial advisory board member, and editorial board member for a number of professional publications. In addition to working in the area of engagement, his research focuses on advanced polytomous models for computerized adaptive testing and the measurement of clinical judgment in entry-level nursing.

Christopher Boyle, BSc (Hons), MSc, BA, PGCE, MSc EdPsych, PhD, is Professor of Inclusive Education and Educational Psychology at the University of Adelaide, Australia. He is a fellow of the British Psychological Society and a senior fellow of the Higher Education Academy. Chris was previously Editor-in-Chief of *The Educational and Developmental Psychologist* (2012–2017) and is the co-inaugural founding editor of *Belonging and Human Connection* (with Kelly-Ann Allen) launched in 2022. He recently co-edited *Research for Sustainable Quality Education: Inclusion, Belonging, and Equity* (2022, Springer Nature).

Tara M. Brown is Associate Professor in the Urban Education specialization at the University of Maryland, College Park. Tara's research focuses on how disciplinary exclusion, high school non-completion, and involvement with the criminal legal system impact the experiences of Black and Latinx adolescents and young adults in low-income, urban communities. She specializes in qualitative, community-based, and participatory action research (PAR) methodologies.

Kristen L. Bub is a professor and coordinator of the Applied Cognition and Development program in the Department of Educational Psychology, University of Georgia. Her research interests include social-emotional development, early education, and research methods. Her research lies at the intersection of development and learning and aims to understand the processes by which young children's cognitive and behavioral regulation skills develop. Her work also centers on evaluating the impact of these skills on subsequent learning outcomes among understudied and at-risk populations of children to develop prevention/intervention programs and to inform policy for young children.

Matthew K. Burns is the College of Education Herbert H. Schooling Professor and Professor of Special Education at the University of Missouri. He is also the director of the Center for Collaborative Solutions for Kids, Practice, and Policy, and interim co-director of the Missouri Partnership for Educational Renewal. Dr. Burns's research interests include the use of assessment data to determine individual or small-group interventions, response to intervention, academic interventions, and facilitating problem-solving teams. He received the 2020 Senior Scientist Award from Division 16 (School Psychology) of the American Psychological Association.

Chun Chen is an Assistant Professor in Applied Psychology in the School of Humanities and Social Science at the Chinese University of Hong Kong - Shenzhen. She previously graduated from the Counseling, Clinical, and School Psychology program at the University of California, Santa Barbara. Grounded in the social-ecological context, her research interests focus on identifying risk and resilience factors (e.g., social-emotional learning competencies, school climate, childhood trauma, bullying and victimization) in school functioning and mental health development (e.g., Internet addiction) among marginalized and minority students around the world.

Sandra L. Christenson is Professor Emeritus in the Department of Educational Psychology, University of Minnesota, and continues to research interventions that enhance engagement at school and with learning for marginalized students with and without disabilities. She has been a principal investigator on several federally funded projects in the areas of dropout prevention and family-school partnerships, including Check & Connect, which is in its 32nd year of research and implementation. Recently she co-edited the books *Student Engagement: Effective Academic, Behavioral, Cognitive, and Affective Interventions at School* and the *Handbook of Student Engagement Interventions*.

Timothy J. Cleary, PhD, is a professor in the Graduate School of Applied and Professional Psychology (GSAPP), Rutgers University. His primary research interests include the development and application of self-regulated learning (SRL) and motivation assessment and intervention practices across academic, athletic, medical, and clinical contexts. He has had his research published in over 65 peer-review journal articles, book chapters, and books addressing SRL-related principles and practices. Dr. Cleary has received extensive extramural grant funding as a principal investigator (PI) and co-PI throughout his career, with total funding over $13 million. His work has been supported by the National Science Foundation (NSF), Institute of Education Sciences (IES), Department of Education's Fund for the Improvement of Postsecondary Education, Spencer Foundation, and others. Dr. Cleary teaches doctoral courses in learning theory, academic interventions, and statistics.

Christa B. Copeland is a postdoctoral research fellow at the Missouri Prevention Science Institute, University of Missouri. She is a former K-12 educator with training and experience in the areas of school psychology, educational leadership, and teaching. Her work centers on school capacity-building to effectively meet the social, emotional, and behavioral needs of all students, with a focus on traditionally underserved youth.

Maddie Cordle, MS, is a doctoral candidate in the Minnesota State University, Mankato School Psychology program. She also serves as a university doctoral assistant in School Psychology and Treasurer of the School Psychology Society. Her research interests include school-based behavioral interventions, and she is conducting her dissertation research, which focuses on the behavioral intervention *Class Pass*.

Marcia H. Davis is an associate professor in the School of Education, Johns Hopkins University, and a co-director of the Center for Social Organization of Schools. She teaches courses in mixed methods and evaluation in the Doctor of Education (EdD) degree program. She has conducted research on a range of topics that include supporting struggling adolescent readers, measurement of adolescent reading motivation, and the use of early warning indicators and systems for dropout prevention.

Maria K. DiBenedetto's doctorate is in Educational Psychology from the City University of New York Graduate Center. Her research is focused on self-regulated learning, motivation, self-efficacy, and assessment. Her microanalytic study was the first study to test Zimmerman and Schunk's three phases of self-regulated learning on an academic task. Dr. DiBenedetto works at the Bryan School of Business and Economics, University of North Carolina at Greensboro (UNCG) as a lecturer and Director of Assessment and Reporting, where she oversees assurance of learning for reaccreditation of the business school. Dr. DiBenedetto also teaches preservice teachers as an adjunct at UNCG's School of Education. In addition to several chapters and articles, she has had two books published and does consulting for schools, testing services, and publishers of books focused on student learning throughout the country. Dr. DiBenedetto is collaborating on an interactive research methods textbook for educators in addition to consulting for the Institute of Education Services. She is also a practicing educational therapist, where she applies self-regulated learning skills and strategies to help students succeed in college.

Véronique Dupéré is Associate Professor in Educational Psychology at the *Université de Montréal* (École de psychoéducation), Canada. Her work focuses on adolescent and young adult development in contrasted contexts, and on preventive approaches aimed at reducing educational gaps between children and youth living in disadvantaged communities and their more advantaged peers.

Jacquelynne S. Eccles is a Distinguished Professor of Education at the University of California, Irvine, and formerly the McKeachie/Pintrich Distinguished University Professor of Psychology and Education at the University of Michigan, as well as a senior research scientist and Director of the Gender and Achievement Research Program at the Institute for Social Research, University of Michigan. Professor Eccles has conducted research on a wide variety of topics, including gender-role socialization, teacher expectancies, classroom influences on student motivation, and social development in the family and school context. Her expectancy-value theory of motivation and her concept of stage-environment have served as perhaps the most dominant models of achievement during the school years. Professor Eccles's awards include the Kurt Lewin Memorial Award for "outstanding contributions to the development and integration of psychological research and social action" from the Society for the Psychological Study of Social Issues; lifetime achievement awards from Society for Research on Adolescence (SRA), Division 15 of the American Psychological Association (APA), the American Psychological Society, the Society for the Study of Human Development, and the Self Society; the Bronfenbrenner Award for Research from Division 7 of the APA; the APA Lifetime Award for Service in Supporting Psychological Research; and the APA Gold Medal Award for Life Achievement in Psychology in the Public Interest. Email: jseccles@uci.edu

Guadalupe Espinoza, PhD, is an associate professor in the Child and Adolescent Studies Department, California State University, Fullerton. Her research interests primarily center on how adolescents' peer relationships (e.g., bullying, cyber victimization) shape their psychosocial and school adjustment, particularly among Latino youth.

Elyse M. Farnsworth, PhD, is an assistant professor in the Department of Psychology and School Psychology doctoral training program, Minnesota State University, Mankato. Dr. Farnsworth obtained her PhD in Educational Psychology from the University of Minnesota School Psychology program and is credentialed as a licensed psychologist in Minnesota and a Nationally Certified School Psychologist. She has worked in urban, suburban, and rural school districts, providing school psychological services. She serves on the editorial review board for *Psychology in the Schools* and serves as an ad hoc reviewer *for Perspectives in Early Childhood Psychology and Education*. Dr. Farnsworth's research team examines how public policy, academic enablers (e.g., hope and student engagement), and early intervention influence school-based cognitive and non-cognitive outcomes for PK-12 students.

Jennifer A. Fredricks is Dean of Academic Departments and Programs, and Professor of Psychology at Union College. She has had her research published in over 60 peer-reviewed articles on student engagement, motivation, parental socialization, and out-of-school activity participation. She is the author of *Eight Myths of Student Engagement: Creating Classrooms of Deep Learning* (2014) and co-editor of the *Handbook of Student Engagement Interventions: Working with Disengaged Youth* (2019) with Amy Reschly and Sandra Christenson.

Claudia L. Galindo is an associate professor in the Education Policy program at the University of Maryland, College Park. Her research examines racial/ethnic minority and poor students' academic outcomes and school experiences, paying particular attention to Latina and immigrant populations. Her research also investigates key mechanisms in families and schools that may perpetuate or ameliorate inequalities. She teaches courses related to sociology of education and research methodologies.

Sarah Gillespie is a doctoral student in Developmental Psychology at the Institute of Child Development, University of Minnesota. She studies ethnic-racial identity development and critical consciousness among adolescents and factors that promote resilience in the context of immigration, globalization, and multicultural societies. She also studies digital and school-based interventions to promote mental and physical well-being.

Jessica R. Gladstone is a postdoctoral fellow at the Department of Foundations of Education, Virginia Commonwealth University. In her research she programmatically examines students' STEM motivation, engagement, and self-regulation through three lines of research: (1) How do important socializers (i.e., parents, teachers, peers, role models) impact students' motivation and engagement in STEM? (2) How do motivation and engagement relate over time to predict students' STEM achievement? (3) A critical analysis of how students' STEM self-regulation, motivation, engagement, and achievement relate to the construct grit. Email: gladstonejr@vcu.edu

Amy Jane Griffiths is a licensed psychologist and a Nationally Certified School Psychologist. Dr. Griffiths is an assistant professor at the Attallah College of Educational Studies. Her scholarly and research interests are focused on preparing children from underserved populations for resilient futures.

Ariana Groen, MA, has a Master's in Clinical and Counseling Psychology and is a doctoral student at the Minnesota State University, Mankato School Psychology program. Ariana also serves as an instructor for undergraduate psychology courses at Minnesota State University, Mankato, is President of the School Psychology Society, and has extensive applied clinical and school experience. Her research interests include school neuropsychology, school-based mental health, and the promotion of positive school climate through equity, diversity, and inclusion for all students.

Seung Yon Ha is an educational psychologist with a background in educational intervention and evaluation. She received her PhD and postdoctoral training from The Ohio State University. She uses quantitative and mixed methodologies, and her current research focuses on adolescent academic and social development through culturally responsive educational support.

Keith C. Herman is a Curator's Distinguished Professor in the Department of Education, School, & Counseling Psychology, University of Missouri. He is the co-founder and co-director of the Missouri Prevention Science Institute. He has an extensive grant and publication record, including over 160 peer-reviewed publications in the areas of prevention and early intervention of child emotional and behavior disturbances and culturally sensitive educational interventions.

Tara L. Hofkens, PhD, is a research assistant professor at the Center for the Advanced Study of Teaching and Learning, School of Education and Human Development, University of Virginia. Her research examines how teacher-student relationships and interactions contribute to educational trajectories and well-being from early childhood through adolescence. Specifically, she applies an interdisciplinary perspective that incorporates research from applied developmental science, learning science, and stress physiology to study the dynamics of engagement and social interactions in school, and how instruction and classroom experiences contribute to achievement and educational trajectories from early childhood through adolescence.

Benjamin J. Houltberg is the CEO and President of Search Institute. He is a developmental scientist, former tenured faculty member, and experienced licensed marriage and family therapist. His work is widely published in topics such as the socialization of adolescent emotion regulation, promoting resilience through adversity, and character and identity development in sports. Ben has a strong record of procuring grant funding and leading interdisciplinary research teams. His motivation to pursue his doctoral degree emerged from his clinical experience in schools and desire to empower youth facing tremendous adversity due to socio-economic disadvantage and marginalization. As a result, he is passionate about linking research insights with practitioner wisdom to have maximum impact on the lives of youth.

Hyungshim Jang is a professor at the Department of Education, Hanyang University, Seoul, Korea. She received her PhD from the University of Iowa, USA. Her research focuses on how teachers' dual provision of both structure and autonomy support contributes constructively to students' motivation, engagement, achievement, and well-being. Her work uses a variety of methodologies and has appeared in journals such as the *Journal of Educational Psychology* and *Contemporary Educational Psychology*.

Michel Janosz Professor at the School of Psychoeducation at the University of Montreal and Dean of the Faculty of Continuing Education, is an internationally recognized scholar on the development and the prevention of youth psychosocial adjustment. A fellow of the Royal Society of Canada, he is mostly renowned for his research and knowledge mobilization activities regarding school improvement and effectiveness, school dropout, and student violence. He is regularly consulted by policymakers and administrators in education and public health.

Shane R. Jimerson is a professor at the Gevirtz Graduate School of Education, University of California, Santa Barbara. Dr. Jimerson is a Nationally Certified School Psychologist and recognized by the American Academy of Experts in Traumatic Stress as a Board Certified Expert and Diplomat, and is included in their international registry of Experts in Traumatic Stress, with specialization in working with children, families, and schools. His international professional and scholarly activities aim to advance and promote science, practice, and policy relevant to education and school psychology, in an effort to benefit children, families, and communities across the country and throughout the world.

Jaana Juvonen, PhD, is a professor in the Department of Psychology, University of California, Los Angeles. Her research examines peer relationships and social experiences (e.g., friendships, bullying) in adolescence. Most of her studies focus on school context.

Casey A. Knifsend, PhD, is an associate professor in the Department of Psychology, California State University, Sacramento. Her research interests include examining how extracurricular activities (e.g., sports, clubs) are linked with academic success and psychosocial well-being during adolescence and emerging adulthood.

Justine H. Lee is a postdoctoral fellow at the University of Maryland, College Park, where she obtained a PhD from the Department of Teaching and Learning, Policy and Curriculum. Her scholarship examines the intersections of race, class, and gender in school-based curriculum and educational policy.

Lisa Linnenbrink-Garcia is Professor of Educational Psychology in the Department of Counseling, Educational Psychology, and Special Education, Michigan State University, and a fellow of the American Psychological Association. She obtained her PhD in Education and Psychology from the University of Michigan, Ann Arbor. Dr. Linnenbrink-Garcia's research focuses on the development of achievement motivation in school settings and the interplay among motivation, emotions, and learning, especially in the domains of science, engineering, and mathematics.

Angela M. Lui, PhD, is a research project manager for the Diagnostic Assessment and Achievement of College Skills (DAACS) (daacs.net) at the CUNY School of Professional Studies. DAACS is an Institute of Education Sciences (IES) grant-funded project that aims to improve college students' retention and academic success. Dr. Lui has conducted research on classroom assessment, responses to feedback, self-regulated learning, and the quality of assessments and instruments.

Andrew J. Martin, PhD, is Scientia Professor, Professor of Educational Psychology, and Chair of the Educational Psychology Research Group at the School of Education, University of New South Wales, Australia. He specializes in student motivation, engagement, achievement, and quantitative research methods.

Ann S. Masten is a Regents Professor at the Institute of Child Development, University of Minnesota. She studies resilience in human development, particularly in the context of homelessness, poverty, war, disaster, and migration. Dr. Masten is a past President of the Society for Research in Child Development, recipient of numerous honors, and author of more than 200 publications, including the book *Ordinary Magic: Resilience in Development*. She offers a free Massive Open Online Course (MOOC) on "Resilience in Children Exposed to Trauma, Disaster and War" taken by thousands of participants from over 180 countries.

Kayla M. Nelson is a doctoral student in Developmental Psychopathology and Clinical Science at the Institute of Child Development, University of Minnesota. She studies models of risk and resilience for development and well-being during adolescence, specifically the role of the family system in promoting resilience during this period of development. She also studies the development and trajectory of depression and other internalizing disorders during adolescence.

Stacey Neuharth-Pritchett is Professor of Educational Psychology and Associate Dean for Academic Programs, with research interests that center on the contexts of early educational intervention, children's transition to school (particularly the Head Start population), and intervention for children with chronic health problems. She has served as the principal investigator and co-investigator on a number of externally funded research projects on Head Start, early literacy, and teacher quality. She teaches courses in educational research methodology, applied educational measurement, and seminars on psychological issues for young children placed at risk. She is a Distinguished Scholar at the Owens Institute for Behavioral Research, University of Georgia.

Elizabeth Olivier is an assistant professor at Université de Montréal. Her research focuses on the impact of teaching practices and student mental health on school motivation, engagement, and success.

Janise Parker, PhD, is an assistant professor and university practicum coordinator in the School Psychology program, William & Mary. She received her PhD in School Psychology from the University of Florida in 2015. She is a licensed psychologist in the states of Florida and Virginia and a Nationally Certified School Psychologist. Dr. Parker also provides and supervises school-based mental health services to youth in the Hampton Roads area of Virginia. Her research focuses on (a) culturally responsive mental and behavioral health services, (b) sociocultural contexts and positive Black youth development, and (c) social-emotional and behavioral health implications for serving religiously and spiritually diverse youth from marginalized backgrounds.

Helen Patrick, PhD, is a professor of educational psychology in the College of Education at Purdue University, USA. Her research includes associations of classroom contexts and teacher practices with student motivation, engagement, and achievement.

Kent Pekel, EdD, is an educational leader who has worked at the school, district, state, federal, and university levels. Throughout his diverse career, he has sought to bridge research, practice, and policy to help all young people thrive. Pekel is the Superintendent of the growing and increasingly diverse urban school district in Rochester, Minnesota, the home of the Mayo Clinic. Prior to joining Rochester Public Schools, Dr. Pekel spent 9 years as President and CEO of Search Institute. During his tenure at Search Institute, Dr. Pekel led the design of the Developmental Relationships Framework, which is now being used across the United States and around the world to build positive and powerful connections between young people and adults in schools, out-of-school time programs, and other settings. Prior to joining Search Institute in 2012, Dr. Pekel led the College Readiness Consortium at the University of Minnesota and served as a K-12 teacher and administrator.

Reinhard Pekrun is Professor of Psychology at the University of Essex, UK, and a professorial fellow at the Institute of Positive Psychology and Education, Australian Catholic University, Sydney, Australia. He is a highly cited scientist who pioneered research on emotions in education, originated the Control-Value Theory of Achievement Emotions, and has more than 350 published books, articles, and chapters to his credit.

Robert C. Pianta, PhD, is Dean of the UVA School of Education and Human Development, Batten Bicentennial Professor of Early Childhood Education, Professor of Psychology, and founding director of the Center for Advanced Study of Teaching and Learning at the University of Virginia. Dr. Pianta's research and policy interests focus on the intersection of education and human development. In particular, his work has been influential in advancing the conceptualization of teacher-student interactions and relationships, and documenting their contributions to students' learning and development. He has authored or co-authored more than 300 articles, 50 chapters, and 10 books, and led research and training grants totaling over $60 million. Dr. Pianta has led research and development on measurement and improvement tools that help teachers interact with students more effectively. He is past editor of the *Journal of School Psychology* and associate editor of *AERA Open*. An internationally recognized expert in both early childhood education and K-12 teaching and learning, Dr. Pianta regularly consults with federal agencies, foundations, universities, and governments. He was named a fellow of the American Education Research Association and received the Distinguished Alumni Award from the University of Minnesota in 2016, and his scholarly accomplishments led to his election to the National Academy of Education.

Hannah J. Puttre is a doctoral student at the Boston University Wheelock College of Education and Human Development studying Applied Human Development. She is a recipient of a National Science Foundation Graduate Research Fellowship and her research interests broadly focus on informal learning and how to capitalize on everyday learning opportunities and children's inherent curiosities in early STEM learning, as well as the practical applications of these types of research.

Kristen E. Raine is a doctoral student in Applied Developmental Psychology at Portland State University. Her research interests primarily concern the reciprocal relationship between interpersonal contexts and children's academic coping, and how this shapes students' motivational resilience, including their engagement, re-engagement, and persistence, in school settings. She is also interested in how these dynamic systems between social partners are embedded in higher-order contexts, and how to improve structural conditions to promote healthy family and academic functioning.

Johnmarshall Reeve is a professor at the Institute for Positive Psychology and Education, Australian Catholic University in Sydney, Australia. He received his PhD from Texas Christian University and completed postdoctoral work at the University of Rochester. His research focuses on all aspects of human motivation and emotion, but mostly on autonomy-supportive teaching, students' agentic engagement, and the neuroscience of intrinsic motivation. He has had his research published in 86 articles in peer-reviewed journals such as the *Journal of Educational Psychology* and authored four books, including *Understanding Motivation and Emotion and Supporting Students' Motivation* (February 2022). Prof. Reeve served as the Editor-in-Chief of the journal *Motivation and Emotion* (2011–2017). Additional information is available at http://www.johnmarshallreeve.org

Wendy M. Reinke is a Curator's Distinguished Professor in the Department of Education, School, & Counseling Psychology, University of Missouri. She is a co-founder and co-director of the Missouri Prevention Science Institute. She has an extensive grant and publication record, including over 130 peer-reviewed publications in the area of prevention and intervention of social emotional and behavior challenges among children and youth, teacher consultation, classroom management, and school mental health.

Amy L. Reschly, PhD, is a professor and Department Head of Educational Psychology at the University of Georgia. Her scholarly work focuses on student engagement, dropout prevention, and working with families to promote student success. She co-edited the *Handbook of Student Engagement Interventions* and *Student Engagement: Effective Academic, Behavioral, Cognitive, and Affective Interventions at School.*

Katariina Salmela-Aro is an academy professor at the Faculty of Educational Sciences, University of Helsinki, Finland, and visiting professor at the Institute of Education, University College London, UK, and Michigan State University, USA. She received her doctorate in Psychology from the University of Helsinki. She is President-Elect of International Association of Applied Psychology (IAAP) (Division 5). Her major interest includes longitudinal studies, motivation, engagement, burnout, well-being, and educational transitions.

Peter C. Scales, PhD, is a developmental psychologist internationally known for his research and writing in positive youth development, developmental assets, and developmental relationships, and is the senior fellow for Search Institute, where he has conducted studies in more than 30 countries worldwide. Over his nearly 50-year career, Dr. Scales has been committed to promoting equitable thriving for all children and youth, through his work as a researcher, direct youth and family services provider, sought-after youth advocate and speaker, and adviser to national youth organizations, foundations, media, and local, state, and federal policymakers. He has more than 250 published books, book chapters, peer-reviewed papers, articles in the popular press, and other publications to his credit, and served as a reviewer or consulting editor for dozens of journals. His most recent work has focused on how student-teacher relationships contribute to school success, and how coaches can help student-athletes maintain mental and emotional wellness while competing at their personal best level in sports. Dr. Scales also works with youth directly as a US Professional Tennis Association-certified tennis teaching pro and long-time high school tennis coach of both boys and girls teams. His mental-emotional game advice column appears regularly in *Racquet Sports Industry* magazine.

Dale H. Schunk is a professor at the Department of Teacher Education and Higher Education, School of Education, University of North Carolina (UNC) at Greensboro. From 2001 to 2011 he served as Dean of the School of Education. He received his PhD in Educational Psychology from Stanford University. Previously he was a faculty member at the University of Houston and the University of North Carolina at Chapel Hill. Prior to his move to UNC Greensboro in 2001 he was Head of the Department of Educational Studies at Purdue University. His research focuses on the effects of social and instructional factors on students' cognitive processes, learning, self-regulation, and motivation, with special emphasis on the application of social cognitive theory. He teaches graduate courses in learning, motivation, and educational psychology, and undergraduate courses in educational psychology and self-regulated learning. He has over 120 published articles and chapters to his credit, is the author of *Learning Theories: An Educational Perspective* (8th edition) and (with Judith Meece and Paul Pintrich) *Motivation in Education: Theories, Research, and Applications* (4th edition), and has edited 12 books on self-regulation and motivation. His awards include the Barry J. Zimmerman Award for Outstanding Contributions from the American Educational Research Association Studying and Self-Regulated Learning Special Interest Group, the Senior Distinguished Research Scholar Award from the University of North Carolina at Greensboro School of Education, the Distinguished Service Award from the Purdue University School of Education, the Early Contributions Award in Educational Psychology from the American Psychological Association, and the Albert J. Harris Research Award from the International Reading Association. He is listed in "Who's Who in America."

David J. Shernoff, PhD, is director of the Center for Mathematics, Science, and Computer Education (CMSCE) and an associate professor in the Department of School Psychology, Graduate School of Applied and Professional Psychology, Rutgers University. He conducts applied research in schools, universities, after-school settings, technology-supported environments, teacher professional development settings, and other learning environments. His research interests are in student engagement, flow, relationships, mentoring, integrative STEM, STEAM, and maker education.

Ellen A. Skinner is a leading expert on the development of children's motivation, coping, and academic identity in school. She is a professor in the Psychology Department, Portland State University, Portland, Oregon. As part of Psychology's concentration in Developmental Science and Education, her research explores ways to promote students' constructive coping, ongoing classroom engagement (marked by hard work, interest, and enthusiasm), and perseverance in the face of obstacles and setbacks. She is especially focused on two ingredients that shape motivational resilience: (1) close relationships with teachers, parents, and peers; and (2) academic work that is authentic and intrinsically motivating.

Crystal L. Spring is a doctoral student at the School of Education, Johns Hopkins University. Her research interests include classroom discussion in middle and high school classrooms, engagement and motivation in English Language Arts, and school culture.

Mallory A. Stevens is a fourth-year doctoral candidate in the School Psychology program at the University of Missouri. Her research and practice interests include evaluating evidence-based reading interventions and whether they meet the unique needs of students with intellectual and developmental disabilities.

Shannon M. Suldo, PhD, is a professor and Director of Clinical Training in the School Psychology program at the University of South Florida. She received her PhD in School Psychology from the University of South Carolina in 2004. She is a licensed psychologist in the state of Florida, and provides and supervises school-based mental health services to youth in the Tampa area. Her research involves conceptualizing and measuring student mental health in a dual-factor model that considers psychopathology and well-being, and evidence-based positive psychology interventions for promoting positive indicators of student well-being.

Xin Tang, PhD, Docent (Associate Professor), is a university researcher at the Faculty of Educational Sciences, University of Helsinki, Finland. He received his doctorate in Psychology from the University of Jyväskylä, Finland, in 2017. His research interests include motivation, engagement, social emotional skills (e.g., grit and curiosity), academic well-being, and classroom practices. He has expertise in advanced statistical methods (e.g., mixture modeling, growth modeling, network analysis) and conducted research using longitudinal data and experience sampling data.

Linda Taylor, PhD, is co-director of the national Center for MH in Schools & Student/Learning Supports at the University of California, Los Angeles (UCLA, which operates under the auspices of the School Mental Health Project). In her early career, Linda was involved in community agency work. From 1973 to 1986, she co-directed the Fernald Laboratory School and Clinic at UCLA. In 1986, she became co-director of the School Mental Health Project. From 1986 to 2000, she also held a clinical psychologist position in the Los Angeles Unified School District and directed several large-scale projects for the school district. Taylor and Howard Adelman have worked together for over 40 years with a constant focus on improving how schools and communities address barriers to learning and teaching, reengage disconnected students, and promote healthy development. Over the years, they have led major projects focused on dropout prevention, enhancing the mental health facets of school-based health centers, and developing comprehensive, school-based approaches for students with learning, behavior, and emotional problems. Their work has involved them in schools and communities across the country. Their focus is on policies, practices, and large-scale systemic transformation. This work includes facilitating the National Initiative for Transforming Student and Learning Supports.

Vincent Tinto is Distinguished University Professor Emeritus at Syracuse University and the former Chair of the Higher Education program. He has carried out research and written extensively on student persistence and the actions institutions can take to promote student success. His book *Leaving College* lays out a theory and policy perspective on student success that is considered the benchmark by which work on these issues are judged. His book *Completing College* lays out a framework for institutional action for student success, describes the range of programs that have been effective in enhancing student success, and the types of policies institutions should follow to successfully implement programs in ways that endure and scale up over time. His most recent work explores what is learned about persistence and policies to address it when seen through the eyes of students. Doing so opens other areas where institutional action can promote student success. Dr. Tinto has received numerous recognitions and awards and has spoken widely throughout the United States, Europe, South America, Australia, and New Zealand. He has worked with a number of organizations, foundations, and government agencies on issues of student success and has sat on a number of advisory boards, including the Community College Survey of Student Engagement, the Bill and Melinda Gates Foundation, and the Lumina Foundation.

Christopher Tran is a practicing K-12 school psychologist. He is pursuing a doctoral degree in Education at Chapman University. His research interests revolve around the impact of youth incarceration on student outcomes.

Katja Upadyaya, PhD, is an associate professor at the Faculty of Educational Sciences, University of Helsinki, Finland. Her research interests include student engagement, academic motivation, research methodology, and lifelong learning. She is also interested in conducting research on teacher-student and parent-child interaction, and teachers' and school principals' well-being. She is conducting research on students' situational experiences while learning, socio-emotional skills, and parental burnout.

Rachel Wiegand is a third-year EdS student, an Licensed Professional Clinical Counselor (LPCC) trainee, and a Warne scholar in the School Psychology program at Chapman University. Her research interests include school-based mental health and developing trauma-informed interventions and practices.

Allan Wigfield is Professor Emeritus in the Department of Human Development and Quantitative Methodology, and also Distinguished Scholar-Teacher at the University of Maryland. Dr. Wigfield has authored more than 160 peer-reviewed journal articles and book chapters on the development of children's motivation and how to improve it. He also has edited six scholarly books and seven special issues of journals devoted to the understanding of students' motivation. Dr. Wigfield has won numerous awards for his research, including most recently the 2019 Sylvia Scribner Award from Division C of the American Educational Research Association. His work has been cited over 85,000 times. Email: awigfiel@umd.edu

Shira Wolff is a doctoral candidate in School Psychology at Rutgers Graduate School of Applied and Professional Psychology. Her research interests focus on human development, specifically identity formation and parental impacts. Clinically, Shira plans to have a career in family and couples counseling.

Cathy Wylie is a chief researcher with the New Zealand Council for Educational Research. Her recent research has focused on school leadership, and the relationships between policy and school capability to engage students in productive learning. She was a member of the New Zealand government's 2018–2019 independent taskforce to review its schooling system. She was a co-editor and contributor to the first *Handbook of Research on Student Engagement*.

James Ysseldyke is an Emeritus Birkmaier Professor of Educational Leadership in the School Psychology program, Department of Educational Psychology, University of Minnesota. He has directed multiple national centers and conducted extensive research in a number of areas, including identifying specific learning disabilities, assessing and modifying instructional environments, and school-based accountability testing. He is a fellow in multiple divisions of the American Psychological Association, and received the 2009 Council for Exceptional Children, J. E. Wallace Wallin Lifetime Achievement Award.

Part I

Defining Student Engagement: Models and Related Constructs

Jingle-Jangle Revisited: History and Further Evolution of the Student Engagement Construct

Amy L. Reschly and Sandra L. Christenson

Abstract

This chapter describes the history and evolution of the student engagement construct, with origins in time-on-task, high school dropout, and school reform to its current status as a meta-construct and framework for interventions to promote positive outcomes among youth. We review and compare three integrative models of student engagement: the Check & Connect Model of Student Engagement, the Development-in-Sociocultural-Context Model, and the Study Demands Resources Model of Student Engagement and Burnout. We reflect on the status of prominent issues in the field—jingle-jangle; motivation and engagement; and, the continuum vs. continua of engagement and disengagement/disaffection—and identify enduring themes and directions for the study of student engagement.

What Is Student Engagement?

We are often struck by the overwhelming acknowledgment/agreement/understanding of the importance of student engagement to learning and the everyday experience of schooling—we *know* when students are engaged or disengaged at school and with learning. Yet, when asked about what student engagement is, beyond, *I know it when I see it*, answers often center on student behavior, typically in terms of participation (e.g., showing up at school, paying attention), and include something about how students feel or think (e.g., we perceive that the student wants to be there, enjoys learning). It is here, from the universality of student engagement to the operationalization of the construct, that things get messy.

The first comprehensive review of the student engagement literature was published almost 40 years ago (i.e., Mosher & McGowan, 1985). The authors concluded, "What is meant by student engagement was (and continues to be) less than clear" (p. 12). They found little in terms of definitions or even published work on the topic and yet, the impetus to conduct such a review is evidence then, as now, of the clear importance of student engagement to those who work with students and its role in accomplishing the goals of schooling.

The question, *what is student engagement?*, is one that we and other scholars sought to address in the first edition of this *Handbook* (Christenson

A. L. Reschly (✉)
University of Georgia, Athens, GA, USA
e-mail: reschly@uga.edu

S. L. Christenson
University of Minnesota, Minneapolis, MN, USA
e-mail: chris002@umn.edu

et al., 2012; Reschly & Christenson, 2012). After careful consideration of the work in that volume, we offered the following definition:

> Student engagement refers to the student's active participation in academic and co-curricular or school-related activities and commitment to educational goals and learning. Engaged students find learning meaningful and are invested in their learning and future. It is a multidimensional construct that consists of behavioral (including academic), cognitive, and affective subtypes. Student engagement drives learning; requires energy and effort; is affected by multiple contextual influences; and can be achieved for all learners (pp. 816–817).

Most scholars endorse the three dimensions or subtypes of student engagement proposed by Fredricks, Blumfeld, and Paris (2004) in their seminal review of the literature: emotion (affective), cognition (cognitive), and behavior (behavioral). What was clear in the first edition of this *Handbook* is that across these three dimensions, which constructs and indicators are included and how they are classified vary greatly. We previously used the jingle-jangle[1] terminology to describe this definitional melee wherein the same term is sometimes used for different indicators of student engagement and different terms may be used for the same indicator (Reschly & Christenson, 2012). The jingle-jangle issue is naggingly persistent in this second edition of the *Handbook*, not only in the definitions and indicators offered by authors but also in the extensive reviews of the literature included herein. Throughout this volume, we asked authors to provide detailed information about how student engagement was measured and the strength of results, where appropriate—one of our recommendations from the first edition for advancing the study of student engagement. This greater precision in the reporting of how student engagement is conceptualized and measured helps address the barrier of the lack of a common language and difficulty integrating results that has plagued the literature. Thus, the exactitude in conceptualization and reporting of results remains a key recommendation in this edition of the *Handbook* as well (Epilogue, Reschly &

Christenson, chapter "Advances in Student Engagement: Conceptual, Empirical, and Applied Considerations", this volume), a particularly important step in light of the proliferation of additional subtypes of student engagement in the last 10 years (e.g., social, social-behavioral, agentic).

However, discussion of a lack of consensus regarding the subtypes and indicators of student engagement may be misleading in terms of the state of the field. There has been considerable progress in the study of student engagement in the last 10 years. This progress spans countries, cultures, and languages (Jimerson & Chen, 2022), as well as measurement (See Fredricks, 2022a, b) and intervention (e.g., Fredricks, Reschly, & Christenson, 2019a; Reschly, Pohl, & Christenson, 2020). Notably, there has been an increase in longitudinal studies, long considered necessary for understanding student engagement and development (Mosher & McGowan, 1985; Christenson et al., 2012), an expansion of person-centered studies of student engagement (e.g., Fredricks et al., 2019b; Lawson & Masyn, 2015; Salmela-Aro et al., 2016) to better understand engagement and disengagement and more efficiently link students to intervention, and further elaboration of the many and varied associations between indicators of student engagement and the development of children and adolescents across academic, social-emotional, and behavioral domains. As ever, student engagement is widely agreed and shown to be essential to student success and well-being.

The purpose of this chapter is to provide a history of the study of student engagement with the premise that understanding the current status of the field requires attention to the historical origins. We review the origins of the student engagement construct, present three integrated models of student engagement, and revisit past and current debates in the field.

Origins of Student Engagement

On-Task/Engaged Time

One underpinning of contemporary work in student engagement is drawn from models of learning and research on time and achievement. One

---

[1] Jingle/Jangle distinction was used to describe personality psychology by Block (2000).

of the first and most important of such models is John Carroll's Model of School Learning (1963). Carroll delineated five classes of variables that accounted for student achievement: aptitude (amount of time needed to learn), opportunity to learn (amount of time allocated for learning), perseverance (time a student is willing to devote to learning; motivation), quality of instruction, and ability to understand instruction (1989). The latter two variables—quality of instruction and ability to understand—have an inverse association with time wherein poorer quality of instruction or lower ability to understand instruction results in more time required to learn. Similarly, higher quality instruction or a student with higher ability requires less time needed to learn.

Carroll noted, "It has always been a matter of some astonishment to me that I am credited with directing attention to time in learning, an exceedingly obvious variable that must have been in the minds of educators over the centuries and that has figured heavily in the work of theorists and experimenters on learning" (p. 27, 1989). Perhaps what was novel about Carroll's model is that it drew attention to characteristics of individual learners (aptitude, ability to understand, motivation), the instructional context in terms of how time is allocated for learning and the quality of instruction provided to students, and the interaction between student and context in producing learning. These concepts (context, existence of individual differences, and interaction/fit between the two) endure in the current, broader conceptualizations of student engagement as a meta-construct and are well suited to intervention. Notably, Carroll (1989) also defined motivation in terms of time (i.e., the amount that a student is willing to invest or spend in learning). From this view, motivation leads to engagement (defined here as academic engaged time (AET) or time-on-task; Gettinger & Walther, 2012).

Carroll's model was influential in others' subsequent work and conceptualizations of learning (see Carroll, 1989, and Gettinger & Walther, 2012 for a review). In particular, Carroll's model advanced study in two areas: Bloom's work in mastery learning (e.g., students who do not pass an instructional unit are provided additional time

and support to reach mastery; Carroll, 1989; Rosenshine, 1986) and the study of time-on-task (Rosenshine, 1986). Of course, it had long been understood that the more time students spend engaged with learning, the greater their achievement. Uncovering the nuances of the associations between time and accomplishment, however, requires the delineation of several time-related concepts.

Academic time and learning may be conceptualized on a continuum (Gettinger & Walther, 2012). At the broadest level is the time that is available for learning, such as the number of hours in a school day or the number of days in an academic year. Policies or efforts that seek to lengthen the school day or year to increase students' opportunities to learn target *available time*. Next is the time that is *scheduled* or *allocated* for learning. The extent to which scheduled time is used productively depends on educators' instruction and management practices, as well as student characteristics (Gettinger & Walther, 2012). Effective instruction increases students' academic engagement and decreases the likelihood of misbehavior. Further, productive instructional time is often lost in transitions between activities and to the management of students' behavior. There are also numerous external interruptions to instruction that undermine instructional time and students' academic engagement and learning. For example, Kraft and Monti-Nussbaum (2021) estimated that a typical classroom is interrupted 2000 times each year, resulting in a loss between 10 and 20 days of instruction. Thus, several current interventions and instructional models target maximizing the amount of productive instructional time by improving (a) individual and classroom behavior management (e.g., reducing disruptions, time in transition and managing misbehavior), (b) the quality of instruction, and (c) climate and relationships to enhance students' academic engagement and, in turn, their achievement (see Burns et al., 2022; Hofkens & Pianta, 2022; Martin, 2022; Reinke et al., 2022).

One additional distinction remains: engaged time/time-on-task and academic engaged time (AET; Gettinger & Walther, 2012). According to

Rosenshine (1986), interest in time-on-task first emerged in educational research in the 1920s and re-emerged in the 1970s with Wiley and Harnischfeger's work examining the amount of allocated/scheduled time as a source of achievement differences between socioeconomic and demographic groups and the subsequent work of Berliner and Fisher on the Beginning Teacher Evaluation Study.

Engagement in academic activities—typically coded as being on-task or as passive (e.g., looking at the teacher) or active (e.g., asking a question) engagement in various educational observational systems—is central to understanding how time is translated into learning. It is also a universal target in the field of education, with observations of individual and classroom-level data of students' on-task academic engagement collected frequently by educators and school psychologists to evaluate the effectiveness of academic and behavioral interventions or document the need for additional support for students and/ or educators (Fredricks, 2022a, b; Reschly & O'Donnell, in press). On-task behavior or academic engagement is also a common outcome variable of many school, classroom, small group, and individual academic and behavioral interventions, including the Good Behavior Game (e.g., Fallon et al., 2020; Ford et al., 2020), Peer-Assisted Learning Strategies (e.g., Barton-Arwood, Wehby, & Falk, 2005; Sinclair, Gesel, & Lemons, 2019), SSIS Classwide Intervention Program (e.g., Diperna, Lei, Bellinger, & Cheng, 2016), Positive Greetings at the Door (Cook et al., 2018), Check, Connect, and Expect (e.g., McDaniel, Houchins, & Robinson, 2016).

However, not all engaged time is created equal: the *quality* of academic engagement matters as well. It should be noted that students' characteristics or individual differences, such as their current skill in a particular area, age, or their ability to sustain attention, influence both academic engagement and AET. AET is a particular subset of academic engagement and time-on-task in which students are undertaking relevant academic activities that are appropriate for their level with a moderate to high level of success (Gettinger & Walther, 2012). With respect to relevance and level, students could be engaged in academic activities that are not appropriately difficult (too easy, too hard) or perhaps not related to the content area under study, thus, appearing engaged or on-task, but such activities are unlikely to result in gains in student achievement.

In sum, there are levels to the connection between time and learning—time available to learn, how time is allocated, the conversion of allocated time to instructional and non-instructional time, maximizing instructional time for optimal active student engagement, and engaged time/time-on-task and its subset, AET. Policy and intervention efforts may target any part of this learning-time continuum (e.g., extending the school year, maximizing how allocated time is used, limiting interruptions to the classroom, engaging students actively in relevant activities). In the current, broader student engagement framework, academic engagement, defined as paying attention, following directions, or participating in instruction and instructional activities, is typically embedded within the behavioral engagement subtype (e.g., Fredricks et al., 2004) or kept as a separate subtype of academic engagement that also includes homework completion, grades, and credits earned (Appleton, Christenson, Kim, & Reschly, 2006; Christenson & Anderson, 2002; Reschly & Christenson, 2006, 2012). The work conducted with time-on-task/academic engagement is an important historical underpinning to the current student engagement conceptualizations, in particular: (a) that time and how it is used is alterable, (b) the role of how contexts influence students' engagement, individual differences, and the interaction between student and context, and (c) linking students' involvement and participation in academic tasks and activities to their achievement and long-term outcomes. However, we have long noted that academic engagement or academic engaged time is not enough to accomplish the broader goals of schooling or to re-engage those students who are at greatest risk of dropping out (Reschly & Christenson, 2006, 2012, 2019). Thus, we shift now to the expanded views of student engagement that emerged from the dropout prevention and school reform literatures.

Dropout Prevention and Intervention

Student engagement, and disengagement in particular, has long been central to conceptualizing and addressing both high school (see Reschly & Christenson, 2006, 2012, 2019) and college noncompletion (Tinto, 1975, 1982, 2022). Our focus here is on the high school literature; however, there are notable similarities across the two literatures, including the importance of relationships with teachers and peers, perceived relevance and significance of schoolwork, attendance, and work completion (in other words, behavioral, affective, and cognitive subtypes), as well as the view that dropout is a process of disengagement that occurs over time (Fraysier et al., 2020; Waldrop et al., 2019).

In the earliest descriptions of student engagement and dropout in the K12 literature, the focus was largely on disengagement as the underlying explanatory mechanism of dropping out, with engagement, then, conceptualized primarily as its opposite (e.g., lack of participation in school vs. participation in school; Mosher & McGowan, 1985). In what may be the first published definitions of engagement and disengagement in this literature, Natriello (1982) defined engagement and disengagement as mirror images in three domains: those activities associated with academics, those that could be described as citizenship or scholarship behaviors needed for a well-functioning school, and participation in extracurricular activities. Disengagement occurred when active engagement in any of those three areas was low (i.e., low levels of effort in school, participation in delinquent activities, withdrawal from or non-participation in school activities, absenteeism). According to Natriello, scholarly interest in disengagement from school could be linked to earlier work on concepts of alienation and organizational estrangement. As Newmann et al. (1992) noted, "[the] Alienation literature does not identify a single term to characterize its opposite, but if one term were chosen, engagement seems to capture many of these missing qualities in relation to people, work or the physical environment" (pp. 16–17).

Although Natriello's work focused on the role of student evaluation and feedback practices as a factor in students' disengagement, it was recognized that student engagement and disengagement had multiple, interactive determinants (e.g., individual, family, and school) and was intermediary to educational outcomes (Mosher & McGowan, 1985). Other enduring premises of student engagement in the dropout literature include: (a) dropout is a long-term process of disengagement (Mosher & McGowan, 1985), (b) school policies and practices affect the likelihood of student disengagement (Natriello, 1982), (c) disengagement can be task specific in that students may be engaged or disengaged from some tasks or classes and not in others (Natriello, 1982), and (d) there were no simple or easy fixes for dropout but rather, addressing it requires "multiple and systemic" processes (Mosher & McGowan, 1985). Then, as now, it was also thought that student engagement was both a "state of mind and a way of being/behaving" (p. 12) and that students' perceptual data were a clear indicator of their engagement (Mosher & McGowan, 1985).

In 1989, Jeremy Finn proposed the influential Participation-Identification Model that conceptualized both the processes of engagement and disengagement/withdrawal that result in school completion or dropout, respectively. The basic engagement processes included participation in school and activities, the experience of success, and subsequent identification with school and learning, which then facilitated students' ongoing participation. The participation-success-identification cycle sustains most students through to graduation, despite occasional setbacks (Finn, 1989; Finn & Zimmer, 2012).

Consistent with the academic engagement literature described previously, Finn and Zimmer (2012) noted the importance of the quality of instruction for students' participation and success, as well as the contribution of student ability to students' successful performance. Thus, as with the academic engagement literature, there was recognition of individual characteristics and the interaction with context. They also called attention to the developmental period prior to school entry, with some students having experiences (e.g., preschool, support and encouragement from home) that better equip them with attitudes, behaviors, and skills necessary to successfully participate at entry to schooling, thereby facilitating the participation-success-identification cycle (Reschly & Christenson, 2012).

Finn and Zimmer (2012) opined that both the requirements for successful participation and opportunities for involvement become greater as students progress in school. With this as background information, the disengagement-withdrawal cycle may best be explained: students who do not have the requisite attitudes, skills, or behaviors to successfully participate are less likely to establish or sustain the participation-success-identification cycle as the demands and opportunities afforded by schooling increase, instead falling into a cycle of non-participation, poor school performance, and emotional withdrawal (dropout). Even with an established participation-success-identification cycle, individual students' family or work experiences or other obstacles may lead to early school departure (Finn & Zimmer, 2012).

Notably, in this model, student engagement and disengagement are also described as opposites of a single continuum and that engagement is comprised of behavioral and affective dimensions. One of the most novel aspects of the Participation-Identification Model is that student engagement and disengagement were situated within a developmental cycle (Finn & Zimmer, 2012). In addition, the model not only reflected the shift in linking disengagement to dropping out but also explicated the processes of engagement that result in the positive outcome of high school completion. However, the Participation-Identification Model does not address how schools influence participation and identification (Rumberger & Larson, 1998) or the broader contexts—families, schools, peers, or communities—that serve as targets of intervention (Reschly & Christenson, 2012).

The Participation-Identification Model remains prominent in current discussions of high school dropout and efforts to promote school completion (Archambault et al., 2022; Reschly, 2020; Reschly & Christenson, 2019).

Furthermore, it is apparent in models and theories of dropout (see Archambault et al., 2022) that student engagement and disengagement are featured in frameworks for both conceptualizing processes and prevention and intervention efforts. Wehlage, Rutter, Smith, Lesko, and Fernandez (1989), for example, proposed a dropout prevention model focused on the school's role in addressing student engagement in terms of educational engagement and school membership, which seem to align with behavioral and affective engagement, respectively (Archambault et al., 2022). Similarly, Rumberger and Larson (1998) described student engagement in terms of academic engagement in learning (e.g., expectations, class preparation) and engagement with social aspects of school (e.g., attendance, misbehavior, school activities) that would be reflected in both students' attitudes and behaviors, in line with earlier postulation by Mosher and McGowan (1985) and Finn (1989).

Connecting Predictive Studies to an Engagement Framework As interest in dropout grew, studies identified dozens of variables that were predictive of dropout or completion. Christenson et al. (2001) argued for shifting focus from the prediction of a negative outcome, dropout, to the promotion of school completion with competence. The authors underscored the importance of a systemic approach, linking with schools, families, and community resources to provide personalized interventions in support of school completion.

In this vein, scholars began to offer distinctions or categorizations of predictive variables, such as those that were demographic or status-oriented in nature (e.g., socioeconomic status) and those that were alterable (e.g., attendance, homework completion, participation). Of those that were alterable or non-demographic, variables were further categorized in terms of proximity of the indicator relative to the event of dropping out (*proximal* vs. *distal*; Rumberger, 1995). In addition, the terms *push* and *pull* were used to describe how schools and outside factors influence a student's decision to leave prematurely (Jordan et al., 1999). We offered a categorization of whether the indicator was a risk or protective factor at the student, family, and school levels (Reschly & Christenson, 2006), and so forth (see also Archambault et al., 2022, and Rosenthal, 1998). Many of the alterable variables reflected students' engagement at school and with learning and aspects of developmental contexts that were appropriate targets of intervention (Reschly & Christenson, 2012; Reschly, 2020).

Building on this and the intervention literatures, Christenson (2008) offered a critical distinction for linking this research to intervention: that is, a distinction between what she termed demographic and functional risk. This distinction built upon research that demonstrated certain sociodemographic groups were less likely to successfully complete high school (e.g., those of low socioeconomic status, students from Black or Latinx racial-ethnic groups in the United States); however, within any of these subgroups, many students did successfully complete. Thus, using demographic risk to identify those in need of additional support would lead to wasted and unnecessary resources (e.g., 74% of American Indian/Alaska Native students who completed high school on-time in the 2018–2019 school year; NCES, 2021). Rather, it is students' *engagement* that is directly associated with current and future school performance, including completion, within various sociodemographic groups (Reschly & Christenson, 2012).

In the next section, we describe a National Academies Panel report (National Research Council & Institute of Medicine [NRC], 2004) as a major impetus for linking student engagement with school reform and the increasing popularity of student engagement; however, it would be misleading to ignore the roots of dropout research and connection to whole-school strategies here as well. It is a logical progression from noting that school policies and practices influence student engagement and disengagement to studies of school-level variables that predict dropout or promote school completion and discussion of efforts to promote engagement for all students. As stated by Wehlage and Rutter (1986),

Certainly public schooling in a democratic society is obligated to respond constructively to children from all backgrounds and social conditions. It may be that some kinds of children are more difficult to teach than others, but the school has no less of a mandate to do its best to provide all the schooling such children can profitably use. (p. 381).
…while most of the literature on dropouts is directed only at the deficiencies found in the marginal student, we see those same characteristics as a reflection on the institution. (p. 389).

Wehlage and Rutter (1986) based their policy recommendations on students' perceptions of the lack of teacher interest and the ineffectiveness and unfairness of school discipline and widespread truancy. They described their findings as, "grounds for recommending general policy and practice reforms that would make school more responsive not only to those who drop out, but also to a large body of students who now stay in school reluctantly" (p. 389).

Student engagement clearly provided a framework for intervention to re-engage students at risk of dropping out or who had dropped out of school, a pathway away from predictive studies of dropout, which dominated the field (Christenson et al., 2001), and a bridge from assessment to intervention (e.g., McPartland, 1994). It was understood by scholars that schools could either positively or negatively influence student engagement and disengagement, which undergirds the reasoning for the necessity of school-wide strategies. Furthermore, the many and varied associations between aspects of student engagement provide a direct link to performance for all students. Together, this sets the stage for the expansion of student engagement to a meta-construct and basis of school reform.

Meta-Construct and School Reform

Dominant concerns in the educational reform movement have neglected one of the problems most critical to the improvement of high schools: how to engage students in academic work. (p. 33, Newmann et al., 1992).
Learning and succeeding in school requires active engagement – whether students are rich or poor, black, brown, or white. The core principles that underlie engagement are applicable to all schools – whether they are in urban, suburban, or rural communities. (p. 1, NRC, 2004).

In the early 2000s, interest in student engagement was spilling over into other areas of study. Two seminal publications in this time period signaled growing interest in student engagement and were harbingers of what would be explosive awareness of the construct among practitioners and educators around the world. In describing the origins of student engagement, we have often grouped these publications together both because of the similar timing of publication (2004) and the shared focused on the larger system and engagement of all students, not just those at risk of dropping out of high school (e.g., Christenson et al., 2008; Reschly & Christenson, 2012).

An esteemed group of educators and scholars, with expertise in motivation, child development, school reform, high school dropout, school climate, and social inequities, comprised the panel that was convened by the National Academies to offer solutions for the declining academic motivation and disengagement from school that occurs as students progress from elementary to high school (NRC, 2004). The Panel's recommendations encompassed curriculum, instruction, and organization of schools from the perspective of meeting students' needs for autonomy, competence, and relatedness (Self-Determination Theory, "I can, I want to, and I belong"). Their recommendations are well summarized in the following excerpt:

> A common theme among effective practices is that they address underlying psychological variables related to motivation, such as competence and control, beliefs about the value of education, and a sense of belonging. In brief, engaging schools and teachers promote students' confidence in their ability to learn and succeed in school by providing challenging instruction and support for meeting high standards, and they clearly convey their own high expectations for their students' success. They provide choices for students and they make curriculum and instruction relevant to adolescents' experiences, cultures, and long-term goals, so that students see some value in the high school curriculum (pp. 2–3).

The Panel described how learning requires students' engagement, the relevance of student engagement for all students, including those of different racial-ethnic and socioeconomic groups and schools (e.g., suburban, urban, rural), and

suggested that promoting or maintaining students' engagement is particularly important for those students who are at greater risk for poor educational outcomes, consistent with the premise that student engagement is a protective factor for those placed at higher risk for poor educational outcomes (Finn & Zimmer, 2012; Masten et al., 2022). Their work centered on motivation and student engagement within the context of social relationships that are critical to student success, a consistent theme in these literatures. Their purpose was arguably action- or intervention-oriented. Interestingly, the seemingly interchangeable use of the terms motivation and engagement portends what continues to be a point of confusion, and sometimes contention, among scholars. That is: what is the association between the two constructs and the relative importance, or lack thereof, of differentiating the two in theory- vs. more applied-work (Christenson et al., 2012).

Another seminal work in student engagement, "Student Engagement: Potential of the Concept, State of the Evidence," was authored by Fredricks, Blumenfeld, and Paris and published the same year as the NRC volume. The authors described student engagement as comprised of three dimensions: behavior, emotion, and cognition. Behavioral engagement was defined in terms of participation in academic, social, and extracurricular activities, which were recognized as necessary for academic success and dropout prevention. Emotional engagement referred to, "positive and negative reactions to teachers, classmates, academics, and school" (p. 60), which promotes students' willingness to complete academic tasks. Lastly, cognitive engagement, drawing from work in motivation, was described in terms of investment and related to students' "willingness to exert the effort necessary to comprehend complex ideas and master difficult skills" (p. 60). These three dimensions or subtypes of student engagement were the primary categorization endorsed by scholars in the first edition of this *Handbook* and remain so in this edition (see Epilogue, this volume).

The authors observed the inherent appeal of student engagement to educators, thereby underscoring its applied nature. Here, too, was the alterability of student engagement, influence of contexts on students' engagement, and ties to important academic outcomes, as well as the notion that student engagement across these dimensions may vary in terms of intensity and duration wherein it may be short-term or situation specific (e.g., a novel task, a method of lesson delivery the student finds interesting) or long-term and stable. The authors noted that a foundation of student engagement is additive in nature (e.g., engagement begets engagement; Reschly, 2010).

Another enduring and especially novel contribution of this work was to propose that student engagement could be viewed as a meta-construct, merging typically independent or separate areas of study under the broad construct of student engagement (Fredricks et al., 2004). Viewing student engagement in this way allowed for a more nuanced understanding of students and their experiences at school, accepting the complexity and interrelated nature of thoughts, emotions, and behavior. However, the student engagement as a meta-construct idea further exacerbated tensions and questions about the associations between engagement and motivation, particularly due to the overlap between cognitive engagement and traditional study of academic motivation.

Models of Student Engagement

In this section, we review three integrated or comprehensive models of student engagement to highlight commonalities and distinctions among scholars that relate to the current and future study of the construct. We refer the reader to Skinner & Raine (2022) for a comprehensive list of models.

Check & Connect Model of Student Engagement We have written extensively about our work with Check & Connect for promoting student engagement and school completion (e.g., Christenson & Pohl, 2020; Christenson & Reschly, 2010; Reschly & Christenson, 2006, 2012), the model of student engagement based on our work with Check & Connect (e.g., Christenson et al., 2008, Reschly, Pohl, Christenson, &

Appleton, 2017; Reschly & Christenson, 2012; Fig. 1), and the self-report measure, the Student Engagement Instrument (SEI), we developed to supplement the observable engagement data (e.g., attendance, behavior, homework completion rate) readily available to Check & Connect intervention staff and educators (e.g., Appleton et al., 2006; Betts et al., 2010; Lovelace et al., 2014, 2017; Reschly, Betts, & Appleton, 2014).

Initially developed as a dropout prevention program for middle school students with learning and emotional and behavior disorders, Check & Connect quickly shifted to a focus on student engagement and the promotion of competence for school completion, a necessary shift to ensure students have more promising career and employment opportunities. In designing Check & Connect, developers drew broadly from both theory and research in development, dropout, resilience, motivation, and cognitive-behavior therapy. The intervention model consists of four main components: (1) a mentor who works with students and their families over an extended period of time; (2) regular monitoring or "checking" of alterable, observable indicators of students' connection and engagement with school (e.g., attendance, behavior, grades); (3) the implementation of timely interventions at the earliest signs of disengagement and more general promotion of social, behavioral, and academic competence; and (4) work with families to foster positive relationships between home and school and to connect families with resources facilitating the home–school relationship and connection of families with resources (Christenson & Pohl, 2020). Check & Connect is one of only a handful of interventions rated by the What Works Clearinghouse as having potentially positive or positive effects in any of the three areas related to school completion (staying in school, progressing in school, completing school; Reschly, 2020).

In the almost 30 years since Check & Connect began, we learned several lessons relative to intervention design and implementation and the promotion of student engagement. We highlight a few of these lessons here but refer the reader to Christenson and Pohl (2020) for more compre-

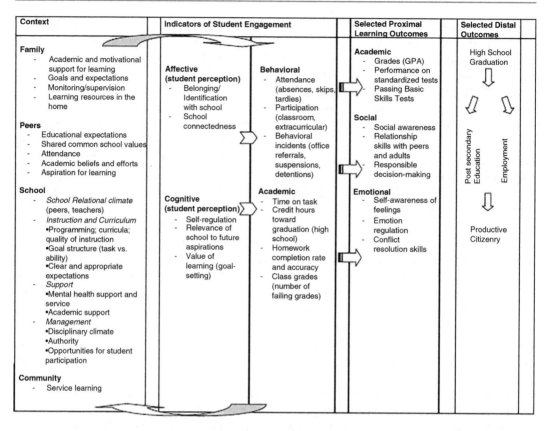

Context	Indicators of Student Engagement		Selected Proximal Learning Outcomes	Selected Distal Outcomes
Family - Academic and motivational support for learning - Goals and expectations - Monitoring/supervision - Learning resources in the home **Peers** - Educational expectations - Shared common school values - Attendance - Academic beliefs and efforts - Aspiration for learning **School** - *School Relational climate* (peers, teachers) - *Instruction and Curriculum* •Programming; curricula; quality of instruction •Goal structure (task vs. ability) •Clear and appropriate expectations - *Support* •Mental health support and service •Academic support - *Management* •Disciplinary climate •Authority •Opportunities for student participation **Community** - Service learning	**Affective (student perception)** - Belonging/ Identification with school - School connectedness **Cognitive (student perception)** - Self-regulation - Relevance of school to future aspirations - Value of learning (goal-setting)	**Behavioral** - Attendance (absences, skips, tardies) - Participation (classroom, extracurricular) - Behavioral incidents (office referrals, suspensions, detentions) **Academic** - Time on task - Credit hours toward graduation (high school) - Homework completion rate and accuracy - Class grades (number of failing grades)	**Academic** - Grades (GPA) - Performance on standardized tests - Passing Basic Skills Tests **Social** - Social awareness - Relationship skills with peers and adults - Responsible decision-making **Emotional** - Self-awareness of feelings - Emotion regulation - Conflict resolution skills	High School Graduation Post secondary Education Employment Productive Citizenry

Fig. 1 Model of associations between context, engagement, and student outcomes. (*Source*: Figure from Reschly & Christenson et al. 2012)

hensive coverage. First, in our work with students at high risk of dropping out, we realized that meeting academic and behavioral standards was not enough to re-engage students for school completion (Christenson & Reschly, 2010; Reschly & Christenson, 2012). Instead, we needed to connect with students and through the mentor–student relationship, we could work to foster interest in the relevance of education to students' futures, their motivation, and self-regulation—or in other words, winning students' hearts and minds (Reschly, 2020). In this vein, some indicators of students' engagement and connection to school were readily available to us—attendance, participation in extracurricular activities, conduct at school, homework completion, etc.—whereas we recognized we could not determine students' perceptions regarding relevance of education to their futures, social support from or relationships with teachers and peers,

feelings of belonging or identification, and so forth without querying their perspectives. Thus, we developed the SEI to specifically measure students' perceptions of their cognitive and affective engagement.

We also recognized that our efforts were at times thwarted by school policies and practices that undermined attempts to re-engage students and by disjointed programs that were not integrated within the broader school community. We concluded that school completion efforts were most effectively implemented within a system that is geared toward the engagement, competence, and school completion of all students. Furthermore, the developmental nature of student engagement and disengagement requires attention and coordination across levels of schooling, from early childhood through high school and into college (Reschly, 2020; Reschly & Christenson, 2019; Reschly, Pohl, & Christenson,

2020). In this broad, developmental view, efforts to improve school discipline and climate, more effectively manage classrooms or provide more interesting and effective curricula and instruction, screen and provide early intervention for academic or mental health difficulties, and so forth may be viewed as school completion efforts. In fact, we argue that student engagement and school completion is a unifying construct or frame of reference across levels of schooling and tiered intervention models (Reschly, 2020).

The influence of Check & Connect and the scholarly traditions it drew from are apparent in the model of student engagement presented in Fig. 1. Elements from Ecological Systems Theory (Bronfenbrenner, 1977) and Self-Systems Processes (Connell & Wellborn, 1991), for example, are evident in the conception of interactions between important developmental contexts (family, peers, school, and community) and individual students, their engagement, and both proximal and distal educational outcomes (i.e., across development). Drawing from these traditions, and consistent with other models of student engagement, students' engagement serves as a mediator between context and outcomes and these interactions have a Matthew effect wherein engagement at one point begets greater engagement at another (e.g., Reschly, 2010; Reschly & Christenson, 2012). Furthermore, person–environment fit is also a crucial element to understanding context–student interactions across time. Person–environment fit is uniquely individual: how students experience contexts differs, what is an excellent fit for one individual may not meet another's needs in the same way. It also buttresses the argument for querying students' own perceptions of their school environment, instruction, support for learning, etc. An applied corollary from the school completion literature is that students disengage for different reasons: there is no one right intervention strategy that works for every student, all of the time.

Our discussion of developmental processes and school levels also draws from Finn's Participation-Identification Model and early childhood research. In particular, pathways to dropout and completion have been identified

from early childhood (e.g., Neuharth-Pritchett & Bub, 2022; Reschly & Christenson, 2012; Reschly, 2020). In addition, studies of early childhood education programs demonstrate long-term effects on students' academic outcomes, likely through influence on the participation-success-identification cycle. In short, students' early school experiences are integral to the cycles of engagement and disengagement or pathways that formed when students enter formal schooling.

In line with the conceptualization of student engagement as a meta-construct, motivational concepts are embedded within the context (e.g., goal structure) and student engagement (e.g., self-regulation, goal setting). Similarly, dropout prevention program strategies, such as the provision of academic and mental health support or opportunities for participation, are also included in the model. Perhaps the clearest illustration of student engagement as a meta-construct is underscored by the interrelated nature of students' thoughts, emotions, and behaviors and the broad range of interventions that may be included within this framework. An intervention that addresses teacher–student relationships, for example, may also affect students' academic or behavioral engagement and, in turn, their achievement (see Reschly, Pohl, & Christenson, 2020).

Development-in-Sociocultural-Context Model

According to Wang et al. (2019), the Development-in-Sociocultural-Context Model for Children's Engagement in Learning delineates five broad categories ordered in terms of direction of effects: External Factors, Internal Factors, Engagement, Resilience Mechanisms, and Distal Outcomes. Similar to other models, external factors include the family, school, and peer contexts. The model uniquely adds the cultural milieu (e.g., cultural capital, stereotypes/prejudice), social position and family characteristics, and the nature of academic work as external or contextual influences. These external factors influence students' developmental competencies (e.g., emotion regulation) and self-appraisals (e.g., attributions), which in turn affect students' behavioral, emotional-affective, and cognitive engagement. Similar to other models, students' engagement is directly related to educational and developmental outcomes; however, the authors added the influence of student engagement on resilience mechanisms (i.e., coping and appraisal, social support), which also influence student outcomes. There are several reciprocal effects noted in the model, such as between the family context and both developmental competencies and self-appraisals and between educational and developmental outcomes and students' ongoing engagement (Wang et al., 2019).

The model draws broadly and integrates theories and research from the educational and psychological literatures. For example, the authors elegantly describe the inclusion of motivational theories in their model, such as Self-System Processes, Expectancy-Value, and Mindset theories, as processes that influence students' self-appraisals and, in turn, their engagement.

Study Demands-Resources Model of Student Engagement and Burnout

The Study Demands-Resources Model (SD-R) is a comprehensive model of student engagement that explicitly incorporates both the processes of engagement and burnout, or disaffection, into the model (Salmela-Aro et al., 2022). The SD-R draws from the workplace engagement literature with the premise that school is the workplace of adolescents. Similar to other models, school engagement is described as a multidimensional construct. Burnout is also multidimensional with components of exhaustion (e.g., tiredness, sleep difficulties), cynicism (e.g., indifference toward school), and feelings of inadequacy in school. Research by Salmela-Aro and others demonstrates that engagement and burnout are distinct states such that students may be simultaneously high or low in both; the presence or absence of one does not indicate the same in the other (e.g., Salmela-Aro, Moeller, Schneider, Spicer, 2016). In addition, burnout uniquely contributes to students' outcomes (Salmela-Aro et al., 2022).

Contextual and individual influences in this model are described in terms of demands and resources. Demands and resources emanate from the school/classroom, family, social (teachers, peers), or the student (personal). Demands, such as a harsh school climate, student perceptions of poor teacher responsiveness or task quality, the experience of harsh parenting, or poor social relationships, may thwart students' engagement. School or classroom resources may include perceptions of school safety or the experience of support from teachers. Family resources include such elements as the affective quality of parent–child relationships and effective parental monitoring and autonomy support. Social resources include the range of positive social relationships (e.g., positive teacher–student relationships, peer relationships) that facilitate healthy youth development and students' engagement (Salmela-Aro et al., 2022).

Students' individual characteristics are represented in the model as personal demands and resources and reserves. Students' mental health difficulties are an example of personal demands whereas individual social skills and cognitive resources are examples of personal resources. Personal resources, which include motivational constructs (e.g., self-efficacy, grit, goal orientation), serve as mediators between the context and demands and students' engagement. Further, it is recognized how an individual student responds to or appraises a situation determines the effect it has on their engagement and burnout (Salmela-Aro et al., 2022). In addition to the independent influence of demands and resources on student engagement, these elements also interact such that as demands increase and overcome the student's resources, the experience of burnout and poorer psychological and academic outcomes increases.

Similar to other comprehensive models, SD-R recognizes that engagement and burnout exist at different levels and over time (e.g., in the moment, day, week). Further, the authors describe gain and loss spirals, similar to concepts of spiraling or Matthew effects (Furrer et al., 2006; Reschly, 2010), wherein contexts, resources, and demands amplify or dampen students' resources and reserves (e.g., greater resources may lead to more resources and increased reserves; high demands diminish resources, leading to loss of reserves; Salmela-Aro et al., 2022).

Summary There are a number of similarities across these broad or integrated models of student engagement. Contexts are conceptualized as including family, school, and peer influences. These contexts may either hinder or facilitate students' engagement. Student engagement, in turn, is directly associated with outcomes of interest. In addition, each model also draws from and seeks to integrate several theories and domains of research. Further, all are developmental in the sense that each considers the interaction between individuals and contexts over time.

There are unique features of each as well. The Check & Connect Model is pragmatic with links to assessment of student engagement and intervention (e.g., Reschly et al., 2020). The model also connects different developmental periods to high school, college, and post-college outcomes. The Wang et al. model (2019) explicitly incorporates relevant and important sociocultural factors as influences on engagement and disengagement. The Check & Connect and Development-in-Sociocultural-Context Models acknowledge that disengagement is separate from student engagement but the processes of disengagement are not well defined. In contrast, Salmela-Aro et al. (2022) draw from a unique literature (i.e., occupational literature) to define burnout and provide the most complete description of how engagement and burnout co-exist and the processes through which contexts and individuals interact toward engagement–competence or burnout–ill-being over time.

Revisiting the Past and Current Status of the Student Engagement Construct

As editors, this second volume allows us an opportunity to consider past issues in the field and reflect upon current state. In this section, we revisit the jingle-jangle phenomenon, the distinction between motivation and engagement, and the

status of the continuum–continua (engagement–disengagement/disaffection) differentiation.

Jingle-Jangle Revisited
Engagement is the linchpin connecting energy, purpose, and enjoyment.
(p. 1087; Wang et al., 2019)
Engagement stands for active involvement, commitment, and concentrated attention, in contrast to superficial participation, apathy, or lack of interest.
(p. 11, Newmann, Wehlage, & Lamborn, 1992)

In the first edition, we noted the issue of jingle-jangle with the terms, subtypes, and indicators commonly used in the study of student engagement. As we noted earlier, this issue is still present in this edition; however, there is increasingly a pattern or order to this phenomenon such that the core of what is meant by student engagement is more readily discerned and able to be compared across scholars and studies.

School/Student/Academic Engagement One source of jingle-jangle is the term that is used to refer to the construct of student engagement as it relates broadly to learning and school-related developmental outcomes, irrespective of subtypes. Although student engagement is currently the most widely used term, school engagement (e.g., Fredricks et al., 2004; Jimerson, Campos, & Grief, 2003; Salmela-Aro et al., 2022) and academic engagement (e.g., Martin, 2022; Skinner & Raine, 2022) are also used. We have argued that student engagement should be the preferred term because it is *students* who are engaged or disengaged at school and with learning. Schools may affect student engagement and disengagement through policies, practices, and school climate; however, families, communities, peers both inside and outside of school, relationships with teachers, etc. also influence students' engagement at school and with learning; therefore, students—not schools—are the appropriate level and focus (Appleton, Christenson, & Furlong, 2008).

The use of academic engagement as the term for the global engagement construct is more recent and is meant to convey the academic focus of students' emotional, behavioral, or cognitive engagement (e.g., Martin, 2022). In our view, this is problematic in that the term academic engagement has been used to refer to on-task behavior or engaged time with academic tasks for several decades. It is also used as a subtype of student engagement (Appleton et al., 2006; Christenson et al., 2008; Reschly & Christenson, 2012).

Subtypes and Indicators As in the first edition, most scholars endorse the three dimensions of student engagement proposed by Fredricks et al. (2004): emotion, cognition, and behavior. Indicators of each dimension or subtype continue to vary across scholars. For example, is cognitive engagement represented by the use of deep learning strategies, investment, effort, self-regulation, students' motivation, and/or perceived relevance of education to one's future? (Table 1). Behavioral engagement is sometimes narrowly conceived of as participation in class and academic tasks while at school or broadly conceived to include tasks outside of school, such as homework, and conduct while in school. Scholars also differ in terms of the inclusion of participation in extracurricular activities, such as band or sports, in the behavioral engagement subtype. Affective engagement may be narrowly defined as emotional state while learning and/or in terms of more global feelings of connectedness and belonging at school and in students' perceptions of their relationships and support from teachers, peers, and their families. Csikszentmihalyi's concept of flow is another example of the inclusion of independent lines of research under the student engagement meta-construct and is one that could be cast both as affective and cognitive engagement. The concepts utility, effort, interest, and investment are particularly difficult to categorize.

There are several likely reasons for the continued jingle-jangle of student engagement indicators. As a meta-construct, student engagement draws from several theoretical perspectives and sometimes disparate lines of research and scholars study engagement at different levels and

times: more narrowly as the visible manifestation of motivation perhaps within a specific subject or broadly as a driver of positive youth development and long-term academic, well-being, and employment outcomes. A study with a focus on learning within a subject or classroom may tap self-regulation and learning strategy use as indicators of cognitive engagement whereas a study with a long-term developmental view might instead use perceived relevance of education to one's future as an indicator of cognitive engagement. Further, the premise that students' engagement is comprised of interrelated thoughts, feelings, and emotions indicates the complexity of the human experience and the difficulty in separating these aspects for study. For example, effort or investment could include visible behavior, emotion, and internal thoughts. In addition, there is a great deal of similarity in the elements of student engagement regardless of the terms used. For instance, if affective engagement is defined in terms of emotional states while learning, scholars may add another subtype to represent the social connectedness that is a major part of students' school experiences and their engagement or disengagement (e.g., Davis, Spring, & Balfanz, 2022) that is embedded in some conceptualizations as affective engagement (e.g., Reschly & Christenson, 2012; Jimerson & Chen, 2022).

Motivation and Engagement
In the first edition of this *Handbook*, we asked authors to offer their definitions of student engagement and motivation and how they differentiated the two constructs. Many scholars endorsed the view that motivation precedes engagement wherein motivation is the will and engagement is the action (Christenson et al., 2012). As we noted then, the problem with this distinction is the internal nature of motivation, affective engagement, and cognitive engagement. It is apparent in this edition that scholars continue to wrestle with the relationship between student engagement and motivation.

There are those that suggest motivation and engagement are synonymous or interchangeable

Table 1 Representative examples of Student Engagement Subtypes and Indicators

	Behavioral	Emotional/affective	Cognitive	Other
Fredricks	Involvement and participation in learning and school contexts (e.g., extracurriculars); positive conduct; absence of disruptive behaviors	Positive and negative reactions to teachers, classmates, academics, or school; sense of belonging; identification with school or subject areas	Investment in learning; includes self-regulation and use of deep learning strategies	
Christensen, Reschly, Appleton et al.	Attendance; participation (classroom, extracurricular); behavioral incidents	Belonging/identification with school; school connectedness *measured as student perceptions of relationships with teachers and peers, family support	Self-regulation; relevance of school to future; value of learning (e.g., goal setting)	**Academic** Time-on-task/ engaged time; credits earned toward graduation; homework completion rate; grades
Salmela-Aro et al. Schoolwork engagement	*Dedication* Students' involvement in schoolwork; perceptions of its meaningfulness; and students' sense of significance, enthusiasm, and inspiration	*Energy* *Vigor with respect to learning, investment of effort*	*Absorption* *High concentration in learning*	
Jimerson and Chen	Observable actions or performance (e.g., extracurricular activities); homework completion; grades; GPA; achievement test scores	Students' feelings about school, teachers, and/or peers	Student's perceptions and beliefs about self, school, teachers, and peers (e.g., self-efficacy, motivation, aspirations)	
Reeve and Jang	Observable action students take to be on-task and exerting effort and persistence **Behavioral disengagement**: Doing just enough to get by	Quality of affective connections students have with task *measured as interest and enjoyment **Emotional disengagement**: Task-rejecting emotions (e.g., boredom, discouragement)	Actions undertaken to enhance thinking (e.g., how to focus attention, understand what one is learning, problem-solving) *measured as concentration, attentional control, problem-solving, use of self-regulation strategies and learning strategies **Cognitive disengagement**: Mental disorganization	**Agentic** Student's constructive contribution to instruction; what students say and do to improve learning

(continued)

Table 1 (continued)

	Behavioral	Emotional/affective	Cognitive	Other
Martin	Participation and involvement		Thoughtful, willing, and strategic to invest in academics; exertion of necessary effort	**Social-emotional** Positive and negative emotional and interpersonal responses to learning and instruction
Archambault et al.	Observable actions in the classroom; participation in activities; collaborate with peers; follow instructions; attendance	Emotional state and reaction to school and classroom contexts and activities	Self-regulation and deep processing while learning	
Davis, Spring, and Balfanz	Active participation in academic activities	Physical display of emotion	Mental investment in learning	**Social** Interaction with peers about academics

terms (e.g., NRC, 2004), which may not be unreasonable from a school or applied intervention perspective in that it underscores the idea that both are essential to accomplish the goals of schooling. Indeed, there likely are reciprocal associations between engagement and motivation such that the associations between the two constructs vary at the time and level each are captured (e.g., Martin et al., 2017). On the other hand, the student engagement meta-construct may subsume motivation as part of student engagement (Fredricks et al., 2004; Christenson et al., 2012), which is further supported by the inclusion of several motivational concepts as indicators of student engagement (see Table 1). Still others suggest that engagement is more than motivation (Newmann et al., 1992) and that engagement begets motivation (Salmela-Aro et al., 2022).

The nexus of this tension is understandable. Motivation has a long, rich history with several well-developed sub-theories. The idea that a field such as motivation or belonging could be subsumed by another, more recent construct is sure to be met with some skepticism (e.g., Allen & Boyle, 2022; Gladstone, Wigfield, & Eccles, 2022; Skinner & Raine, 2022). However, there are also concerns about the fragmentation of

various motivational theories and concomitant waning usefulness (e.g., Anderman, Patrick, & Ha, 2022; Skinner & Raine, 2022).

As Eccles and Wang (2012) noted in the first edition, there are issues with being too broad or too narrow in conceptualizations of phenomena. Broad conceptualizations work well for communicating with policymakers and other stakeholders, such as educators and parents, whereas narrower conceptualizations are more useful for research and theory-testing. Admittedly, as student engagement and school completion scholars, we cannot underscore emphatically enough how useful the student engagement framework is for conceptualizing and communicating the interactions among contexts and individuals that produce engagement and related outcomes, the role of developmental processes, the rich characterization of students' school experiences as comprising their emotions, cognitions, and behavior inherent in the student engagement meta-construct, and as a framework for comprehensive interventions.

However, to paraphrase Skinner and Raine (2022), student engagement cannot be everything to everyone. The authors offer a comprehensive and thoughtful review of both literatures and recommendations for integrating motivation and student engagement research. We agree that student engagement and motivation are not incompatible, and, as others have noted, perhaps the differences between motivation and engagement are a matter of focus (Finn & Zimmer, 2012).

Our reading of the literature and chapters in this second edition has led us to the following conclusions. A useful distinction might be between a developmental view of student engagement and a motivational view. The integrated models of engagement described earlier in this chapter clearly draw from developmental theories and there are examinations of student engagement from early childhood through college (Neuharth-Pritchett & Bub, 2022; Tinto, 2022). Schooling includes a number of developmental tasks and milestones that are important in most cultures and societies (Masten et al., 2022). Furthermore, dropout and completion scholars increasingly approach the topic from a life course perspective (Archambault et al., 2022; Rumberger & Rotermund, 2012).

Conversely, from a motivational viewpoint, student engagement may be conceptualized in the way described by many motivational scholars with motivation as intent and student engagement as action. The motivational view on student engagement is narrower, more amenable to theory testing, and better integrated with existing motivational theories. Thus, motivation is central to students' engagement but it is just one part of the broader construct: it also exists as an independent and worthy area of study. This distinction in developmental and motivational views also captures another difference in the two perspectives in that the primary outcome of academic motivation research is achievement whereas achievement is one of many outcomes of interest in student engagement. Given this distinction, it is understandable that much motivation research is conducted with high school and college students while student engagement is more likely to cover the range of schooling (e.g., Archambault et al., 2022; Neuharth-Pritchett & Bub, 2022; Tinto, 2022). Finally, as Tinto (2022) noted, it may be more appropriate to refer to student engagement as a framework or model given its broad, interdisciplinary, integrated nature whereas motivation

and sub-theories are more accurately described as theories.

The distinction between model and theory is just one of the areas in which we recommend student engagement scholars consider greater precision with their language. Another is clear reporting of scholars' operationalization of student engagement and indicators so that results may be better integrated and nuances identified across studies. Also imperative to clearer conceptualizations of student engagement is the recognition that student engagement may be studied at different levels, such as with learning activities, within the classroom, with school, and with prosocial institutions (Skinner & Raine, 2022) or at either the classroom or school levels (Martin, 2022). Specification of level may also bring greater organization/clarity among measures of student engagement (e.g., engagement within a specific class vs. a global measure of engagement with school).

Engagement-Disengagement Versus Engagement and Disaffection (Continuum Versus Continua)

In the first edition of this *Handbook*, we noted that one way in which models of engagement differed was in their conceptualization of engagement and disengagement as existing on a single continuum ranging from high to low or as two separate continua (Reschly & Christenson, 2012). We agree with Wang et al. (2019) and Salmela-Aro et al. (2022) that there is now compelling evidence that these are two separate continua. However, there is little clarity as to whether the "other" continuum is best described as disengagement (Wang et al., 2019), disaffection (Skinner et al., 2008, 2009), or burnout (Salmela-Aro et al., 2022). Skinner et al. characterized disaffection as having emotional (e.g., boredom, disinterest, frustration) and behavioral (e.g., passivity, withdrawal, distraction) components whereas Salmela-Aro et al. use the term burnout to refer to exhaustion, a cynical attitude toward school, and feelings of inadequacy. Among current indicators, how does one differentiate low engagement from disaffection/disengagement/burnout? Where would indicators such as disciplinary incidents, a low rate of work completion, skipping classes, and absences fall? Although the processes of disengagement and withdrawal were described in Finn's Participation-Identification Model (1989), disengagement and engagement are cast as ends of a single continuum. From the continua perspective, how do disaffection and burnout emerge?

Past, Present, and Future

"...the promotion of student engagement should bring benefits to quality of life that are more fundamental than increases in school achievement." (p. 17, Newmann, Wehlage, & Lamborn 1992)

In this chapter, we revisited the history and origins of the student engagement construct and offered our thoughts on past and current issues in the field. We are struck by two enduring themes in our work with student engagement and in the scholarship of others. The first is the importance of student perceptions and voice. The dropout literature is clear that it is *students' perceptions* of discipline, fairness, relevance, support, etc. that are tied to outcomes of interest. Indeed, one of the earliest reviews of student engagement noted students' perceptual data were an indicator of their engagement (Mosher & McGowan, 1985). Tinto (2022) reaches a similar conclusion when he noted that it is "...not engagement per se that matters, as it is students' perceptions of their engagements and the meanings they draw from them as to their self-efficacy, sense of belonging, and the relevance of their studies." That is not to say that others' perceptions are not relevant to school intervention and improvement efforts or that these data should not be supplemented with observations, the views of others, or considered in aggregate (e.g., teacher support at the classroom level, classroom goal students) but rather, simply, that students cannot be overlooked. Support for this notion could likely be garnered from several areas, including the role of context–individual interactions that are inherent in developmental models (e.g., Bronfenbrenner, 1977) and the principle/notion of person–environment fit. Essentially, how an individual experiences the context is at least somewhat unique to that individual.

The second theme is the importance of relationships to students' development in general and relative to student engagement and both proximal and distal outcomes. The primacy of relationships is not a new revelation in development (Pianta & Walsh, 1996), resilience (Masten & Reed, 2002), or school completion literatures (e.g., Anderson, Christenson, Sinclair, & Lehr, 2004; McPartland 1994). We recently reached a similar conclusion regarding relationships and promising interventions to promote student engagement and positive developmental outcomes (Fredricks, Reschly & Christenson, 2019a), and yet, throughout this volume, we are stuck by the extent to which relationships—teacher–student and among students—serve as the core of students' experiences at school, with influences on their motivation, self-regulation, learning, engagement in risky health behaviors, and overall student engagement at school and with learning, among other things. Thus, support for the development and sustainability of positive relationships is a key to the developmental outcomes that are of interest to educators and scholars around the world.

It is the promise of student engagement for promoting positive development among youth—from early childhood through college—that was a focus of this edition of the *Handbook of Research on Student Engagement*. The student engagement framework is essential for promoting academic, social, emotional, and behavioral learning among all youth.

References

Allen, K.-A., & Boyle, C. (2022). School belonging and student engagement: The critical overlap, similarities, and implications for student outcomes. In A. L. Reschly & S. L. Christenson (Eds.), *Handbook of research on student engagement* (2nd ed.). Springer.

Anderman, E. M., Patrick, H., & Ha, S. Y. (2022). Achievement goal theory and engagement. In A. L. Reschly & S. L. Christenson (Eds.), *Handbook of research on student engagement* (2nd ed.). Springer.

Anderson, A. R., Christenson, S. L., Sinclair, M. F., & Lehr, C. A. (2004). Check & connect: The importance of relationships for promoting engagement with school. *Journal of School Psychology, 42*, 95–113. https://doi.org/10.1016/j.jsp.2004.01.002

Appleton, J. J., Christenson, S. L., Kim, D., & Reschly, A. L. (2006). Measuring cognitive and psychological engagement: Validation of the student engagement instrument. *Journal of School Psychology, 44*, 427–445. https://doi.org/10.1016/j.jsp.2006.04.002

Appleton, J. J., Christenson, S. L., & Furlong, M. J. (2008). Student engagement with school: Critical conceptual and methodological issues of the construct. *Psychology in the Schools, 45*, 369–386. https://doi.org/10.1002/pits.20303

Archambault, A., Janosz, M., Olivier, E., & Dupéré, V. (2022). Student engagement and school dropout: Theories, evidence, and future directions. In A. L. Reschly & S. L. Christenson (Eds.), *Handbook of research on student engagement* (2nd ed.). Springer.

Barton-Arwood, S. M., Wehby, J. H., & Falk, K. B. (2005). Reading instruction for elementary-age students with emotional and behavioral disorders: Academic and behavioral outcomes. *Exceptional Children, 72*, 7–27. https://doi.org/10.1177/001440290507200101

Betts, J., Appleton, J. J., Reschly, A. L., Christenson, S. L., & Huebner, E. S. (2010). A study of the reliability and construct validity of the school engagement instrument across multiple grades. *School Psychology Quarterly, 25*, 84–93. https://doi.org/10.1037/a0020259

Bronfenbrenner, U. (1977). Toward an experimental ecology of human development. *American Psychologist, 32*, 513–531.

Burns, M. K., Stevens, M., & Ysseldyke, J. (2022). Instruction and student engagement: Implications for academic engaged time. In A. L. Reschly & S. L. Christenson (Eds.), *Handbook of research on student engagement* (2nd ed.). Springer.

Carroll, J. B. (1963). A model of school learning. *Teachers College Record, 64*, 723–733.

Carroll, J. B. (1989). The carroll model: A 25-year retrospective and prospective view. *Educational Researcher, 18*, 26–31.

Christenson, S. L. (2008, January 22). Engaging students with school: The essential dimension of dropout prevention programs. [webinar] National Dropout Prevention Center for Students with Disabilities.

Christenson, S. L., & Pohl, A. (2020). The relevance of student engagement: The impact of and lessons learned implementing Check & Connect. In A. L. Reschly, A. Pohl, & S. L. Christenson (Eds.), *Student engagement: Effective academic, behavioral, cognitive, and affective interventions at school.* Springer.

Christenson, S. L., & Reschly, A. L. (2010). Check & Connect: Enhancing school completion through student engagement. In E. Doll & J. Charvat (Eds.), *Handbook of prevention science* (pp. 327–348). Routledge/Taylor and Francis.

Christenson, S. L., Sinclair, M. F., Lehr, C. A., & Godber, Y. (2001). Promoting successful school completion: Critical conceptual and methodological guidelines. *School Psychology Quarterly, 16*, 468–484. https://doi.org/10.1521/scpq.16.4.468.19898

Christenson, S. L., & Anderson, A. R. (2002). Commentary: The centrality of the learning context for students' academic enabler skills. *School Psychology Review, 31*(3), 378–393. https://doi.org/10.1080/02796015.2002.12086162

Christenson, S. L., Reschly, A. L., Appleton, J. J., Berman, S., Spanjers, D., & Varro, P. (2008). Best practices in fostering student engagement. In A. Thomas & J. Grimes (Eds.), *Best practices in school psychology* (5th ed., pp. 1099–1119). National Association of School Psychologists.

Christenson, S., Reschly, A. L., & Wylie, C. (2012). Epilogue. In S. L. Christenson, A. L. Reschly, & C. Wylie (Eds.), *Handbook of research on student engagement* (pp. 813–817). Springer.

Cook, C. R., Fiat, A., Larson, M., Daikos, C., Slemrod, T., Holland, E. A., Thayer, A. J., & Renshaw, T. (2018). Positive greetings at the door: Evaluation of a low-cost, high-yield proactive classroom management strategy. *Journal of Positive Behavior Interventions, 20*, 149–159. https://doi.org/10.1177/1098300717753831

Connell, J. P., & Wellborn, J. G. (1991). Competence, autonomy, and relatedness: A motivational analysis of self-system processes. In M. R. Gunnar & L. A. Sroufe (Eds.), *Self processes and development: The Minnesota symposia on child psychology* (Vol. 23, pp. 43–77).

Davis, M. H., Spring, C. L., & Balfanz, R. W. (2022). Engaging high school students in Learning. In A. L. Reschly & S. L. Christenson (Eds.), *Handbook of research on student engagement* (2nd ed.). Springer.

Diperna, J. C., Lei, P., Bellinger, J., & Cheng, W. (2016). Effects of a universal positive classroom behavior program on student learning. *Psychology in the Schools, 53*, 189–203. https://doi.org/10.1002/pits

Eccles, J. S., & Wang, M. T. (2012). Part 1 commentary: So what is student engagement anyway? In S. L. Christenson, A. L. Reschly, & C. Wylie (Eds.), *Handbook of research on student engagement* (pp. 133–145). Springer. https://doi.org/10.1007/978-1-4614-2018-7_6

Fallon, L. M., Marcotte, A. M., & Ferron, J. M. (2020). Measuring academic output during the Good Behavior Game: A single case design study. *Journal of Positive Behavior Interventions, 22*, 246–258. https://doi.org/10.1177/1098300719872778

Finn, J. D. (1989). Withdrawing from school. *Review of Educational Research, 59*(2), 117–142.

Finn, J. D., & Zimmer, K. S. (2012). Student engagement: What is it? Why does it matter? In S. L. Christenson, A. L. Reschly, & C. Wylie (Eds.), *Handbook of research on student engagement* (pp. 97–131). Springer. https://doi.org/10.1007/978-1-4614-2018-7

Ford, W. B., Radley, K. C., Tingstrom, D. H., & Dufrene, B. A. (2020). Efficacy of a no-team version of the Good Behavior Game in high school classrooms. *Journal of Positive Behavior Interventions, 22*, 181–190. https://doi.org/10.1177/1098300719890059

Fraysier, K., Reschly, A. L., & Appleton, J. J. (2020). Predicting postsecondary enrollment and persistence with secondary student engagement data. *Journal of*

Psychoeducational Assessment, 38, 882–899. https://doi.org/10.1177/0734282920903168

Fredricks, J. A. (2022a). The measurement of student engagement: Methodological advances and comparison of new self-report instruments. In A. L. Reschly & S. L. Christenson (Eds.), *Handbook of research on student engagement* (2nd ed.). Springer.

Fredricks, J. A. (2022b). Measuring Student engagement with observational techniques. In A.L. Reschly and S.L. Christenson (Eds.), *Handbook of research on student engagement* (2nd ed.). Springer.

Fredricks, J. A., Blumenfeld, P. C., & Paris, A. H. (2004). School engagement: Potential of the concept, state of the evidence. *Review of Educational Research, 74*, 59–109.

Fredricks, J. A., Reschly, A. L., & Christenson, S. L. (2019a). *Handbook of student engagement interventions: Working with disengaged youth.* Elsevier. https://doi.org/10.1016/C2016-0-04519-9

Fredricks, J. A., Ye, F., Wang, M.-T., & Brauer, S. (2019b). Profiles of school disengagement: Not all disengaged students are alike. *Handbook of Student Engagement Interventions*, 31–43. https://doi.org/10.1016/b978-0-12-813,413-9.00003-6

Furrer, C. J., Skinner, E., Marchand, G., & Kindermann, T. A. (2006, March). *Engagement vs. disaffection as central constructs in the dynamics of motivational development.* Paper presented at the annual meeting of the Society for Research on Adolescence, San Francisco, CA.

Gettinger, M., & Walther, M. J. (2012). Classroom strategies to enhance academic engaged time. In S. L. Christenson, A. L. Reschly, & C. Wylie (Eds.), *Handbook of research on student engagement* (pp. 653–673). Springer.

Gladstone, J. R., Wigfield, A., & Eccles, J. S. (2022). Situated expectancy value theory, dimensions of engagement, and academic outcomes. In A. L. Reschly & S. L. Christenson (Eds.), *Handbook of research on student engagement* (2nd ed.). Springer.

Hofkens, T. L., & Pianta, R. C. (2022). Teacher-student relationships, engagement in school, and student outcomes. In A. L. Reschly & S. L. Christenson (Eds.), *Handbook of research on student engagement* (2nd ed.). Springer.

Jimerson, S. R., & Chen, C. (2022). Multicultural and cross-cultural considerations in understanding student engagement in schools: Promoting the development of diverse students around the world. In A. L. Reschly & S. L. Christenson (Eds.), *Handbook of research on student engagement* (2nd ed.). Springer.

Jimerson, S., Campos, E., & Greif, J. (2003). Towards an understanding of definitions and measures of school engagement and related terms. *The California School Psychologist, 8*, 7–28. https://doi.org/10.1007/bf03340893

Jordan, W. J., McPartland, J. M., & Lara, J. (1999). Rethinking the causes of high school dropout. *The Prevention Researcher, 6*, 1–4.

Kraft, M. A., & Monti-Nussbaum, M. (2021). The big problem with little interruptions to classroom learning. *AERA Open, 7*, 1–17. https://doi.org/10.1177/23328584211028856

Lawson, M. A., & Masyn, K. E. (2015). Analyzing profiles, predictors, and consequences of student engagement dispositions. *Journal of School Psychology, 53*(1), 63–86. https://doi.org/10.1016/j.jsp.2014.11.004

Lovelace, M. D., Reschly, A. L., Appleton, J. J., & Lutz, M. E. (2014). Concurrent and predictive validity of the student engagement instrument. *Journal of Psychoeducational Assessment, 32*(6), 509–520. https://doi.org/10.1177/0734282914527548

Lovelace, M. D., Reschly, A. L., & Appleton, J. J. (2017). Beyond school records: The value of cognitive and affective engagement in predicting dropout and on-time graduation. *Professional School Counseling: 2017–2018, 21*(1), 70–84. https://doi.org/10.5330/1096-2409-21.1.70

Martin, A. J. (2022). The role of academic engagement in students' educational development: Insights from load reduction instruction and the 4 M academic engagement framework. In A. L. Reschly & S. L. Christenson (Eds.), *Handbook of research on student engagement* (2nd ed.). Springer.

Martin, A. J., Ginns, P., & Papworth, B. (2017). Motivation and engagement: Same or different? Does it matter? *Learning and Individual Differences, 55*, 150–162.

Masten, A. S., & Reed, M. J. (2002). Resilience in development. In C. R. Snyder & S. J. Lopez (Eds.), *Handbook of positive psychology* (pp. 74–88). Oxford University Press.

Masten, A., Nelson, K.M., & Gillespie, S. (2022). Resilience and student engagement: Promotive and protective processes in schools. In A. L. Reschly, & S.L. Christenson (Eds.). *Handbook of research on student engagement* (2nd ed.). Springer.

McDaniel, S. C., Houchins, D. E., & Robinson, C. (2016). The effects of check, connect, and expect on behavioral and academic growth. *Journal of Emotional and Behavioral Disorders, 24*, 42–53. https://doi.org/10.1177/1063426615573262

McPartland, J. M. (1994). Dropout prevention in theory and practice. In R. J. Rossi (Ed.), *Schools and students at risk: Context and framework for positive change* (pp. 255–276). Teachers College.

Mosher, R., & McGowan, B. (1985). Assessing student engagement in secondary schools: Alternative conceptions, strategies of assessing, and instruments. University of Wisconsin, Research and Development Center. (ERIC Document Reproduction Service No. ED 272812).

National Center for Education Statistics. (2021, May). Public High School Graduation Rates. Retrieved from: nces.ed.gov/programs/coe/indicator/coi

National Research Council and the Institute of Medicine. (2004). *Engaging Schools: Fostering High School Students' Motivation to Learn.* Committee on Increasing High School Students' Engagement and Motivation to Learn. Board on Children, Youth, and

Families, Division of Behavioral and Social Sciences and Education. Washington, DC: The National Academies Press.

Natriello, G. (1982). Organizational evaluation systems and student disengagement in secondary schools. Final Report.

Neuharth-Pritchett, S., & Bub, K. L. (2022). Early childhood engagement. In A. L. Reschly & S. L. Christenson (Eds.), *Handbook of research on student engagement* (2nd ed.). Springer.

Newmann, F. M., Wehlage, G. G., & Lamborn, S. D. (1992). The significance and sources of student engagement. In F. M. Newmann (Ed.), *Student engagement and achievement in American secondary schools* (pp. 11–39). Teachers College Press.

Pianta, R. C., & Walsh, D. J. (1996). *High-risk children in the schools: Creating sustaining relationships*. Routledge.

Reinke, W. M., Herman, K. C., & Copeland, C. (2022). Student engagement: The importance of classroom context. In A. L. Reschly & S. L. Christenson (Eds.), *Handbook of research on student engagement* (2nd ed.). Springer.

Reschly, A. L. (2010). Reading and school completion: Critical connections and Matthew effects. *Reading & Writing Quarterly, 26*, 67–90. https://doi.org/10.1080/10573560903397023

Reschly, A. L. (2020). Dropout prevention and student engagement. In A. L. Reschly, A. Pohl, & S. L. Christenson (Eds.), *Student engagement: Effective academic, behavioral, cognitive, and affective interventions at school* (pp. 31–54). Springer.

Reschly, A. L., & Christenson, S. L. (2006). Promoting school completion. In G. Bear & K. Minke (Eds.), *Children's needs III: Understanding and addressing the developmental needs of children*. National Association of School Psychologists.

Reschly, A. L., & Christenson, S. L. (2012). *Jingle, jangle, and conceptual haziness: Evolution and future directions of the engagement construct*. In S. L. Christenson, A. L. Reschly, & C. Wylie (Eds.), *Handbook of research on student engagement* (pp. 3–19). Springer Science + Business Media. https://doi.org/10.1007/978-1-4614-2018-7_1

Reschly, A. L. & Christenson, S. L. (2019, September). *Lowering the high school dropout rate: Lessons from the research* (PDK Primer #2). Phi Delta Kappa.

Reschly, A. L., & O'Donnell, K. C. (in press). Best practices in promoting academic engagement. In P. L. Harrison, S. L. Proctor, & A. Thomas (Eds.), *Best practices in school psychology* (7th ed.) National Association of School Psychologists.

Reschly, A. L., Betts, J., & Appleton, J. J. (2014). An examination of the validity of two measures of student engagement. *International Journal of School and Educational Psychology, 2*, 106–114. https://doi.org/10.1080/21683603.2013.876950

Reschly, A. L., Pohl, A., Christenson, S. L., & Appleton, J. J. (2017). Engaging adolescents in secondary schools. In B. Schultz, J. Harrison, & S. Evans (Eds.), *School mental health services for adolescents*. Oxford University Press. https://doi.org/10.1093/med-psych/9780199352517.003.0003

Reschly, A. L., Pohl, A., Christenson, S. L., & (Eds). (2020). *Student engagement: Effective academic, behavioral, cognitive, and affective interventions at school*. Springer. https://doi.org/10.1007/978-3-030-37285-9

Rosenthal, B. S. (1998). Non-school correlates of dropout: An integrative review of the literature. *Children and Youth Services Review, 20*, 413–433. https://doi.org/10.1016/S0190-7409(98)00015-2

Rosenshine, B. (1986). Reviewed work(s): Perspectives on instructional time by Charles W. Fisher and David C. Berliner. *Instructional Science, 15*, 169–173.

Rumberger, R. W. (1995). Dropping out of middle school: A multilevel analysis of students and schools. *American Educational Research Journal, 32*, 583–625.

Rumberger, R. W., & Larson, K. A. (1998). Student mobility and the increased risk of high school dropout. *American Journal of Education, 107*, 1–35. https://doi.org/10.1086/444201

Rumberger, R. W., & Rotermund, S. (2012). The relationship between engagement and high school dropout. In S. L. Christenson, A. L. Reschly, & C. Wylie (Eds.), *Handbook of research on student engagement* (pp. 491–514). Springer Science. https://doi.org/10.1007/978-1-4614-2018-7_24

Salmela-Aro, K., Moeller, J., Schneider, B., & Spicer, J. (2016). Integrating the light and dark sides of student engagement using person-oriented and situation-specific approaches. *Learning and Instruction, 43*, 61– In A.L. Reschly and S.L. Christenson (Eds.). *Handbook of research on student engagement* (2nd ed.). Springer. 70. https://doi.org/10.1016/j.learninstruc.2016.01.001

Salmela-Aro, K., Tang, X., & Upadyaya, K. (2022). Study demands- resources model of student engagement and burnout. In A. L. Reschly & S. L. Christenson (Eds.), *Handbook of research on student engagement* (2nd ed.). Springer.

Sinclair, A. C., Gesel, S. A., & Lemons, C. (2019). The effects of peer-assisted learning on disruptive behavior and academic engagement. *Journal of Positive Behavior Interventions, 21*, 238–248. https://doi.org/10.1177/1098300719851227

Skinner, E. A., & Raine, K. E. (2022). Unlocking the positive synergy between engagement and motivation. In A. L. Reschly & S. L. Christenson (Eds.), *Handbook of research on student engagement* (2nd ed.). Springer.

Skinner, E., Furrer, C., Marchand, G., & Kindermann, T. (2008). Engagement and disaffection in the classroom: Part of a larger motivational dynamic? *Journal of Educational Psychology, 100*(4), 765–781. https://doi.org/10.1037/a0012840

Skinner, E., Kindermann, T., & Furrer, C. (2009). A motivational perspective on engagement and disaffection: Conceptualization and assessment of children's behavioral and emotional participation in academic activities in the classroom. *Educational and Psychological Measurement, 69*(3), 493–525. https://doi.org/10.1177/0013164408323233

Tinto, V. (1975). Dropout from higher education: A theoretical synthesis of recent research. *Review of Educational Research, 45*(1), 89–125.

Tinto, V. (1982). Defining dropout: A matter of perspective. *New Directions for Institutional Research, 1982*(36), 3–15.

Tinto, V. (2022). Exploring the character of student persistence in high education: The impact of perception, motivation, and engagement. In A. L. Reschly & S. L. Christenson (Eds.), *The handbook of research on student engagement* (2nd ed.). Springer.

Waldrop, D., Reschly, A. L., Fraysier, K., & Appleton, J. J. (2019). Measuring the engagement of college students: Administration format, structure, and validity of the Student Engagement Instrument-College. *Measurement and Evaluation in Counseling and Development, 52*, 90–107. https://doi.org/10.1080/07481756.2018.1497429

Wang, M.-T., Degol, J. L., & Henry, D. A. (2019). An integrative development-in-sociocultural-context model for children's engagement in learning. *American Psychologist, 74*, 1086–1102. https://doi.org/10.1037/amp0000522

Wehlage, G. G., & Rutter, R. A. (1986). Dropping out: how much do schools contribute to the problem? *Teacher's College Record, 87*(3), 375–392.

Wehlage, G. G., Rutter, R. A., Smith, G. A., Lesko, N., & Fernandez, R. R. (1989). *Reducing the risk: Schools as communities of support.* The Falmer Press.

Unlocking the Positive Synergy Between Engagement and Motivation

Ellen A. Skinner and Kristen E. Raine

Abstract

Scholarship on engagement and motivation presents complementary profiles. This enables the strengths of each to help compensate for the shortcomings of the other. The strengths of work on academic motivation are its deep roots in multiple generative traditions and its rich body of well-researched theories; its corresponding limitations are its overarching fragmentation and lack of coherence. In contrast, the strengths of student engagement as a field are its wholistic appreciation for factors from many levels that contribute to school success, combined with its focus on a malleable observable process that is a primary engine of academic functioning; its corresponding limitations are its overarching confusion about the core construct itself and uncertainty about its place in a full explanatory model. We identify three ways that conceptualizations of engagement can support efforts to create a more integrated and coherent account of academic motivation: (1) engagement as "energy in action" provides a point of convergence for all theories of motivation; (2) it highlights the central role of action in processes of motivation; and (3) engagement as a "meta-construct" encourages a more wholistic and comprehensive conceptualization of academic motivation. We also explore three insights from the field of motivation that may help work on engagement make progress in clarifying conceptualizations and building out more complete explanatory models: (1) theories of motivation confirm the power of engagement as "energy in action"; (2) they help differentiate components within the meta-construct of engagement and allow each to be more fully realized; and (3) they suggest a common horizontal structure for theories of engagement that highlight the sequential functioning of their components as a dynamic and recursive explanatory process. We end by identifying three insights taken from the intersection of motivation and engagement to illustrate their utility in guiding efforts to promote competence and positive youth development. Our goal is to help unlock the synergy between these two areas, so researchers in both fields have the opportunity to learn from each other, and together to create richer, more comprehensive, nuanced, and coherent accounts of both motivation and engagement.

E. A. Skinner (✉) · K. E. Raine
Psychology Department, Portland State University, Portland, OR, USA
e-mail: ellen.skinner@pdx.edu; raine@pdx.edu

© The Author(s), under exclusive license to Springer Nature Switzerland AG 2022
A. L. Reschly, S. L. Christenson (eds.), *Handbook of Research on Student Engagement*,
https://doi.org/10.1007/978-3-031-07853-8_2

Engagement represents one of the most active and fastest growing areas of research in education and educational psychology today. From its inception, however, questions have been raised about its connections to academic motivation, both specific motivational constructs and the field as a whole. Starting with the seminal review of engagement almost two decades ago (Fredricks et al., 2004) and continuing with landmark handbooks (Christenson et al., 2012; Fredricks et al., 2019), integrative conceptualizations (Lawson & Lawson, 2013; Wang, Degol, & Henry, 2019; Wong & Liem, 2021), special sections, and definitive reviews of achievement motivation (Wentzel & Wigfield, 2009; Wentzel & Miele, 2016; Wigfield et al., 2015), a range of opinions have been offered: engagement subsumes motivation; motivation subsumes engagement; motivation is a component of the meta-construct of engagement; engagement is a behavioral manifestation of motivation; motivation is the precursor, engagement the outcome; motivation is the intent, engagement the resultant action; motivation is the private inner psychological process, engagement the publicly observable outward behavior; motivation influences engagement; engagement influences motivation; they reciprocally influence each other. Although it is accurate to summarize these alternatives by noting that "most scholars assume that engagement and motivation are related, but distinct constructs" (Fredricks et al., 2016, p. 1), we believe that underneath this general consensus is a more interesting and complex set of possibilities.

The central question can be found in the title of a recent article: "Motivation and Engagement: The Same or Different? Does it Matter?" (Martin et al., 2017). We try to deconstruct this question and provide one set of answers, which could be summarized as, "Motivation and Engagement: Not Identical, Not Distinct, and It Does Matter." We argue that important overlap exists between the two areas of study (meaning they are not distinct), but that they also offer complementary perspectives (meaning they are not identical). Our view is that the seemingly contradictory positions listed above are mostly correct but also mostly incomplete. Moreover, when they are all

considered together in a serial string, they sound confusing, at least in part because we do not always have an integrated understanding of the nature of motivation or a differentiated vocabulary for talking about the multiple meanings of engagement.

We argue that engagement and motivation are inextricably intertwined. They offer complementary perspectives and this tension creates the potential for great synergy between the two areas of study. Each has something of value to offer the other, so that each can shore up the other's weaknesses and fill gaps in the other's blind spots. Working together, researchers can create richer, more comprehensive, nuanced, and coherent accounts of both motivation and engagement, and so provide better foundations for future work in both areas. In this chapter, we start by providing an overview of each field, including their strengths and limitations, analyze the structures underlying each, and then suggest key places where each can make complementary contributions to the other (summarized in Table 1). In keeping with the focus of this *Handbook*, we end by identifying three insights taken from the intersection of these two fields to illustrate their utility in guiding efforts to promote competence and positive youth development. Following in the footsteps of previous scholars (see Christenson et al., 2012, for multiple examples), our goal is to help unlock the positive synergy between engagement and motivation.

The Fields of Academic Motivation and Student Engagement

The Field of Academic Motivation

The study of academic motivation is part of the older larger field of human motivation (Ryan, 2012). From the Latin root *movere*, meaning "to move," *motivation* takes as its central subject matter the processes underlying the energy, direction, and durability of action. Hence, the study of motivation in school examines how much effort students invest in their academic work, the emotional quality and authenticity of their participa-

Table 1 Positive synergy between work on engagement and motivation

How insights about engagement can strengthen work on motivation
1. Identifies "energy in action" as a core point of convergence among all theories of motivation
Targeting motivated behavior, emotion, and cognitive orientation
Organized by multidimensional constructs of engagement and disaffection
Place to begin integrating current motivational theories and studies
2. Highlights "energy in action" as a manifestation of motivation
As a site of learning and development; as a mediator of self and context
As an entry point for teachers' observation and understanding of student motivation
As messages to the developing self and academic identity
3. Encourages a more wholistic examination of academic motivation
Highlights involvement of multiple psychological processes (i.e., self-appraisals)
Points to utility of umbrella constructs like academic identity
Suggests broadening of action component to consider motivational resilience
How insights about motivation can strengthen work on engagement
1. Highlights core components of engagement with learning activities as "energy in action"
Provides evidence that interactions with educational activities are engines of learning and development
Offers coherent definitions of behavioral, emotional, and cognitive dimensions of "energy in action"
Needs disaffection, which also incorporates multiple dimensions
2. Helps differentiate components within the meta-construct of engagement and allows each to be more fully realized
Distinguishes action from self, context, perceived context, and outcomes
Highlights the central role of self-appraisals and how they can be used to derive contextual provisions that support action
Encourages consideration of engagement as part of arc of motivational resilience
3. Offers a common framework for models of engagement as a "meta-construct"
Highlights the sequential functioning of their components as a recursive causal process
Views alternative theories of engagement as nested
Suggests ways in which multiple models can be integrated

tion in learning activities, their choices about the interests they pursue and the courses in which they enroll, and their tenacity in the face of obstacles, setbacks, and demanding scholastic tasks. At its core, academic motivation focuses on the "fire" that fuels students' choices, participation, and persistence in the educational process. The field's primary strengths lie in its richness and depth. It is home to a wide range of generative and empirically tested theories (Brophy, 2013; Schunk et al., 2012; Wentzel & Miele, 2016; Wigfield et al., 2015), each of which represents decades of careful study and refinement. Typically grounded in larger frameworks that are applied in multiple domains, these bodies of work provide dense and detailed accounts of academic motivation.

However, such long traditions of separate investigation have also produced relatively isolated islands of deep understanding (Eccles, 2016). In principle, all these theories are focused on the same target—student motivation—but not in a way that has produced a cohesive or coherent account. It is as if each owes its primary allegiance to the larger and more general motivational framework from which it was derived. To date, as pictured in Fig. 1, these isolated islands make the field seem more like an archipelago than a common continuous territory. As a result, the field of academic motivation as a whole is often described as complex, fragmented, and resistant to integration (Anderman, 2020; Ford & Smith, 2009; Hattie et al., 2020; Koenka, 2020; Pintrich, 2003; Martin, 2009; Wigfield & Koenka, 2020). This creates problems for the field and all those who attempt to apply it. Researchers new to the area find it difficult to identify a set of core predictors or indicators to anchor their studies. Alternative constructs and measures are not examined for overlap or distinctiveness. Investigations from different traditions often produce findings that are not comparable and so cannot be integrated, slowing the accumulation of empirical evidence. Interventionists find it difficult to create comprehensive programs that incorporate all the essential ingredients needed to improve motivation. Parents and teachers find it difficult to construct comprehensive mental mod-

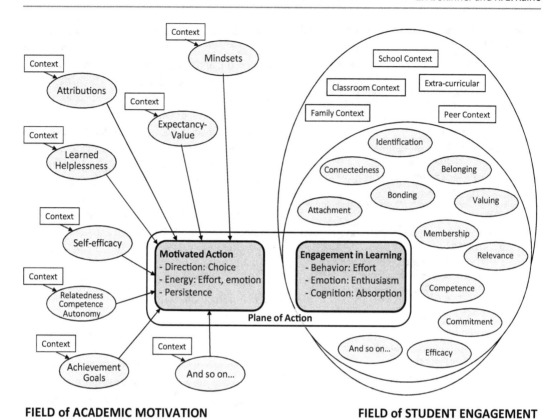

Fig. 1 A schematic representation of the current state of the fields of motivation and engagement, in which theories of motivation represent multiple islands of deep understanding and theories of engagement represent a single rich land mass

els of student motivation based on the field as a whole, even though that is what they would need in order to do their parts in supporting its development. Hence, the strengths of work on academic motivation are its deep roots in multiple generative traditions and its rich body of well-researched theories. Its corresponding limitations are its overarching fragmentation and lack of integration and coherence.

The Field of Student Engagement

The field of student engagement (Eccles, 2016; Fredricks et al., 2004; Jimerson et al., 2003; aka school engagement, Fredricks et al., 2004) stems from multiple traditions, most centrally the study of school participation and dropout (i.e., Finn, 1989; Finn & Zimmer, 2012; Mosher &

McGowan, 1985; Newmann, 1991). It is younger, inherently domain specific, and focuses largely on the educational arena, although arguments have been advanced for expanding it into other domains (e.g., Lawson & Lawson, 2013; Wang & Hofkens, 2020). At its most general, student engagement refers to the quality of students' participation, involvement, and connections to schooling (Christenson et al., 2012; Fredricks et al., 2004; Fredricks et al., 2019). Research in this area has exploded over the last two decades, based on its three interlocking strengths. First, engagement is a strong predictor of key academic outcomes, including student learning, performance, and achievement, as well as retention and graduation (e.g., Lei et al., 2018; Upadyaya & Salmela-Aro, 2013). Second, engagement also exerts a protective effect, buffering students from many of the typical risks of adolescence, including dropout and delinquency (e.g., Li & Lerner, 2011; Virtanen et al., 2021; Wang & Fredricks, 2014). Second, unlike most of the status predictors of academic outcomes (like gender, socioeconomic status, and ethnicity), engagement has proven to be a malleable state that can be influenced by many factors under the control of schools and parents. This makes it an ideal target for intervention efforts (Appleton et al., 2008; Fredricks, 2014; Fredricks et al., 2019; Lawson & Lawson, 2013). Third, some features of engagement are visible in the classroom. In fact, its antithesis, student disengagement or disaffection, is a major stressor for teachers (e.g., Fredricks, 2014). As a result, educators and school leaders immediately understand its importance (Finn & Zimmer, 2012).

As work on the construct has progressed, however, its limitations have also become increasingly clear. Disagreements persist about the core meaning of "engagement," as well as its dimensions, its opposite (described with terms like withdrawal, disengagement, disaffection, or burnout), and perhaps, most importantly, its boundaries, that is, specification of the features that should be considered indicators of engagement proper versus its facilitators or consequences (Azevedo, 2015; Boekaerts, 2016; Fredricks et al., 2016; Lawson & Lawson, 2013; Sinatra et al., 2014; Sinclair et al., 2003; Wang, Degol, & Henry, 2019; Wang, Fredricks, et al., 2019; Wang, Tian, & Huber, 2019; Wong & Liem, 2021). Leaders in the field rightly worry that haziness about central constructs is slowing conceptual and empirical progress (Fredricks et al., 2016; Reschly & Christenson, 2012). A thicket of different constructs and definitions has grown up around the term itself. Lack of clarity creates downstream problems for measurement; results from studies using different operationalizations cannot be integrated. Ambiguity also impedes the construction of the kinds of multi-step process-oriented theories that are needed to guide explanatory research and intervention efforts.

If the field of motivation can be likened to an archipelago of isolated islands of understanding, the corresponding metaphor for the field of engagement, also pictured in Fig. 1, is that of a single high-value island surrounded by a fence with a sign that says "Only engagement constructs beyond this point." Many researchers want to claim real estate on that island, so to gain entry they are renaming all the constructs in the neighborhood—including those studied as antecedents, psychological mediators, and other action components—as "engagement." At this point, the island is so crowded that the field "runs the risk of explaining almost everything related to students' experiences in school, and as a result not really explaining anything at all" (Fredricks et al., 2016, p. 2). Educators who are attracted to the potential inherent in the construct find it difficult to construct comprehensible mental models of the area as a whole. In sum, the strengths of student engagement as a field are its wholistic appreciation for factors from many levels that contribute to school success, combined with its focus on a malleable observable process that is a primary engine of academic functioning. Its corresponding shortcomings are its overarching confusion about the core construct itself and uncertainty about its place in a coherent explanatory model.

Basics of Motivational Theories and Conceptualizations of Student Engagement

In order to understand how work from each area can help strengthen the other, it is useful to first consider the underlying structure of theories in these fields.

Theories of Academic Motivation

The field is populated by precise and well-researched theories, nine of which are summarized in Table 2 (for overviews, see Brophy, 2013; Schunk et al., 2012; Wentzel & Miele, 2016; Wigfield et al., 2015). This table illustrates the richness and density of the field. Most explanatory theories of academic motivation, because they provide process-oriented accounts of motivated action, are horizontal and work with at least

Table 2 Synopses of nine major theories of motivation in school (in alphabetical order)

1. Achievement goal theory (Urdan & Kaplan, 2020): Students' views of the purpose or reasons for engaging in school-related tasks: whether they are focused on learning and self-improvement, or instead on demonstrating their abilities (if they are considered high) or protecting their abilities (if they are considered low), producing different patterns of effort, engagement, preference for challenge, and responses to failure or criticism
2. Attribution theory (Graham, 2020): Explanations for the causes of academic performances (like effort, ability, task difficulty, or chance) that differ on their internality, controllability, and stability, and that act as filters through which the meaning of success and failure are interpreted, and so shape their effects on emotional reactions and subsequent actions. Interpersonal version, too, involving causal explanations for other people's behavior that act as filters when interpreting their meaning, and so shape responses
3. Effectance and intrinsic motivation (Gottfried, 1985; White, 1959): Innate inborn desire to produce effects; underlies human curiosity, interest in novelty, desire to seek out opportunities to explore, experiment, and figure out how to make things happen, without any expectation of reward or reinforcement; includes a joyful response to feelings of efficacy and dejection in the face of impotence
4. Expectancy-value theory (Eccles & Wigfield, 2020): Multiplicative combination of how confident an individual is in his/her ability to succeed on a task mixed with how important, useful, or enjoyable the individual perceives the task to be (derived from a variety of societal, familial, and interpersonal sources, individual perceptions, and previous experiences) that together influence subsequent achievement choices, engagement, effort, persistence, and performance on these tasks
5. Learned helplessness and mastery (Seligman, 1975): Prolonged exposure to non-contingency or failure produces motivational, emotional, and cognitive deficits, especially when explanations for the failure rely on causes that are internal, stable, and global
6. Mindsets (Dweck, 2017): Assumptions about whether the nature of one's attributes (like ability and personality) are stable and cannot be changed or instead can develop and improve through the application of effort, practice, and the acquisition of effective strategies; shapes preference for challenge, willingness to exert effort, reactions to obstacles and setbacks, and interpretations of struggles, criticism, and others' successes
7. Self-determination theory (Ryan & Deci, 2017, 2020): Strong organismic position on intrinsic human needs as the source of energy and development, especially the need to experience oneself as the author of one's own actions. Integrated theories of intrinsic and extrinsic motivation, showing how extrinsic motivations can be internalized and regulated autonomously. Also incorporated a theory of the differential functions of rewards: as controlling or as informational
8. Self-efficacy (Schunk & DiBenedetto, 2020): Judgments of personal capacity to enact effective actions (based on successful performances, vicarious experiences, social persuasion, and physiological reactions) that, combined with judgments about action-outcome connections, influence motivational outcomes (task choice, effort, persistence), learning, achievement, and self-regulation.
9. Self-system model of motivational development (Connell & Wellborn, 1991): Students come with the desire to feel connected to others, effective in their interactions, and the source of their own actions; when needs are met at school, students are energized to participate constructively, which promotes learning and development; when needs are not met, students become disaffected

Adapted from Skinner (2019) with permission

four basic functional steps: (1) context, (2) self, (3) action, and (4) outcomes (Connell & Wellborn, 1991). Theories typically posit that: (1) social contexts, including pedagogical, interpersonal, and curricular contexts, shape (2) students' motivationally relevant psychological processes, typically referred to as self-system processes, self-appraisals, self-perceptions, or social cognitions. These psychological processes underlie and fuel (3) students' motivationally relevant patterns of action, including their choice, effort, participation, emotional reactions, and self-regulation; which in turn provide one path- way through which social contexts and self-appraisals influence (4) important educational outcomes, such as learning, academic functioning, achievement, and development. Both action and academic outcomes, in turn, feed back to influence subsequent contextual responses and shape developing self-systems and other psychological processes. Taken together, these feedforward and feedback effects comprise a "motivational dynamic" hypothesized to contribute to short- and long-term academic development (Lawson & Lawson, 2013; Reeve, 2012; Skinner & Pitzer, 2012).

This common underlying structure can be used to graph any explanatory motivational theory. Figure 2 illustrates this notion with three theories: expectancy-value theory (Wigfield & Eccles, 2020), attribution theory (Graham, 2020), and self-efficacy theory (Schunk & DiBenedetto, 2020). Each conceptualization takes a different set of appraisals (for which theories are typically named) as its target. To show that these self-appraisals have motivational power, each theory also specifies their consequences for motivated actions, and through these for academic outcomes. These well-documented causally efficacious functions qualify each as a major theory of motivation and as directly relevant to the achievement domain. All major theories have also undertaken a careful analysis of the antecedents of

their target self-appraisals, focusing on social, contextual, and personal factors that shape the construction and revision of self-systems. These portions of theories have also been tested empirically and figure prominently in efforts to design programmatic interventions and educational reforms (e.g., Wigfield & Wentzel, 2007).

Prioritizing self-appraisals As seen in Fig. 1, motivational theories are most centrally concerned with the self-systems or self-appraisals for which core theories are named (e.g., expectancies and values, attributions, self-efficacy, achievement goals, mindsets). These comprise the theories' unwavering conceptual and empirical commitments, their flags. Because many researchers have their eyes primarily on these tar-

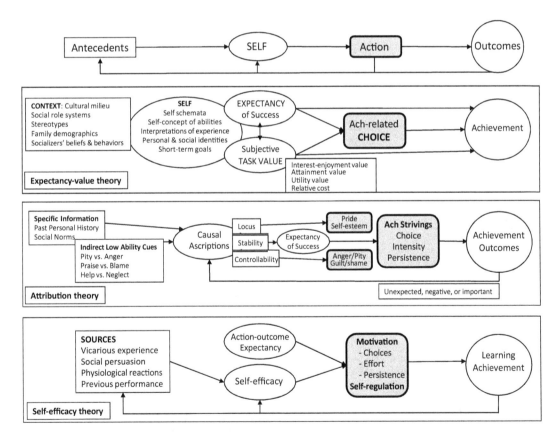

Fig. 2 The structure of explanatory theories of academic motivation, characterized wholistically as the study of (1) how social contexts, including pedagogical, interpersonal, and curricular contexts, shape (2) students' motivationally relevant appraisal processes, which underlie and fuel (3) their patterns of motivated action; which in turn provide one pathway through which social contexts and self-appraisals influence (4) important educational outcomes. The utility of this schematic is illustrated by diagramming three major theories of motivation

get self-appraisals, it is easy to see why each theory keeps to its own island, where those cognitive constructions rule. To some extent, these divisions are also strengthened by underlying meta-theoretical differences. Some theories (e.g., self-efficacy) view self-appraisals as temporary assessments arising from local interactions and experiences. Other theories (most notably self-determination theory) posit that self-systems (i.e., sense of relatedness, perceived competence, or autonomy orientations) are much more: They arise from, reflect, and are organized around fundamental organismic psychological needs (Ryan & Deci, 2017, 2020). In sum, explanatory theories of motivation comprise process-oriented accounts that privilege their target self-appraisals while also including social contexts, action, and outcomes.

Conceptualizations of Student Engagement

The field is populated by a variety of overlapping conceptualizations and theories of engagement, about a dozen of which are summarized in Table 3 (for overviews, see Appleton et al., 2008; Christenson et al., 2012; Lawson & Lawson, 2013; Wang, Degol, & Henry, 2019; Wang, Fredricks, et al., 2019; Wang, Tian, & Huebner, 2019; Wong & Liem, 2021). Theories of engagement also have their own underlying structure,

Table 3 Synopses of 11 theories and conceptualizations of student engagement (in alphabetical order)

1. *Check & Connect* (Reschly & Christenson, 2012*)*: Model of context, engagement, and outcomes underlying a structured mentoring intervention designed to promote student success and engagement at school and with learning. School, family, and peer contexts shape four aspects of engagement: (a) affective (belonging/identification, connectedness), (b) cognitive (self-regulation, relevance, value), (c) behavioral (attendance, participation, disciplinary incidents), and (d) academic (time-on-task, credits earned, homework, class grades), which in turn influence proximal learning and distal outcomes (e.g., graduation, college enrollment, employment)
2. *Dual Component Framework of Student Engagement* (Wong & Liem, 2021): Differentiates (a) learning engagement (psychological state of activity during learning tasks when students exert effort, are emotionally activated and absorbed) versus learning disengagement (state of inactivity during learning tasks when students feel deactivated, withdraw effort, and are distracted); from (b) school engagement (students' state of connection with the school community, characterized by relational attachment to people at school, cooperative participation in school activities, and psychological identification as a member of the school) versus school disengagement (state of alienation entailing a sense of disconnection from the school community, characterized by relational detachment, resistant participation, and psychological disidentification)
3. *Engagement in Academic Work* (Newmann, 1991): "the student's psychological investment in and effort directed toward learning, understanding, or mastering the knowledge, skills, or crafts that academic work is intended to promote," fostered by a need for competence, a sense of school membership, and the opportunity to participate in authentic academic work
4. *Integrative Development-in-Sociocultural-Context Model* (Wang, Degol, & Henry, 2019): A dynamic model of engagement as energized, sustained, and directed actions toward learning (versus disengagement, that is, withdrawal from and avoidance of learning), which is shaped by students' developmental competencies (e.g., cognitive and socioemotional skills) and self-appraisals (e.g., self-efficacy, task value, and mindsets). These in turn are influenced by external factors, including social position and family characteristics, cultural milieu, family, school, and peer context, and the nature of academic work. Engagement influences resilience mechanisms (coping, appraisal, and social support) as well as educational and developmental outcomes (e.g., achievement, educational aspirations, behavioral problems, psychological adjustment, retention, and college enrollment)
5. *Motivation and Engagement Wheel* (Martin, 2007): A use-inspired integrative framework comprising four higher-order dimensions: (a) adaptive cognitions/motivation (self-efficacy, valuing, mastery orientation), (b) adaptive behaviors/engagement (planning, task management, persistence), (c) impeding/maladaptive cognitions/motivation (anxiety, failure avoidance, uncertain control), and (d) maladaptive behaviors/engagement (self-handicapping, disengagement)

Table 3 (continued)

6. *Participation-Attachment-Commitment-Membership Model* (Furlong et al., 2003): Engagement as a developmental continuum that follows the progression from (a) participation (i.e., behavioral engagement in the classroom, extracurricular, and school environment), which facilitates the formation of (b) interpersonal attachments with people in the school (i.e., affective engagement—bonding, attachment, belonging—toward school, teachers, and peers), which leads students to develop (c) a sense of personal commitment to the school community (i.e., cognitive engagement or identification with school), and ultimately incorporating (d) school membership as part of their self-identity

7. *Participation-Identification* (Finn, 1989): Early engagement and academic success lead students to bond with school (develop feelings of valuing and belonging), and engage with school more deeply as they progress through their academic careers (from simple attendance and compliance to active initiation and ownership to participation in extracurricular and then self-governance activities)

8. *School/Student Engagement* (Fredricks et al., 2004): Multidimensional construct tapping students' commitment to, or investment in, school and school activities, including three different but related forms: (a) behavioral (i.e., participation, involvement in academic and social or extracurricular activities, positive conduct, effort, persistence, concentration, and attention), (b) emotional (affective responses to teachers, classmates, academics, and school), and (c) cognitive (investment in learning, thoughtfulness and willingness to exert the effort necessary to comprehend complex ideas and master difficult skills)

9. *Schoolwork Engagement Versus Burnout Model* (Salmela-Aro & Upadaya, 2012): Derived from the concept of work engagement in occupational psychology, an enduring state of work-related fulfillment characterized by energy (feelings of vigor during school-related tasks), dedication (positive cognitive attitude and sense of significance toward schoolwork), and absorption (full attention and concentration while working); versus burnout (i.e., exhaustion due to study demands, a cynical attitude toward school, and feelings of inadequacy as a student)

10. *Self-Determination Model of Engagement* (Reeve, 2012): Extent of a student's active involvement in a learning activity, comprised of four interrelated aspects: (a) behavioral (concentration, attention, and effort), (b) emotional (task-facilitating emotions such as interest and the absence of task-withdrawing emotions such as distress), (c) cognitive (use of strategic and sophisticated learning strategies, seeking conceptual understanding rather than surface knowledge, and active self-regulation), and (d) agentic engagement (students' constructive contribution into the flow of the instruction they receive by intentionally and somewhat proactively trying to personalize and otherwise enrich what is to be learned)

11. *Transactional View of Student Engagement* (Lawson & Lawson, 2013): Engagement as a dynamic, social, and synergistic process defined by a host of recursive elements including (a) acts of engagement (various states of experience of individuals as they participate in discrete activities at particular moments in time, including emotional, behavioral, cognitive, agentic as well as attentional, positional, and social-cultural features of engagement), (b) benefits/competencies (and/or consequences) of engagement (social-cultural, cognitive, affective, behavioral, academic, extracurricular), (c) conditions and contexts of engagement (surrounding organizational conditions and ecologies, including population demography, organizational ecology, and social geography), and (d) dispositions and drivers of engagement (students' perceptions of the "will" and "skill" they bring to activity, including social agency, interests, prior experiences, identities, motivations, attachments, future aspirations, initiative, investment)

largely vertical to date, which can be represented in two ways (see also Martin, 2012). The first focuses on the *objects* of engagement or exactly what students are engaged *with* (see also Wong & Liem, 2021). As depicted in Fig. 3, broad definitions of engagement suggest a nested hierarchy. At the top would be engagement with school as an example of participation in larger prosocial institutions, such as extended family, church, and community organizations (e.g., Lawson & Lawson, 2013). This kind of multi-arena engagement both marks and promotes healthy development and wellbeing for youth, and also protects them from risky behaviors that otherwise can emerge during adolescence. Nested within this broad umbrella is student engagement itself, which encompasses participation in school as an organization, including involvement in extracurricular activities, clubs, sports teams, student government, and so on. Student engagement both reflects and fosters students' retention, graduation, and educational aspirations, and protects adolescents from alienation and dropout.

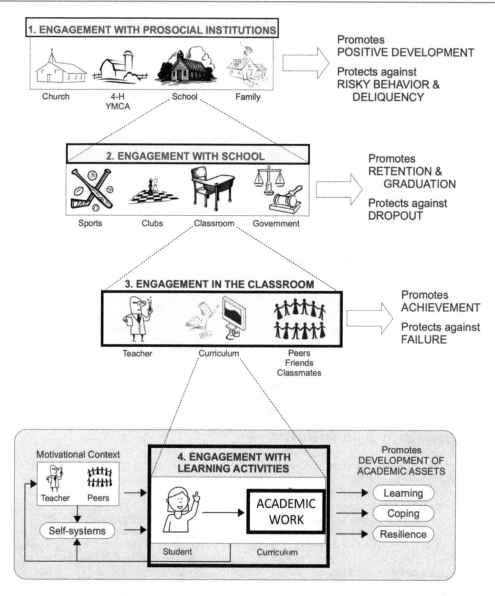

Fig. 3 A hierarchical perspective on engagement with school that depicts four nested levels of conceptualizations, starting at the highest level with engagement with school as one among many prosocial contexts, and ending with moment-to-moment engagement with learning activities. (Adapted from Skinner & Pitzer, 2012, with permission)

At the third level, nested within the larger school, is classroom engagement, which includes involvement with a community of learners in a specific class or classes. Here social partners include teachers, friends, and other classmates, as well as the curriculum. Finally, at the lowest level is academic engagement with learning activities themselves; here social partners are educational tasks or schoolwork. High-quality engagement of this kind promotes deep understanding and mastery. (For additional levels, see Azevedo, 2015; Lawson, 2017; or Martin, 2012.) Some confusion in the field is the result of misspecification about where in the hierarchy particular constructs and measures are located (Fredricks et al., 2011, 2016; Sinatra et al., 2014; Wong & Liem, 2021).

Prioritizing Action The second way that the field of engagement is structured can be seen by looking down into the construct itself and identifying its subcomponents (Wong & Liem, 2021). Scholars seem to agree that engagement is multidimensional and incorporates components that are affective/emotional, behavioral, and cognitive (Fredricks et al., 2004). However, that seems to be where agreement ends. One way of making sense of the heterogeneity among conceptualizations is to divide them into two main branches, which we label: (1) engagement as "energy in action," which views engagement as a multidimensional action construct, and (2) engagement as a "meta-construct," which views engagement as an umbrella for a variety of different constructs (see also Wong & Liem, 2021). These branches understand the internal structure of engagement in two very different ways, and both can trace their lineages back more than 30 years (e.g., Connell & Wellborn, 1991; Finn, 1989; Newmann, 1991).

Engagement as energy in action For many educational and motivational theorists (e.g., Lam et al., 2012; Reeve, 2012; Skinner & Pitzer, 2012; Wang, Degol, & Henry, 2019; Wang, Fredricks, et al., 2019; Wang, Tian, & Huebner, 2019), the most important way of defining academic engagement is as "energy in action" (Russell et al., 2005)—as pictured in Fig. 3 at the lowest level in the hierarchy. From this perspective, the core of the construct is high-quality participation in educational activities, which is why it is also called "engagement in learning" (Wang, Degol, & Henry, 2019; Wang, Fredricks, et al., 2019; Wang, Tian, & Huebner, 2019) or "learning engagement" (Wong & Liem, 2021). Hence, *behavioral engagement* includes on-task behavior, effort, exertion, attention, and hard work (examples from survey items: "When I'm in class, I listen very carefully," "In my class, this student works as hard as he/she can"). *Emotional engagement* focuses on affective states, like enthusiasm, enjoyment, excitement, interest, curiosity, and fun, experienced during participa-

tion in learning activities (e.g., "I am interested in the work at school," "When we start something new in class, this student is enthusiastic"). *Cognitive engagement* comprises "heads-on" investment, commitment, and absorption during interactions with learning activities where students think deeply about ideas and make meaning of the material presented to them (Blumenfeld et al., 2006; Greene, 2015; e.g., "If I don't understand what I read, I go back and read it over again," "I try to connect what we are learning now to things I know already").

These three dimensions—all facets of energy in action—are inherent aspects of the learning process (Boekaerts, 2016), which is why this kind of engagement is considered a necessary condition for learning and a robust predictor of academic performance. These three dimensions have their own internal dynamics, which helps explain why profiles of engagement are greater than the sum of their parts (Eccles & Wang, 2012; Lawson & Lawson, 2013; Reeve, 2012). Behavioral and cognitive engagement power progress in learning. Emotional states provide energy that activates and sustains ongoing behavioral and cognitive involvement (Pekrun & Linnenbrink-Garcia, chapter "Academic Emotions and Student Engagement", this volume; Skinner et al., 2008). The puzzlement, discovery, and aha! experiences inherent in cognitive engagement funnel effortful enthusiastic involvement toward deep understanding and mastery. As Wang and colleagues (2019) explain in their recent integrative review,

[E]ngagement provides a holistic lens for understanding how children interact with learning activities, with distinct behavioral, emotional-affective, and cognitive components forming a multidimensional engagement profile for each child (Fredricks et al., 2004; Wang & Degol, 2014). At its core, engagement involves making a concerted effort toward a goal and employing the necessary tactics to achieve that goal. Engagement is also the linchpin connecting energy, purpose, and enjoyment. Hence, children who are engaged not only are able to recover after setbacks and accomplish their goals but also are more likely to find these tasks to be satisfying. (p. 1087)

Engagement as a meta-construct The second branch of the field entails conceptualizations of engagement from higher up in the hierarchy, typically at the second level in Fig. 3. These formulations trace their roots to concerns with dropout as a protracted process of withdrawal from school, interventions for at-risk students, and school reform efforts (e.g., Finn, 1989; Finn & Voelkl, 1993; Finn & Zimmer, 2012; Fredricks et al., 2004; Reschly & Christenson, 2012). Scholars aimed to critique simplistic and static notions of dropout as a one-time event that happens to at-risk students. They wanted to broaden then current views—in terms of both time horizons and intervention levers—explaining that "engagement is more than just time-on-task" and "school success is more than just staying in school" (Reschly & Christenson, 2012). If "energy in action" is described as a single multidimensional construct, this branch can be described as a "meta-construct" that includes multiple different constructs under its umbrella.

One way to examine the alternatives formulated as part of this branch is to ignore terminology and consider the different constructs (i.e., theoretical concepts) that theories incorporate. Most of them retain the behavioral subcomponent of energy in action described previously, which incorporates effortful constructive participation in educational activities. In many ways, this dimension anchors the entire field because it gives engagement its claim to fame as a robust predictor of crucial academic outcomes like learning and performance. In some formulations, "participation" also extends to activities outside of schoolwork (such as extracurricular sports, clubs, or band); the quality of students' participation is considered to unfold sequentially and signify progressively greater connection to school (Finn, 1989; Finn & Zimmer, 2012). In other formulations, participation incorporates other academic markers, like grades, and credit hours earned; and in yet others, it is distinguished from mere attendance, compliance with classroom norms, and lack of behavior problems (see Table 3).

To this core, alternative conceptualizations of engagement add different components. For example, participation-identification models add the construct of "identification" (Finn & Zimmer, 2012; Voelkl, 2012), defined as a positive bond with school that includes (1) belonging or "feelings of being a significant member of the school community, having a sense of inclusion in school…" and (2) valuing or the "recognition of school as both a social institution and a tool for facilitating personal development" (Voelkl, 1997, p. 296). Some formulations include a component focused on investment (called cognitive engagement in conceptualizations of engagement as energy in action described previously); others also add future aspirations. However, it is also relatively common for researchers to incorporate self-regulated learning (e.g., Wang & Eccles, 2012) and some conceptualizations have added students' perceptions of close relationships with people at school, including teachers, classmates, and peers (e.g., Furlong et al., 2003).

Much confusion has been created because conceptualizations and measures use a variety of different labels to refer to all of these constructs (Azevedo, 2015; Boekaerts, 2016; Fredricks et al., 2016; Lawson & Lawson, 2013; Reschly & Christenson, 2012; Sinatra et al., 2014; Sinclair et al., 2003; Wong & Liem, 2021). For example, effort is typically part of "behavioral engagement" (Wang, Degol, & Henry, 2019; Wang, Fredricks, et al., 2019; Wang, Tian, & Huebner, 2019), but some consider it "cognitive engagement" (Eccles, 2016), because effort is often mental in nature. Identification, which includes belonging and valuing, has been called "affective engagement" (Voelkl, 2012); but "belonging" has also been referred to as "school membership," "bonding," "school connectedness," or "attachment." In some formulations, belonging and value are considered "psychological engagement" (since they reflect psychological processes; Appleton et al., 2006, now renamed as "affective engagement") and in others, "cognitive engagement" (because they are cognitive constructions or representations; Reschly & Christenson, 2012). In some conceptualizations, close relationships are called "bonding" or "attachment" (e.g., Furlong et al., 2003), and in others "emotional engagement" or "social engagement" (e.g., Linnenbrink-Garcia et al., 2011). In some formulations, "cognitive engagement" comprises investment (e.g., Fredricks et al., 2004); in others self-regulated learning (e.g., Cleary & Zimmerman, 2012); and in yet others, future aspirations (e.g., Appleton et al., 2006; see Table 3).

In sum, to the core idea of high-quality participation in academic work, these higher-level more elaborated conceptualizations of engagement as a meta-construct use a variety of labels (i.e., student, school, behavioral, affective, emotional, cognitive, academic, psychological, and social engagement) to add a range of different components, including participation in extracurricular activities; psychological processes like belonging, membership, bonding, connectedness, attachment, value, relevance, and educational aspirations; strategies of self-regulated learning; positive and negative reactions to and relationships with teachers, classmates, peers, and family; and attendance, credit hours, and grades. Building on these ideas, the remainder of this chapter explores ways that insights and knowledge from each field can help clarify, enrich, and fill in gaps for the other.

What the Field of Student Engagement Offers Work on Academic Motivation

As enumerated in Table 1, we first explore three ways that conceptualizations of engagement can support efforts to create a more integrated and coherent account of academic motivation as a whole. For this task, we focus first on the branch that conceptualizes engagement as "energy in action," arguing that it: (1) identifies a core point of convergence for all theories of motivation; and (2) highlights the central role of action in processes of motivation. We then turn to conceptualizations of "engagement as a meta-construct" and show how they (3) encourage a more wholistic and comprehensive conceptualization of academic motivation.

1. *Engagement as "energy in action" provides a core point of convergence for theories of motivation.*

The limitations of the field of motivation are visualized in Fig. 4, which lists the primary constructs of all the explanatory theories listed in Table 2 according to the four process steps identified previously (i.e., context, self, action, outcome). This figure illustrates the field's overall lack of coherence. This wall of constructs is what new researchers, interventionists, and educators face when they approach the field for the first time, seeking guidance for their studies, programs, or classrooms. A second glance at Fig. 4, however, also suggests much potential for integration among theories. Within each block of constructs, both overlap and distinctiveness are apparent. Because most motivational theories are centered on their designated self-appraisals, it may seem logical for integrative efforts to begin with them. However, because these represent the die-hard commitments of each mainland theory, this column of constructs is where theorists are most likely to insist upon exceedingly fine distinctions.

A potentially less controversial starting place might be inside the common ground staked out by engagement as "energy in action." Listed in Fig. 4 under "action," these constructs could also be called "motivated actions" because they can be considered the observable manifestations of motivation (Martin, 2009; Reeve, 2012; Skinner, Kindermann, Connell, & Wellborn, 2009; Wang, Degol, & Henry, 2019; Wang, Fredricks, et al., 2019; Wang, Tian, & Huebner, 2019; Wigfield et al., 2015; Wong & Liem, 2021). "Action" is defined here as a complex construct that, following the long European tradition of action theory (e.g., Brandtstädter, 2006; Heckhausen & Heckhausen, 2018), entails not only goal-directed behavior, but also intentions, emotions, and cognitions. All motivational theories target such actions; these manifestations tie core self-appraisals to the larger field of motivation. From this perspective, engagement can serve as a crucial point of convergence for motivational theories because they all have as one of their target

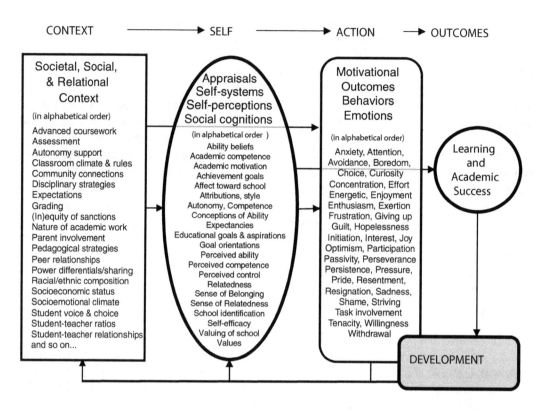

Fig. 4 A compendium of constructs utilized by major theories of academic motivation, organized according to (1) the contextual factors that shape motivation, (2) the self-system appraisals that underlie motivation, (3) expressions of motivated action, and (4) outcomes of motivational processes. (Adapted from Skinner, Kindermann, Connell, & Wellborn, 2009 with permission)

outcomes the kinds of actions studied under this conceptualization of engagement.

To illustrate this idea, Table 4 lists multiple major motivational theories and identifies the motivated actions targeted by each (see Skinner, Kindermann, Connell, & Wellborn, 2009; Skinner, Kindermann, & Furrer, 2009 for details; or Lawson & Lawson, 2013; Christenson et al., 2012, especially Part II, for multiple examples). These motivated actions include precisely the same behaviors (action, initiation, effort exertion, persistence), emotions (enthusiasm, interest, discouragement, boredom), and cognitive orientations (preference for challenge, flexibility of action, absorption) that are considered hallmarks of engagement as energy in action. Motivation is not identical with these actions; it is underneath them, providing the energy, desire, and passion

that galvanize them, guide their direction, and endow them with durability and persistence (Reeve, 2012). Sometimes motivation is enacted (i.e., realized on the plane of action) and sometimes not, but engagement, as defined by this branch, is a motivational process. It is not *only* a motivational process, in that engagement can also mark regulatory processes (Filsecker & Kerres, 2014; Wong & Liem, 2021), especially in the absence of spontaneous motivation (Ryan & Deci, 2020). However, high-quality engagement signals motivation—its manifestation on the plane of action (Reeve, 2012). Thus, engagement as energy in action provides common ground for all explanatory theories of motivation and can serve as a starting point for their integration.

2. *Engagement highlights the plane of action as crucial for theories of motivation.*

Table 4 Motivational theories and examples of the constructs that correspond to engagement and disaffection

Motivational theory (in alphabetical order)	Examples of behavioral engagement	Examples of emotional engagement	Examples of engaged orientation
Achievement goal orientations (Urdan & Kaplan, 2020)	Effort, exertion, persistence, task involvement, procrastination	Enthusiasm, enjoyment, anxiety	Selection of challenging tasks
Causal attributions (Graham, 2020)	Effort, persistence vs. giving up, withdrawal	Joy, anger, pride, shame, guilt	
Effectance motivation (Harter, 1978; White, 1959)	Energized participation	Enthusiasm, joy	Preference for challenge
Expectancy-value (Wigfield & Eccles, 2020)	Achievement strivings, effort exertion, persistence		
Intrinsic motivation (Gottfried, 1985; Gottfried et al., 2001)	Task involvement, persistence	Enjoyment, interest, curiosity	Preference for challenging, difficult, novel tasks
Learned helplessness (Abramson et al. 1978; Peterson et al., 1993; Seligman, 1975)	Passivity, apathy, avoidance, giving up, failure to respond	Sadness, dejection	Hopelessness
Mastery (Dweck & Molden, 2005)	Effort, persistence, concentration	Determination, enthusiasm, enjoyment	Preference for challenge, hypothesis testing, optimism
Self-determination (Reeve, 2012)	Participation, persistence vs. withdrawal	Enthusiastic, joyful, energetic vs. anxious, angry, rote	Willing, flexible, spontaneous vs. rigid, pressured
Self-efficacy (Schunk & Mullen, 2012)	Initiation of action, expenditure of effort, performance attempts	Anxiety, resignation	
Self-system model of motivational development (Connell & Wellborn, 1991)	Effort, hard work, persistence vs. withdrawal, passivity	Enthusiasm, interest, liking vs. boredom, sadness, frustration	Attention, concentration, preference for challenge, beyond the call

Adapted from Skinner, Kindermann, Connell, & Wellborn, 2009 with permission

Engagement as motivated action serves many functions in theories of motivation. As pictured in Fig. 5, engagement and disaffection are primary mediators between the self-appraisals privileged in motivational theories and the achievement outcomes that demonstrate their importance to the academic domain. In fact, because engagement is not only a central outcome of motivational appraisals, but also a necessary condition for learning (i.e., students can learn from an educational task only if they engage with it), it can be considered a *primary* pathway for motivationally relevant processes. Moreover, as shown in Fig. 5, engagement is important to motivation because it can serve as a gateway to other actions—like choice and perseverance—that are also central to motivational theories. That is, enthusiastic heads-on participation in particular educational activities may lead students, when they have a choice, to select those subjects they have found to be engaging in the past. Or, engagement may serve as an energetic resource when students encounter academic challenges, providing momentum for constructive self-regulation and adaptive coping, so students can persist or re-engage.

Engagement and disaffection also serve social functions. They may provide portals through which teachers and others get a glimpse into students' inner motivational workings. In other words, engagement may be an entry point for teachers' observation and understanding of student motivation. If teachers and parents use engagement to make decisions about whether students are "motivated" or "unmotivated," and

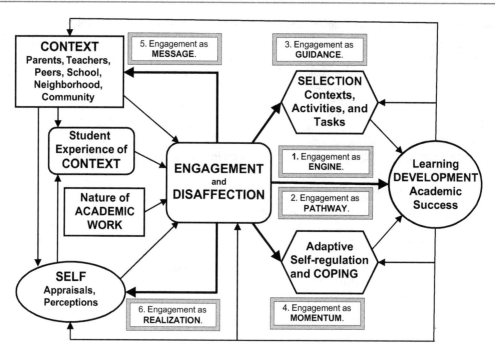

Fig. 5 Six functions of engagement and disaffection in motivational processes: (1) as a necessary condition for learning; (2) as a mediator of the effects of actual contexts, students' experiences, and views of the self on academic success; (3) as contributors to students' choices about contexts and activities; (4) as energetic resources for constructive coping and self-regulation; (5) as motivational communications that evoke reactions from social partners; and (6) as ongoing information that shapes the developing self. (Adapted from Skinner, 2016, with permission)

to diagnose and treat motivational problems, then a deeper analysis of the actual connections between engaged states and underlying motivational processes would be very useful. Accurate mappings could help practitioners formulate responses in ways that are more effective in counteracting student disaffection and fostering engagement (Furrer et al., 2014). Engagement may also play an important role in shaping students' own self-appraisals. Motivational theories exploring this possibility can build on participation-identification models that examine how the interactions between students and learning activities embodied in engagement (as well as resultant learning and academic success) carry messages to students about their belonging and the value of the larger school enterprise. Belonging/relatedness and value are two of the self-appraisals central to motivational theories, suggesting that high-quality engagement may also convey messages to students about other aspects of their academic identities, such as their

self-efficacy, autonomy, mastery goals, or mindsets. In fact, situative meta-theories (e.g., Nolen et al., 2015), which assume that beliefs and behaviors emerge from people's participation in social, cultural, and historical contexts or systems, insist that these patterns of culturally mediated activity are the primary grist from which identities are co-constructed. Identifying engagement as an outcome of all motivational theories highlights the many common pathways along which motivational influences flow.

3. *Engagement as a meta-construct encourages a more wholistic examination of academic motivation.*

The meta-construct of engagement (see Fig. 1) serves as an umbrella for a range of actions, psychological processes, and contextual affordances that contribute to students' short-term investment and commitment to school, and their long-term retention, graduation, and readiness for secondary education and employment. This wholistic quest reminds theorists that all motivational theories (e.g., Table 2) and all motivational constructs (e.g., Fig. 4) are parts of the same puzzle. This insight can encourage researchers to formulate more integrative models that extend beyond motivated actions (i.e., engagement) to include the self and contextual constructs. We note that efforts at integration are not likely to be undertaken by leaders in the field, nor should they be expected to. Many of them are leaders by virtue of their pursuit of the application of their chosen theories in the educational domain. It is for others (e.g., those who wish to design comprehensive interventions or help teachers construct comprehensible working models) to grapple with the task of integrating the field as a whole (e.g., Anderman, 2020; Dweck, 2017; Ford, 1992; Martin, 2009, 2012; Pintrich, 2003; Skinner, in press; Wigfield & Koenka, 2020).

Once it is ready, the field can turn its attention to the block of constructs in Fig. 4 under the heading of "Self," and begin to identify themes or families of constructs and then sort motivationally relevant psychological processes into these categories. Even if distinctions among these family members are initially sharpened (e.g., theorists may highlight subtle differences between "expectancies of success," "self-efficacy," and "perceived competence"), the broader families or themes, while at a coarser grain size, may provide sufficient resolution for educators, parents, or interventionists to make sense of their general tenor and function in students' motivation (Anderman, 2020; Martin, 2009; Skinner, in press).

Theoreticians can then work backward from these themes to locate the range of contextual attributes and practices that communicate messages to students about each of them (e.g., Lin-Siegler et al., 2016; Wentzel & Skinner, in press). A good example of how to do this can be found in work on mindsets, where researchers have located the communiques about fixed versus growth mindsets embodied by a variety of pedagogical, management, and interpersonal practices (Dweck & Yeager, 2019). An important lesson learned from this research is that students are influenced less by what teachers and parents *think* (i.e., their own mindsets) and more by what they *do* (i.e., practices and behaviors; Haimovitz & Dweck, 2017), a lesson relevant to achievement goal theorists who tend to prioritize the achievement goals held by social partners rather than their behaviors.

Finally, the centrality of engagement in motivational theories also encourages researchers to begin to distinguish and organize other facets of "action." It is possible to highlight categories of motivationally relevant action that are *not* parts of academic engagement—like choice, initiation, self-regulation, coping, tenacity, and persistence. As these constructs are teased out from multiple motivational theories (and the blocks of constructs in Fig. 4), and with the help of action theory, it is possible to view these actions as representing a series of steps through which students seek out, encounter, engage, manage, and deal with learning activities over time. One possible sequence has been described as *motivational resilience and vulnerability* (e.g., Skinner et al., 2020): Students' (1) choices and preference for challenging activities and coursework place them in settings with affordances for advanced learning, which supports (2) high-quality ongoing engagement that, when they (3) encounter problems and setbacks in their schoolwork, can minimize (4) emotional reactivity and other negative reactions. As a result, students have greater access to (5) constructive ways of coping and regulating their behaviors, emotions, and cognitions that allow them to (6) rebound and (7) re-engage with and persist in demanding academic work. All of these action steps, and not just the ones focused on engagement, can be used as points of convergence for motivational theories. Their analysis not only reveals common constructs, but also differentiates motivational theories according to the step(s) that each prioritizes. From a bird's eye view, conceptualizations of engagement help motivational theorists see that the field, which we have argued looks like an archipelago made up of isolated islands of understanding, is actually connected to the same solid ground.

What the Field of Academic Motivation Offers Work on Student Engagement

As summarized in Table 1, there are three ways insights from motivational theories may be helpful to engagement as researchers make progress in clarifying conceptualizations and building out more complete explanatory models: (1) theories of motivation confirm the power of engagement as "energy in action"; (2) they help differentiate components within the meta-construct of engagement and allow each to be more fully realized; and (3) they suggest a common horizontal structure for theories of engagement that highlight the sequential functioning of their components as a dynamic and recursive explanatory process. Many of these ideas have been articulated already by other engagement researchers (e.g., Wong & Liem, 2021), especially those who, like us, are working at the intersection of motivation and engagement (e.g., Connell & Wellborn, 1991; Eccles, 2016; Reeve, 2012; Wang, Degol, & Henry, 2019; Wang, Fredricks, et al., 2019; Wang, Tian, & Huebner, 2019).

1. *Theories of motivation encourage conceptualizations of engagement to distinguish and prioritize "energy in action."*

Motivational theories have a strong opinion about where the "bang" in the student engagement "buck" is located. It is centered on definitions of engagement as "energy in action" (Connell & Wellborn, 1991; Reeve, 2012; Skinner, Kindermann, Connell, & Wellborn, 2009; Skinner, Kindermann, & Furrer, 2009 Wang, Degol, & Henry, 2019; Wang, Fredricks, et al., 2019; Wang, Tian, & Huebner, 2019), also referred to as "academic engagement" to specify that the objects are curricular or academic tasks. From a motivational perspective, these emotionally charged heads-on participatory actions represent a force powerful enough to fuel learning and counteract dropout and other risky adolescent behaviors (e.g., Reeve, 2012; Skinner & Pitzer, 2012). This suggests that engagement researchers can begin to clarify core definitions by wading into the pile of constructs surrounding their meta-construct and extract those that target

the plane of action, that is, the quality of students' participation in educational activities (Finn & Zimmer, 2012; Newmann, 1991; Reeve, 2012). Two recent integrative reviews target exactly this component, which researchers label "engagement in learning" (Wang, Degol, & Henry, 2019; Wang, Fredricks, et al., 2019; Wang, Tian, & Huebner, 2019) and "learning engagement" (Wong & Liem, 2021). As made clear by definitions that use phrases such as "participation," "interact with learning activities," and "state of activity/inactivity," these are *action* constructs: They represent students' actual *interactions* with educational tasks and activities on the plane of action.

Motivational theories help draw lines around this component because it represents "patterns of motivated action." Moreover, the empirical base accumulated by motivational researchers provides robust evidence that this component of engagement serves the important functions enumerated in Fig. 5. They are: (1) necessary conditions for learning; (2) mediators of the effects of actual and perceived contexts and students' views of the self on their academic success; (3) contributors to students' choices about contexts and activities; (4) resources for adaptive coping and self-regulation; (5) motivational communications that evoke reactions from social partners; and (6) ongoing information that shapes the developing self.

Antithesis of engagement Motivational theories also encourage conceptualizations to incorporate the opposite of engagement, variously labeled as withdrawal, disengagement, burnout, alienation, switching off, or disaffection (Connell & Wellborn, 1991; Fredricks, 2014; Hascher & Hadjar, 2018; Martin, 2012; Wong & Liem, 2021). Perhaps because the field arose as a reaction to researchers' narrow focus on risk and dropout, conceptualizations of engagement seem uncertain about whether to include a "dark side" (Salmela-Aro et al., 2016). The field of motivation, which has always considered lack or loss of motivation as prime material for its theories, highlights the benefits of conceptualizations that extend into this territory. Theoretically, they are richer. Disaffection is more than lack of engagement. Measures that incorporate both have shown that the two are distinguishable but closely related and that each adds predictive power over and above the other (e.g., Martin et al., 2011; Salmela-Aro et al., 2016; Skinner, Kindermann, Connell, & Wellborn, 2009; Skinner, Kindermann, & Furrer, 2009; Wang, Fredricks, et al., 2019). Such conceptualizations give researchers and interventionists the flexibility to consider them separately or in combination, and to be explicit about whether contextual and psychological factors are hypothesized to foster engagement, counteract disaffection, or both. Concepts and measures that capture both encourage explicit consideration of how to reach both goals, as well as providing information about the location of problems should interventions fall short in bolstering engagement or in reducing disaffection. These broader views also suggest that there are multiple profiles that combine different features of engagement and disaffection (e.g., Wang & Peck, 2013), and these alternatives can be used to diagnose targeted remedies that may not be the same for all students (Furrer et al., 2014). For example, students whose academic engagement is faltering due to boredom need different kinds of supports than students who are cognitively overwhelmed by task demands or those experiencing anxiety or academic burnout. Hence, assessments of disaffection may be useful in designing multi-pronged programs that create differentiated pathways back to engagement.

If the field heeds this advice, conceptualizations of *disaffection* would mirror the internal structure of engagement as energy in action (Skinner, Kindermann, Connell, & Wellborn, 2009; Skinner, Kindermann, & Furrer, 2009; Wang, Degol, & Henry, 2019; Wang, Fredricks, et al., 2019; Wang, Tian, & Huebner, 2019; Wong & Liem, 2021). *Behavioral disaffection* entails passivity and lack of effort or exertion as well as more active off-task or disruptive behavior; *emotional disaffection* ranges from the most common deactivating academic emotion, boredom, to worry, sadness, discouragement, irritation, and frustration while working on academic tasks; and *cognitive disaffection* includes inattention, mind-wandering, lack of concentration, and thoughts of escape. All three dimensions of disaffection are active parts of internal causal dynamics. Deactivating emotions can exert a downward pressure on behavioral participation, sapping energy and will, and, if they occupy working memory, can interfere with cognitive engagement. Cognitive disaffection potentially undermines behavioral participation and aggravates negative emotions. Together these create a multi-dimensional profile of disaffection that can add depth, scope, and power to engagement, and enable more well-rounded and nuanced accounts of patterns of action.

2. *Motivational theories help differentiate components within the meta-construct of engagement, and suggest ways individual components can be enriched with insights from work on motivation and regulation*

Motivational theories can help conceptualizations of engagement find a useful place for all the components that have been nominated to date as part of the meta-construct. Using the horizontal structure underlying theories of motivation (see Fig. 2), constructs can be sorted according to whether they correspond to "context," "self," "action," or "outcomes." First, constructs relevant to the behavioral, emotional, and cognitive dimensions of "energy in action" can be grouped as parts of a component labeled "action." Then a second set, including constructs like valuing, belonging, identification, and self-efficacy, can be grouped as parts of a component relevant to "self." Motivational theories insist that these self-appraisals (aka self-perceptions, self-system processes, self-relevant representations, or internal working models) should be distinguished from actions. They represent internal psychological processes or social cognitions that *influence* action readiness or actions themselves. As documented by motivational research over many decades, individuals use these appraisals to interpret past exchanges and guide future action (Brophy, 2013; Schunk et al., 2012; Wentzel & Miele, 2016; Wigfield et al., 2015).

Constructs within this component could also collectively be called "identification" or "academic identity." As described by participation-identification models, also over many decades, these are the psychological processes whose development is *influenced* by academic success and patterns of action. In conceptualizations of engagement as "energy in action," action components are indicators of engagement, whereas constructs in the self-component are facilitators (e.g., Skinner, 2016; Wang, Degol, & Henry, 2019; Wang, Fredricks, et al., 2019; Wang, Tian, & Huebner, 2019). In conceptualizations of engagement as a meta-construct, both action *and* self-constructs fall under the umbrella of engagement. They are both indicators; contexts are the facilitators (e.g., Reschly & Christenson, 2012). Whether or not self-appraisals are considered *parts* of engagement, however, conceptualizations must distinguish between self and action if studies are to examine whether and how these two processes are (reciprocally) causally related.

Those aspects of the meta-construct of engagement that reflect actual external conditions can be grouped together as parts of a third component labeled "Context." Sometimes called "engagement contexts" (e.g., Furlong et al., 2003), interpersonal contexts are marked by the quality of students' actual relationships with teachers, classmates, friends, and other social partners at school. Contexts also include pedagogical, disciplinary, climate, and even discriminatory practices. Aspects of "Context" are observable, since they reflect what is actually going on in the classroom or other relevant settings, and can be assessed via observations in the classroom (e.g., Pianta & Hamre, 2009) or other settings where engagement takes place. A component labeled "Perceived Context" can hold constructs that reflect students' subjective take on these objective contextual affordances, messages, and interactions. This component would include, for example, students' perceptions of whether their teachers and peers like and care about them. These can be contrasted with actual contextual conditions (i.e., whether teachers or peers really do like a specific student) and self-appraisals (i.e., whether a student feels she belongs and is worthy of love). Compared to actual contextual conditions that can be mapped with observations,

these experiential constructs can be captured only via self-reports because they reflect the cumulative meaning students make out of their actual experiences in particular social and physical environments.

Finally, the proximal and distal consequences of engagement can be included as parts of the component labeled "Outcomes," ranging from actual learning, grades, and achievement to development of competencies and attitudes, retention, graduation, enrollment in college, employment, and productive citizenry; as well as all the risks averted, such as dropout, delinquency, and gang involvement. Differentiating the components of engagement allows researchers to consider each one more carefully or to call on motivational and volitional research that has already done so.

Central role of self Motivational theories prioritize self-appraisals, since these psychological processes are at the heart of their theories. Hence, the field encourages work on engagement to take seriously the task of determining the social cognitions that are most important in influencing the action components of engagement, rather than just declaring them a priori as *parts* of the meta-construct of engagement. As shown in Table 3, current conceptualizations already include some important psychological processes—like belonging and valuing. Explanatory theories of engagement can test and build out on these, or scrutinize research on motivation, which has accumulated relatively detailed bodies of evidence about such appraisal processes.

These are some of the most powerful predictors of student engagement as energy in action, but for theories of engagement, they represent something more—they can help researchers systematically derive the causally efficacious contextual factors that will serve as levers in successful interventions designed to promote engagement. As explained by Lin-Siegler and colleagues, this step is part of "a promising but underexplored approach to improving students' motivation and learning in schools: the design and implementation of psychologically informed instructional activities to change students' attitudes and beliefs" (Lin-Siegler et al., 2016, p. 295). Just as engagement serves as a portal through which teachers can view student motivation, so too can the motivational messages contained in self-appraisals act as diagnostic tools for interventionists (and teachers and parents) in formulating strategies to bolster engagement.

Without a full understanding of these mediational processes, engagement researchers are left to search for direct contextual effects or to rely on generically "good" contexts characterized by high-quality relationships and best pedagogical and management practices. It is always a good idea to promote generically positive contextual conditions, of course, but a focus on specific self-appraisals allows educators and interventionists to think more broadly and deeply. For example, the focus on a sense of belonging has galvanized educators from pre-Kindergarten to college to think about the messages their institutional practices send, especially to students from underrepresented and minoritized backgrounds, where the default implicit communication is "You are not welcome here" (see Galindo, Brown, & Lee, chapter "Expanding an Equity Understanding of Student Engagement: The Macro (Social) and Micro (School) Contexts", this volume). Coming to grips with the thousands of ways these messages are transmitted, ranging from enrollment processes, to the languages of signs in the hall, to the contents of curricula and discipline practices, has enabled schools to begin a culture shift guided by the goal of reversing those default messages for all students. At this point, motivational theories can provide a menu of options for self-appraisals that could be relevant to explanatory theories of engagement; a list of examples is included in the "Self" block in Fig. 4. As motivational theorists identify core families of self-appraisals (e.g., Dweck, 2017; Ford, 1992; Martin, 2009: Skinner, in press), this menu of options should become clearer and more focused.

Richer views of the action components of engagement The field of motivation has found it productive to incorporate insights from work on regulation, deepening its understanding, for example, of what happens when the "fire" of intrinsic motivation dims (e.g., Reeve, 2012; Ryan & Deci, 2020) or academic tasks become too demanding (e.g., Skinner & Saxton, 2019, 2020). Motivational theories have returned the favor, showing, for example, how normative losses in motivation can help explain why the use of certain self-regulatory strategies declines across adolescence even though cognitive and meta-cognitive capacities are advancing (e.g., Karabenick & Newman, 2013; Van der Veen & Peetsma, 2009). The two areas share a common interest in targets on the plane of action (i.e., participation in activities for which there is no intrinsic motivation, self-regulated learning, adaptive help-seeking, academic coping) and both understand that these processes all have underpinnings that are both motivational and regulatory.

Such cross-area fertilization suggests that research on regulation may also hold keys to understanding the roots of engagement (Cleary & Liu, chapter "Using Self-Regulated Learning (SRL) Assessment Data to Promote Regulatory Engagement in Learning and Performance Contexts", this volume; Cleary & Zimmerman, 2012; Filsecker & Kerres, 2014; Fredricks et al., 2004; Schunk & Mullen, 2012). These examples also indicate *where* in episodes of engagement such regulatory processes are likely to matter most: when motivational processes falter or when the actions of engagement need to be managed intentionally (Boekaerts, 2016). Following this train of thought, processes of self-regulation are likely to be activated when students are confronted by uncertainty (e.g., key choice points), lack of motivation (e.g., boredom), or demands that overwhelm their automatic responses (e.g., challenges, setbacks, problems). If self-regulatory capacities and autonomous motivation are available, students should show tenacity (i.e., durability in engagement) as well as strategies of adaptive coping that allow them to re-engage constructively. To explore these possibilities, however, conceptualizations of engagement will first have to extract self-regulated learning from *inside* the meta-construct itself (Boekaerts,

2016), where it has often been considered part of cognitive engagement.

From this perspective, as mentioned previously, engagement would be considered *both* a motivational and a regulatory process (Boekaerts, 2016; Cleary & Zimmerman, 2012; Filsecker & Kerres, 2014; Schunk & Mullen, 2012), with the idea that these two subprocesses are continuously in play, and it is the balance between the two that gives engagement its vigor, quality, and tenacity. Just as with research on motivation, conceptualizations of engagement may wish to consider its role in the arc of motivational resilience (e.g., Skinner et al., 2020), where motivated actions like choice may create differential opportunities for high-quality engagement; and regulatory strategies (e.g., self-regulated learning, help-

seeking, coping) may help explain how engagement can be sustained during demanding academic activities. Moreover, when engagement falters, this umbrella construct also focuses on how it can be regained through processes both regulatory and motivational, called buoyancy, bounce back, or re-engagement.

3. *Motivational theories offer a view of meta-constructs of engagement that highlight the sequential functioning of their components as a dynamic recursive causal process*

The structure that underlines explanatory theories of motivation can also be used to map meta-constructs of engagement. This notion is illustrated in Fig. 6 with three prominent models: the Participation-Identification model (Finn, 1989; Finn & Zimmer, 2012; Finn & Voelkl,

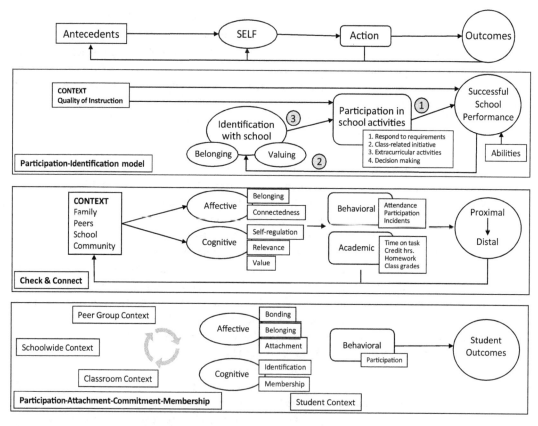

Fig. 6 The structure of explanatory theories of engagement, characterized wholistically as the study of (1) how the social contexts of engagement, including pedagogical, interpersonal, and curricular contexts, shape (2) students' engagement-relevant appraisal processes, which underlie and fuel (3) their patterns of learning engagement, which influence (4) important educational outcomes. Learning engagement and school success in turn feedback to shape subsequent self-appraisals. The utility of this schematic is illustrated by diagraming three major theories of engagement

1993; Voelkl, 2012), the Check & Connect model (Reschly & Christenson, 2012), and the Participation-Attachment-Commitment-Membership model (Furlong et al., 2003). However, these components could be used to map any of the models of engagement summarized in Table 3. Of special note are the many direct and indirect feedforward and feedback arrows that connect components in these models. These arrows indicate that such connections are not "part-whole" relationships (as implied by the term "meta-construct"), but instead reflect "cause-effect" relationships that indicate explanatory processes. Such differentiation allows engagement researchers to think through whether their models can best be described as "conceptualizations" of engagement—which refer to definitions and dimensions of a single construct (like academic or learning engagement)—or as full-blown "theories" of engagement, which not only

specify target phenomena, but also antecedents, consequences, and mediators. Many "meta-constructs," when unpacked, likely represent explanatory theories in their own right.

Mapping meta-constructs of engagement This underlying framework might also provide a basis for beginning to integrate different perspectives on engagement. A general model of multi-component theories of engagement—what Wong and Liem (2021) referred to as "mixed models" because they include both learning and school engagement—is depicted in Fig. 7 (see also Wang, Degol, & Henry, 2019; Wang, Fredricks, et al., 2019; Wang, Tian, & Huebner, 2019). It has as its core "engagement in action," also called academic engagement (Connell & Wellborn, 1991), engagement in learning (Wang, Degol, & Henry, 2019; Wang, Fredricks, et al., 2019; Wang, Tian, & Huebner, 2019), or learning

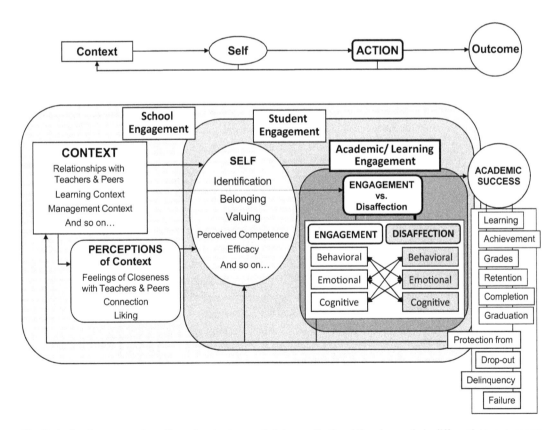

Fig. 7 A visual representation of how the structure underlying motivational theories can help differentiate components of engagement into multi-step process-oriented explanatory theories

engagement (Wong & Liem, 2021). Although we hesitate to state anything definitive about how engagement terms have been parsed (based on widespread inconsistencies), it might be possible to speculate that some theories that incorporate self-appraisals refer to their meta-constructs as "student engagement" (e.g., Reschly & Christenson, 2012), whereas theories that also incorporate contextual conditions, like the quality of interpersonal relationships with people at school, refer to their meta-constructs as "school engagement" (e.g., Wong & Liem, 2021).

Nested models From a bird's eye view, motivational theories can help the field of engagement see more clearly that, living on their island are two camps with competing proposals for how to build out that high-value real estate (Wong & Liem, 2021). On the one hand, engagement can be viewed as "energy in action," that is, defined as a pattern of action during learning activities, complemented by disaffection, where both have behavioral, emotional, and cognitive facets. This multidimensional construct has its own internal dynamics among these subcomponents (e.g., the effects of emotional disaffection on behavioral engagement), and also calls on underlying motivational and regulatory processes to explain its emergence, quality, direction, and durability on the plane of action. This kind of engagement is one component of a larger explanatory theory, which could be called the external dynamics of engagement, because it contains elements outside of engagement proper, specifically, self-appraisals, experienced and actual contextual conditions, and learning outcomes (see Fig. 6 for similar mappings of other theories, such as Reschly & Christenson, 2012). These internal and external dynamics explain the recursive processes that influence its functioning and development (e.g., Finn & Zimmer, 2012; Green et al., 2012; Martin et al., 2017; Wang, Tian, & Huebner, 2019). Consistent with other scholars (e.g., Connell & Wellborn, 1991; Lam et al., 2012; Reeve, 2012; Wang, Degol, & Henry, 2019; Wang, Fredricks, et al., 2019; Wang, Tian, & Huebner, 2019), that is the perspective we use in our own research.

On the other hand, there is a larger and more wholistic understanding of engagement as a meta-construct (Christenson et al., 2012; Fredricks et al., 2004), of which students' enthusiastic participation in learning activities is only a narrow and visible slice. From this perspective, psychological processes, like sense of belonging, valuing school, and identifying with its goals, are not predictors; they are additional slices, as are close and caring relationships with members of the school community. These are all considered parts of the *internal* dynamics of engagement. Engagement at all these levels is a cumulative process, and without this "glue" (Lawson & Lawson, 2013) at multiple levels of school, a student's future can be considered at risk. Here, external dynamics are the contexts, both institutional (e.g., teacher working conditions, principal leadership, school district supports) and societal (e.g., teaching training, parental involvement), that promote or impede the task of creating a school culture where this kind of engagement is the right of every student.

Motivational theories suggest that some of the confusion in the area of engagement, while currently causing real problems, may reflect relatively superficial disagreements. On the one hand, scholars are using the term engagement for the more complex multifaceted whole (i.e., the entire engagement system) as well as for some or all of its parts. On the other, scholars are attempting to find labels that involve the term "engagement" (i.e., behavioral, affective, emotional, cognitive, academic, psychological, or social engagement) for constructs that refer to "context," "perceived context," "self," and "action." It would be possible to conceptualize engagement in a way that allows for both, as long as researchers use terminology that clarifies the differences between them. This would allow conceptualizations of engagement as energy in action to be fully nested within larger explanatory theories of engagement as a meta-construct, in ways that would also allow a seamless integration with motivational theories.

Promoting Youth Competence and Positive Development: Three Lessons Located at the Intersection of Engagement and Motivation

To contribute to the focus of this *Handbook* and to highlight the potential synergy between engagement and motivation, we close by selecting three insights taken from the intersection between these fields, and show how they can contribute to efforts to promote youth competence and positive development. These synergistic ideas entail: (1) a focus on *motivational resilience* as a protective factor and powerful developmental force for youth; (2) the notion of *academic identity* as a lever for strengthening competence and resilience; and (3) a broader consideration of contexts as *complex social ecologies* that include multiple microsystems and social partners (e.g., parents, teachers, and peers) as well as the pedagogical practices, management strategies, and community connections at school.

Motivational resilience as a target of intervention Efforts The organizational construct of motivational resilience, defined broadly as "patterns of action that allow students to constructively deal with, overcome, recover, and learn from encounters with academic challenges, obstacles, and failures" (Skinner et al., 2020, p. 290), brings together work from the areas of engagement, motivation, and regulation (e.g., self-regulated learning, academic coping) within a frame of everyday academic resilience and buoyancy (Martin & Marsh, 2009; Skinner & Pitzer, 2012; Yeager & Dweck, 2012). As described previously, motivational resilience represents students' desire to choose and undertake challenging tasks, to fully engage, and, when they encounter difficulties, to cope thoughtfully and strategically (e.g., via problem-solving or seeking help), allowing them to rebound, recover, and re-engage. Such competencies can be contrasted with the state of motivational vulnerability, when students avoid challenge, become disaffected, and so are more likely to encounter difficulties and react to them with negative emotions, contributing to reliance on maladaptive ways of coping or dysregulation (e.g., concealment or blaming others), and so making it more likely they will give up or disengage.

A focus on motivational resilience allows interventions to target these patterns of action as important protective factors, while drawing on explanatory research from the many areas that share an interest in motivational resilience (e.g., mindsets, engagement, self-regulation, help-seeking, academic coping, and buoyancy). These areas of work have all identified social contextual factors and practices that support students' dealings with problems and setbacks, and the umbrella construct encourages interventionists and practitioners to bring them all together in one place in order to design learning contexts that promote resilience (e.g., Fredricks et al., 2019; Wigfield & Wentzel, 2007). Such supports may be especially important during the years of late childhood and the run up to the transition to middle school, which some students experience as challenging and stressful. Motivational resilience can set students up with the tools they will need to deal effectively with these new demands, while strengthening their competencies in multiple areas, both academic and non-academic. Moreover, motivational resilience (like its subcomponent engagement) unfolds on the plane of action, which means that it is visible to parents and practitioners—if they know what they are looking for. Such access allows them to monitor their efforts to support students, and to fine tune or pull back their own actions or task characteristics (e.g., difficulty level) based on whether they are enabling resilience (e.g., engagement or help-seeking) or pushing students toward responses that indicate more vulnerability (e.g., self-deprecation or desistance).

Academic identity as a Lever for Promoting Competence and Resilience While constructs of motivational resilience underscore the important role of actions on the ground, theories of both engagement and motivation highlight the internal working models students are constructing based on these interactions and encounters, which engagement researchers sometimes consider as parts of engagement and which motivational researchers prioritize as their target self-appraisals. As shown in Figs. 1 and 4, motivational theories offer a menu of such appraisals, and as seen in Figs. 6 and 7, theories of engagement encourage interventionists to consider these processes wholistically instead of in isolation. Both areas suggest that these self-appraisals reflect students' "academic identities," which are central to youth because they are part of the larger identity project early adolescents undertake during this developmental period (Erikson, 1950). Both motivation and engagement can nominate themes around which to organize the many self-appraisals at play in their theories. For example, engagement theories highlight the theme of "belonging" (e.g., attachment, bonding, relatedness, connectedness) while motivation theories suggest "mastery" (e.g., self-efficacy, perceived competence, mastery learning orientations, mindsets). Self-determination theory incorporates both of these self-appraisals while highlighting the theme of "autonomy" (authenticity, authorship, purpose, relevance). Taken together, these themes suggest that interventions will promote positive youth development to the extent they support all students in constructing views of themselves as competent, authentic, well-respected, and valued members of a purpose-driven learning community.

Such appraisals and identities are key to intervention efforts because they represent the meaning students make of their experiences at home and at school (Spencer, 2006). As a result, they are crucial phenomenological mediators between external environmental events and the actions students take. They also provide essential information to practitioners and interventionists as they try to transform environments to become more supportive. No matter how well intentioned, it is students' interpretations of their experiences that will have the last word about the effects of interventions. But they can be hard to access: Such indicators of the student experience are largely internal and so invisible unless social contexts ask students directly or bring out their views in honest conversation. The questions that

underlie these themes (e.g., "Am I welcome here?" "Do I have what it takes to do well?" "What is our purpose here?") can be used to evaluate (current or future) programs, practices, and contextual features for the messages they communicate to students about these core aspects of their identities. Especially important is the design of social contexts that send positive messages about *all* these questions at the same time, and do not create trade-offs between, for example, mastery and belonging to a specific (ethnic, gender, or peer) group. Such appraisals are key levers in promoting competence, resilience, and positive development. Some theories also posit that these self-appraisals are more than cognitive constructions—they derive their energetic power because they represent the extent to which students' fundamental psychological needs are being met in the school or classroom context (Connell & Wellborn, 1991; Reeve, 2012; Ryan & Deci, 2017).

Complex social ecologies of positive youth development Theories of engagement and motivation concur that the social contexts that support students' development are multi-level, nested, and embedded in higher-order societal systems of social hierarchy, resources, and constraints (e.g., Bronfenbrenner & Morris, 2006). These can be called the complex social ecologies of engagement and motivation (e.g., Lawson & Lawson, 2013; Skinner et al., in press). From such conceptualizations of the context, theories from both fields prioritize interpersonal relationships—the social contexts provided by families and parents, teachers and school personnel, peers, classmates, and friends. All have been implicated in the development of engagement (e.g., Upadyaya & Salmela-Aro, 2013) and motivation (Wentzel & Ramani, 2016; Wigfield et al., 2015), and these relationships seem to provide both the glue and the "proximal processes" (or repeated daily social interactions; Bronfenbrenner & Morris, 2006) that shape all aspects of functioning and development.

Pattern-centered approaches suggest that the relationships and interactions with these many kinds of social partners can be considered together to create wholistic ecologies, niches, "lifespaces" (Roeser & Peck, 2003), or "worlds" (Phelan et al., 1998) that differ among students in the supports, resources, and affordances they provide. There are many different ways in which these microsystems (e.g., family, schools, neighborhoods) and the social partners and relationships they contain (e.g., parents, teachers, peers) can be organized and work together (Skinner et al., in press). The concept of "niche" may be especially important in describing the social ecologies to which many students from minoritized and racialized groups are relegated (Spencer, 2006). Macrosystem factors that create poverty and marginalization divert resources and force risk into all the microsystems youth inhabit, and so must be transformed together to create social ecologies that support the positive development of competence and resilience of all youth (see Galindo, Brown, & Lee, chapter "Expanding an Equity Understanding of Student Engagement: The Macro (Social) and Micro (School) Contexts", this volume).

Conclusion

The goal of this chapter is to help unlock the positive synergy between engagement and motivation. Our read of both fields is that what is currently holding them back from this goal is the same thing: their successes. The field of motivation has been wildly successful in creating precise and exquisite theories and research on academic motivation; so generative, in fact, that each of these theories has created its own isolated local climate and ecology. Hence, the current archipelago, and the field's next task: integration. The field of engagement, in contrast, has gotten its arms around a wildly powerful idea, so powerful, in fact, that it is now overrun with an abundance of constructs, definitions, and measures; in this exuberance; however, the roots of these ideas are no longer clear or even visible. Hence, the current overcrowded island, and the field's next task: differentiation.

We believe that the solutions to both fields' biggest problems are also the same: a sober reconsideration of their own gaps, blind spots, and areas for improvement. These reflections call for a bird's eye view, some aerial reconnaissance that will reveal that the isolated islands of motivational theories are all connected to the territory encompassed by engagement as well as other core action constructs. In addition, some of these islands are closer to each other than motivational theories seem to realize; they may even share common territory. Moreover, the crowd on the high-value real estate claimed by engagement can be thinned by moving some occupants, specifically those that refer to sets of self-relevant beliefs, qualities of interpersonal relationships and contexts, and strategies of self-regulated learning. However, they should not be moved far—just to neighboring territory, so they can be connected by hypothesized causal bridges tested for their efficacy in leading to and from engagement as energy in action. Some of these occupants will find themselves on islands already inhabited by theories of motivation and self-regulation. Taken together, we envision a thriving interdisciplinary domain, encouraging rich cross-border cooperation, migration, and deep mutual learning. As part of these reflections and reconnaissance, we think that each field will naturally come to see the other as a friendly and helpful neighbor—an ally, advocate, and trusted source of insights and advice. We believe that together, work at the intersection of these fields has much to offer future conceptual, empirical, and applied efforts, as illustrated by the joint insights they provide about the study and promotion of competence and positive youth development. We hope that the respect and admiration we hold for both fields are evident in our attempts to aid in this forward movement.

References

Abramson, L. Y., Seligman, M. E., & Teasdale, J. D. (1978). Learned helplessness in humans: Critique and reformulation. *Journal of Abnormal Psychology, 87*(1), 49–74. https://doi.org/10.1037/0021-843X.87.1.49

Anderman, E. M. (2020). Achievement motivation theory: Balancing precision and utility. *Contemporary Educational Psychology, 101864.* https://doi.org/10.1016/j.cedpsych.2020.101864

Appleton, J. J., Christenson, S. L., Kim, D., & Reschly, A. L. (2006). Measuring cognitive and psychological engagement: Validation of the student engagement instrument. *Journal of School Psychology, 44*(5), 427–445. https://doi.org/10.1016/j.jsp.2006.04.002

Appleton, J. J., Christenson, S. L., & Furlong, M. J. (2008). Student engagement with school: Critical conceptual and methodological issues of the construct. *Psychology in the Schools, 45*(5), 369–386. https://doi.org/10.1002/pits.20303

Azevedo, R. (2015). Defining and measuring engagement and learning in science: Conceptual, theoretical, methodological, and analytical issues. *Educational Psychologist, 50,* 84–94. https://doi.org/10.1080/00461520.2015.1004069

Blumenfeld, P. C., Kempler, T. M., & Krajcik, J. S. (2006). Motivation and cognitive engagement in learning environments. In R. K. Sawyer (Ed.), *The Cambridge handbook of the learning sciences* (pp. 475–484). Cambridge University Press. https://doi.org/10.1017/CBO9780511816833.029

Boekaerts, M. (2016). Engagement as an inherent aspect of the learning process. *Learning and Instruction, 43,* 76–83. https://doi.org/10.1016/j.learninstruc.2016.02.001

Brandtstädter, J. (2006). Action perspectives on human development. In W. Damon (Series Ed.) & R. M. Lerner (Vol. Ed.), *Handbook of child psychology: Vol. 1. Theoretical models of human development* (pp. 51–568). Wiley. https://doi.org/10.1002/9780470147658.chpsy0110.

Bronfenbrenner, U., & Morris, P. A. (2006). The bioecological model of human development. In W. Damon (Series Ed.) & R. M. Lerner (Vol. Ed.), *Handbook of child psychology: Vol. 1. Theoretical models of human development* (6th ed., pp. 793–828). Wiley. https://doi.org/10.1002/9780470147658.chpsy0114.

Brophy, J. E. (2013). *Motivating students to learn.* Routledge. https://doi.org/10.4324/9781410610218

Christenson, S. L., Reschly, A. L., & Wylie, C. (Eds.). (2012). *Handbook of research on student engagement.* Springer. https://doi.org/10.1007/978-1-4614-2018-7

Cleary, T. J., & Zimmerman, B. J. (2012). A cyclical self-regulatory account of student engagement: Theoretical foundations and applications. In S. L. Christenson, A. L. Reschly, & C. Wylie (Eds.), *Handbook of research on student engagement* (pp. 237–257). Springer. https://doi.org/10.1007/978-1-4614-2018-7_11

Connell, J. P., & Wellborn, J. G. (1991). Competence, autonomy, and relatedness: A motivational analysis of self-system processes. In M. R. Gunnar & L. A. Sroufe (Eds.), *Self processes and development* (pp. 43–77). Lawrence Erlbaum Associates, Inc.

Dweck, C. S. (2017). From needs to goals and representations: Foundations for a unified theory of motivation, personality, and development. *Psychological Review, 124*(6), 689–719. https://doi.org/10.1037/rev0000082

Dweck, C. S., & Molden, D. C. (2005). Self-theories: Their impact on competence motivation and acquisition. In A. J. Elliot & C.S. Dweck (Eds.), *Handbook of competence and motivation* (pp. 122–140). Guilford Publications.

Dweck, C. S., & Yeager, D. S. (2019). Mindsets: A view from two eras. *Perspectives on Psychological Science, 14*(3), 481–496. https://doi.org/10.1177/1745691618804166

Eccles, J. S. (2016). Engagement: Where to next? *Learning and Instruction, 43,* 71–75. https://doi.org/10.1016/j.learninstruc.2016.02.003

Eccles, J. S., & Wang, M. (2012). Part I commentary: So what is student engagement anyway? In S. L. Christenson, A. L. Reschly, & C. Wylie (Eds.), *Handbook of research on student engagement* (pp. 133–145). Springer. https://doi.org/10.1007/978-1-4614-2018-7_6

Eccles, J. S., & Wigfield, A. (2020). From expectancy-value theory to situated expectancy value theory: A developmental, social cognitive, and sociocultural perspective on motivation. *Contemporary Educational Psychology, 61,* 101859. https://doi.org/10.1016/j.cedpsych.2020.101859

Erikson, E. H. (1950). *Childhood and society.* Norton.

Filsecker, M., & Kerres, M. (2014). Engagement as a volitional construct: A framework for evidence-based research on educational games. *Simulation & Gaming, 45,* 450–470. https://doi.org/10.1177/1046878114553569

Finn, J. D. (1989). Withdrawing from school. *Review of Educational Research, 59,* 117–142. https://doi.org/10.3102/00346543059002117

Finn, J. D., & Voelkl, K. E. (1993). School characteristics related to school engagement. *Journal of Negro Education, 62,* 249–268. https://doi.org/10.2307/2295464

Finn, J. D., & Zimmer, K. S. (2012). Student engagement: What is it? Why does it matter? In S. L. Christenson, A.L. Reschly, & C. Wylie (Eds.), *Handbook of research on student engagement* (pp. 97–131). Springer. https://doi.org/10.1007/978-1-4614-2018-7_5

Ford, M. E. (1992). *Motivating humans: Goals, emotions, and personal agency beliefs.* Sage. https://doi.org/10.4135/9781483325361.n1

Ford, M. E., & Smith, P. R. (2009). Commentary: Building on a strong foundation: Five pathways to the next level of motivational theorizing. In K. R. Wenzel & A. Wigfield (Eds.), *Handbook of motivation at school* (pp. 267–275). Routledge. https://doi.org/10.4324/9780203879498

Fredricks, J. A. (2014). *The eight myths of student disengagement: Creating classrooms of deep learning.* Corwin Press. https://doi.org/10.4135/9781483394534

Fredricks, J. A., Blumenfeld, P. C., & Paris, A. H. (2004). School engagement: Potential of the concept, state of the evidence. *Review of Educational Research, 74*(1), 59–109. https://doi.org/10.3102/00346543074001059

Fredricks, J., McColskey, W., Meli, J., Mordica, J., Montrosse, B., & Mooney, K. (2011). Measuring student engagement in upper elementary through high school: A description of 21 instruments (Issues & Answers Report, REL 2011–No. 098). Washington, DC: U.S.

Fredricks, J. A., Filsecker, M., & Lawson, M. A. (2016). Student engagement, context, and adjustment: Addressing definitional, measurement, and methodological issues. *Learning and Instruction, 43*, 1–4. https://doi.org/10.1016/j.learninstruc.2016.02.002

Fredricks, J. A., Reschly, A. L., & Christenson, S. L. (2019). *Handbook of student engagement interventions*. Academic Press. https://doi.org/10.1016/c2016-0-04519-9

Furlong, M. J., Whipple, A. D., Jean, G. S., Simental, J., Soliz, A., & Punthuna, S. (2003). Multiple contexts of school engagement: Moving toward a unifying framework for educational research and practice. *The California School Psychologist, 8*(1), 99–113. https://doi.org/10.1007/BF03340899

Furrer, C. J., Skinner, E. A., & Pitzer, J. R. (2014). The influence of teacher and peer relationships on students' classroom engagement and everyday resilience. In D. J. Shernoff & J. Bempechat (Eds.), *National Society for the Study of Education Yearbook. Engaging youth in schools: Empirically-based models to guide future innovations* (Vol. 113, pp. 101–123). Columbia University: Teachers's College.

Graham, S. (2020). An attributional theory of motivation. *Contemporary Educational Psychology, 61*, 101861. https://doi.org/10.1016/j.cedpsych.2020.101861

Green, J., Liem, G. A. D., Martin, A. J., Colmar, S., Marsh, H. W., & McInerney, D. (2012). Academic motivation, self-concept, engagement, and performance in high school: Key processes from a longitudinal perspective. *Journal of Adolescence, 35*(5), 1111–1122.

Greene, B. A. (2015). Measuring cognitive engagement with self-report scales: Reflections from over 20 years of research. *Educational Psychologist, 50*(1), 14–30. https://doi.org/10.1016/j.adolescence.2012.02.016

Gottfried, A. E. (1985). Academic intrinsic motivation in elementary and junior high school students. *Journal of Educational Psychology, 77*(6), 631–645. https://doi.org/10.1037/0022-0663.77.6.631

Gottfried, A. E., Fleming, J. S., & Gottfried, A. W. (2001). Continuity of academic intrinsic motivation from childhood through late adolescence: A longitudinal study. *Journal of Educational Psychology, 93*(1), 3–13. https://doi.org/10.1037/0022-0663.93.1.3

Haimovitz, K., & Dweck, C. S. (2017). The origins of children's growth and fixed mindsets: New research and a new proposal. *Child Development, 88*(6), 1849–1859. https://doi.org/10.1111/cdev.12955

Harter, S. (1978). Effectance motivation reconsidered. Toward a developmental Model. *Human Development, 21*(1), 34–64. https://doi.org/10.1159/000271574

Hascher, T., & Hadjar, A. (2018). School alienation—Theoretical approaches and educational research. *Educational Research, 60*(2), 171–188. https://doi.org/10.1080/00131881.2018.1443021

Hattie, J., Hodis, F. A., & Kang, S. H. (2020). Theories of motivation: Integration and ways forward. *Contemporary Educational Psychology, 101865*. https://doi.org/10.1016/j.cedpsych.2020.101865

Heckhausen, J., & Heckhausen, H. (2018). *Motivation and action*. Springer. https://doi.org/10.1017/CBO9780511499821

Jimerson, S. R., Campos, E., & Greif, J. L. (2003). Toward an understanding of definitions and measures of school engagement and related terms. *The California School Psychologist, 8*, 7–27. https://doi.org/10.1007/BF03340893

Karabenick, S. A., & Newman, R. S. (Eds.). (2013). *Help seeking in academic settings: Goals, groups, and contexts*. Routledge. https://doi.org/10.4324/9780203726563

Koenka, A. C. (2020). Academic motivation theories revisited: An interactive dialog between motivation scholars on recent contributions, underexplored issues, and future directions. *Contemporary Educational Psychology, 101831*. https://doi.org/10.1016/j.cedpsych.2019.101831

Lam, S. F., Wong, B. P., Yang, H., & Liu, Y. (2012). Understanding student engagement with a contextual model. In S. L. Christenson, A. L. Reschly, & C. Wylie (Eds.), *Handbook of research on student engagement* (pp. 403–419). Springer. https://doi.org/10.1007/978-1-4614-2018-7_19

Lawson, M. A. (2017). Commentary: Bridging student engagement research and practice. *School Psychology International, 38*(3), 221–239. https://doi.org/10.1177/0143034317708010

Lawson, M. A., & Lawson, H. A. (2013). New conceptual frameworks for student engagement research, policy, and practice. *Review of Educational Research, 83*(3), 432–479. https://doi.org/10.3102/0034654313480891

Lei, H., Cui, Y., & Zhou, W. (2018). Relationships between student engagement and academic achievement: A meta-analysis. *Social Behavior and Personality: An International Journal, 46*(3), 517–528. https://doi.org/10.2224/sbp.7054

Li, Y., & Lerner, R. M. (2011). Trajectories of school engagement during adolescence: Implications for grades, depression, delinquency, and substance use. *Developmental Psychology, 47*(1), 233–247. https://doi.org/10.1037/a0021307

Linnenbrink-Garcia, L., Rogat, T. K., & Koskey, K. L. (2011). Affect and engagement during small group instruction. *Contemporary Educational Psychology, 36*(1), 13–24. https://doi.org/10.1016/j.cedpsych.2010.09.001

Lin-Siegler, X., Dweck, C. S., & Cohen, G. L. (2016). Instructional interventions that motivate classroom learning. *Journal of Educational Psychology, 108*(3), 295–299. https://doi.org/10.1037/edu0000124

Martin, A. J. (2007). Examining a multidimensional model of student motivation and engagement using a construct validation approach. *British Journal of Educational Psychology, 77*(2), 413–440. https://doi.org/10.1348/000709906X118036

Martin, A. J. (2009). Motivation and engagement across the academic lifespan: A developmental construct validity study of elementary school, high school, and university/college students. *Educational and Psychological Measurement, 69*, 794–824. https://doi.org/10.1177/0013164409332214

Martin, A. J. (2012). Part II commentary: Motivation and engagement: Conceptual, operational, and empirical clarity. In S. L. Christenson, A. L. Reschly, & C. Wylie (Eds.), *Handbook of research on student engagement* (pp. 303–311). Springer. https://doi.org/10.1007/978-1-4614-2018-7_14

Martin, A. J., Anderson, J., Bobis, J., Way, J., & Vellar, R. (2011). Switching on and switching off in mathematics: An ecological study of future intent and disengagement amongst middle school students. *Journal of Educational Psychology, 104*, 1–18. https://doi.org/10.1037/a0025988

Martin, A. J., Ginns, P., & Papworth, B. (2017). Motivation and engagement: Same or different? Does it matter? *Learning and Individual Differences, 55*, 150–162. https://doi.org/10.1016/j.lindif.2017.03.013

Martin, A. J., & Marsh, H. W. (2009). Academic resilience and academic buoyancy: Multidimensional and hierarchical conceptual framing of causes, correlates and cognate constructs. *Oxford Review of Education, 35*(3), 353–370. https://doi.org/10.1080/03054980902934639

Mosher, R., & McGowan, B. (1985). *Assessing student engagement in secondary schools: Alternative conceptions, strategies of assessing, and instruments.* University of Wisconsin, Research and Development Center (ERIC Document No. ED 272812).

Newmann, F. M. (1991). Student engagement in academic work: Expanding the perspective of secondary school effectiveness. In J. R. Bliss & W. A. Firestone (Eds.), *Rethinking effective schools: Research and practice* (pp. 58–76). Teachers College Press.

Nolen, S. B., Horn, I. S., & Ward, C. J. (2015). Situating motivation. *Educational Psychologist, 50*(3), 234–247. https://doi.org/10.1080/00461520.2015.1075399

Peterson, C., Maier, S. F., & Seligman, M. E. (1993). *Learned helplessness: A theory for the age of personal control.* Oxford University Press.

Phelan, P., Davidson, A. L., & Yu, H. C. (1998). *Adolescents' worlds: Negotiating family, peers, and school.* Teachers College Press.

Pianta, R. C., & Hamre, B. K. (2009). Conceptualization, measurement and improvement of classroom processes. *Educational Researcher, 38*, 109–119. https://doi.org/10.3102/0013189X09332374

Pintrich, P. R. (2003). A motivational science perspective on the role of student motivation in learning and teaching contexts. *Journal of Educational Psychology, 95*, 667–686. https://doi.org/10.1037/0022-0663.95.4.667

Reeve, J. (2012). A self-determination theory perspective on student engagement. In S. Christenson, A. Reschly, & C. Wylie (Eds.), *Handbook of research on student engagement* (pp. 149–172). Springer. https://doi.org/10.1007/978-1-4614-2018-7_7

Reschly, A. L., & Christenson, S. L. (2012). Jingle, jangle, and conceptual haziness: Evolution and future directions of the engagement construct. In S. Christenson, A. Reschly, & C. Wylie (Eds.), *Handbook of research on student engagement* (pp. 3–19). Springer. https://doi.org/10.1007/978-1-4614-2018-7_1

Roeser, R. W., & Peck, S. C. (2003). Patterns and pathways of educational achievement across adolescence: A holistic-developmental perspective. *New Dir Child Adolesc Dev*, 39–62. https://doi.org/10.1002/cd.81

Russell, J., Ainley, M., & Frydenberg, E. (2005). *Schooling issues digest: Student motivation and engagement.* Australian Government, Department of Education Science and Training.

Ryan, R. M. (Ed.). (2012). *The Oxford handbook of human motivation.* Oxford University Press. https://doi.org/10.1093/oxfordhb/9780195399820.001.0001

Ryan, R. M., & Deci, E. L. (2017). *Self-determination theory: Basic psychological needs in motivation, development, and wellness.* The Guilford Press. https://doi.org/10.1521/978.14625/28806

Ryan, R. M., & Deci, E. L. (2020). Intrinsic and extrinsic motivation from a self-determination theory perspective: Definitions, theory, practices, and future directions. *Contemporary Educational Psychology, 61*, 101860. https://doi.org/10.1016/j.cedpsych.2020.101860

Salmela-Aro, K., Moeller, J., Schneider, B., Spicer, J., & Lavonen, J. (2016). Integrating the light and dark sides of student engagement using person-oriented and situation-specific approaches. *Learning and Instruction, 43*, 61–70. https://doi.org/10.1016/j.learninstruc.2016.01.001

Salmela-Aro, K., & Upadaya, K. (2012). The Schoolwork Engagement Inventory: Energy, dedication, and absorption (EDA). *European Journal of Psychological Assessment, 28*(1), 60–67. https://doi.org/10.1027/1015-5759/a000091

Schunk, D. H., & DiBenedetto, M. K. (2020). Motivation and social cognitive theory. *Contemporary Educational Psychology, 61*, 101832. https://doi.org/10.1016/j.cedpsych.2019.101832

Schunk, D. H., & Mullen, C. A. (2012). Self-efficacy as an engaged learner. In S. Christenson, A. Reschly, & C. Wylie (Eds.), *Handbook of research on student engagement* (pp. 219–235). Springer. https://doi.org/10.1007/978-1-4614-2018-7_10

Schunk, D. H., Meece, J. R., & Pintrich, P. R. (2012). *Motivation in education: Theory, research, and applications.* Pearson Higher Ed.

Seligman, M.E.P. (1975) *Helplessness: On depression, development, and death.* W.H. Freeman.

Sinatra, G. M., Heddy, B. C., & Lombardi, D. (2014). The challenge of defining and measuring student engagement in science. *Educational Psychologist, 50*, 1–13. https://doi.org/10.1080/00461520.2014.1002924

Sinclair, M. F., Christenson, S. L., Lehr, C. A., & Anderson, A. R. (2003). Facilitating student engagement: Lessons learned from check & connect longitudinal studies. *The California School Psychologist, 8*, 29–41. https://doi.org/10.1007/BF03340894

Skinner, E. A. (2016). Engagement and disaffection as central to processes of motivational resilience and development. In K. Wentzel & D. Miele (Eds.), *Handbook of motivation at school* (2nd ed., pp. 145–168). Erlbaum. https://doi.org/10.4324/9781315773384-14

Skinner, E. A. (2019). Engagement and motivation during childhood. In S. Hupp & J. Jewell (Eds.), *Encyclopedia of Child and Adolescent Development* (pp. 1-14). New York: Wiley. https://doi.org/10.1002/9781119171492.wecad170

Skinner, E. A. (in press). Four guideposts on the journey toward a comprehensive and coherent model of academic motivation: Motivational resilience, academic identity, social contexts, and development. *Educational Psychology Review*.

Skinner, E. A., & Pitzer, J. R. (2012). Developmental dynamics of student engagement, coping, and everyday resilience. In S. L. Christenson, A. L. Reschly, & C. Wylie (Eds.), *Handbook of Research on Student Engagement* (pp. 21–44). Springer US. https://doi.org/10.1007/978-1-4614-2018-7_2

Skinner, E. A., & Saxton, E. A. (2019). The development of academic coping in children and youth: A comprehensive review and critique. *Developmental Review, 53*, 100870. https://doi.org/10.1016/j.dr.2019.100870

Skinner, E., & Saxton, E. (2020). The development of academic coping across late elementary and early middle school: Do patterns differ for students with differing motivational resources? *International Journal of Behavioral Development, 44*(4), 339–353. https://doi.org/10.1177/0165025419896423

Skinner, E. A., Kindermann, T. A., Connell, J. P., & Wellborn, J. G. (2009). Engagement as an organizational construct in the dynamics of motivational development. In K. Wentzel & A. Wigfield (Eds.), *Handbook of motivation at school* (pp. 223–245). Routledge. https://doi.org/10.4324/9780203879498

Skinner, E. A., Kindermann, T. A., & Furrer, C. (2009). A motivational perspective on engagement and disaffection: Conceptualization and assessment of children's behavioral and emotional participation in academic activities in the classroom. *Educational and Psychological Measurement, 69*, 493–525. https://doi.org/10.1177/0013164408323233

Skinner, E., Furrer, C., Marchand, G., & Kindermann, T. (2008). Engagement and disaffection in the classroom: Part of a larger motivational dynamic? *Journal of Educational Psychology, 100*(4), 765–781. https://doi.org/10.1037/a0012840

Skinner, E. A., Graham, J. P., Brule, H., Rickert, N., & Kindermann, T. A. (2020). "I get knocked down but I get up again": Integrative frameworks for studying the development of motivational resilience in school. *International Journal of Behavioral Development, 44*(4), 290–300. https://doi.org/10.1177/0165025420924122

Skinner, E. A., Kindermann, T. A., Vollet, J. W., & Rickert, N. P. (in press). Motivation in the wild: Capturing the complex social ecologies of academic motivation. In M. Bong, S.-I. Kim, & J. Reeve (Eds.), *Motivation science: Controversies and insights*. Oxford University Press.

Spencer, M. B. (2006). Phenomenology and ecological systems theory: Development of diverse groups. In R. M. Lerner & W. Damon (Eds.), *Handbook of child psychology: Theoretical models of human development* (Vols. 1, 6th ed., pp. 829–893). John Wiley & Sons Inc.

Upadyaya, K., & Salmela-Aro, K. (2013). Development of school engagement in association with academic success and well-being in varying social contexts: A review of empirical research. *European Psychologist, 18*(2), 136–147. https://doi.org/10.1027/1016-9040/a000143

Urdan, T., & Kaplan, A. (2020). The origins, evolution and future directions of achievement goal theory. *Contemporary Educational Psychology, 61*, 101862. https://doi.org/10.1016/j.cedpsych.2020.101862

Van der Veen, I., & Peetsma, T. T. D. (2009). The development in self-regulated learning behaviour of first-year students in the lowest level of secondary school in the Netherlands. *Learning and Individual Differences, 19*, 34–46. https://doi.org/10.1016/j.lindif.2008.03.001

Virtanen, T. E., Räikkönen, E., Engels, M. C., Vasalampi, K., & Lerkkanen, M. K. (2021). Student engagement, truancy, and cynicism: A longitudinal study from primary school to upper secondary education. *Learning and Individual Differences, 86*, 101972. https://doi.org/10.1016/j.lindif.2021.101972

Voelkl, K. E. (1997). Identification with school. *American Journal of Education, 105*(3), 294–318. https://doi.org/10.1086/444158

Voelkl, K. E. (2012). School identification. In S. L. Christenson, A. L. Reschly, & C. Wylie (Eds.), *Handbook of research on student engagement; handbook of research on student engagement* (pp. 193–218). Springer. https://doi.org/10.1007/978-1-4614-2018-7_9

Wang, M. T., & Fredricks, J. A. (2014). The reciprocal links between school engagement and youth problem behavior during adolescence. *Child Development, 85*, 722–737. https://doi.org/10.1111/cdev.12138

Wang, M. T., & Hofkens, T. L. (2020). Beyond classroom academics: A school-wide and multi-contextual perspective on student engagement in school. *Adolescent Research Review, 5*(4), 419–433. https://doi.org/10.1007/s40894-019-00115-z

Wang, M. T., & Peck, S. C. (2013). Adolescent educational success and mental health vary across school engagement profiles. *Developmental Psychology, 49*(7), 1266–1276. https://doi.org/10.1037/a0030028

Wang, M. T., Degol, J. L., & Henry, D. A. (2019). An integrative development-in-sociocultural-context model for children's engagement in learning. *American Psychologist, 74*(9), 1086–1102. https://doi.org/10.1037/amp0000522

Wang, M.-T., & Eccles, J. S. (2012). Social support matters: Longitudinal effects of social support on three dimensions of school engagement from middle to high school. Child Development, 83(3), 877-895.

Wang, M.-T., Fredricks, J., Ye, F., Hofkens, T., & Linn, J. S. (2019). Conceptualization and assessment of adolescents' engagement and disengagement in school: A multidimensional school engagement scale. *European Journal of Psychological Assessment, 35*(4), 592–606. https://doi.org/10.1027/1015-5759/a000431

Wang, Y., Tian, L., & Huebner, E. S. (2019). Basic psychological needs satisfaction at school, behavioral school engagement, and academic achievement: Longitudinal reciprocal relations among elementary school students. *Contemporary Educational Psychology, 56*, 130–139. https://doi.org/10.1016/j.cedpsych.2019.01.003

Wentzel, K., & Miele, D. (2016). *Handbook of motivation at school* (2nd ed.). Erlbaum. https://doi.org/10.4324/9781315773384

Wentzel, K. R., & Ramani, G. B. (Eds.). (2016). *Handbook of social influences in school contexts: Social-emotional, motivation, and cognitive outcomes.* Routledge. https://doi.org/10.4324/9781315769929

Wentzel, K., & Skinner, E. (co-editors, in press). The other half of the story: The role of social relationships and social contexts in the development of academic motivation. Special issue in *Educational Psychology Review*.

Wentzel, K., & Wigfield, A. (2009). *Handbook of motivation at school.* Routledge. https://doi.org/10.4324/9780203879498

White, R. W. (1959). Motivation reconsidered: The concept of competence. *Psychological Review, 66*(5), 297–333. https://doi.org/10.1037/h0040934

Wigfield, A., & Eccles, J. S. (2020). 35 years of research on students' subjective task values and motivation: A look back and a look forward. In A. J. Elliot (Ed.), *Advances in motivation science* (pp. 161–198). Elsevier Academic Press. https://doi.org/10.1016/bs.adms.2019.05.002

Wigfield, A., & Koenka, A. C. (2020). Where do we go from here in academic motivation theory and research? Some reflections and recommendations for future work. *Contemporary Educational Psychology, 101872.* https://doi.org/10.1016/j.cedpsych.2020.101872

Wigfield, A., & Wentzel, K. R. (2007). Introduction to motivation at school: Interventions that work. *Educational Psychologist, 42*(4), 191–196. https://doi.org/10.1080/00461520701621038

Wigfield, A., Eccles, J. S., Fredricks, J. A., Simpkins, S., Roeser, R., & Schiefele, U. (2015). Development of achievement motivation and engagement. In R. M. Lerner (Series Ed.) & M. Lamb (Volume Ed.), *Handbook of child psychology and developmental science*, 7th ed., *Vol. 3., Socioemotional processes* (pp. 657–700). Wiley. https://doi.org/10.1002/9781118963418.childpsy316.

Wong, Z. Y., & Liem, G. A. D. (2021). Student engagement: Current state of the construct, conceptual refinement, and future research directions. *Educational Psychology Review*, 1–32. https://doi.org/10.1007/s10648-021-09628-3

Yeager, D. S., & Dweck, C. S. (2012). Mindsets that promote resilience: When students believe that personal characteristics can be developed. *Educational Psychologist, 47*(4), 302–314. https://doi.org/10.1080/00461520.2012.722805

Situated Expectancy-Value Theory, Dimensions of Engagement, and Academic Outcomes

Jessica R. Gladstone, Allan Wigfield, and Jacquelynne S. Eccles

Abstract (✉)

In this chapter, we examine the relations between constructs found within expectancy-value theory (EVT), now called situated expectancy-value theory (SEVT), and engagement dimensions. We first discuss the various definitions of the five proposed dimensions of engagement and discuss how some of these definitions share overlap with how constructs in SEVT are defined. We then provide an overview of EVT, the constructs that are central to predicting achievement-related outcomes, and the reason and implications of renaming it SEVT. After reflecting on the comments and issues raised by Eccles and Wang (2012) in the first edition of this *Handbook*, we summarize work that has examined the relations between students' expectancies, values, and engagement. Our summary of this research allowed the first author to provide a formal proposal for where the various dimensions of engagement and disaffection might fit within the SEVT model. We follow this with a discussion of how the various dimensions of engagement can promote positive student outcomes, such as achievement, course intentions, and well-being. Finally, we provide several important future directions for researchers to consider to further progress the study of student engagement.

J. R. Gladstone (✉)
Virginia Commonwealth University, Richmond, VA, United States
e-mail: gladstonejr@vcu.edu

A. Wigfield
University of Maryland, College Park, MD, USA
e-mail: awigfiel@umd.edu

J. S. Eccles
University of California, Irvine, Irvine, CA, USA

Australian Catholic University, Brisbane, QLD, Australia
e-mail: jseccles@uci.edu

As illustrated by the various chapters of this *Handbook*, over the last 30 years many researchers have studied student engagement. This surge of interest in the study of student engagement has been accompanied by researchers varying in their conceptualizations and operationalizations of what it means for a student to be engaged. At the same time, there also has been much work on the nature and development of students' motivation. Additionally, some researchers have connected these two research areas and discuss how engagement and motivation relate to each other and various outcomes (Fredricks et al., 2018; Gladstone, 2020).

One theoretical model that has connected students' motivation and engagement is Eccles and colleagues' expectancy-value theory (EVT), now called situated expectancy-value theory (SEVT). This model has been an influential one in the field, guiding much work on the development of motivation and how individuals' motivation impacts their performance on and engagement with different tasks, activities, or domains along with choices of which activities to continue (Eccles, 1993, 2005; Eccles (Parsons) et al., 1983; Eccles & Wigfield, 2020; Wigfield & Eccles, 2020). SEVT posits that individuals' expectancies for success, or how well they think they will do on an upcoming activity, and valuing of it, the purposes or incentives for engaging in it, are the strongest proximal predictors of both performance and choice. Individuals' expectancies and values are influenced by various other self-beliefs, affective reactions to achievement outcomes, and a host of social, socialization, and cultural factors. As discussed in more detail later, Eccles and Wigfield changed the name of the theory to SEVT to emphasize the central role the particular situations individuals are in have in their choices and their performance.

In the first edition of this *Handbook*, Eccles and Wang (2012) provided a commentary on the set of chapters discussing "what is student engagement." In their commentary, they provided a brief overview of EVT before commenting on the different chapters. However, in that edition, there was not a chapter on EVT in the set of chapters linking engagement and motivation. In this chapter, we provide a more detailed discussion of SEVT and provide proposals for how engagement "fits" into the theoretical model.

Purpose of this Chapter

We begin this chapter by discussing definitions of the major proposed dimensions of engagement: behavioral, cognitive, emotional or affective, agentic, and social. We then present an overview of EVT and the implications of renaming it SEVT. From there, we turn to a consideration of issues Eccles and Wang (2012) raised in their discussion of how motivation and engagement relate, and summarize the work examining how students' expectancies and values relate to their engagement. The next section presents a formal proposal for placing the different dimensions of engagement into the SEVT model, to illustrate the complex interplay of the two constructs. We close with a brief discussion of how (from the perspective of this chapter) engagement relates to positive student outcomes and recommendations for future research.

Defining Student Engagement

At least since Fredricks et al.'s (2004) landmark review, there is a general consensus that student engagement is comprised of at least three dimensions: behavioral, cognitive, and emotional engagement. However, there is growing evidence that student engagement also includes an agentic engagement dimension (Reeve, 2012) and a social engagement dimension (Wang et al., 2016). In this section, we will briefly summarize some of the most widely used definitions of the various dimensions of student engagement. We will then discuss how some of these definitions and dimensions share considerable overlap with constructs found within expectancy-value theory (EVT).

Behavioral Engagement

Behavioral engagement is one of the most easily observable dimensions of engagement and has become one of the most frequently studied dimensions of student engagement. Researchers have defined behavioral engagement in different ways. Finn's (1989) interest in student engagement was premised on understanding and preventing student dropout and ensuring students graduated from high school. Because Finn was interested in understanding how engagement may predict the likelihood of students continuing their education, Finn's original definition of behavioral engagement emphasized students' *participation* in various activities. Finn stated that students' behavioral engagement included four separate components: (1) responding to school requirements (e.g., teacher's instructions); (2) participating in and taking the initiative in class-related activities; (3) being involved in extracurricular activities; and (4) setting goals.

Skinner and colleagues provide a different definition and model of engagement that they derived from their self-system model of motivational development grounded in self-determination theory (Connell & Wellborn, 1991; Skinner & Pitzer, 2012; Skinner & Wellborn, 1997). In this model, Skinner and colleagues purposefully contrast engagement and disaffection as disaffection is not necessarily the absence of engagement (Skinner & Belmont, 1993; Skinner et al., 2008; Skinner et al., 2009). Skinner and colleagues defined behavioral engagement as students' positive effort, attention, and involvement in school. In contrast, they defined behavioral disaffection as students giving up, being distracted, and unprepared for class. Thus, behavioral disaffection is maladaptive in terms of student development in the classroom compared to behavioral engagement,

Martin (2007, 2009, 2010) developed the Motivation and Engagement Wheel to integrate motivation and engagement. Martin developed this model based on Pintrich's (2003) thinking, who emphasized the importance of creating a model that integrates themes from multiple theoretical frameworks. Martin's Motivation and Engagement Wheel represents adaptive and maladaptive behavior and cognition. Thus, Martin conceptualized and divided behavioral engagement into adaptive and maladaptive dimensions. Martin defines adaptive behavioral engagement as students being persistent and staying on task, whereas maladaptive behavioral engagement comprises students purposefully not putting forth effort (see also Martin, chapter "The Role of Academic Engagement in Students' Educational Development: Insights from Load Reduction Instruction and the 4M Academic Engagement Framework", this volume).

Martin's (2007) conceptualization of behavioral engagement is very similar to Skinner and colleagues' (Skinner & Belmont, 1993; Skinner et al., 2008, 2009). These definitions emphasize the importance of students participating in various school and classroom activities as an indicator that they are behaviorally engaged. Later, we will discuss how students' motivation, as defined

by EVT, may help lead to students being behaviorally engaged in the classroom.

Cognitive Engagement

There is a general consensus among researchers studying engagement that cognitive engagement is an important dimension of student engagement. However, as discussed by Sinatra et al. (2015), the definition of cognitive engagement is not clear. There are two broad ways in which researchers have defined cognitive engagement: (a) beliefs and values about the importance of school and learning (Appleton et al., 2006; Martin, 2007); (b) self-regulation, strategy use, goals, and exerting effort (Appleton et al., 2006; Connell & Wellborn, 1991; Corno & Mandinach, 1983; Greene, 2015; Martin, 2007; Meece et al., 1988; Pintrich & De Groot, 1990; Zimmerman & Martinez-Pons, 1988).

To further illustrate this, Appleton et al. (2006) define cognitive engagement in terms of students' valuing of learning, their self-regulation, and their goal setting. According to Appleton and colleagues, students' valuing of learning includes how important and relevant a student thinks what they are learning is to their future. As will be discussed later, this definition overlaps considerably with some task value constructs found within EVT. They further describe self-regulation in terms of actions such as whether a student checks over their homework and define goal setting in terms of how important students perceive school to be to their future goals. Similar to Appleton and colleagues, Martin (2007) defines adaptive cognitive engagement in terms of students' valuing of academic tasks, having a mastery goal orientation, and high self-efficacy toward school. On the other hand, Martin defines maladaptive cognitive engagement as students engaging in maladaptive processes such as self-handicapping or not studying until the last minute to have a reason if they fail at a task.

Regarding the second conceptualization, Greene (2015) defined cognitive engagement as students' use of cognitive strategies, self-regulation, and exerting mental effort. Greene further conceptualizes cognitive engagement by contrasting deep versus shallow engagement. Deep engagement involves using prior knowledge and strategies to learn new material, and shallow engagement involves rote processing and more simple strategies, such as memorization. Greene's definition of cognitive engagement is similar to the construct of self-regulation because Greene derived her definition from Pintrich and De Groot's (1990) conceptualization of cognitive engagement, which was called self-regulated learning strategies, and from Zimmerman and Martinez-Pons' (1988) work on self-regulation and goal setting.

We agree with Sinatra et al. (2015) about the lack of definitional clarity of cognitive engagement. Further adding to this confusion is that some of these definitions overlap with definitions of constructs found within EVT, and some share similarities with definitions of behavioral engagement (i.e., emphasizing effort). We discuss below how some also share similarities with definitions of emotional engagement.

Emotional Engagement

Emotional engagement, or sometimes referred to as affective engagement, is generally conceptualized as comprised of positive and negative feelings toward school, teachers, and peers (Fredricks et al., 2004). Skinner and colleagues (2008, 2009; Skinner and Wellborn (1997)) include positive and negative dimensions of emotional engagement. They describe emotional engagement as students' enthusiasm, pride, interest, and enjoyment in school and emotional disaffection as students' boredom, frustration, anxiety, and disinterest in school.

However, other researchers define emotional engagement in terms of students' identification with school, teachers, peers, and/or academics (Appleton et al., 2006; Finn, 1989). Finn (1989, 2006) has further suggested that identification is an appropriate way to capture student's emotional engagement because if students feel they belong in the school and value it, they are much more likely to remain engaged when things do not go as planned. The emphasis on the *perceived value of school* does share similarities with how Appleton et al. (2006) and Martin (2007) define cognitive engagement and as mentioned previously, share a clear overlap with task value constructs found within SEVT. As we will dis-

cuss in later sections, the definition used for emotional engagement can have implications for how it relates to and is predicted by constructs found within SEVT.

Agentic Engagement

Reeve and his colleagues have proposed agentic engagement as another important dimension of student engagement and define it as individuals trying to actively enrich their learning experiences and taking responsibility for them (Reeve, 2012; Reeve & Tseng, 2011; Reeve & Jang, chapter "Agentic Engagement", this volume). Example activities include students expressing their opinions in class and letting the teacher know when something is interesting to them. Reeve (2012) argued for the inclusion of agentic engagement as a core dimension of student engagement because students who are engaged do not only *react* to the learning activity but also are *proactive* with the learning activity, meaning they take agency over their learning.

Reeve (2013) demonstrated that agentic engagement is conceptually distinct from behavioral, cognitive, and emotional engagement through confirmatory factor analysis. Patall et al. (2019) extended Reeve's work on agentic engagement by examining agentic engagement and motivation (i.e., need satisfaction) in science among US high school students. They found evidence that agentic engagement can be a powerful pathway for enhancing students' motivation but that it is also important to take into account teachers' support for motivation. However, compared to the other three dimensions, the work on agentic engagement is limited and little is still known about how agentic engagement relates to important outcomes in students outside of Korea. Further, there is limited work on how prominent motivation constructs, such as those found within EVT, predict agentic engagement. Interestingly, Eccles and Wang (2012) discussed the importance of agency for motivation in their commentary in the first edition of this *Handbook*. They mentioned that they believed motivation would be highest when the demands of the task fit well with students' sense of agency, in this case their expectancies of success and their values. Therefore, it is possible that agentic engagement and students' expectancies for success are related. In later sections, we will discuss how agentic engagement may be related to constructs found within EVT.

Social Engagement

Social engagement is another proposed dimension of engagement, but less research has been done on this dimension, so it is not as established as behavioral, cognitive, and emotional engagement. Finn and Zimmer (2012) provided the first definition of social engagement, and it shared considerable overlap with behavioral engagement. They defined social engagement in terms of the extent to which students follow classroom rules or the social norms of the classroom. Due to this overlap with behavioral engagement, Pekrun and Linnenbrink-Garcia (2012) refer to social engagement as social-behavioral engagement. Their definition of social-behavioral engagement includes students having high-quality social relationships with their peers; such relationships can positively impact students' learning. These high-quality relationships include students working cohesively together and supporting one another.

Fredricks et al. (2016) interviewed students and teachers to determine how they conceptualize engagement in math and science courses, and one theme that emerged was a social component. Thus, they developed a definition of social engagement that emphasizes the quality of students' social interactions with their peers and teachers. These interactions include students working with their peers and whether they enjoyed working with their peers.

Now that we have discussed the various definitions of the proposed dimensions of engagement, we will turn to an overview of expectancy-value theory.

From Expectancy-Value Theory to Situated Expectancy-Value Theory

In this section, we present a detailed overview of expectancy-value theory and Eccles and Wigfield's (2020) recent renaming of it to SEVT.

We define key constructs in the model and then discuss the implications of changing its name from EVT to SEVT. Figure 1 presents the most recent version of the model.

Eccles (Parsons) et al.'s Expectancy-Value Theory of Performance and Choice

In expectancy-value models, individuals' expectancies for success and valuing of the activities they do are key predictors of performance and choice. Eccles (Parsons) et al. (1983) initially developed their expectancy-value model to help explain gender differences in adolescents' achievement choices, such as why girls do not take as many advanced high school math courses or pursue math and science careers. Researchers basing their work in this model have shown that students' expectancies and values indeed do predict their choices in a variety of domains. Researchers using this model have also looked at the developmental course of individuals' expectancies and values and other constructs in the model (e.g., Durik et al., 2006; Gaspard et al., 2020; Jacobs et al., 2002). We focus here on the right side of the model (Fig. 1), beginning with the box containing affective memories, because that is where engagement constructs can be located. For discussion of the left (socialization) side of the model, see Eccles (1993) and Simpkins et al. (2015). We start by defining key terms in the boxes on the right side of the model.

Definitions of Key Terms in the Model

Expectancies for Success and Self-Concept of Ability Building on earlier work by Atkinson (1957), Bandura (1977), Lewin (1938), and Tolman (1932), Eccles (Parsons) et al. (1983) defined expectancies for success as children's beliefs about how well they will do on an upcoming task (e.g., how well do you think you will do in math next year?). They distinguished expectancies for success from the individual's self-concept of abilities (SCAs). These latter beliefs refer to children's domain-specific assessment of their current competence or ability, both in terms of their assessments of their own ability and how they think they compare to

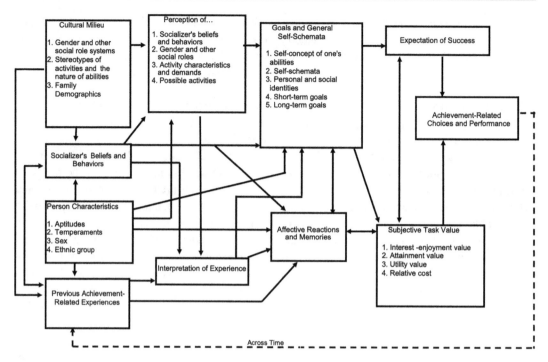

Fig. 1 Eccles and Wigfield's (2020) situated expectancy-value model of achievement choices

other students and other achievement domains. Although SCAs and expectations for success are theoretically distinct, they strongly overlap empirically and thus are often treated as a single construct in statistical analyses (Eccles & Wigfield, 1995).

Subjective Task Values Eccles and her colleagues defined values with respect to the qualities of different achievement tasks and how those qualities influence the individual's desire to do the tasks (Eccles, 2005; Eccles (Parsons) et al., 1983; Wigfield & Eccles, 1992, 2020). Further, in EVT, task values are *subjective* because various individuals assign different values to the same activity; math achievement is valuable to some students but not to others. We, therefore, use the label subjective task values (STVs) in discussing them throughout this article.

Eccles (Parsons) et al. (1983) initially proposed three components of task value—attainment value, intrinsic or interest value, and utility value—and described perceived cost as an impor-

tant influence on overall task value. They defined attainment value as the personal importance of doing well on a given task. More recently, Eccles (2005, 2009) has discussed attainment value in relation to different activities to individuals' social and personal identities and the extent to which tasks allow or do not allow them to express or confirm important aspects of self.

Intrinsic value is the enjoyment one gains from doing the task. This component is similar in certain respects to notions of intrinsic motivation and interest (see Hidi & Renninger, 2006; Ryan & Deci, 2009, 2016; Schiefele, 2009), but it is more specific because of its focus on tasks or domains (see Eccles, 2005, and Wigfield et al., 2017, for discussion of distinctions among these constructs). When children intrinsically value an activity, they often become deeply engaged in it and can persist at it for a long time. This characteristic of engagement also typifies engagement in tasks with a high positive attainment value.

Utility value or usefulness refers to how a task fits into an individual's present or future plans, such as taking a math class to fulfill a requirement for a science degree. In certain respects, utility value is similar to extrinsic motivation because when doing an activity out of utility value, the activity is a means to an end rather than an end in itself (see Ryan & Deci, 2017). However, the activity also can reflect important goals that the person holds deeply, such as attaining a certain occupation, which means it can connect closely to attainment value. Gaspard et al. (2015) expanded the attainment and utility value constructs initially defined by Eccles (Parsons) et al. by proposing subcomponents of it (e.g., utility for future life, utility for job).

Eccles (Parsons) et al. (1983) conceptualized cost as what is lost or given up or suffered when doing any particular task. Engaging in any specific task or activity has costs as well as benefits. If an activity "costs" too much, the individual likely will not do it (see also Eccles, 1984, 2005; Wigfield & Eccles, 2020). Eccles (Parsons) et al. initially described different kinds or types of costs: Individuals' perceptions of how much effort they would need to exert to complete a task and whether it is worth doing so (effort cost), how much engaging in one activity means that other valued activities cannot be done (e.g., Do I do my math homework or check Instagram?), and the emotional or psychological costs of pursuing the task, particularly the cost of failure (e.g., Will taking this advanced course make me feel emotionally drained?). Research on cost has burgeoned in the last several years, and researchers have both proposed new dimensions of cost and developed new measures of it. Wigfield and Eccles (2020) and Wigfield et al. (2017) provide detailed reviews of this work, including discussion of a proposal made by Barron and Hulleman (2015) that the theory be renamed expectancy-value-*cost* theory.

Eccles and Wang (2012) stated that task values both lead to engagement and are influenced by the kinds of activities in which one engages; we return to this point below.

Affective Memories Eccles (Parsons) et al. (1983) primarily focused on three aspects of affective memories. First were basic conditioning effects; when people succeed on something, they have positive emotional/affective reactions to that activity; when they fail, their emotional reactions are negative (see also Pekrun, 2009; Weiner, 1985). These affective memories can accumulate, leading individuals to value or de-value different activities. Second, negative affective reactions can produce anxiety, which also dissuades individuals from engaging in the tasks or activities causing anxiety. As we will see, these affective reactions can connect quite directly to emotional engagement and the other aspects of engagement as well. Third, individuals' interpretations of the outcomes they experience are key to the affective reactions they have. Eccles (Parsons) et al. (1983) connected these "objective" experiences to the kinds of attributions individuals make about the reasons why they did well or poorly (Weiner, 1985). When individuals attribute success to ability and effort, they have positive affective reactions. When they attribute failure to lack of ability, however, affective reactions can be negative and debilitating.

From EVT to SEVT: Rationale and Implications

There are some key reasons why Eccles and Wigfield (2020) decided to change the name of the theory and implications that emerge from this change. First and most importantly, they wanted to emphasize that the processes in the model are dynamic, and the relations among the constructs in the model are both developmental (that is, they change over time) and situationally sensitive (that is, influenced by the immediate situation). With respect to the "situative" aspect, they stated, "In the EVT model we have always considered the situation's impact on children's developing motivation to be an important aspect of the model… further, we believe all aspects of the model are situative, even if the model (in Fig. 1) does not fully capture that" (p. 101859). Second, concerning decisions individuals make, they stated, "Each person will arrive at each decision point with their own set of available options that operate either in the moment or over longer time frames. They will only be familiar with a very limited subset of all possible behaviors and options. They will only have a small subset of the skills and resources that could be drawn on in enacting whatever decision they make. Both their own view and the view of those around them of what is going on and the available options will be limited" (p. 101859). Third, the dynamic aspect of the model is illustrated by the connections between performance and choice shown at the far right in the model, back to beliefs and processes at the far left. Relations among the constructs in different parts of the model are recursive rather than unidirectional and linear. These implications all impact how expectancies and values relate to engagement—the topic we turn to next.

Connecting SEVT to Engagement: Issues, Findings, and a Formal Proposal

We begin this section with a discussion of some of the points Eccles and Wang (2012) raised in their commentary on several chapters on engagement in the first edition of this *Handbook:* (a) challenges for the field regarding definitions of engagement and its relation to motivation; (b) specific ways in which constructs from EVT link to engagement; and (c) how the "fit" between students' developing needs and the educational circumstances that they are in can impact their motivation and engagement.

Eccles and Wang (2012) pointed out that the first challenge for the field is defining engagement clearly and indicating its different levels (the individual, the classroom, the school). The second challenge they noted is how broadly or narrowly engagement is defined; in making this comment, they noted that the authors of the chapters they discussed took different approaches to this issue. Third and what we will elaborate on in this section, they discussed the relations of motivation and engagement, beginning by stating that in the motivation literature, researchers have discussed how children's motivation is comprised of a variety of components or aspects and that these components of motivation influence students' achievement in different ways. These motivation components are influenced by a variety of personal, social, and cultural factors, and the components of children's motivation show different patterns of change across childhood and adolescence.

From there, Eccles and Wang (2012) linked motivation to engagement, initially stating that (apparently) at the general level, the links are clear and straightforward: motivation leads to behavior (or engagement), which leads to learning/performance. But then they pointed out that if affective engagement is substituted for behavioral engagement, then the links get harder to keep distinct, with engagement preceding motivation in some models (see in particular Finn & Zimmer, 2012). This challenge is compounded further when one takes developmental, iterative approaches to both motivation and engagement, with motivation leading to some forms of engagement, which enhances performance, which can then boost subsequent motivation. Further, and again as we noted in our discussion of the definitions of the different engagement components, as researchers define different aspects of motivation and different types and subtypes of engagement then questions can arise regarding which constructs might fit better under the engagement umbrella, and which in motivation. Clarifying this has important implications not just for our understanding of motivation and engagement but also for our understanding of whether interventions designed to increase engagement (or motivation) indeed do so and pinpoint the reasons for the effects, or the lack thereof.

Eccles and Wang (2012) then moved to a discussion of how engagement relates to the constructs in EVT, now SEVT, that we discussed in the previous section. They first discussed how Eccles and colleagues' purpose in developing the model, "to explain individual and group differences in individuals' decisions to engage in, and the extent of their engagement in, various achievement-related activities" (p. 141), relates to the engagement literature. They first noted that the EVT (now SEVT) model always included notions of engagement given its focus on activity (e.g., in which activities I should engage in), persistence, and performance. That is, they see these forms of engagement as outcomes of children's developing expectancies for success and subjective task values. They further stated (or Eccles, 2012, stated) that she sees emotional engagement either as a *precursor* to cognitive and behavioral engagement or as emotional reactions to doing different tasks/being engaged in different tasks.

Building further on this latter point, Eccles and Wang (2012) noted that they believe that the role of affective reactions and memories, which are also determinants of subjective task value, may be one aspect of EVT that overlaps the most with engagement. In Eccles (Parsons) et al.'s (1983) chapter that initially described the model and in subsequent writings, Eccles and colleagues described how children's successes or failures/challenges at different achievement activities produce affective reactions (see also Weiner, 1985). Depending upon their consistency, these can grow into relatively positive or negative affect toward those activities (e.g., "I HATE history"). As depicted in the model in Fig. 1, these affective reactions impact children's developing task values—their interest in the activity, its importance to them, and utility, as well as the activity's perceived cost. Ultimately, the extent to which these affective reactions and values are incorporated into individuals' broader sense of themselves can lead students to identify with the settings in which the activities occur (such as schools), or disidentify, in ways Finn (1989; Finn & Zimmer, 2012) describes. We would add that given the bidirectional links of an individual's task values and expectancies for success, affective memories also can impact children's developing expectancies. Finally, because the model has recursive paths back to the left side of the model, engagement leads to the boxes at the left side of the model, and after more performance outcomes, to new affective memories about different school tasks, activities, and even broader outcomes like beliefs about and identification with schooling.

Eccles and Wang (2012) also discussed how Eccles and Midgley's (1989) extension of the EVT model in their stage-environment fit theory could impact how we think about students' engagement. Eccles and Midgley discussed that the "fit" between students' developing motivational beliefs, values, goals, and needs and the school environments they face could strongly impact their motivation and engagement. Eccles and Midgley discussed how many junior high schools/middle schools do not meet students' developing needs for autonomy and control, among other things. The broader point here is that researchers need to consider not only individuals' own motivation and engagement but also how the situations they are in either facilitate or debilitate both.

Relations of Students' Competence-Related Beliefs and Values to Their Engagement

There is a growing body of work examining how students' competence-related beliefs and subjective task values and student engagement relate. Wang and Eccles (2013) examined how middle school students' perceptions of the school environment, motivation, and engagement (behavioral, emotional, and cognitive) related over time. They used adapted versions of Finn and Voelkl's (1993) measure, Pintrich's (2000) measure, and Skinner and Wellborn's (1994) measures to assess students' behavioral engagement with five items (e.g., "How often do you participate in class discussion actively?"), emotional engagement with six items (e.g., "I find schoolwork interesting."), and cognitive engagement with five items (e.g., "How often do you make academic plans for solving problems?"). They found that adolescents who highly valued school (comprised of attainment and intrinsic value) also reported being behaviorally, cognitively, and emotionally engaged in school. Further, they found that students' self-concept of ability beliefs were stronger predictors of behavioral and cognitive engagement in school than their subjective task value of school. However, students' subjective task value was a stronger predictor of their emotional engagement than their self-concept of ability beliefs in school.

Marchand and Gutierrez (2016) examined how graduate students' attainment, intrinsic, and utility value for their introductory research methods course predicted their self-reported perceived cognitive and behavioral engagement for the course. They measured cognitive engagement using Greene and colleagues' (2004) measure of meaningful strategy use (e.g., "Before a quiz or exam, I plan out how I will study.") and measured behavioral engagement using an adapted version of Skinner et al.'s (2008) behavioral engagement scale (e.g., "I work as hard as I can in my research methods course."). They found each of the components of task value, measured at mid-semester using Eccles and Wigfield's (1995) scale, predicted their semester-end reports of behavioral and cognitive engagement (β = 0.20– 0.23, $p < 0.05$). However, they did not examine how competence-related beliefs may have predicted students' behavioral and cognitive engagement in their research methods course.

Further building upon this work, Guo et al. (2016) examined how adolescents attainment value, intrinsic value, utility value, cost, and self-concept of ability beliefs predicted teacher-reported behavioral engagement. Teacher-reported behavioral engagement was measured using a scale comprised of one item measuring students classroom engagement (e.g., This student participates in math lessons as well as he/she can) and one item measuring student effort (e.g., This student works on all of his/her tasks and homework thoroughly). Task values and cost were measured using Gaspard et al. (2015) value facets questionnaire and self-concept of ability beliefs were measured using the German adaptation (Schwanzer et al., 2005) of the Self-Description Questionnaire III (Marsh et al., 2005). They found that students attainment value (β = 0.23, $p < 0.001$), intrinsic value (β = 0.22, $p < 0.001$), and perceptions of low cost[1] (β = 0.22, $p < 0.05$) positively and uniquely predicted teacher-reported behavioral engage-

ment, but utility value did not ($\beta = 0.01, p < 0.05$). Students self-concept of ability beliefs predicted their behavioral engagement when subjective task value was controlled for in the analyses ($\beta = 0.29, p < 0.001$).

In another study, Fredricks et al. (2018), using a mixed-methods design, examined how attainment value, utility value, and expectancies for success predicted 7th–12th graders' engagement in math and science. They assessed students' behavioral (e.g., "I put effort into math/science"), emotional (e.g., "I look forward to math/science class"), cognitive (e.g., "I think about different ways to solve a problem"), and social engagement (e.g., "I build on others' ideas") using the Math and Science Engagement Scales (see Wang et al., 2016, for more information). Students' task values and expectancies for success were measured using Trautwein et al.'s (2012) scales of students' value and expectancy beliefs. They found that students' attainment value predicted their behavioral, cognitive, emotional, and social engagement in math and science classes ($\beta = 0.18 - 0.35, p < 0.001$). Their utility value predicted math ($\beta = 0.13, p < 0.001$) and science behavioral engagement ($\beta = 0.12, p < 0.001$), science cognitive engagement ($\beta = 0.11, p < 0.001$), and science social engagement ($\beta = 0.08, p < 0.05$). Students' expectancies for success predicted their math ($\beta = 0.20, p < 0.001$) and science behavioral engagement ($\beta = 0.21, p < 0.001$), math ($\beta = 0.30, p < 0.001$) and science emotional engagement ($\beta = 0.31, p < 0.001$), and science cognitive engagement ($\beta = 0.23, p < 0.001$). Through qualitative interviews, they found that participants reported feeling more engaged when they saw the relevance of what they were doing in their math and science class and how it could be applied to their lives outside of class, when they were able to demonstrate their ability to their teachers, when they perceived they had the skills to solve challenging problems, and when they felt they could be successful in their math and science classes.

In summary, these studies show that different-aged individuals' expectancies for success, self-concept of ability, and the different aspects of their subjective task value relate to different types

---

[1]Low cost was measured by reverse coding items from Perez and colleagues (2014) and Wigfield and Eccles (2002) that measured opportunity cost, effort required, and emotional cost.

of engagement. In general, the correlations/predictive relations of self-concept of ability or expectancies to engagement appear somewhat stronger than those of the different aspects of subjective task value, although the researchers in the studies just described did not test for the significance of these differences. For the most part the various aspects of subjective task value relate to engagement in about the same way, except for utility value in Guo et al.'s (2016) study.

To date, research examining the links between EVT constructs and student engagement is limited in that researchers have (for the most part) only examined certain aspects of students' values and certain aspects of engagement and have not included all subjective task values and proposed engagement dimensions. This is particularly true for perceived cost, which remains understudied in terms of its relationship with the various engagement dimensions. Further, researchers have predominately examined how competence-related beliefs and subjective task values are associated with and predict dimensions of engagement and have not examined in much detail how these constructs relate over time.

Gladstone (2020) conducted a study to begin to fill these gaps. She examined how undergraduate students' competence-related beliefs and multiple facets of students' subjective task values (i.e., attainment, intrinsic, utility, utility for future, task effort cost, outside effort cost, loss of valued alternatives, and emotional costs) are associated with and predict all five proposed dimensions of student engagement and behavioral and emotional disaffection in math and science courses. Undergraduate students' behavioral (eight items; e.g., "I stay focused."), cognitive (eight items; e.g., "I think about different ways to solve a problem."), emotional (ten items; e.g., "I look forward to science/math class."), and social engagement (seven items; e.g., "I try to work with others who can help me in science/math.") were measured using Wang et al.'s (2016) Math and Science Engagement Scales. Agentic engagement was measured with five items using an adapted version of Reeve's (2013) Agentic Engagement Scale (e.g., "During class, I ask questions." [see Reeve & Jang, chapter "Agentic

Engagement", this volume]). Behavioral (e.g., "When I'm in class, I just act like I'm working.") and emotional disaffection (e.g., "When I'm in class, I feel worried.") were measured with five items each using an adapted version of Skinner et al.'s (2009) Engagement versus Disaffection with Learning Scale. Gladstone further examined whether these constructs related reciprocally or not and whether engagement dimensions might mediate the relationship between motivational beliefs, values, and domain-specific achievement as measured by students' final grade in the math or science course they reported on.

Gladstone (2020) found that undergraduate students' competence-related beliefs, attainment value, utility value, utility for future life, and intrinsic value were positively associated with behavioral, cognitive, and emotional engagement ($*\hat{\beta} = 0.22 - 0.56, p < 0.001$); cost perceptions (measured as task, effort, emotional, and loss of valued alternative) were negatively associated with them and ranged from $*\hat{\beta} = -0.17 \text{ to } \hat{\beta} = -0.69 (p < 0.001)$. Students' competence-related beliefs, attainment value, utility value, utility for future, and intrinsic value were negatively associated with behavioral and emotional disaffection and ranged from $*\hat{\beta} = -0.12 \text{ to } \hat{\beta} = -0.71 (p < 0.01)$; cost perceptions were positively associated with them ($*\hat{\beta} = 0.12 - 0.85, p < 0.001$).

Gladstone (2020) also examined how different demographic variables related to engagement dimensions. She found that students who self-identified as Asian or Asian American perceived themselves to be more agentic ($*\hat{\beta} = 0.10, p = 0.032$). Much of the work done on agentic engagement, including scale development and validity, was conducted in Asian countries (Reeve, 2013; Reeve & Tseng, 2011; see Patall et al., 2019, for an exception). Thus, agentic engagement may be particularly relevant to students who identify as Asian or identify as someone from an Eastern culture. Clearly, more work is needed on agentic engagement in other groups.

Another important issue Gladstone (2020) investigated is where the different engagement dimensions might fit within the SEVT model. To do so she first examined, using cross-lagged panel analyses, how students' competence-related beliefs and subjective task values predict engagement dimensions and vice versa over time. Gladstone (2020) found several significant unidirectional paths from motivation constructs to engagement dimensions and vice versa, indicating that motivation is not always the driving force of engagement, and that engagement can sometimes be the driving force of motivation among older students. To illustrate this, Gladstone found that emotional engagement (i.e., students' positive emotional reactions to teachers, peers, and classroom activities as well as their valuing of learning and interest in their math/science class) was more predictive of SEVT constructs than vice versa. This suggests, at least among college students in STEM classes, that emotional engagement may be one driving force of students' motivational beliefs and subjective task values rather than the other way around. She also found a number of reciprocal effects, in which both SEVT variables and engagement dimension at time one were significant predictors of the other at time two, for the following pairs of variables: students' intrinsic value and behavioral disaffection, utility value and behavioral disaffection, utility for future life and emotional disaffection, and finally for utility for future life and social engagement. These findings illustrate the complex interplay between different aspects of motivation and engagement. Future research should continue to examine the complexities of these relationships and whether this finding remains among younger students who may not have as much autonomy to choose in which courses to enroll.

Gladstone (2020) also began to address where the different engagement dimensions might fit within the SEVT model by examining whether the dimensions of engagement mediate the relations of student's motivational beliefs and subjective task values to achievement. Examining whether engagement could be a mediator was important because researchers have treated engagement dimensions as both an outcome and a predictor of academic achievement (Reschly & Christenson, 2012). Therefore, when examining the SEVT model, it is important to consider

whether engagement dimensions should go into the "Achievement-Related Choices and Performance" box (as Eccles has suggested in personal communications with the first author and in her commentary with Wang in the first edition of this *Handbook*), or if engagement may mediate the relationship between students' motivational beliefs, subjective task values, and achievement.

Interestingly, Gladstone (2020) found that students' behavioral (i.e., students' involvement in math/science class-based activities) and cognitive engagement (i.e., students' use of deep cognitive strategies in order to understand what is being taught in their math/science class) mediated the relations of all the SEVT constructs to domain-specific grades, except for that between competence-related beliefs and grades. Much previous work shows that competence-related beliefs directly predict students' achievement outcomes (such as test scores and GPA; Durik et al., 2006; Eccles [Parsons] et al., 1983; Guo et al., 2016; Meece et al., 1990; Tonks et al., 2017; Wigfield et al., 2015). Gladstone's findings illustrate a mechanism by which their subjective task values impact grades: they foster behavioral and emotional engagement.

Gladstone (2020) also found that students' emotional engagement was a significant mediator of many of the relations between students' subjective task values and their grades. She argued that because in Eccles (Parsons) et al.'s (1983) model affect is included in the "Individual's Affective Reactions and Memories" box, which precedes subjective task value, emotional engagement should be considered a precursor rather than as a consequence of motivational beliefs and values.

Social engagement, agentic engagement, and behavioral disaffection were not significant mediators of the relations between students' competence beliefs and subjective task values to their grades. These results suggest that (at least among college students) these variables may not be strong predictors of achievement (although see Wang et al., 2016, who showed that social engagement was a significant negative predictor of math and science achievement among high school students). There is limited evidence that agentic engagement relates to achievement. Reeve (2013) found that agentic engagement is uniquely predictive of course achievement among college students enrolled in an education course in Seoul, South Korea. The differences in the results of these studies could be due to subject area differences and the population used for each study (US sample compared to South Korean sample; undergraduates compared to middle and high school students).

A Proposal for Placing Engagement and Disaffection into SEVT

So, given these results, where might we position the various dimensions of engagement into the SEVT model? As noted above, in recent conversations, Eccles stated that she has always considered engagement to be an outcome that belongs in the achievement-related choices box (see Fig. 1). There also is consensus in the motivational literature that *in general* engagement should be considered an outcome of motivation. However, results from more recent work discussed in this chapter suggest that there might be an alternative and more nuanced model that considers the unique dimensions that make up student engagement, as these different dimensions have been found to be predictors and mediators of various other achievement-related outcomes. Therefore, in Fig. 2, we provide a version of the SEVT model that includes *suggested* placements for the various dimensions of engagement. Given that research has found that individuals' subjective task values consistently predict their behavioral and cognitive engagement and mediate the relations of subjective task value and STEM achievement, the first author suggests placing behavioral and cognitive engagement in their own box in between the "Subjective Task Values" box and the "Achievement-Related Choices and Performance" box. Because emotional engagement predicts the motivational beliefs and subjective task values in SEVT, it could be placed in the "Affective Reactions and Memories" box, along with a double-headed

across-time arrow from that box to the "Subjective Task Value" box to account for the mediation effects.

Gladstone also proposes that the limited research on social engagement in relation to the SEVT constructs suggests it should be placed in its own box with arrows coming from "Expectation of Success" and "Subjective Task Value" but not an arrow from its own box to the "Achievement-Related Choices and Performance" box. Finally, we are uncertain whether agentic engagement should be incorporated into the model given its self-determination theory roots. However, if it were to be, Gladstone suggests that agentic engagement should be placed in its own box with an arrow coming from the "Expectation of Success" box but not an arrow from its own box to the "Achievement-Related Choices and Performance" box as agentic engagement was not a significant mediator of the relationships between competence-related beliefs, subjective task values, and domain-specific grades.

Turning to Skinner and colleagues' (Skinner & Pitzer, 2012) behavioral and emotional disaffection constructs, both conceivably could be put into the SEVT model. Behavioral disaffection might be best placed within its own box with arrows leading to it from the "Expectation of Success" box and the "Subjective Task Value" box. Given the overlap of emotional disaffection, Gladstone (2020) found, we propose that emotional disaffection and emotional cost are essentially the same things, and therefore we would include emotional disaffection in the "Subjective Task Value" box.

The authors all agree that further empirical work is needed to test these suggestions. The studies' designs need to be longitudinal and include students varying in age, cultural background, and school domain.

Engagement and Positive Developmental Outcomes

A major reason student engagement has become such a popular construct to study is that it relates

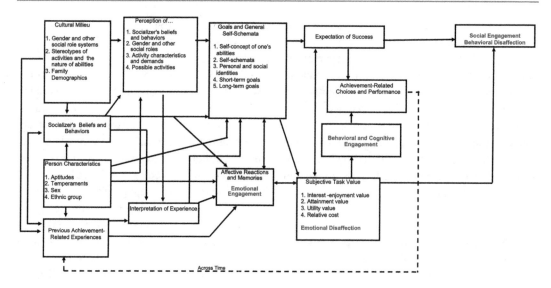

Fig. 2 Gladstone proposal for placing engagement and disaffection dimensions into the SEVT model

to various positive outcomes. Because we are most interested in achievement motivation from the perspective of SEVT, we have focused primarily on the outcomes of achievement and choice to continue taking different school subjects. Students who are engaged in their schoolwork are more likely to have high achievement and continue pursuing an education (Finn & Zimmer, 2012; Fredricks et al., 2004; Wang & Eccles, 2013). Of course, there are other positive developmental outcomes associated with engagement; we briefly discuss how the various dimensions of engagement relate to positive outcomes.

Wang et al. (2016) examined how different aspects of math and science engagement related to STEM achievement and career aspirations. They found that general engagement was the strongest positive predictor of math and science achievement and career aspirations. However, each of the four engagement factors differentially predicted math and science achievement and career aspirations. They found that behavioral engagement was the strongest predictor of math and science achievement. Interestingly, it was a statistically significant negative predictor of math and science career aspirations. Emotional engagement was the only dimension that was a significant positive predictor of math and science career aspirations. Cognitive engagement did not

predict either math or science achievement and cognitive engagement was surprisingly a statistically significant negative predictor of students' math career aspirations. Students' social engagement was a statistically significant negative predictor of their math and science achievement and a non-significant negative predictor of their math and science career aspirations.

The research examining the relationship between agentic engagement and positive outcomes continues to grow, although still limited (Reeve & Jang, chapter "Agentic Engagement", this volume). Reeve (2013) tested the predictive validity of agentic engagement. To do this, Reeve included five items from the Engagement versus Disaffection with Learning measure (Skinner et al., 2009) to measure behavioral engagement (e.g., "I pay attention in this class.") and five items from this scale to measure emotional engagement (e.g., "This class is fun."). Reeve also measured cognitive engagement using four items from the Metacognitive Strategies Questionnaire (Wolters, 2004; e.g., "When I study for this class, I try to connect what I am learning with my own experiences."). Reeve found that Korean college students' agentic engagement predicted their course-specific grades when controlling for students' behavioral, cognitive, and emotional engagement. These results provide some evidence that agentic engagement can be a unique predictor of students' academic achievement.

More recently, Patall et al. (2019) built upon Reeve's (2013) work and conducted a study using the same measures as above and found that agentic engagement predicts positive outcomes in science for US high school students. Their longitudinal analyses showed that agentic engagement predicted an increase in perceived teacher autonomy support, need satisfaction, and behavioral, cognitive, and emotional engagement. They further found through mediation analyses that agentic engagement can dynamically shape the classroom environment by emerging from an autonomy-supportive context to predict subsequent motivation in the course.

Because behavioral and emotional disaffection each represent negative dimensions of engagement, one would expect that the presence of either of these dimensions would result in negative academic outcomes. In their chapter in the first edition of this *Handbook*, Skinner and Pitzer (2012) discussed how behavioral and emotional disaffection could lead to negative achievement outcomes, which then have implications for their developing motivation (see also Martin, 2012, for discussion of this point). Gladstone (2020) found some evidence of this when she examined the reciprocal relationships between motivational beliefs, values, and disaffection. Gladstone found that behavioral and emotional disaffection at the start of the semester was a negative predictor of some of the subjective task values at the end of the semester. These results demonstrate the importance of how interventions at the beginning of the semester could help promote the development of positive engagement rather than disaffection.

More broadly, researchers have found that engagement predicts students' well-being. Salmela-Aro and Read (2017) found that engaged students reported the most positive well-being, whereas students experiencing burnout, which can be considered disengagement, had the lowest reported well-being. Salmela-Aro and Read measured engagement using the schoolwork engagement scale (e.g., "I am enthusiastic about my studies"; Salmela-Aro & Upadaya, 2012), which

was adapted from the Utrecht Work Engagement Scale (Schaufeli et al., 2002). Further, Watt et al. (2019) examined how different motivational profiles among adolescents in mathematics and science were related to academic outcomes, including well-being. They identified three different profiles among tenth grade students' expectancies, values, and perceived costs for mathematics and science. They found that students in what they called the "Positively Engaged" profile (i.e., high perceived talent, intrinsic and utility values, and low costs) had more pronounced positive well-being compared to students in the "Struggling Ambitious" (i.e., high perceived talent, intrinsic and utility values, and costs) and "Disengaged" (i.e., low perceived talent, intrinsic and utility values, and high costs) profiles.

Although this work shows important links between engagement and different outcomes, more work is needed to examine which aspects of engagement relate to which developmental outcomes. We close this chapter with some suggestions for future research in this and other areas.

Future Directions

We have made suggestions for future research throughout this chapter; in this section, we highlight what we think are the most crucial next steps in research in this area.

First, given the conceptual/definitional and, in some cases, empirical overlap of motivation and engagement, more work is needed to continue to examine how distinct they are as constructs. This is particularly true for certain of the proposed dimensions of engagement and some of the variables in SEVT, such as cost and emotional disaffection, but it can be extended to other constructs as well. Looking at relations over time in these constructs and subconstructs will help clarify how they relate to each other, and which may take "causal priority."

More specifically, longitudinal research is needed to understand better the dynamic and reciprocal relationship between motivational beliefs, values, and dimensions of engagement. Although Gladstone (2020) found some evidence of a dynamic relationship between motivational beliefs, subjective task values, and dimensions of engagement and disaffection among college students, these relationships were examined over two time points. Additional time points would have allowed for stronger conclusions about their reciprocal relations. Future research should examine the relationship between motivational beliefs, subjective task values, and engagement dimensions across multiple age groups and time points to better understand when motivation is the driving force of engagement and when engagement may lead to subsequent motivation. This will also help clarify whether engagement, or dimensions of engagement, fully mediates the relationship between motivation and achievement-related outcomes.

We also think it is important for future research to examine the relationships between motivational beliefs, subjective task values, and dimensions of engagement developmentally. We know there are declines in many students' motivational beliefs and values as students move through school (see Wigfield et al., 2015, for review). To date there is little research on how these declines relate to or impact changes in engagement. Mahatmya et al. (2012) discussed in the first edition of this *Handbook* how there are opportunities and challenges that are unique to different developmental periods, and these differences can lead to nuanced differences in the development of engagement and its relations to outcomes. Important developmental questions to explore include: Are there important differences in the relationship between motivation and engagement in different grades? What do these relationships look like during major transition periods, such as middle school to high school? Will motivation interventions aimed at slowing down the typical decline we see in motivation across the school years have implications for developing engagement?

As in many areas of research, we still do not know a great deal about possible gender, race, and ethnic differences in the relations of motivation and engagement. Relatedly, we know little about factors in the school environment that inhibit and support the development of motivation and engagement among students from different gender, racial, and ethnic backgrounds (Bingham & Okagaki, 2012). We suggest that it is particularly important to examine the factors that promote or reduce the positive development of student motivation and engagement among students from marginalized groups that may experience discrimination (See Galindo et al., chapter "Expanding an Equity Understanding of Student Engagement: The Macro (Social) and Micro (School) Contexts", this volume).

Much of the research examining the relationships between motivational beliefs, values, and engagement dimensions we discussed here has focused on science and mathematics domains. Future research is needed to know how these relationships may be similar or different in other domains, such as History or Language Arts. Science and mathematics domains are highly stereotyped domains, and so one might expect that females and students from typically marginalized groups who are more likely to experience negative stereotypes in these courses may have differing levels of motivation and engagement in other domains. This could have implications for where engagement dimensions should be placed within the SEVT model given that constructs found within SEVT focus on the level of the task.

Finally, future work should continue to examine the relationships between motivational beliefs, subjective task values, and agentic and social engagement because there is much less research examining how motivation is related to and predicts these more recently proposed dimensions.

Conclusion

In this chapter, we reviewed work on the relations between students' expectancies, subjective task values, and the five proposed dimensions of engagement. As is clear from our chapter and the other chapters in this *Handbook,* students' engagement is an important precursor for academic outcomes and many other outcomes as well. Finding ways to promote the positive development of engagement will be important to ensure the success of all students. We want to end this chapter by suggesting that one way to help ensure success for all of our students is by continuing collaborative efforts among motivation and engagement researchers. This *Handbook* is an excellent step toward convergence and sharing of ideas among motivation and engagement researchers, which will eventually develop more fruitful interventions to help our students achieve. The next step will be for engagement and motivation researchers to seek out opportunities to work in tandem so that more progress can be made across the two fields of study rather than working in separate camps.

References

Appleton, J. J., Christenson, S. L., Kim, D., & Reschly, A. L. (2006). Measuring cognitive and psychological engagement: Validation of the student engagement instrument. *Journal of School Psychology, 44*, 427–445. https://doi.org/10.1016/j.jsp.2006.04.002

Atkinson, J. W. (1957). Motivational determinants of risk-taking behavior. *Psychological Review, 64*, 359–372. https://doi.org/10.1037/h0043445

Bandura, A. (1977). Self-efficacy: Toward a unifying theory of behavioral change. *Psychological Review, 84*(2), 191–215. Google Scholar.

Barron, K. E., & Hulleman, C. S. (2015). The expectancy-value-cost model of motivation. In J. D. Wright (Ed.), *International encyclopedia of the social and behavioral sciences (2nd)*. Elsevier Ltd.

Bingham, G. E., & Okagaki, L. (2012). Ethnicity and student engagement. In S. L. Christenson, A. L. Reschly, & C. Wylie (Eds.), *Handbook of research on student engagement* (pp. 65–95). Springer.

Connell, J. P., & Wellborn, J. G. (1991). Competence, autonomy, and relatedness: A motivational analysis of self system processes. In M. R. Gunnar & L. A. Sroufe (Eds.), *Self processes and development: The Minnesota symposia on child psychology* (Vol. 23, pp. 43–77). L. Erlbaum Associates.

Corno, L., & Mandinach, E. B. (1983). The role of cognitive engagement in classroom learning and motivation. *Educational Psychologist, 18*, 88–108. https://doi.org/10.1080/00461528309529266 .

Durik, A. M., Vida, M., & Eccles, J. S. (2006). Task values and ability beliefs as predictors of high school literacy choices: A developmental analysis. *Journal of Educational Psychology, 98*, 382–393. https://doi.org/10.1037/0022-0663.98.2.382

Eccles, J. S. (1984). Sex differences in achievement patterns. In T. Sonderegger (Ed.), *Nebraska sympo-sium on motivation* (Vol. 32, pp. 97–132). Univ. of Nebraska Press.

Eccles, J. S. (1993). School and family effects on the ontogeny of children's interests, self-perceptions, and activity choice. In J. Jacobs (Ed.), *Nebraska symposium on motivation, 2992: Developmental perspectives on motivation* (pp. 145–208). University of Nebraska Press.

Eccles, J. S. (2005). Subjective task value and the Eccles et al. model of achievement-related choices. In A. J. Elliot & C. S. Dweck (Eds.), *Handbook of competence and motivation* (pp. 105–121). Guildford.

Eccles, J. S. (2009). Who am I and what am I going to do with my life? Personal and collective identities as motivators of action. *Educational Psychologist, 44*, 78–89. https://doi.org/10.1080/00461520902832368

Eccles (Parsons), J. S., Adler, T. F., Futterman, R., Goff, S. B., Kaczala, C. M., Meece, J., & et al. (1983). Expectancies, values and academic behaviors. In J. T. Spence (Ed.), *Achievement and achievement motives: Psychological and sociological approaches* (pp. 75–146). Freeman.

Eccles, J. S., & Midgley, C. (1989). Stage/environment fit: Developmentally appropriate classrooms for early adolescents. In R. Ames & C. Ames (Eds.), *Research on motivation in education* (Vol. 3, pp. 139–181). Academic Press.

Eccles, J. S., & Wang, M. T. (2012). Part 1 commentary: So what is student engagement anyway? In S. L. Christenson, A. L. Reschly, & C. Wylie (Eds.), *Handbook of research on student engagement* (pp. 133–145). Springer.

Eccles, J. S., & Wigfield, A. (1995). In the mind of the actor: The structure of adolescents' achievement task values and expectancy-related beliefs. *Personality and Social Psychology Bulletin, 21*, 215–225. https://doi.org/10.1177/0146167295213003

Eccles, J. S., & Wigfield, A. (2020). From expectancy-value theory to situated expectancy-value theory: A developmental, social cognitive, and sociocultural perspective on motivation. *Contemporary Educational Psychology, 61*, 101859. https://doi.org/10.1016/j.cedpsych.2020.101859

Finn, J. D. (1989). Withdrawing from school. *Review of Educational Research, 59*, 117–142. https://doi.org/10.3102/00346543059002117

Finn, J. D. (2006). *The adult lives of at-risk students: The roles of attainment and engagement in high school* (NCES 2006–328). Washington, DC: U.S. Department of Education, National Center for Education Statistics.

Finn, J. D., & Voelkl, K. E. (1993). School characteristics related to school engagement. *Journal of Negro Education, 62*, 249–268. https://doi.org/10.2307/i314505

Finn, J. D., & Zimmer, K. (2012). Student engagement: What is it? Why does it matter? In S. L. Christenson, A. L. Reschly, & C. Wylie (Eds.), *Handbook of research on student engagement* (pp. 97–131). Springer.

Fredricks, J. A., Blumenfeld, P. C., & Paris, A. H. (2004). School engagement: Potential of the concept, state of the evidence. *Review of Educational Research, 74*, 59–109. https://doi.org/10.3102/00346543074001059

Fredricks, J. A., Wang, M. T., Schall Linn, J., Hofkens, T. L., Sung, H., Parr, A., & Allerton, J. (2016). Using qualitative methods to develop a survey measure of math and science engagement. *Learning and Instruction, 43*, 5–15. https://doi.org/10.1016/j.learninstruc.2016.01.009

Fredricks, J. A., Hofkens, T., Wang, M. T., Mortenson, E., & Scott, P. (2018). Supporting girls' and boys' engagement in math and science learning: A mixed methods study. *Journal of Research in Science Teaching, 55*, 271–298. https://doi.org/10.1002/tea.21419

Gaspard, H., Dicke, A. L., Flunger, B., Schreier, B., Häfner, I., Trautwein, U., & Nagengast, B. (2015). More value through greater differentiation: Gender differences in value beliefs about math. *Journal of Educational Psychology, 107*, 663–677. https://doi.org/10.1037/edu0000003

Gaspard, H., Lauermann, F., Rose, N., Wigfield, A., & Eccles, J. S. (2020). Cross-domain trajectories of students' ability self-concepts and intrinsic values in math and language arts. *Child Development, 91*(5), 1800–1818. https://doi.org/10.1111/cdev.13343

Gladstone, J. R. (2020). *Uncovering the relations among college students' expectancies, task values, engagement, and STEM course outcomes* (Doctoral dissertation). https://doi.org/10.13016/qgsc-opvx

Greene, B. A., Miller, R. B., Crowson, H. M., Duke, B. L., & Akey, C. L. (2004). Predicting high school students' cognitive engagement and achievement: Contributions of classroom perceptions and motivation. Contemporary Educational Psychology, 29, 462–482. https://doi.org/10.1016/j.cedpsych.2004.01.006

Greene, B. A. (2015). Measuring cognitive engagement with self-report scales: Reflections from over 20 years of research. *Educational Psychologist, 50*, 14–30. https://doi.org/10.1080/00461520.2014.989230

Guo, J., Nagengast, B., Marsh, H. W., Kelava, A., Gaspard, H., Brandt, H., Cambria, J., Flunger, B., Dicke, A. L., Hafner, I., Brisson, B., & Trautwein, U. (2016). Task values, and their interactions using multiple value facets and multiple academic outcomes. *AERA Open, 2*, 1–20. https://doi.org/10.1177/2332858415626884

Hidi, S., & Renninger, K. A. (2006). The four-phase model of interest development. *Educational Psychologist, 41*, 111–127. https://doi.org/10.1207/s15326985ep4102_4

Jacobs, J., Lanza, S., Osgood, D. W., Eccles, J. S., & Wigfield, A. (2002). Ontogeny of children's self-beliefs: Gender and domain differences across grades one through 12. *Child Development, 73*, 509–527. https://doi.org/10.1111/1467-8624.00421

Lewin, K. (1938). *The conceptual representation and the measurement of psychological forces.* Durham, NC: Duke University Press.

Mahatmya, D., Lohman, B. J., Matjasko, J. L., & Farb, A. F. (2012). Engagement across developmental periods. In S. L. Christenson, A. L. Reschly, & C. Wylie (Eds.), *Handbook of research on student engagement* (pp. 45–63). Springer. https://doi.org/10.1007/978-1-4614-2018-7_3

Marchand, G. C., & Gutierrez, A. P. (2016). Processes involving perceived instructional support, task value, and engagement in graduate education. *The Journal of Experimental Education, 85*, 87–106. https://doi.org/10.1080/00220973.2015.1107522

Marsh, H. W., Trautwein, U., Lüdtke, O., Köller, O., & Baumert, J. (2005). Academic self-concept, interest, grades, and standardized test scores: Reciprocal effects models of causal ordering. *Child Development, 76*(2), 397–416. https://doi.org/10.1111/j.1467-8624.2005.00853.x

Martin, A. J. (2007). Examining a multidimensional model of student motivation and engagement using a construct validation approach. *British Journal of Educational Psychology, 77*, 413–440. https://doi.org/10.1348/000709906X118036

Martin, A. J. (2009). Motivation and engagement across the academic lifespan: A developmental construct validity study of elementary school, high school, and university/college students. *Educational and Psychological Measurement, 69*, 794–824. https://doi.org/10.1177/0013164409332214

Martin, A. J. (2010). *Building classroom success: Eliminating academic fear and failure.* Continuum.

Martin, A. J. (2012). The motivation and engagement scale (11th ed.). Sydney: Lifelong Achievement Group (www.lifelongachievement.com).

Meece, J. L., Blumenfeld, P. C., & Hoyle, R. H. (1988). Student's goal orientations and cognitive engagement in classroom activities. *Journal of Educational Psychology, 80*, 514–523. Google Scholar

Meece, J. L., Wigfield, A., & Eccles, J. S. (1990). Predictors of math anxiety and its influence on young adolescents' course enrollment intentions and performance in mathematics. *Journal of Educational Psychology, 82*, 60–70. https://doi.org/10.1037/0022-0663.82.1.60

Patall, E. A., Pituch, K. A., Steingut, R. R., Vasquez, A. C., Yates, N., & Kennedy, A. A. (2019). Agency and high school science students' motivation, engagement, and classroom support experiences. *Journal of Applied Developmental Psychology, 62*, 77–92. https://doi.org/10.1016/j.appdev.2019.01.004

Pekrun, R. (2009). Emotions at school. In K. R. Wentzel & A. Wigfield (Eds.), *Handbook of motivation at school* (pp. 575–604). Routledge.

Pekrun, R., & Linnenbrink-Garcia, L. (2012). Academic emotions and student engagement. In S. L. Christenson, A. L. Reschly, & C. Wylie (Eds.), *Handbook of research on student engagement* (pp. 259–282). Springer. https://doi.org/10.1007/978-1-4614-2018-7_12

Pintrich, P. R. (2000). An achievement goal theory perspective on issues in motivation terminology, theory, and research. Contemporary Educational Psychology, 25, 92–104. https://doi.org/10.1006/ceps.1999.1017

Pintrich, P. R. (2003). A motivational science perspective on the role of student motivation in learning and teaching contexts. *Journal of Educational Psychology, 95*, 667–686. https://doi.org/10.1037/0022-0663.95.4.667

Pintrich, P. R., & De Groot, E. V. (1990). Motivational and self-regulated learning components of classroom academic performance. *Journal of Educational Psychology, 82*, 33–40. https://doi.org/10.1037/0022-0663.82.1.33

Reeve, J. (2012). A self-determination theory perspective on student engagement. In S. L. Christenson, A. L. Reschly, & C. Wylie (Eds.), *Handbook of research on student engagement* (pp. 149–172). Springer.

Reeve, J. (2013). How students create motivationally supportive learning environments for themselves: The concept of agentic engagement. *Journal of Educational Psychology, 105*, 579. https://doi.org/10.1037/a0032690

Reeve, J., & Tseng, C. M. (2011). Agency as a fourth aspect of students' engagement during learning activities. *Contemporary Educational Psychology, 36*, 257–267. https://doi.org/10.1016/j.cedpsych.2011.05.002

Reschly, A. L., & Christenson, S. L. (2012). Jingle, jangle, and conceptual haziness: Evolution and future directions of the engagement construct. In S. L. Christenson, A. L. Reschly, & Wylie, C. (Eds.), Handbook of research on student engagement (pp. 3-19). New York: NY, Springer.

Ryan, R. M., & Deci, E. L. (2009). Promoting self-determined school engagement: Motivation, learning, and Well-being. In K. R. Wentzel & A. Wigfield (Eds.), *Handbook of motivation at school* (pp. 171–195). Routledge.

Ryan, R. M., & Deci, E. L. (2016). Facilitating and hindering motivation, learning, and Well-being in schools: Research and observations from self-determination theory. In K. R. Wentzel & D. B. Miele (Eds.), *Handbook of motivation at school* (2nd ed., pp. 96–119). Erlbaum.

Ryan, R. M., & Deci, E. L. (2017). *Self-determination theory: Basic psychological needs in motivation, development, and wellness.* Guildford Press.

Salmela-Aro, K., & Read, S. (2017). Study engagement and burnout profiles among Finnish higher education students. *Burnout Research, 7*, 21–28. https://doi.org/10.1016/j.burn.2017.11.001

Salmela-Aro, K., & Upadaya, K. (2012). The school-work engagement inventory. *European Journal of Psychological Assessment, 28*(1), 60–67. https://doi.org/10.1027/1015-5759/a000091

Schaufeli, W. B., Salanova, M., González-Romá, V., & Bakker, A. B. (2002). The measurement of engagement and burnout: A two sample confirmatory factor analytic approach. *Journal of Happiness Studies, 3*(1), 71–92. https://doi.org/10.1023/A:1015630930326.

Schiefele, U. (2009). Situational and individual interest. In K. R. Wentzel & A. Wigfield (Eds.), *Handbook of motivation at school* (pp. 197–222). Routledge.

Schwanzer, A. D., Trautwein, U., Lüdtke, O., & Sydow, H. (2005). Entwicklung eines instruments zur Erfassung des Selbstkonzepts junger Erwachsener [development of a questionnaire on young adults'

self-concept]. *Diagnostica, 51*, 183–194. https://doi.org/10.1026/0012-1924.51.4.183

Simpkins, S. D., Fredricks, J., & Eccles, J. S. (2015). The role of parents in the ontogeny of achievement-related motivation and behavioral choices. *Monographs of the Society for the Study of Child Development, 80*(2), 1–22. https://doi.org/10.1111/mono.12157

Sinatra, G. M., Heddy, B. C., & Lombardi, D. (2015). The challenges of defining and measuring student engagement in science. *Educational Psychologist, 50*, 1–13. https://doi.org/10.1080/00461520.2014.1002924

Skinner, E. A., & Belmont, M. J. (1993). Motivation in the classroom: Reciprocal effects of teacher behavior and student engagement across the school year. *Journal of Educational Psychology, 85*, 571–581. https://doi.org/10.1037/0022-0663.85.4.571

Skinner, E. A., & Pitzer, J. R. (2012). Developmental dynamics of student engagement, coping, and everyday resilience. In S. L. Christenson, A. L. Reschly, & C. Wylie (Eds.), *Handbook of research on student engagement* (pp. 21–44). Springer.

Skinner, E. A., & Wellborn, J. G. (1994). Coping during childhood and adolescence: A motivational perspective. In D. Featherman, R. Lerner, & M. Perlmutter (Eds.), *Life-span development and behavior* (Vol. 12, p. 91e133). Erlbaum.

Skinner, E. A., & Wellborn, J. G. (1997). Children's coping in the academic domain. In S. A. Wolchik & I. N. Sandler (Eds.), *Handbook of children's coping with common stressors: Linking theory and intervention* (pp. 387–422). Plenum Press.

Skinner, E., Furrer, C., Marchand, G., & Kinderman, T. (2008). Engagement and disaffection in the classroom: Part of a larger motivational dynamic? *Journal of Educational Psychology, 100*, 765–781. https://doi.org/10.1037/a0012840

Skinner, E. A., Kinderman, T. A., & Furrer, C. J. (2009). A motivational perspective on engagement and disaffection: Conceptualization and assessment of children's behavioral and emotional participation in academic activities in the classroom. *Educational and Psychological Measurement, 69*, 493–525. https://doi.org/10.1177/0013164408323233

Tolman, E. C. (1932). *Purposive behavior in animals and men.* Century.

Tonks, S., Wigfield, A., & Eccles, J. S. (2017). Expectancy-value theory in cross-cultural perspective: What have we learned in the last 15 years? In G. A. De Liem & D. McInerney (Eds.), *Recent advances in sociocultural influences on motivation and learning: Big theories revisited* (2nd ed.). Information Age Press.

Trautwein, U., Marsh, H. W., Nagengast, B., Lüdtke, O., Nagy, G., & Jonkmann, K. (2012). Probing for the multiplicative term in modern expectancy-value theory: A latent interaction modeling study. *Journal of Educational Psychology, 104*, 763–777. https://doi.org/10.1037/a0027470

Wang, M. T., & Eccles, J. S. (2013). School context, achievement motivation, and academic engagement: A longitudinal study of school engagement using a multidimensional perspective. *Learning and Instruction, 28*, 12–23. https://doi.org/10.1016/j.learninstruc.2013.04.002

Wang, M. T., Fredricks, J. A., Ye, F., Hofkens, T. L., & Schall Linn, J. (2016). The math and science engagement scales: Scale development, validation, and psychometric properties. *Learning and Instruction, 43*, 16–26. https://doi.org/10.1016/j.learninstruc.2016.01.008

Watt, H. M., Bucich, M., & Dacosta, L. (2019). Adolescents' motivational profiles in mathematics and science: Associations with achievement striving, career aspirations and psychological wellbeing. *Frontiers in Psychology, 10*, 990. https://doi.org/10.3389/fpsyg.2019.00990

Weiner, B. (1985). An attributional theory of achievement motivation and emotion. *Psychological Review, 92*(4), 548–573. https://doi.org/10.1037/0033-295X.92.4.548

Wigfield, A., & Eccles, J. S. (1992). The development of achievement task values: A theoretical analysis. *Developmental Review, 12*(3), 265–310. https://doi.org/10.1016/0273-2297(92)90011-P

Wigfield, A., & Eccles, J. S. (2020). 35 years of research on students' subjective task values and motivation: A look back and a look forward. In *In advances in motivation science* (Vol. 7, pp. 161–198). Elsevier.

Wigfield, A., Eccles, J. S., Fredericks, J., Roeser, R., Schiefele, U., & Simpkins, S. (2015). Development of achievement motivation and engagement. In R. Lerner (series Ed.) & C. Garcia Coll & M. lamb (volume Eds.), *Handbook of child psychology*, 7th ed. Vol. 3, social and emotional development.

Wigfield, A., Rosenzweig, E., & Eccles, J. (2017). Achievement values. In A. J. Elliot, C. S. Dweck, & D. S. Yeager (Eds.), *Handbook of competence and motivation: Theory and application* (2nd ed., pp. 116–134). Guilford Press.

Wolters, C. A. (2004). Advancing achievement goal theory: Using goal structures and goal orientations to predict students' motivation, cognition, and achievement. Journal of Educational Psychology, 96, 236–250. https://doi.org/10.1037/0022-0663.96.2.236

Zimmerman, B., & Martinez-Pons, M. (1988). Construct validation of a strategy model of student self-regulated learning. *Journal of Educational Psychology, 80*, 284–290. https://doi.org/10.1037/0022-0663.80.3.284

Study Demands-Resources Model of Student Engagement and Burnout

Katariina Salmela-Aro, Xin Tang, and Katja Upadyaya

Abstract

To piece empirical studies on student engagement together, this chapter uses the framework presented in the Study Demands-Resources (SD-R) model. The SD-R model offers a comprehensive view on engagement, demands, resources, and outcomes, and on the interplay of various antecedents. Unlike previous frameworks, the SD-R model endorses the duality of the contextual, personal, and social features (i.e., demands and resources), and the following processes leading from engagement to high motivation, performance, and well-being (i.e., motivational process) or from student burnout and exhaustion to decreased well-being (i.e., energy-depleting process), and thus highlights the synergistic relationships among the different features of the model. In addition, this chapter sheds light on the role of socio-emotional skills as resources of student engagement. Moreover, some future directions in the field of engagement research using the SD-R framework will be addressed.

Introduction

Engagement in the academic domain, particularly student engagement, has been described as academic engagement (Furrer & Skinner, 2003), agentic engagement (Reeve & Tseng, 2011), student engagement (Christenson et al., 2012), school engagement (Fredricks et al., 2004), and schoolwork engagement (Salmela-Aro & Upadyaya, 2012). Researchers have been interested in how and why students focus at school, invest in their studies, how students behave and interact with peers and other people around them while learning, and how students learn in diverse educational activities and settings over time. Because engagement is a core mechanism of knowledge building in and out of educational contexts (Howard-Jones et al., 2018), engagement has been called the "holy grail of learning" (Sinatra et al., 2015).

Conceptualization of Engagement

Student engagement has mostly been conceptualized as a multidimensional construct (Christenson et al., 2012; Schmidt et al., 2018; Wang et al., 2015, 2019a). The main dimensions of engagement have included emotional engagement (feelings about school, learning, and/or a task; Fredricks et al., 2004), cognitive engagement (mental effort and strategies employed while

K. Salmela-Aro (✉) · X. Tang · K. Upadyaya
Faculty of Educational Sciences, University of Helsinki, Helsinki, Finland
e-mail: katariina.salmela-aro@helsinki.fi;
xin.tang@helsinki.fi; katja.upadyaya@helsinki.fi

A. L. Reschly, S. L. Christenson (eds.), *Handbook of Research on Student Engagement*,
https://doi.org/10.1007/978-3-031-07853-8_4

learning; Wang et al., 2019b), behavioral engagement (observable participation in activities; Wang et al., 2019b), social engagement (cooperation with others; Wang & Hofkens, 2019; Tuovinen et al., 2020), and agentic engagement (students' active contribution in shaping their academic activities; Reeve & Tseng, 2011). During the past decade, the most dominant perspective on engagement has been the concept of multidimensional engagement, aspects of which include emotions, cognitions, and behaviors (Fredricks et al., 2004; for an overview, see Salmela-Aro et al., 2021a). This multidimensional perspective has advanced our understanding of the complex nature of engagement.

Emotional engagement encompasses the positive affective reactions attributed to school activities, such as flow experiences, enjoyment, and happiness (Csikszentmihalyi, 1990; Salmela-Aro et al., 2016; Wang et al., 2015). Cognitive engagement refers to the degree to which students invest in their learning, exert the effort needed to understand complex ideas and master difficult skills, and show a desire to go beyond the requirements, including willingness to expend the effort required to do high-quality work (Fredricks et al., 2004; Wang et al., 2019a).

Behavioral engagement refers to productive and proactive participation in academic activities, whereas behavioral disengagement is manifested in giving up schoolwork (Fredricks et al., 2004; Wang et al., 2019a). Behavioral engagement refers to the degree to which students participate in academic, social, and extracurricular activities at school. Students with high behavioral engagement do their best in their classwork and homework, turn in assignments on time, show positive school and classroom behavior, and maintain good attendance.

Agentic engagement refers to engagement that includes agency. In agentic engagement, students are involved in shaping their experience of a task, acting either independently or as co-agents (Salmela-Aro, 2009) with their peers and other people involved in the learning process (see Reeve & Jang, chapter "Agentic Engagement", this volume). For individual students, agency can influence the internal dynamics of engagement,

for example self-regulating the co-actions between emotion, motivation, and action (Schunk & Zimmerman, 2012). In addition, new literature is emerging on social engagement (Tuovinen et al., 2020; Wang et al., 2019b), which refers to students' engagement in social processes at school.

In line with the work engagement literature, student engagement has also been conceptualized as energy, dedication, and absorption in studies/school (i.e., schoolwork engagement, Salmela-Aro & Upadyaya, 2012). In general, *energy* is characterized by high levels of vigor in the learning process, and a willingness to invest effort in learning. *Dedication*, in turn, refers to being strongly involved in schoolwork and perceiving it as meaningful, and experiencing a sense of significance, enthusiasm, inspiration, and challenge. *Absorption* is characterized by high concentration on learning, whereby time passes quickly. Recent research has also described energy, dedication, and absorption as correspondents of widely used emotional, cognitive, and behavioral components of engagement (Upadyaya & Salmela-Aro, 2013a; Wong & Liem, 2021; see also Salmela-Aro et al., 2016). However, the most significant feature of this conceptual approach is that it emphasizes students' deep engagement in an activity; for example, instead of classroom participation, the approach examines students being deeply engrossed in an activity.

The Role of School Burnout

In addition to school engagement, the SD-R framework takes into account students' experiences of exhaustion, cynicism, and feelings of inadequacy in their studies, defined as symptoms of school burnout (Salmela-Aro & Upadyaya, 2014). School is a central context in adolescents' lives. In fact, school can be seen as the primary workplace of adolescents, characterized as it is by features similar to those in adult workplaces, such as standard tasks and activities, deadlines, work responsibility, and feedback routines (Eccles & Roeser, 2011; Salmela-Aro, 2009). As in adult workplaces, adolescents contend with experiences that induce anxiety or stress, thereby impairing their well-being. Recently, based on the rationale that school is a place where students work (Salmela-Aro & Tynkkynen, 2012), the concept of burnout has been extended to the school and education contexts (Salmela-Aro, 2017; Walburg, 2014). School burnout as a new research topic has quickly gained international attention during the last decade, testifying to its perceived relevance across countries (e.g., Herrmann et al., 2019; May et al., 2015; Yang & Chen, 2016). School burnout can be observed among students in countries with different educational systems and academic policies, indicating that it is neither a culturally nor geographically restricted phenomenon (Walburg, 2014).

School burnout can be defined as a school-related syndrome with three components: exhaustion, negative cynical attitude toward school, and feelings of inadequacy as a student, referring, respectively, to the emotional, cognitive, and behavioral components of school burnout (Salmela-Aro et al., 2009, 2017). Exhaustion refers to being tired, ruminating on school-related issues, and experiencing sleep problems; cynicism refers to an indifferent or distal attitude toward studying in general, a loss of interest in studying, and not seeing studying as meaningful; and sense of inadequacy as a student refers to a diminished feeling of academic competence, achievement, and accomplishment. A recent study revealed that about two-thirds of high school students suffer from school-related stress or even burnout (Salmela-Aro & Upadyaya, 2020).

Whereas some studies have approached engagement as the opposite of burnout, a large number of studies have suggested that burnout should be perceived as a separate and distinct psychological process that makes a unique contribution to academic learning (Salmela-Aro, 2017). Research using person-oriented approach has challenged the assumption of engagement and burnout as opposite poles of the same construct by showing that engagement co-exists with high exhaustion and amotivation (Salmela-Aro et al., 2016, 2018; Tuominen-Soini & Salmela-Aro, 2014). For example, 30% of higher educa-

tion students simultaneously experience high engagement and exhaustion especially during the first 2 years of their studies (Salmela-Aro et al., 2018). Even engaged-exhausted students often have resources and do well in their studies; they feel more stressed with possible failures (Tuominen-Soini & Salmela-Aro, 2014). Latest research using growth modeling also showed that engagement increases, rather than reduces, the likelihood of being exhausted (Junker et al., 2021). These findings imply that burnout is not simply the opposite of engagement, but it is a distinct psychological factor that contributes independently to academic and psychological outcomes: a student can be engaged and burned-out at the same time.

Study Demands-Resources Model

Originally, the conceptualization of demands-resources stems from the literature on occupational psychology and work engagement (Bakker et al., 2003; Bakker & Demerouti, 2017; Demerouti et al., 2001), and has successfully been used to describe students' engagement while learning (Salmela-Aro & Upadyaya, 2014; Schaufeli et al., 2002; Upadyaya & Salmela-Aro, 2013a). Study Demands-Resources (SD-R) model conceptualizes engagement and burnout as positive and negative aspects of students' school-related well-being and psychological functioning (Klusmann et al., 2008). However, absence of one aspect does not necessarily indicate the presence of other, that is, students without burnout symptoms do not necessarily experience high engagement (see also Klusmann et al., 2008), and different combinations of engagement and burnout indicate more complexity related to students' well-being and socioemotional skills (Salmela-Aro et al., 2021b). In addition, the SD-R model proposes a motivational process, which leads from resources to engagement and well-being, and an energetic process originating from high demands and leading to wearing out and burnout. As mentioned above, school can be seen as the main environment for students' achievements, performing daily tasks and assignments, and collaborating with peers; and thus the school demands-resources model can integrate the energetic and motivational processes by combining simultaneous engagement and burnout among students (Salmela-Aro & Upadyaya, 2014).

Although there are a few contextual models of engagement in the literature (Lam et al., 2012; Skinner & Pitzer, 2012; Wang et al., 2019a), the SD-R model has several unique contributions and offers a more comprehensive framework on the contextual, personal, and social influences. The first unique feature of the SD-R model lies on the understanding of the duality of the pathways between various demands, resources, and student engagement, unlike previous models that mostly focus on the promotive factors (Lam et al., 2012; Wang et al., 2019a). The SD-R model describes various psychological, social, and environmental demands and resources that can either hinder or promote engagement. Demands are factors that often challenge students to learn and to engage in school (e.g., difficult assignments) or factors that may hinder learning and engagement (e.g., study-related stress), while resources are factors that typically support students' learning and engagement (e.g., teacher support; Salmela-Aro & Upadyaya, 2014). Both demands and resources encompass factors that are present at multiple levels such as situational (e.g., demands and resources related to the learning situation or characteristics of a task), intra-individual (e.g., psychological demands and resources), and interindividual levels (e.g., social demands and resources), and at the school level (e.g., environmental demands and resources). Concerning the various types of demands and resources, SD-R model uniquely posits that, apart from the independent effects of demands and resources, interaction between them plays an influential role in engagement and study-related burnout. When demands overtake resources, it is more likely to lead to the energy-depleting process of wearing out to occur leading to burnout and decreases in well-being, even if the level of resources is relatively high (Bakker & Demerouti, 2017). Also, in highly demanding situations, a strong support from the environment can promote students to engage in learning (Bakker & Demerouti, 2017). In some complicated situations, high demands and wealthy resources may lead to increases or decreases in engagement in the long run (Salmela-Aro, 2017; Salmela-Aro et al., 2016). Therefore, SD-R model does not only cover different levels of antecedents but also suggests synergistic relationships between them that further determine engagement and burnout.

In this chapter, we propose an expanded SD-R model on the basis of the previous SD-R model (presented by Salmela-Aro & Upadyaya, 2014). According to the expanded model (see Fig. 1), high levels of school, family, social, and personal demands are often positively related to school burnout, whereas high levels of school, family, social, and personal resources are associated with student engagement (Salmela-Aro & Upadyaya, 2014).

In the following section, using the SD-R model, we will review demands and resources presented in previous literature in association with student engagement. First, school, family, social (teachers and peers), and personal demands are reviewed, followed by school, family, social (teachers and peers), and personal resources and reserves.

Demands

School Demands Numerous school-related factors, such as harsh school climate or large school size, can act as demands and hinder engagement. In addition, during challenging periods, such as school transitions, engagement often decreases drastically, which may be due to various demands related to the school environment (Wang & Eccles, 2012). For example, high school has been described as more rigid, structured, and less mastery-oriented compared to middle school, and after the transition to high school students' engagement has been found to decline (Wang & Eccles, 2012). Another significant school demand that affects adolescents' engagement in learning is the lack of safety students may experience in the school environment. In schools where victimization behaviors and violence are high, adoles-

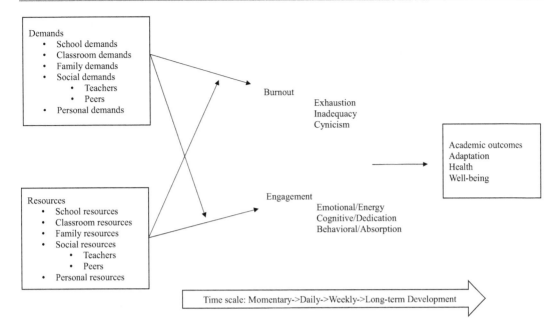

Fig. 1 Study Demands-Resources model

cent students' classroom engagement (i.e., teacher-reported schoolwork behaviors) is often low ($r = -0.24$; Côté-Lussier & Fitzpatrick, 2016), and the proportion of low performers is high (Herrero Romero et al., 2019). Moreover, among ethnic minority students, experiences of racial discrimination at school impede their academic engagement (e.g., academic curiosity and persistence; $\beta = -0.07$ to -0.30; Leath et al., 2019; see also Galindo et al., chapter "Expanding an Equity Understanding of Student Engagement: The Macro (Social) and Micro (School) Contexts", this volume).

Finnish and US adolescents demonstrated that, compared to other classroom activities, students in science classrooms reported lower levels of engagement (i.e., report of being interested, skilled, and challenged) when they were writing, being tested, or listening (Inkinen et al., 2019). Moreover, engagement may vary by academic domains and the level of challenge they present to each student. For example, in highly demanding domains such as mathematics, students report less behavioral/cognitive and emotional engagement than in less demanding domains such as physical education (Pöysä et al., 2018).

Classroom Demands In the classrooms, demands related to schoolwork and teachers' instruction may prevent adolescents from engaging in learning. For example, students' perceptions concerning the general level of challenge in their assignments and obstructive behaviors by teachers (e.g., failing to respond to students, poor lesson plans) reduce students' engagement (i.e., situational cognitive and emotional engagement) in the classroom ($\beta = -0.11$ to -0.14 under emotional obstruction; Strati et al., 2017). Some classroom activities may also manifest as demands in learning situations. A cross-national study among

Family Demands Families are embedded within larger structural contexts that influence engagement directly and indirectly through parental beliefs and expectations concerning their children (Reschly & Christenson, 2019). Several parental behaviors, such as parental monitoring and involvement, often serve as resources for students' engagement (Upadyaya & Salmela-Aro, 2013b; Wilder, 2014). However, some parental behaviors may manifest as demands. For example, adolescents who experience harsh parenting behaviors often report low self-control capabilities, manifested as difficulties in engaging in learning (i.e., behavioral/cognitive/emotional/agentic engagement; $r = -0.15$ to -0.24; Wang et al., 2018b). High pressure placed by parents on their children is associated with low emotional and behavioral engagement ($r = -0.06$ to -0.18; Raufelder et al., 2015).

Some family demographic factors may also present as demands for engagement. Immigrant status, low achievement, and social adversity have been found to be risk factors for engagement (Motti-Stefanidi et al., 2015), suggesting that young immigrants may disengage from school to protect themselves from academic failure. For example, immigrant students were found to disengage from their studies more often than their nonimmigrant/native peers (Motti-Stefanidi & Masten, 2013). In Finland, a cynical attitude toward school (i.e., cynicism), often similar to disengagement, has become more common toward the end of comprehensive education, and among recently immigrated boys (Salmela-Aro et al., 2018). Li and Lerner (2011) also found that immigrant and minority students followed problematic behavioral and emotional engagement paths. Moreover, family social-economic status (SES) can also influence adolescents' engagement. Studies have consistently found that adolescents from low SES families are less likely engaged in schoolwork (Park et al., 2012; Tang et al., 2019).

Social Demands Social demands at school include poor relationships and difficult social situations, and may involve multiple players such as teachers and peers.

Teachers as Social Demands Teachers are influential actors in determining students' engagement. Apart from the instructional and management demands mentioned above, socioemotional demands related to teachers are another factor affecting academic engagement. Hughes and Cao (2018) followed the same group of adolescents and teachers for 7 years, including during the transition to middle school. They found that, in general, teachers reported a decline in affective behaviors and an increase in conflicts with students. Moreover, the slope of the changes mattered. A positive growth in conflict predicted lower behavioral engagement ($\beta = -0.13$ to -0.77). Thus, this study implied that to keep students engaged it is not enough to consider the initial levels of warmth and conflict but also their rate of change.

Peers as Social Demands Recent research has sought to understand how peer contexts influence engagement through selection and socialization processes, social acceptance, and peer rejection processes. Students tend to adjust their engagement to the levels of their peer group (Wang et al., 2018b; see also Knifsend et al., chapter "The Role of Peer Relationships on Academic and Extracurricular Engagement in School", this volume). Moreover, adolescents often select peers who share similar levels of behavioral engagement (Kindermann, 2016). Peer interactions among adolescents are complex and multidimensional and can take many forms from best friend dyads to large friendship groups (e.g., Seo & Huang, 2012). Peer similarity extends to learning, well-being, school engagement, and academic achievement (Kindermann, 2016; Li et al., 2011). A recent study showed how a student's position in his/her ego network was associated with indicators of disengagement: adolescents who experienced social exclusion or, in some cases, rejection were at increased risk for school burnout (Rimpelä et al., 2020).

Contrary to a common belief, friendships do not always protect adolescents. Friendships also induce stress, and friend-related stress is significantly associated with low level of cognitive and behavioral engagement in schoolwork ($r = -0.04$ to -0.21, except one case at 0.04) and high-risk behaviors (Benner et al., 2020). Moreover, instability of adolescent friendship creates tensions between peers, thus hampering students' cognitive/behavioral engagement in schoolwork ($\beta = -0.17$), and finally impairing their academic achievement (Lessard & Juvonen, 2018). Furthermore, victimization behaviors by peers, such as kicking/pushing/hitting, name calling, teasing, socially isolating others, are detrimental to adolescents' engagement (i.e., an aggregated score of behavioral, cognitive, and emotional engagement; $r = -0.06$, $\beta = -0.16$; Totura et al., 2014), particularly for emotional engagement (Forster et al., 2019).

Personal Demands Personal demands are individual factors that create difficulties for adolescents' learning and engagement at school. Those factors may include cognitive/learning difficulties, mental health problems, misconduct, or challenging personality traits. For example, students with attention/deficit hyperactivity disorder (ADHD) have been found to be less engaged in school (i.e., less school and peer connectedness, lower motivation) and more likely to be suspended from school than those without ADHD (Zendarski et al., 2017). For regular students without learning difficulties, they are also likely to have low levels of school engagement (i.e., behavioral and emotional engagement), when suffering from internalizing symptoms such as depression ($\beta = -0.08$ to -0.09; Stiles & Gudiño, 2018), externalizing symptoms ($\beta = -0.11$ to -0.13; Stiles & Gudiño, 2018), and problem behaviors ($\beta = -0.03$ to -0.12; particularly for behavioral engagement, $\beta = -0.10$ to -0.12; Archambault et al., 2017).

Notes on Demands As we have emphasized in this chapter, the relationships between demands and engagement/burnout are not always straightforward. Idiosyncratic appraisal processes can also play an important role in deciding whether a demand is beneficial or detrimental. For example, Putwain et al. (2017) studied students' reactions toward a stressful event, passing an important course. Their study showed that students are more likely to learn when a demanding event was appraised as an opportunity than when it was appraised as a threat. In addition, Verkuyten et al. (2019) theorized that ethnic/racial minority students may, in certain situations, pursue academic engagement as an instrumental way to escape a discriminatory environment. For those students, being exposed to discrimination may, unexpectedly, promote academic engagement.

These studies remind us that attention should also be paid to individuals' perceptions and evaluations of specific demanding factors.

Resources

Resources are factors that generally facilitate student engagement and include multilayered factors that range from the school level to personal level.

School and Classroom Resources Resources at the school level mostly refer to structural factors such as facilities and infrastructure, or to school services, instructional and management factors, and the psychological atmosphere. Most recent studies have focused on the latter group. A few studies have tapped into the structural aspects. School safety has been a prominent topic: two studies unanimously showed that perceived school safety helped students to engage in schoolwork ($r = 0.24$; Côté-Lussier & Fitzpatrick, 2016) and generally in school (i.e., behavioral, emotional, and cognitive engagement; $r = 0.18$–0.35; Storlie & Toomey, 2020). In the school context, students' behavioral, emotional, and cognitive engagement are associated with school emotional atmosphere ($r = 0.33$–0.44; Datu & Park, 2019), and teachers' academic and emotional support ($r = 0.31$–0.38; Liu et al., 2018). In addition, teachers who provide clear instructions, constructive feedback, and strong guidance have often engaged students in terms of behavioral, emotional, and cognitive engagement ($r = 0.30$–0.36; Jang et al., 2010). High-quality pedagogy, and learning tasks that incorporate hands-on activities and real-world applications also tend to keep students engaged (i.e., being momentarily engaged in schoolwork; Maestrales et al., 2021; Shernoff et al., 2016).

Family Resources Family is an environment that can provide ample resources, including financial, cultural, social, emotional, and educational resources. Adolescents from wealthy or high SES families are more likely to have good academic, cultural, and recreational environments thus rendering them less likely to burnout at school ($r = -0.18$ to -0.26; Luo et al., 2016). Parents also have a role in shaping student engagement. Several studies have shown that parental involvement, affection, monitoring, and support all promote student engagement with school (Im et al., 2016; Upadyaya & Salmela-Aro, 2013b; Wang & Eccles, 2012; Wilder, 2014). Parental involvement, whether in the form of parents' knowledge of school activities ($\beta = 0.21–0.32$ for behavioral engagement; Im et al., 2016) or parent-teacher communication and autonomy support ($r = 0.45–0.50$ for three engagement components; Li et al., 2019), has been found to be a significant factor increasing student engagement. Close and supportive relationships, including parental affection in general (i.e., affective support and warmth from one's parents), typically increase adolescents' engagement (i.e., energy, dedication, absorption) in schoolwork ($r = 0.15–0.27$; Upadyaya & Salmela-Aro, 2013b) and behavioral, emotional, and cognitive engagement ($r = 0.29–0.31$; Sun et al., 2020). Parental autonomy support may serve as an environmental protective factor, while the more sources of autonomy support one has, the lower one's school burnout particularly at the high school ($\beta = -0.12$ to -0.13; Duineveld et al., 2017). Multiple sources of support may serve adolescent students as ecological assets that, together with high student engagement, promote positive youth development and a successful school-to-work transition, which in turn is a precursor of successful career development (Lerner et al., 2015).

Social Resources Social connections and relatedness with parents, teachers, peers, and supervisors serve as sources of support for students/young adults by promoting high engagement, adjustment to transitions, and positive educational and vocational success (King, 2015; Upadyaya & Salmela-Aro, 2013a; Wang & Eccles, 2012). In fact, this has been one of most studied themes during the past decade. Wang and Eccles (2012) found that social support provided

by teachers, parents, and peers all contributed to students' engagement measured by school compliance, school identification, participation in extracurricular activities, and perceived value of learning. More specifically, the study demonstrated that the effects of social support on school engagement differed by the sources of social support and domain of engagement. For example, teachers' social support had greater impact on school identification and the perceived value of learning, whereas peer social support was stronger in determining participation in extracurricular activities. King (2015) further demonstrated that perceived peer relatedness, in comparison to perceived parent and teacher relatedness, was the strongest factor predicting behavioral and emotional engagement ($r = 0.23–0.43$) and disaffection ($r = -0.22$ to -0.46). However, only perceived parent relatedness contributed to the development of disaffection ($\beta = -0.11$). These results indicate that the complex relationships between multidimensional engagement and the ecological-social support systems that adolescents have in their life merit further study.

Teachers as Social Resources Social resources provided by teachers can refer to the relationships between teachers and adolescents (Martin & Collie, 2019; Roorda et al., 2017), the support adolescents receive from teachers (Quin et al., 2018), teacher characteristics such as enthusiasm or affection (Keller et al., 2014), or to emotional support and transmission embedded in knowledge instruction in classroom practices (Pöysä et al., 2019; Reyes et al., 2012). In one large-scale longitudinal study, Martin and Collie (2019) focused on the relative balance of positive and negative teacher-student relationships and their effects on students' behavioral, emotional, and cognitive engagement. They found that a positive teacher-student relationship was beneficial for three types of engagement. When positive relationships outweighed negative relationships, engagement increased significantly ($\beta = 0.13–0.16$). These effects also held for curvilinear associations. Thus, the results showed that there is no point along the curve that counteracts the beneficial effect of a positive relationship. The message is straightforward: the better the relationship between teachers and students, the better their students' engagement (i.e., behavioral, emotional, and cognitive engagement). Other studies have unanimously supported these findings on the important role of teachers' social and emotional support in adolescent students' behavioral, cognitive, and emotional engagement (Liu et al., 2018; Pöysä et al., 2019; Quin et al., 2018).

Peers as Social Resources One of the most researched topics in recent engagement literature has been peer influence (Salmela-Aro et al., 2021a). Many studies have examined the role of peer influence on student engagement and shown that such influences become more prominent during adolescence. In general, good peer relationships ($r = 0.11$–0.32; Mikami et al., 2017), quality friendships ($r = 0.23$–0.43; King, 2015), high peer-nominated popularity ($r = 0.07$–0.11; Zhang et al., 2019), and a high amount of peer support ($r = 0.09$–0.12; Wang & Eccles, 2012) promote students' behavioral, emotional, and cognitive engagement in school and in learning. Studies using social-network analysis also found that socially active and popular students were more engaged (i.e., energy, dedication, absorption) in schoolwork and were at lower risk for burnout than less active and less popular students (Rimpelä et al., 2020; Wang et al., 2018a). Two adolescents were more likely to become friends if both were engaged in learning; this, in turn, reinforced their engagement in studying. This study thus indicates a feedback loop of peer influence on engagement. It may also remind us of the negative feedback loop in which adolescents whose friends are disengaged are also likely to disengage from school, thus making it hard to escape a disadvantaged environment (Schwartz et al., 2016; see more discussions in the Demands section).

Personal Resources Personal resources are individual factors that promote student engagement and hinder burnout. Such factors include

cognitive resources, emotional/motivational resources, socio-emotional skills, and personality traits. Many studies have focused on these factors during the past decade (Salmela-Aro et al., 2021a). For example, socio-cognitive factors such as achievement goal orientations (Tuominen et al., 2020) have been found to increase student engagement (i.e., energy, dedication, absorption; $r = 0.34$–0.48) and reduce school burnout ($r = -0.03$ to -0.44). Even general well-being, for example, life satisfaction (Heffner & Antaramian, 2016) as personal affective resources, has been found to increase behavioral, emotional, and cognitive student engagement ($\beta = 0.24$–0.28). Personal resources can also act as mediators on the pathways between contextual and social demands-resources and student engagement, including, for example, self-efficacy ($r = 0.49$; Sun et al., 2020) and grit/perseverance ($r = 0.44$–0.46; Tang et al., 2019). One recent large-scale study (over 60,000 secondary school students) also demonstrated growth goal as a personal resource can act as a mediator and a moderator (Martin et al., 2021). The study showed that, first, teacher's instructional support as a classroom resource affects the development of engagement directly (i.e., behavioral and cognitive engagement; Martin et al., 2021). Second, students' growth goal mediates the pathways between instructional support and engagement (indirect effect = 0.08–0.24, except for organization and clarity; Martin et al., 2021). The same study further showed that growth goal can motivate the students who are from low socio-economic status families (i.e., high family demands) to have better engagement than those from high SES families (Martin et al., 2021).

Socio-emotional Skills The OECD (2021) has identified key socio-emotional skills, which serve as personal resources of students' well-being and engagement (Salmela-Aro & Upadyaya, 2020; Guo et al., 2022). Socio-emotional skills can be described within five broader clusters or "Big Five" domains, each of them referring to a set of underlying socio-emotional skills. These five domains include task performance (e.g., persistence, self-control, grit), emotional regulation (e.g., optimism, stress resistance, academic buoyancy), engaging with others (e.g., social engagement, belongingness, lack of loneliness), collaboration (e.g., cooperation, trust), and open-mindedness (e.g., curiosity, creativity; Kankaraš et al., 2019; OECD, 2021). Relying on self-report measures, recent research has shown that socio-emotional skills support engagement in schoolwork (i.e., energy, dedication, absorption; $r = 0.20–0.36$) and protect against burnout ($r = -0.03$ to -0.56) among high school students (Salmela-Aro & Upadyaya, 2020). In addition, changes in schoolwork engagement (i.e., energy, dedication, absorption) and school burnout during COVID-19 were associated with changes in socio-emotional skills (Salmela-Aro et al., 2021b). Especially, increases in schoolwork engagement are associated with increases in curiosity, grit, and academic buoyancy, whereas decreases in school burnout are associated with decreases in social engagement and belongingness, and increases in loneliness (Salmela-Aro & Upadyaya, 2020; Salmela-Aro et al., 2021b). Moreover, besides serving as important personal resources, the role of socio-emotional skills is especially highlighted during school transitions when demands related to socio-emotional regulation increase and students need to navigate through changing school environments (Salmela-Aro & Upadyaya, 2020), as well as during challenging societal times, such as the COVID-19 pandemic, which drastically changed the educational environment of millions of students worldwide (Salmela-Aro et al., 2021b).

Interaction and Accumulation of Demands and Resources

As we described earlier, one of the strengths of the SD-R model is its contribution to theorizing on the multiplicative effects of demands and resources in affecting engagement. These effects, however, have largely been neglected in other models (Lam et al., 2012; Wang et al., 2019a). Recent research has witnessed a broad range of studies in search of synergistic effects between demands and resources. For example, students' behavioral, emotional, and cognitive engagement were better in classrooms where teachers provided more structure (e.g., imposing high expectation, providing strong guidance) and more autonomy support ($r = 0.33–0.44$; Hospel & Galand, 2016). These results illustrate a *boosting effect* that often occurs between two resources, when one resource boosts the effect of the other resource (here structure and autonomy support) leading to high engagement. Similarly, *buffering effects* often occur when one resource buffers against the negative impact of demands on academic well-being. For instance, a study with high school students found that both emotional intelligence and teachers' emotional support can reduce the level of burnout ($r = -0.36$ to -0.40; Romano et al., 2020). However, when students simultaneously experienced academic anxiety, the protective role of resources was significantly weakened (Romano et al., 2020).

Demands-resources interaction has often been found in the social domain. For instance, Moses and Villodas (2017) studied adversity among adolescents (e.g., living in poverty, being maltreated by caregivers) and found that high-quality peer relationships reduced the negative effects of adversities on student engagement in prosocial activities. Similarly, among adolescents who are victims of bullying, the better their school climate (operationalized as good teacher-student relationships, student-student relationships, fairness of rules, clarity of expectations, school safety, and respect for diversity), the more likely they are to have high emotional and cognitive-behavioral engagement compared to counterparts in a negative school climate (Yang et al., 2018). In addition, parents' racial socialization protects ethnic/racial minority adolescents who experience discrimination from low achievement and low educational aspirations (Wang & Huguley, 2012). The aforementioned studies highlight the importance of further examining the multiplicative effects of demands and resources. Demands-resources interaction may occur in the same environment (e.g., school demands × school resources) or spillover to different contexts (e.g., family demands × personal resources; personal resources × school demands).

When examining demands and resources it is important to note that demands and resources do not occur in vacuum but interact with each other and accumulate over time (Bakker & Demerouti, 2017). Building on the conservation of resources (COR) theory (Hobfoll, 2001; Hobfoll et al., 2018), students with high initial resources tend to gain more resources later on (often called *gain spirals*), whereas constant high demands may lead to losses of one's finite personal resources leading to *loss spirals*. Accumulation of resources (gain spirals) helps in building one's resource reserves that serve for confronting future demands, whereas loss spirals may weaken existing resource reserves (Bakker & Demerouti, 2017). Thus, people do not employ key resources solely as a response to demands but also in order to build reserves of resources for future use (Hobfoll et al., 2018). For example, students who have multiple sources of support (teachers, parents, peers) show high motivation and behavioral engagement in science (Simpkins et al., 2020). Further, students have an active role in building their own resources and confronting demands, and just as employees craft their jobs, students can make their studies more manageable by crafting the demands and resources they have. For example, whenever possible, university students can make decisions about the amount and periodic timing of their study courses, and whether and how much they choose to work and have other extracurricular activities simultaneously with their studies. In order to support students with such decisions, universities could provide introductory lectures on time management and self-care. Among younger students, parents can help in building a sustainable study schedule and environment.

Outcomes of Engagement and Burnout

Both engagement and burnout have notable interconnections with academic and psychological functioning (Lam et al., 2012; Madigan & Curran, 2020; Wang et al., 2019a). Experiencing a high level of engagement (e.g., schoolwork engagement) is beneficial for students' academic performance, well-being, and future success in life (Upadyaya & Salmela-Aro, 2013a). Students scoring higher on schoolwork engagement are more likely to have higher GPA (e.g., $r = 0.20$–0.26, Tang et al., 2019; $r = 0.19$–0.46, Wang et al., 2015) and educational aspirations ($r = 0.26$–0.32, Tang et al., 2019), and fewer depressive symptoms ($r = -0.03$ to -0.24; Wang et al., 2015). Students who experience positive trajectories of behavioral and emotional engagement are less depressed ($r = -0.12$ to -0.29) and less likely to be involved in delinquency and substance abuse ($r = -0.07$ to -0.33), and have better academic outcomes ($r = 0.09$–0.41; Li & Lerner, 2011). In turn, school burnout is linked to negative indicators, such as high rates of substance use and problem behaviors ($\beta = 0.03$–0.22; Henry et al., 2012) and psychological symptoms ($r = 0.28$–0.51; Tang et al., 2021). A recent meta-analysis (Madigan & Curran, 2020), with more than 100,000 students, showed that academic burnout was negatively associated with academic achievement ($r = -0.24$). In particular, feelings of inadequacy and academic attainment were negatively associated ($r = -0.39$).

In support of the SD-R model, longitudinal studies have shown that engagement spills over from the domain-specific school context to general ill- and well-being (Salmela-Aro & Upadyaya, 2014). Student burnout predicts later depressive symptoms, whereas student engagement predicts later life satisfaction (see also Upadyaya & Salmela-Aro, 2017). Moreover, student burnout and engagement not only spillover to well-being but also to further educational choices, achievements, and pathways. Longitudinal studies show that student engagement predicts higher grades (Kiuru et al., 2020), a successful transition from high school to tertiary studies (Vasalampi et al., 2018) and onward (Upadyaya & Salmela-Aro, 2013b), and later satisfaction with choice of career and educational pathways (Upadyaya & Salmela-Aro, 2015). Student burnout, in turn, predicts involuntary gap years after high school, decreases in educational aspirations, and a fourfold greater likelihood of dropping out (Bask & Salmela-Aro, 2013). In line with the stage-environment fit theory (Eccles & Roeser, 2009), the risk for school burnout is greater when the school context does not support student's psychological needs.

Conclusion

In this chapter, we propose a new framework, the Study Demands-Resources model, to integrate what we have found in the literature and to indicate new directions for the field. The SD-R model highlights the interplay of demands and resources in determining engagement and burnout. This is important as more studies move into momentary-level and digital/online research. In these situations, there is a need to examine the dynamic process of engagement and the dynamic interplay between environmental and individual factors. As we write this chapter, the world is experiencing the COVID-19 pandemic that has forced millions of students to study online or at a distance. Remote learning will inevitably set new demands but will also provide new resources to support adolescents' engagement. It is foreseeable that remote learning will be further integrated into the regular school day and thus have profound implications for engagement research in the future.

References

Archambault, I., Vandenbossche-Makombo, J., & Fraser, S. L. (2017). Students' oppositional behaviors and engagement in school: The differential role of the student-teacher relationship. *Journal of Child and Family Studies, 26*(6), 1702–1712. https://doi.org/10.1007/s10826-017-0691-y

Bakker, A. B., & Demerouti, E. (2017). Job demands–resources theory: Taking stock and looking forward. *Journal of Occupational Health Psychology, 22*(3), 273–285. https://doi.org/10.1037/ocp0000056

Bakker, A. B., Demerouti, E., de Boer, E., & Schaufeli, W. B. (2003). Job demands and job resources as predictors of absence duration and frequency. *Journal of Vocational Behavior, 62*(2), 341–356. https://doi.org/10.1016/S0001-8791(02)00030-1

Bask, M., & Salmela-Aro, K. (2013). Burned out to drop out: Exploring the relationship between school burnout and school dropout. *European Journal of Psychology of Education, 28*(2), 511–528. https://doi.org/10.1007/s10212-012-0126-5

Benner, A. D., Hou, Y., & Jackson, K. M. (2020). The consequences of friend-related stress across early adolescence. *The Journal of Early Adolescence, 40*(2), 249–272. https://doi.org/10.1177/0272431619833489

Christenson, S. L., Wylie, C., & Reschly, A. L. (2012). Handbook of research on student engagement. In S. L. Christenson, A. L. Reschly, & C. Wylie (Eds.), *Handbook of research on student engagement.* Springer. https://doi.org/10.1007/978-1-4614-2018-7

Côté-Lussier, C., & Fitzpatrick, C. (2016). Feelings of safety at school, socioemotional functioning, and classroom engagement. *Journal of Adolescent Health, 58*(5), 543–550. https://doi.org/10.1016/j.jadohealth.2016.01.003

Csikszentmihalyi, M. (1990). *Flow: The psychology of optimal experience.* Harper and Row.

Datu, J. A. D., & Park, N. (2019). Perceived school kindness and academic engagement: The mediational roles of achievement goal orientations. *School Psychology International, 40*(5), 456–473. https://doi.org/10.1177/0143034319854474

Demerouti, E., Bakker, A. B., De Jonge, J., Janssen, P. P., & Schaufeli, W. B. (2001). Burnout and engagement at work as a function of demands and control. *Scandinavian Journal of Work, Environment & Health, 27*(4), 279–286.

Duineveld, J. J., Parker, P. D., Ryan, R. M., Ciarrochi, J., & Salmela-Aro, K. (2017). The link between perceived maternal and paternal autonomy support and adolescent well-being across three major educational transitions. *Developmental Psychology, 53*(10), 1978–1994. https://doi.org/10.1037/dev0000364

Eccles, J. S., & Roeser, R. W. (2009). Schools, academic motivation, and stage-environment fit. In R. M. Lerner & L. Steinberg (Eds.), *Handbook of adolescent psychology.* Wiley. https://doi.org/10.1002/9780470479193.adlpsy001013

Eccles, J. S., & Roeser, R. W. (2011). Schools as developmental contexts during adolescence. *Journal of Research on Adolescence, 21*(1), 225–241. https://doi.org/10.1111/j.1532-7795.2010.00725.x

Forster, M., Gower, A. L., Gloppen, K., Sieving, R., Oliphant, J., Plowman, S., Gadea, A., & McMorris, B. J. (2019). Associations between dimensions of school engagement and bullying victimization and perpetration among middle school students. *School Mental Health, 12*(2), 296–307. https://doi.org/10.1007/s12310-019-09350-0

Fredricks, J. A., Blumenfeld, P. C., & Paris, A. H. (2004). School engagement: Potential of the concept, state of the evidence. *Review of Educational Research, 74*(1), 59–109. https://doi.org/10.3102/00346543074001059

Furrer, C., & Skinner, E. (2003). Sense of relatedness as a factor in children's academic engagement and performance. *Journal of Educational Psychology, 95*(1), 148–162. https://doi.org/10.1037/0022-0663.95.1.148

Guo, J., Tang, X., Marsh, H., Parker, P., Basarkod, G., Baljinder, S., Ranta, M. & Salmela-Aro, K. (2022). The roles of social–emotional skills in students' academic and life success: A multi-informant and multicohort perspective. *Journal of Personality and Social Psychology.* http://dx.doi.org/10.1037/pspp0000426

Heffner, A. L., & Antaramian, S. P. (2016). The role of life satisfaction in predicting student engagement and achievement. *Journal of Happiness Studies, 17*(4), 1681–1701. https://doi.org/10.1007/s10902-015-9665-1

Henry, K. L., Knight, K. E., & Thornberry, T. P. (2012). School disengagement as a predictor of dropout, delinquency, and problem substance use during adolescence and early adulthood. *Journal of Youth and Adolescence, 41*(2), 156–166. https://doi.org/10.1007/s10964-011-9665-3

Herrero Romero, R., Hall, J., & Cluver, L. (2019). Exposure to violence, teacher support, and school delay amongst adolescents in South Africa. *British Journal of Educational Psychology, 89*(1), 1–21. https://doi.org/10.1111/bjep.12212

Herrmann, J., Koeppen, K., & Kessels, U. (2019). Do girls take school too seriously? Investigating gender differences in school burnout from a self-worth perspective. *Learning and Individual Differences, 69*, 150–161. https://doi.org/10.1016/j.lindif.2018.11.011

Hobfoll, S. E. (2001). The influence of culture, community, and the nested-self in the stress process: Advancing conservation of resources theory. *Applied Psychology, 50*(3), 337–421. https://doi.org/10.1111/1464-0597.00062

Hobfoll, S. E., Halbesleben, J., Neveu, J.-P., & Westman, M. (2018). Conservation of resources in the organizational context: The reality of resources and their consequences. *Annual Review of Organizational Psychology and Organizational Behavior, 5*(1), 103–128. https://doi.org/10.1146/annurev-orgpsych-032117-104640

Hospel, V., & Galand, B. (2016). Are both classroom autonomy support and structure equally important for students' engagement? A multilevel analysis. *Learning and Instruction, 41*, 1–10. https://doi.org/10.1016/j.learninstruc.2015.09.001

Howard-Jones, P., Ioannou, K., Bailey, R., Prior, J., Yau, S. H., & Jay, T. (2018). Applying the science of learning in the classroom. *Impact: Journal of the Chartered College of Teaching, 18*(19). https://impact.chartered.college/article/howard-jones-applying-science-learning-classroom/

Hughes, J. N., & Cao, Q. (2018). Trajectories of teacher-student warmth and conflict at the transition to middle school: Effects on academic engagement and achievement. *Journal of School Psychology, 67*, 148–162. https://doi.org/10.1016/j.jsp.2017.10.003

Im, M. H., Hughes, J. N., & West, S. G. (2016). Effect of trajectories of friends' and parents' school involvement on adolescents' engagement and achievement.

Journal of Research on Adolescence, 26(4), 963–978. https://doi.org/10.1111/jora.12247

Inkinen, J., Klager, C., Schneider, B., Juuti, K., Krajcik, J., Lavonen, J., & Salmela-Aro, K. (2019). Science classroom activities and student situational engagement. *International Journal of Science Education, 41*(3), 316–329. https://doi.org/10.1080/09500693.2018.1549372

Jang, H., Reeve, J., & Deci, E. L. (2010). Engaging students in learning activities: It is not autonomy support or structure but autonomy support and structure. *Journal of Educational Psychology, 102*(3), 588–600. https://doi.org/10.1037/a0019682

Junker, N. M., Kaluza, A. J., Häusser, J. A., Mojzisch, A., Dick, R., Knoll, M., & Demerouti, E. (2021). Is work engagement exhausting? The longitudinal relationship between work engagement and exhaustion using Latent Growth Modeling. *Applied Psychology, 70*(2), 788–815. https://doi.org/10.1111/apps.12252

Kankaraš, M., Drasgow, F., & Chernyshenko, O. S. (2019). Social and emotional skills for student success and well-being. *OECD Education Working Papers, 173*(January), 1–134.

Keller, M. M., Goetz, T., Becker, E. S., Morger, V., & Hensley, L. (2014). Feeling and showing: A new conceptualization of dispositional teacher enthusiasm and its relation to students' interest. *Learning and Instruction, 33*, 29–38. https://doi.org/10.1016/j.learninstruc.2014.03.001

Kindermann, T. A. (2016). Peer group influences on students' academic motivation. In *Handbook of social influences in school contexts: Social-emotional, motivation, and cognitive outcomes.* https://doi.org/10.4324/9781315769929

King, R. B. (2015). Sense of relatedness boosts engagement, achievement, and well-being: A latent growth model study. *Contemporary Educational Psychology, 42*, 26–38. https://doi.org/10.1016/j.cedpsych.2015.04.002

Kiuru, N., Wang, M.-T., Salmela-Aro, K., Kannas, L., Ahonen, T., & Hirvonen, R. (2020). Associations between adolescents' interpersonal relationships, school well-being, and academic achievement during educational transitions. *Journal of Youth and Adolescence, 49*(5), 1057–1072. https://doi.org/10.1007/s10964-019-01184-y

Klusmann, U., Kunter, M., Trautwein, U., Lüdtke, O., & Baumert, J. (2008). Engagement and emotional exhaustion in teachers: Does the school context make a difference? *Applied Psychology, 57*(s1), 127–151. https://doi.org/10.1111/j.1464-0597.2008.00358.x

Lam, S., Wong, B. P. H., Yang, H., & Liu, Y. (2012). Understanding student engagement with a contextual model. In *Handbook of research on student engagement* (pp. 403–419). Springer. https://doi.org/10.1007/978-1-4614-2018-7_19

Leath, S., Mathews, C., Harrison, A., & Chavous, T. (2019). Racial identity, racial discrimination, and classroom engagement outcomes among black girls and boys in predominantly black and predominantly white school districts. *American Educational Research Journal, 56*(4), 1318–1352. https://doi.org/10.3102/0002831218816955

Lerner, R. M., Lerner, J. V., Bowers, E. P., & Geldhof, G. J. (2015). Positive youth development and relational-developmental-systems. In *Handbook of child psychology and developmental science* (pp. 1–45). Wiley. https://doi.org/10.1002/9781118963418.childpsy116

Lessard, L. M., & Juvonen, J. (2018). Losing and gaining friends: Does friendship instability compromise academic functioning in middle school? *Journal of School Psychology, 69,* 143–153. https://doi.org/10.1016/j.jsp.2018.05.003

Li, R., Yao, M., Liu, H., & Chen, Y. (2019). Chinese parental involvement and adolescent learning motivation and subjective well-being: More is not always better. *Journal of Happiness Studies, 21*(7), 2527–2555. https://doi.org/10.1007/s10902-019-00192-w

Li, Y., & Lerner, R. M. (2011). Trajectories of school engagement during adolescence: Implications for grades, depression, delinquency, and substance use. *Developmental Psychology, 47*(1), 233–247. https://doi.org/10.1037/a0021307

Li, Y., Lynch, A. D., Kalvin, C., Liu, J., & Lerner, R. M. (2011). Peer relationships as a context for the development of school engagement during early adolescence. *International Journal of Behavioral Development, 35*(4), 329–342. https://doi.org/10.1177/0165025411402578

Liu, R.-D., Zhen, R., Ding, Y., Liu, Y., Wang, J., Jiang, R., & Xu, L. (2018). Teacher support and math engagement: Roles of academic self-efficacy and positive emotions. *Educational Psychology, 38*(1), 3–16. https://doi.org/10.1080/01443410.2017.1359238

Luo, Y., Wang, Z., Zhang, H., & Chen, A. (2016). The influence of family socio-economic status on learning burnout in adolescents: Mediating and moderating effects. *Journal of Child and Family Studies, 25*(7), 2111–2119. https://doi.org/10.1007/s10826-016-0400-2

Madigan, D. J., & Curran, T. (2020). Does burnout affect academic achievement? A meta-analysis of over 100,000 students. *Educational Psychology Review, 33*(2), 387–405. https://doi.org/10.1007/s10648-020-09533-1

Maestrales, S., Marias Dezendorf, R., Tang, X., Salmela-Aro, K., Bartz, K., Juuti, K., Lavonen, J., Krajcik, J., & Schneider, B. (2021). U.S.and Finnish high school science engagement during the COVID-19 pandemic. *International Journal of Psychology, 57*(1), 73–86. https://doi.org/10.1002/ijop.12784

Martin, A. J., Burns, E. C., Collie, R. J., Bostwick, K. C. P., Flesken, A., & McCarthy, I. (2021). Growth goal setting in high school: A large-scale study of perceived instructional support, personal background attributes, and engagement outcomes. *Journal of Educational Psychology.* https://doi.org/10.1037/edu0000682

Martin, A. J., & Collie, R. J. (2019). Teacher–student relationships and students' engagement in high school: Does the number of negative and positive relation-ships with teachers matter? *Journal of Educational Psychology, 111*(5), 861–876. https://doi.org/10.1037/edu0000317

May, R. W., Bauer, K. N., & Fincham, F. D. (2015). School burnout: Diminished academic and cognitive performance. *Learning and Individual Differences, 42,* 126–131. https://doi.org/10.1016/j.lindif.2015.07.015

Mikami, A. Y., Ruzek, E. A., Hafen, C. A., Gregory, A., & Allen, J. P. (2017). Perceptions of relatedness with classroom peers promote adolescents' behavioral engagement and achievement in secondary school. *Journal of Youth and Adolescence, 46*(11), 2341–2354. https://doi.org/10.1007/s10964-017-0724-2

Moses, J. O., & Villodas, M. T. (2017). The potential protective role of peer relationships on school engagement in at-risk adolescents. *Journal of Youth and Adolescence, 46*(11), 2255–2272. https://doi.org/10.1007/s10964-017-0644-1

Motti-Stefanidi, F., Masten, A., & Asendorpf, J. B. (2015). School engagement trajectories of immigrant youth. *International Journal of Behavioral Development, 39*(1), 32–42. https://doi.org/10.1177/0165025414533428

Motti-Stefanidi, F., & Masten, A. S. (2013). School success and school engagement of immigrant children and adolescents. *European Psychologist, 18*(2), 126–135. https://doi.org/10.1027/1016-9040/a000139

OECD. (2021). *Beyond academic learning: First results from the survey of social and emotional skills.* OECD. https://doi.org/10.1787/92a11084-en

Park, S., Holloway, S. D., Arendtsz, A., Bempechat, J., & Li, J. (2012). What makes students engaged in learning? A time-use study of within- and between-individual predictors of emotional engagement in low-performing high schools. *Journal of Youth and Adolescence, 41*(3), 390–401. https://doi.org/10.1007/s10964-011-9738-3

Pöysä, S., Vasalampi, K., Muotka, J., Lerkkanen, M.-K., Poikkeus, A.-M., & Nurmi, J.-E. (2018). Variation in situation-specific engagement among lower secondary school students. *Learning and Instruction, 53,* 64–73. https://doi.org/10.1016/j.learninstruc.2017.07.007

Pöysä, S., Vasalampi, K., Muotka, J., Lerkkanen, M.-K., Poikkeus, A.-M., & Nurmi, J.-E. (2019). Teacher–student interaction and lower secondary school students' situational engagement. *British Journal of Educational Psychology, 89*(2), 374–392. https://doi.org/10.1111/bjep.12244

Putwain, D. W., Symes, W., & Wilkinson, H. M. (2017). Fear appeals, engagement, and examination performance: The role of challenge and threat appraisals. *British Journal of Educational Psychology, 87*(1), 16–31. https://doi.org/10.1111/bjep.12132

Quin, D., Heerde, J. A., & Toumbourou, J. W. (2018). Teacher support within an ecological model of adolescent development: Predictors of school engagement. *Journal of School Psychology, 69,* 1–15. https://doi.org/10.1016/j.jsp.2018.04.003

Raufelder, D., Hoferichter, F., Ringeisen, T., Regner, N., & Jacke, C. (2015). The perceived role of parental support and pressure in the interplay of test anxiety and school engagement among adolescents: Evidence for gender-specific relations. *Journal of Child and Family Studies, 24*(12), 3742–3756. https://doi.org/10.1007/s10826-015-0182-y

Reeve, J., & Tseng, C.-M. (2011). Agency as a fourth aspect of students' engagement during learning activities. *Contemporary Educational Psychology, 36*(4), 257–267. https://doi.org/10.1016/j.cedpsych.2011.05.002

Reschly, A. L., & Christenson, S. L. (2019). The intersection of student engagement and families: A critical connection for achievement and life outcomes. In *Handbook of student engagement interventions* (pp. 57–71). Elsevier. https://doi.org/10.1016/B978-0-12-813413-9.00005-X

Reyes, M. R., Brackett, M. A., Rivers, S. E., White, M., & Salovey, P. (2012). Classroom emotional climate, student engagement, and academic achievement. *Journal of Educational Psychology, 104*(3), 700–712. https://doi.org/10.1037/a0027268

Rimpelä, A., Kinnunen, J. M., Lindfors, P., Soto, V. E., Salmela-Aro, K., Perelman, J., Federico, B., & Lorant, V. (2020). Academic well-being and structural characteristics of peer networks in school. *International Journal of Environmental Research and Public Health, 17*(8), 2848. https://doi.org/10.3390/ijerph17082848

Romano, L., Tang, X., Hietajärvi, L., Salmela-Aro, K., & Fiorilli, C. (2020). Students' trait emotional intelligence and perceived teacher emotional support in preventing burnout: The moderating role of academic anxiety. *International Journal of Environmental Research and Public Health, 17*(13), 4771. https://doi.org/10.3390/ijerph17134771

Roorda, D. L., Jak, S., Zee, M., Oort, F. J., & Koomen, H. M. Y. (2017). Affective teacher–student relationships and students' engagement and achievement: A meta-analytic update and test of the mediating role of engagement. *School Psychology Review, 46*(3), 239–261. https://doi.org/10.17105/SPR-2017-0035.V46-3

Salmela-Aro, K. (2009). Personal goals and well-being during critical life transitions: The four C's—Channelling, choice, co-agency and compensation. *Advances in Life Course Research, 14*(1–2), 63–73. https://doi.org/10.1016/j.alcr.2009.03.003

Salmela-Aro, K. (2017). Dark and bright sides of thriving – School burnout and engagement in the Finnish context. *European Journal of Developmental Psychology, 14*(3), 337–349. https://doi.org/10.1080/17405629.2016.1207517

Salmela-Aro, K., Kiuru, N., Leskinen, E., & Nurmi, J.-E. (2009). School burnout inventory (SBI). *European Journal of Psychological Assessment, 25*(1), 48–57. https://doi.org/10.1027/1015-5759.25.1.48

Salmela-Aro, K., Moeller, J., Schneider, B., Spicer, J., & Lavonen, J. (2016). Integrating the light and dark sides of student engagement using person-oriented and situation-specific approaches. *Learning and Instruction, 43*, 61–70. https://doi.org/10.1016/j.learninstruc.2016.01.001

Salmela-Aro, K., Read, S., Minkkinen, J., Kinnunen, J. M., & Rimpelä, A. (2018). Immigrant status, gender, and school burnout in Finnish lower secondary school students. *International Journal of Behavioral Development, 42*(2), 225–236. https://doi.org/10.1177/0165025417690264

Salmela-Aro, K., Tang, X., Symonds, J., & Upadyaya, K. (2021a). Student engagement in adolescence: A scoping review of longitudinal studies 2010–20. *Journal of Research on Adolescence, 31*(2), 256–272. https://doi.org/10.1111/jora.12619

Salmela-Aro, K., & Tynkkynen, L. (2012). Gendered pathways in school burnout among adolescents. *Journal of Adolescence, 35*(4), 929–939. https://doi.org/10.1016/j.adolescence.2012.01.001

Salmela-Aro, K., & Upadyaya, K. (2012). The schoolwork engagement inventory. *European Journal of Psychological Assessment, 28*(1), 60–67. https://doi.org/10.1027/1015-5759/a000091

Salmela-Aro, K., & Upadyaya, K. (2014). School burnout and engagement in the context of demands-resources model. *British Journal of Educational Psychology, 84*(1), 137–151. https://doi.org/10.1111/bjep.12018

Salmela-Aro, K., & Upadyaya, K. (2020). School engagement and school burnout profiles during high school – The role of socio-emotional skills. *European Journal of Developmental Psychology, 17*(6), 1–22. https://doi.org/10.1080/17405629.2020.1785860

Salmela-Aro, K., Upadyaya, K., Hakkarainen, K., Lonka, K., & Alho, K. (2017). The dark side of internet use: Two longitudinal studies of excessive internet use, depressive symptoms, school burnout and engagement among Finnish early and late adolescents. *Journal of Youth and Adolescence, 46*(2), 343–357. https://doi.org/10.1007/s10964-016-0494-2

Salmela-Aro, K., Upadyaya, K., Vinni-Laakso, J., & Hietajärvi, L. (2021b). Adolescents' longitudinal school engagement and burnout before and during COVID-19—The role of socio-emotional skills. *Journal of Research on Adolescence, 31*(3), 796–807. https://doi.org/10.1111/jora.12654

Schaufeli, W. B., Martínez, I. M., Pinto, A. M., Salanova, M., & Bakker, A. B. (2002). Burnout and engagement in university students. *Journal of Cross-Cultural Psychology, 33*(5), 464–481. https://doi.org/10.1177/0022022102033005003

Schmidt, J. A., Rosenberg, J. M., & Beymer, P. N. (2018). A person-in-context approach to student engagement in science: Examining learning activities and choice. *Journal of Research in Science Teaching, 55*(1), 19–43. https://doi.org/10.1002/tea.21409

Schunk, D. H., & Zimmerman, B. J. (2012). In D. H. Schunk & B. J. Zimmerman (Eds.), *Motivation and self-regulated learning*. Routledge. https://doi.org/10.4324/9780203831076

Schwartz, D., Kelly, B. M., Mali, L. V., & Duong, M. T. (2016). Exposure to violence in the community predicts friendships with academically disengaged peers during middle adolescence. *Journal of Youth and Adolescence, 45*(9), 1786–1799. https://doi.org/10.1007/s10964-016-0485-3

Seo, D.-C., & Huang, Y. (2012). Systematic review of social network analysis in adolescent cigarette smoking behavior. *Journal of School Health, 82*(1), 21–27. https://doi.org/10.1111/j.1746-1561.2011.00663.x

Shernoff, D. J., Kelly, S., Tonks, S. M., Anderson, B., Cavanagh, R. F., Sinha, S., & Abdi, B. (2016). Student engagement as a function of environmental complexity in high school classrooms. *Learning and Instruction, 43*, 52–60. https://doi.org/10.1016/j.learninstruc.2015.12.003

Simpkins, S. D., Liu, Y., Hsieh, T.-Y., & Estrella, G. (2020). Supporting Latino high school students' science motivational beliefs and engagement: Examining the unique and collective contributions of family, teachers, and friends. *Educational Psychology, 40*(4), 409–429. https://doi.org/10.1080/01443410.2019.1661974

Sinatra, G. M., Heddy, B. C., & Lombardi, D. (2015). The challenges of defining and measuring student engagement in science. *Educational Psychologist, 50*(1), 1–13. https://doi.org/10.1080/00461520.2014.1002924

Skinner, E. A., & Pitzer, J. R. (2012). Developmental dynamics of student engagement, coping, and everyday resilience. In *Handbook of research on student engagement* (pp. 21–44). Springer. https://doi.org/10.1007/978-1-4614-2018-7_2

Stiles, A. A., & Gudiño, O. G. (2018). Examining bidirectional associations between school engagement and mental health for youth in child welfare. *School Mental Health, 10*(4), 372–385. https://doi.org/10.1007/s12310-018-9248-5

Storlie, C. A., & Toomey, R. B. (2020). Facets of career development in a new immigrant destination: Exploring the associations among school climate, belief in self, school engagement, and academic achievement. *Journal of Career Development, 47*(1), 44–58. https://doi.org/10.1177/0894845319828541

Strati, A. D., Schmidt, J. A., & Maier, K. S. (2017). Perceived challenge, teacher support, and teacher obstruction as predictors of student engagement. *Journal of Educational Psychology, 109*(1), 131–147. https://doi.org/10.1037/edu0000108

Sun, Y., Liu, R.-D., Oei, T.-P., Zhen, R., Ding, Y., & Jiang, R. (2020). Perceived parental warmth and adolescents' math engagement in China: The mediating roles of need satisfaction and math self-efficacy. *Learning and Individual Differences, 78*, 101837. https://doi.org/10.1016/j.lindif.2020.101837

Tang, X., Upadyaya, K., & Salmela-Aro, K. (2021). School burnout and psychosocial problems among adolescents: Grit as a resilience factor. *Journal of Adolescence, 86*, 77–89. https://doi.org/10.1016/j.adolescence.2020.12.002

Tang, X., Wang, M.-T., Guo, J., & Salmela-Aro, K. (2019). Building grit: The longitudinal pathways between mindset, commitment, grit, and academic outcomes.

Journal of Youth and Adolescence, 48(5), 850–863. https://doi.org/10.1007/s10964-019-00998-0

Totura, C. M. W., Karver, M. S., & Gesten, E. L. (2014). Psychological distress and student engagement as mediators of the relationship between peer victimization and achievement in middle school youth. *Journal of Youth and Adolescence, 43*(1), 40–52. https://doi.org/10.1007/s10964-013-9918-4

Tuominen, H., Niemivirta, M., Lonka, K., & Salmela-Aro, K. (2020). Motivation across a transition: Changes in achievement goal orientations and academic well-being from elementary to secondary school. *Learning and Individual Differences, 79*, 101854. https://doi.org/10.1016/j.lindif.2020.101854

Tuominen-Soini, H., & Salmela-Aro, K. (2014). Schoolwork engagement and burnout among Finnish high school students and young adults: Profiles, progressions, and educational outcomes. *Developmental Psychology, 50*(3), 649–662. https://doi.org/10.1037/a0033898

Tuovinen, S., Tang, X., & Salmela-Aro, K. (2020). Introversion and social engagement: Scale validation, their interaction, and positive association with self-esteem. *Frontiers in Psychology, 11*, 3241. https://doi.org/10.3389/fpsyg.2020.590748

Upadyaya, K., & Salmela-Aro, K. (2013a). Development of school engagement in association with academic success and well-being in varying social contexts: A review of empirical research. *European Psychologist, 18*(2), 136–147. https://doi.org/10.1027/1016-9040/a000143

Upadyaya, K., & Salmela-Aro, K. (2013b). Engagement with studies and work. *Emerging Adulthood, 1*(4), 247–257. https://doi.org/10.1177/2167696813484299

Upadyaya, K., & Salmela-Aro, K. (2015). Development of early vocational behavior: Parallel associations between career engagement and satisfaction. *Journal of Vocational Behavior, 90*, 66–74. https://doi.org/10.1016/j.jvb.2015.07.008

Vasalampi, K., Kiuru, N., & Salmela-Aro, K. (2018). The role of a supportive interpersonal environment and education-related goal motivation during the transition beyond upper secondary education. *Contemporary Educational Psychology, 55*, 110–119. https://doi.org/10.1016/j.cedpsych.2018.09.001

Verkuyten, M., Thijs, J., & Gharaei, N. (2019). Discrimination and academic (dis)engagement of ethnic-racial minority students: A social identity threat perspective. *Social Psychology of Education, 22*(2), 267–290. https://doi.org/10.1007/s11218-018-09476-0

Walburg, V. (2014). Burnout among high school students: A literature review. *Children and Youth Services Review, 42*, 28–33. https://doi.org/10.1016/j.childyouth.2014.03.020

Wang, M., Deng, X., & Du, X. (2018b). Harsh parenting and academic achievement in Chinese adolescents: Potential mediating roles of effortful control and classroom engagement. *Journal of School Psychology, 67*, 16–30. https://doi.org/10.1016/j.jsp.2017.09.002

Wang, M.-T., Chow, A., Hofkens, T., & Salmela-Aro, K. (2015). The trajectories of student emotional engagement and school burnout with academic and psychological development: Findings from Finnish adolescents. *Learning and Instruction, 36*, 57–65. https://doi.org/10.1016/j.learninstruc.2014.11.004

Wang, M.-T., Degol, J. L., & Henry, D. A. (2019a). An integrative development-in-sociocultural-context model for children's engagement in learning. *American Psychologist, 74*(9), 1086–1102. https://doi.org/10.1037/amp0000522

Wang, M.-T., & Eccles, J. S. (2012). Social support matters: Longitudinal effects of social support on three dimensions of school engagement from middle to high school. *Child Development, 83*(3), 877–895. https://doi.org/10.1111/j.1467-8624.2012.01745.x

Wang, M.-T., Fredricks, J., Ye, F., Hofkens, T., & Linn, J. S. (2019b). Conceptualization and assessment of adolescents' engagement and disengagement in school. *European Journal of Psychological Assessment, 35*(4), 592–606. https://doi.org/10.1027/1015-5759/a000431

Wang, M.-T., & Hofkens, T. L. (2019). Beyond classroom academics: A school-wide and multi-contextual perspective on student engagement in school. *Adolescent Research Review, 5*(4), 419–433. https://doi.org/10.1007/s40894-019-00115-z

Wang, M.-T., & Huguley, J. P. (2012). Parental racial socialization as a moderator of the effects of racial discrimination on educational success among African American adolescents. *Child Development, 83*(5), 1716–1731. https://doi.org/10.1111/j.1467-8624.2012.01808.x

Wang, M.-T., Kiuru, N., Degol, J. L., & Salmela-Aro, K. (2018a). Friends, academic achievement, and school engagement during adolescence: A social network approach to peer influence and selection effects. *Learning and Instruction, 58*, 148–160. https://doi.org/10.1016/j.learninstruc.2018.06.003

Wilder, S. (2014). Effects of parental involvement on academic achievement: A meta-synthesis. *Educational Review, 66*(3), 377–397. https://doi.org/10.1080/00131911.2013.780009

Wong, Z. Y., & Liem, G. A. D. (2021). Student engagement: Current state of the construct, conceptual refinement, and future research directions. *Educational Psychology Review, 2021*, 1–32. https://doi.org/10.1007/s10648-021-09628-3

Yang, C., Sharkey, J. D., Reed, L. A., Chen, C., & Dowdy, E. (2018). Bullying victimization and student engagement in elementary, middle, and high schools: Moderating role of school climate. *School Psychology Quarterly, 33*(1), 54–64. https://doi.org/10.1037/spq0000250

Yang, H., & Chen, J. (2016). Learning perfectionism and learning burnout in a primary school student sample: A test of a learning-stress mediation model. *Journal of Child and Family Studies, 25*(1), 345–353. https://doi.org/10.1007/s10826-015-0213-8

Zendarski, N., Sciberras, E., Mensah, F., & Hiscock, H. (2017). Early high school engagement in students with attention/deficit hyperactivity disorder. *British Journal of Educational Psychology, 87*(2), 127–145. https://doi.org/10.1111/bjep.12140

Zhang, X., Pomerantz, E. M., Qin, L., Logis, H., Ryan, A. M., & Wang, M. (2019). Early adolescent social status and academic engagement: Selection and influence processes in the United States and China. *Journal of Educational Psychology, 111*(7), 1300–1316. https://doi.org/10.1037/edu0000333

Agentic Engagement

Johnmarshall Reeve and Hyungshim Jang

Abstract

Agentic engagement is one type of engagement, but it may be the most important type for students of the twenty-first century. Agentic engagement is what students say and do to create a more supportive learning environment for themselves (e.g., offer their input, express a preference, find interesting things to do). Through their agency and initiative, students personalize and upgrade the quality of their surrounding learning environment. This upgrade (e.g., teachers become more supportive, activities become more interesting, resources surface) catalyzes students' motivational satisfactions, positive development, and academic progress. Given these benefits, we consider the possible design and implementation of student-focused agentic engagement interventions. We outline what a possible intervention might look like, and we offer our recommendations for how to design and implement such future intervention work.

J. Reeve (✉)
Institute for Positive Psychology and Education,
Australian Catholic University, Sydney, NSW,
Australia
e-mail: johnmarshall.reeve@acu.edu.au

H. Jang
Department of Education, Hanyang University, Seoul,
South Korea
e-mail: janghs@hanyang.edu.kr

To be truly educated means to be in a position to inquire and create on the basis of the resources available to you, to know where to look, to know how to formulate serious questions, to question standard doctrine, to find your own way, to shape the questions that are worth pursuing, and to develop the path to pursue them.

That means knowing and understanding many things, but also much more importantly than what you have stored in your mind, to know where to look, how to look, how to question, how to challenge, how to proceed independently to deal with the challenges that the world presents to you and that you develop in the course of your self-education and inquiry and investigations in cooperation and in solidarity with others—that's what an educational system should cultivate from kindergarten to graduate school.

– Noam Chomsky

For 100 years—from Dewey to Bloom—educators have contrasted two visions for an educational system. The traditional system is curricular- and teacher-centric in which an expert presents information for students to digest, while a progressive system encourages students to question everything and think through things for themselves. To date, engagement scholars have nicely explained how to promote student engagement within a traditional system. Essentially, the teacher presents a valued learning activity and then encourages students to behaviorally, emotionally, and cognitively engage in that activity. Then, through their effort (behavioral engagement), interest (emotional engagement), and deep information processing (cognitive engagement), students profit from that learning experience (e.g., they learn, develop skill, improve their performance). However, engagement scholars have not yet explained how to promote student engagement within a progressive system.

This is a major omission, as the engagement literature too much treats students as recipients of education and less as agents who, in the words of Chomsky, know how "to inquire and create on the basis of the resources available to you, to know where to look, to know how to formulate serious questions, to question standard doctrine, to find your own way, to shape the questions that are worth pursuing, and to develop the path to pursue them." In this chapter, we turn our attention toward twenty-first century youth and twenty-first century instruction to help educators appreciate agentic engagement and understand how to catalyze and support it.

Before turning to student engagement in the twenty-first century, it is helpful to pause and assess where we see the engagement research literature today. In the first edition of this *Handbook* (Christenson et al., 2012), we defined engagement as "the extent of student's active involvement in a learning activity" (Reeve, 2012, p. 150). We further suggested that students displayed this "active involvement" in three interconnected ways—behaviorally (effort, persistence), emotionally (interest, enjoyment), and cognitively (elaboration, critical thinking). *Behavioral engagement* refers to the observable action students take to be on-task and exerting effort. It is typically conceptualized and measured in terms of students' on-task attention, effort, and persistence (Skinner et al., 2009b). *Emotional engagement* refers to the quality of the affective connection students have with the task at hand. It is typically conceptualized and measured in terms of students' interest and enjoyment (Skinner et al., 2009a). *Cognitive engagement* refers to action taken to optimize one's thinking processes—usually to focus one's attention, understand what one is trying to learn, or to problem-solve through an obstacle. It is typically conceptualized and measured in terms of concentration, attentional control, problem-solving,

critical thinking, the use of self-regulatory strategies, and the use of sophisticated and strategic learning strategies (e.g., elaboration; Senko & Miles, 2008).

Since that publication, we expanded our thinking to focus on engagement's dark side—namely, disengagement (Jang et al., 2016). Like others (Skinner et al., 2009b), we conceptualized engagement and disengagement as two distinct classroom phenomena with behavioral disengagement reflecting doing just enough to get by (but no more), emotional disengagement reflecting task-rejecting emotions such as boredom and discouragement, and cognitive disengagement capturing mental disorganization (e.g., "I don't know what to study or where to start" (Elliot et al., 1999, p. 563). This dual-process model is warranted because engagement best predicts students' extent of academic flourishing (e.g., learning, performance, skill development), while disengagement best predicts students' extent of academic floundering (e.g., absenteeism, dropout, defiance; Jang et al., 2016).

Today, students not only react to the learning activities their teachers and textbooks provide with varying levels of behavioral, emotional, and cognitive engagement and disengagement. Students of the twenty-first century are much more likely to proact—to create, enrich, and pursue their own learning goals and their own learning activities. Learning and developing in the twenty-first century take place in the age of information. Students still have their teachers and textbooks, but they further seek out information and resources of their own (e.g., Duolingo app), as well as their own teachers and role models (e.g., YouTube videos). The twenty-first century is not only the age of information; it is the age of agency. Empowered with a sense of agency, students identify for themselves what matters, they explore and influence the world around them, and they become authors of their own learning, development, and life. Because of this, we suggest that engagement researchers need to expand and extend their existing conceptualization of engagement and disengagement as rooted not just in behavior, emotion, and cognition but also in agency.

Agent, Agency, and Agentic Engagement

An *agent* is someone who takes action to improve his or her circumstances and surroundings (Bandura, 2006, 2018). An agent initiates a causal, intentional change in the surrounding environment. In the context of education, an agent is someone who takes action to improve their learning conditions.

Agency is motivation—the motivation to intentionally influence and produce desired effects on the environment. Agency as motivation includes desire, intention, and a sense of purpose to produce intentional and strategic changes in the environment. This motivation is multisourced, as it arises from the students' self-efficacy beliefs, psychological needs (autonomy, competence, and relatedness), intrinsic motivation, personal goals, and personal growth strivings (Reeve & Shin, 2020). For a student, agency means wanting and desiring to go beyond just passively receiving the instruction one is exposed to and, instead, contributing constructively into that instruction to improve it in some important way, such as by rendering it more interesting and more personally relevant. Agency motivation fuels agentic engagement.

Agentic engagement is action and behavior. Agentic engagement represents all those behaviors the student initiates to change their circumstances for the better (Reeve, 2013). Formally defined, agentic engagement is the student's constructive contribution into the flow of instruction they receive; it is what students say and do to create a more motivationally supportive learning environment for themselves (Matos et al., 2018; Reeve, 2013). Less formally, it is simply what students say and do from one moment to the next to improve their learning conditions. Its opposite is passivity (or "agentic disengagement"; Reeve et al., 2020b). The passive student simply receives and accepts "as is" whatever instruction, activities, resources, assigned goals, learning opportunities, learning partners, mentors, events, and circumstances happen to come his or her way. In contrast, the agentically engaged learner is full of personal initiative (agency motivation) and action

(agentic engagement) to optimize those same learning conditions—or to make sure that better conditions come his or her way.

Agentic engagement (one type of engagement) is the proactive, reciprocal, and educationally constructive action students initiate to catalyze their own learning and personal development (Bandura, 2006; Reeve, 2013). It is *proactive* in the sense the student takes action before, and during, a learning experience begins (e.g., make a suggestion, offer some input, express a preference) in the hope that the provider of the learning environment (the teacher) will adjust the lesson so that it more aligns with the student's interests and goals. The agentically engaged student speaks up to "make a difference" in the flow of instruction they receive, often by making a choice (selecting a book or YouTube video) or expressing a preference ("I'm interested in Mars! Can we talk about that?").

It is *reciprocal* in that the student seeks a pattern of teacher–student interaction in which the student's input and suggestions affect and transform what the teacher says, does, and provides (Fitzpatrick et al., 2018), just as what the teacher says and does affects and transforms what the student says and does (Sameroff, 2009). The agentically engaged student sees the teacher as an interpersonal resource and source of support to create highly favorable and motivationally supportive learning conditions.

It is educationally *constructive* in that the purpose of agentic engagement is to make academic progress (e.g., learn, develop skill, improve performance; Reeve, 2013; Reeve et al., 2020a; Reeve & Tseng, 2011). If the student's input, suggestions, and preferences are off topic (i.e., not constructive toward academic progress), then such activity is something other than agentic engagement (e.g., distraction, avoidance, complaining, disruption, entertainment, defiance).

To communicate the essence of agentic engagement and disengagement, Table 1 provides the five items to assess agentic engagement and the five items to assess agentic disengagement from the Agentic Engagement Questionnaire (AEQ; Jang et al., 2016; Reeve, 2013). When the AEQ has been used in classroom-based research

Table 1 The 10-item, 2-scale Agentic Engagement Questionnaire (AEQ)

AEQ

Instructions. Please respond to each of the following statements by indicating the degree to which you agree or disagree with the statement as it applies to your experience in this particular class.

	Strongly disagree			Agree and disagree equally			Strongly agree
Agentic engagement items							
1. I let my teacher know what I need and want.	1	2	3	4	5	6	7
2. I let my teacher know what I am interested in.	1	2	3	4	5	6	7
3. During this class, I express my preferences and opinions.	1	2	3	4	5	6	7
4. During class, I ask questions to help me learn.	1	2	3	4	5	6	7
5. When I need something in this class, I'll ask the teacher for it.	1	2	3	4	5	6	7
Agentic disengagement items							
1. Most of the time in this class, I am passive.	1	2	3	4	5	6	7
2. Most of the time in this class, I am silent and unresponsive.	1	2	3	4	5	6	7
3. During this class, I hide from the teacher what I am thinking about.	1	2	3	4	5	6	7
4. In this class, I avoid asking any questions.	1	2	3	4	5	6	7
5. In this class, I do only what I am told to do—nothing more.	1	2	3	4	5	6	7

Table 2 Illustrative examples of students' agentic engagement

Act of agentic engagement	Illustrative student quotation
Let the teacher know what you want.	"I want to learn about life on Mars."
Let the teacher know what you are interested in.	"Creativity—I am interested in creativity."
Express a preference.	"Reading Shakespeare is nice, but I would prefer to watch the movie version. May we do that?"
Offer input.	"Could we practice this language in a real setting, and not just memorize note cards?"
Make a suggestion.	"A trip to the computer lab would be helpful; could we do that?"
Make a recommendation.	"Can we start with a demonstration?"
Ask for a say in what to do and how to do it.	"May we work with a partner?"
Generate options.	"I would like to add a drawing to my essay; may I do that?"
Ask "why?" questions.	"Why do we need to wear these safety goggles?"
Ask a question to help you learn.	"I don't get it; why is the periodic table arranged in these columns and rows?"
Ask for support and guidance.	"Could you show me how to do this?" "Could you give an example?"
Ask the teacher for needed resources.	"Could we have a little more time?"
Recommend a goal to pursue.	"I want to learn all 12 cranial nerves."
Personalize the learning experience.	"Learning about the economy is interesting. Can I do a special project on the stock market?"
Communicate likes and dislikes.	"What I like most about painting is mixing the olors."

(most often with Korean adolescents), it has shown strong psychometric properties (internal consistency [αs > 0.80], discriminant validity vs. measures of behavioral, emotional, and cognitive engagement), and a reliable capacity to predict important student outcomes (e.g., achievement, teacher-provided autonomy support; Jang et al., 2016; Reeve et al., 2020a). In addition, Table 2 provides 15 specific examples of what agentically engaged K-12 students say and do during classroom instruction. Each example is paired with an illustrative student quotation (adapted from Reeve & Shin, 2020).

Essentially, what agentically engaged students do in a classroom setting is speak up to give voice to their interests, preferences, priorities, and goals. They do this not only to change their learning conditions for the better but also to "take ownership over their own learning" (Mynard & Shelton-Strong, 2022). What this looks like outside of the classroom (e.g., trying to learn a foreign language on one's own) involves selecting a preferred environment, finding peers with similar interests and goals, securing helpful resources, setting and pursuing intrinsic goals, choosing which activities and materials to spend time with, exploring one's surroundings for new opportunities, asking competent others for guidance and support, finding expert role models to observe and emulate, developing personal standards of what constitutes progress, finding new technologies, prioritizing one's time to do one thing rather than another, and basically taking ownership over one's own learning and developing.

Agentic Engagement Within the Larger Engagement Framework

Engagement has a special place in educational practice because of its close predictive relation to important educational outcomes, such as achievement and graduation (Abbott-Chapman et al., 2014; Ladd & Dinella, 2009). And, among the antecedent conditions that predict these important educational outcomes, engagement warrants a special status because it is a malleable, even a highly malleable, predictor. For instance, when students experience a spike in their confidence or interest, a corresponding spike in engagement typically follows (Tsai et al., 2008), and when teachers more support students' autonomy and self-determination, greater engagement typically follows in kind (Patall et al., 2019). This means that engagement can rise and fall in a moment's time (i.e., highly malleable), and that it is respon-

sive to gains in motivation (e.g., efficacy, interest) and interpersonal support (e.g., autonomy support).

Behavioral, emotional, and cognitive engagement predict various indicators of academic progress, such as learning, skill, talent, grades, standardized test scores, and educational and occupational attainment (Abbott-Chapman et al., 2014; Alexander et al., 1993; Jang et al., 2016; Ladd & Dinella, 2009; Skinner et al., 2016). But even after considering the contribution from these three engagement components, the further consideration of how agentically engaged the student is adds additional predictive power to these positive student outcomes (Reeve et al., 2020a; Reeve & Tseng, 2011). This is because, over the course of a semester, agentically engaged Korean adolescents (grades 7–12) take the action necessary (see Table 2) to develop their skills and achievements (Reeve, 2013; Reeve et al., 2020a). Longitudinal studies with middle schoolers and high schoolers further confirm that, through their acts of agentic engagement, students find, create, or discover their own student-initiated pathway to academic progress, as Korean students (grades 7–12) who are agentically engaged at the beginning of the semester subsequently show increased end-of-semester achievement outcomes, such as course grades and course-specific skill development (Reeve et al., 2020a, 2020b)—even after controlling for how behaviorally, emotionally, and cognitively engaged they were throughout the semester.

When agentic engagement is added as a fourth dimension, the explanatory capacity of engagement to predict important educational outcomes increases (Patall et al., 2019; Reeve, 2013; Reeve et al., 2020a, 2020b); Reeve & Tseng, 2011). For instance, in two longitudinally designed classroom-based studies, secondary-grade Korean students self-reported their course-specific behavioral, emotional, cognitive, and agentic engagement, and these scores were used to predict their objectively scored course achievement (i.e., grades; Study 1) and end-of-semester gains in perceived academic progress (Study 2). In both studies, after accounting for the positive effects of students' behavioral, emotional, and cognitive engagement, students' agentic engagement was able to predict and explain a significantly higher proportion of the variance in these two student outcomes (F-change and R^2 change, $p < 0.001$; Reeve et al., 2020a, 2020b)). So, agentic engagement adds explanatory power to the traditional three-component notion of engagement.

To illustrate the (a) additive and (b) unique role of agentic engagement in the larger engagement construct, we provide Fig. 1, which is based on Skinner's (2016) "Context ➔ Self ➔ Action ➔ Outcomes" self-system model. The "a" path shows engagement's capacity to catalyze various indicators of academic progress. But the figure adds an important new element to this "Social context ➔ Motivation ➔ Engagement ➔ Achievement" model—namely, agentic engagement. Agentic engagement is more important than "just another dimension of engagement." Unlike behavioral, emotional, and cognitive engagement, agentic engagement catalyzes two additional important educational processes. These two additional effects (discussed next) are that agentically engaged students recruit a more supportive learning environment for themselves (path "b") and experienced greater motivational satisfactions (path "c").

Agentic Engagement Produces a More Supportive Learning Environment (Path "b" in Fig. 1)

The more agentically engaged students are, the greater longitudinal gains they report in how autonomy-supportive their teachers become (e.g., greater perspective-taking, offer students more interesting and personally relevant learning activities; Matos et al., 2018; Patall et al., 2018, 2019; Reeve, 2013; Reeve et al., 2020a). When Peruvian university students speak up to express their interests and preferences, they change how their teacher interacts with them (Matos et al., 2018). When students offer constructive input, then teachers become increasingly aware of what students want, need, and are interested in doing and therefore are better positioned to bend (i.e., adjust, calibrate) their lessons in those directions that are increasingly relevant to and supportive of their students' expressed interests, preferences, and goals. In this way, agentically engaged students become architects of their own learning environments.

In contrast, when students are quiet and passive during instruction—even if they are working hard (behaviorally), enthusiastically (emotionally), and smart (cognitively)—teachers lose an important means to come to know and appreciate what their students want, are interested in, and prefer to do (or not to do). The more silent students are, the less likely it becomes that their teachers will become autonomy-supportive toward them. Thus, among Korean middle and high school students, student passivity (i.e., agentic disengagement) begets minimal, longitudinally lesser autonomy-supportive teaching (Reeve et al., 2020b).

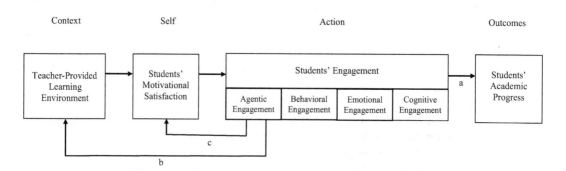

Fig. 1 Three hypothesized functions of agentic engagement: Create a supportive learning environment (path "b"); generate motivational satisfaction (path "c"); and increase effective functioning (path "a")

Agentic Engagement Produces Motivational Satisfactions (Path "c" in Fig. 1)

The more agentically engaged students are, the greater longitudinal gains they report in their course-related interest, need satisfactions (e.g., autonomy), and self-efficacy (Patall et al., 2019; Patall et al., 2022; Reeve et al., 2020a; Reeve & Lee, 2014). Agentically engaged students are more likely than their nonagentically engaged counterparts to take the action necessary to satisfy their curiosity (e.g., ask the teacher a question, search on the computer), develop their interests (e.g., volunteer for the school play, explore school resources), build their sense of competence and efficacy (e.g., search for an online video of a skilled performance), and attain their personal goals (e.g., spend their free time pursuing that personal goal; Jang et al., 2016). In this way, agentically engaged students contribute to their own motivational satisfactions.

Sitting passively, on the other hand, students do little to interact with the environment in ways that might otherwise yield interesting, need-satisfying, and efficacy-building experiences. Being quiet, silent, and passive tends to create deprivation-like conditions (motivationally speaking) in which students become susceptible to experiences of autonomy dissatisfaction (e.g., "I don't have a say in what I do," "I am not pursuing goals that are my own," "I don't feel free to be myself"; Bhavsar et al., 2020). Passive students go home at the end of the day to realize that they did little or nothing at school that was interesting or worthwhile.

Agentic disengagement does not have to be a chronic condition (i.e., it too is malleable). When teachers learn how to teach in more autonomy-supportive ways, they become increasingly able to nudge agentically disengaged students out of their classroom passivity (Reeve et al., 2020b). When agentically disengaged students (measured at the beginning of the academic year) are placed into a classroom with a highly autonomy-supportive teacher, these students become increasingly able during the academic year to create need-satisfying learning experiences for themselves. These autonomy-supportive teachers provide learning activities in autonomy-satisfying ways that awaken or vitalize their Korean secondary grade level students' need for autonomy. Once students experience autonomy satisfaction, they then begin to leave behind their passivity to instead speak up and show some personal initiative (i.e., agentic engagement; Reeve et al., 2020a, 2020b).

Implications

Recruiting greater autonomy support (path "b" in Fig. 1) and generating motivational satisfactions for oneself (path "c" in Fig. 1) are particularly important functions of agentic engagement. By recruiting support and by generating motivational satisfactions, agentically engaged students are able to create the very conditions that promote their own future (a) classroom engagement (and prevent their own future classroom disengagement) and (b) agentic engagement in particular (and prevent their own future agentic disengagement). That is, agentic engagement begets the very conditions for its future development and growth.

What We Learned About Engagement Interventions by Conducting Autonomy-Supportive Teaching Interventions

We have conducted and published 20 teacher-focused autonomy-supportive teaching interventions (for the full list, see Reeve & Cheon, 2021a, b). What we have learned from 20 years of helping K-12 teachers in several different nations improve their classroom motivating style offers some unique insights for helping students improve their classroom agentic engagement.

A teacher's motivating style includes everything the teacher says and does to motivate the students' classroom engagement. In conducting these workshop-based interventions, we help teachers develop the skill they need to support students' engagement in two core ways. The first is to offer students an *engagement invitation*. Here, we help K-12 teachers learn how to provide instruction in a way that supports students' intrinsic motivation. To do this, teachers in an experimental condition develop and refine the two instructional behaviors: "invite students to pursue their personal interests" and "present learning activities in need-satisfying ways." When teachers learn how to do this, their students report greater intrinsic motivation and show greater classroom engagement. Teachers who offer their students interesting, need-satisfying things to do, essentially provide their students with an engagement invitation (e.g., "What are you interested in? What would you like to do?").

The second is to make an *engagement request*. Here, we help K-12 teachers learn how to provide instruction in a way that supports students' internalization of teacher-valued behaviors, activities, and requirements. To do this, teachers in an experimental condition develop and refine the four instructional behaviors: "provide explanatory rationales for teacher requests" (e.g., "Doing this activity is useful because…"), "acknowledge and accept negative feelings" (e.g., "Okay, I understand…"), "rely on invitational language" (e.g., "You might want to consider this alternative…"), and "display patience" (i.e., listening and understanding, rather than directing and rushing in to solve the problem). When teachers learn how to do this, their students report greater value (internalization) for learning activities and show greater classroom engagement. Teachers who help students work through the internalization process—even during relatively uninteresting activities and requirements—essentially learn how to make an effective engagement request (e.g., "I am going to ask you to revise your essay. Why? Because…").

Greater autonomy-supportive teaching enhances students' behavioral, emotional, and cognitive engagement (Cheon et al., 2019, 2020), but it also enhances students' agentic engagement in particular (Reeve et al., 2020b). When students receive autonomy support day-after-day, agentic engagement begins to take on a life of its own, as students become fully capable of engaging themselves in classroom learning activities—by regulating their own attention and generating their own effort and persistence (behavioral engagement), by generating task-facilitating emotions such as interest and curiosity (emotional engagement), by deeply processing task- and goal-related information, as by problem-solving, mental simulations, and critical thinking (cognitive engagement), and by speaking up, showing initiative, and taking ownership over their own learning (agentic engagement; Reeve et al., 2020b). In this way, promoting student-initiated agentic engagement becomes *a third way* that K-12 teachers can support their students' classroom engagement (in addition to engagement invitations and engagement requests).

After conducting all these autonomy-supportive teaching interventions, a key insight is that it is best for teachers to focus on students' motivation, rather than on students' engagement per se. When teachers focus directly on students' engagement (e.g., "read the book, revise your paper"), two problems typically occur. First, with a direct focus on students' engagement, teachers are at risk of slipping into a counterproductive controlling motivating style (e.g., uttering directives, offering means–end incentives, displaying impatience, and focusing only on the teacher's priorities). Second, engagement is the behavioral manifestation of students' underlying motivational states. So, teachers need to focus more on the horse (motivation) and less on the cart (engagement). Moving the cart is what matters, but the cart does not move until the horse moves first. So, what we have learned after conducting all these teacher-focused interventions is that agentic engagement arises out of autonomous motivation, and autonomous motivation arises out of autonomy-supportive teaching. This suggests to us that engagement interventions probably work best by starting (intervening) on the left side of Fig. 1, rather than by directly targeting anything on the right side of Fig. 1.

Interventions

Successful student engagement interventions are surprisingly rare. There have been several successful engagement interventions published in the literature, but a close inspection of many of these interventions reveals that they typically focus on "improve the social context" (e.g., provide greater teacher, school, or family support) or "improve student motivation" (e.g., boost students' efficacy, interest, goal setting) rather than on "improve student engagement" per se (e.g., Fredricks et al., 2019). In other words, student engagement is often treated as a dependent measure, rather than as an independent variable that can be manipulated, changed, and strengthened (e.g., a cart, rather than a horse). This raises the question of the causal status of engagement. Can manipulated agentic engagement produce a causal beneficial effect? It also raises the question of what "manipulated agentic engagement" might look like in the context of an intervention study. If one were to try to intervene to change (i.e., increase, enhance) students' agentic engagement, what would one do? If one were to do this, would such an intervention work? We discuss these questions next.

Causal Status of Agentic Engagement

A prerequisite to the conduct of an intervention is an initial experimental study to confirm that manipulated agentic engagement does indeed produce causal benefits. The hope for a possible, future, student-focused agentic engagement intervention would be that, if students could be taught how to express their interests and preferences and let the teacher know what they needed, then they could become proactive, constructive "agents" (Bandura, 2006) or "origins" (deCharms, 1976) who could enrich their own learning experiences.

We conducted such an experimental investigation by randomly assigning Korean university students to receive a brief (12-min) tutorial to encourage them to display agentically engaged behaviors during an upcoming learning activity.

Compared to students randomly assigned to receive a neutral tutorial, students in the experimental group did display more agentic engagement during that learning activity, as scored by objective raters and as self-reported by the students themselves (Reeve et al., 2021). This means that greater agentic engagement can be experimentally manipulated (i.e., it is malleable). Importantly, these agentically engaged students recruited greater support from their teacher (i.e., as scored by objective raters and as self-reported by students), and they experienced greater motivational satisfactions (i.e., autonomy satisfaction, task interest). Overall, what these findings mean is that level of agentic engagement can be manipulated, and greater agentic engagement has a direct, causal effect on (a) creating a more (autonomy) supportive learning environment (path "b" in Fig. 1) and (b) boosting personal motivation (path "c" in Fig. 1).

Unfortunately, however, this brief experimental manipulation did not significantly increase these students' task performance (e.g., performance on that same task during a follow-up assessment). This means that manipulated agentic engagement did not increase path "a" in Fig. 1. This is a major limitation because much of the excitement and promise of an engagement intervention is the idea that greater engagement should boost performance/achievement. In the only other experimental manipulation of agentic engagement that we are aware of, Patall et al., (2022) conducted an experimental study in which university students in the USA were provided with an online session to teach an "agentic mindset" (i.e., think of their motivation and the teacher's motivational support as malleable and as responsive to agentic engagement strategies). The intervention did boost an agentic mindset (i.e., motivation) but it did not boost performance (i.e., grades).

Apparently, what is needed in a successful agentic engagement intervention is to help students learn *both* agency motivation and agentic engagement behaviors (i.e., the will and the way). That is, it is insufficient to teach students how to offer their input and make suggestions unless they also have the motivation (interest, efficacy, goals) to energize these behaviors in the first place. Similarly, it is insufficient to teach students agency motivation unless they also have the behavioral repertoire capable of translating that motivation into effective functioning and positive outcomes. Thus, we suggest that a successful future intervention needs to help students develop both agentically engaged behaviors and the motivation to energize it (i.e., the cart and the horse working together).

What Would Students Be Taught to Do in an Agentic Engagement Intervention?

The primary purpose of an agentic engagement intervention should be to teach students how to recruit a more supportive learning environment for themselves (path "c" in Fig. 1). That is, the essence of an agentic engagement intervention would be to encourage students to act on, improve, and negotiate with their learning environment to render its interpersonal and task-related elements more motivationally supportive.

This recommendation is rooted not only in the findings from the earlier-mentioned experimental investigation, but also in the consistent track record showing that students who receive instruction from an autonomy-supportive teacher thrive in multiple ways, including greater motivation (i.e., need satisfaction, intrinsic motivation, and internalization of school values; Reeve & Cheon, 2021a). So, even if an agentic engagement intervention "only" helped students learn how to recruit greater autonomy-supportive teaching, this benefit would also help students become motivationally enriched "agents" and "origins," because that is what greater autonomy-supportive teaching does so well (Reeve & Cheon, 2021a).

Would Such an Agentic Engagement Intervention Work?

For any engagement intervention to work (i.e., produce educationally important benefits), we suggest that engagement should not be separated from the motivation that produces it. This is true for behavioral, emotional, and cognitive engagement, and it is similarly true to agentic engagement. We suspect that agentic engagement needs to be closely aligned with and emanate out of an energizing motivational catalyst (e.g., autonomy need satisfaction, self-efficacy, or a mastery goal orientation) to yield its gains. If students experienced gains in both their agency motivation and their capacity to enact agentically engaged behaviors, then such an intervention would likely produce educational benefits. We have already seen that it is not enough to promote agentically engaged behaviors only (Reeve et al., 2021) or agentically engaged motivation only (Patall et al., 2022).

What Do We Recommend?

We suggest that a successful agentic engagement intervention requires two essential components. First, students need help in becoming agents or origins in terms of their course-related motivation. That is, to energize students' agentic engagement, students first need to build a motivation catalyst such as a personal goal to pursue, interest in the course, or an agentic mindset. Second, students need skill-based training in how to initiate agentically engaged behaviors. That is, students need modeling, guidance, scaffolding, practice, and feedback to the sort of agentic behaviors listed in Table 2. The order of these two accomplishments is probably important as well—first the horse, then the cart. Overall, we suggest a successful student-focused agentic engagement intervention needs to consist of two parts: (1) enhance students' motivation (e.g., agentic mindset, need satisfaction, self-efficacy, personal goals), and (2) provide the skill-based training students will need to translate their agency into behaviors that actually produce academic progress.

There is a possibility that a successful agentic engagement intervention needs a third critical ingredient as well—namely, exposure to an autonomy-supportive teacher. Once students learn how to act in a highly agentically engaged way, there is every reason to expect that they would successfully "pull" greater autonomy-supportive teaching out of their teacher. But it is also possible that expressions of students' classroom agentic engagement might "backfire" (as suggested by Patall et al., 2022). When teachers adopt a controlling motivating style or are resistant to students' attempts to introduce agentically engaged behaviors into the classroom, such efforts may not only *not* support such agency but may actually suppress such behaviors—thereby producing more harm than benefits. A controlling teacher might take a hardline stance to suppress such student-initiated agency. So, while we do not believe that a priori access to an autonomy-supportive teacher is necessary (because agentic engagement itself brings out greater autonomy-supportive teaching), we acknowledge that access to an autonomy-supportive teacher is helpful—an interaction partner who will accept, value, and be responsive to one's voice, initiative, and personal strivings.

The Role of Agentic Engagement in Youth Development

For every individual, development is a story waiting to be told. If youth want to be the author of their own development and life course, it serves them well to become active agents who are willing and able to agentically engage with all those environmental events that impact their development. In the classroom, such authorship comes as youth speak up, express their interests and preferences, and engineer constructive changes in the circumstances that surround them. In doing so, the environment in which one develops becomes more interesting and supportive. During that developmental journey, such agency puts the wind at one's back.

Conclusion

Academic progress does not just happen. To make progress (e.g., learn a foreign language, become a better writer), students need to leave

behind their passivity (i.e., agentic disengagement) to take on the personal initiative needed to learn and develop skill. When students show a little initiative, they become constructive causal agents in their own learning. Because this is so, educators now have a proverbial green light to create and implement student-focused agentic engagement interventions.

But just as academic progress does not just happen, neither do successful, theoretically sound, methodologically rigorous, and classroom-applicable interventions. To spark such future research, we explained why we find existing engagement interventions a bit lacking, and we provided our thoughts on the causal status of agentic engagement, what students in an agentic engagement would be taught to do, whether (and why) such an intervention would work to produce important student benefits, and, finally, what we recommend overall for the researcher who is considering the design and implementation of a future agentic engagement intervention.

References

Abbott-Chapman, J., Martin, K., Ollington, N., Venn, A., Dwyer, T., & Gall, S. (2014). The longitudinal association of childhood school engagement with adult educational and occupational achievement: Findings from an Australian national study. *British Educational Research Journal, 40*(1), 102–120. https://doi.org/10.1002/berj.3031

Alexander, K. L., Entwisle, D. R., & Dauber, S. L. (1993). First-grade classroom behavior: Its short and long-term consequences for school performance. *Child Development, 64*, 801–814. https://doi.org/10.1111/j.1467-8624.1993.tb02944.x

Bandura, A. (2006). Toward a psychology of human agency. *Perspectives on Psychological Science, 1*, 164–180.

Bandura, A. (2018). Toward a psychology of human agency: Pathways and reflections. *Perspectives on Psychological Science, 13*(2), 130–136.

Bhavsar, N., Bartholomew, K. J., Quested, E., Gucciardi, D. F., Thøgersen-Ntoumani, C., Reeve, J., Sarrazin, P., & Ntoumanis, N. (2020). Measuring psychological need states in sport: Theoretical considerations and a new measure. *Psychology of Sport and Exercise*, Article 101617.

Cheon, S. H., Reeve, J., Lee, Y., Ntoumanis, N., Gillet, N., Kim, B. R., & Song, Y.-G. (2019). Expanding autonomy psychological need states from two (satisfaction, frustration) to three (dissatisfaction): A classroom-based intervention study. *Journal of Educational Psychology, 111*(4), 685–702. https://doi.org/10.1037/edu0000306

Cheon, S. H., Reeve, J., & Vansteenkiste, M. (2020). Expanding a traditional autonomy-supportive intervention into a multiple motivating styles intervention for PE teachers: Benefits to students, benefits to teachers. *Teaching and Teacher Education.*

Christenson, S. L., Reschly, A., & Wylie, C. (Eds.). (2012). *Handbook of research on student engagement.* Springer.

deCharms, R. (1976). *Enhancing motivation: Change in the classroom.* Irvington.

Elliot, A. J., McGregor, H. A., & Gable, S. (1999). Achievement goals, study strategies, and exam performance: A mediation analysis. *Journal of Educational Psychology, 91*(3), 549–563.

Fitzpatrick, J., O'Grady, E., & O'Reilly, J. (2018). Promoting student agentic engagement through curriculum: Exploring the negotiated integrated curriculum initiative. *Irish Educational Studies, 37*(4), 453–473.

Fredricks, J. A., Christenson, S. L., & Reschly, A. L. (Eds.). (2019). *Handbook of student engagement interventions: Working with disengaged youth.* Elsevier.

Jang, H., Kim, E.-J., & Reeve, J. (2016). Why students become more engaged or more disengaged during the semester: A self-determination theory dual-process model. *Learning and Instruction, 43*, 27–38.

Ladd, G. W., & Dinella, L. M. (2009). Continuity and change in early school engagement: Predictive of children's achievement trajectories from first to eighth grade? *Journal of Educational Psychology, 101*, 190–206. https://doi.org/10.1037/a0013153

Matos, L., Reeve, J., Herrera, D., & Claux, M. (2018). Students' agentic engagement predicts longitudinal increases in perceived autonomy-supportive teaching: The squeaky wheel gets the grease. *Journal of Experimental Education, 86*(4), 592–609.

Mynard, J., & Shelton-Strong, S. (Eds.). (2022). *Autonomy support beyond the language learning classroom: A self-determination theory perspective.* Multilingual Matters.

Patall, E. A., Zambrano, J., Kennedy, A. A. U., Yates, N., & Vallin, J. A. (2022). Promoting an agentic orientation: An intervention in university psychology and physical science courses. *Journal of Educational Psychology, 114*(2), 368–392. https://doi.org/10.1037/edu0000614

Patall, E. A., Steingut, R. R., Vasquez, A. C., Trimble, S. S., Pituch, K. A., & Freeman, J. L. (2018). Daily autonomy supporting or thwarting and students' motivation and engagement in the high school science classroom. *Journal of Educational Psychology, 110*(2), 269–288.

Patall, E. A., Pituch, K. A., Steingut, R. R., Vasquez, A. C., Yates, N., & Kennedy, A. A. U. (2019). Agency and high school science students' motivation, engage-ment, and classroom experiences. *Journal of Applied Developmental Psychology, 62*(1), 77–92.

Reeve, J. (2012). A self-determination theory perspective on student engagement. In S. L. Christenson, A. Reschly, & C. Wylie (Eds.), *Handbook of research on student engagement.* (Chapter 7) (pp. 149–172). Springer.

Reeve, J. (2013). How students create motivationally supportive learning environments for themselves: The concept of agentic engagement. *Journal of Educational Psychology, 105*, 579–595.

Reeve, J., & Cheon, S. H. (2021a). Autonomy-supportive teaching: Its malleability, benefits, and potential to improve educational practice. *Educational Psychologist, 56*, 54–77.

Reeve, J., & Cheon, S. H. (2021b). Sociocultural influences on teachers' reactions to an intervention to help them become more autonomy supportive. In G. A. D. Liem & D. M. McInerney (Eds.), *Promoting motivation and learning in contexts: Sociocultural perspectives on educational interventions* (pp. 13–36). Information Age Publishing.

Reeve, J., & Lee, W. (2014). Students' classroom engagement produces longitudinal changes in classroom motivation. *Journal of Educational Psychology, 106*, 527–540.

Reeve, J., & Shin, S. H. (2020). How teachers can support students' agentic engagement. *Theory Into Practice, 59*(2), 150–161.

Reeve, J., & Tseng, C.-M. (2011). Agency as a fourth aspect of students' engagement during learning activities. *Contemporary Educational Psychology, 36*, 257–267.

Reeve, J., Cheon, S. H., & Jang, H. (2020a). How and why students make academic progress: Reconceptualizing the student engagement construct to increase its explanatory power. *Contemporary Educational Psychology*, Article 101899. https://doi.org/10.1016/j.cedpsych.2020.101899

Reeve, J., Cheon, S. H., & Yu, T. H. (2020b). An autonomy-supportive intervention to develop students' resilience by boosting agentic engagement. *International Journal of Behavioral Development, 44*(4), 325–338.

Reeve, J., Jang, H.-R., Ahn, S., Shin, S., Matos, L., & Gargurevich, R. (2021). When students show some initiative: Two experiments on the benefits of increased agentic engagement.. Manuscript under review.

Sameroff, A. (Ed.). (2009). *The transactional model of development: How children and contexts shape each other.* American Psychological Association.

Senko, C., & Miles, K. M. (2008). Pursuing their own learning agenda: How mastery-oriented students jeopardize their class performance. *Contemporary Educational Psychology, 33*, 561–583. https://doi.org/10.1016/j.cedpsych.2007.12.001

Skinner, E. A. (2016). Engagement and disaffection as central to processes of motivational resilience and development. In K. R. Wentzel & D. B. Miele (Eds.), *Handbook of motivation at school* (pp. 145–168). Routledge. (Chapter 8).

Skinner, E. A., Kindermann, T. A., Connell, J. P., & Wellborn, J. G. (2009a). Engagement as an organizational construct in the dynamics of motivational development. In K. Wentzel & A. Wigfield (Eds.), *Handbook of motivation in school* (pp. 223–245). Erlbaum.

Skinner, E. A., Kindermann, T. A., & Furrer, C. (2009b). A motivational perspective on engagement and disaffection: Conceptualization and assessment of children's behavioral and emotional participation in academic activities in the classroom. *Educational and Psychological Measurement, 69*, 493–525.

Skinner, E. A., Pitzer, J. R., & Steele, J. S. (2016). Can student engagement serve as a motivational resource for academic coping, persistence, and learning during late elementary and early middle school? *Developmental Psychology, 52*, 2099–2117. https://doi.org/10.1037/dev0000232

Tsai, Y.-M., Kunter, M., Ludtke, O., Trautwein, U., & Ryan, R. M. (2008). What makes lessons interesting? The role of situational and individual factors in three school subjects. *Journal of Educational Psychology, 100*(2), 460–472.

Academic Emotions and Student Engagement

Reinhard Pekrun and Lisa Linnenbrink-Garcia

Abstract

Emotions are ubiquitous in academic settings, and they profoundly affect students' academic engagement and performance. In this chapter, we summarize the extant research on academic emotions and their linkages with students' engagement. First, we outline relevant concepts of academic emotion, including achievement, epistemic, topic, and social emotions. Second, we discuss the impact of these emotions on students' cognitive, motivational, behavioral, cognitive-behavioral, and social-behavioral engagement, and on their academic performance. Next, we examine the origins of students' academic emotions in terms of individual and contextual variables. Finally, we highlight the complexity of students' emotions, focusing on reciprocal causation as well as regulation and treatment of these emotions. In conclusion, we discuss directions for future research, with a special emphasis on the need for educational design and intervention research targeting emotions.

R. Pekrun (✉)
University of Essex, Colchester, UK

Australian Catholic University, North Sydney, NSW, Australia
e-mail: pekrun@lmu.de

L. Linnenbrink-Garcia
Michigan State University, East Lansing, MI, USA
e-mail: llgarcia@msu.edu

Emotions are ubiquitous in academic settings. Remember the last time you studied some learning material? Depending on your goals and the contents of the material, you may have enjoyed learning or been bored, experienced flow forgetting time or been frustrated about never-ending obstacles, felt proud of your progress or ashamed of lack of accomplishment. Furthermore, these emotions affected your effort, motivation to persist, and strategies for learning—even if you were unaware of these effects. Similarly, think of the last time you took an important exam. You may have hoped for success, been afraid of failure, or felt desperate because you were unprepared, but you likely did not feel indifferent about it. Again, these emotions likely had profound effects on your motivation, concentration, and strategies used when taking the exam.

Empirical findings corroborate that students experience a wide variety of emotions when attending class, doing homework, and taking tests and exams. For example, in exploratory research on emotions experienced by university students, emotions reported frequently included enjoyment, hope, pride, anger, anxiety, frustration, and boredom in academic settings (Pekrun et al., 2002). Traditionally, these emotions did not receive much attention by researchers, except for studies on test anxiety (Zeidner, 1998) and on causal attributions of success and failure as antecedents of emotions (Weiner, 1985). During the past 25 years, however, there has been growing recognition that emotions are central to human achievement strivings. Emotions are no longer regarded as epiphenomena that may occur in academic settings but lack any instrumental relevance. Increasingly, affect and emotions are recognized as being of critical importance for students' academic learning, achievement, personality development, and health (Linnenbrink, 2006; Linnenbrink-Garcia & Pekrun, 2011; Camacho-Morles et al., 2021; Loderer et al., 2020a; Pekrun & Linnenbrink-Garcia, 2014).

In this chapter, we consider academic emotions and their functions for students' engagement. As noted by Fredricks et al. (2004), student engagement is multifaceted. In line with this view, we define student engagement as a multicomponent construct, the common denominator being that all the components (i.e., types of engagement) comprise active, energetic, approach-oriented involvement with academic tasks. We distinguish the following types of engagement: *cognitive* (attention and memory processes), *motivational* (intrinsic/extrinsic motivation, achievement goals), *behavioral-effort investment* (effort and persistence), *cognitive-behavioral* (strategy use and self-regulation), and *social-behavioral* (social on-task behavior). Given our focus on emotions as precursors to these forms of engagement, emotional engagement (e.g., enjoyment of learning) is considered as an antecedent of other components of engagement in this chapter.

These five categories of engagement overlap with the three broad categories of cognitive, behavioral, and emotional engagement traditionally considered (Fredricks et al., 2004); however, we have expanded this framework to clarify the unique ways in which emotions relate to engagement. Specifically, within Fredricks et al.'s category of cognitive engagement, we differentiate between cognitive and cognitive-behavioral engagement. Our conceptualization of behavioral engagement is similar to that proposed by Fredricks et al. However, we take a more specific view focusing on effort and persistence. Regarding the broad category of affective or emotional engagement originally proposed by Fredricks and her colleagues, we differentiate

between emotions and motivational engagement. Finally, we extend the Fredricks et al. framework to include social-behavioral engagement to better capture forms of engagement related to peer-to-peer learning.

We begin by outlining different concepts describing students' emotions, including affect, mood, achievement emotions, epistemic emotions, topic emotions, and social emotions. Next, the impact of emotions on the five types of student engagement and resulting academic achievement are addressed. In the third section, we discuss the individual and social origins of students' emotions, including a brief discussion of the relative universality of mechanisms of emotions and engagement across contexts. We conclude by considering principles of reciprocal causation of emotion and engagement and their implications for emotion regulation, treatment of emotions, and the design of learning environments.

Concepts of Academic Emotions

Emotion, Mood, and Affect

Emotions are defined as multifaceted phenomena involving sets of coordinated psychological processes, including affective, cognitive, physiological, motivational, and expressive components (Scherer & Moors, 2019). For example, a student's anxiety before an exam can be comprised of nervous, uneasy feelings (affective); worries about failing the exam (cognitive); increased heart rate or sweating (physiological); impulses to escape the situation (motivation); and an anxious facial expression (expressive). As compared to intense emotions, *moods* are of lower intensity and lack a specific referent. Different emotions and moods are often compiled in more general constructs of *affect*. In the educational literature, the term "affect" is often used to denote a broad variety of noncognitive constructs including emotion, but also including self-concept, beliefs, and motivation (e.g., Alsop & Watts, 2003). In contrast, in emotion research, "affect" refers to emotions and moods more specifically. In this research, the term is often used to denote omnibus variables of positive versus negative emotions or moods, with *positive affect* being compiled of various positive states (e.g., enjoyment, pride, satisfaction) and *negative affect* consisting of negative states (e.g., anger, anxiety, frustration).

Valence and Arousal

Two important dimensions describing emotions, moods, and affect are *valence* and *arousal*. In terms of valence, positive (i.e., pleasant) states, such as enjoyment and happiness, can be differentiated from negative (i.e., unpleasant) states, such as anger, anxiety, or boredom. In terms of arousal, physiologically activating states can be distinguished from deactivating states, such as activating excitement versus deactivating relaxation. These two dimensions are orthogonal, making it possible to organize affective states in a two-dimensional space. In *circumplex models* of affect, affective states are grouped along the dimensions of valence and arousal (e.g., Barrett & Russell, 1998; see Fig. 1). By classifying affective states as positive or negative, and as activating or deactivating, the circumplex can be transformed into a 2 × 2 taxonomy including four broad categories of emotions and moods (*positive activating:* e.g., enjoyment, hope, pride; *positive deactivating:* relief, relaxation; *negative*

activating: anger, anxiety, shame; *negative deactivating:* hopelessness, boredom; Pekrun, 2006).

Academic Emotions

In addition to valence and activation, emotions can be grouped according to their object focus (Pekrun, 2006, 2021). For explaining the psychological functions of emotions, this dimension is no less important than valence and activation. Specifically, regarding the functions of emotions for students' academic engagement, object focus is critical because it determines if emotions pertain to the academic task at hand or not. In terms of object focus, the following broad groups of emotions may be most important in the academic domain.

Achievement Emotions We define achievement emotions as emotions that relate to activities or outcomes that are judged according to competence-based standards of quality. In the academic domain, achievement emotions can relate to activities like studying or taking exams, and to the success and failure outcomes of these activities. Accordingly, two groups of achievement emotions are activity-related emotions, such as enjoyment or boredom during learning, and outcome-related emotions, such as hope and pride related to success, or anxiety and shame

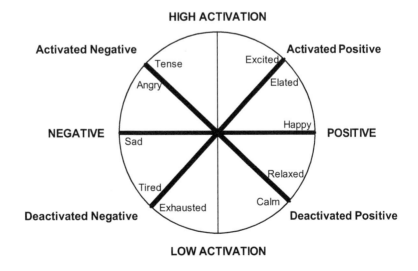

Fig. 1 Affective circumplex. (Model adapted from Barrett and Russell (1998))

related to failure. Within the latter category, an important distinction is between prospective emotions related to future success and failure, such as hope and anxiety, and retrospective emotions related to success and failure that already occurred, such as pride, shame, relief, and disappointment. Combining the valence, activation, and object focus (activity vs. outcome) dimensions renders a three-dimensional taxonomy of achievement emotions (Pekrun, 2006; see Table 1).

Epistemic Emotions Emotions related to the generation of knowledge are referred to as *epistemic*. These emotions are caused by cognitive qualities of task information, such as cognitive incongruity triggering surprise and curiosity. As suggested by Pekrun and Stephens (2012), these emotions are considered epistemic because they pertain to the epistemic aspects of learning and cognitive activities. A typical sequence of epistemic emotions induced by a cognitive problem may involve (1) surprise; (2) curiosity if the surprise is not dissolved; (3) anxiety in case of severe incongruity and information that deeply disturbs existing cognitive schemas; (4) enjoyment and delight experienced when recombining information such that the problem gets solved; or (5) frustration when this seems not possible.

Topic Emotions Emotions can be triggered by the contents covered by learning material. Examples are the empathetic emotions pertaining to a protagonist's fate when reading a novel, the emotions triggered by political events dealt with in political lessons, or the emotions related to topics in science class, such as the frustration experienced by American children when they were informed by their teachers that Pluto was reclassified as a dwarf planet (Broughton et al., 2013). In contrast to achievement and epistemic emotions, topic emotions do not directly pertain to learning and problem solving. However, they can strongly influence students' engagement by affecting their interest and motivation in an academic domain.

Social Emotions Academic learning is situated in social contexts. Even when learning alone, students do not act in a social vacuum; rather, the goals, contents, and outcomes of learning are socially constructed. By implication, academic settings induce a multitude of emotions related to other persons. These emotions include social achievement emotions, such as admiration, envy, contempt, or empathy related to the success and failure of others, as well as nonachievement emotions, such as love or hate in the relationships with classmates and teachers. Social emotions can directly influence students' engagement with academic tasks, especially so when learning is situated in teacher–student or student–student interactions. They can also indirectly influence learning by motivating students to engage or disengage in task-related interactions with teachers and classmates (Linnenbrink-Garcia et al., 2011).

Table 1 A three-dimensional taxonomy of achievement emotions

	Positive[a]		Negative[b]	
Object focus	Activating	Deactivating	Activating	Deactivating
Activity	Enjoyment	Relaxation	Anger Frustration	Boredom
Outcome/prospective	HopeJoy[c]	Relief[c]	Anxiety	Hopelessness
Outcome/retrospective	Joy Pride Gratitude	Contentment Relief	Shame Anger	Sadness Disappointment

[a]Positive = pleasant emotion
[b]Negative = unpleasant emotion
[c]Anticipatory joy/relief

Functions for Students' Engagement and Achievement

Cognitive and neuroscientific research has shown that emotions are fundamentally important for human learning and development. Specifically, experimental mood studies have found that affect influences a broad variety of cognitive processes that contribute to learning, such as perception, attention, social judgment, cognitive problem solving, decision making, and memory processes (Barrett et al., 2016). However, one fundamental problem with much of this research is that it used global constructs of positive versus negative affect or mood, but did not attend to the specific qualities of different kinds of affects. This implies that it may be difficult and potentially misleading to use the findings for explaining students' emotions and learning in real-world academic contexts. Specifically, as argued both in Pekrun's (1992a, 2006) cognitive/motivational model of emotion effects and in Linnenbrink-Garcia's research on affect and engagement (Linnenbrink, 2007; Linnenbrink & Pintrich, 2004; Linnenbrink-Garcia et al., 2011; Linnenbrink-Garcia, Patall, et al., 2016; Linnenbrink, Wormington, et al., 2016), it is not sufficient to differentiate positive from negative affective states, but imperative to also attend to the degree of arousal implied.

As such, the minimum necessary is to distinguish between the four groups of emotions outlined earlier (positive activating, positive deactivating, negative activating, and negative deactivating). For example, both anxiety and hopelessness are negative (unpleasant) emotions; however, their effects on students' engagement can differ dramatically, as anxiety can motivate a student to invest effort in order to avoid failure, whereas hopelessness undermines any kind of engagement. Even within each of the four categories, it may be necessary to further distinguish between distinct emotions. For example, both anxiety and anger are activating negative emotions; however, paradoxically, whereas anxiety is associated with avoidance, anger is related to approach motivation (Carver & Harmon-Jones, 2009).

Emotions can influence students' engagement, which in turn impacts their academic learning and achievement. By implication, we regard engagement as a mediator between students' emotions and their achievement. In the following sections, we first summarize research on the relation of emotions to the five types of engagement outlined at the outset. This research comprises both experimental studies and correlational field research. In experimental studies, emotions were typically induced via mood induction procedures; in field studies, self-report scales such as Pekrun et al.'s (2011) Achievement Emotions Questionnaire (AEQ) were used. We then outline implications for the effects of different emotions on students' achievement.

Cognitive Engagement

In our discussion of cognitive engagement, we focus on cognitive processes of attention, mood-congruent memory recall, and memory storage and retrieval that imply active involvement with academic tasks. Specifically, cognitive engagement refers to the way in which emotions shape cognitive resources and memory processes that are activated automatically (for intentional cognitive processes, see the section on cognitive-behavioral engagement).

Attention and Flow Emotions consume cognitive resources (i.e., resources of the working memory) by focusing attention on the object of emotion. This effect was first addressed in interference models of test anxiety, which posited that anxiety reduces performance on complex and difficult tasks; this occurs because anxiety involves worries and produces task-irrelevant thoughts that interfere with task completion (e.g., Wine, 1971). For example, while preparing for an exam, a student may fear failure and worry about the consequences of failure, which in turn may distract their attention away from the task. Interference models of anxiety were expanded by resource allocation models, which postulated that any negative and positive emotions can consume cognitive resources and reduce task-related attention (Meinhardt & Pekrun, 2003; Mikels & Reuter-Lorenz, 2019).

However, the resource consumption effect likely is bound to emotions that have task-extraneous objects and generate task-irrelevant thinking, such as affective pictures in experimental mood research, or worries about impending failure on an exam in test anxiety. In contrast, in positive task-related emotions such as curiosity and enjoyment of learning, the task is the object of emotion. In these emotions, attention is focused on the task, and working memory resources can be used for task completion. However, it is possible that some positive task-related emotions, such as pride or overexcitement, may also distract attention away from the task.

Corroborating these expectations, empirical evidence from correlational studies with K-12 and university students shows that negative academic emotions, such as anger, anxiety, shame, boredom, and hopelessness, were associated with task-irrelevant thinking and reduced flow, whereas enjoyment related negatively to irrelevant thinking and positively to flow (Pekrun et al., 2010, 2011; Zeidner, 1998). A similar pattern was observed with more global measures of positive and negative affect (Linnenbrink & Pintrich, 2002a; Linnenbrink et al., 1999) and those using a circumplex approach (Ranellucci et al., 2021). These findings suggest that students' emotions have profound effects on their attentional engagement with academic tasks.

Mood-Congruent Memory Recall Memory research has shown that emotions influence storage and retrieval of information. Mood-congruent retrieval (Parrott & Spackman, 2000) implies that mood facilitates the retrieval of like-valenced material, with positive mood facilitating the retrieval of positive self- and task-related information, and negative mood facilitating the retrieval of negative information. Mood-congruent recall can impact students' motivation. For example, positive mood can foster positive self-appraisals and thus benefit

motivation to learn and performance; in contrast, negative mood can promote negative-self appraisals and thus hamper motivation and performance.

Retrieval-Induced Forgetting and Facilitation Retrieval-induced forgetting implies that practicing some learning material impedes later retrieval of related material that was not practiced, presumably so because of inhibitory processes in memory networks. In contrast, retrieval-induced facilitation implies that practicing enhances memory for related, but unpracticed material (Kuhbandner & Pekrun, 2013). With learning material consisting of disconnected elements, such as single words, retrieval-induced forgetting has been found to occur. For example, after learning a list of words, practicing half of the list can impede memory for the other half. In contrast, facilitation has been shown to occur for connected materials consisting of elements that show strong interrelations. For example, after learning coherent text material, practicing half of the material leads to better memory for the nonpracticed half.

Emotions have been shown to influence retrieval-induced forgetting. Specifically, negative mood can undo forgetting, likely because it can inhibit spreading activation in memory networks which underlies retrieval-induced forgetting. Conversely, positive emotions activate associative memory networks (Madan et al., 2019). As such, they can facilitate retrieval-induced facilitation since they promote the relational processing of information underlying such facilitation (Kuhbandner & Pekrun, 2013). These findings suggest that negative emotions might be helpful for learning lists of unrelated material (such as lists of foreign language vocabulary), whereas positive emotions should promote learning of coherent material. However, caution should be taken when interpreting these mechanisms of retrieval-induced forgetting and facilitation observed in the psychological laboratory. Studies are needed to explore if these mechanisms operate under natural conditions as well.

Motivational Engagement

Motivation refers to processes shaping goal direction, intensity, and persistence of behavior (see Pekrun, in press). Given the active, energetic, and approach-oriented role of these processes in initiating and sustaining academic effort, it is important to consider motivation directed toward task involvement as a form of engagement. Furthermore, motivational engagement can shape other forms of engagement (e.g., behavioral engagement). As such, it is important to consider how emotions shape motivational engagement.

As compared to cognitive effects, the influence of emotions on motivational engagement has been less well studied. However, it is generally acknowledged that specific emotions function to trigger impulses for specific action and thus play a role in initiating behaviors. Specifically, each of the major negative emotions is associated with distinct action impulses and serves to prepare the organism for action (or non-action), such as fight, flight, and behavioral withdrawal in anger, anxiety, and hopelessness, respectively. For positive emotions, motivational consequences are less specific. Likely, one of the functions of positive emotions such as enjoyment is to motivate exploratory behavior and an enlargement of one's action repertoire, as addressed in Fredrickson's (2001) broaden-and-build model of positive emotions.

In the academic domain, emotions can profoundly influence students' motivational engagement. The available evidence suggests that affect influences students' adoption of achievement goals, as addressed in Linnenbrink and Pintrich's (2002b) bidirectional model of affect and achievement goals. Specifically, it has been shown that pleasant emotions can have positive effects, and unpleasant emotions negative effects, on undergraduate students' adoption of mastery-approach goals (Linnenbrink & Pintrich, 2002b). In line with this evidence, positive achievement emotions such as enjoyment of learning, hope, and pride have been shown to relate positively to K-12 and university students' interest and intrinsic motivation, whereas nega-

tive emotions like anger, anxiety, shame, hopelessness, and boredom related negatively to these variables (Pekrun et al., 2010, 2011; Zeidner, 1998).

However, as addressed in Pekrun's (1992a, 2006) cognitive/motivational model of emotion and performance, motivational effects may be different for activating versus deactivating emotions. This model posits that activating positive emotions (e.g., joy, hope, and pride) promote motivational engagement, whereas deactivating emotions (e.g., hopelessness and boredom) undermine motivational engagement. In contrast, effects are posited to be more complex for deactivating positive emotions (e.g., relief and relaxation) and activating negative emotions (e.g., anger, anxiety, and shame). For example, relaxed contentment following success can be expected to reduce immediate motivation to reengage with learning contents, but strengthen long-term motivation to do so. Regarding activating negative emotions, anger, anxiety, and shame have been found to reduce intrinsic motivation, but strengthen extrinsic motivation to invest effort in order to avoid failure, especially so when expectations to prevent failure and attain success are favorable (Turner & Schallert, 2001; von der Embse et al., 2018). Due to these variable effects on different kinds of motivation, the effects of these emotions on students' overall motivation to learn can be variable as well.

Behavioral Engagement: Investment of Effort

Behavioral engagement includes effort and persistence (Fredricks et al., 2004). Several psychological models suggest that positive affect leads to behavioral disengagement in terms of reduced effort, either because one is progressing at a sufficient rate toward one's goals (Carver et al., 1996), or because it signals that all is well and there is no need to engage (Schwartz, 2012). For example, when academic tasks are easy, students may enjoy success and infer that there is no need to put forth more effort. Other models question this perspective and instead suggest that positive affect frees resources away from a threat, allowing more expansive task-related action (Fredrickson, 2001). Negative emotions such as sadness (for approach goals) and anxiety (for avoidance goals) may signal that one is not making sufficient progress toward one's goals or that there is a threat in the environment, suggesting that they may also contribute to intensified effort (Carver et al., 1996).

However, these perspectives do not consider the interplay between valence and arousal and thus may not fully capture the way in which emotions shape behavioral engagement. As noted, activating versus deactivating emotions can exert different effects on students' motivation. By implication, the effects on resulting effort and persistence can differ as well. From studies with K-12 and university students, there is general support that positive activating emotions such as enjoyment of learning are positively associated with effort, and that negative deactivating emotions such as hopelessness and boredom are negatively associated with effort (e.g., Linnenbrink, 2007; Pekrun et al., 2010, 2011).

In contrast, effects have been shown to be more variable for negative activating emotions such as anger, anxiety, and shame. These emotions often show negative overall correlations with effort, but in some cases, they may support behavioral engagement as they can serve to energize students (Linnenbrink, 2007; Turner & Schallert, 2001). Furthermore, when studying emotion profiles (i.e., patterns of multiple emotions), Robinson et al. (2017) found that students who experienced negative deactivating affect (e.g., feeling tired and exhausted) had either lower or high behavioral disengagement depending on whether they also experienced positive activating affect (e.g., excited) or negative activating affect (e.g., angry and irritated), respectively.

Cognitive-Behavioral Engagement

Cognitive-behavioral engagement refers to complex cognitive processes that are intentionally instigated by the learner, including cogni-tive problem solving, use of cognitive and metacognitive learning strategies, and self-regulation of learning. These processes are similar to what Fredricks et al. (2004) referred to as cognitive engagement. We use the term cognitive-behavioral engagement to differentiate these processes both from automatic cognitive processes described earlier and from pure quantity of effort as reflected by behavioral engagement.

Problem Solving Experimental evidence from laboratory research with university students suggests that positive mood promotes flexible, creative, and holistic ways of solving problems and a reliance on generalized, heuristic knowledge structures (Fredrickson, 2001; Fiedler & Beier, 2014; Bohn-Gettler, 2019). Conversely, negative mood has been found to promote focused, detail-oriented, and analytical ways of thinking (Forgas, 2017). To explain these findings, mood-as-information approaches assume that positive affective states signal that all is well (e.g., sufficient goal progress), whereas negative states signal that something is wrong (e.g., insufficient goal progress; Schwartz, 2012). "All is well" conditions imply safety and the discretion to creatively explore the environment, broaden one's cognitive horizon, and build new actions. In contrast, "all is not well" conditions may imply a threat to well-being, thus making it necessary to focus on these problems in analytical, cognitively cautious ways.

Learning Strategies Judging from the experimental evidence on problem solving, positive activating emotions such as enjoyment of learning should facilitate use of flexible, holistic learning strategies like elaboration and organization of learning material or critical thinking. Negative emotions, on the other hand, should sustain more rigid, detail-oriented learning, like simple rehearsal of learning material. Correlational evidence from studies with university students generally supports this view (Linnenbrink & Pintrich, 2002a; Pekrun et al., 2011). However, for deactivating positive and negative emotions, these effects may be less pronounced. Deactivating emotions, like relaxation or boredom, may produce shallow information processing rather than any more intensive use of learning strategies.

Meta-Strategies and Self-Regulation Self-regulation of learning includes the use of meta-cognitive, meta-motivational, and meta-emotional strategies (Miele & Scholer, 2018; Wolters, 2003) making it possible to adopt goals, monitor and regulate learning activities, and evaluate their results in flexible ways, such that learning activities can be adapted to task demands. An application of these strategies presupposes cognitive flexibility. Therefore, it can be assumed that positive emotions foster self-regulated learning and use of meta-strategies, whereas negative emotions can motivate the student to rely on external guidance. Correlational evidence from studies with university students is in line with these propositions (Linnenbrink & Pintrich, 2002a; Pekrun et al., 2011). However, the reverse causal direction may also play a role—self-regulated learning may be enjoyable, and external directions for learning may trigger anxiety.

Social-Behavioral Engagement

With the growing emphasis on constructivist forms of learning, student–student interactions have become increasingly important in shaping students' learning and achievement. Socially engaging with one's peers includes behavioral engagement, such as participating in discussion or listening to other students (Fredricks et al., 2004), but it can also include higher-order quality forms of social participation such as working cohesively and supporting other students' learning. Thus, we use the term social-behavioral engagement to refer to a range of social forms of engagement with academic tasks, including actively participating with peers on academic tasks as well as affective and motivational interactions geared toward supporting positive social dynamics within the group and peers' participation in academic tasks (Linnenbrink-Garcia et al., 2011). Instructional settings that require interac-tions with peers may present unique emotional challenges and evoke strong emotional responses (Jarvenoja & Jarvela, 2009; Rogat & Linnenbrink-Garcia, 2011). This is not surprising, especially given the key role that social agents play in shaping emotions across time (Frenzel et al., 2018). As such, we consider the interplay between emotions and social-behavioral engagement, in terms of both direct peer-to-peer interactions and online peer interactions.

Direct Interaction There is growing evidence that emotions relate to social-behavioral engagement in direct peer interaction, in both laboratory and field-based research involving small groups and class discussion. Research conducted with upper elementary-aged children participating in small group work during mathematics instruction found that positive emotions, such as feeling happy or calm, helped to support social-behavioral engagement including active listening, supporting one's peers, and general group cohesion, while negative deactivating states such as feeling tired undermined it (Linnenbrink-Garcia et al., 2011). Linnenbrink-Garcia et al. (2011) also found that both activated (tense) and deactivated (tired) neg-ative affective states were associated with decreased social-behavioral engagement in the form of social loafing, or allowing the other stu-dents during small group work to do all the work. Moreover, within small group settings, negative emotions seemed to sustain negative cycles of interactions such as disrespecting others and dis-couraging their participation. However, this research also suggests that the interplay between emotions and social-behavioral engagement is complex, such that negative emotions can at times support rather than undermine engagement (Do & Schallert, 2004; Linnenbrink-Garcia et al., 2011; Rogat & Linnenbrink-Garcia, 2011). For instance, in their study of college students engaged in dis-cussion during a weekly seminar course, Do and Schallert (2004) found that while positive emo-tions were associated with engagement, negative emotions were associated with both engagement and disengagement, as negative emotions could spur students to dive into the discussion to express their views.

Online Interaction Studies analyzing online discussions and group work also suggest that emotions and social engagement are related (Bakhtiar et al., 2018; Nummenmaa & Nummenmaa, 2008; Wosnitza & Volet, 2005). For example, in a study of undergraduates working in an asynchronous web-environment (e.g., students post comments and discuss ideas but are not required to interact in real-time), social interactions were more likely than other aspects of the learning environment to evoke emotional responses (Vuorela & Nummenmaa, 2004). There was no relation between mean levels of emotion with social-behavioral engagement; however, students who had more variability in experienced emotions were found to engage more in the online exchange.

In sum, there is growing evidence that emotions emerge from, and likely strongly contribute to social-behavioral engagement when students work with their peers on academic tasks, at both the upper elementary and postsecondary levels. Broadly speaking, positive emotions seem to support social-behavioral engagement, while negative emotions can undermine it. However, with social-behavioral engagement as well, it is important to note that the nature of these relations is complex, suggesting the need to consider variable effects of emotions as well as reciprocal and cyclical relations between emotions and engagement. Moreover, additional research is needed among a broader range of students from different age groups to better understand the connection between emotions and social-behavioral engagement across development.

Academic Achievement

Since many different mechanisms of engagement can contribute to the influence of emotions, the overall effects on students' achievement are inevitably complex and may depend on the interplay between different mechanisms, as well as between these mechanisms and task demands. Nevertheless, it is possible to derive inferences from theory and the existing evidence.

Positive Emotions Traditionally it was assumed that positive emotions, notwithstanding their potential to foster creativity, are often maladaptive for performance as a result of inducing unrealistically positive appraisals triggered by mood-congruent retrieval, fostering nonanalytical information processing, and making effort expenditure seem unnecessary by signaling that everything is going well. From this perspective, "our primary goal is to feel good, and feeling good makes us lazy thinkers who are oblivious to potentially useful negative information and unresponsive to meaningful variations in information and situation" (Aspinwall, 1998, p. 7).

However, as noted, positive mood has typically been regarded as a unitary construct in experimental research. As argued above, such a view is inadequate because it fails to distinguish between activating and deactivating emotions. *Deactivating* positive emotions, like relief or relaxation, may well have the negative performance effects described for positive mood, whereas *activating* positive emotions, such as task-related enjoyment or pride, should have positive effects. The evidence cited above suggests that enjoyment focuses attention on the task; promotes relational processing of information; induces intrinsic motivation; and facilitates use of flexible learning strategies and self-regulation, thus likely exerting positive effects on overall performance under many task conditions. In contrast, deactivating positive emotions, such as relief and relaxation, can reduce task attention, can have variable motivational effects, and can lead to superficial information processing, thus making effects on overall achievement more variable.

Empirical evidence confirms that activating positive emotions can enhance achievement. Specifically, enjoyment of learning correlates positively with K-12 and college students' academic performance. In a recent meta-analysis of 57 studies, the average correlation of enjoyment and academic achievement, as measured by grades or test scores, was $\rho = 0.27$ (Camacho-Morles et al., 2021; see also Loderer et al., 2020a), representing a moderately strong association (based on the benchmarks of $\rho = 0.15$, 0.25, and 35 as small, moderate, and strong for latent correlations, Gignac & Szodorai, 2016). Furthermore, students' enjoyment, hope, and pride correlated positively with college students' interest, effort invested in studying, elaboration of learning material, and self-regulation of learning, in line with the view that these activating positive emotions can be beneficial for students' academic agency (Pekrun et al., 2011).

Consistent with this evidence, general positive affect has been found to correlate positively with students' cognitive engagement (Linnenbrink, 2007). Interestingly, Robinson et al. (2017) found that students who reported high positive deactivating emotions (coupled either with positive activating emotions *or* negative deactivating emotions) during an undergraduate anatomy class also had high behavioral engagement and subsequent achievement, suggesting that positive deactivating emotions may also support engagement and learning, at least when coupled with other forms of emotions.

In explaining correlations with measures of achievement, reciprocal causation of emotion and achievement has to be considered. Linkages between emotions and achievement may be caused by effects of emotion on achievement, but also by reverse effects of success and failure on the development of emotions. Longitudinal studies with secondary school students in the domain of mathematics have confirmed that the correlations for positive emotions are due to effects of these emotions on achievement, in addition to effects of achievement on these emotions (Forsblom et al., 2022; Pekrun, Lichtenfeld, et al., 2017; Pekrun et al., in press).

Negative Activating Emotions As noted, emotions such as anger, anxiety, and shame produce task-irrelevant thinking and undermine intrinsic motivation. On the other hand, these emotions can induce motivation to avoid failure and facilitate the use of more rigid learning strategies. By implication, the effects on resulting academic performance depend on task conditions and may well be variable, similar to the proposed effects

of positive deactivating emotions. The available evidence supports this position. Specifically, it has been shown that anxiety impairs performance on complex or difficult tasks that demand cognitive resources, such as difficult intelligence test items, whereas performance on easy, less complex, and repetitive tasks may not suffer or is even enhanced (Zeidner, 1998). In line with experimental findings, field studies have documented that anxiety shows moderate to strong negative correlations with students' academic achievement across age groups (e.g., average $r = -0.28$ for students' anxiety and achievement in mathematics, Barroso et al., 2021; see also Hembree, 1988; Loderer et al., 2020a; von der Embse et al., 2018). Again, in explaining the evidence, reciprocal causation has to be considered. Evidence from studies with upper elementary and secondary school students suggests that anxiety and students' achievement are in fact linked by reciprocal causation across school years (e.g., Meece et al., 1990; Pekrun, Lichtenfeld, et al., 2017; Pekrun, Muis, et al., 2017).

Few studies have addressed the effects of negative activating emotions other than anxiety. Similar to anxiety, self-reported *shame* related to failure showed negative overall correlations with university students' academic achievement and negatively predicted their exam performance (Pekrun et al., 2009, 2011). However, as with anxiety, shame likely exerts variable effects (Turner & Schallert, 2001). Similarly, while achievement-related *anger* correlated negatively with academic performance (strong negative correlation of $\rho = -0.35$ across studies; Camacho-Morles et al., 2021), the underlying mechanisms may be complex and imply more than just negative effects. In a study by Lane et al. (2005), depressed mood interacted with anger experienced before an academic exam, such that anger was related to improved performance in undergraduates who reported no depressive mood symptoms—presumably because they were able to maintain motivation. In the study by Robinson et al. (2017) cited earlier, composite variables assessing multiple forms of negative activating emotions (annoyed, irritated, agitated, and angry) were used. The results showed that undergraduates who experienced high negative activating (along with high negative deactivating) emotions had low levels of achievement. In sum, the findings for anxiety, shame, and anger support the notion that performance effects of negative activating emotions are complex, although relationships with overall performance are negative for many task conditions and students.

Negative Deactivating Emotions Negative deactivating emotions, such as boredom and hopelessness, are posited to uniformly impair performance by reducing cognitive resources, undermining both intrinsic and extrinsic motivation, and promoting superficial information processing (Pekrun, 2006). Supporting this view, there is cumulative evidence that self-reported boredom correlates negatively with K-12 and undergraduate students' achievement (average correlation $\rho = -0.25$; Camacho-Morles et al., 2021). Evidence for hopelessness is scarce, but also shows negative correlations with achievement (e.g., Pekrun et al., 2011). Again, longitudinal evidence suggests that these correlations are due to reciprocal effects linking emotion and achievement, including effects of boredom and hopelessness on students' achievement over the school years as well as reverse effects of achievement on these emotions (Forsblom et al., 2022; Pekrun, Lichtenfeld, et al., 2017).

In sum, theoretical expectations, experimental evidence, and findings from field studies suggest that students' emotions have profound effects on their engagement and academic achievement. Engagement and achievement, in turn, shape students' personality development, educational careers, and future prospects, implying that emotions also affect students' development more broadly. As such, administrators and educators should pay attention to the emotions experienced by students. According to the available evidence, the effects of enjoyment of learning are beneficial, whereas hopelessness and boredom are detrimental for engagement. The effects of emotions like anger, anxiety, or shame are more complex,

but for the average student, these emotions also have negative overall effects.

Origins of Academic Emotions

Given the relevance of students' emotions for their engagement, it is important to consider their origins as well. While a more detailed review is beyond the scope of this chapter, we provide a short overview of current research (for more comprehensive treatments, see Pekrun & Linnenbrink-Garcia, 2014; Pekrun, 2018; Pekrun, Muis, et al., 2017). We first address appraisals and achievement goals as individual antecedents of students' emotions, and subsequently the role of learning tasks and social environments.

Appraisals as Proximal Antecedents

Emotions can be caused and modulated by numerous individual factors, such as situational perceptions, cognitive appraisals, neurohormonal processes, and sensory feedback from expressive behavior (Barrett et al., 2016). However, the emotions experienced in an academic context pertain to culturally defined demands in settings that are a recent product of civilization. In these settings, the individual has to learn how to adapt to situational demands while preserving individual autonomy—inevitably a process guided by appraisals. As such, cognitive appraisals of task demands, personal competences, the probability of success and failure, and the value of these outcomes likely play a major role in the arousal of academic emotions, and research on the determinants of academic emotions from early on has focused on such appraisals.

Research on Achievement Anxiety Studies on test anxiety and other types of achievement anxiety (e.g., math anxiety) were the first to address the appraisal antecedents of students' emotions. In these studies, appraisals concerning threat of failure have been addressed as causing anxiety. In terms of R. S. Lazarus' transactional stress model

(Lazarus & Folkman, 1984), threat in a given achievement setting is evaluated in terms of the likelihood and subjective importance of failure ("primary appraisal") and possibilities to cope with this threat ("secondary appraisal"). Students may experience anxiety when their primary appraisal indicates that failure on an important exam is likely, and when their secondary appraisal indicates that this threat is not sufficiently controllable. Empirical research confirms that achievement anxiety is closely related to perceived lack of control over performance. Specifically, numerous studies have shown that K-12 and postsecondary students' academic self-concepts, control beliefs, and self-efficacy expectations correlate negatively with their test and math anxiety (von der Embse et al., 2018; Zeidner, 1998; e.g., correlations around $r = -0.50$ between secondary school students' self-concept and anxiety in mathematics in Pekrun et al., 2019).

Attributional Theory In attributional theories explaining emotions following success and failure, perceived control plays a central role as well. In B. Weiner's (1985, 2018) approach, attributions of success and failure to various causes are held to be primary determinants of these emotions. Pride is assumed to be aroused by attributions of success to internal causes (i.e., causes located within the person, such as ability and effort). Shame is seen to be instigated by failure attributed to internal causes that are uncontrollable (like lack of ability), and gratitude and anger by attributions of success and failure, respectively, to external causes that are under control by others. The stability of perceived causes is posited to be important for hopefulness and hopelessness regarding future performance. Findings from scenario studies asking students how they, or others, might react to success and failure were largely in line with Weiner's propositions, as were findings from field studies investigating links between university students' achievement attributions and their emotions (Pekrun & Marsh, 2018; Weiner, 1985, 2018).

Control-Value Theory While test anxiety theories and attributional theories have addressed outcome emotions pertaining to success and failure, they have neglected activity-related emotions. In Pekrun's (2006, 2018, 2021) control-value theory (CVT), core propositions of the transactional stress model and attributional theories are revised and expanded to explain a broader variety of emotions. CVT originally focused on achievement emotions (Pekrun, 2006). The current, generalized version of the theory also considers epistemic and social emotions (Pekrun, 2021). CVT posits that emotions are induced when the individual feels in control of, or out of control of, activities and outcomes that are subjectively important—implying that appraisals of control and value are important proximal determinants of emotions (e.g., Forsblom et al., 2022; Shao et al., 2020). Control appraisals pertain to the perceived controllability of actions and outcomes, as implied by causal expectations (self-efficacy expectations and outcome expectations), causal attributions, and competence appraisals. Value appraisals relate to the subjective importance of these activities and outcomes.

Different combinations of control and value appraisals are proposed to instigate different emotions (Table 1). In terms of outcome-related achievement emotions, prospective, anticipatory joy and hopelessness are expected to be triggered when there is high perceived control (joy) or a complete lack of perceived control (hopelessness). For example, students who believe they have the necessary resources to get an A+ on an important exam may feel joyous about the prospect of receiving such a grade. Conversely, if they believe they are incapable of preventing failure on an exam, they may experience hopelessness. Prospective hope and anxiety are instigated when there is uncertainty about control, the attentional focus being on anticipated success in the case of hope, and on anticipated failure in the case of anxiety. For example, a student who is unsure about being able to master an important exam may hope for success, fear failure, or both.

Similarly, retrospective pride, shame, gratitude, and anger are also induced by appraisals of control and value.

Regarding activity emotions, enjoyment of achievement activities is proposed to depend on a combination of positive competence appraisals and positive appraisals of the intrinsic value of the action (e.g., studying) and its reference object (e.g., learning material). For example, students are expected to enjoy learning if they feel competent to meet the demands of the task and value the learning material. If they feel incompetent, or are disinterested in the material, studying is not enjoyable. Anger and frustration are aroused when the intrinsic value of the activity is negative (e.g., when working on a difficult project is perceived as taking too much effort which is experienced as aversive). Finally, boredom is experienced when the activity lacks any intrinsic incentive value (Pekrun et al., 2010).

For epistemic and social emotions, additional appraisals play a role as well. For example, epistemic emotions are prompted by appraisals of cognitive incongruity. CVT considers three types of incongruity: Current information can be inconsistent with prior information (e.g., prior expectations and beliefs); it can differ from desired knowledge that is not yet available; and it can be contradictory in itself (e.g., when reading contradictory texts). The first type of incongruity is posited to prompt surprise, the second type curiosity, and the third one confusion. All three types of incongruity can lead to frustration if the incongruity is not resolved. Appraisals of control and value modulate the intensity of these emotions (except for surprise which is an immediate response to violations of expectations; Reisenzein et al., 2019). For example, students will be more curious about learning materials they are interested in.

Nonreflective Induction of Emotions Recurring appraisal-based induction of emotions can become automatic and nonreflective over time. When academic activities are repeated over and over again, appraisals and the induction of emotions can become routinized to the extent that there is no longer any conscious

mediation of emotions (Reisenzein, 2001). In the procedural emotion schemata established by routinization, situation perception and emotion are directly linked such that perceptions can automatically induce the emotion (e.g., the mere smell of a chemistry lab inducing joy). However, when the situation changes or attempts are made to change the emotion (as in psychotherapy), appraisals come into play again.

The Role of Achievement-Related Goals and Orientations

To the extent that cognitive appraisals are proximal determinants of emotions, more distal antecedents should affect emotions by first influencing appraisals (Fig. 2; Pekrun, 2006). An example is achievement-related goals and goal orientations, which direct attentional focus in the course of achievement activities. Specifically, these goals and orientations provide a lens through which individuals interpret achievement-related settings. *Achievement goals* are defined as the competence-relevant aims that individuals strive for in achievement settings (Elliot & McGregor, 2001), with different goals being related to different definitions of achievement. In mastery goals, achievement is judged by intraindividual standards or absolute criteria; in performance goals, achievement is judged by normative standards comparing performance across individuals. *Achievement goal orientations* are broader cognitive schemas that comprise achievement goals as well as reasons to pursue these goals (Pintrich, 2000). Mastery goal orientations focus on developing competence, whereas performance goal orientations focus on demonstrating competence. These primary goals and orientations can be further differentiated into approach and avoidance dimensions (Elliot & McGregor, 2001; Pintrich, 2000). Students can strive toward success or away from failure, resulting in four possible goals and goal orientations (mastery-approach, mastery-avoidance, performance-approach, performance-avoidance; for further differentiation, see Elliot et al., 2011).

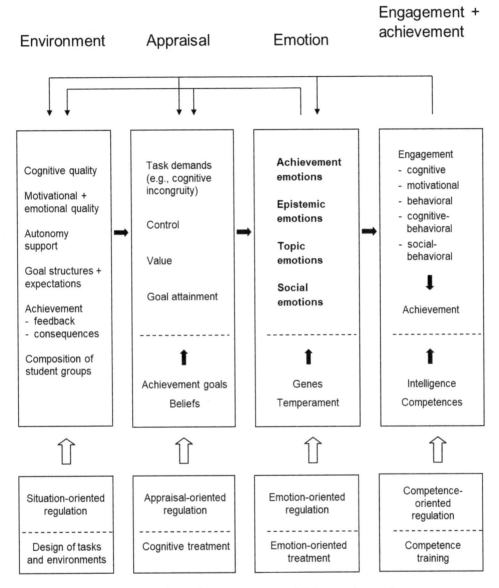

Fig. 2 Reciprocal causation of academic emotions, engagement, and their antecedents and outcomes

Different goals and orientations focus attention on different aspects of current academic activities, thus promoting different kinds of appraisals and emotions. Specifically, goals can promote appraisals of the controllability and value of achievement, and of the rate of progress toward goal attainment. Furthermore, they can differentially focus the individual on the task versus the self. In terms of controllability and value, CVT suggests that mastery goals should focus attention on the controllability and positive value of task activities, thus promoting positive activity emotions such as enjoyment of learning, and reducing negative activity emotions such as boredom (Pekrun et al., 2009). Performance-approach goals should focus attention on the controllability and positive value of success, thus facilitating positive outcome emotions such as hope and pride, and performance-avoidance goals focus attention on the uncontrollability and negative value of failure, thus inducing negative outcome emotions such as anxiety, shame, and hopelessness.

In terms of the rate of progress, Linnenbrink and Pintrich's bidirectional model of goals and affect (Linnenbrink and Pintrich's 2002b; Linnenbrink, 2007; Linnenbrink-Garcia & Barger, 2014) proposes that mastery goals promote perceptions of progress toward success since progress is judged relative to one's own improvement, thus facilitating emotions such as elation and happiness. Performance-approach goals promote emotions such as sadness for the many individuals who perceive insufficient progress toward success due to competition with others, and happiness for those who do perceive sufficient progress. Performance-avoidance goals promote perceptions of moving away from or toward failure, thus facilitating relief or anxiety, respectively. Both performance-approach and avoidance goals are proposed to prompt anxiety, due to the heightened focus on the self. As such, performance-approach goal orientations in particular should be associated with a range of both positive and negative emotions including elation, happiness, sadness, and anxiety, depending both on perceived progress and the salience of the self.

The predictions from the two models are complementary and largely consistent, with few exceptions such as differences in the proposed links for hopelessness and sadness (Tyson et al., 2009; Pekrun & Stephens, 2009). Empirical evidence from samples across schooling levels supports these predictions (see Linnenbrink-Garcia & Barger, 2014, for a review). The relation between performance-avoidance goals and achievement anxiety is best documented, but research also shows clear relations for mastery goals and activity emotions (positive for enjoyment and negative for boredom), and for performance goals and outcome emotions other than anxiety, such as pride, shame, and hopelessness (e.g., Linnenbrink, 2007; Linnenbrink & Pintrich, 2002b; Pekrun et al., 2009). The relation between achievement goals and emotions also implies that emotions can function as mediators in the effects of achievement goals on engagement and achievement. For example, in a laboratory study by Linnenbrink et al. (1999), general negative affect was a mediator of mastery goal effects on task performance among undergraduates completing a working memory task.

Similarly, in the study by Pekrun et al. (2009), students' performance-avoidance goals in a university course predicted their self-reported anxiety before the mid-term exam which, in turn, was a negative predictor of exam performance, suggesting that anxiety mediated the effects of these goals on performance.

The Influence of Tasks and Environments

The impact of task design and learning environments primarily has been investigated for students' test anxiety (Zeidner, 1998; Putwain et al., 2017). Lack of structure and clarity, excessively high task demands, competitive goal structures in the classroom, negative feedback after performance, and negative consequences of poor performance (e.g., public humiliation) relate positively to students' anxiety, likely because these factors reduce expectancies for success and increase the importance of avoiding failure (Pekrun, 1992b). Open-ended formats of tasks (e.g., essay questions) may induce more anxiety than multiple-choice formats, likely due to higher working memory demands which are difficult to meet when memory capacity is used for worrying about failure. In contrast, giving individuals the choice between tasks, relaxing time constraints, and giving second chances in terms of retaking tests can reduce anxiety, presumably because perceived control is enhanced under these conditions (Zeidner, 1998).

Recent research has expanded the perspective by considering other emotions as well. For example, Linnenbrink-Garcia, Patall, et al. (2016) identified five instructional design principles that help to promote positive emotions (as well as motivation): support students' feelings of competence, enhance autonomy, use personally relevant and active tasks, emphasize learning and de-emphasize social comparison, and encourage feelings of belonging. Studies on the design of multimedia learning environments have shown that emotions conveyed in these environment (e.g., through human-like agents), the provision of autonomy, standards for achievement, and feedback about achievement influence learners' emotions and engagement (Loderer et al., 2020b; Plass & Kaplan, 2016). The following factors in traditional as well as online learning environments may be most relevant for a broad variety of academic emotions (see Fig. 2).

Cognitive Quality The cognitive quality of instruction and tasks as defined by their structure, clarity, and potential for cognitive stimulation likely has a positive influence on perceived competence and the perceived value of tasks, thus positively influencing students' emotions and engagement. Specifically, inducing appropriate levels of cognitive incongruity may be of primary importance for the arousal of epistemic emotions such as surprise and curiosity. In addition, the relative difficulty of tasks can influence perceived control, and the match between task demands and competences can influence subjective task value, thus also influencing emotions. If demands are too high or too low, the incentive value of tasks may be reduced to the extent that boredom is experienced (Pekrun et al., 2010; see Martin, chapter "The Role of Academic Engagement in Students' Educational Development: Insights from Load Reduction Instruction and the 4M Academic Engagement Framework", this volume, for a discussion of instruction, cognitive load, and student engagement).

Motivational and Emotional Quality Teachers and peers, as well as virtual agents in multimedia learning deliver direct and indirect messages conveying academic values. Two ways of inducing emotionally relevant values may be most important. First, if tasks and environments are shaped such that they meet students' needs, positive activity-related emotions should be fostered. For example, learning environments that support cooperation should help students fulfill their needs for social relatedness, thus making working on academic tasks more enjoyable and promoting their social engagement as discussed earlier. Second, teachers' own enthusiasm in dealing with tasks can facilitate the adoption of achievement values and related emotions (Frenzel et al., 2018). We assume that observational learning and emotional contagion are prime mechanisms mediating these effects (Hatfield et al., 1994).

Autonomy Support Tasks and environments supporting autonomy can increase perceived control and, by meeting needs for autonomy, the value of related achievement activities (for empirical evidence, see Tsai et al., 2008; Loderer et al., 2020b). However, these beneficial effects likely depend on the match between individual competences and needs for academic autonomy, on the one hand, and the affordances of these environments, on the other. In case of a mismatch, loss of control and negative emotions could result.

Goal Structures and Social Expectations Different standards for defining achievement can imply individualistic (mastery), competitive (normative performance), or cooperative goal structures (Johnson & Johnson, 1974). The goal structures provided in academic settings conceivably influence emotions in two ways. First, they can influence the achievement goals adopted by the individual student and any emotions mediated by these goals as outlined earlier. Second, goal structures determine opportunities for experiencing success and perceiving control, thus influencing control-dependent emotions. Specifically, competitive goal structures imply, by definition, that some students have to experience failure, thus inducing negative outcome emotions such as anxiety and hopelessness in these students. Similarly, the demands implied by an important other's unrealistic expectancies for achievement can lead to negative emotions resulting from reduced subjective control.

Feedback and Consequences of Achievement Cumulative success can strengthen perceived control, and cumulative failure can undermine control. In environments involving frequent assessments, performance feedback is likely of primary importance for the development of academic emotions (for empirical evidence, see Forsblom et al., 2022; Pekrun, Lichtenfeld, et al., 2017; Pekrun et al., in press). In addition, the perceived consequences of success and failure are important, since these consequences affect the instrumental value of achievement outcomes. Positive outcome emotions (e.g., hope for success) can be increased if success produces beneficial long-term outcomes (e.g., future career opportunities). Negative consequences of failure (e.g., unemployment), on the other hand, may increase achievement-related anxiety and hopelessness (Pekrun, 1992b).

Composition of Student Groups It follows from CVT that the composition of student groups is also critically important. The ability level of the classroom determines the likelihood of performing well relative to one's classmates. All else being equal, chances for performing well relative to others are reduced when being in a high-achieving class, thus students' perceived control and competence also tend to be reduced. In contrast, being in a low-achieving class offers more chances to be successful, enabling a sense of control. Due to these effects on perceived control, positive emotions such as enjoyment can be reduced, and negative emotions such as anxiety exacerbated, when a student is in a high-achieving class ("happy-fish-little-pond effect"; Pekrun et al., 2019).

In sum, individual antecedents as well as learning environments can shape students' academic emotions and, consequently, any emotion-dependent engagement with learning. Environments, goals, and appraisals can induce, prevent, and modulate students' emotions, and they can shape their objects and contents. Depending on individual goals and the learning environment, students' academic life can be infused with positive affect and joyful task engagement, or with anxiety, frustration, and boredom. However, the strong impact of the environment does not imply that basic mechanisms linking students' emotions with their engagement vary as a function of social context. Rather, these mechanisms seem to be stable across contexts (see Loderer et al., 2020b; Pekrun et al., 2009; Pekrun, 2018).

For example, in a cross-cultural comparison of Chinese and German high school students' emotions in mathematics, Frenzel et al. (2007) found that mean levels of emotions differed between cultures, with Chinese students reporting more achievement-related enjoyment, pride,

anxiety, and shame, and less anger in mathematics. However, the functional linkages of these emotions with perceived control, important others' expectations, and academic achievement in mathematics were equivalent across cultures. Similarly, in the OECD's Programme of International Student Assessment (PISA) 2015 cycle, students' schoolwork-related anxiety showed negative correlations with their science performance in 52 of 55 countries participating in the assessment of anxiety, and the relation between students' enjoyment and performance in science was positive in all of the 68 countries for which this relation was examined (OECD, 2016). Most likely, the general functions of emotions for students' engagement and achievement described earlier are universal across different learning environments and cultural contexts.

Reciprocal Causation, Emotion Regulation, and Treatment Interventions

Academic emotions influence students' engagement and achievement, but achievement outcomes can reciprocally influence appraisals, emotions, and the environment (Pekrun, 2006, 2021; see Fig. 2). As such, academic emotions, their antecedents, and their effects can be linked by reciprocal causation over time. Reciprocal causation may involve a number of feedback loops, including the following three that may be especially important. First, learning environments shape students' appraisals and emotions, but these emotions reciprocally affect students' learning environments and the behavior of teachers and classmates. For example, teachers' and students' enjoyment of classroom instruction are likely linked in reciprocal ways (see Frenzel et al., 2018). Second, emotions impact students' engagement, and engagement affects students' emotions. For example, enjoyment of learning can facilitate students' self-regulation and use of creative learning strategies, and self-directed involvement with tasks can, in turn, promote students' enjoyment. Similarly, emotions influence students' motivational engagement in terms of adopting various achievement goals, but these goals reciprocally influence students' emotions (Linnenbrink & Pintrich, 2002b). Third, by impacting engagement, students' emotions have an influence on their achievement. Academic achievement outcomes and feedback on these outcomes, however, are primary forces shaping students' emotions, again suggesting reciprocal causation.

In line with perspectives of dynamic systems theory (Turner & Waugh, 2007), we assume that such reciprocal causation can take different forms and can extend over fractions of seconds (e.g., in linkages between appraisals and emotions), days, weeks, months, or years. Positive feedback loops likely are commonplace. To explain, positive feedback loops are defined by effects in both directions having the same sign—either positive as in reciprocal linkages between teachers' and students' enjoyment as cited earlier, or negative as in reciprocal effects linking hopelessness or boredom and achievement. However, negative feedback loops can also be important. In negative feedback loops, effects in the two directions bear opposite signs; for example, when failure on an exam induces anxiety in a student, and anxiety motivates the student to successfully avoid failure on the next exam.

Reciprocal causation has implications for the regulation of academic emotions, for the treatment of excessively negative emotions, and for the design of learning environments. Since emotions, their antecedents, and their effects can be reciprocally linked over time, emotions can be regulated and changed by addressing any of the elements involved in these cyclic feedback processes (Ben-Eliyahu, 2019; Harley et al., 2019; Lobczowski, 2020; Pekrun & Stephens, 2009). Regulation and treatment can target (a) the emotion itself (*emotion-oriented* regulation and treatment, such as using drugs and relaxation techniques to cope with anxiety or employing interest-enhancing strategies to reduce boredom); (b) the control and value appraisals underlying emotions (*appraisal-oriented* regulation and treatment); (c) the competences determining individual agency (*competence-oriented* regula-

tion and treatment; e.g., training of learning skills); and (d) tasks and learning environments (*design of tasks and environments*).

Emotion regulation and ways to treat excessive negative academic emotions have mainly been studied for test anxiety (e.g., Davis et al., 2008). Specifically, test anxiety treatment is among the most successful psychological therapies available, effect sizes in randomized controlled trials often being around $d = 1$ (von der Embse et al., 2013; Zeidner, 1998). However, evidence on motivational treatment interventions suggests that interventions promoting students' adaptive control and value beliefs can have a positive influence on other emotions as well (e.g., attributional retraining, Perry et al., 2014).

Moreover, Ben-Eliyahu and Linnenbrink-Garcia (2015) examined how high school and college students' self-reported emotion regulation strategies, including reappraisal (e.g., cognitively reframing the situation to regulate emotions) and suppression (e.g., inhibiting emotional expression), related to their self-reported cognitive learning strategies (e.g., deep self-regulatory learning strategies, organizational self-regulated strategy use) and behavioral engagement in students' favorite and least favorite classes. While results varied across contexts, reappraisal was generally positively related to learning strategies for high school students. Suppression was negatively associated with learning strategies across favorite and least favorite classes for high school students and favorite classes for college students.

Conclusion

As argued in this chapter, emotions are critically important for students' engagement with academic tasks and resulting learning outcomes. Engagement and achievement, in turn, are drivers for students' personality development, career trajectories, and psychological health. As such, due to their influence on engagement, academic emotions are also critically important for positive development in youth more broadly. Emotions likely influence all major types of cognitive, motivational, and behavioral engagement contributing to students' academic success. Much of the initial research supporting this conclusion was conducted by cognitive psychologists and neuroscientists in laboratory studies, far removed from the reality of academic contexts. Research on students' emotions in real-world academic settings has grown substantially during the past 25 years but is clearly still in a nascent stage.

To better understand the role of emotions for students' engagement, we suggest several areas for future research. First, researchers should investigate a variety of forms of emotions (achievement, epistemic, topic, and social) that may be relevant in educational contexts. There is a growing body of research on achievement emotions, but relatively little research on epistemic emotions or social emotions. We still know little about how emotions emerge in response to specific task elements or in relation to social interactions in classroom. Given the close proximity of epistemic and social emotions to the learning activity itself, studying emotions at this level may be especially fruitful for understanding how emotions shape engagement in school.

Second, the diversity of theoretical definitions has plagued emotion research in other fields. Thus, we urge researchers conducting research on emotions in educational settings to be clear about how they define emotions within the context of education, and to carefully match the theoretical conceptualization of emotions with their assessment instruments. Third, within affective neuroscience, great strides have been made in understanding the neurological bases for emotions and their link to other aspects of psychological functioning (e.g., Immordino-Yang et al., 2009). Researchers studying emotions in the classroom should be aware of the implications of this research, especially with respect to the implicit aspects of emotions and the way in which emotions shape cognitive processing.

Furthermore, the reciprocal aspects of emotions are often neglected. Yet the models we discussed highlight the dynamic quality of emotions and engagement. Future research needs to develop better methods for unpacking these dynamic relations across time, including intensive longitudinal studies and use of within-person analytic designs (Murayama et al., 2017). Finally, if we are to truly understand the role of emotions in classroom settings, we need to design learning environments that are emotionally adaptive for students and test the effectiveness of these environments. Instructional design researchers have made a promising start in creating virtual learning environments that help to reach this aim (see Lajoie et al., 2020; Loderer et al., 2020b). Further, we have also made recommendations for instructional design principles to be used in the classroom (Linnenbrink-Garcia, Patall, et al., 2016), but these have yet to be more widely tested with respect to emotions.

References

Alsop, S., & Watts, M. (2003). Science education and affect. *International Journal of Science Education, 25*(9), 1043–1047. https://doi.org/10.1080/0950069032000052180

Aspinwall, L. (1998). Rethinking the role of positive affect in self-regulation. *Motivation and Emotion, 22*(1), 1–32.

Bakhtiar, A., Webster, E. A., & Hadwin, A. F. (2018). Regulation and socio-emotional interactions in a positive and negative group climate. *Metacognition and Learning, 13*(1), 57–90. https://doi.org/10.1007/s11409-017-9178-x

Barrett, F. L., Lewis, M., & Haviland-Jones, J. M. (Eds.). (2016). *Handbook of emotions* (4th ed.). Guilford.

Barrett, L. F., & Russell, J. A. (1998). Independence and bipolarity in the structure of current affect. *Journal of Personality and Social Psychology, 74*(4), 967–984. https://doi.org/10.1037/0022-3514.74.4.967

Barroso, C., Ganley, C. M., McGraw, A. L., Geer, E. A., Hart, S. A., & Daucourt, M. C. (2021). A meta-analysis of the relation between math anxiety and math achievement. *Psychological Bulletin, 147*(2), 134–168. https://doi.org/10.1037/bul000030

Ben-Eliyahu, A. (2019). Academic emotional learning: A critical component of self-regulated learning in the emotional learning cycle. *Educational Psychologist, 54*(2), 84–105. https://doi.org/10.1080/00461520.2019.1582345

Ben-Eliyahu, A., & Linnenbrink-Garcia, L. (2015). Integrating the regulation of affect, behavior, and cognition into self-regulated learning paradigms among secondary and post-secondary students. *Metacognition and Learning, 10*(1), 15–42. https://doi.org/10.1007/s11409-014-9129-8

Bohn-Gettler, C. M. (2019). Getting a grip: The PET framework for studying how reader emotions influence comprehension. *Discourse Processes, 56*(5–6), 386–401. https://doi.org/10.1080/0163853x.2019.1611174

Broughton, S. H., Sinatra, G. M., & Nussbaum, E. M. (2013). "Pluto has been a planet my whole life!" Emotions, attitudes, and conceptual change in elementary students learning about Pluto's reclassification. *Research in Science Education, 43*(2), 529–550. https://doi.org/10.1007/s11165-011-9274-x

Camacho-Morles, J., Slemp, G. R., Pekrun, R., Loderer, K., Hou, H., & Oades, L. G. (2021). Activity achievement emotions and academic performance: A meta-analysis. *Educational Psychology Review, 33*(3), 1051–1095. https://doi.org/10.1007/s10648-020-09585-3

Carver, C. S., & Harmon-Jones, E. (2009). Anger is an approach-related affect: Evidence and implications. *Psychological Bulletin, 135*(2), 183–204. https://doi.org/10.1037/a0013965

Carver, C. S., Lawrence, J. W., & Scheier, M. F. (1996). A control-process perspective on the origins of affect. In L. L. Martin & A. Tesser (Eds.), *Striving and feeling: Interactions among goals, affect, and self-regulation* (pp. 11–52). Lawrence Erlbaum.

Davis, H. A., DiStefano, C., & Schutz, P. A. (2008). Identifying patterns of appraising tests in first-year college students: Implications for anxiety and emotion regulation during test taking. *Journal of Educational Psychology, 100*(4), 942–960. https://doi.org/10.1037/a0013096

Do, S. L., & Schallert, D. L. (2004). Emotions and classroom talk: Toward a model of the role of affect in students' experiences of classroom discussions. *Journal of Educational Psychology, 96*(4), 619–634. https://doi.org/10.1037/0022-0663.96.4.619

Elliot, A. J., & McGregor, H. A. (2001). A 2 × 2 achievement goal framework. *Journal of Personality and Social Psychology, 80*(3), 501–519. https://doi.org/10.1037/0022-3514.80.3.501

Elliot, A. J., Murayama, K., & Pekrun, R. (2011). A 3 × 2 achievement goal model. *Journal of Educational Psychology, 103*(3), 632–648. https://doi.org/10.1037/a0023952

Fiedler, K., & Beier, S. (2014). Affect and cognitive processes in educational contexts. In R. Pekrun & L. Linnenbrink-Garcia (Eds.), *International handbook of emotions in education* (pp. 36–55). Taylor & Francis.

Forgas, J. P. (2017). Can sadness be good for you? *Australian Psychologist, 52*(1), 3–13. https://doi.org/10.1111/ap.12232

Forsblom, L., Pekrun, R., Peixoto, F., & Loderer, K. (2022). Cognitive appraisals, achievement emotions, and students' math achievement: A longitudinal analysis. *Journal of Educational Psychology, 114*(2), 346.

Fredricks, J. A., Blumenfeld, P. C., & Paris, A. H. (2004). School engagement: Potential of the concept, state of the evidence. *Review of Educational Research, 74*(1), 59–109. https://doi.org/10.3102/00346543074001059

Frederickson, B. L. (2001). The role of positive emotions in positive psychology: The broaden-and-build theory of positive emotions. *American Psychologist, 56*(3), 218–226. https://doi.org/10.1037/0003-066x.56.3.218

Frenzel, A. C., Becker-Kurz, B., Pekrun, R., Goetz, T., & Lüdtke, O. (2018). Emotion transmission in the classroom revisited: A reciprocal effects model of teacher and student enjoyment. *Journal of Educational Psychology, 110*(5), 628–639. https://doi.org/10.1037/edu0000228

Frenzel, A. C., Thrash, T. M., Pekrun, R., & Goetz, T. (2007). Achievement emotions in Germany and China: A cross-cultural validation of the Academic Emotions Questionnaire-Mathematics (AEQ-M). *Journal of Cross-Cultural Psychology, 38*(3), 302–309. https://doi.org/10.1177/0022022107300276

Gignac, G. E., & Szodorai, E. T. (2016). Effect size guidelines for individual differences researchers. *Personality and Individual Differences, 102, 74–78, S0191886916308194.* https://doi.org/10.1016/j.paid.2016.06.069

Harley, J. M., Pekrun, R., Taxer, J. L., & Gross, J. J. (2019). Emotion regulation in achievement situations: An integrated model. *Educational Psychologist, 54*(2), 106–126. https://doi.org/10.1080/00461520.2019.1587297

Hatfield, E., Cacioppo, J. T., & Rapson, R. L. (1994). *Emotional contagion.* Cambridge University Press.

Hembree, R. (1988). Correlates, causes, effects, and treatment of test anxiety. *Review of Educational Research, 58*(1), 47–77. https://doi.org/10.3102/00346543058001047

Immordino-Yang, M., McColl, A., Damasio, H., & Damasio, A. (2009). Neural correlates of admiration and compassion. *Proceedings of the National Academic of Sciences, 106*(19), 8021–8026. https://doi.org/10.1073/pnas.0810363106

Jarvenoja, H., & Jarvela, S. (2009). Emotion control in collaborative learning situations: Do students regulate emotions evoked by social challenges? *British Journal of Educational Psychology, 79*(3), 463–481. https://doi.org/10.1348/000709909x402811

Johnson, D. W., & Johnson, R. T. (1974). Instructional goal structure: Cooperative, competitive or individualistic. *Review of Educational Research, 44*(2), 213–240. https://doi.org/10.3102/00346543044002213

Kuhbandner, C., & Pekrun, R. (2013). Affective state influences retrieval-induced forgetting for integrated knowledge. *PLoS One, 8*(2), e56617. https://doi.org/10.1371/journal.pone.0056617

Lajoie, S. P., Azevedo, R., Pekrun, R., & Leighton, J. (2020). Emotions in technology-based learning environments [Special issue]. *Learning and Instruction, 70*(6), 101272.

Lane, A. M., Whyte, G. P., Terry, P. C., & Nevill, A. M. (2005). Mood, self-set goals and examination performance: The moderating effect of depressed mood.

Personality and Individual Differences, 39(1), 143–153. https://doi.org/10.1016/j.paid.2004.12.015

Lazarus, R. S., & Folkman, S. (1984). *Stress, appraisal, and coping.* Springer.

Linnenbrink, E. A. (2006). Emotion research in education: Theoretical and methodological perspectives on the integration of affect, motivation, and cognition [Special issue]. *Educational Psychology Review, 18*(4), 307–314.

Linnenbrink, E. A. (2007). The role of affect in student learning: A multi-dimensional approach to considering the interaction of affect, motivation, and engagement. In P. A. Schutz & R. Pekrun (Eds.), *Emotion in education* (pp. 107–124). Academic Press.

Linnenbrink, E. A., & Pintrich, P. R. (2002a). The role of motivational beliefs in conceptual change. In M. Limon & L. Mason (Eds.), *Reconsidering conceptual change: Issues in theory and practice* (pp. 115–135). Kluwer Academic Publishers.

Linnenbrink, E. A., & Pintrich, P. R. (2002b). Achievement goal theory and affect: An asymmetrical bidirectional model. *Educational Psychologist, 37*(2), 69–78. https://doi.org/10.1207/s15326985ep3702_2

Linnenbrink, E. A., & Pintrich, P. R. (2004). Role of affect in cognitive processing in academic contexts. In D. Dai & R. Sternberg (Eds.), *Motivation, emotion, and cognition: Integrative perspectives on intellectual functioning and development* (pp. 57–87). Lawrence Erlbaum.

Linnenbrink, E. A., Ryan, A. M., & Pintrich, P. R. (1999). The role of goals and affect in working memory functioning. *Learning and Individual Differences, 11*(2), 213–230. https://doi.org/10.1016/s1041-6080(00)80006-0

Linnenbrink-Garcia, L., & Barger, M. M. (2014). Achievement goals and emotions. In R. Pekrun & L. Linnenbrink-Garcia (Eds.), *International handbook of emotions in education* (pp. 142–161). Taylor & Francis.

Linnenbrink-Garcia, L., Patall, E. A., & Pekrun, R. (2016). Adaptive motivation and emotion in education: Research and principles for instructional design. *Policy Insights from Behavioral and Brain Sciences, 3*(2), 228–236. https://doi.org/10.1177/2372732216644450

Linnenbrink-Garcia, L., & Pekrun, R. (2011). Students' emotions and academic engagement [special issue]. *Contemporary Educational Psychology, 36*(1), 1–3.

Linnenbrink-Garcia, L., Rogat, T. M., & Koskey, K. L. (2011). Affect during small group interaction: Implications for students' engagement. *Contemporary Educational Psychology, 36*(1), 13–24. https://doi.org/10.1016/j.cedpsych.2010.09.001

Linnenbrink-Garcia, L., Wormington, S. V., & Ranellucci, J. (2016). Measuring affect in educational contexts: A circumplex approach. In M. Zembylas & P. A. Schutz (Eds.), *Methodological advances in research on emotion and education* (pp. 165–178). Springer.

Lobczowski, N. G. (2020). Bridging gaps and moving forward: Building a new model for socioemotional formation and regulation. *Educational Psychologist,* 55(2), 53–68. https://doi.org/10.1080/00461520.2019.1670064

Loderer, K., Pekrun, R., & Lester, J. C. (2020a). Beyond cold technology: A systematic review and meta-analysis on emotions in technology-based learning environments. *Learning and Instruction, 70*, 101162. https://doi.org/10.1016/j.learninstruc.2018.08.002

Loderer, K., Pekrun, R., & Plass, J. L. (2020b). Emotional foundations of game-based learning. In J. L. Plass, B. D. Homer, & R. E. Mayer (Eds.), *Handbook of game-based learning* (pp. 111–151). MIT Press.

Madan, C. R., Scott, S. M., & Kensinger, E. A. (2019). Positive emotion enhances association-memory. *Emotion, 19*(4), 733–740. https://doi.org/10.1037/emo0000465

Meece, J. L., Wigfield, A., & Eccles, J. S. (1990). Predictors of math anxiety and its influence on young adolescents' course enrolment intentions and performance in mathematics. *Journal of Educational Psychology, 82*(1), 60–70. https://doi.org/10.1037/0022-0663.82.1.60

Meinhardt, J., & Pekrun, R. (2003). Attentional resource allocation to emotional events: An ERP study. *Cognition and Emotion, 17*(3), 477–500. https://doi.org/10.1080/02699930244000039

Miele, D. B., & Scholer, A. A. (2018). The role of meta-motivational monitoring in motivation regulation. *Educational Psychologist, 53*(1), 1–21. https://doi.org/10.1080/00461520.2017.1371601

Mikels, J. A., & Reuter-Lorenz, P. A. (2019). Affective working memory: An integrative psychological construct. *Perspectives on Psychological Science, 14*(4), 543–559. https://doi.org/10.1177/1745691619837597

Murayama, K., Goetz, T., Malmberg, L.-E., Pekrun, R., Tanaka, A., & Martin, A. J. (2017). Within-person analysis in educational psychology: Importance and illustrations. In D. W. Putwain & K. Smart (Eds.), *British journal of educational psychology monograph series II: Psychological aspects of education – Current trends: The role of competence beliefs in teaching and learning* (pp. 71–87). Wiley.

Nummenmaa, M., & Nummenmaa, L. (2008). University students' emotions, interest and activities in a web-based learning environment. *British Journal of Educational Psychology, 78*(1), 163–178. https://doi.org/10.1348/000709907x203733

Organization for Economic Cooperation and Development. (2016). *PISA 2015 results (volume 1): Excellence and equity in education.* Author.

Parrott, W. G., & Spackman, M. P. (2000). Emotion and memory. In M. Lewis & J. M. Haviland-Jones (Eds.), *Handbook of emotions* (2nd ed., pp. 476–490). Guilford.

Pekrun, R. (1992a). The impact of emotions on learning and achievement: Towards a theory of cognitive/motivational mediators. *Applied Psychology, 41*(4), 359–376. https://doi.org/10.1111/j.1464-0597.1992.tb00712.x

Pekrun, R. (1992b). Expectancy-value theory of anxiety: Overview and implications. In D. G. Forgays, T. Sosnowski, & K. Wrzesniewski (Eds.), *Anxiety:*

Recent developments in self-appraisal, psychophysiological and health research (pp. 23–41). Hemisphere.

Pekrun, R. (2006). The control-value theory of achievement emotions: Assumptions, corollaries, and implications for educational research and practice. *Educational Psychology Review, 18*(4), 315–341. https://doi.org/10.1007/s10648-006-9029-9

Pekrun, R. (2018). Control-value theory: A social-cognitive approach to achievement emotions. In G. A. D. Liem & D. M. McInerney (Eds.), *Big theories revisited 2: A volume of research on sociocultural influences on motivation and learning* (pp. 162–190). Information Age Publishing.

Pekrun, R. (2021). Self-appraisals and emotions: A generalized control-value approach. In T. Dicke, F. Guay, H. W. Marsh, R. G. Craven, & D. M. McInerney (Eds.), *Self – A multidisciplinary concept* (pp. 1–30). Information Age Publishing.

Pekrun, R. (in press). Jingle-jangle fallacies in motivation science: Towards a definition of core motivation. In M. Bong, S. Kim, & J. Reeve (Eds.), *Motivation science: Controversies and insights*. Oxford University Press.

Pekrun, R., Elliot, A. J., & Maier, M. A. (2009). Achievement goals and achievement emotions: Testing a model of their joint relations with academic performance. *Journal of Educational Psychology, 101*(1), 115–135. https://doi.org/10.1037/a0013383

Pekrun, R., Goetz, T., Daniels, L. M., Stupnisky, R. H., & Perry, R. P. (2010). Boredom in achievement settings: Control-value antecedents and performance outcomes of a neglected emotion. *Journal of Educational Psychology, 102*(3), 531–549. https://doi.org/10.1037/a0019243

Pekrun, R., Goetz, T., Frenzel, A. C., Barchfeld, P., & Perry, R. P. (2011). Measuring emotions in students' learning and performance: The Achievement Emotions Questionnaire (AEQ). *Contemporary Educational Psychology, 36*(1), 36–48. https://doi.org/10.1016/j.cedpsych.2010.10.002

Pekrun, R., Goetz, T., Titz, W., & Perry, R. P. (2002). Academic emotions in students' self-regulated learning and achievement: A program of quantitative and qualitative research. *Educational Psychologist, 37*(2), 91–106. https://doi.org/10.1207/s15326985ep3702_4

Pekrun, R., Lichtenfeld, S., Marsh, H. W., Murayama, K., & Goetz, T. (2017). Achievement emotions and academic performance: Longitudinal models of reciprocal effects. *Child Development, 88*(5), 1653–1670. https://doi.org/10.1111/cdev.12704

Pekrun, R., & Linnenbrink-Garcia, L. (Eds.). (2014). *International handbook of emotions in education.* Francis & Taylor/Routledge.

Pekrun, R., & Marsh, H. W. (2018). Weiner's attribution theory: Indispensable – But is it immune to crisis? *Motivation Science, 4*(1), 19–20. https://doi.org/10.1037/mot0000096

Pekrun, R., Marsh, H. W., Suessenbach, F., Frenzel, A. C., & Goetz, T. (in press). School grades and students' emotions: Longitudinal models of within-person reciprocal effects. Learning and Instruction.

Pekrun, R., Muis, K. R., Frenzel, A. C., & Goetz, T. (2017). *Emotions at school.* Taylor & Francis/Routledge.

Pekrun, R., Murayama, K., Marsh, H. W., Goetz, T., & Frenzel, A. C. (2019). Happy fish in little ponds: Testing a reference group model of achievement and emotion. *Journal of Personality and Social Psychology, 117*(1), 166–185. https://doi.org/10.1037/pspp0000230

Pekrun, R., & Stephens, E. J. (2009). Goals, emotions, and emotion regulation: Perspectives of the control-value theory of achievement emotions. *Human Development, 52*(6), 357–365. https://doi.org/10.1159/000242349

Pekrun, R., & Stephens, E. J. (2012). Academic emotions. In K. R. Harris, S. Graham, T. Urdan, J. M. Royer, & M. Zeidner (Eds.), *APA educational psychology handbook* (Vol. 2, pp. 3–31). American Psychological Association.

Perry, R. P., Chipperfield, J. G., Hladkyj, S., Pekrun, R., & Hamm, J. M. (2014). Attribution-based treatment interventions in some achievement settings. In S. Karabenick & T. C. Urdan (Eds.), *Advances in motivation and achievement* (Vol. 18, pp. 1–35). Emerald.

Pintrich, P. R. (2000). The role of goal orientation in self-regulated learning. In M. Boekarts, P. R. Pintrich, & M. Zeidner (Eds.), *Handbook of self-regulation: Theory, research and applications* (pp. 451–502). Academic Press.

Plass, J. L., & Kaplan, U. (2016). Emotional design in digital media for learning. In S. Y. Tettegah & M. Gartmeier (Eds.), *Emotions, technology, design, and learning* (pp. 131–161). Elsevier.

Putwain, D. W., Symes, W., & Wilkinson, H. M. (2017). Fear appeals, engagement, and examination performance: The role of challenge and threat appraisals. *British Journal of Educational Psychology, 87*(1), 16–31. https://doi.org/10.1111/bjep.12132

Ranellucci, J., Robinson, K. A., Rosenberg, J. M., Lee, Y.-k., Roseth, C. J., & Linnenbrink-Garcia, L. (2021). Comparing the roles and correlates of emotions in class and during online video lectures in a flipped anatomy classroom. *Contemporary Educational Psychology, 65*, 101966.

Reisenzein, R. (2001). Appraisal processes conceptualized from a schema-theoretic perspective. In K. R. Scherer, A. Schorr, & T. Johnstone (Eds.), *Appraisal processes in emotion* (pp. 187–201). Oxford University Press.

Reisenzein, R., Horstmann, G., & Schützwohl, A. (2019). The cognitive-evolutionary model of surprise: A review of the evidence. *Topics in Cognitive Science, 11*(1), 50–74. https://doi.org/10.1111/tops.12292

Robinson, K. A., Ranellucci, J., Lee, Y.-K., Wormington, S. V., Roseth, C. J., & Linnenbrink-Garcia, L. (2017). Affective profiles and academic success in a college science course. *Contemporary Educational Psychology, 51*, 209–221. https://doi.org/10.1016/j.cedpsych.2017.08.004

Rogat, T. K., & Linnenbrink-Garcia, L. (2011). Socially shared regulation in collaborative groups: An analysis of the interplay between quality of social regulation and group processes. *Cognition & Instruction, 29*(4), 375–415. https://doi.org/10.1080/07370008.2011.607930

Scherer, K. R., & Moors, A. (2019). The emotion process: Event appraisal and component differentiation. *Annual Review of Psychology, 70*(1), 719–745. https://doi.org/10.1146/annurev-psych-122216-011854

Schwartz, N. (2012). Feelings-as-information theory. In P. A. M. Van Lange, A. Kruglanski, & E. T. Higgins (Eds.), *Handbook of theories of social psychology* (pp. 289–308). Sage.

Shao, K., Pekrun, R., Marsh, H. W., & Loderer, K. (2020). Control-value appraisals, achievement emotions, and foreign language performance: A latent interaction analysis. *Learning and Instruction, 69*, 101356. https://doi.org/10.1016/j.learninstruc.2020.101356

Tsai, Y.-M., Kunter, M., Lüdtke, O., & Trautwein, U. (2008). What makes lessons interesting? The role of situational and individual factors in three school subjects. *Journal of Educational Psychology, 100*(2), 460–472. https://doi.org/10.1037/0022-0663.100.2.460

Turner, J. E., & Schallert, D. L. (2001). Expectancy-value relationships of shame reactions and shame resiliency. *Journal of Educational Psychology, 93*(2), 320–329. https://doi.org/10.1037/0022-0663.93.2.320

Turner, J. E., & Waugh, R. M. (2007). A dynamical systems perspective regarding students' learning processes: Shame reactions and emergent self-organizations. In P. A. Schutz & R. Pekrun (Eds.), *Emotions in education* (pp. 125–145). Academic Press.

Tyson, D. F., Linnenbrink-Garcia, L., & Hill, N. E. (2009). Regulating debilitating emotions in the context of performance: Achievement goal orientations, achievement-elicited emotions, and socialization contexts. *Human Development, 52*(6), 329–356. https://doi.org/10.1159/000242348

von der Embse, N., Barterian, J., & Segool, N. (2013). Test anxiety interventions for children and adolescents: A systematic review of treatment studies from 2000-2010. *Psychology in the Schools, 50*(1), 57–71. https://doi.org/10.1002/pits.21660

von der Embse, N., Jester, D., Roy, D., & Post, J. (2018). Test anxiety effects, predictors, and correlates: A 30-year meta-analytic review. *Journal of Affective Disorders, 227*, 483–493. https://doi.org/10.1016/j.jad.2017.11.048

Vuorela, M., & Nummenmaa, L. (2004). Experienced emotions, emotion regulation and student activity in a web-based learning environment. *European Journal of Psychology of Education, 19*(4), 423–436. https://doi.org/10.1007/bf03173219

Weiner, B. (1985). An attributional theory of achievement motivation and emotion. *Psychological Review, 92*(4), 548–573. https://doi.org/10.1037/0033-295x.92.4.548

Weiner, B. (2018). The legacy of an attribution approach to motivation and emotion: A no-crisis zone. *Motivation Science, 4*(1), 4–14. https://doi.org/10.1037/mot0000082

Wine, J. D. (1971). Test anxiety and the direction of attention. *Psychological Bulletin, 76*(2), 92–104. https://doi.org/10.1037/h0031332

Wolters, C. A. (2003). Regulation of motivation: Evaluating an underemphasized aspect of self-regulated learning. *Educational Psychologist, 38*(4), 189–205. https://doi.org/10.1207/s15326985ep3804_1

Wosnitza, M., & Volet, S. (2005). Origin, direction and impact of emotions in social online learning. *Learning and Instruction, 15*(5), 449–464. https://doi.org/10.1016/j.learninstruc.2005.07.009

Zeidner, M. (1998). *Test anxiety: The state of the art.* Plenum.

School Belonging and Student Engagement: The Critical Overlaps, Similarities, and Implications for Student Outcomes

Kelly-Ann Allen ⓘ and Christopher Boyle ⓘ

Abstract

The theoretical and empirical literature has long included belonging as central to student engagement. Some conceptualizations and approaches have suggested that a student's sense of belonging is a central and foundational principle underpinning engagement. Engagement also contributes to a sense of belonging. Two distinct literatures have developed insights around the importance of, pathways to, and outcomes associated with each construct. This chapter narratively explores similarities and differences between belonging and student engagement, identifying areas of overlap as well as helpful distinctions, with implications for research and educational practice. Although the two are closely connected, these two friends are more effectively treated as complementary constructs, both of

K.-A. Allen (✉)
School of Educational Psychology and Counselling, Faculty of Education, Monash University, Clayton, Australia

Centre for Wellbeing Science, Melbourne Graduate School of Education, Melbourne University, Parkville, Australia
e-mail: Kelly-Ann.Allen@Monash.edu

C. Boyle
School of Education, University of Adelaide, Adelaide, Australia
e-mail: chris.boyle@adelaide.edu.au

which are essential components for positive development in young people.

School Belonging and Student Engagement: The Critical Overlaps, Similarities, and Implications for Student Outcomes

The controversial "Two Pretty Best Friends" meme began when Jordan Scott (also known as @jayrscottyy) recorded a video post and posted it on the social media platform TikTok (www.tiktok.com). The well-connected Scott shared a cryptic phrase: "I ain't ever seen 2 pretty best friends, always one of em gotta [sic.] be ugly." The words quickly became a meme that went viral, spreading across various social media platforms. The saying could imply that two things of equal beauty rarely work together side by side.

Although the meme was met with significant backlash, to some degree, this modern saying resonates with psychological research around assets and deficits. To justify relevance, positive psychological assets are often contrasted with negative psychological deficits. For instance, engagement in learning is contrasted with boredom. Happiness is contrasted with mental illness. Belonging and prosociality are contrasted with loneliness and antisocial behavior. But can two pretty best friends walk hand-in-hand?

This chapter highlights one example of two pretty best friends: belonging and engagement. At times these are viewed as the same construct; at other times one is seen as critical to the other, or they are competing priorities for the limited time and resources within schools. Extensive research indicates that student engagement and school belonging matter (e.g., Korpershoek et al., 2019; Li, 2011; St-Amand et al., 2017). Voelkl (2012), in the first edition of the *Handbook of Research on Student Engagement*, reviewed the role of school identification in influencing the social and learning behaviors of students. The assumptions were that school identification mainly involves emotions rather than cognitions, consists of a specific set of attitudes which ultimately define student behavior at school, and takes time. It is worth noting that the focus of Voelkl's (2012) perspective drew from Finn's participation-identification model (Finn, 1989). Despite the model being represented as a relatively simple two-component model, it afforded engagement dimensions to be grouped into either those which involve behavior (participation component) or those which relate to emotions (identification component). According to Voelkl, student identification was likely to influence social as well as learning behaviors in a way that was yet to be clarified.

In the framework proposed by Voelkl (2012), two main components of identification in Finn's model, namely belonging and valuing, were first introduced. With belonging set to be defined later in this chapter, here it suffices to mention that this first component has been recognized as a basic human necessity which needs to be fulfilled. As students strive to fulfill their need to belong, they form relationships with teachers and peers and may even become active participants in school activities, including academic work. When students succeed, their achievements not only become a source of motivation but also encourage positive behavior which, in turn, can further improve academic performance. Similarly, people have a need to feel that they are of value. Within the school context, *valuing*, the second component of Finn's model, can be either of personal importance, where students show interest and enjoyment from school tasks or satisfaction

at good grades, or of practical importance (i.e., recognizing that schools are important to obtain good qualifications or to secure a good job). In this case, by building on well-established theories as well as empirical data, Voelkl pointed out that efforts, engagement, and persistence in learning were more likely to be observed when students value school work, with academic success also more likely to follow. Hence, giving high importance to certain tasks can be a major source of motivation.

Considering the assumptions of the proposed framework by Voelkl (2012) in the previous edition of the Handbook, it was assumed that once school identification was achieved (i.e., the need for belonging and valuing were fulfilled), students would be more engaged and have more positive attitudes toward school, with the latter eventually shaping student behavior in a positive manner. Voelkl's (2012) framework, therefore, seeks to make clear that school identification is "an intrinsic form of achievement motivation that encourages students to engage in appropriate learning behaviors" (Voelkl, 2012, p. 194), however, it was also recognize that positive behavior was not a spontaneous process. That is, when students enter schools, they already have certain feelings toward school as well as some early forms of behavior. But as they progress through different grades, the action of external motivators, such as specific behaviors being imposed or encouraged by parents and teachers (e.g., learning, doing homework), may reinforce certain attitudes. Eventually these students, especially those with an increased sense of belonging and those who give value to academic activities, adopt these externally motivated behaviors as their own, which turn into a form of intrinsic motivation. In fact, this whole process may be encouraged by certain school conditions such as a safe environment or a supportive classroom, which are referred to as "contextual facilitating conditions." Taken together, it can be said that the main concept behind Voelkl's proposed framework was to consider school identification and student engagement mainly in terms of emotions generated through school experiences (i.e., emotions produced by a feeling of connectedness with the school, or felt when successfully completing tasks which are believed to be important).

In this chapter, a different approach is used where school belonging and student engagement will be viewed as distinct and independent constructs that intertwine and complement one another. As such, this chapter narratively synthesizes theory and research on belonging and engagement, including historical considerations, examination of terminology, definitions, theories, and frameworks appearing in the literature in order to identify areas of similarity and distinction. As a whole, our review illustrates that belonging is very much needed for engagement and vice versa. For the sake of educational outcomes, the two constructs of belonging and engagement are indeed best friends that together should be emphasized in schools, not viewed as competing. We conclude with implications for research and educational practice.

Beginning with Belonging

The need to belong is considered to be a universal need which is innate and common to most human beings (Allen, 2020a; Allen, Kern et al., 2021). Although a sense of belonging is, in a general way, important to the social lives of people, it is particularly valuable within a school setting (Allen & Kern, 2017, 2019). School belonging has been recognized by many researchers as being associated with academic motivation and positive school outcomes such as participation in extracurricular activities and school attendance (Anderman & Freeman, 2004; Irvin et al., 2011; Shochet et al., 2011). Interestingly, such positive associations can even be found for students across different grades, thereby further indicating that school belonging is an important component of students' school lives (Korpershoek et al., 2019). Despite its importance in education, school belonging has been studied and defined in numerous ways (Allen & Bowles, 2012; Libbey, 2004; O'Brien & Bowles, 2013). Allen and Bowles (2012) described the field of school belonging as "unsystematic and diluted" (p. 108) due to disparities in definition and terminology.

Despite the absence of a universal definition for school belonging, St-Amand et al. (2017) identified three key attributes of school belonging. First, it is a major factor which contributes to the psychological development of an individual in a positive way. This has also been recognized by other researchers who have pointed to findings that school belonging is essential for personal identification and a social identity—which are key development processes of adolescence (Allen & Bowles, 2012; Verhoeven et al., 2019). The second key attribute of a sense of belonging is that it is a basic need that leads to social bonding between people as well as affiliations with members of a group (Hagerty et al., 1996). This attribute, explained in the specific context of school settings by Langevin (1999), emphasises the importance of social relationships in both the formal and informal aspects of school life. Similarly, while suggesting that friendships are important components of belonging, Williams and Downing (1998, p. 103) state:

> Students thought that being a part of the class meant that they had a place in the classroom, felt welcomed, wanted, and respected by their classmates and teachers. Being familiar with their classmates and having friends who understood them made the student feel as if he or she belonged to a group and/or to a class as a whole.

The final defining attribute involves four key terms or characteristics which clearly differentiate school belonging from other concepts: positive emotions, positive social relations, involvement, and harmonization (i.e., "individuals must adapt and adjust by changing personal aspects to align with any situations or people" St-Amand et al., 2017, p. 109). Altogether, these defining features and characteristics not only help to better define school belonging but also to identify its main components so as to develop more accurate means of measuring the concept.

School or Student Engagement

School engagement and student engagement are terms that have become widely used in educational settings. Before proceeding, it is worth noting that although the two terms are often used interchangeably, they may actually refer to two distinct concepts. In this context, Appleton et al. (2008) noted that the former places emphasis on the importance of school contexts, hence the name school engagement. On the other hand, since the focus of student engagement is on an individual, it takes into account the psychology, behavior, and academic achievement as well as the influence of families and friends on the students. However, for the purpose of this work, despite prior distinctions, the two terms will be used interchangeably or referred to as the general term "engagement." The concept of engagement is intricately linked to that of school belonging. It refers to "students' expression of opinions or attitudes and behaviors" (Wonglorsaichon et al., 2014, p. 1749). However, Bakadorova and Raufelder (2017), basing their definition on the work of previous researchers, have provided a more comprehensive definition of school engagement as being that of a complex and multidimensional construct consisting of two or three components, namely:

- *Behavioral engagement*—involves active participation in school-related activities (both curricular and extracurricular), good conduct and absence of disobedience to school regulations (Engels et al., 2016; Finn, 1993; Skinner & Belmont, 1993).
- *Emotional engagement*—refers to students' relationships and emotions toward their peers, academics, and the school in general (Skinner, Kindermann, & Furrer, 2009), thereby allowing students to identify themselves with their schools (Finn, 1989; Skinner & Belmont, 1993).
- *Cognitive engagement*—[also referred to as "psychological investment"] where students display learning motivation and are willing to put in the required efforts to learn or develop their own learning process, especially when new or complex ideas are concerned (Fredricks et al., 2004; Newmann et al., 1992).

More recently, the inclusion of a fourth component known as *agentic engagement* was proposed (Dincer et al., 2019; see also Reeve & Jang, chapter "Agentic Engagement", this volume). According to Reeve (2013), it refers to the active and constructive contributions demonstrated by students during the learning process. However, it is also recognized that more research is needed in order to determine whether it is, indeed, a distinct concept, which has different predictive value when compared to the three components of engagement (i.e., behavioral, emotional, cognitive) (Eccles, 2016). From this definition, it is clear that engagement can play an important role in influencing students' achievement. Indeed, as pointed out by Lippman and Rivers (2008) who described similar components, school engagement can improve academic performance and promote attendance in school while inhibiting risky or negative youth behaviors. However, it would be remiss not to point out that this concept was not always recognized as a valuable part of youth development. This is described by Li (2011) who stated that although it was known that children's enthusiasm for learning deteriorated as they went through the school system—elementary to middle to high school (Skinner, Kindermann, Connell, & Wellborn, 2009; Wigfield et al., 2006)—this reduced motivation was mostly attributed to undesirable behaviors such as smoking, drinking, drug use, unsafe sex, teenage pregnancy, and violence among young people. As such, a great deal of research focused on preventing these negative behaviors from manifesting so as to ensure a smoother transition through students' lives. Eventually, it became clear that this simplistic view was limited and not cognizant of the wider issues of school belonging and engagement. Active school contributions through school engagement is now a widely accepted possible solution to decreasing academic motivation and achievement (Bosnjak et al., 2017; Chodkiewicz & Boyle, 2016; Fredricks et al., 2004).

A Definitional Overlap

Although the two terms of school belonging and student engagement are clearly distinguished, they are intricately linked to each other. Indeed, the two concepts often overlap at different levels whether in terms of definitions, constructs or the measures used. For instance, some definitions of school engagement are still akin to descriptions of school belonging and, therefore, it is not surprising to note that the two terms have been used interchangeably in some research (O'Brennan & Furlong, 2010), with disengagement being used to describe not belonging to school (Willms, 2000). Moreover, in The Organisation for Economic Co-operative Development (OECD)'s Programme for International Student Assessment (PISA) report, Willms referred to school belonging as:

> A psychological component pertaining to students' sense of belonging at school and acceptance of school values, and a behavioral component pertaining to participation in school activities . . . the term disengaged from school is used to characterize students who do not feel they belong at school and have withdrawn from school activities in a significant way (Willms, 2000, p. 8).

Similarly, when considering the individual components of engagement, it will be noted that the concept of emotional engagement, as defined before, encompasses students' relationships and emotions toward their peers and teachers and, therefore, it is concerned with feelings toward the school or school characteristics in general (Skinner, Kindermann, & Furrer, 2009). According to Sciarra and Seirup (2008), this feeling represents a form of care for the school and can be translated into a feeling of belongingness. As such, it is not surprising that this has led Korpershoek et al. (2019) to consider both terms (school belonging and emotional engagement) to be similar, at least in the way in which they have been conceptualized. In fact, as it will be noted later, it is this similarity between belongingness and emotional engagement which is often highlighted when considering how the two terms overlap, although to some extent, similarities with behavioral or cognitive forms of engagement may also be observed.

Furlong et al. (2013) tried to disentangle the overlap between school belonging (and its regular synonyms of school connectedness, school bonding, sense of school membership) and school engagement. In their research, they present the notion that there are two types of engagement that explains why sometimes school belonging and school engagement are used to mean the same construct. Furlong et al. (2013) proposed that the first type of engagement used by researchers relates to academic outcomes and the second type relates more to the affective state and relationships which a student experiences—the latter being more akin to school belonging.

Furlong et al. (2013) also focused on the behavioral aspect of school belonging and engagement by considering a gratitude component as being highly influential in affecting the cognitive component such as self-esteem. Gratitude is a crucial aspect of belonging where both teachers and students can appreciate the roles that others play in the school environment, thereby understanding that engagement can be seen in the effort of others. This can increase social cohesion and "...teachers can encourage appreciative responding in students by emphasizing and reinforcing kind acts in the classroom, and teachers and staff can model reciprocity and thankfulness in coordinated activities with students" (Furlong et al., 2013, p. 71). Understanding the roles that school staff plays in the school and how much commitment is invested is crucial to being able to appreciate the gratitude component. If gratitude is used well, it could facilitate a place where young people feel valued leading to a greater sense of belonging benefiting all members of the school community. Furlong et al. (2003) are straightforward and suggest that engagement is over a long rather than short period and if used appropriately it is about "...inoculating students against the consequences of poor school bonding" (p. 111).

Theories and Frameworks

Models and Frameworks of School Engagement

School engagement is undoubtedly an important factor that influences a student's academic achievements, thereby exerting a direct influence on his or her school career (Appleton et al., 2008;

Fredricks et al., 2004). As such, this concept has been widely investigated by different researchers who eventually came up with different models or theoretical frameworks in order to gain a better understanding of school engagement as well as ways through which it could be fostered. However, through these frameworks, school engagement is not only regarded as the final objective but also as a means of promoting or predicting positive outcomes (e.g., high academic achievement) or preventing negative ones (e.g., school dropout) (Frydenberg et al., 2005; Ryan & Deci, 2009). Li (2011) identified four key frameworks of engagement which can be applied within the school setting. An overview of these models indicates that they are often derived from general theories but each focuses on constructs which attempt to explain how certain variables influence school engagement in general or its individual components (i.e., behavioral, emotional, or cognitive engagement). Hence, a common feature of engagement models is that they consider school engagement as malleable and that, by identifying its predictors, engagement can be promoted.

School Reform and Motivational Models

According to Finn and Zimmer (2012), one of the earliest models recognizes that school engagement is influenced by the school setting. Based on this, Newmann (1981) suggested that only important reforms to those settings could lead to an increase in school engagement and for this purpose, six possible changes or guiding principles were proposed. This concept was later taken up by Wehlage et al. (1989) who also advocated the need for school reforms, but instead of promoting engagement, these reforms were viewed as a means of preventing dropouts. However, it should be noted that in order to implement reforms, prior knowledge of the type of school settings which influence engagement is required. In this context, Fredricks et al. (2004) noted that the school settings being referred to in this model can be of two types. First, they can occur at the school-level which basically represents certain school characteristics that can alter school

engagement. For instance, in one historical study, it was found that schools of small sizes provided students with more opportunities to participate in extracurricular activities while developing social relationships (Barker & Gump, 1964). Similarly, in terms of school practices, it was assumed, despite conflicting results, that adopting fair and flexible rules could decrease risks of disengagement (Finn & Voelkl, 1993; Natriello, 1984). Therefore, educational reforms should occur beyond the classroom and school leadership should have a central role.

The classroom context, itself, is a multidimensional construct involving different components which can broadly be classified as being organizational, instructional, or social (Dotterer & Lowe, 2011). In the case of classroom structure, this refers to the expectations which teachers have regarding the social and academic behavior of students, the extent to which these expectations are made clear and the establishment of rules or norms which are applied when these expectations are not met (Connell, 1990; Fredricks et al., 2004). Although not many studies examine the link between classroom structure and engagement, evidence has shown that clearer expectations and work rules were positively associated with higher cognitive, emotional and behavioral engagement, with the latter being especially visible in the form of less disciplinary issues (Connell & Wellborn, 1991; Doyle, 1986; Fredricks et al., 2002).

The concepts of autonomy support and task characteristics are identified as potentially increasing engagement in the classroom environment. According to researchers, autonomy is supported when students are offered the opportunity to choose and participate in decision-making processes while not being pressured into doing schoolwork or displaying good behavior by control measures such as rewards and punishments (Connell, 1990; Deci & Ryan, 1985). Although such conditions are believed to enhance engagement, only limited research has examined this link (Connell, 1990). For instance, it was observed that students from elementary schools showed higher levels of cognitive engagement when provided with the opportunity to choose the type of tasks which they wished to do as well as the place and time to perform them (Perry, 1998; Turner, 1995). However, in a different study, the same link between autonomy support and engagement was not visible for junior high school students. However, it should be noted that in that study the authors identified the lack of more opportunities and the presence of more control measures as possible reasons for these observations (Midgley & Feldlaufer, 1987; Moos, 1979).

As far as task characteristics are concerned, it is worth noting that, within the classroom context, repetitive tasks or those based on memorization strategies are considered to be common, but they are ineffective in developing cognitive engagement as they involve less effort or learning commitments from the students (Newmann et al., 1992). As a result, Newmann proposed changes by suggesting five characteristics which were needed for tasks to be engaging (e.g., authentic tasks, tasks which allow students to be autonomous in terms of conceptualization, execution, and evaluation, tasks which allow students to collaborate, tasks which allow students to express different types of talents, and tasks which provide opportunities for fun) (Newmann, 1991; Newmann et al., 1992). Some of these features were investigated, with one study showing that students who collaborated with their peers on new but personally meaningful tasks were more likely to use certain gestures, expressions, and behaviors which were indicative (linguistic and behavioral indicators) of higher cognitive engagement (Helme & Clarke, 2001). Similarly, higher cognitive engagement was observed when students received teachers' support and encouragement after being given complex tasks to complete (Blumenfeld & Meece, 1988). Although the last two characteristics are not often the subject of studies, the results clearly show which type of tasks are likely to sustain student engagement and, in doing so, they not only support the hypothesis regarding the importance of task characteristics but also highlight the value of relationships (with peers and teachers). This leads us to the third component of the classroom context which is its social aspect.

As evidenced by the large body of literature, social relationships in classrooms are arguably one of the most studied concepts as far as engagement is concerned. These studies also include the influence of peers in shaping the engagement levels of students. Research, in this case, has been focused on the predictive effects of peer acceptance, with results demonstrating both higher emotional (e.g., satisfaction at school) and behavioral engagements (e.g., prosocial behaviors, pursuing academic goals) for students who felt accepted by their peers (Berndt & Keefe, 1995; Wentzel, 1994). This was especially evident if the group already involved highly engaged individuals (Kindermann, 1993). However, peer rejection is also a reality, and it is not surprising that it was shown to lead to opposite effects in the form of reduced levels of both types of engagement as well as higher risks of dropout (Buhs & Ladd, 2001; DeRosier et al., 1994; French & Conrad, 2001). After peers, the influence of teachers in the form of teacher support is another factor which shapes student engagement within classrooms. The effects of supportive teachers have been positively associated with all forms of engagement, namely, behavioral, emotional, as well as cognitive (Battistich et al., 1997; Blumenfeld & Meece, 1988; Croninger & Lee, 2001; Skinner & Belmont, 1993) and the fact that these results were consistent not only for students from elementary up to high schools but also across different ethnic groups further shows the importance of this factor (Marks, 2000). Furthermore, in addition to creating a socially supportive environment, it will be recalled from earlier descriptions, that teachers play a central role in supporting students' autonomy, creating appropriate task characteristics as well as providing clear classroom structures. Hence, they are arguably the most important component of all the previously described factors within the classroom context. Overall, it can be said that there is enough evidence to show that school characteristics influence student engagement, thereby supporting the reform model.

Closely related to the reform model is that of Connell's self-system theory (Connell, 1990; Connell & Wellborn, 1991). According to this model, children have three basic psychological requirements, namely, the need for competence, the need for autonomy, and the need for relatedness, with the level of school engagement being dependent on the extent to which students feel that those needs are being fulfilled. This direct link between students' needs and engagement levels is widely accepted by researchers but interestingly, as pointed out by Fredricks et al. (2004), the self-system model also takes into account the continuous influence of contextual factors, that is, the social environment within which students evolve and which was described in the previous model. Therefore, while acknowledging the influence of those social factors on school engagement, this model also stipulates that the fulfillment of students' needs act as the link between the two. For instance, in one study it was found that teachers considered students to be more engaged when they thought they shared a high-quality emotional relationship (a measure of high relatedness) (Connell & Wellborn, 1991) and this relatedness was itself more likely to occur when a supportive and caring environment was provided both by the teachers as well as peers.

Similarly, in another study, relatedness was found to be linked to emotional engagement (Furrer & Skinner, 2003), with Ryan et al. (1994) suggesting that the behavioral component of engagement could also be involved. In terms of the second need, that of autonomy, Ryan and Connell (1989) described it as students' "desire to do things for personal reasons, rather than doing things because their actions are controlled by others" (p. 81) and it is believed that in cases where students can contribute to decision-making processes or have the freedom to make choices, this need for autonomy is fulfilled, hence leading to a higher level of school engagement (Connell & Wellborn, 1991). As an example, many studies have reported that performing activities out of pleasure or interest (considered to be autonomous reasons) was positively linked with both emotional (e.g., happiness) and behavioral (e.g., higher participation) engagement (Connell & Wellborn, 1991; Patrick et al., 1993). However, unlike the need for relatedness, there are no stud-

ies which examine the above assumption that social contexts can contribute to engagement by supporting autonomy (Fredricks et al., 2004).

A similar observation can be made regarding the need for competence which is met when students start to believe that they control their own success while believing in their own abilities to succeed and understanding the means to attain it. Again, despite evidence of the link between perceived competence and engagement (Rudolph et al., 2001; Skinner et al., 1990), no studies have examined the involvement of factors such as school structure in fulfilling that need for competence. There is no doubt that further research is, therefore, required in order to find more evidence which supports the self-system model. Nevertheless, it can be concluded that, through the conceptualization of needs, this model has the merit of explaining why engagement is promoted under certain social contexts.

It is worth noting that the concept of needs is not necessarily exclusive to the self-system model. Similar constructs can be found within the motivational model (Li, 2011), itself based on the Self-Determination Theory of Ryan and Deci (2000). As the name suggests, compared to the previous model, the only difference is the inclusion of the concept of motivation. Hence, in this case, the model stipulates that the fulfillment of the psychological need determines the quality of motivation which eventually influences the level of school engagement (Eccles, 2004). Motivation, in this case, is regarded as an important intermediate requirement for engagement (Saeed & Zyngier, 2012) and this is observed not only in the fact that highly motivated students tend to perform better at schools (Pintrich, 2003), but also that it is considered to be one of the most important factors which need to be targeted by teachers in order to improve learning (Williams & Williams, 2011). While motivation is clearly a useful way of measuring engagement levels, it is not considered in the self-system model. In the same way, the motivation model excludes the influence of social contexts. As such, it is not surprising to note the proposal of a more general one, the self-system model of motivational development (SSMMD), in an attempt to reconcile the two (Nouwen & Clycq, 2020), as through this integrated model, engagement can be visualized both in terms of the motivation processes and the continuous interactions with social contexts (Fig. 1).

Participation–Identification Model

A second model which is commonly applied in the engagement literature is Finn's participation–identification model (Finn, 1989). According to this theory, the first step in building success is when a willing student starts to participate in school activities which basically are classified into four main types, namely, social tasks, class-related initiatives, extracurricular activities, and responsive behaviors (Archambault et al., 2009; Finn & Zimmer, 2012). Participation in any of these activities are considered to reflect different levels of a student's engagement, thereby suggesting that, based on this model, the development of behavioral engagement is the first requirement for success. While continuous participation is believed to lead to some form of academic success, it may also subsequently lead to a form of school bonding, that is the identification part of the model which actually reflects a student's emotional engagement (Finn & Zimmer, 2012). Eventually, being cyclic in nature, these types of interactions can encourage further participation, success, and bonding. However, the converse is also true and, therefore, Finn's participation–identification model explains school dropouts as being due to a lack of encouragement in the early participation in school activities which will gradually lead to disengagement. This model is depicted in Fig. 2.

Models and Frameworks of School Belonging

Despite the importance of school belonging for healthy psychological development of students, very few models or frameworks provide guidance on the best ways to support or encourage school belonging (Allen et al., 2019; Allen, Vella-Brodrick et al., 2016; Libbey, 2004). Allen, Vella-Brodrick and colleagues (2016) found that some frameworks had been previously developed (e.g., Brendtro et al., 2002; Connell & Wellborn, 1991; Malti & Noam, 2009; Ryan & Deci, 2000) but these were of limited focus. Thus, they ignored the contribution of certain factors or did not consider the concept as a multidimensional construct based on empirical evidence (e.g., Rowe et al., 2007; Waters et al., 2009). Hence a new framework was proposed based on Bronfenbrenner's (1979) ecological framework for human development, whereby school belonging was viewed as a "multilayered socio-ecological phenomenon" (Allen, Vella-Brodrick et al., 2016), not dissimilar to Anderson et al.'s (2014) adaptation for inclusive education. In Allen and colleagues' approach, children are considered to be at the center of a broader system, surrounded by multiple layers of influence (the microsystem, mesosystem, exosystem, and macrosystem), which interact to shape development and psychosocial adjustment (Allen, Kern et al., 2016; Allen, Vella-Brodrick et al., 2016), as depicted in Fig. 3. This framework, unlike others which are only based on constructs involving an individual, is not only concerned with the importance of social relationships but it also takes into account other variables such as ecological, environmental, or even physical factors which are likely to influence a student.

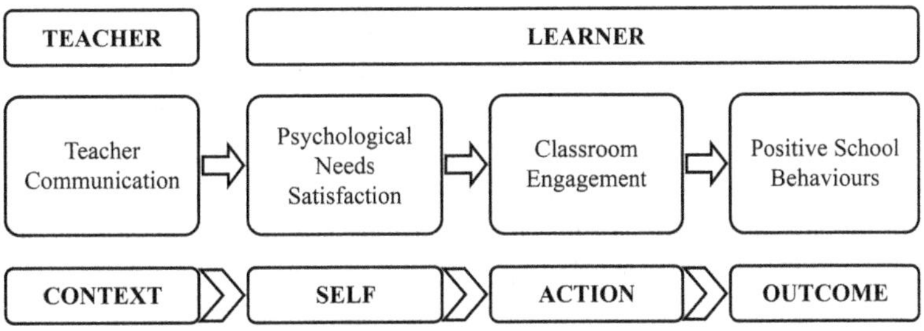

Fig. 1 The self-system model of motivational development (SSMMD) (Source: Dincer et al., 2019)

TEACHER | LEARNER

Teacher Communication → Psychological Needs Satisfaction → Classroom Engagement → Positive School Behaviours

CONTEXT ⟫ SELF ⟫ ACTION ⟫ OUTCOME

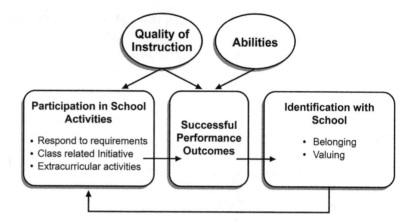

Fig. 2 The participation–identification model as conceptualized by Finn. (Source: Finn & Zimmer, 2012)

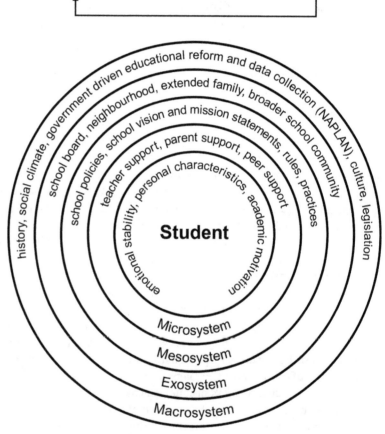

Fig. 3 The socio-ecological model proposed by Allen et al. 2016 for school belonging (Source: Allen, Vella-Brodrick et al., 2016)

Such a multilayered framework, therefore, provides different levels at which decision-makers such as educators, school leaders, and school psychologists can choose to intervene in order to improve school belonging. Additionally, this framework provides a means of organizing and categorizing research results according to the levels to which they apply in order to determine those which deserve more focus.

Closely related to the above framework is the rainbow model of school belonging (see Allen, 2020b). This model visually captures seven systems concerned with school belonging: a student's individual characteristics, primary social groups, the school climate, the local village, the environment, the culture, and the ecosystem. These systems clearly resemble the different levels of the socio-ecological framework. However, this model also possesses some unique features which make it particularly useful for portraying the concept of school belonging. For instance, the rainbow is a spectrum of colors which reflects the spectrum of belonging. The different layers might be brighter or lighter, depending on how much influence that layer has. On some days, the feeling of belongingness can be intense and this can be visualized by the rainbow range moving from the rainclouds (low sense of belonging) to bright sunshine (high sense of belonging). Experiences of belonging to school are unique to the individual—just like each rainbow is unique (e.g., different sizes, times, and places). Among its other features, the rainbow model also reflects the bidirectional nature of the influences exerted by each layer. Finally, the final outcome of belonging can also be conceived in the form of the pot of gold under the rainbow as school belonging is positively associated with a range of good outcomes for students who last well into adulthood. At the same time, since it is not possible to have rainbows without rain, challenges and stressors which can hinder belongingness are appropriately represented by the clouds.

Overlaps and Similarities of School Belonging and Engagement

Apart from their definitions, the two concepts are related at the framework level in that they both attempt to achieve the same result of academic success. Unlike previous theories where school belonging and engagement were viewed as empirical constructs (i.e., as measurable or dependent/mediating variables which would explain observations or theories), they are now considered as outcomes in their own right (i.e., they are themselves a product of the interaction of different factors). Hence, they are both recognized as objectives which need to be targeted in order to attain that result (Bouchard & Berg, 2017; Fredricks et al., 2004). Furthermore, the different models used for each concept take into account the continuous influence of several external variables to explain the dynamic nature of school belonging and engagement. In this case, overlap of the two terms is obvious not only in

similarities in terms of the variables but also in the constructs used to define the relationships between those variables and the two concepts.

For instance, let us consider the socio-ecological framework for school belonging. A closer view of the different layers described by Allen, Vella-Brodrick et al. (2016) suggests that the proposed framework is based on constructs which can also be found in the concept of school engagement. This is especially obvious for the innermost layer—the individual, which basically focuses on the factors which are specifically related to a student and which are likely to influence his or her sense of belonging. At this level, three major individual factors can be identified although it is noted that the contribution of "demographic characteristics" as a fourth factor, also have been mentioned (Allen, Kern et al., 2016). This may be due to the fact that characteristics such as gender, race, or even ethnicity have been reported to influence a sense of school belonging (Bonny et al., 2000; Sánchez et al., 2005). However, for this chapter, the focus will be mainly on the main three factors as they represent those which are most related to the concept of school engagement.

One of the attributes which is influenced by a sense of school belonging is academic motivation which Libbey (2004) describes as the "extent to which students are motivated to learn and do well in school" (p. 278). The importance of this factor was reflected in the study by Neel and Fuligni (2013) who found that the feeling of being connected to the school was positively associated with higher levels of academic motivation. Interestingly, as previously discussed, this concept of motivation is also often associated with school engagement, especially in the motivational model or its most recent alternative the self-system model of motivational development (SSMMD) (Nouwen & Clycq, 2020). Furthermore, the earlier definition of school engagement in this chapter is that one of its components is cognitive engagement whereby young people display a willingness to learn which is referred to as "psychological investment." Many authors, in their definitions of school engagement, have recognized this investment as being important to learn, master, and understand the knowledge and skills taught at schools (Newmann et al., 1992; Wehlage et al., 1989). Based on the descriptions of these authors, Fredricks et al. (2004) rightly pointed out that the psychological investment had similarities with the concept of motivation, especially with specific constructs such as motivation to learn as it is this which allows students to value learning and inspires them to make the necessary efforts for this purpose. This similarity was further highlighted in a report where the terms engagement and motivation were used interchangeably (National Research Council and Institute ·of Medicine, 2004), with some researchers even suggesting that engagement was a form of motivation (Wigfield et al., 2006). Hence, while school belonging is considered to be one of the greatest sources of motivation (Fiske, 2004), the latter can itself be a measure of school engagement levels, thereby acting as a common link between the two concepts. Moreover, it is worth pointing out that motivation, as conceptualized in the different models of engagement, is believed to be an intermediate psychological state which will not only determine the level of engagement but which is itself dependent on a number of external variables such as contextual factors (Dincer et al., 2019). As such, it is not unlikely that those same factors or models could also be applied to explain school belonging through motivational constructs.

The other two factors which influence school belonging at an individual level are personal characteristics and emotional stability (Allen, Vella-Brodrick et al., 2016), with the latter also referred to as negative personal factors in a different review (Allen, Kern et al., 2016). The first one is concerned with the specific nature of students such as their personal qualities (e.g., coping and problem-solving skills) or social and emotional characteristics (e.g., ability to control behavior and emotions when faced with stresses or being friendly and getting along with peers and teachers). On the other hand, emotional stability mostly involves the absence of mental illness or other negative factors such as persistent anxiety,

depression and negative emotions (e.g., sadness and gloomy) as in many studies, these were found to be linked to a low sense of school belonging (McMahon et al., 2008; Shochet et al., 2007; Shochet et al., 2011). Again, these two factors, despite being considered in the context of school belonging, also show some degree of overlap with school engagement. More specifically, the similarity occurs with reference to the emotional engagement component which has been described as "students' affective reactions in the classroom" (Connell & Wellborn, 1991; Skinner & Belmont, 1993). As such, emotional engagement involves a wide range of emotions which, in the context of school belonging, is considered as part of a student's emotional stability. This is probably why authors such as Finn (1989), in describing emotional engagement as identification with school, also defined belonging as one of its dimensions. To a lesser extent, some overlap also occurs with the behavioral component of school engagement since one of the three definitions provided by Fredricks et al. (2004) involves positive behavior as well as the absence of disruptive conduct and both of these, being a student's personal characteristics, are recognized as important variables within the socio-ecological framework of school belonging.

Similarity with emotional engagement can also be observed for the second layer of the framework. For this level, referred to as the microsystem (Fig. 3), the focus is basically on relationships and according to Brophy's systematic review (Brophy, 2004), this layer is closely linked to the previous one because the building of positive personal characteristics can, in turn, improve the relational skills of students, thereby allowing them to strengthen their relationships, whether with parents, peers or teachers. The importance of this concept is clearly evident from the number of studies which sought to determine how relationships influenced school belonging (Anderman, 2003; Garcia-Reid, 2007; Hamm & Faircloth, 2005; Johnson, 2009; Reschly et al., 2008; Wang & Eccles, 2012). However, it should be noted that the importance of relationships is not limited to school belonging but is also included within the concept of school engagement (Appleton et al., 2008). In engagement theories, the value of relationships is mentioned as part of the classroom environment where connections with peers and teachers have been reported to exert a strong influence on engagement levels (Battistich et al., 1997).

The mesosystem represents the third layer of the socio-ecological framework for which some of the elements overlap with constructs of school engagement. Broadly speaking, this level involves the school environment and its associated features such as the organizational structure, school policies or school practices which together are known to affect school belonging (Loukas et al., 2010; Waters et al., 2010). This description of the mesosystem clearly bears similarities with the contextual factors mentioned in the engagement literature, especially those which outline the influence of school-level factors (e.g., Fredricks et al., 2004). More specifically, at the mesosystem level, multiple group memberships and participation in extracurricular activities have been shown to influence school belonging in a positive way (Dotterer et al., 2007; Drolet & Arcand, 2013). Interestingly, these same features are also recognized as promoting behavioral and emotional engagement (Finn, 1993; Finn et al., 1995; Wehlage & Smith, 1992), hence these may be considered as a common measure for both school belonging and school engagement. In addition, engagement theories also distinguish between school-level factors and classroom contexts and even though the same distinction is not made in belonging models, the same features such as task characteristics or even autonomy support are also accepted as being important for fostering school belonging (Vaz et al., 2015). It can be concluded, therefore, that the environmental context acts as a common variable for both engagement, and school belonging concepts.

It will be observed that as we move away from the outermost circle depicted in Fig. 1, the similarity or overlap with other constructs is reduced, and this is particularly obvious with the exo- and the macrosystem of the socio-ecological framework. The former involves surrounding communities such as local businesses and community groups while the latter consists of wider legal and public policies (e.g., government-driven initiatives and regulations) (Saab, 2009). Therefore, a common aspect of these two levels is that they are not directly associated with students (Allen, Vella-Brodrick et al., 2016) but instead, they affect school belonging by influencing school activities, policies, and objectives. This could be the main reason for the absence of overlapping constructs as school engagement is more specifically focused on students. Nevertheless, the exosystem and mesosystem remain two important levels at which decision- or policy-makers may intervene in an attempt to foster school belonging.

In a similar way, in the two-dimensional model of student engagement described by Finn, two components of engagement were identified, namely, participation and identification (Finn, 1989, 1993; Finn & Rock, 1997). These components were related to those suggested by Brewster and Bowen (2004), with the participation component referring to the behavioral dimension and the identification part involving the affective side, which eventually relates to a student's sense of belonging to school, thereby showing some degree of overlap of the two terms.

Another way of viewing this overlap is through the measures used for school belonging. In this case, when investigating school connectedness based on these measures, Libbey (2004) identified common constructs such as academic engagement, discipline and fairness, students' liking of school, student voice, involvement in extracurricular activities, peer relations, safety, and teacher support which altogether represent important themes in a large number of measures and terms used to describe school belonging. As noted earlier, some of these constructs are also common in defining school engagement and hence further highlights how this concept is closely related to that of school belonging. Nevertheless, it should be remembered that both represent clearly defined terms and should therefore be used appropriately.

Outcomes of School Belonging and Engagement

From a historical perspective, it has been generally observed that students tend to show less enthusiasm as they progress through the school system, with increasing numbers either leaving or being almost uninterested by the time they reach higher schools (Skinner, Kindermann, Connell et al., 2009; Steinberg et al., 1996). The concepts of school belonging and engagement were, therefore, developed as a means of understanding this declining process, with the main outcome being to achieve academic success. This outcome was considered to be the primary objective which had to be attained but over time, the concepts evolved such that each concept now has a defined set of outcomes which, in a general way, can be classified as either positive or negative. For instance, based on the results of previous studies, Fredricks et al. (2004), like other researchers (Dotterer & Lowe, 2011; Finn & Zimmer, 2012), describe the positives under the broad category of academic achievement and found that they were positively related with both emotional and behavioral engagement (Connell & Wellborn, 1991; Skinner et al., 1990). Conversely, school dropout is considered as the main negative outcome which occurs as a result of low engagement levels. In fact, preventing school dropouts may be considered to be the main objective behind the different theoretical frameworks of engagement (Reschly & Christenson, 2012), particularly the one developed by Finn (1989). However, other authors took a different approach although the ultimate outcome remains of promoting academic success or avoiding dropouts, a number of intermediate objectives have also been recognized, depending on which component of engagement was encouraged. One example is behavioral engagement where three types of targeted results can be identified. These include following school regulations while avoiding repeated absences or lateness as well as trouble-making (Finn, 1993; Finn & Rock, 1997), being involved in academic learning in the form of efforts, showing attention or completion of homework (Birch & Ladd,

1997; Finn et al., 1995) and finally, participation in activities, both academic and nonacademic ones (Finn et al., 1995). Similarly, results of emotional engagement could take the form of positive emotions or showing interest (Connell & Wellborn, 1991) while developing good relationships with peers and teachers (Lee & Smith, 1995). On the other hand, being conceptualized as a student's psychological investment, the outcome of cognitive engagement may be more difficult to assess. However, some researchers consider visible markers such as the ability to solve problems, a particular preference for hard work as well as work commitments as indicative of successful cognitively engaged students (Connell & Wellborn, 1991).

As previously discussed, academic success is also a major outcome which is shared by school belonging, and achieving this has been the main focus of many studies (e.g., Mai et al., 2015). Similarly, the main negative outcome due to the absence of belongingness is school dropout (Hascher & Hagenauer, 2010) but at the same time, a number of intermediate outcomes are also targeted. For instance, as explained by the socio-ecological framework, school belonging is highly influenced by individual characteristics, relationships, and school factors. Hence, positive outcomes often involve improved self-characteristics such as higher self-esteem or self-discipline (Dotterer & Wehrspann, 2016; Mai et al., 2015). Furthermore, better relationships with teachers and peers promote higher social skills (Mai et al., 2015) while encouraging higher school participation (Finn, 1989). More importantly though, school belonging also helps to promote high levels of engagement (Lam et al., 2012; Roorda et al., 2011) and therefore, being connected to the school promotes positive student well-being.

Interventions for School Belonging and Student Engagement

Since school belonging and student engagement are clearly important within the educational context, it is, therefore, not surprising that a genuine attempt has been made to identify and apply interventions to foster both of them. In this respect, through randomized control trials as well as systematic reviews, many researchers have assessed the suitability of interventions which are often guided by well-established theories to identify ideal points of intervention (Allen, Jamshidi et al., 2021a, 2021b; Christenson & Pohl, 2020; Fredricks et al., 2019; Greenwood & Kelly, 2019). For instance, Finn's participation–identification model (1989) helps to understand the process which causes students to leave school early; this was applied in the design and implementation of the Check & Connect projects (C & C) that sought to increase school completion (Christenson & Pohl, 2020). In this case, engagement was promoted in a number of ways by, for example, recognizing early warning signs of disengagement, monitoring students' attendance, academic performances and progress, and even involving parents in order to strengthen family–school relationships. In fact, the multidimensional nature of engagement makes it possible to identify different types of interventions which may be aimed at promoting specific components of engagement (i.e., behavioral, emotional, and cognitive) (Fredricks et al., 2019). Similarly, based on other models (e.g., the self-system motivational model), some interventions have considered contextual factors as a means of fostering engagement, while others (e.g., the Positive-Activity Model or the Synergistic Change Model) have, instead, focused on positive psychology interventions to foster well-being (Fredricks et al., 2019; Lyubomirsky & Layous, 2013; Rusk et al., 2018).

As far as belonging is concerned, Greenwood and Kelly's (2019) systematic review pointed out the different ways in which belonging could be fostered. They identified providing support, whether academic or personal, the school culture and classroom practices as those features which were most likely to encourage connectedness. While these features are often part of normal practice within schools, they may also be implemented as part of intervention programs. In a similar way to engagement interventions, empirically supported theories form the basis of belonging interventions. These may be focused on the positive development of young people as well as the enhancement of their social skills, especially by establishing positive relationships with teachers and peers while encouraging teacher–student communication (Chapman et al., 2013). By building on the results of previous studies, Allen, Jamshidi et al. (2021a, 2021b) also identified other types of school interventions, such as those targeting social skills, problem-solving, and goal planning which were aimed at improving students' behavior for better connectedness. Similarly, interventions involving the regulation of students' emotions and those displayed toward teachers or peers were also found to be effective at promoting well-being, with positive effects even observed in the cases of disabled students, those who need mental health support as well as those who are likely to have low academic performance. Although the above-mentioned measures are by no means exhaustive, they do represent examples where theoretical knowledge was successfully translated into practice.

Future Research and Practice

There is no doubt that, since their conceptualization, we have now come a long way in our understanding of belonging and engagement. However, the avenues for further research are as numerous as before, as we seek to improve our current knowledge regarding these concepts. One key issue is that there are many discrepancies and inconsistencies in the way belonging and engagement have been described and defined in literature (Allen, Jamshidi et al., 2021a, 2021b; Slaten et al., 2016), leading to the overlap and differences mentioned previously. Furthermore, this can be particularly problematic when devising measurement scales aimed at providing empirical data in support of a theoretical framework, as results may not be easily comparable. More recently, Wong and Liem (2021) have elaborated on the risks associated with overgeneralization of terms such as student engagement. Hence working toward the standardization of constructs might help in overcoming such issues in the future. More precise measurements and careful use of terminology are needed to clearly distinguish terms like belonging and engagement (Allen et al., 2021).

Future research may also be directed toward the implementation of new interventions as despite the positive outcomes, there have been a number of shortcomings. One key issue is that of implementation, which refers to how successfully a particular program is applied within a context. The implementation of school measures to foster belonging and engagement is dependent on a number of factors (Sanetti & Luh, 2020), but as noted by Fredricks et al. (2019), such information is often absent despite its importance for interpreting results. In fact, many reported interventions may also not be of high quality, thereby preventing researchers from drawing appropriate conclusions from available data (Allen, Jamshidi et al., 2021a, 2021b). Fredricks et al. (2019) further identified a number of other issues with reported measures but one which deserves mention is that of variability among students. Although a multitiered approach (from general to specific subgroups of students) for belonging and engagement interventions can be used, they are often uniformly applied, albeit to specific class levels or age groups. As such, they often do not consider that the levels of belonging and engagement can be highly variable among students. However, since individualized approaches might also not be a plausible option, having measures targeted at specific groups (e.g., socio-economic

background, special needs, family issues) might, in the future, provide alternative options for reliably assessing the suitability of measures aimed at fostering school belonging and student engagement.

Conclusion

This chapter has presented a narrative synthesis that has explored the similarities and differences between school engagement and belonging. Our review reveals that the two concepts are often confused or used interchangeably despite being distinct terms which examine the different psychological needs of students. However, they show unmistakable similarities in terms of their constructs, especially when considering the various models which explain how they are influenced by surrounding factors (see Table 1). The differences and similarities identified in this review are presented in Table 1.

Based on our review, it can be concluded that school belonging and engagement are intricately linked and may even be considered to be symbiotic, requiring each other to exist. However, it is also widely accepted that even though there is enough empirical evidence to show how they encourage positive outcomes and reduce negative ones, further research is still required to build on the available knowledge. In short, the concepts of belonging and student engagement can be con-

Table 1 Similarities and differences of school belonging and engagement

Features and themes	School belonging	School engagement
As a mediator of academic outcomes	Less evidence for grade improvement and more evidence for academic related outcomes like hardiness and motivation	Highly associated with improved academic performance and emotional well-being
Interventions	Limited interventions that specifically aim to increase school belonging	Higher number of interventions aimed at improving behavioral, emotional and cognitive engagement
Feature	Manifested at an emotional level	Can be of different subtypes (i.e., behavioral, emotional, and cognitive) and hence, not limited to emotional traits
As an outcome	Influenced by a number of factors grouped at different levels	Influenced by various factors identified through different theoretical models
Influential factors	Can be fostered through positive emotions and building relationships	Positive emotions and relationships are particularly important for emotional engagement

sidered two best friends—needed for one another and essential for students in educational contexts.

References

Allen, K. A., Jamshidi, N., Berger, E., Reupert, A., Wurf, G., & May, F. (2021a). Effective school-based interventions for building school belonging in adolescence: A systematic review. *Educational Psychology Review*, 1–29. https://doi.org/10.1007/s10648-021-09621-w

Allen, K. A., Gray, D., Baumeister, R., & Leary, M. (2021). The need to belong: A deep dive into the origins, implications, and future of a foundational construct. *Educational Psychology Review*. https://doi.org/10.1007/s10648-021-09633-6

Allen, K. A. (2020a). *The psychology of belonging*. Routledge (Taylor and Francis Group).

Allen, K. A. (2020b). Do you feel like you belong? *Frontiers for Young Minds, 8*, 99. https://doi.org/10.3389/frym.2020.00099

Allen, K. A., & Bowles, T. (2012). Belonging as a guiding principle in the education of adolescents. *Australian Journal of Educational and Developmental Psychology, 12*, 108–119.

Allen, K. A., & Kern, M. L. (2017). *School belonging in adolescents: Theory, research, and practice*. Springer Social Sciences. ISBN 978-981-10-5996-4.

Allen, K. A., & Kern, P. (2019). *Boosting school belonging in adolescents: Interventions for teachers and mental health professionals*. Routledge.

Allen, K. A., Jamshidi, N., Berger, E., Reupert, A., Wurf, G., & May, F. (2021b). Impact of school-based interventions for building school belonging in adolescence: A systematic review. *Educational Psychology Review*. https://doi.org/10.1007/s10648-021-09621-w

Allen, K. A., Kern, M. L., Rozek, C. S., McInerney, D. M., & Slavich, G. M. (2021). Belonging: A review of conceptual issues, an integrative framework, and directions for future research. *Australian Journal of Psychology, 73*(5), 1–16. https://doi.org/10.1080/00049530.2021.1883409

Allen, K. A., Kern, M. L., Vella-Brodrick, D., Hattie, J., & Waters, L. (2016). What schools need to know about fostering school belonging: A meta-analysis. *Educational Psychology Review, 30*(1), 1–34. https://doi.org/10.1007/s10648-016-9389-8

Allen, K. A., Vella-Brodrick, D., & Waters, L. (2016). Fostering school belonging in secondary schools using a socio-ecological framework. *The Educational and Developmental Psychologist, 33*(1), 1–25. https://doi.org/10.1017/edp.2016.5

Allen, K., Boyle, C., & Roffey, S. (2019). Creating a culture of belonging in a school context. *Educational and Child Psychology, 36*(4), 5–7.

Anderman, L. H. (2003). Academic and social perceptions as predictors of change in middle school students' sense of school belonging. *The Journal of Experimental Education, 72*(1), 5–22. https://doi.org/10.1080/00220970309600877

Anderman, L. H., & Freeman, T. M. (2004). Students' sense of belonging in school. *Advances in Motivation and Achievement, 13*, 27–63. https://doi.org/10.1016/S0749-7423(03)13002-6

Anderson, J., Boyle, C., & Deppeler, J. (2014). The ecology of inclusive education: Reconceptualising Bronfenbrenner. In Z. Zhang, P. W. K. Chan, & C. Boyle (Eds.), *Equality in education: Fairness and inclusion* (pp. 23–34). Sense Publishers.

Appleton, J. J., Christenson, S. L., & Furlong, M. J. (2008). Student engagement with school: Critical conceptual and methodological issues of the construct. *Psychology in the Schools, 45*(5), 369–386. https://doi.org/10.1002/pits.20303

Archambault, I., Janosz, M., Fallu, J. S., & Pagani, L. S. (2009). Student engagement and its relationship with early high school dropout. *Journal of Adolescence, 32*(3), 651–670. https://doi.org/10.1016/j.adolescence.2008.06.007

Bakadorova, O., & Raufelder, D. (2017). The interplay of students' school engagement, school self-concept and motivational relations during adolescence. *Frontiers in Psychology, 8*, 2171. https://doi.org/10.3389/fpsyg.2017.02171

Barker, B. G., & Gump, P. V. (1964). *Big school, small school: High school size and student behavior*. Press.

Battistich, V., Solomon, D., Watson, M., & Schaps, E. (1997). Caring school communities. *Educational Psychologist, 32*(3), 137–151. https://doi.org/10.1207/s15326985ep3203_1

Berndt, T. J., & Keefe, K. (1995). Friends' influence on adolescents' adjustment to school. *Child Development, 66*(5), 1312–1329. https://doi.org/10.2307/1131649

Birch, S. H., & Ladd, G. W. (1997). The teacher-child relationship and children's early school adjustment. *Journal of School Psychology, 35*(1), 61–79. https://doi.org/10.1016/S0022-4405(96)00029-5

Blumenfeld, P. C., & Meece, J. L. (1988). Task factors, teacher behavior, and students' involvement and use of learning strategies in science. *The Elementary School Journal, 88*(3), 235–250. https://doi.org/10.1086/461536

Bonny, A. E., Britto, M. T., Klostermann, B. K., Hornung, R. W., & Slap, G. B. (2000). School disconnectedness: Identifying adolescents at risk. *Pediatrics, 106*(5), 1027–1021. https://doi.org/10.1542/peds.106.5.1017

Bosnjak, A., Boyle, C., & Chodkiewicz, A. R. (2017). An intervention to retrain attributions using CBT: A pilot study. *The Educational and Developmental Psychologist, 34*(1), 21–32. https://doi.org/10.1017/edp.2017.1

Bouchard, K. L., & Berg, D. (2017). Students' school belonging: Juxtaposing the perspectives of teachers and students in the late elementary school years (grades 4–8). *School Community Journal, 27*(1), 107–136.

Brendtro, L. K., Brokenleg, M., & van Bockern, S. (2002). *Reclaiming youth at risk: Our hope for the future.* National Educational Service.

Brewster, A., & Bowen, G. L. (2004). Teacher support and the school engagement of Latino middle and high school students at risk of school failure. *Child and Adolescent Social Work Journal, 21*(1), 47–67. https://doi.org/10.1023/B:CASW.0000012348.83939.6b

Bronfenbrenner, U. (1979). *The ecology of human development.* Harvard University Press.

Brophy, J. (2004). *Motivating students to learn* (2nd ed.).

Buhs, E. S., & Ladd, G. W. (2001). Peer rejection as antecedent of young children's school adjustment: An examination of mediating processes. *Developmental Psychology, 37*(4), 550–560. https://doi.org/10.1037/0012-1649.37.4.550

Chapman, R. L., Buckley, L., Sheehan, M., & Shochet, I. (2013). School-based programs for increasing connectedness and reducing risk behavior: A systematic review. *Educational Psychology Review, 25*(1), 95–114. https://doi.org/10.1007/s10648-013-9216-4

Chodkiewicz, A. R., & Boyle, C. (2016). Promoting positive learning in students aged 10–12 years using attribution retraining and cognitive behavioural therapy: A pilot study. *School Psychology International, 37*(5), 519–535. https://doi.org/10.1177/0143034316667114

Christenson, S. L., & Pohl, A. J. (2020). The relevance of student engagement: The impact of and lessons learned implementing check & connect. In A. Reschly, A. Pohl, & S. Christenson (Eds.), *Student Engagement* (pp. 3–30). Springer. https://doi.org/10.1007/978-3-030-37285-9_1

Connell, J. P. (1990). Context, self, and action: A motivational analysis of self-system processes across the life span. In D. Cicchetti & M. Beeghly (Eds.), *The John D. and Catherine T. MacArthur foundation series on mental health and development. The self in transition: Infancy to childhood* (pp. 61–97). University of Chicago Press.

Connell, J. P., & Wellborn, J. G. (1991). Competence, autonomy, and relatedness: A motivational analysis of self-system processes. In M. R. Gunnar & L. A. Sroufe (Eds.), *The Minnesota symposia on child psychology* (Vol. 23, pp. 43–77). Lawrence Erlbaum Associates, Inc..

Croninger, R. G., & Lee, V. E. (2001). Social capital and dropping out of high school: Benefits to at-risk students of teachers' support and guidance. *Teachers College Record, 103*(4), 548–581. https://doi.org/10.1111/0161-4681.00127

Deci, E., & Ryan, R. M. (1985). *Intrinsic motivation and self-determination in human behavior.* Plenum.

DeRosier, M. E., Kupersmidt, J. B., & Patterson, C. J. (1994). Children's academic and behavioral adjustment as a function of the chronicity and proximity of peer rejection. *Child Development, 65*(6), 1799–1813. https://doi.org/10.2307/1131295

Dincer, A., Yeşilyurt, S., Noels, K. A., & Vargas Lascano, D. I. (2019). Self-determination and classroom engagement of EFL learners: A mixed-methods study

of the self-system model of motivational development. *SAGE Open, 9*(2), 215824401985391. https://doi.org/10.1177/2158244019853913

Dotterer, A. M., & Lowe, K. (2011). Classroom context, school engagement, and academic achievement in early adolescence. *Journal of Youth and Adolescence, 40*(12), 1649–1660. https://doi.org/10.1007/s10964-011-9647-5

Dotterer, A. M., & Wehrspann, E. (2016). Parent involvement and academic outcomes among urban adolescents: Examining the role of school engagement. *Educational Psychology, 36*(4), 812–830. https://doi.org/10.1080/01443410.2015.1099617

Dotterer, A. M., McHale, S. M., & Crouter, A. C. (2007). Implications of out-of-school activities for school engagement in African American adolescents. *Journal of Youth and Adolescence, 36*(4), 391–401. https://doi.org/10.1007/s10964-006-9161-3

Doyle, W. (1986). Classroom management techniques and student discipline. *ERIC*. Clearinghouse.

Drolet, M., & Arcand, I. (2013). Positive development, sense of belonging, and support of peers among early adolescents: Perspectives of different actors. *International Education Studies, 6*(4), 29–38. https://doi.org/10.5539/ies.v6n4p29

Eccles, J. S. (2004). Schools, academic motivation, and stage-environment fit. In R. M. Lerner & L. D. Steinberg (Eds.), *Handbook of adolescent psychology* (pp. 125–153). Wiley.

Eccles, J. S. (2016). Engagement: Where to next? *Learning and Instruction, 43*, 71–75. https://doi.org/10.1016/j.learninstruc.2016.02.003

Engels, M. C., Colpin, H., van Leeuwen, K., Bijttebier, P., van den Noortgate, W., Claes, S., Goossens, L., & Verschueren, K. (2016). Behavioral engagement, peer status, and teacher–student relationships in adolescence: A longitudinal study on reciprocal influences. *Journal of Youth and Adolescence, 45*(6), 1192–1207. https://doi.org/10.1007/s10964-016-0414-5

Finn, J. D. (1989). Withdrawing from school. *Review of Educational Research, 59*(2), 117–142. https://doi.org/10.2307/1170412

Finn, J. D. (1993). *School engagement & students at risk.* National Center for Education Statistics (ED).

Finn, J. D., & Rock, D. A. (1997). Academic success among students at risk for school failure. *Journal of Applied Psychology, 82*(2), 221–234. https://doi.org/10.1037/0021-9010.82.2.221

Finn, J. D., & Voelkl, K. E. (1993). School characteristics related to student engagement. *Journal of Negro Education, 62*(3), 249–268. https://doi.org/10.2307/2295464

Finn, J. D., & Zimmer, K. S. (2012). Student engagement: What is it? Why does it matter? In S. L. Christenson, A. L. Reschly, & C. Wylie (Eds.), *Handbook of research on student engagement* (pp. 97–131). Springer Science + Business Media. https://doi.org/10.1007/978-1-4614-2018-7_5.

Finn, J. D., Pannozzo, G. M., & Voelkl, K. E. (1995). Disruptive and inattentive-withdrawn behavior and achievement among fourth graders. *The Elementary School Journal, 95*(5), 421–434. https://doi.org/10.1086/461853

Fiske, S. T. (2004). *Social beings: A core motives approach to social psychology*. Wiley.

Fredricks, J. A., Blumenfeld, P. C., & Paris, A. H. (2004). School engagement: Potential of the concept, state of the evidence. *Review of Educational Research, 74*(1), 59–109. https://doi.org/10.3102/00346543074001059

Fredricks, J. A., Blumenfeld, P. B., Friedel, J., & Paris, A. (2002). *Increasing engagement in urban settings: An analysis of the influence of the social and academic context on student engagement*. Annual Meeting of the American Educational Research Association.

Fredricks, J. A., Reschly, A. L., & Christenson, S. L. (2019). Interventions for student engagement: Overview and state of the field. *Handbook of student engagement interventions* (pp. 1–11). https://doi.org/10.1016/b978-0-12-813413-9.00001-2.

French, D. C., & Conrad, J. (2001). School dropout as predicted by peer rejection and antisocial behavior. *Journal of Research on Adolescence, 11*(3), 225–244. https://doi.org/10.1111/1532-7795.00011

Frydenberg, E., Ainley, M., & Russell, J. (2005). *Student motivation and engagement: Schooling issues digest*. Department of Education.

Furlong, M. J., Froh, J. J., Muller, M. E., & Gonzalez, V. (2013). The role of gratitude in fostering school bonding. *National Society for the Study of Education, 113*(1), 58–79.

Furlong, M. J., Whipple, A. D., Jean, G. S., Simental, J., Soliz, A., & Punthuna, S. (2003). Multiple contexts of school engagement: Moving toward a unifying framework for educational research and practice. *California School Psychologist, 8*, 99–113. https://doi.org/10.1007/BF03340899

Furrer, C., & Skinner, E. (2003). Sense of relatedness as a factor in children's academic engagement and performance. *Journal of Educational Psychology, 95*(1), 148–162. https://doi.org/10.1037/0022-0663.95.1.148

Garcia-Reid, P. (2007). Examining social capital as a mechanism for improving school engagement among low income Hispanic girls. *Youth & Society, 39*, 164–181. https://doi.org/10.1177/0044118X07303263

Greenwood, L., & Kelly, C. (2019). A systematic literature review to explore how staff in schools describe how a sense of belonging is created for their pupils. *Emotional and Behavioural Difficulties, 24*(1), 3–19. https://doi.org/10.1080/13632752.2018.1511113

Hagerty, B. M., Williams, R. A., Coyne, J. C., & Early, M. R. (1996). Sense of belonging and indicators of social and psychological functioning. *Archives of Psychiatric Nursing, 10*(4), 235–244. https://doi.org/10.1016/S0883-9417(96)80029-X

Hamm, J. V., & Faircloth, B. S. (2005). The role of friendship in adolescents' sense of school belonging. *New Directions for Child and Adolescent Development, 107*, 61–78. https://doi.org/10.1002/cd.121

Hascher, T., & Hagenauer, G. (2010). Alienation from school. *International Journal of Educational Research, 49*(6), 220–232. https://doi.org/10.1016/j.ijer.2011.03.002

Helme, S., & Clarke, D. (2001). Identifying cognitive engagement in the mathematics classroom. *Mathematics Education Research Journal, 13*(2), 133–153. https://doi.org/10.1007/BF03217103

Irvin, M. J., Meece, J. L., Byun, S. Y., Farmer, T. W., & Hutchins, B. C. (2011). Relationship of school context to rural youth's educational achievement and aspirations. *Journal of Youth and Adolescence, 40*(9), 1225–1242. https://doi.org/10.1007/s10964-011-9628-8

Johnson, L. S. (2009). School contexts and student belonging: A mixed methods study of an innovative high school. *The School Community Journal, 19*(1), 99–118.

Kindermann, T. A. (1993). Natural peer groups as contexts for individual development: The case of children's motivation in school. *Developmental Psychology, 29*(6), 970–977. https://doi.org/10.1037/0012-1649.29.6.970

Korpershoek, H., Canrinus, E. T., Fokkens-Bruinsma, M., & de Boer, H. (2019). The relationships between school belonging and students' motivational, social-emotional, behavioural, and academic outcomes in secondary education: A meta-analytic review. *Research Papers in Education, 35*(6), 641–680. https://doi.org/10.1080/02671522.2019.1615116

Lam, S., Wong, B. P. H., Yang, H., & Liu, Y. (2012). Understanding student engagement with a contextual model. In S. L. Christenson, A. L. Reschly, & C. Wylie (Eds.), *Handbook of research on student engagement* (pp. 403–419). Springer. https://doi.org/10.1007/978-1-4614-2018-7_19

Langevin, L. (1999). L'abandon scolaire. In *On ne naît pas décrocheur!* Logiques.

Lee, V. E., & Smith, J. B. (1995). Effects of high school restructuring and size on early gains in achievement and engagement. *Sociology of Education, 68*(4), 241–270. https://doi.org/10.2307/2112741

Li, Y. (2011). School engagement: What it is and why it is important for positive youth development. *Advances in Child Development and Behavior, 41*, 131–160. https://doi.org/10.1016/B978-0-12-386492-5.00006-3

Libbey, H. P. (2004). Measuring student relationships to school: Attachment, bonding, connectedness, and engagement. *Journal of School Health, 74*(7), 274–283. https://doi.org/10.1111/j.1746-1561.2004.tb08284.x

Lippman, L., & Rivers, A. (2008). Assessing school engagement: A guide for out-of-school time program practitioners. *Child Trends.* http://www.childtrends.org/files/child_Trends-2008_10_29_rb_Schoolengage.pdf

Loukas, A., Roalson, L. A., & Herrera, D. E. (2010). School connectedness buffers the effects of negative family relations and poor effortful control on early adolescent conduct problems. *Journal of Research on Adolescence, 20*(1), 13–22. https://doi.org/10.1111/j.1532-7795.2009.00632.x

Lyubomirsky, S., & Layous, K. (2013). How do simple positive activities increase Well-being? *Current*

Directions in Psychological Science, 22(1), 57–62. https://doi.org/10.1177/0963721412469809

Mai, M. Y. M., Yusuf, M., & Saleh, M. (2015). Motivation and engagement as a predictor of students' science achievement satisfaction of Malaysian of secondary school students. *European Journal of Social Sciences Education and Research, 2*(4), 25–33.

Malti, T., & Noam, G. G. (2009). A developmental approach to the prevention of adolescent's aggressive behavior and the promotion of resilience. *International Journal of Developmental Science, 3*(3), 215–217. https://doi.org/10.3233/DEV-2009-3303

Marks, H. M. (2000). Student engagement in instructional activity: Patterns in the elementary, middle, and high school years. *American Educational Research Journal, 37*(1), 153–184.

McMahon, S. D., Parnes, A. L., Keys, C. B., & Viola, J. J. (2008). School belonging among low-income urban youth with disabilities: Testing a theoretical model. *Psychology in the Schools, 45*(5), 387–401. https://doi.org/10.1002/pits.20304

Midgley, C., & Feldlaufer, H. (1987). Students' and teachers' decision-making fit before and after the transition to junior high school. *The Journal of Early Adolescence, 7*(2), 225–241. https://doi.org/10.1177/0272431687072009

Moos, R. H. (1979). *Evaluating educational environments.* Jossey-Bass.

National Research Council and Institute of Medicine. (2004). *Engaging schools: Fostering high school students' motivation to learn.* The National Academies Press.

Natriello, G. (1984). Problems in the evaluation of students and student disengagement from secondary schools. *Journal of Research and Development in Education, 17*(4), 14–24.

Neel, C. G. O., & Fuligni, A. (2013). A longitudinal study of school belonging and academic motivation across high school. *Child Development, 84*(2), 678–692. https://doi.org/10.1111/j.1467-8624.2012.01862.x

Newmann, F. M. (1981). Reducing student alienation in high schools: Implications of theory. *Harvard Educational Review, 51*(4), 546–564. https://doi.org/10.17763/haer.51.4.xj67887u87l5t66t

Newmann, F. M. (1991). Linking restructuring to authentic student achievement. *Phi Delta Kappan, 72*(6), 458–463.

Newmann, F. M., Wehlage, G. G., & Lamborn, S. D. (1992). The significance and sources of student engagement. In F. M. Newmann (Ed.), *Student engagement and achievement in American secondary schools* (pp. 11–39). Teachers College Press.

Nouwen, W., & Clycq, N. (2020). Assessing the added value of the self-system model of motivational development in explaining school engagement among students at risk of early leaving from education and training. *European Journal of Psychology of Education, 36*, 243–261. https://doi.org/10.1007/s10212-020-00476-3

O'Brennan, L. M., & Furlong, M. J. (2010). Relations between students' perceptions of school connectedness and peer victimization. *Journal of School Violence, 9*(4), 375–391. https://doi.org/10.1080/15388220.2010.509009

O'Brien, K. A., & Bowles, T. V. (2013). The importance of belonging for adolescents in secondary school settings. *The European Journal of Social & Behavioural Sciences, 5*(2), 976–984.

Patrick, B. C., Skinner, E. A., & Connell, J. P. (1993). What motivates children's behavior and emotion? Joint effects of perceived control and autonomy in the academic domain. *Journal of Personality and Social Psychology, 65*(4), 781–791. https://doi.org/10.1037/0022-3514.65.4.781

Perry, N. E. (1998). Young children's self-regulated learning and contexts that support it. *Journal of Educational Psychology, 90*(4), 715–729. https://doi.org/10.1037/0022-0663.90.4.715

Pintrich, P. R. (2003). A motivational science perspective on the role of student motivation in learning and teaching contexts. *Journal of Educational Psychology, 95*(4), 667–686. https://doi.org/10.1037/0022-0663.95.4.667

Reeve, J. (2013). How students create motivationally supportive learning environments for themselves: The concept of agentic engagement. *Journal of Educational Psychology, 105*(3), 579–595. https://doi.org/10.1037/a0032690

Reschly, A. L., & Christenson, S. L. (2012). Jingle, jangle, and conceptual haziness: Evolution and future directions in the engagement construct. In S. L. Christenson, A. L. Reschly, & C. A. Wylie (Eds.), *Handbook of research on student engagement* (pp. 3–19). Springer Science.

Reschly, A. L., Huebner, E. S., Appleton, J. J., & Antaramian, S. (2008). Engagement as flourishing: The contribution of positive emotions and coping to adolescents' engagement at school and with learning. *Psychology in the Schools, 45*(5), 419–431. https://doi.org/10.1002/pits.20306

Roorda, D. L., Koomen, H. M. Y., Spilt, J. L., & Oort, F. J. (2011). The influence of affective teacher–student relationships on students' school engagement and achievement. *Review of Educational Research, 81*(4), 493–529. https://doi.org/10.3102/0034654311421793

Rowe, F., Stewart, D., & Patterson, C. (2007). Promoting school connectedness through whole school approaches. *Health Education, 107*(6), 524–542. https://doi.org/10.1108/09654280710827920

Rudolph, K. D., Lambert, S. F., Clark, A. G., & Kurlakowsky, K. D. (2001). Negotiating the transition to middle school: The role of self-regulatory processes. *Child Development, 72*(3), 929–946. https://doi.org/10.1111/1467-8624.00325

Rusk, D. R., Vella-Brodrick, D. A., & Waters, L. (2018). A complex dynamic systems approach to lasting positive change: The synergistic change mode. *The Journal of Positive Psychology, 13*(4), 406–418. https://doi.org/10.1080/17439760.2017.1291853

Ryan, R. M., & Connell, J. P. (1989). Perceived locus of causality and internalization: Examining reasons for acting in two domains. *Journal of Personality and Social Psychology, 57*(5), 749–761. https://doi.org/10.1037/0022-3514.57.5.749

Ryan, R. M., & Deci, E. L. (2000). Intrinsic and extrinsic motivations: Classic definitions and new directions. *Contemporary Educational Psychology, 25*(1), 54–67. https://doi.org/10.1006/ceps.1999.1020

Ryan, R. M., & Deci, E. L. (2009). Promoting self-determined school engagement: Motivation, learning, and Well-being. In R. Wenzel & A. Wigfield (Eds.), *Educational psychology handbook series. Handbook of motivation at school* (pp. 171–195). Routledge/Taylor & Francis Group.

Ryan, R. M., Stiller, J. D., & Lynch, J. H. (1994). Representations of relationships to teachers, parents, and friends as predictors of academic motivation and self-esteem. *The Journal of Early Adolescence, 14*(2), 226–249. https://doi.org/10.1177/027243169401400207

Saab, H. (2009). *The school as a setting to promote student health.* https://Qspace.Library.Queensu.Ca/

Saeed, S., & Zyngier, D. (2012). How motivation influences student engagement: A qualitative case study. *Journal of Education and Learning, 1*(2), 252–267. https://doi.org/10.5539/jel.v1n2p252

Sánchez, B., Colón, Y., & Esparza, P. (2005). The role of sense of school belonging and gender in the academic adjustment of latino adolescents. *Journal of Youth and Adolescence, 34*(6), 619–628. https://doi.org/10.1007/s10964-005-8950-4

Sanetti, L. M. H., & Luh, H. J. (2020). Treatment fidelity in school-based intervention. In A. Reschly, A. Pohl, & S. Christenson (Eds.), *Student Engagement* (pp. 77–87). Springer. https://doi.org/10.1007/978-3-030-37285-9_4

Sciarra, D. T., & Seirup, H. J. (2008). The multidimensionality of school engagement and math achievement among racial groups. *Professional School Counseling, 11*(4), 218–228. https://doi.org/10.1177/2156759X0801100402

Shochet, I. M., Smith, C. L., Furlong, M. J., & Homel, R. (2011). A prospective study investigating the impact of school belonging factors on negative affect in adolescents. *Journal of Clinical Child & Adolescent Psychology, 40*(4), 586–595. https://doi.org/10.1080/15374416.2011.581616

Shochet, I. M., Smyth, T. L., & Homel, R. (2007). The impact of parental attachment on adolescent perception of the school environment and school connectedness. *Australian and New Zealand Journal of Family Therapy, 28*(2), 109–118. https://doi.org/10.1375/anft.28.2.109

Skinner, E. A., & Belmont, M. J. (1993). Motivation in the classroom: Reciprocal effects of teacher behavior and student engagement across the school year. *Journal of Educational Psychology, 85*(4), 571–581. https://doi.org/10.1037/0022-0663.85.4.571

Skinner, E. A., Kindermann, T. A., & Furrer, C. J. (2009). A motivational perspective on engagement and disaffection. *Educational and Psychological Measurement, 69*(3), 493–525. https://doi.org/10.1177/0013164408323233

Skinner, E. A., Kindermann, T., Connell, J. P., & Wellborn, J. G. (2009). Engagement and disaffection as organizational constructs in the dynamics of motivational development. In K. R. Wenzel & A. Wigfield (Eds.), *Educational psychology handbook series: Handbook of motivation at school* (pp. 223–245). Routledge/Taylor & Francis Group.

Skinner, E. A., Wellborn, J. G., & Connell, J. P. (1990). What it takes to do well in school and whether I've got it: A process model of perceived control and children's engagement and achievement in school. *Journal of Educational Psychology, 82*(1), 22–32. https://doi.org/10.1037/0022-0663.82.1.22

Slaten, C. D., Ferguson, J. K., Allen, K. A., Brodrick, D. V., & Waters, L. (2016). School belonging: A review of the history, current trends, and future directions. *The Educational and Developmental Psychologist, 33*(1), 1–15. https://doi.org/10.1017/edp.2016.6

St-Amand, J., Girard, S., & Smith, J. (2017). Sense of belonging at school: Defining attributes, determinants, and sustaining strategies. *IAFOR Journal of Education, 5*(2), 105–119. https://doi.org/10.22492/ije.5.2.05

Steinberg, L. D., Brown, B. B., & Dornbusch, S. M. (1996). *Beyond the classroom: Why school reform has failed and what parents need to do.* Simon and Schuster.

Turner, J. C. (1995). The influence of classroom contexts on young children's motivation for literacy. *Reading Research Quarterly, 30*(3), 410–441. https://doi.org/10.2307/747624

Vaz, S., Falkmer, M., Ciccarelli, M., Passmore, A., Parsons, R., Tan, T., & Falkmer, T. (2015). The personal and contextual contributors to school belongingness among primary school students. *PLoS One, 10*(4), e0123353. https://doi.org/10.1371/journal.pone.0123353

Verhoeven, M., Poorthuis, A. M. G., & Volman, M. (2019). The role of school in adolescents' identity development. A literature review. *Educational Psychology Review, 31*, 35–63. https://doi.org/10.1007/s10648-018-9457-3

Voelkl, K. E. (2012). School identification. In S. L. Christenson, A. L. Reschly, & C. Wylie (Eds.), *Handbook of research on student engagement* (pp. 193–218). Springer.

Wang, M. T., & Eccles, J. S. (2012). Social support matters: Longitudinal effects of social support on three dimensions of school engagement from middle to high school. *Child Development, 83*(3), 877–895. https://doi.org/10.1111/j.1467-8624.2012.01745.x

Waters, S. K., Cross, D. S., & Runions, K. (2009). Social and ecological structures supporting adolescent connectedness to school: A theoretical model. *Journal of School Health, 79*(11), 516–524. https://doi.org/10.1111/j.1746-1561.2009.00443.x

Waters, S., Cross, D., & Shaw, T. (2010). Does the nature of schools matter? An exploration of selected school ecology factors on adolescent perceptions of school connectedness. *British Journal of Educational Psychology, 80*(3), 381–402. https://doi.org/10.1348/000709909X484479

Wehlage, G. G., & Smith, G. A. (1992). Building new programs for students at risk. In F. M. Newmann (Ed.), *Student engagement and achievement in American secondary schools.* Teachers College Press.

Wehlage, G. G., Rutter, R. A., Smith, G. A., Lesko, N. L., & Fernandez, R. R. (1989). *Reducing the risk: Schools as communities of support.* The Falmer Press.

Wentzel, K. R. (1994). Relations of social goal pursuit to social acceptance, classroom behavior, and perceived social support. *Journal of Educational Psychology, 86*(2), 173–182. https://doi.org/10.1037/0022-0663.86.2.173

Wigfield, A., Eccles, J. S., Schiefele, U., Roeser, R. W., & Davis-Kean, P. (2006). Development of achievement motivation. In N. Eisenberg & W. Damon (Eds.), *Handbook of child psychology: Social, emotional, and*

personality development (Vol. 3, 6th ed., pp. 933–1002). Wiley.

Williams, K. C., & Williams, C. C. (2011). Five key ingredients for improving student motivation. *Research in Higher Education Journal, 12*, 121–123.

Williams, L. J., & Downing, J. E. (1998). Membership and belonging in inclusive classrooms: What do middle school students have to say? *Journal of the Association for Persons with Severe Handicaps, 23*(2), 98–110. https://doi.org/10.2511/rpsd.23.2.98

Willms, J. D. (2000). A sense of belonging and participation: Results from PISA 2000. *OECD.* http://www.Oecd.Org/Edu/School/Programmeforinternationalstudentassessmentpisa/33689437.Pdf.

Wong, Z. Y., & Liem, G. A. D. (2021). Student engagement: Current state of the construct, conceptual refinement, and future research directions. *Educational Psychology Review.* https://doi.org/10.1007/s10648-021-09628-3

Wonglorsaichon, B., Wongwanich, S., & Wiratchai, N. (2014). The influence of students school engagement on learning achievement: A structural equation modeling analysis. *Procedia – Social and Behavioral Sciences, 116*, 1748–1755. https://doi.org/10.1016/j.sbspro.2014.01.467

Self-Efficacy and Engaged Learners

Dale H. Schunk and Maria K. DiBenedetto

Abstract

Student engagement bears an important relation to motivation and other positive outcomes. *Engagement* refers to how learners' cognitions, behaviors, and affects are energized, directed, and sustained during academic activities. According to Bandura's social cognitive theory, *self-efficacy* (perceived capabilities for learning or performing actions at designated levels) is a key cognitive variable influencing motivation and engagement. The conceptual framework of social cognitive theory is described to include the roles played by vicarious, symbolic, and self-regulatory processes. We discuss how self-efficacy affects motivation through goals and self-evaluations of progress and how various contextual factors may influence self-efficacy. Research is described that relates self-efficacy to motivation and engagement. This chapter concludes with educational implications and recommendations for future research.

D. H. Schunk (✉) · M. K. DiBenedetto
Bryan School of Business & Economics, University
of North Carolina at Greensboro, Greensboro, NC,
USA
e-mail: dhschunk@uncg.edu; m_dibene@uncg.edu

Self-Efficacy and Engaged Learners

Since the publication of the first edition of this handbook (Christenson et al., 2012), research and applied interest in student engagement has increased dramatically. Although historically many researchers and practitioners were interested in the topic as a means of lessening negative outcomes (e.g., school dropout), today there is growing interest in engagement as a means of promoting students' positive outcomes such as motivation, learning, interest, and enjoyment (Schunk & DiBenedetto, 2014).

As used in this chapter, *student engagement* refers to the manifestation of students' motivation, or how their cognitions, behaviors, and affects are energized, directed, and sustained during learning and other academic activities (Reschly & Christenson, 2012; Skinner et al., 2009). *Motivation* refers to internal processes that energize, direct, and sustain goal-directed activities (Schunk et al., 2014). This emphasis on engagement is well founded, with increasing evidence showing its positive influence on myriad student outcomes including learning, achievement, and adjustment (Christenson et al., 2012).

Our thesis is that motivation is a key driving force behind engagement and that motivation and engagement can be enhanced. Although various theoretical principles can explain student motivation and engagement, we utilize Bandura's (1977b, 1986, 1997, 2001) *social cognitive the-*

ory, which emphasizes that much human learning and behavior occur in social environments. By interacting with others live or virtually, people learn knowledge, skills, strategies, beliefs, norms, and attitudes. Students act in accordance with their beliefs about their capabilities and the expected outcomes of their actions. Social cognitive researchers have explored the operation and outcomes of cognitive and affective processes hypothesized to underlie motivation (Schunk & DiBenedetto, 2016, 2020).

We focus particularly on the key social cognitive motivational variable of *self-efficacy,* defined as one's perceived capabilities for learning or performing actions at designated levels (Bandura, 1977a, 1997). Researchers have shown that a higher sense of self-efficacy can positively affect learning, achievement, self-regulation, and motivational outcomes such as individuals' choices of activities, effort, persistence, and interests (Bandura, 1997; Schunk & DiBenedetto, 2016; Schunk & Usher, 2019). Self-efficacious students are motivated and engaged in learning, which promotes their competence as learners. Thus, self-efficacy influences motivation, which affects engagement. As students are engaged in learning, they see that they are making progress, which helps sustain their self-efficacy and motivation (Fig. 1). Teachers who help students experience success by fostering their development of skills, learning strategies, and a positive outlook on their capabilities and future, can positively impact self-efficacy in their classrooms (Schunk & DiBenedetto, 2016).

We next describe the conceptual framework of social cognitive theory including vicarious, symbolic, and self-regulatory processes. We then discuss self-efficacy and the process whereby self-efficacy affects motivation through goals and self-evaluations of progress, as well as how self-efficacy can affect student engagement and how contextual factors may influence self-efficacy. The research evidence presented relates self-efficacy to student success. We conclude with recommendations for future research and implications for educational practice.

Conceptual Framework

Bandura's social cognitive theory is based on a model of reciprocal interactions and vicarious, symbolic, and self-regulatory processes.

Reciprocal Interactions

Bandura (1977b, 1986, 1997, 2001) postulated that human activity operates within a framework of *reciprocal interactions* involving personal (e.g., cognitions, beliefs, skills, affects), behavioral, and social/environmental factors. For example, self-efficacy can influence achievement behaviors such as task choice, effort, persistence, and self-regulatory strategies (person → behavior; Schunk & DiBenedetto, 2016). These behaviors also affect self-efficacy. As students work on tasks and observe their learning progress, self-efficacy for continued learning is enhanced (behavior → person). The links between self-efficacy, motivation, and engagement demonstrate this reciprocality.

Fig. 1 The interrelation of self-efficacy, motivation, and engagement

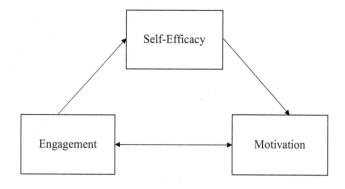

The connection between personal and social/environmental factors is often seen with students with learning disabilities who often hold low self-efficacy for performing well (Schunk & DiBenedetto, 2020). Persons may react to these students based on attributes typically associated with them (e.g., low skills) rather than based on their actual capabilities (person → social/environment). Environmental feedback can affect self-efficacy, as when teachers encourage students by communicating, "I know you can do this" (social/environment → person).

The influence between behavioral and social/environmental factors is evident in many instructional sequences. For example, when teachers point to a display and say, "Look here," students may do that with little conscious attention (social/environment → behavior). Behaviors can alter learners' instructional environments. When students give incorrect answers, teachers may stop the lesson and reteach the material (behavior → social/environment).

Social cognitive theory contends that individuals strive to develop a sense of *agency*, or the belief that they can exert a large degree of control over important events in their lives (Schunk & Usher, 2019). They hold beliefs that allow them to exert control over their thoughts, feelings, and actions. In reciprocal fashion, people influence and are influenced by their actions and environments. The scope of this reciprocal influence is broader than individuals because they live in social environments. *Collective agency* refers to people's shared beliefs about what they are capable of accomplishing as a group. Groups affect and are affected by their actions and environments as well.

Vicarious, Symbolic, and Self-Regulatory Processes

Vicarious, symbolic, and self-regulatory processes influence people's desire to attain a sense of agency.

Vicarious processes Much human learning occurs *vicariously* through observing others (e.g., live, filmed, virtual; Bandura, 1977b). This capability allows individuals to acquire beliefs, cognitions, affects, skills, strategies, and behaviors from their social environments, media, the Internet, and the like, which saves time because learning is not demonstrated when it occurs. This capability also allows people to select environmental features (e.g., individuals, materials) to which they want to attend. Learners who strive to become musicians enroll in music lessons and classes and put themselves in situations where they can learn vicariously, such as by observing and working with musicians.

Symbolic processes Symbolic processes involve language, mathematical and scientific notation, iconography, and cognition. These processes help people adapt to and alter their environments (Bandura, 1986). They use symbolic processes when they formulate thoughts to guide their actions. People do not just react to events. Rather, they plan, solve problems, and alter their self-regulatory strategies as needed. Symbolic processes also foster verbal and written communications and thereby promote learning.

Self-regulatory processes Self-regulation refers to the processes people use to activate and sustain their behaviors, cognitions, and affects to attain goals (Zimmerman, 2000). People regulate their behaviors to conform to their internal standards and goals. Before they begin a task, individuals determine their goals and which strategies to use, and they feel self-efficacious about performing well. As they engage in tasks, they monitor their performances, assess their goal progress, and decide whether their strategy needs adjusting. During breaks in learning and when tasks are completed, they reflect, make modifications, and determine next steps. Believing they have learned and made progress strengthens their self-efficacy and motivates learning. Highly engaged learners also are apt to be self-regulated (Usher & Schunk, 2018; Zimmerman & Cleary, 2009).

Self-Efficacy

Self-efficacy is a key personal factor and motivational variable in Bandura's (1986, 1997) social cognitive theory (Schunk & DiBenedetto, 2020). Self-efficacy can affect choice of activities, effort, persistence, and achievement. Research in academic settings shows that students who feel efficacious about learning tend to be engaged and set learning goals, use effective learning strategies, monitor learning, evaluate goal progress, and create supportive environments (Usher & Schunk, 2018). In turn, self-efficacy is influenced by behavioral outcomes (e.g., goal progress, achievement) and environmental inputs (e.g., teacher feedback, comparisons with peers). Self-efficacy impacts motivation and learning, as well as decisions and events that affect one's life (Schunk & Usher, 2019).

Sources of Self-Efficacy Information

Information for assessing one's self-efficacy is acquired from actual performances, vicarious experiences, forms of persuasion, and physiological indexes (e.g., anxiety, stress; Bandura, 1997). Because performances are tangible indicators of individuals' capabilities, they are the most reliable source (Schunk & DiBenedetto, 2016). Interpretations of one's performances as successful raise self-efficacy whereas perceived failures may lower it, although an occasional failure or success may not have much impact. Self-efficacious learners are apt to view difficulties as challenges that they can overcome, whereas lower-efficacy learners may believe that they lack the capabilities to succeed (Bandura, 1997).

Individuals acquire much information about their capabilities through social comparisons with others (Bandura, 1997). Similarity to others is a cue for gauging self-efficacy (Schunk & DiBenedetto, 2016). Observing others succeed can raise observers' self-efficacy and motivate them to try the task because they are apt to believe that if others can succeed, they can as well. But a vicarious increase in self-efficacy can be negated by subsequent difficulties. Persons who observe peers

fail may believe they lack competence, which can dissuade them from attempting the task.

People also assess self-efficacy based on persuasive information from others (e.g., "I know you can do this"; Bandura, 1997); however, such persuasion must be credible for people to believe that success is attainable. Although positive feedback can raise individuals' self-efficacy, the effects will not endure if they subsequently perform poorly (Schunk & DiBenedetto, 2016).

Physiological and emotional reactions such as anxiety and stress provide input about self-efficacy (Bandura, 1997). Strong emotional reactions can signal anticipated success or failure. When people experience negative thoughts and fears about their capabilities (e.g., feeling nervous when thinking about taking a test), those affective reactions can lower self-efficacy (Zajacova et al., 2005). Conversely, when people feel less stressful (e.g., anxiety subsides while taking a test), they may experience higher self-efficacy.

These sources do not operate automatically (Bandura, 1997). Individuals interpret the results of events and use these interpretations to gauge self-efficacy (Schunk & DiBenedetto, 2016). Some ways that research has shown to effectively build students' self-efficacy are to have students set difficult but attainable goals and assess their own goal progress (mastery experiences), allow students to observe models similar to themselves learning skills (vicarious experiences), and provide students with feedback that links their learning progress to their diligently applying a learning strategy (social persuasion; Schunk & Usher, 2019).

Although important, self-efficacy is not the only influence on behavior. Self-efficacy will not produce competent performances when requisite skills are absent. Also important are *outcome expectations* (beliefs about the likely consequences of actions; Bandura, 1997), and *values* (perceptions of the importance and utility of learning and acting in given ways (Wigfield et al., 2016). Even students who feel efficacious about performing well in school may not be academically engaged if they do not value it or believe that negative outcomes may result, such as rejection by peers. Assuming requisite skills and positive values and outcome expectations, self-efficacy is a key determinant of motivation, learning, self-regulation, and achievement (Schunk & DiBenedetto, 2016).

Consequences of Self-Efficacy

Self-efficacy can affect various motivational outcomes relevant to student engagement, including task choice, effort, and persistence (Bandura, 1997; Schunk & DiBenedetto, 2020). Individuals typically choose to engage in tasks at which they feel competent. Self-efficacy also can affect how much cognitive and physical effort they expend on task, how long they persist when they encounter difficulties, and how well they learn and achieve. Students with high self-efficacy tend to set challenging goals, work diligently, persist in the face of difficulty, and recover their sense of self-efficacy after setbacks. Those with low self-efficacy may set easier goals, expend minimal effort, quit when they encounter difficulties, and feel dejected by failure, all of which negatively affect engagement and learning (Bandura, 1997).

Goals and Self-Evaluations of Progress

Social cognitive theory highlights the importance of various symbolic processes for motivation. In addition to self-efficacy, goals and self-evaluations of goal progress are critical.

Goals can instigate and sustain actions, assuming that learners make a commitment to attempt to attain the goals (Locke & Latham, 2015). As learners work on a task, they compare their performances with their goals. Self-evaluations of progress strengthen self-efficacy and sustain motivation. A perceived discrepancy between present performance and the goal may create dissatisfaction, which can increase effort. Goals motivate learners to expend the effort necessary and persist at the task (Locke & Latham, 2015), resulting in enhanced engagement and performance (Zimmerman et al., 2015).

Goals are important, but their motivational effects depend on the properties of specificity, proximity, and difficulty. Goals that denote specific performance standards (e.g., "Work 20 math problems.") are more likely to lead to self-evaluations of progress and enhance self-efficacy and motivation than are general goals (e.g., "Work some math problems"; Bandura, 1986). Goals also are distinguished by how far they project into the future. Because it is easier to determine progress toward goals that are closer at hand (e.g., "Study math tonight."), proximal (short-term) goals enhance self-efficacy and motivation better than do distant (long-term) goals (e.g., "Study math by the end of the week."; Zimmerman et al., 2015).

Goal difficulty refers to the level of task proficiency required. People tend to work harder to attain challenging goals, although people may not be motivated to attempt to attain very difficult goals because they hold low self-efficacy for attaining them. Learners are apt to feel self-efficacious when they perceive as goals as challenging but attainable (Zimmerman et al., 2015).

Goals also can be distinguished on the basis of intended outcome. A *learning goal* refers to which knowledge, behavior, skill, or strategy students hope to acquire, whereas a *performance goal* refers to which task is to be completed. These goals can have differential effects on motivation and achievement (Anderman & Wolters, 2006). Learning goals motivate by focusing and sustaining attention on processes and strategies that help learners acquire competence and skills. Self-efficacy is substantiated as learners work on the task and assess their progress (Zimmerman et al., 2015).

In contrast, performance goals focus attention on completing tasks. They may not highlight the value of the processes and strategies underlying task completion or raise self-efficacy for learning. As they engage in tasks, learners may not compare their present and past performances to determine progress. Performance goals can lead to social comparisons with others to determine progress. These comparisons can lower self-efficacy when students experience learning difficulties, which adversely affects motivation and engagement.

Research supports these hypothesized effects. Schunk and Ertmer (1999) conducted two studies with teacher education college undergraduates as they worked on computer projects. Students received the goal of learning computer applications or the goal of performing them. In the first study, half of the students in each goal condition evaluated their learning progress midway through the instructional program. The learning goal led to higher self-efficacy, self-judged progress, and self-regulatory competence and strategy use. The opportunity to self-evaluate progress promoted self-efficacy. In the second study, self-evaluation students assessed their progress after each instructional session. Frequent self-evaluation produced comparable results when linked with a learning or performance goal. These results suggest that multiple self-evaluations of progress can raise motivation, engagement, and achievement.

Self-Efficacy and Student Engagement

Characteristics of Engaged Learners

Student engagement in learning reflects cognitive, behavioral, and affective variables that include motivation and self-regulation (Schunk & Usher, 2019; Zimmerman, 2000). Among cognitive variables, students engaged in learning hold a sense of self-efficacy that they are capable of learning. They also value the learning and believe that positive outcomes will result from learning. They set goals and decide to use strategies that they believe will help them learn.

Engaged learners also display productive achievement behaviors. They create physical and social environments conducive to learning that include necessary materials and equipment. While engaged in tasks, they focus their attention, expend effort, persist when they encounter difficulties, and evaluate their progress. They seek help from teachers, parents, peers, the Internet, and so on, when they are unsure of what to do. Engaged learners self-monitor their use of

time. They may keep records of what they have done and what remains to be done (e.g., by using a planner).

Affective variables include creating and maintaining a positive attitude toward learning. Engaged learners value learning; by succeeding, they experience a sense of pride. They are strategic about learning and know how to keep themselves from becoming discouraged. For example, if they cannot answer the first few questions on a test, they answer other questions to gain a sense of progress. If they become stuck on difficult content, they seek help (e.g., from teachers) rather than sit idly and become anxious.

Self-efficacy comes into play at all points in engaged learning. Prior to beginning a task, students hold a sense of self-efficacy for learning (Schunk & Usher, 2019). Their self-efficacy is substantiated as they work on tasks and observe their goal progress. Self-efficacy helps to keep students motivated and engaged in learning activities. Similar to how they handle difficulties, students who feel efficacious about learning but perceive that their progress is inadequate make adjustments to improve their learning (e.g., change strategy, seek help, enhance one's environment). Such modifications promote continued engagement.

Contextual Influences

Contextual variables affect self-efficacy, motivation, and engagement. Some of the most prominent are familial, sociocultural, and educational variables (Table 1).

Familial variables Families influence self-efficacy through their *capital,* which includes resources and assets (Bradley & Corwyn, 2002). Resources may be material (e.g., income), human (e.g., education), and social/cultural (e.g., networks). These resources include knowledge and skills that are valued in school settings (e.g., technological resources such as computers in the home; Yosso, 2005). Children are motivated to learn when the home has activities and materials that arouse and hold their interest and that pro-

Table 1 Contextual variables affecting self-efficacy, motivation, and engagement

Contextual variables	Examples
Familial	Family capital
	Family environment
	Role models
Sociocultural	Socioeconomic status
	Possible selves
	Peers
	Culture related stress
Educational	Methods of instruction
	Modeling
	Social feedback

vide attainable challenges (Schunk & Usher, 2019). Parents who are better educated and have social connections are apt to stress education and enroll their children in school and extramural programs that foster self-efficacy, engagement, and learning.

Families that foster a responsive and supportive environment, encourage exploration and stimulate interest, and facilitate learning experiences, accelerate their children's intellectual development. Because mastery experiences constitute a powerful source of self-efficacy information, parents who arrange for their children to experience mastery in their interests (e.g., music, sports) are apt to develop efficacious youngsters (Schunk & Usher, 2019). In contrast, parents may negatively affect their children's academic motivation, engagement, and achievement through various practices. For example, providing extrinsic rewards that are not tied to learning progress may decrease motivation when rewards are not given. Parents who make unrealistic demands may create anxiety in learners. Those who do not encourage self-regulated learning may not prepare students to meet academic challenges.

Another means of influence is vicariously through role models. Family members who model ways to cope with difficulties, persistence, and effort, strengthen their children's self-efficacy. Family members also provide persuasive information. Parents who encourage their children to try different activities facilitate their capability for addressing challenges.

Families also are influential with adult children. Western societies are characterized by a longer transition to adulthood and a prolonged time to finish school, become employed, and start families (Settersten & Ray, 2010). Children from impoverished backgrounds may not attain these points at the same rate as their more privileged peers. Modern families can experience undue stress where children remain semi-dependent for different types of assistance. Those from low-income families receive approximately 70% less material assistance than those in the top quarter of the income distribution (Settersten & Ray, 2010).

Sociocultural variables Socioeconomic status (SES) is positively related to self-efficacy and achievement. Borkowski and Thorpe (1994) reviewed empirical studies and found that lower-SES students often lack positive visions of and long-term goals for themselves in school, career, and life.

Learners who view school subjects in light of who they want to become (e.g., lawyer, teacher) improve their capabilities, motivation, and engagement (Shell & Husman, 2001). Based on their study involving almost 200 primarily White undergraduate students, Shell and Husman (2001) found that students' future time beliefs (i.e., relative importance of attaining immediate versus long-term future outcomes) were associated with higher self-efficacy, achievement, and study time and effort.

Children can be guided to develop future-oriented conceptions (possible selves; (Borkowski & Thorpe, 1994). Short- and long-range goals are critical for their development (Borkowski & Thorpe, 1994; Oyserman & James, 2009). Teachers who have a future time perspective can influence engagement and motivate students by explaining the importance of present behavior on future actions and identity (Simons et al., 2004). Although short-term and specific goals are strong motivators, long-term goals also are important (Bandura, 1986).

Teachers engage their students by taking into account their capacities to think about the future

(Husman & Lens, 1999). Teachers exert socio-cultural influence as role models when they help students understand what possibilities can be acted upon in their environment and when they assist with problem solving and goal setting for achieving future goals (Miller & Brickman, 2004). Teachers can exert a positive influence by changing the classroom environment, modifying their instructional and interpersonal strategies, and addressing students' individual goals (Miller & Brickman, 2004).

In a 5-year study of the motivational levels of Native Americans and White Americans, McInerney et al. (1998) found that middle schoolers experienced difficulty in imagining the future (e.g., employability and other long-term goals). Students may need to be encouraged to connect their present and future goals by determining an instrumental route to the future (McInerney, 2004). Developmental changes may make a difference. McInerney et al. (1998) found that when they reached high school, middle schoolers often became more receptive to imagining their futures and projecting themselves into colleges and jobs. Adolescents are better able to do this than younger children.

Peers constitute another sociocultural influence. With development, peers become important influences on self-efficacy (Schunk et al., 2014). Parents who steer their children toward efficacious peers provide opportunities for vicarious increases in self-efficacy. When children observe their peers succeed, they are likely to experience higher self-efficacy and motivation.

Peer influence also operates through *networks*, or groups of friends and others with whom students associate. Students who belong to networks tend to be similar (Cairns et al., 1989), which enhances the likelihood of influence by modeling. Networks help define students' opportunities for interactions and observations of others' interactions, as well as their access to activities. Over time, network members tend to become even more similar. Arroyo and Zigler (1995) studied African American and White peer groups in urban high schools and found that racial identification can affect achievement when members believe that others hold a negative per-ception of their group. The African American participants reported lower identification with their racial group, instead being concerned about jeopardizing the approval of nonmembers.

Peer groups promote motivational socialization. Changes in children's motivation across the school year are predicted by their peer group membership (Kindermann et al., 1996). Children affiliated with highly motivated groups change positively, whereas those in less motivated groups change negatively. Steinberg et al. (1996) tracked students throughout their high school years, finding that those with similar grades but affiliated with academically oriented crowds achieved more than those affiliated with less academically inclined peers. Peer group academic socialization can influence academic self-efficacy (Schunk & Usher, 2019).

Another influence on academic self-efficacy is perceived stress and anxiety. Stress has the potential to depress students' self-efficacy, especially among disadvantaged college populations (e.g., nontraditional, immigrant, and minority; Zajacova et al., 2005) and urban high school students (Gillock & Reyes, 1999). Pajares and Kranzler (1995) found that mathematics anxiety exerted a weaker influence than self-efficacy on high school students' mathematical performances. Zajacova et al. (2005) assessed self-efficacy and stress among freshmen immigrant and minority college students and found that academic self-efficacy and stress were negatively correlated.

Minority and immigrant students experience culture-related stress, making them more susceptible to social stress than native-born and White students (Zajacova et al., 2005). Despite increasing diversity within classrooms, many African American and Hispanic students feel disengaged and culturally segregated.

Educational variables The role of self-efficacy in student engagement has been explored by researchers in diverse educational domains with students differing in age, developmental level, and cultural background. Researchers have established that self-efficacy influences individuals' motivation, achievement, and self-regulation in both correlational and empirical studies (Bandura, 1997; Pajares, 1997; Schunk & DiBenedetto, 2016; Stajkovic & Luthans, 1998). A recent study with 881 urban, primarily minority and low income, first-to-third graders, identified by teachers as at-risk for reading, examined the role of self-efficacy in predicting achievement (Lee & Jonson-Reid, 2016). Students' reading skills were tested at both the beginning and the end of the school year and students, parents, and teachers were administered surveys assessing students' reading, self-efficacy, behavior, and global-reading self-concept. Surveys were developed by obtaining questions from previously established assessment scales of self-efficacy and self-concept and then modified to be more appropriate for this sample's age. Findings revealed that young students were able to differentiate between self-efficacy and self-concept and that self-efficacy predicted students' motivation and performance. Reading self-efficacy had a significant and positive impact on standardized reading achievement measures whereas the effect of reading self-concept on reading achievement was not significant.

The relationship between self-efficacy, engagement, and performance has also been shown in high school and college students. In a study with 220 suburban high school students, researchers examined the impact of self-efficacy and other variables on cognitive engagement and achievement (Greene et al., 2004). A series of questionnaires were distributed over a three-month period. Results showed that self-efficacy and meaningful strategy use were the strongest predictors of academic achievement. Percentage grade was significantly and positively predicted by self-efficacy ($B = :38$, $t = 5:29$) and strategy use ($B = :15$, $t = 2:08$). DiBenedetto and Bembenutty (2013) examined changes in science self-efficacy over a semester for 113 college students enrolled in intermediate level science courses. Findings revealed self-efficacy beliefs at the end of the semester declined and yet were more closely related to final term averages than they were at the start of the semester (pre-assessment $M = 6.30$, $SD = 0.78$ and postassess-

ment $M = 6.02$, SD 0.94, $t = -3.68$). These results suggest that students' beliefs about their performance became better calibrated as the semester progressed.

Experimental research also has shown that instructional and social practices that convey to students that they are making progress and becoming competent learners raise self-efficacy, motivation, and achievement (Schunk & DiBenedetto, 2016). Some beneficial practices are having students pursue proximal and specific goals, using social models in instruction, providing feedback indicating competence, having students self-monitor and evaluate their learning progress, and teaching students to use metacognitive strategies while learning (Coutinho, 2008; Schunk & Ertmer, 1999; Schunk & DiBenedetto, 2016). Other benefits on students' self-efficacy occur from role models who provide encouragement and high expectations for achievement, a feeling of control over and empowerment within one's environment, and rewards for doing well in school (Jonson-Reid et al., 2005; Miller & Brickman, 2004).

Falco and Summers (2019) conducted an intervention study incorporating the four sources of self-efficacy on high school girls' STEM (science, technology, engineering, mathematics) career self-efficacy beliefs. Ethnically diverse high school girls received nine 50-minute counseling sessions targeted at building students' self-efficacy for making intentional career decisions and for building self-efficacy for careers in STEM. The four sources to build self-efficacy included focusing on performance accomplishments, modeling, strategies for controlling anxiety, and verbal persuasions and encouragement. Results showed positive moderate-to-large effect sizes for the impact of the intervention on both students' career decision making self-efficacy and self-efficacy for careers in STEM.

Ramdass and Zimmerman (2011) examined the influence of modeling and social feedback on 76 sixth- and seventh-grade students' self-efficacy and mathematical achievement. Students observed coping models with or without social feedback, or mastery models with or without social feedback. Mastery models demonstrate faultless performance from the outset; coping models initially experience difficulties but gradually improve and eventually perform as well as mastery models. Findings revealed that students in the coping model conditions surpassed those in the mastery model conditions on the posttests mathematics performance ($F(1, 71) = 14.83$, $p < 0.001$), and on self-efficacy ($F(1, 71) = 5.04$, $p < 0.05$). Thus, the sources of self-efficacy can be used to foster competency beliefs, motivation, and engagement in learners.

Self-Efficacy and Positive Development and Outcomes

The role of self-efficacy in engagement has been studied extensively in underachievement and dropout (Alexander et al., 2001; Christenson et al., 2012; Hardre & Reeve, 2003; Lee & Burkam, 2003; Rumberger & Thomas, 2000). Factors contributing to underachievement and dropout include under-developed academic and social skills, little interest in school subjects, classrooms that stress competition and ability social comparisons, low perceived value of school learning, little sense of belonging or relatedness to the school environment, and inadequate vision of the future (Alexander et al., 2001; McInerney, 2004; Meece et al., 2006; Wentzel, 2005).

In recent years, researchers have increasingly turned their attention toward how self-efficacy may promote positive student development, adjustment, and other outcomes (Furlong et al., 2014). The latter depend heavily on students' involvement and participation in school; in particular, how much the environment promotes their perceptions of autonomy and relatedness (Suldo et al., 2014), which in turn can influence self-efficacy and achievement. Students who feel a sense of belonging at school are more apt to be engaged academically, socially, and physically in school activities (Ryan & Deci, 2016). Parents, teachers, and peers affect students' feelings of belongingness, and peer groups exert increasing influence during adolescence (Kindermann, 2007; Steinberg et al., 1996).

High self-efficacy can promote student engagement, but by itself does not guarantee motivation and engagement. It is possible to feel efficacious about learning but show little interest if students place little value on school learning or show low interest in it. It is important that teachers, parents, and peers build self-efficacy in learners through the sources mentioned earlier: performance accomplishments, vicarious experiences, social persuasions, and physiological indexes. The perception of progress in learning is a reliable indicator of capabilities because progress conveys to students that they are capable of learning. Such self-referential feedback that others might provide can raise students' self-efficacy and motivation for school (Schunk & DiBenedetto, 2016). Especially for learners who have disadvantaged backgrounds it is critical that they receive positive information in school that they can be successful.

Interventions can be simple such as class-based programs, but they also can involve school district policies and entire schools. Social policies and second-chance programs have been in effect for years; however, many of these are restrictive in scope and problem-based, not developmental (Bloom, 2010). They often have not assessed students' self-efficacy, but this is necessary. Increased research is needed on such programs and a focus on ethnic identity and prevention at the high school level or earlier (Bloom, 2010). Engagement strategies for assisting high-risk dropout populations (e.g., immigrants, disabled, young mothers, foster care youth, youth offenders) include identity development, paid work, internships, job training, community service, and life skills. Research shows that these types of experiences can promote academic self-efficacy of diverse first-generation students (Majer, 2009).

Future Research Directions

The principles of social cognitive theory add value to understanding student engagement. There are several self-efficacy research areas that should be addressed. Among these are contextual influences, cross-cultural relevance, collective self-efficacy, and integration with technology.

Contextual Influences

Self-efficacy can affect and be influenced by social/environmental variables that often are context specific. Enhancing students' self-efficacy, motivation, and engagement requires an understanding of how contextual variables operate.

For example, an area needing to be addressed is the role of school transitions (e.g., middle school to high school) because these produce many contextual changes that can affect self-efficacy. It is not unusual for students' self-efficacy to decline after a transition (Wigfield & Cambria, 2010). Material to be learned typically becomes more difficult and students' comparison groups shift membership. Researchers should address how students perceive these changes and how they might affect self-efficacy. A key question is how social/environmental variables might be structured to not only prevent a decline but also provide efficacy-strengthening experiences.

Another research emphasis should be on how self-efficacy interacts with students' perceptions of school climate and sense of belonging—variables that are key predictors of school engagement (Ryan & Deci, 2016; Suldo et al., 2014). Learners who experience positive emotions in school and feel a sense of belonging in a positive environment are less at risk for underachieving and dropping out (Suldo et al., 2014). Research on students' perceptions will suggest ways to improve their self-efficacy and engagement in learning. For example, imaging a future goal and how school might contribute to that can enhance self-efficacy and engagement (Borkowski & Thorpe, 1994; Jonson-Reid et al., 2005). Knowing how classroom factors contribute to perceptions of climate can lead to improvements in environmental factors. Research also can investigate self-conceptions and possible selves, as well as experiences of academic identification (Kerpelman et al., 2008).

Cross-Cultural Relevance

Most social cognitive research has been conducted in Western societies, but this situation is changing as researchers are testing principles of social cognitive theory globally. The topics of self-efficacy and self-regulation have much international appeal. And cross-cultural research has yielded differences (McInerney, 2008). For example, Klassen (2004) found that individuals in individualistic (Western) cultures tend to judge self-efficacy higher than do learners in collectivist cultures. The correspondence between self-efficacy and skills is better for those in collectivist cultures.

These are important findings because people who overestimate their self-efficacy may attempt tasks beyond their means and perform poorly, whereas those who underestimate may be reluctant to engage in tasks and thereby preclude opportunities for learning (Schunk & DiBenedetto, 2020). These results suggest that collectivist cultures may promote modest self-efficacy judgments and that in some cultures collective self-efficacy (self-efficacy of what a group can accomplish; discussed next) may predict learning outcomes better than individual self-efficacy.

Although social cognitive theory has been found to be cross-culturally relevant, more needs to be known about students from different cultures and countries. Most educational self-efficacy studies have focused on students from the United States without sufficient attention on issues of diversity, especially as related to learning and engagement. This is especially important today as schools become more diverse including within cultures. Cross-cultural studies will expand understanding of the operation and generality of self-efficacy.

Research that focuses on culturally ethnic students' experiences at different types of institutions is also needed. Hand in hand with this focus is that of social policies and programs that can address in a specific way not only the lower achievement and higher attrition for African American college students but also what types of interventions and resources foster ethnic students' self-efficacy and success. Given that research on self-efficacy has mostly focused on White students at predominately White institutions, we need a better understanding of African American youths' sense of self-efficacy, in addition to strategies that foster a belief in the value of education (Jonson-Reid et al., 2005).

Collective Self-Efficacy

As noted previously, cultural dimensions such as individualism and collectivism may influence the relation of self-efficacy to academic outcomes (Oettingen & Zosuls, 2006). Kim and Park (2006) argued that theories that emphasize individualistic values—such as self-efficacy—cannot explain the high achievement of East Asian students. Instead, the Confucian-based socialization practices that promote close parent–child relationships seem responsible for high levels of self-regulatory, relational, and social efficacy. In these cultures, relational efficacy (i.e., perceived competence in family and social relations), as well as social support from parents, may influence students' academic performances. Self-efficacy may be more other-oriented in some non-Western (particularly Asian) cultures than in Western cultures (Klassen, 2004), a point that needs further research.

Many educational contexts are structured for group work. It makes sense to ask how to create and sustain engaged groups. These groups display the same features as engaged individuals. *Collective self-efficacy* (perceived capabilities of the group, team, or larger social entity) is not the average of individuals' self-efficacy but rather members' perceived capabilities to attain a common goal by working together (Bandura, 1997).

As noted earlier in this chapter, collective self-efficacy may predict group performance better than individual self-efficacy and especially among persons in collectivist cultures. But even in more individualistic cultures, working in groups is considered important in- and outside-of-school.

In a similar vein, *collective teacher self-efficacy* is the belief of a group of teachers that they can enhance students' achievement and well-being (Bandura, 1997). Collective self-efficacy and collective teacher self-efficacy are influenced by the same sources as is individual self-efficacy. Collective efficacy can be developed when group members work together to achieve common goals (performance accomplishments), learn from one another and from mentors (vicarious experiences), receive encouragement and support from others (forms of persuasion), and work together to cope with difficulties and alleviate stress (physiological indexes). Cantrell and Hughes (2008), for example, found that sixth- and ninth-grade teachers' collective self-efficacy improved after a year-long professional development program involving a team approach to teaching literacy.

Relative to individual self-efficacy, there is far less research on collective efficacy. But researchers have shown that collective self-efficacy is positively related to teacher job satisfaction and retention (Caprara et al., 2003). Teachers and students who remain engaged are less likely to drop out of teaching or school. We recommend enhanced research on collective self-efficacy both to clarify its operation within groups and suggest implications for educational practices.

Integration with Technology

Social cognitive theory was largely developed prior to technological advances. Most research has been face-to-face. The theory does not need major revisions because the principles are intended to be generic and apply across different contexts. But the role of technology requires some theoretical adaptations.

Social cognitive research is needed with social media. These media offer ways for learners to be engaged with others, and we know little about how such engaged interactions may influence self-efficacy and other variables. Learning from others is a source of self-efficacy information, and this should be true regardless of whether the interactions are live or virtual. Social media fit well with a social cognitive theory.

Such research has implications for teaching and learning. There are many educational uses for technologies such as Facebook and Zoom. How might these and other forms of media be used to help students set goals, monitor progress, assess self-efficacy for learning, and the like? How might instruction be designed to incorporate social media that take self-efficacy of learners and teachers into account? Research is needed to expand the generality of the theory beyond its original formulation.

Educational Applications

There are several applications of self-efficacy theory and research for student engagement, especially using the four sources of self-efficacy information. Mastery experiences are powerful influences on self-efficacy, especially when learners set challenging but attainable goals and practice and refine skills. As they observe their goal and learning progress, their self-efficacy for continued learning is strengthened. Teachers also can provide vicarious experiences by indicating how other similar students have mastered skills, as well as persuasive information through realistic encouragement. Encouraging students to attempt very difficult tasks may prove demoralizing and lower self-efficacy. Teachers can use physiological indicators, such as when they tell students that they are reacting in a less-stressful way to completing assignments.

Teachers want students to be successful and may be tempted to assist them. Assistance often is necessary in the early stages of learning. But success with help does not build strong self-efficacy because students may attribute the success to the teacher's help. Allowing learners to succeed on their own strengthens self-efficacy better.

Another idea is to use an appropriate instructional model that allows for differentiation. Students do not learn at the same rate or in the same way. Nonindividualized assignments mean some will succeed but others will not. The latter

students, when they compare their performances to those of students who have done well, may doubt their capabilities. Individualized instruction minimizes social comparisons. Teachers can provide individualized feedback, such as by telling them, "See how much better you're doing on these now?"

Students can be encouraged to evaluate their learning and gauge their progress. For example, teachers could give students a scale ranging from 1 (low) to 10 and ask them to assess their progress in solving different types of mathematical problems. Such assessments are good indicators of where students may need additional instruction and practice.

A key goal is for learners to have a sense of realistic optimism about what they can learn or accomplish, which can motivate them to improve (Bandura, 1997). A sense of realistic optimism gives learners goals to strive for and makes for enjoyable environments in which to learn.

Conclusion

Research evidence supports the point that self-efficacy is a significant influence on learners' motivation and engagement (Schunk & DiBenedetto, 2016, 2020). Self-efficacy helps to create a sense of agency and contributes to learners' positive development in- and out-of-school (Schunk & DiBenedetto, 2016).

Social cognitive theory stresses learning from the social environment. The conceptual focus of Bandura's theory postulates reciprocal interactions among personal, behavioral, and social/environmental factors. Self-efficacy is a critical personal factor that can affect motivation, engagement, learning, and achievement. Self-efficacy is shaped by personal, cultural, and social factors.

Attention to ways of building students' skills and self-efficacy will help learners become academically motivated and stay engaged in learning. These outcomes should help diminish underachievement and dropout, as well as provide learners with a sense of realistic optimism about their capabilities. Important research questions remain that will help refine the theory and have implications for teaching and learning.

References

Alexander, K., Entwisle, D., & Kabbani, N. (2001). The dropout process in life course perspective: Early risk factors at home and school. *Teachers College Record, 103*, 760–822. https://doi.org/10.1111/0161-4681.00134

Anderman, E. M., & Wolters, C. A. (2006). Goals, values, and affects: Influences on student motivation. In P. A. Alexander & P. H. Winne (Eds.), *Handbook of educational psychology* (2nd ed., pp. 369–389). Erlbaum.

Arroyo, C. G., & Zigler, E. (1995). Racial identity, academic achievement, and the psychological Well-being of economically disadvantaged adolescents. *Journal of Personality and Social Psychology, 69*(5), 903–914. https://doi.org/10.1037/0022-3514.69.5.903

Bandura, A. (1977a). Self-efficacy: Toward a unifying theory of behavioral change. *Psychological Review, 84*, 191–215.

Bandura, A. (1977b). *Social learning theory*. Prentice Hall.

Bandura, A. (1986). *Social foundations of thought and action: A social cognitive theory*. Prentice Hall.

Bandura, A. (1997). *Self-efficacy: The exercise of control*. Freeman.

Bandura, A. (2001). Social cognitive theory: An agentic perspective. *Annual Review of Psychology, 52*, 1–26.

Bloom, D. (2010). Programs and policies to assist high school dropouts in the transition to adulthood. *The Future of Children, 20*(1), 89–108. https://doi.org/10.1353/foc.0.0039

Borkowski, J. G., & Thorpe, P. K. (1994). Self-regulation and motivation: A life-span perspective on underachievement. In D. H. Schunk & B. J. Zimmerman (Eds.), *Self regulation of learning and performance: Issues and educational applications* (pp. 45–73). Erlbaum.

Bradley, R. H., & Corwyn, R. F. (2002). Socioeconomic status and child development. *Annual Review of Psychology, 53*, 371–399. https://doi.org/10.1146/annurev.psych.53.100901.135233

Cairns, R. B., Cairns, B. D., & Neckerman, J. J. (1989). Early school dropout: Configurations and determinants. *Child Development, 60*, 1437–1452. https://doi.org/10.1111/j.1467-8624.1989.tb04015.x

Cantrell, S. C., & Hughes, H. K. (2008). Teacher efficacy and content literacy implementation: An exploration of the effects of extended professional development with coaching. *Journal of Literacy Research, 40*, 95–127. https://doi.org/10.1080/10862960802070442

Caprara, G. V., Barbaranelli, C., Borgogni, L., & Steca, P. (2003). Efficacy beliefs as determinants of teachers' job satisfaction. *Journal of Educational Psychology, 95*, 821–832. https://doi.org/10.1037/0022-0663.95.4.821

Christenson, S. L., Reschly, A. L., & Wylie, C. (Eds.). (2012). *Handbook of research on student engagement*. Springer.

Coutinho, S. (2008). Self-efficacy, metacognition, and performance. *North American Journal of Psychology, 10*(1), 165–172.

DiBenedetto, M., & Bembenutty, H. (2013). Within the pipeline: Self-regulated learning, self-efficacy, and socialization among college students in science courses. *Learning and Individual Differences, 23*(1), 218–224. https://doi.org/10.1016/j.lindif.2012.09.015

Falco, L. D., & Summers, J. J. (2019). Improving career decision self-efficacy and STEM self-efficacy in high school girls: Evaluation of an intervention. *Journal of Career Development, 46*(1), 62–76. https://doi.org/10.1177/0894845317721651

Furlong, M. J., Gilman, R., & Huebner, E. S. (Eds.). (2014). *Handbook of positive psychology in schools* (2nd ed.). Routledge.

Greene, B. A., Raymond, B. M., Crowson, M. H., Duke, B. L., & Akey, K. L. (2004). Predicting high school students' cognitive engagement and achievement: Contributions of classroom perceptions and motivation. *Contemporary Educational Psychology, 29*(4), 462–482.

Gillock, K. L., & Reyes, O. (1999). Stress, support, and academic performance of urban, low-income, Mexican–American adolescents. *Journal of Youth and Adolescence, 28*(2), 259–282. https://doi.org/10.1016/j.cedpsych.2004.01.006

Hardre, P., & Reeve, J. (2003). A motivational model of rural students' intentions to persist in, versus drop out of, high school. *Journal of Educational Psychology, 95*, 347–356. https://doi.org/10.1037/0022-0663.95.2.347

Husman, J., & Lens, W. (1999). The role of the future in student motivation. *Educational Psychologist, 34*(2), 113–125. https://doi.org/10.1207/s15326985ep3402_4

Jonson-Reid, M., Davis, L., Saunders, J., Williams, T., & Williams, J. H. (2005). Academic self-efficacy among African American youths: Implications for school social work practice. *Children & Schools, 27*(1), 5–14. https://doi.org/10.1093/cs/27.1.5

Kerpelman, J. L., Eryigit, S., & Stephens, C. J. (2008). African American adolescents' future education orientation: Associations with self-efficacy, ethnic identity, and perceived parental support. *Journal of Youth Adolescence, 37*, 997–1008. https://doi.org/10.1007/s10964-007-9201-7

Kim, U., & Park, Y. S. (2006). Factors influencing academic achievement in collectivist societies: The role of self-, relational, and social efficacy. In F. Pajares & T. Urdan (Eds.), *Self-efficacy beliefs of adolescents* (pp. 267–286). Information Age Publishing.

Kindermann, T. A. (2007). Effects of naturally existing peer groups on changes in academic engagement in a cohort of sixth graders. *Child Development, 78*, 1186–1203. https://doi.org/10.1111/j.1467-8624.2007.01060.x

Kindermann, T. A., McCollam, T. L., & Gibson, E., Jr. (1996). Peer networks and students' classroom engagement during childhood and adolescence. In J. Juvonen & K. R. Wentzel (Eds.), *Social motivation: Understanding children's school adjustment* (pp. 279–312). Cambridge University Press.

Klassen, R. M. (2004). Optimism and realism: A review of self-efficacy from a cross-cultural perspective. *International Journal of Psychology, 39*, 205–230. https://doi.org/10.1080/00207590344000330

Lee, V. E., & Burkam, D. T. (2003). Dropping out of high school: The role of school organization and structure. *American Educational Research Journal, 40*, 353–393. https://doi.org/10.3102/00028312040002353

Lee, Y. W., & Jonson-Reid, M. (2016). The role of self-efficacy in reading achievement of young children in urban schools. *Child & Adolescent Social Work Journal, 33*(1), 79–89. https://doi.org/10.1007/S10560-015-0404-6

Locke, E. A., & Latham, G. P. (2015). Breaking the roles: A historical overview of goal setting theory. In A. J. Elliot (Ed.), *Advances in motivation science* (Vol. 2, pp. 99–126). Elsevier.

Majer, J. M. (2009). Self-efficacy and academic success among ethnically diverse first-generation community college students. *Journal of Diversity in Higher Education, 2*(4), 243–250. https://doi.org/10.1037/a0017852

McInerney, D. M. (2004). A discussion of future time perspective. *Educational Psychology Review, 16*(2), 141–151. https://doi.org/10.1023/B:EDPR.0000026610.18125.a3

McInerney, D. M. (2008). The motivational role of cultural differences and cultural identity in self-regulated learning. In D. H. Schunk & B. J. Zimmerman (Eds.), *Motivation and self-regulated learning: Theory, research, and applications* (pp. 369–400). Taylor & Francis.

McInerney, D. M., Hinkley, J., Dowson, M., & Van Etten, S. (1998). Aboriginal, Anglo, and immigrant Australian students' motivational beliefs about personal academic success: Are there cultural differences? *Journal of Educational Psychology, 90*, 621–629. https://doi.org/10.1037/0022-0663.90.4.621

Meece, J. L., Anderman, E. M., & Anderman, L. H. (2006). Classroom goal structure, student motivation, and academic achievement. *Annual Review of Psychology, 57*, 487–503. https://doi.org/10.1146/annurev.psych.56.091103.070258

Miller, R. B., & Brickman, S. J. (2004). A model of future-oriented motivation and self-regulation. *Educational Psychology Review, 16*(1), 9–33. https://doi.org/10.1023/B:EDPR.0000012343.96370.39

Oettingen, G., & Zosuls, C. (2006). Self-efficacy of adolescents across culture. In F. Pajares & T. Urdan (Eds.), *Self-efficacy beliefs of adolescents* (pp. 245–266). Information Age Publishing.

Oyserman, D., & James, L. (2009). Possible selves: From content to process. In K. D. Markman, W. M. P. Klein, & J. A. Suhr (Eds.), *Handbook of imagination and mental simulation* (pp. 373–394). Psychology Press.

Pajares, F. (1997). Current directions in self-efficacy research. In M. Maehr & P. R. Pintrich (Eds.), *Advances in motivation and achievement,10* (pp. 1–49). JAI Press.

Pajares, F., & Kranzler, J. (1995). Self-efficacy beliefs and general mental ability in mathematical problem-solving. *Contemporary Educational Psychology, 20*(4), 426–443. https://doi.org/10.1006/ceps.1995.1029

Ramdass, D., & Zimmerman, B. J. (2011). The effects of modeling and social feedback on middle-school students' math performance and accuracy judgments. *The International Journal of Educational and Psychological Assessment, 7*(1), 4–23.

Reschly, A. L., & Christenson, S. L. (2012). Jingle, jangle, and conceptual haziness: Evolution and future directions of the engagement construct. In S. L. Christenson, A. L. Reschly, & C. Wylie (Eds.), *Handbook of research on student engagement* (pp. 3–19). Springer.

Rumberger, R. W., & Thomas, S. L. (2000). The distribution of dropout and turnover rates among urban and suburban high schools. *Sociology of Education, 73*(1), 39–67. https://doi.org/10.2307/2673198

Ryan, R. M., & Deci, E. L. (2016). Facilitating and hindering motivation, learning, and Well-being in schools: Research and observations from self-determination theory. In K. R. Wentzel & D. B. Miele (Eds.), *Handbook of motivation at school* (2nd ed., pp. 96–119). Routledge.

Schunk, D. H., & DiBenedetto, M. K. (2014). Academic self-efficacy. In M. J. Furlong, R. Gilman, & E. S. Huebner (Eds.), *Handbook of positive psychology in schools* (2nd ed., pp. 115–130). Routledge.

Schunk, D. H., & DiBenedetto, M. K. (2016). Self-efficacy theory in education. In K. R. Wentzel & D. B. Miele (Eds.), *Handbook of motivation at school* (2nd ed., pp. 34–54). Routledge.

Schunk, D. H., & DiBenedetto, M. K. (2020). Social cognitive theory, self-efficacy, and students with disabilities: Implications for students with learning disabilities, reading disabilities, and attention-deficit/hyperactivity disorder. In A. J. Martin, R. A. Sperling, & K. J. Newton (Eds.), *Handbook of educational psychology and students with special needs* (pp. 243–261). Routledge.

Schunk, D. H., & Ertmer, P. A. (1999). Self-regulatory processes during computer skill acquisition: Goal and self-evaluative influences. *Journal of Educational Psychology, 91*, 251–260. https://doi.org/10.1037/0022-0663.91.2.251

Schunk, D. H., Meece, J. L., & Pintrich, P. R. (2014). *Motivation in education: Theory, research, and applications* (4th ed.). Pearson Education.

Schunk, D. H., & Usher, E. L. (2019). Social cognitive theory and motivation. In R. M. Ryan (Ed.), *The Oxford handbook of human motivation* (2nd ed., pp. 11–26). Oxford University Press.

Settersten, R. A., Jr., & Ray, B. (2010). What's going on with young people today? The long and twisting path to adulthood. *The Future of Children, 20*(1), 19–41. https://doi.org/10.1353/foc.0.0044

Shell, D. F., & Husman, J. (2001). The multivariate dimensionality of personal control and future time perspective beliefs in achievement and self-regulation. *Contemporary Educational Psychology, 26*, 481–506. https://doi.org/10.1006/ceps.2000.1073

Simons, J., Vansteenkiste, M., Lens, W., & Lacante, M. (2004). Placing motivation and future time perspective theory in a temporal perspective. *Educational Psychology Review, 16*(2), 121–139. https://doi.org/10.1023/B:EDPR.0000026609.94841.2f

Skinner, E. A., Kindermann, T. A., Connell, J. P., & Wellborn, J. G. (2009). Engagement and disaffection as organizational constructs in the dynamics of motivational development. In K. R. Wentzel & A. Wigfield (Eds.), *Handbook of motivation at school* (pp. 223–245). Routledge.

Stajkovic, A. D., & Luthans, F. (1998). Self-efficacy and work-related performances: A meta-analysis. *Psychological Bulletin, 124*, 240–261. https://doi.org/10.1037/0033-2909.124.2.240

Steinberg, L., Brown, B. B., & Dornbusch, S. M. (1996). *Beyond the classroom: Why school reform has failed and what parents need to do.* Simon & Schuster.

Suldo, S. M., Bateman, L. P., & Gelley, C. D. (2014). Understanding and promoting school satisfaction in children and adolescents. In M. J. Furlong, R. Gilman, & E. S. Huebner (Eds.), *Handbook of positive psychology in schools* (2nd ed., pp. 365–380). Routledge.

Usher, E. L., & Schunk, D. H. (2018). Social cognitive theoretical perspective of self-regulation. In D. H. Schunk & J. A. Greene (Eds.), *Handbook of self-regulation of learning and performance* (2nd ed., pp. 19–35). Routledge.

Wentzel, K. R. (2005). Peer relationships, motivation, and academic performance at school. In A. J. Elliot & C. S. Dweck (Eds.), *Handbook of competence and motivation* (pp. 279–296). Guilford Press.

Wigfield, A., & Cambria, J. (2010). Students' achievement values, goal orientations, and interest: Definitions, development, and relations to achievement outcomes. *Developmental Review, 30*, 1–35. https://doi.org/10.1016/j.dr.2009.12.001

Wigfield, A., Tonks, S., & Klauda, S. L. (2016). Expectancy-value theory. In K. R. Wentzel & D. B. Miele (Eds.), *Handbook of motivation at school* (2nd ed., pp. 55–74). Routledge.

Yosso, T. J. (2005). Whose culture has capital? A critical race theory discussion of community cultural wealth. *Race, Ethnicity, and Education, 8*(1), 69–91. https://doi.org/10.1080/1361332052000341006

Zajacova, A., Lynch, S. M., & Espenshade, T. J. (2005). Self-efficacy, stress, and academic success in college. *Research in Higher Education, 46*(6), 677–706. https://doi.org/10.1007/s11162-004-4139-z

Zimmerman, B. J. (2000). Attaining self-regulation: A social cognitive perspective. In M. Boekaerts, P. R. Pintrich, & M. Zeidner (Eds.), *Handbook of self-regulation* (pp. 13–39). Academic Press.

Zimmerman, B. J., & Cleary, T. J. (2009). Motives to self-regulate learning: A social cognitive account. In K. R. Wentzel & A. Wigfield (Eds.), *Handbook of motivation at school* (pp. 247–264). Routledge.

Zimmerman, B. J., Schunk, D. H., & DiBenedetto, M. K. (2015). A personal agency view of self-regulated learning: The role of goal setting. In F. Guay, H. Marsh, D. M. McInerney, & R. G. Craven (Eds.), *Self-concept, motivation, and identity: Underpinning success with research and practice* (pp. 83–114). Information Age Publishing.

Using Self-Regulated Learning (SRL) Assessment Data to Promote Regulatory Engagement in Learning and Performance Contexts

Timothy J. Cleary and Angela M. Lui

Abstract

Applications of self-regulated learning (SRL) processes in school contexts continue to rise in popularity and sophistication. In addition to intervention programs and initiatives, researchers have begun examining the effects of professional development programming and the role of SRL assessment practices in promoting optimal functioning and development. This chapter focuses on both SRL intervention and assessment practices, with particular emphasis on the emerging role of various SRL measures as formative assessment tools. Specifically, we review research and illustrate how SRL microanalysis and the Diagnostic Assessment and Achievement of College Students (DAACS) self-report questionnaire can be used in a formative fashion by researchers and/or practitioners to promote optimal feedback that can enhance student engagement and overall learning as well as teachers' instructional approaches or interactions with students. Implications for practice and suggested areas for future research are also presented and discussed.

T. J. Cleary (✉) · A. M. Lui
Rutgers, The State University of New Jersey,
New Brunswick, NJ, USA
e-mail: timothy.cleary@rutgers.edu;
angela.lui@rutgers.edu

Student engagement represents one of the most important constructs that school-based researchers and educators can address in their professional roles and activities, given its strong relation to students' behavioral and academic outcomes (Cleary & Kitsantas, 2017; Lovelace et al., 2017; Reschly, 2020). Defined by Christenson et al. (2012) as "[…] active participation in academic and cocurricular or school-related activities, and commitment to educational goals and learning" (pp. 816–817), student engagement is often viewed as a multi-dimensional construct with multiple subtypes: academic, behavioral, cognitive, and affective categories (Fredericks et al., 2004; Reschly & Christenson et al., 2012). Linked to each subtype are several indicators, such as task completion, productivity, or performance (i.e., academic engagement), class participation and attendance (i.e., behavioral engagement), self-regulatory processes like self-reflection or goal-setting (i.e., cognitive engagement), and feelings of connectedness and belongingness to school and peers (i.e., affective or emotional engagement).

Many scholars assert that models of student engagement and self-regulated learning (SRL) overlap conceptually, at least to some degree (Cleary et al., 2021; Cleary & Zimmerman, 2012; Reschly & Christenson et al., 2012). From an engagement perspective, regulatory and motivational processes (e.g., goal-setting, monitoring, and evaluation) are subsumed within cognitive engagement. Pohl (2020) underscored this premise, noting that "cognitive engagement can be defined as students' investment in their learning, valuing of their learning, directing effort toward learning, and using learning strategies to understand material, accomplish tasks, master skills, and achieve goals" (p. 254). In the first edition of this Handbook, Cleary and Zimmerman (2012) also discussed SRL specifically with regard to cognitive engagement. They argued that most SRL models are discussed in terms of a *cyclical feedback loop*; that is, an internal, largely cognitively driven cyclical process that is central to understanding the ways through which individuals optimize their overall engagement and learning in school. They also underscored additional areas of overlap between these two constructs, namely with respect to the role of situational dependence or context in understanding students' engagement or regulation.

The primary objectives of this chapter are (1) to stretch the boundaries of current thinking about the link between student engagement and SRL processes and (2) to underscore recent research focusing on innovative applications of SRL intervention and assessment practices that promote student engagement. To begin, we provide a general overview of the definitions and descriptions of both student engagement and SRL, emphasizing areas of overlap and divergence. While we still concur with Cleary and Zimmerman (2012) regarding the close correspondence between cognitive engagement and SRL, we emphasize a more expansive viewpoint of SRL that underscores an integration of cognitive, affective, behavioral, and contextual factors (Cleary & Callan, 2018; Zimmerman, 2000). With respect to this comprehensive conceptualization and our desire to underscore the close connection between engagement and regulation concepts, we use the term *regulatory engagement* and SRL interchangeably throughout this chapter.

We then shift our focus to recent trends in the SRL literature, highlighting research on emerging and innovative attempts to optimize students' achievement and regulatory engagement in learning contexts. Although we consider initiatives

from both direct (i.e., SRL interventions) and indirect (i.e., SRL professional development with teachers) service delivery perspectives, our primary objective is to discuss how SRL assessment practices and tools (e.g., self-report questionnaires, SRL microanalysis) can be used in a formative fashion by researchers and/or practitioners to promote optimal feedback that can enhance student engagement and overall learning. We end this chapter with implications for practice and areas for future research.

Conceptual Overview of SRL and Student Engagement

Educators have long been interested in understanding the determinants of student engagement and/or SRL processes in school contexts. From the perspectives of various school personnel, such as school psychologists and teachers, these constructs are critical to student success and thus are often the topic of professional development initiatives (Cleary et al., 2010; Cleary & Zimmerman, 2006; Coalition for Psychology in Schools and Education, 2006; Wehmeyer et al., 2000). The focus of this section involves examining the conceptual overlap (i.e., similarities and distinctions) between models of student engagement and SRL frameworks. Our goal in conducting this broad level analysis is not to draw any conclusions regarding the relative effectiveness or superiority of a given model, perspective, or approach to enhancing student engagement in school. We simply hope to provide some commentary for readers to more clearly understand the nature of SRL processes, or what we term *regulatory engagement*.

In reviewing the engagement literature, it is clear that most models depict engagement as a mega-construct consisting of different subtypes (i.e., academic, behavioral, cognitive, and affective), and with each subtype having associated indicators and facilitators (Christenson et al., 2012; Fredericks et al., 2004; Skinner et al., 2008). *Academic engagement* entails one's overall investment or participation in school-related work, tasks, or classroom activities (Reschly,

2020). When students are academically engaged, they will often complete their classwork and homework on time, have opportunities to respond during class, and sustain efforts to complete coursework. In contrast, *behavioral engagement* refers to student conduct and their overall participation in school-related events or activities (Fredericks et al., 2004). If a teacher describes their students as behaviorally engaged, one would likely observe these students attending school on a regular basis and showing up on time, actively listening during classroom instruction or taking notes, or perhaps getting involved in extracurricular school activities (e.g., theatre, sports). Christenson and colleagues' model of student engagement also posits that academic and behavioral engagement tend to reflect observable indicators, while the other two dimensions—affective and cognitive—reflect internal processes.

Affective engagement is conceptualized as the emotions or feelings that have a motivational effect for engaging in an activity or task (Cook et al., 2020). Affective engagement typically emphasizes interpersonal factors and feelings of connectedness or belongingness in students (Christenson et al., 2012). Thus, students who are affectively engaged will likely feel connected to school, supported by teachers and peers, and have positive, stable friendships. The fourth dimension, *cognitive engagement*, has often been equated with or described in terms of self-regulatory and motivational processes, such as perception of task value, goal orientation, or use of regulatory strategies. Overall, there is much research showing that each of these four engagement subtypes plays a critical role in students' academic success, whether success is defined in terms of grades, persistence, behavioral functioning, or even dropout rates (Reschly, 2020).

Over the past few decades, several SRL theoretical frameworks have also been developed (Panadero, 2017; Schunk & Greene, 2018; Zimmerman & Schunk, 2001). Collectively, these models have provided a fertile foundation from which to examine and understand essential processes that promote students' strategic thinking and behaviors in learning or performance sit-

uations (Panadero, 2017; Schunk & Greene, 2018). Although there are important distinctions across models in terms of the processes that are emphasized, sources of motivation, and the perceived role of the social environment, there is also considerable overlap among them (Puustinen & Pulkkinen, 2001; Panadero, 2017). In fact, in a recent review of several theoretical frameworks frequently cited in the SRL literature, Panadero (2017) noted that among other things, virtually all of the models converge on the premise that SRL is a dynamic, fluid, cyclical process consisting of different phases and subprocesses.

Most contemporary SRL researchers are interested in detailing the task-specific, dynamic, goal-directed aspects of the regulatory processes than they are in discussing stable traits or regulatory dispositions of students. In other words, SRL researchers and interventionists typically strive to target the malleable and teachable regulatory skills and processes that enable students to manage their lives in pursuit of personal goals. Cleary and Zimmerman (2004) aptly capture this contextualized, dynamic aspect of SRL in terms of a guiding regulatory question relevant for assessment and intervention practices, "To what extent does *this* student have the knowledge of, select, and regulate the use of *these* specific study and self-regulation strategies to enhance his or her performance on *these* performance outcomes in *that* particular class?" (p. 541). Central to most contemporary models of SRL is the focus on accomplishing and adapting behaviors and strategies to reach one's goals.

It is important to note, however, that outside of learning and academic situations, other researchers use the term *self-regulation* (SR), or in some cases *self-control* (Barkley, 2016; Greene, 2018). SR models are similar to SRL perspectives in their focus on the management and monitoring of cognition, behavior, and emotional arousal to achieve goals. However, SR researchers tend to address topics or situations outside of academic learning, such as addictions, behavioral control, dieting, or interpersonal interactions, and focus on individuals' ability to resist temptations, to delay gratification or impulses, or to think in flexible adaptable ways during problem-solving

(Barkley, 2016; Vohs & Baumeister, 2016). We recognize the importance of such models in a broad sense, but focus this chapter exclusively on SRL models and their applications in academic or learning contexts.

Another commonality across SRL models is a focus on the operation and structure of the *cyclical feedback loop* (Panadero, 2017; Schunk & Greene, 2018). Conceptually, a feedback loop refers to a goal-directed process whereby information or feedback about behavior or performance is used to evaluate goal progress and to facilitate decision-making regarding adaptations needed to attain goals. The basic idea is that individuals will be motivated to reduce a discrepancy between their performance and a standard (i.e., goal). After an initial goal is achieved, students will stop engagement or shift their engagement efforts toward new goals or activities. Self-regulatory feedback loops also tend to operate in a temporal sequence (i.e., before, during, and after dimensions) that mirrors the temporal characteristics of learning activities. For example, to understand the regulatory engagement of students attempting to write a persuasive essay, researchers or practitioners would examine how the students plan or approach the task (before), use and monitor the effectiveness of specific strategies while writing (during), and use internal or external feedback to evaluate the strategy effectiveness relative to their goals (after). Although different labels have been used to describe this temporal process (Schmitz & Wiese, 2006; Winne & Perry, 2000), we focus on Zimmerman's three-phase model of SRL, which is grounded in social-cognitive theoretical principles (Bandura, 1986; Zimmerman, 2000).

Zimmerman's (2000) cyclical model of SRL is represented by three sequential, interrelated phases—forethought, performance control, and self-reflection. His theoretical framework is one of the most widely cited in the SRL literature and has been used as the theoretical foundation for both assessment and intervention programming (Cleary et al., 2021; Cleary et al., 2017; Panadero, 2017). It is also quite useful from a practical perspective in that it provides an organizational structure for researchers and practitioners alike to understand the operation, influence, and relation among motivational, metacognitive, behavioral, and affective processes as individuals engage in learning-related activities, such as taking notes in class, completing homework assignments, or studying for exams.

Before engaging in a learning activity, highly regulated learners plan and think about an appropriate course of action. In the SRL model, these preparatory actions and thoughts reflect *forethought processes*, such as identifying the demands and expectations of a learning task (task analysis), setting specific goals for that activity (goal setting), and developing plans or approaches on how best to achieve one's goals (strategic planning). Because SRL is an effortful process, this model also underscores the deterministic role of motivation beliefs, such as self-efficacy and task values, in stimulating students to engage in the learning process (Cleary et al., 2018).

During attempts to learn in the *performance control* phase, students will purposefully and intentionally use specific self-control strategies to optimize their learning, behaviors, and emotions. For example, when studying for a mathematics test, students may use concept mapping and self-quizzing (i.e., learning strategies), deep breathing and mindfulness (i.e., anxiety control), or positive self-talk to sustain high levels of motivation. Regulated learners do not rigidly use the same strategies in all situations; they tend to be flexible and nimble in their strategic behaviors and are willing to adapt or change their approach based on emerging challenges or difficulties in a given situation (Wolters, 2003; Zimmerman, 2000). In addition to deploying effective strategies during learning, highly regulated learners engage in self-observation, a process entailing tracking one's task performance and the conditions surrounding it. From a regulatory engagement perspective, self-monitoring or observation is a hallmark feature of the cyclical feedback loop because it facilitates error analysis and enhances the likelihood that individuals will make fine-grained adjustments to their strategies when not learning effectively.

In the final phase of this cyclical feedback loop, regulated learners will often reflect on particular aspects of their learning or performance including *how well did I do?* (i.e., self-evaluation); *why did I perform that way?* (i.e., causal attributions), *how do I feel about my performance?* (satisfaction/affect), and *what do I need to do now?* (i.e., adaptive inferences). Thus, highly regulated learners will first compare self-monitored or externally provided feedback to their personal goals or other standards to determine their level of success. They then search for the most tenable reasons for their performance, and ideally attribute their performance to controllable factors, such as the strategies used during learning. Of particular importance from a regulatory perspective, however, are the conclusions or adaptive inferences that individuals make about how to improve performance or their behaviors when they are not reaching their goals.

When comparing Christenson and colleagues' model of student engagement and Zimmerman's three phase model of SRL, there are clear similarities (see Table 1). Both perspectives focus on multi-dimensional aspects of student functioning, specifically across academic, cognitive, behavioral, and affective aspects of functioning. Christenson and colleagues' model is quite explicit in terms of the operational definitions and indicators for the four subtypes. SRL models are similar in that they consider these four areas when conceptualizing or defining the regulatory processes, although these descriptions are narrower in focus. Zimmerman (2000) aptly captured the multi-dimensional focus of SRL in stating, "Self-regulation refers to self-generated *thoughts*, *feelings*, and *actions* that are *planned* and *cyclically adapted* to the attainment of personal goals" (italics added for emphasis, p. 14). SRL models do not label the terms cognitive, affective, and behaviors as distinct subtypes of regulation; rather, they conceive of them as interrelated domains of functioning that become integrated as individuals perform specific academic or learning activities.

Both models also recognize the importance of the reciprocal relations between contextual influences and student engagement. For example, Reschly and Christenson et al. (2012) highlighted myriad contextual facilitators that play a role in student engagement, such as family supports, peer relations, school-based initiatives and supports, and even community impacts. These contextual facilitators are intertwined with engagement-related interventions and can be adapted or changed to best meet student needs (Reschly et al., 2020). Zimmerman's model is largely grounded in Bandura's (1986) premise of reciprocal determinism; that is, human functioning can be described in terms of the reciprocal relations among personal and environmental factors as well as behavior. Similar to engagement models, social-cognitive theorists recognize that contexts are dynamic entities that can directly influence but also be influenced by students operating in that context. Similarly, both engagement and SRL perspectives appear to support the premise that student perceptions and perspectives are central in understanding student functioning; when devising interventions to enhance student engagement, their perceptions might even serve as a key mediator between contextual influences and enhanced engagement (Cleary & Kitsantas, 2017; Reschly & Christenson, 2012).

Table 1 Broad comparison of student engagement and SRL frameworks

Engagement	Point of comparison	SRL
Yes	Considers academic, behavioral cognitive, and affective aspects of functioning	Yes
Yes	Emphasizes the importance of social, contextual, or cultural milieu	Yes
Yes	Emphasizes importance of student perceptions for engagement	Yes
No	Described and operationalized as a task-specific process	Yes
No	Defined by the goals that individuals set for themselves	Yes

From our perspective, SRL and engagement models can be most easily distinguished in terms of the specificity in focus on particular academic tasks and the explicitness of a goal-directed process. That is, although both models clearly address similar aspects of functioning (i.e., academic, behavioral, cognitive, affective), SRL models are more fine-grained and narrower in their description of these areas of functioning and explicitly explicate particular regulatory processes and their intersecting influences on student learning and performance. For example, if school psychologists are interested in optimizing students' regulatory engagement, they typically will be most concerned with assessing and providing interventions that simultaneously consider students' cognitive (including metacognitive), affective, and behavioral processes during engagement in specific learning tasks or activities, such as writing an essay, studying for an exam, or completing a science investigation. This "in the moment" type of regulatory engagement is not only defined by the nature of the activity in which students engage but also the goals students possess relative to that activity. Thus, as students' goals shift and change within the short and long term, so too will the nature of their regulatory engagement.

Trends in Approaches to Optimize SRL Engagement

There is a burgeoning literature focused on SRL applications in school contexts. Central to these "application innovations" are SRL-focused interventions for academically at-risk youth and the provision of SRL professional development (PD) for educators. Most recently, researchers have begun to consider how SRL assessment tools can be used in a formative manner to enhance student functioning and/or to guide instructional efforts. We briefly consider research on SRL and PD innovations, but focus most directly on the use of SRL assessment data as feedback and progress monitoring mechanisms to promote regulatory engagement.

Student-Focused SRL Interventions

There are myriad academic, behavioral, and mental health interventions that incorporate SRL processes, such as goal-setting, self-monitoring, or self-evaluation (Briesch & Briesch, 2016; Reddy et al., 2018; Suveg et al., 2015). For example, a large percentage of interventions designed to help students with ADHD utilize aspects of self-monitoring or self-evaluation (Reddy et al., 2018). Many academic interventions consider SRL principles and processes as primary or central aspects. Collectively, these academic interventions seek to optimize students' metacognitive, strategic, and motivational functioning as they engage in reading texts (Tonks & Taboada, 2011), writing essays (Graham & Harris, 2009; Graham et al., 2012), or solving mathematics problems (Montague et al., 2014). Other school-based SRL interventions focus less on the development of academic skills and more on the optimization of students' strategic skills in managing and overcoming common academic, motivational, and regulatory challenges experienced during learning or the completion of common school-related activities. The Self-Regulation Empowerment Program (SREP) is illustrative of these programs (Cleary et al., 2017).

SREP is a comprehensive intervention program designed to optimize the strategic, motivational, and metacognitive skills of academically at-risk middle school and high school students as they engage in learning and academic activities. SREP sessions are typically presented in small group formats and provide students with structured instructional supports and coaching that enables and empowers student to think and act in cyclical, regulatory ways during learning (Cleary & Platten, 2013; Cleary et al., 2017). In the beginning stages of the SREP instructional process, students are introduced to the importance of *strategic thinking* and *adaptive mindsets* as they learn and evaluate success or failure. The SREP coaches also provide modeling and guided practice experiences so that students learn new and effective strategies to learn course content or to more effectively manage their behaviors (e.g., effort, help seeking) and emotions (e.g., anxiety).

Importantly, the SREP coaches guide students through a highly systematic process of self-reflection about grades for course assignments and tests. Through the use of microanalysis questions (see assessment section; Cleary et al., 2017), the coaches prompt students to respond to critical questions linked to their reflective phase processes: "how well did I do?" (self-evaluation); "why did I perform this way?" (attributions); "am I satisfied with my performance?" (satisfaction/affect); and "what do I need to do to improve?" (adaptive inferences). Both students and SREP coaches use this microanalysis assessment information to stimulate interactive conversations and discussions within the SREP group.

Teacher SRL Professional Development (PD) Experiences

Survey research in education reveals that student SRL and motivational skills are of particular interest to educators and other school personnel (e.g., school psychologists) because such skills are essential to student success and are often raised as areas of concern for students referred for psychoeducational evaluations (Cleary et al., 2010). Interestingly, despite the importance of SRL processes, most educators do not believe they receive enough training or experiences to effectively assess and/or enhance students' regulatory engagement (Cleary et al., 2010; Kremer-Hayon & Tillema, 1999; Lau, 2012; Pauli et al., 2007; Spruce & Bol, 2015). This gap has stimulated efforts by researchers to develop and evaluate the effects of SRL PD programming.

In the literature, SRL PD initiatives can vary in both comprehensiveness and duration. Some PD programs are implemented over several years (e.g., Perry et al., 2007), while others are provided on a continuous basis over the course of a couple of months (e.g., Ganda & Boruchovitch, 2018; Kramarski & Michalsky, 2015; Peters-Burton & Botov, 2017) or even for only one or two sessions (Allshouse, 2016). Despite this variability in SRL PD training duration and the nature of PD experiences, research tends to support its overall effectiveness for both the teachers and

students (Kramarski et al., 2013; Peters-Burton et al., 2020; Spruce & Bol, 2015). Perry et al. (2007) implemented a long-term project emphasizing SRL PD with 18 preservice teachers, and reported important shifts in teachers' ability to develop learning activities that promoted students' regulatory engagement during reading and writing. Peters-Burton and Botov (2017) found that immersing SRL principles within an intensive PD program helped to improve the SRL skills (i.e., goal setting, self-monitoring, learning tactics) of elementary science teachers. Further, Allshouse (2016) reported statistically significant pretest-posttest changes in the knowledge and SRL application skills of middle school and high school teachers following one half-day SRL workshop experience. In short, PD initiatives represent an important SRL application innovation that can better reach a broader set of students than is possible with direct intervention services.

Overview of SRL Measures and Formative Assessment Practices

A contemporary and important issue in educational circles involves the extent to which appropriate decisions regarding resource and service allocation can be made based on assessment data about students' academic and behavioral functioning. In the realm of assessment, there is often a distinction made between summative (i.e., assessment *of* learning) and formative assessments (assessment *for* learning; Stiggins, 2005). Summative assessments are administered at the end of a unit or course, with the purpose of measuring students' achievement, and/or mastery of required content or skills. In contrast, formative assessments are administered on a more frequent and continuous basis, often throughout the instructional or intervention process. The key objective in this approach is to gather data that informs and enhances both learning and teaching processes.

As an example, when students are assigned to write an argumentative essay for summative purposes, teachers focus on reviewing and evaluating the quality of the essay and subsequently assigning a grade, perhaps using a rubric with specified criteria. In this situation, students are less likely to receive much feedback about the writing process because the focus is on evaluating how well students have written their essays and/or their level of learning. On the other hand, if a teacher utilized a formative assessment approach as part of the essay writing process, they would be more interested in structuring the activity to optimize student feedback or to create opportunities for students to evaluate progress and make strategic adaptations, as needed, to their writing. The benefits of a formative assessment framework, however, are not confined to students. In fact, by gathering information about student behavior, work products, or ways of thinking, teachers can develop a deeper and more accurate understanding of student skills and strategic processes; information that can be used to potentially adapt their own instruction and/or approaches when interacting with students.

Feedback is an integral part of formative assessment given that it seeks to "reduce discrepancies between students' current understandings/performance and a desired goal" (Hattie & Timperley, 2007, p. 87). Effective feedback conveys information to the student and/or teacher about the goals to be attained (Where am I going?), goal progress (How am I going?), and likely next steps (Where to next?). While the nature of feedback is critical, it is equally important that students are provided clear standards on how to use that feedback to make appropriate modifications and adaptations. Scholars have argued that for formative assessments to improve student learning: (1) the learning standards should be clear to students, indicating where they need to be (goals); (2) teacher, peer, or self-feedback should reflect these standards so students can more easily self-evaluate or monitor progress; and (3) students and/or teachers need opportunities to use the assessment data to reduce discrepancies between current and expected skill levels (e.g., Andrade, 2016; Butler & Winne, 1995; Hattie & Timperley, 2007; Wiggins, 2012). When feedback reflects these essential components, is delivered in a supportive and timely manner, and is communicated in a way that students can understand, there is an increased likelihood that students will value and use the feedback in productive ways to enhance learning (Andrade, 2013; Hattie & Timperley, 2007; Shute, 2008). Furthermore, formative assessment, when implemented effectively, would naturally engage students in their learning process (Nichols & Dawson, 2012).

From our perspective, there is a natural symmetry between formative assessment practices and SRL assessments. We believe that using SRL assessment data within a formative assessment process can, when implemented effectively, directly inform and improve students' SRL processes and overall learning and performance. Increasingly, efforts have been made to explicitly foster students' regulatory engagement through SRL assessments and feedback of these processes (e.g., Cleary et al., 2017; Osborne et al., 2020; Peters-Burton et al., 2020).

Overview of SRL assessments Broadly speaking, SRL researchers have identified two broad categories of assessment tools: *aptitude* and *event* measures (Cleary et al., 2021; Winne & Perry, 2000). Although assessment tools within each of these categories are similar in their overall focus on SRL, they are actually quite distinct in format, procedure, and overall scope and purpose (Cleary & Callan, 2018; Cleary et al., 2021).

Briefly, *event measures* gather data about SRL processes as they emerge or change in specific moments, situations, or learning activities (Schunk & Greene, 2018). These measures, which include direct observations, think alouds, and SRL microanalysis, are structured to reveal information regarding how individuals plan, engage in, monitor, and/or reflect on and adapt their strategic actions during a *specific activity* in a *given situation* at a particular *moment in time* (Bernacki, 2018; Cleary et al., 2021; Greene, 2018). In most situations, event measures are well-suited to target specific processes within the three-phase cyclical loop as individuals learn, solve mathematic problems, write essays, or engage in other relevant academic tasks.

Conversely, *aptitude measures* capture broader information regarding students' SRL skills and tend to produce scores that reflect a global attribute or stable trait within a person (Cleary et al., 2021; Winne & Perry, 2000). Aptitude measures, which include self-report questionnaires, rating scales, and certain types of interviews, typically entail having respondents provide retrospective ratings about their general tendencies, quality, and/or frequency of their regulatory behaviors, beliefs, and/or processes. Although questionnaire items can reflect a general context (e.g., school) or content area (e.g., mathematics), they are not designed to measure SRL as it unfolds or evolves during specific tasks or academic activities (i.e., as is the case with event measures). In fact, in most instances, scores from multiple items or questions are aggregated into a composite score. It is from these composite scores that inferences are made regarding individuals' regulatory engagement. Given these features, aptitude measures are ideal for targeting aspects within and across the broader dimensions of SRL (i.e., metacognition, strategy use, motivation), while event measures are more appropriate for capturing the dynamic, fluid task-specific processes.

Although most SRL assessments have not traditionally been used in a diagnostic or formative sense, there has been increased interest in such applications. In the next sections, we describe one event measure (i.e., SRL microanalysis) and one aptitude measure (i.e., DAACS SRL Survey) and how they have been provide illustrative examples of how they are used in a formative manner to optimize student skill development or learning and/or to enhance the nature of instruction provided to the students.

SRL Microanalysis The term SRL microanalysis reflects a task-specific structured interview designed to assess myriad SRL processes (e.g., goal-setting, self-observation, attributions) within the three-phase cyclical model as individuals engage in learning or performance-related activities. Although information about this assessment approach is described elsewhere in much detail (see Cleary, 2011; Cleary et al.,

2021), we provide a brief summary to help readers understand its potential as a formative assessment tool.

One of the most important features of SRL microanalysis is that the target questions are directly and intimately linked with tasks or learning activities (e.g., writing an essay, studying for an exam, completing homework) commonly used in schools. Thus, the development of microanalysis tools necessitates one to identify and understand the demands, requirements, and challenges of those activities (i.e., beginning, middle, and end). After selecting the activity, one needs to identify the SRL processes to assess. As revealed in a recent systematic review of the SRL microanalytic literature, over 40 empirical studies utilizing microanalysis procedures across various domains (e.g., academic, sports, clinical) and corresponding domain tasks (e.g., test preparation, basketball free throw shooting, practicing a musical instrument) have been published (Cleary et al., 2021). Some researchers have comprehensively examined SRL processes across all three cyclical phases, while others have adopted a more narrow and selective approach, such as focusing on forethought or reflection phase only.

Regardless of the scope of assessment, microanalysis questions should be simple, brief, and directly linked to a specific regulatory process. Thus, they are often phrased to represent the definitions of SRL sub-processes included within Zimmerman's three-phase model (Cleary, 2011). Further, given that microanalysis questions are directly linked to these activities and domains, they are phrased to reflect such activities. Thus, to assess students' strategic planning and adaptive inferences relative to solving a set of algebra word problems, example questions might include, *"Do you have a plan in mind as you prepare to solve this problem? Tell me about that"* (strategic planning) and *"What do you need to do to sustain or improve your performance when solving similar types of problems in the future?"* (adaptive inferences). Although free response or open-ended formats are often emphasized in microanalysis assessments, the use of metric or quantitative questions (e.g., Likert scale) can be utilized when assessing certain processes, such as motivational beliefs (e.g., self-efficacy).

One of the most important aspects of SRL microanalysis involves the sequence or order with which the specific questions are administered. Given that most target activities reflect some temporal dimension (i.e., before, during, and after the activity), microanalysis assessments are structured so that phase-specific questions (i.e., forethought, performance, self-reflection) are aligned with the before, during, and after dimensions of the activity. Specifically, forethought questions (e.g., goal-setting, planning) are administered as individuals prepare to engage in the target activity, performance questions (e.g., self-observation, monitoring) during the activity, and reflection questions following the activity or after receiving some type of performance feedback. From a formative assessment perspective, this SRL phase-task dimension alignment enables one to draw meaningful inferences from data regarding the nature of students' SRL processes in the context of critical academic activities (Cleary & Callan, 2018).

Self-Report Questionnaires Self-report questionnaires represent one of the most common approaches for assessing learners' SRL skills and processes, and the various dimensions of student engagement. O'Donnell and Reschly (2020) noted that self-report questionnaires and teacher rating scales are often used to assess students' academic, cognitive, and affective engagement, one of which is the Student Engagement Instrument (see Fredericks, chapter "The Measurement of Student Engagement: Methodological Advances and Comparison of New Self-Report Instruments", this volume, for a review of measures). This measure has been used across elementary and secondary school populations. Some of the most common SRL self-report measures include the Motivated Strategies for Learning Questionnaire (MSLQ; Pintrich et al., 1991), Self-Regulation Strategy Inventory (SRSI; Cleary, 2006), Metacognitive Awareness Inventory (MAI; Schraw & Dennison, 1994), and Learning and Study Strategies Inventory (LASSI; Weinstein et al., 2002). Collectively, these measures generate information regarding student perceptions of their regulatory behaviors and strategies, metacognitive processes, and motivational beliefs.

The self-report measure we feature in this chapter is the SRL Survey from the Diagnostic Assessment and Achievement of College Skills (DAACS) assessment-to-feedback system (daacs. net; Bryer et al., 2022). DAACS represents an open-source diagnostic assessment tool designed to assess the reading, writing, mathematics, and SRL skills of newly enrolled college students. As part of this system, students receive actionable, individualized feedback and resources that they can use to enhance their preparation and overall performance in college. There are four primary components of the DAACS system: (1) diagnostic assessments of SRL, reading, writing, and mathematics; (2) automated feedback, recommendations, and links to open educational resources (OERs) based on scores from the diagnostic assessments; (3) a dashboard to guide advisor–student interactions; and (4) predictive modeling. The first three components were designed to directly influence student engagement, while the fourth represents an institutional-level feature for better understanding students' continued matriculation and dropout rates. For the purpose of this chapter, we focus on the SRL survey component of DAACS and the corresponding actionable feedback and recommendations within the DAACS system (Bryer et al., 2022; Lui et al., 2018).

Applications of SRL Measures as Formative Assessment Tools

Use of SRL Microanalysis to Promote Regulatory Engagement

SRL Microanalysis procedures have been applied to diverse domains, settings, and learning activities. We provide an overview of recent attempts to use this assessment approach in a formative way to enhance learning and/or the instructional process. We draw from research focusing on SRL interventions with middle school students in mathematics, SRL PD activities with high school science teachers, and self-directed practice sessions with college musicians. For each of these examples, we focus on two key issues: (a) the use of microanalysis as a formative assessment tool, and (b) the use of microanalysis data as feedback to enhance student learning and/or the nature of teacher instruction.

SRL Microanalysis and Academic Interventions Cleary and colleagues have examined the effects of the Self-Regulation Empowerment Program (SREP) on motivation, SRL skills, and academic achievement of middle school and high school students (Cleary & Platten, 2013: Cleary et al., 2017). As previously mentioned, SREP is a comprehensive SRL program that enables students to become more goal-directed and strategic as they complete assignments and study for exams across different content area classes. Students meet in small groups with trained SREP coaches one or two times per week over the course of several months. Although the majority of the coaching sessions involve modeling and practice in using learning and SRL strategies, the coaches engage students in structured self-reflection activities following each major assignment or test. To begin this reflection activity, each student is asked to complete a self-reflection microanalysis form (with approximately 6–7 questions) and an SRL Graph. On the SRL Graph, students plot their grades and record the nature of the strategies they utilized to complete or prepare for that activity. The microanalysis form includes questions pertaining to the self-reflection phase of the cyclical feedback loop: *self-evaluative judgments* (i.e., perceptions of success or failure), *attributions* (i.e., potential causes of grade), *satisfaction or affect* (i.e., affective reaction to obtained grade), and *adaptive inferences* (i.e., conclusions about how to sustain or enhance future grades on similar assignments or activities; Cleary et al., 2017). The students use the graph and microanalysis questions in an integrated fashion to reflect.

As students reflect on their answer to the microanalysis questions, the SREP coaches encourage peer collaboration and discussion among students to reveal strategies that worked well, and to identify alternative ways of perceiving their performance, the potential causes of their grade, and how best to adapt or change their strategic behaviors, if needed. Thus, the microanalysis data are used in a formative way by individual students (or as a peer group) to help understand "what happened?" regarding the test or assignment grade and to figure out "what now?"; that is, to chart the best pathway forward for enhancing future performance (Cleary et al., 2021).

SREP coaches play a key role in this reflection process as they structure or guide the collaborative exchanges among peers while also prompting students to reflect on the effectiveness of their learning strategies (Cleary et al., 2017). From a formative assessment perspective, SREP coaches will also use student responses to the microanalysis questions to guide their instruction during subsequent SREP sessions. For example, if the coach observes that many of the students believe that they struggle to effectively manage their time and have not yet mastered how to use concept maps or other strategies to learn course materials, they will explore these issues with the students and, if appropriate, teach them the relevant strategies. In short, the data generated from the SRL microanalysis can be directly used by students in their reflections about how to improve but also by the coaches in helping them make decisions about how best to facilitate this improvement.

SRL Microanalysis and PD Activities Peters-Burton and colleagues have conducted a couple of studies that have embedded microanalysis in PD activities in order to optimize teachers' pedagogical skills and to enhance the overall quality of PD sessions. Peters-Burton and Botov (2017) implemented a 15-week (3 hours once a week) PD course for elementary science teachers. As part of this study, microanalysis was used formatively by the PD facilitator to generate data to guide instructional enhancements and to assist teachers in guiding their own behaviors during their learning of pedagogical skills in inquiry-based teaching, and when developing inquiry-based lesson plans. As part of the 15-week PD course, teachers participated in sample inquiry-oriented lessons on earth science topics, watched videos of modeled scientific inquiry, and developed lesson plans for earth science content.

The SRL microanalysis procedure was separated into three parts—forethought, performance, and reflection protocols—which were subsequently administered at three different timepoints (i.e., before, during, after) of the PD process. Thus, the forethought protocol was administered before the start of the PD course. These questions targeted teachers' self-efficacy, task interest, and goal orientation, and their skills in goal setting and strategic planning. The performance protocol, which assessed teachers' attention focusing, self-instruction, and self-monitoring, was administered during different PD activities, but most notably during lesson plan development. Finally, the reflection protocol was administered at the end of the 15-week PD course to examine teachers' self-evaluation, attributions, and self-reactions.

Given the nature of the target activity (i.e., defined as the 15-week PD experience), the PD facilitator was only able to use forethought and performance phase microanalysis data to generate real-time feedback for the participating teachers and for herself as the facilitator. Of particular interest to the authors was examining how microanalysis data informed the facilitator's decisions about how to expand, modify, or enhance the nature of PD activities and scaffolding support. Using forethought microanalysis data, the PD facilitator came to understand that teachers struggled to set process goals. For example, one teacher set a vague and general goal to, "acquire knowledge of what inquiry lessons are and how to teach the lessons" (p. 58), while another teacher set a goal to, "become more comfortable planning inquiry lessons," (p. 61). With this information, the PD instructor learned that teachers needed smaller steps from which to design the inquiry-based lessons. Therefore, the PD instructor created a rubric in collaboration with the teachers, detailing the key characteristics of inquiry-based lessons. This rubric was used as a monitoring tool in subsequent lessons.

The participating teachers also directly used the microanalysis data to reflect on and adapt their approaches to lesson plan development. The rubric, thereafter, provided teachers with clarity in terms of the standards to which they would self-monitor, reflect, and set goals as they revised existing lessons and created new ones. In addition to this evaluative criteria, the teachers' own responses to performance phase (i.e., self-monitoring and self-observation) microanalysis questions enabled them to monitor their progress and work toward these standards. Peters-Burton and Botov (2017) noted, "Two criteria from the rubric [...] resonated with the group and became the touchstones for self-monitoring." (p. 68). As a result, they became aware of what worked well for them and what did not, and made adjustments to self-instruction and improvements to subsequent lesson plans.

SRL Microanalysis and Music Intervention As a final example, we discuss recent research that used SRL microanalysis data to guide students' self-assessment of their regulatory processes during practice of a musical instrument. Multiple studies have been conducted by McPherson and colleagues in this realm (McPherson et al., 2017; Osborne et al., 2020). Most recently, Osborne et al. (2020) designed a five-page microanalysis-embedded diary, Optimal Music Practice Protocol(OMPP), for seven students who were selected from 33 piano students who got accepted into the Bachelor of Music at a prestigious Australian University music program. Unlike Peters-Burton and Botov (2017) and Cleary et al. (2017), this study focused specifically on the use of microanalysis data gathered by students as they engaged in self-directed practice sessions. A coach or teacher did not play a role in the feedback generation or prompting process given the self-directed nature of the target activity.

All of the college musicians were instructed to use the microanalytic diary during self-directed piano practice sessions. For these practice sessions, students focused on a new piece of repertoire to be performed for an end-of-semester examination recital. In alignment with the suggested three-phase design of a microanalysis procedure, the diary was divided into three sections: (1) *Before starting my practice* (forethought). (2) *During my practice* (performance). (3) *After my practice was completed* (self-reflection). The diary consisted of open-ended prompts, Likert-type, and forced-choice items that were designed to target different aspects of students' regulatory engagement. The forethought section of the diary was completed prior to the students initiating their self-directed practice sessions, and targeted their goals and strategic plans for the practice as well as the nature of their self-motivation beliefs (i.e., self-efficacy, outcome expectancies, task interest, and task value). The performance section was completed during the practice sessions when students were able to record their engagement or use of strategic processes, such as self-control (e.g., task strategies, self-instruction, time management, environmental structuring, help-seeking) and self-observations (i.e., metacognitive monitoring, self-recording). After completing a given practice session, the students answered questions regarding their self-judgments (i.e., self-evaluation on practice and strategy effectiveness), self-reactions, and overall satisfaction. All students were asked to complete the diary at three specific timepoints within a 9-week semester (Weeks 4, 8, and 12). Importantly, they were encouraged and prompted by researchers, during a one-on-one meeting before Week 8, to use information from each session to guide behavior in future practice sessions and to self-assess growth in the quality of their regulatory processes over the semester.

Findings from this study suggested that the OMPP provided prompts for students to become more aware of the self-regulatory processes, which, in turn, appeared to stimulate their metacognitive thinking (planning, monitoring, and reflection) relative to their performance or progress at the moment (Where am I?) as well as end of semester goals and expectations (Where do I need to be?). Through enhanced self-awareness and explicit documentation of these processes in the diary, the students' notes became a source of formative self-feedback that could be used to

inform their goals and strategies for subsequent practice sessions (Osborne et al., 2020). Findings from informal interviews with these undergraduate students also suggested that this notebook, designed based on the microanalysis framework, was easy to understand and use to self-assess their learning processes and outcomes. It is important to emphasize that as undergraduates pursuing a Bachelor of Music degree and majoring in piano, these students were experienced in the field of music and piano performance. Instruction or scaffolding directly from a teacher or mentor on how to use the OMPP for formative purposes may be needed to enhance its effectiveness for more novice or inexperienced learners. This is an important area for future research.

Use of Self-Report Assessment Data to Promote Regulatory Engagement

Self-report questionnaires are frequently used by researchers and practitioners, in part, because they are easy to administer and score and because of their potential for targeting covert constructs that might relate to student functioning in school. Unlike SRL microanalysis, self-report questionnaires typically do not reveal task-specific information about students' regulatory engagement. Rather, they produce scores that can lead to inferences regarding students' perceptions of broader aspects of perceived regulatory engagement, such as typical strategy use or level of motivational beliefs (e.g., self-efficacy, interest). Despite a lack of task-specificity, questionnaire data can be used in a formative fashion to help students enhance their functioning; whether directly by using that data themselves or through interactions with others who share access to such information.

DAACS SRL Survey　In this section, we discuss the SRL survey as part of DAACS and detail initial attempts to use it as a formative assessment tool. The DAACS SRL self-report measure focuses on three core dimensions and 11 subscales of self-regulatory processes related to academic success in college: (1) motivation (i.e., measures of mastery orientation, test anxiety, self-efficacy, and mindset); (2) learning strategies (i.e., measures of help seeking behaviors and ability to manage their understanding, time, and environment; and (3) metacognition (i.e., measures of planning, monitoring, and evaluation skills; Efklides, 2011; Lui et al., 2018; Winne & Hadwin, 1998; Zimmerman, 2000). As defined and operationalized by the DAACS SRL Survey, *motivation* is a multidimensional process that "activates and sustains cognitions, emotions, and actions in the interest of one's goals" (Lui et al., 2018, p. 2), including goal orientation, test anxiety, self-efficacy, and mindset. *Metacognition* is the awareness and management of one's thoughts, and involves planning one's learning, monitoring the learning progress, and reflecting on if and how well the learning occurred. The *learning strategies* scale measures the cognitions and behaviors that learners engage in when processing new knowledge and completing academic tasks. There are three to six items per subscale, with internal consistencies ranging between .61 and .91 (Lui et al., 2018).

Consistent with formative assessment principles, the DAACS system was developed to ensure that all assessments (i.e., reading, math, writing, SRL) generate scores and information that: (a) can be used by both individual learners and their advisors, and (b) correspond to actionable feedback with links to relevant open educational resources. For the SRL survey, feedback was generated and provided at the composite level (motivation, strategies, metacognition; Fig. 1), subscales within each composite score (Fig. 2), and item levels (Fig. 3). The feedback that students receive is based on scores across the composite and subscale levels. Using a hypothetical example, suppose Aurora completed the DAACS survey and received feedback as illustrated in Figs. 1, 2, and 3. In Fig. 1, Aurora and her advisor can easily see that Aurora received three stars (maximum rating) for learning strategies and metacognition, indicating a level of mastery or highly frequent use of such strategies. However, she only received two stars for motivation, indicating a less than optimal level. At this composite

level analysis, Aurora would be prompted to explore ways in which her motivation can be improved. If she clicked on the "More Info" tab for Motivation, Aurora would observe a more nuanced profile of her motivational beliefs across the four motivation subscales (i.e., self-efficacy, managing test anxiety, mastery orientation, and mindset). These profiles are useful because they communicate areas of strengths and weaknesses while concurrently offering recommendations and actionable steps that Aurora may perceive as valuable or helpful to improving her skills (Fig. 2).

Suppose Aurora was particularly interested in understanding why her self-efficacy was so low (i.e., one star, indicating the lowest level of development), and more importantly, why improving her overall confidence could help her as a learner. Within the DAACS system, she could click on "More Info" for self-efficacy. She would then have access to information that addresses self-efficacy on a conceptual level (i.e., in written form and videos) and on a practical level (i.e., case scenarios, her responses to individual items on the self-efficacy subscale; see Fig. 3). She also would be directed to use various open educational resources, if desired, such as the SRL Lab (srl.daacs.net), an open educational resource on self-regulated learning.

DAACS is structured so that students and college advisors have access to the same information about students' SRL profiles and skills. In a similar way that Aurora has gone through her feedback, her advisor or instructors can do the same, and use the same information to encourage Aurora to become more engaged in her learning by becoming more self-regulated (Bryer et al., 2022).

Conclusions and Future Directions

SRL and student engagement are critical constructs that researchers and practitioners have increasingly focused on over the past several decades. In this chapter, we operationally defined the term *regulatory engagement* and discussed areas of similarity and divergence relative to

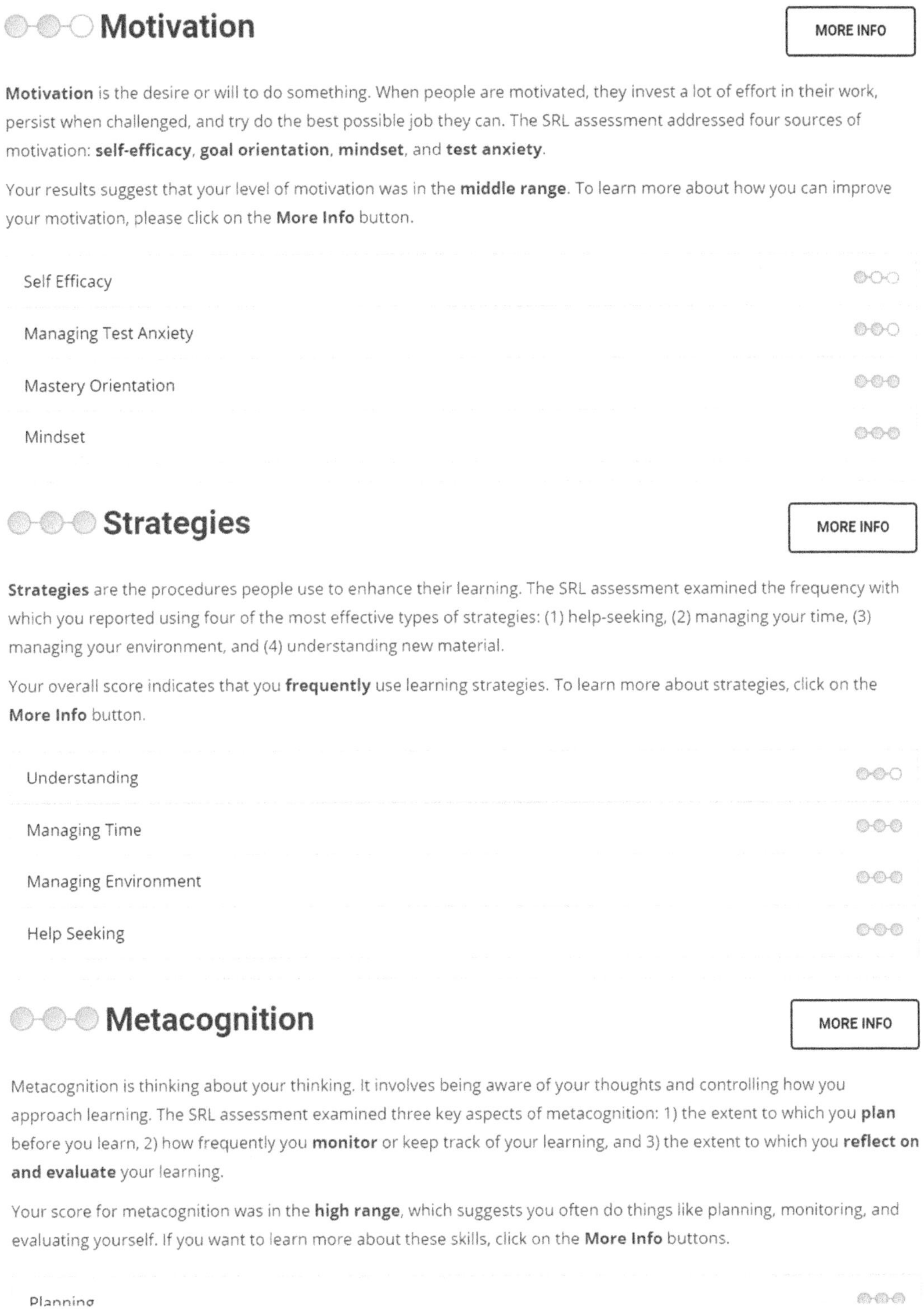

Motivation

MORE INFO

Motivation is the desire or will to do something. When people are motivated, they invest a lot of effort in their work, persist when challenged, and try do the best possible job they can. The SRL assessment addressed four sources of motivation: **self-efficacy**, **goal orientation**, **mindset**, and **test anxiety**.

Your results suggest that your level of motivation was in the **middle range**. To learn more about how you can improve your motivation, please click on the **More Info** button.

Self Efficacy

Managing Test Anxiety

Mastery Orientation

Mindset

Strategies

MORE INFO

Strategies are the procedures people use to enhance their learning. The SRL assessment examined the frequency with which you reported using four of the most effective types of strategies: (1) help-seeking, (2) managing your time, (3) managing your environment, and (4) understanding new material.

Your overall score indicates that you **frequently** use learning strategies. To learn more about strategies, click on the **More Info** button.

Understanding

Managing Time

Managing Environment

Help Seeking

Metacognition

MORE INFO

Metacognition is thinking about your thinking. It involves being aware of your thoughts and controlling how you approach learning. The SRL assessment examined three key aspects of metacognition: 1) the extent to which you **plan** before you learn, 2) how frequently you **monitor** or keep track of your learning, and 3) the extent to which you **reflect on and evaluate** your learning.

Your score for metacognition was in the **high range**, which suggests you often do things like planning, monitoring, and evaluating yourself. If you want to learn more about these skills, click on the **More Info** buttons.

Planning

Fig. 1 Sample DAACS feedback for motivation, strategies, and metacognition scales. (From *Diagnostic Assessment & Achievement of College Skills* by DAACS, 2016 (https://my.daacs.net). CC BY 4.0)

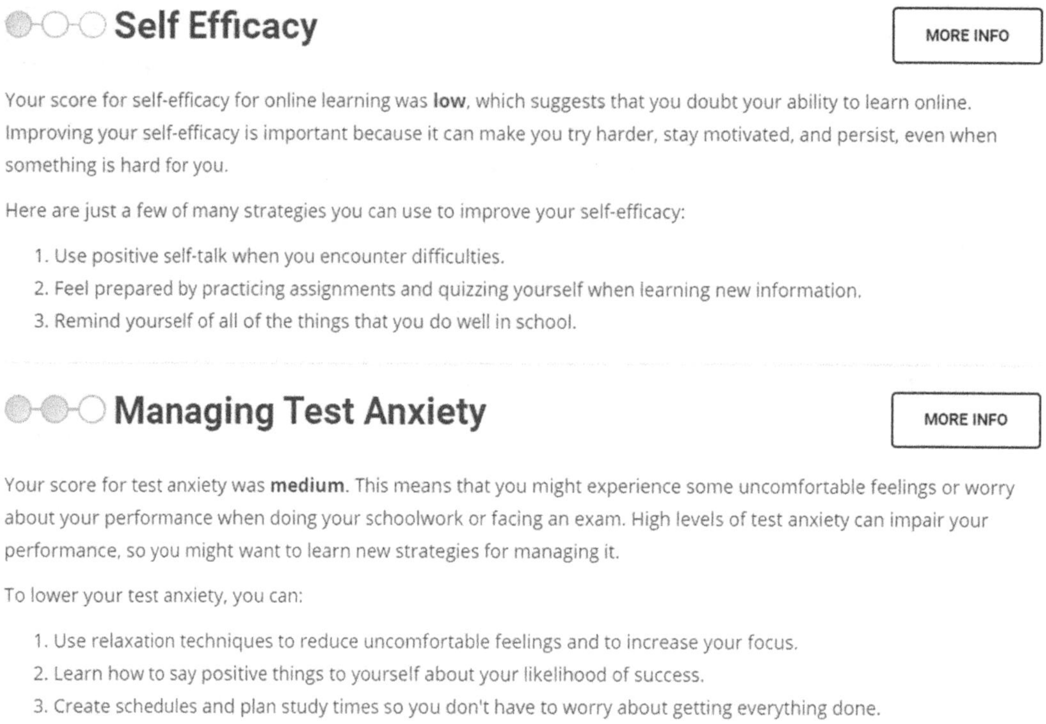

◉-○-○ **Self Efficacy**   [MORE INFO]

Your score for self-efficacy for online learning was **low**, which suggests that you doubt your ability to learn online. Improving your self-efficacy is important because it can make you try harder, stay motivated, and persist, even when something is hard for you.

Here are just a few of many strategies you can use to improve your self-efficacy:

1. Use positive self-talk when you encounter difficulties.
2. Feel prepared by practicing assignments and quizzing yourself when learning new information.
3. Remind yourself of all of the things that you do well in school.

◉-◉-○ **Managing Test Anxiety**   [MORE INFO]

Your score for test anxiety was **medium**. This means that you might experience some uncomfortable feelings or worry about your performance when doing your schoolwork or facing an exam. High levels of test anxiety can impair your performance, so you might want to learn new strategies for managing it.

To lower your test anxiety, you can:

1. Use relaxation techniques to reduce uncomfortable feelings and to increase your focus.
2. Learn how to say positive things to yourself about your likelihood of success.
3. Create schedules and plan study times so you don't have to worry about getting everything done.

Fig. 2 Sample DAACS feedback for self-efficacy and managing test anxiety subscales. (From *Diagnostic Assessment & Achievement of College Skills* by DAACS, 2016 (https://my.daacs.net). CC BY 4.0)

other commonly used engagement constructs in the educational literature. Of particular importance to this chapter, however, was our premise that SRL interventions, SRL PD training initiatives, and SRL formative assessment practices represent a set of potentially valuable approaches for applying SRL principles in school contexts. We briefly addressed the importance of each of these innovations, but focused most heavily on SRL formative assessment (i.e., ongoing assessments of student SRL as they engage in learning activities) and its potential for directly enhancing students' behavioral and academic functioning or indirectly through the promotion of more effective instructional practices.

When reflecting on how best to implement and apply SRL principles to academic contexts, it is critical to understand the development process through which students become independent and strategic regulated learners, as well as the various socialization processes (e.g., modeling, feedback, prompts) that optimize this development.

Zimmerman (2000) presented a model of strategic and regulatory development consisting of four levels: observation, emulation, self-control, and self-regulation. This model is based on the assumption that social and contextual influences predominate in the early stages of learning strategic skills (i.e., observation, emulation) but that over time, students assume greater control and responsibility over the learning process (i.e., self-control and self-regulation; Cleary et al., 2018). At the observational and emulation levels, students learn from watching others (i.e., observation) and from practicing strategies and skills within the context of guided practice sessions and feedback developed and structured by a teacher, parent, or other individual (i.e., emulation). A key aspect of these two levels is the heavy role of social agents on the structuring and organization of "regulatory opportunities" for the students (Cleary et al., 2018; Zimmerman, 2000). In our chapter, this notion of *guided practice sessions* was illustrated in the reflection activities that stu-

Self-Efficacy

Self-efficacy is your confidence in your ability to do something. Self-efficacy is specific to a certain task so, for example, you might have high self-efficacy for a math test but low self-efficacy for public speaking, or vice versa.

The SRL assessment suggests that you have **low** *self-efficacy for online learning*. This might mean that you doubt your abilities, avoid online work, or give up quickly when you encounter challenges. The following scenario illustrates how low self-efficacy can affect a person's thoughts, feelings, and actions.

> Maria, a first year college student, was hesitant about enrolling in an online biology course. Although she has strong self-efficacy for reading, science had never been her strongest subject and she was afraid that she wouldn't understand biology concepts without meeting face-to-face with an instructor. The first class module was difficult for Maria, and she had a hard time understanding the material. "I may as well give up now," she thought, "Maybe this was a mistake."

Students like Maria have many self-doubts when learning, which can cause them to give up prematurely and to avoid things. The key thing that Maria needs are opportunities to practice working online so that she can experience some success. As students become more confident they tend to try harder, persist longer, and perform better in school.

Having low self-efficacy is not ideal—but it is not something to feel badly about. These beliefs can be changed and are somewhat under your control. To learn more about self-efficacy and/or a few strategies to help you become more confident working in an online environment, click on the **Learn**, **See**, and/or **Do** buttons below.

Your Assessment Responses

I am confident I can learn without the physical presence of an instructor to assist me.
Disagree

I am certain I can understand even the most difficult material presented in an online course.
Strongly Disagree

I am confident I can do an outstanding job on the activities in an online course.
Strongly Agree

Even with distractions, I am confident I can learn material presented online. Strongly Disagree

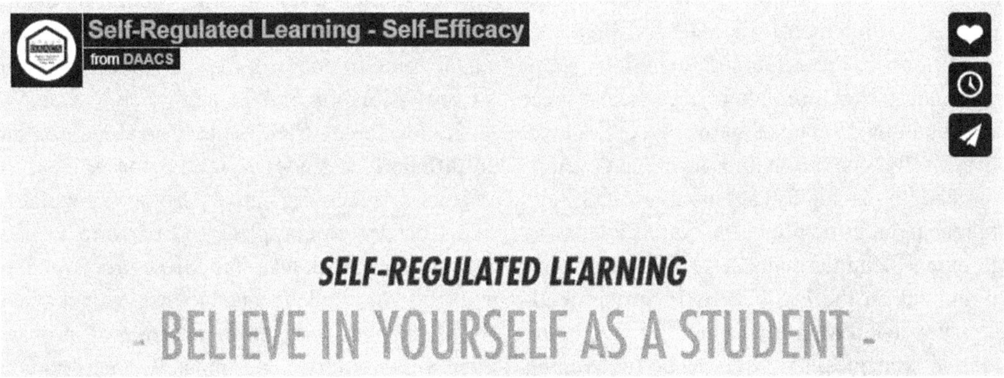

Self-Regulated Learning - Self-Efficacy
from DAACS

SELF-REGULATED LEARNING
- BELIEVE IN YOURSELF AS A STUDENT -

Fig. 3 Sample DAACS feedback for self-efficacy subscale and items. (From *Diagnostic Assessment & Achievement of College Skills* by DAACS, 2016 (https://my.daacs.net). CC BY 4.0)

dents experience as part of SREP. That is, the SREP coaches intentionally and purposefully structure reflective conversations and use micro-analysis approaches to gather information about students' thoughts, behaviors, and reactions. It is within this highly structured practice session that students receive feedback, prompts, or recommendations on how to improve their strategic skills (Cleary et al., 2017).

As students shift to the self-control level of strategy development, the influence of socialization processes, such as modeling and feedback, are less emphasized or needed. At this level, students intentionally practice skills or use strategies, often in the absence of their teachers or others who would typically provide support or feedback. Although students at the self-control level may still seek out help and supports from others, they are more proactive in making their own decisions about how best to learn and practice their skills. The methods used by Osborne et al. (2020) to examine SRL skills of high performing musicians reflect practice sessions operating at the self-control level of development. Although the researchers devised the microanalytic diary and procedures, students were operating at the self-control level given that they initiated and used these procedures on their own, often making their personal decisions and determinations about how to use the microanalysis data to guide behaviors.

The final and most sophisticated level of development, self-regulation, involves learners proactively setting their own goals and standards of performance; these learners are much more likely to adapt and refine their strategies to meet new and unique demands that they face. Students who typically operate at this level of development tend to be highly autonomous and self-sufficient and thus do not need social agents to as large extent (Zimmerman, 2000). Students who read and act on the DAACS SRL Survey feedback independently, perhaps by trying out the suggested strategies, are likely to be functioning at this level.

From an SRL development perspective, it is also important to recognize that the expected level of sophistication of students' SRL and stra-

tegic skills is a function of the demands and expectations of the contexts and settings in which they learn (Cleary et al., 2018; Grolnick & Raftery-Helmer, 2015). Cleary et al. (2018) emphasized this point while noting that SRL skills are most important and functional when students face challenges or obstacles or, more informally, when "the rules of the game change." To understand this latter phrase, consider the example of students transitioning from elementary school to middle school and then on to high school. In most elementary school settings, students have a primary teacher for much of the day and often complete much of the required work and learning during school hours. However, upon entering middle school, students are now faced with a different set of demands and experiences. That is, students will typically have different teachers for each of their academic content areas, all of whom may have different or unique rules and expectations for students. Students in middle school will also be exposed to more complex course content and assignments, with much of the work conducted outside of school hours, such as completing research lab reports, studying for cumulative exams, and writing research papers or essays (Grolnick & Raftery-Helmer, 2015). Thus, as the expectations of the contexts, teachers, and coursework increase in complexity or nuance, students will need to independently draw upon their regulatory capacities to meet such challenges. Conversely, students will not need to engage in high levels of independent, regulatory thinking and action when the situation is not challenging or does not require students to adapt to a new situation or demand.

In developing SRL skills, it is also important to differentiate students' motivation or desire to engage in a learning activity from the regulatory skills needed to complete and perform well on that activity. Because the SRL process is an effortful one, students need to display some level of motivation along with a sense of personal agency to control and manage their actions, thoughts, as well as their learning environment. Social-cognitive theorists underscore the role of various self-motivational beliefs in promoting human agency, but they place particular emphasis on self-efficacy—the belief in one's ability to perform specific actions at a particular level in specific situations and contexts (Bandura, 1997). It is through the developmental process of observation, emulation, and self-control and the corresponding feedback from others that students will begin to experience heightened levels of self-efficacy and a corresponding sense of personal agency (Bandura, 1997; Cleary & Kitsantas, 2017).

There are other important considerations that pertain specifically to the nature of SRL assessments and their use as a feedback-generating or formative assessment tool. One of the most important considerations involves the clarity of expectations and standards for students, teachers, and others who might be using the SRL data. Because goals or self-standards ultimately govern the regulatory engagement process, it is important that all individuals who interact with students, such as parents, teachers, or tutors, be cognizant of their own goals within their respective roles. Another important implication is that SRL assessment data should speak to various aspects of students' functioning, including their cognitive, affective, metacognitive, and behavioral changes. Finally, using SRL assessment data as feedback for students is only one step in the formative assessment process. After SRL assessment data are collected and interpreted, students and/or other individuals (e.g., teachers) need opportunities to use that feedback, while receiving additional guidance, structure, and prompts, to make improvements and promote learning.

Regarding microanalysis, although there is fairly robust evidence (i.e., convergent, concurrent validity) to support the validity of inferences made from microanalysis results, there is a paucity of studies examining other validity issues, such as consequential validity; that is, the intended and unintended consequences of using microanalysis assessments as a formative assessment tool for guiding instructional or intervention initiatives (Cleary et al., 2021). At this point, researchers have used microanalysis in a formative fashion or to inform practice relative to SREP implementation, PD initiatives with teachers, and

structured practice sessions with advanced musicians. It is clear that research in the use of SRL microanalysis formative assessment practices is still in its infancy and thus, many questions remain. Future research needs to expand the range of situations and contexts for applying SRL microanalysis and to examine the sensitivity of microanalysis assessments to intra- and inter-individual differences in measuring SRL processes. Further, as schools increasingly rely on data-based decision-making and service delivery frameworks that emphasize progress monitoring tools, it is critical for researchers to gather evidence on school personnel's perceived acceptability, usability, feasibility, and/or perceived effectiveness of microanalysis assessments. Given the qualitative nature of microanalysis data and the corresponding time intensive nature of data analysis, developers of microanalysis assessments need to also consider how technological supports and innovations can enhance the overall feasibility and scalability of its use in schools for formative purposes. Reducing logistic burdens in assessment implementation will enhance the quality of data obtained and decisions made for improving intervention planning that lead to meaningful educators and student outcomes (Cleary et al., 2021).

As school personnel continue to become more interested in instructional effectiveness and student progress across key academic skill areas, another potentially fruitful line of research involves examining reliable estimates of change or growth in student SRL processes over time. Aligned with formative assessment practices, microanalysis assessment approaches need to be shown to reliably gather information about SRL processes across multiple time points in a school year, with opportunities for students and teachers to use this information to inform revisions and next steps. The degree to which microanalysis scores obtained from repeated measures reflect "true" rates of change in SRL regulatory processes is a key prerequisite for improving educator intervention implementation (fidelity) and student goal attainment.

Several areas of future research that we recommended for SRL microanalysis are also applicable to the DAACS SRL Survey or other types of SRL questionnaires; that is, issues pertaining to feasibility, utility, scalability, and overall effectiveness of these measures as formative assessment tools. Another interesting line of research entails examining the unique and relative effects of SRL microanalysis and DAACS SRL Survey data on student outcomes and overall rates of growth and improvement. It is certainly possible that there are additive effects to using both assessment approaches as part of the formative assessment process. Finally, while the DAACS system is still in its infancy in terms of development and use in applied contexts, it has much potential given that it leverages technology and open resource supports to customize and streamline the nature of data and feedback provided to students. Unfortunately, not much is known regarding how students actually use these survey data to improve their regulatory skills and performance. This is an area in need of more research and investigation.

References

Allshouse, A. D. (2016). *Professional development in self-regulated learning: Effects of a workshop on teacher knowledge, skills, and self-efficacy, and the development of a coaching framework* (Publication No. 10297495) [Doctoral dissertation, Rutgers, The State University of New Jersey]. ProQuest Dissertations and Theses Global.

Andrade, H. (2013). Classroom assessment in the context of learning theory and research. In J. H. McMillan (Ed.), *SAGE handbook of research on classroom assessment* (pp. 17–34). SAGE. https://doi.org/10.4135/9781452218649.n2

Andrade, H. (2016). *Classroom assessment and learning: A selective review of theory and research* [White paper]. National Academy of Sciences.

Bandura, A. (1986). *Social foundations of thought and action: A social cognitive theory.* Prentice-Hall.

Bandura, A. (1997). *Self-efficacy: The exercise of control.* W. H. Freeman.

Barkley, R. A. (2016). Attention-deficit/hyperactivity disorder and self-regulation: Taking an evolutionary perspective on executive functioning. In K. D. Vohs & R. F. Baumeister (Eds.), *Handbook of self-regulation: Research, theory and application* (3rd ed., pp. 497–515). Guilford Press.

Bernacki, M. L. (2018). Examining the cyclical, loosely sequenced, and contingent features of self-regulated learning: Trace data and their analysis. In D. H. Schunk & J. A. Greene (Eds.), *Educational psychology handbook series. Handbook of self-regulation of learning and performance* (pp. 370–387). Routledge/Taylor & Francis Group. https://doi.org/10.4324/9781315697048.ch24

Briesch, A. M., & Briesch, J. M. (2016). Meta-analysis of behavioral self-management interventions in single-case research. *School Psychology Review, 45*(1), 3–18. https://doi.org/10.17105/SPR45-1.3-18

Bryer, J. M., Andrade, H. L., Cleary, T. J., Lui, A. M., Franklin Jr., D., & Akhmedjanova, D. (2022). The efficacy and predictive power of the diagnostic assessment and achievement of college skills on academic success [Manuscript submitted for publication]. Department of Data Sciences and Information Systems, School of Professional Studies – CUNY.

Butler, D. L., & Winne, P. H. (1995). Feedback and self-regulated learning: A theoretical synthesis. *Review of Educational Research, 65*(3), 245–281. https://doi.org/10.3102/00346543065003245

Christenson, S. L., Reschly, A. L., & Wylie, C. (Eds.). (2012). Handbook of research on student engagement. *Guilford Press.* https://doi.org/10.1007/978-1-4614-2018-7

Cleary, T. J. (2006). The development and validation of the Self-Regulation Strategy Inventory—Self-Report. *Journal of School Psychology, 44*(4), 307–322. https://doi.org/10.1016/j.jsp.2006.05.002

Cleary, T. J. (2011). Emergence of self-regulated learning microanalysis: Historical overview, essential features, and implications for research and practice. In B. J. Zimmerman & D. H. Schunk (Eds.), *Handbook of self-regulation of learning and performance* (pp. 329–345). Taylor Francis.

Cleary, T. J., & Callan, G. L. (2018). Assessing self-regulated learning using microanalytic methods. In D. H. Schunk & J. A. Greene (Eds.), *Handbook of self-regulation of learning and performance* (2nd ed., pp. 338–351). Routledge. https://doi.org/10.4324/9781315697048.ch22

Cleary, T. J., & Kitsantas, A. (2017). Motivation and self-regulated learning influences on middle school mathematics achievement. *School Psychology Review, 46*(1), 88–107. https://doi.org/10.1080/02796015.2017.12087607

Cleary, T. J., & Platten, P. (2013). Examining the correspondence between self-regulated learning and academic achievement: A case study analysis [Special issue]. *Educational Research International.* https://doi.org/10.1155/2013/272560

Cleary, T. J., & Zimmerman, B. J. (2004). Self-regulation empowerment program: A school-based program to enhance self-regulated and self-motivated cycles of student learning. *Psychology in the Schools, 41*(5), 537–550. https://doi.org/10.1002/pits.10177

Cleary, T. J., & Zimmerman, B. J. (2006). Teachers' perceived usefulness of strategy microanalytic assessment information. *Psychology in the Schools, 43*(2), 149–155. https://doi.org/10.1002/pits.20141

Cleary, T. J., & Zimmerman, B. J. (2012). A cyclical self-regulatory account of student engagement: Theoretical foundations and applications. In S. Christenson, A. L. Reschly, & C. Wylie (Eds.), *Handbook of research on student engagement* (pp. 237–258). Springer. https://doi.org/10.1007/978-1-4614-2018-7_11

Cleary, T. J., Gubi, A., & Prescott, M. V. (2010). Motivation and self-regulation assessments: Professional practices and needs of school psychologists. *Psychology in the Schools, 47*(10), 985–1002. https://doi.org/10.1002/pits.20519

Cleary, T. J., Velardi, B., & Schnaidman, B. (2017). Effects of the Self-Regulation Empowerment Program (SREP) on middle school students' strategic skills, self-efficacy, and mathematics achievement. *Journal of School Psychology, 64*, 28–42. https://doi.org/10.1016/j.jsp.2017.04.004

Cleary, T. J., Kitsantas, A., Pape, S. L., & Slemp, J. (2018). Integration of socialization influences and the development of self-regulated learning (SRL) skills: A social-cognitive perspective. In G. A. D. Alief & D. McInerney (Eds.), *Big theoriesrevisited* (2nd ed., pp. 269–294). Information Age Publishing.

Cleary, T. J., Slemp. J., Alperin, A., Reddy, L., Alperin, A., Lui, A., Austin, A., & Cedar, T. (2021). Characteristics and uses of SRL microanalysis across diverse contexts, tasks, and populations: A systematic review. *School Psychology Review*, 1–21. https://doi.org/10.1080/2372966X.2020.1862627

Coalition for Psychology in Schools and Education. (2006). *Report on the teacher needs survey*. American Psychological Association, Center for Psychology in Schools and Education. https://www.apa.org/ed/schools/coalition/2006-teacher-needs-report.pdf

Cook, C. R., Thayer, A. J., Fiat, A., & Sullivan, M. (2020). Interventions to enhance affective engagement. In A. L. Reschly, A. J. Pohl, & S. L. Christenson (Eds.), *Student engagement: Effective academic, behavioral, cognitive, and affective interventions at school* (pp. 203–238). SpringerLink. https://doi.org/10.1007/978-3-030-37285-9_12

Efklides, A. (2011). Interactions of metacognition with motivation and affect in self-regulated learning: The MASRL model. *Educational Psychologist, 46*(1), 6–25. https://doi.org/10.1080/00461520.2011.538645

Fredericks, J. A., Blumenfeld, P. C., & Paris, A. H. (2004). School engagement: Potential of the concept, state of the evidence. *Review of Educational Research, 74*(1), 59–109. https://doi.org/10.3102/00346543074001059

Ganda, D. R., & Boruchovitch, E. (2018). Promoting self-regulated learning of Brazilian preservice student teachers: Results of an intervention program. *Frontiers in Education, 3*(5), 1–12. https://doi.org/10.3389/feduc.2018.00005

Graham, S., & Harris, K. R. (2009). Almost 30 years of writing research: Making sense of it all with *The Wrath of Khan*. *Learning Disabilities Research, 24*(2), 58–68. https://doi.org/10.1111/j.1540-5826.2009.01277.x

Graham, S., McKeown, D., Kiuhara, D., & Harris, K. R. (2012). A meta-analysis of writing instruction for students in the elementary grades. *Journal of Educational Psychology, 104*(4), 879–896. https://doi.org/10.1037/a0029185

Greene, J. A. (2018). *Self-regulation in education*. Routledge.

Grolnick, W. S., & Raftery-Helmer, J. N. (2015). Contexts supporting self-regulated learning at school transitions. In T. J. Cleary (Ed.), *Self-regulated learning interventions: Enhancing adaptability, performance, and well-being* (pp. 251–276). American Psychological Association. https://doi.org/10.1037/14641-012

Hattie, J. A. C., & Timperley, H. (2007). The power of feedback. *Review of Educational Research, 77*(1), 81–112. https://doi.org/10.3102/003465430298487

Kramarski, B., & Michalsky, T. (2015). Effect of a TPCK-SRL model on teachers' pedagogical beliefs, self-efficacy, and technology-based lesson design. In C. Angeli & N. Valanides (Eds.), *Technological pedagogical content knowledge* (pp. 89–112). Springer. https://doi.org/10.1007/978-1-4899-8080-9_5

Kramarski, B., Desoete, A., Bannert, M., Narciss, S., & Perry, N. (2013). New perspectives on integrating self-regulated learning at school [Special issue]. *Education Research International.* https://doi.org/10.1155/2013/498214

Kremer-Hayon, L., & Tillema, H. H. (1999). Self-regulated learning in the context of teacher education. *Teaching and Teacher Education, 15*, 507–522. https://doi.org/10.1016/S0742-051X(99)00008-6

Lau, K. L. (2012). Chinese language teachers' perception and implementation of self-regulated learning-based instruction. *Teaching and Teacher Education, 31*, 56–66. https://doi.org/10.1016/j.tate.2012.12.001

Lovelace, M. D., Reschly, A. L., & Appleton, J. J. (2017). Beyond school records: The value of cognitive and affective engagement in predicting dropout and on-time graduation. *Professional School Counseling, 21*, 70–84. https://doi.org/10.5330/1096-2409-21.1.70

Lui, A. M., Franklin, D., Jr., Akhmedjanova, D., Gorgun, G., Bryer, J., Andrade, H. L., & Cleary, T. (2018). Validity Evidence of the Internal Structure of the DAACS Self-Regulated Learning Survey. *Future Review: International Journal of Transition, College, and Career Success, 1*(1), 1–18.

McPherson, G. E., Osborne, M. S., Evans, P., & Miksza, P. (2017). Applying self-regulated learning microanalysis to study musicians' practice. *Psychology of Music*, 1–15. https://doi.org/10.1177/0305735617731614

Montague, M., Enders, C., & Dietz, S. (2014). Effects of cognitive strategy instruction on math problem solving of middle school students with learning disabilities. *Learning Disability Quarterly, 34*(4), 262–272. https://doi.org/10.1177/0731948711421762

Nichols, S. L., & Dawson, H. S. (2012). Assessment as context for student engagement. In S. Christenson, A. L. Reschly, & C. Wylie (Eds.), *Handbook of research on student engagement* (pp. 457–478). Springer. https://doi.org/10.1007/978-1-4614-2018-7_22

O'Donnell and Reschly. (2020). Assessment of student engagement. In A. L. Reschly, A. J. Pohl, & S. L.

Christenson (Eds.), *Student engagement: Effective academic, behavioral, cognitive, and affective interventions at school* (pp. 55–76). Springer. https://doi.org/10.1007/978-3-030-37285-9_3

Osborne, M., McPherson, G. E., Miksza, P., & Evans, P. (2020). Using a microanalysis intervention to examine shifts in musician's self-regulated learning. *Psychology of Music*, 1–17. https://doi.org/10.1177/0305735620915265

Panadero, E. (2017). A review of self-regulated learning: Six models and four directions for research. *Frontiers in Psychology, 8*, 193–316. https://doi.org/10.3389/fpsyg.2017.00422

Pauli, C., Reusser, K., & Grob, U. (2007). Teaching for understanding and/or self-regulated learning? A video-based analysis of reform-oriented mathematics instruction in Switzerland. *International Journal of Educational Research, 46*(5), 294–305. https://doi.org/10.1016/j.ijer.2007.10.004

Perry, J. C., DeWine, D. B., Duffy, R. D., & Vance, K. S. (2007). The academic self-efficacy of urban youth: A mixed-methods study of a school-to-work program. *Journal of Career Development, 34*, 103–126. https://doi.org/10.1177/0894845307307470

Peters-Burton, E. E., & Botov, I. S. (2017). Self-regulated learning microanalysis as a tool to inform professional development delivery in real-time. *Metacognition and Learning, 12*(1), 45–78. https://doi.org/10.1007/s11409-016-9160-z

Peters-Burton, E. E., Rich, P., Cleary, T., Burton, S., Kitsantas, A., Egan, G., & Ellsworth, J. (2020). Using computational thinking for data practices in high school science. *The Science Teacher, 87*(6), 30–36.

Pintrich, P. R., Smith, D. A., Garcia, T., & McKeachie, W. J. (1991). *A manual for the use of the Motivated Strategies for Learning Questionnaire*. The Regents of the University of Michigan.

Pohl, A. J. (2020). Strategies and interventions for promoting cognitive engagement. In A. L. Reschly, A. J. Pohl, & S. L. Christenson (Eds.), *Student engagement: Effective academic, behavioral, cognitive, and affective interventions at school* (pp. 253–280). Springer. https://doi.org/10.1007/978-3-030-37285-9_14

Puustinen, M., & Pulkkinen, L. (2001). Models of self-regulated learning: A review. *Scandinavian Journal of Educational Research, 45*(3), 269–286. https://doi.org/10.1080/00313830120074206

Reddy, L. A., Cleary, T. J., Alperin, A., & Verdesco, A. (2018). A critical review of self-regulated learning interventions for children with attention-deficit hyperactivity disorder. *Psychology in the Schools, 55*(6), 609–628. https://doi.org/10.1002/pits.22142

Reschly, A. L. (2020). Dropout prevention and student engagement. In A. L. Reschly, A. J. Pohl, & S. L. Christenson (Eds.), *Student engagement: Effective academic, behavioral, cognitive, and affective interventions at school* (pp. 31–54). Springer. https://doi.org/10.1007/978-3-030-37285-9_2

Reschly, A. L., & Christenson, S. L. (2012). Jingle, jangle, and conceptual haziness: Evolutions and future directions of the engagement construct. In S. L. Christenson, A. L. Reschly, & C. Wylie (Eds.), *Handbook of research on student engagement* (pp. 3–19). Springer. https://doi.org/10.1007/978-1-4614-2018-7_1

Reschly, A. L., Pohl, A. J., & Christenson, S. L. (Eds.). (2020). *Student engagement: Effective academic, behavioral, cognitive, and affective interventions at school*. Springer International Publishing. https://doi.org/10.1007/978-3-030-37285-9

Schmitz, B., & Wiese, B. S. (2006). New perspectives for the evaluation of training sessions in self-regulated learning: Time-series analyses of diary data. *Contemporary Educational Psychology, 31*(1), 64–96. https://doi.org/10.1016/j.cedpsych.2005.02.002

Schraw, G., & Dennison, R. S. (1994). Assessing metacognitive awareness. *Contemporary Educational Psychology, 19*(4), 460–475. https://doi.org/10.1006/ceps.1994.1033

Schunk, D. H., & Greene, J. A. (2018). *Handbook of self-regulation of learning and performance* (2nd ed.). Routledge. https://doi.org/10.4324/9781315697048

Shute, V. (2008). Focus on formative feedback. *Review of Educational Research, 78*(1), 153–189. https://doi.org/10.3102/0034654307313795

Skinner, E. A., Furrer, C., Marchand, G., & Kindermann, T. (2008). Engagement and disaffection in the classroom: Part of a larger motivational dynamic? *Journal of Educational Psychology, 100*, 765–781. https://doi.org/10.1177/0013164408323233

Spruce, R., & Bol, L. (2015). Teacher beliefs, knowledge, and practice of self-regulated learning. *Metacognition and Learning, 10*(2), 245–277. https://doi.org/10.1007/s11409-014-9124-0

Stiggins, R. (2005). From formative assessment to assessment for learning: A path to success in standards–based schools. *The Phi Delta Kappan, 87*(4), 324–328. https://doi.org/10.1177/003172170508700414

Suveg, C., Davis, M., & Jones, A. (2015). Emotion regulation interventions for youth with anxiety disorders. In T. J. Cleary (Ed.), *Self-regulated learning interventions with at-risk youth: enhancing adaptability, performance, and well-being* (pp. 137–156). American Psychological Association. http://www.jstor.org/stable/j.ctv1chrrn8.12

Tonks, S. M., & Taboada, A. (2011). Developing self-regulated readers through instruction for reading engagement. In B. J. Zimmerman & D. H. Schunk (Eds.), *Handbook of self-regulation of learning and performance* (pp. 173–186). Routledge.

Vohs, K. D., & Baumeister, R. F. (2016). *Handbook of self-regulation: Research, theory, and applications* (3rd ed.). The Guilford Press.

Wehmeyer, M. L., Agran, M., & Hughes, C. A. (2000). National survey of teachers' promotion of self-determination and student-directed learning. *Journal of Special Education, 34*, 56–68. https://doi.org/10.1177/002246690003400201

Weinstein, C. E., Palmer, D. R., & Shulte, A. C. (2002). *LASSI user's manual* (2nd ed.). H & H.

Wiggins, G. (2012). Seven keys to effective feedback. *Educational Leadership, 70*(1), 10–16.

Winne, P. H., & Hadwin, A. F. (1998). Studying as self-regulated learning. In D. J. Hacker, J. Dunlosky, & A. C. Graesser (Eds.), *Metacognition in educational theory and practice* (pp. 27–30). Routledge Taylor & Francis Group.

Winne, P. H., & Perry, N. E. (2000). Measuring self-regulated learning. In M. Boekaerts, P. R. Pintrich, & M. Zeidner (Eds.), *Handbook of self-regulation* (pp. 531–566). Academic Press. https://doi.org/10.1016/B978-012109890-2/50045-7

Wolters, C. A. (2003). Regulation of motivation: Evaluating an underemphasized aspect of self-regulated learning. *Educational Psychologist, 38*(4), 189–205. https://doi.org/10.1207/S15326985EP3804_1

Zimmerman, B. J. (2000). Attaining self-regulation: A social-cognitive perspective. In M. Boekaerts, P. R. Pintrich, & M. Zeidner (Eds.), *Handbook of self-regulation* (pp. 13–39). Academic Press. https://doi.org/10.1016/B978-012109890-2/50031-7

Zimmerman, B. J., & Schunk, D. H. (2001). *Self-regulated learning and academic achievement: Theoretical perspectives* (2nd ed.). Lawrence Erlbaum Associates. https://doi.org/10.1007/978-1-4612-3618-4

Hope and Student Engagement: Keys to School Success

Elyse M. Farnsworth, Maddie Cordle, and Ariana Groen

Abstract

A number of psychological factors contribute to students' capacity to access and benefit from instruction. These include motivation, self-efficacy, agency, social skills, student engagement, and hope. This chapter aims to explore the relationship between student engagement, hope, and student outcomes. Both student engagement and hope serve as psychological facilitators of achievement. That is, students who are actively engaged in learning and who have high levels of hope are likely to benefit from instruction and experience positive academic, social, emotional, and behavioral outcomes at school. In this chapter, we first describe and define our conceptualization of student engagement. Then, we define hope, explore Hope Theory, and describe how hope is measured in children and adolescents. Following this foundational discussion, we provide an integrative review of the extant literature regarding student outcomes associated with hope and student engagement, and we explore how student engagement and hope may interact to impact student outcomes. We also briefly describe interventions which show promise for promoting hope among students. The chapter ends with a discussion of future directions for research from which findings may assist educators in fostering student engagement and hope in order to promote positive outcomes for all students.

E. M. Farnsworth (✉) · M. Cordle · A. Groen
Department of Psychology, Minnesota State University – Mankato,
Mankato, MN, USA
e-mail: elyse.farnsworth@mnsu.edu

Hope and Student Engagement: Keys to School Success

Hope is not equivalent to desire. Hope is a cognitive process involving thinking about one's goals, feeling motivated to accomplish those goals, and understanding the path toward goal attainment (Snyder, 1995). Consider the last time you set a goal. Did you experience high hope related to the likelihood that you would attain your goal, or did you feel a sense of hopelessness? Perhaps your goal was to compete in a 5K run or triathlon. Maybe you identified a number of books you would like to read for pleasure, or you aspired to learn a new skill like cooking or knitting. High hope, and subsequently a greater likelihood of goal attainment, is elicited by engaging in both agency and pathway thinking related to one's goal (Snyder, 1995, 2002). Agency thinking serves as the motivational component of hope, while pathway thinking provides the possible route toward goal attainment as well as alternatives should one need to overcome an obstacle along the way. For example, if you experienced high hope regarding a goal to compete in a 5K run, you might engage in pathway thinking by creating a plausible training plan to prepare for the race. Likewise, you would engage in agency thinking, believing that you are capable of following your training plan, adjusting your plan as needed, and crossing the finish line on race day. Individuals who engage in these cognitive processes indicative of high hope are more likely to attain their goals and experience positive outcomes in areas such as academic achievement, athletics, physical health, psychological adjustment, and human connection (see Snyder et al., 2018).

As with our personal and professional goal attainment as adults, the construct of hope is relevant to educational outcomes for students (see TeramotoPedrotti, 2018). While working in elementary and secondary school settings, we observed students who experienced high levels of hope as well as those who had a sense of hopelessness, lacking agency or a clear direction toward goal attainment. Sometimes students who experienced low hope struggled to articulate clear and achievable goals. During structured student interviews and informal interactions, we began asking students about their goals and what they *hoped* to do in the future. From these conversations, we noticed a pattern. The students who demonstrated behaviors consistent with higher engagement in school (e.g., better attendance, realistic future planning, and connections to peers and teachers; Appleton et al., 2008) also articulated *hopes* for the future. They had clear goals, plans to accomplish their goals, and the motivation or agency to follow through on those plans.

The *hopes* they shared were specific like attending culinary school and opening a restaurant or owning their own auto mechanic business or attending college to become a teacher or nurse. For each of these future aspirations, they were able to describe the steps needed to pursue their goals, including the actions they needed to take as a student to support the accomplishment of these *hopes*. Conversely, the students who demonstrated behaviors correlated with lower levels of engagement (e.g., difficulty maintaining relationships with peers and teachers, lack of active involvement in the learning process, and difficulty setting goals; Appleton et al., 2008) frequently struggled to describe their *hopes* for the future. When asked what they *hoped* to do in the future, this group of students often shrugged, stated "I dunno," or provided a vague, generic response like "probably go to college or something." Students who demonstrated behaviors representative of lower levels of engagement struggled to articulate their *hopes* and were unable to identify what actions they would need to take to pursue the vague goals.

Notably, these observations are anecdotal; however, they led us to wonder whether hope is related to student engagement. Past studies provide empirical evidence for the relationship between hope and several academic, cognitive, affective, and behavioral indicators of student engagement (e.g., Dixson & Stevens, 2018; Marques et al., 2017; Rubens et al., 2020; Snyder, 2002; Wurster et al., 2021). For example, Dixson and Stevens (2018) reported moderate, positive effects with higher levels of hope being associated with increased school belongingness, academic self-concept, goal valuation, attitude toward teachers, academic motivation, and self-regulation. Further, students with high levels of hope were more likely to achieve positive academic outcomes, such as improved grades and higher rates of school completion (Marques et al., 2017; Rubens et al., 2020). Finally, some studies suggest students who experience high hope may be less likely to demonstrate school disengagement and experience negative affect (Dixson, 2019; Marques et al., 2017), while being more likely to feel self-efficacious (Wurster et al., 2021). Collectively, these findings suggest there may be an important relationship between hope and student engagement.

Before examining the relationship between indicators of the four domains of student engagement and hope, we will describe our conceptualization of student engagement and define the construct of hope through a review of Hope

Theory (see Snyder et al., 1991; Snyder, 1994; Snyder et al., 1999; and Snyder, 2002). We will also discuss how hope is measured among students and the educational outcomes that are associated with high versus low levels of hope. After providing this foundational information about hope, we will review selected empirical findings regarding the relationship between hope and indicators of student engagement described in the literature (see Reschly & Christenson, 2012). A brief summary of interventions and supports to foster student hope will also be presented. Finally, since this is an emerging area of interest, we will discuss future directions for research regarding the relationship between hope and student engagement.

Conceptualization of Student Engagement

To begin to understand the relationship between hope and student engagement, it is important to describe our conceptualization of student engagement given the variations in how engagement is defined in the literature. Researchers define student engagement as a multi-dimensional construct (see Appleton et al., 2008 for a review of definitions of student engagement) with varying domains. Most definitions include the behavioral and cognitive domains of engagement, while some scholars have acknowledged the academic and affective domains of engagement (see Appleton et al., 2008). Being an engaged learner is an essential facilitator of positive academic and behavioral outcomes among elementary and secondary students. Namely, studies indicate that disengaged students are more likely to partake in risk and problem behaviors (Wang & Fredericks, 2014), experience peer rejection (Crosnoe, 2002), and dropout of school (Finn, 1989). Further, students who are highly engaged are 2.4 times more likely to graduate from high school and less likely to demonstrate significant absenteeism (Finn & Zimmer, 2012). Clearly, being engaged (e.g., actively participating in class, setting realistic goals, completing assignments, feeling con-

nected to peers and educators) facilitates access to instruction, leading to more positive short- and long-term outcomes for all students.

In this chapter, we conceptualize student engagement as a multi-dimensional construct with four domains (i.e., behavioral, academic, cognitive, and affective engagement), consistent with the model of engagement proposed by Christenson, Appleton, Reschly and colleagues (see Appleton et al., 2006; Christenson et al., 2008; Reschly & Christenson, 2012). In this model of engagement, behavioral engagement is demonstrated via attendance, behavior incidents, class participation, and how well prepared a student is for school, whereas academic engagement is measured by a student's on-task behaviors, work completion, grades, and credits accrued. Cognitive engagement represents the value placed on learning, self-regulatory classroom behaviors, and goals set by a student. Finally, a student's affective engagement is reflective of their feelings of belonging and connectedness to peers, teachers, and school. This model was selected as a tool for describing the relationship between student engagement and hope because the domains align with the outcomes studied by researchers interested in student hope. Namely, many indicators of student engagement described in this model have been investigated as correlates or outcomes associated with student levels of hope.

For instance, the goal-setting indicators of cognitive engagement are reflective of the goal-setting demonstrated by students with high hope. In both theories, students who endorse high levels of hope and students who demonstrate higher levels of student engagement set realistic and attainable goals and participate in future-directed thinking. Likewise, the indicators of behavioral and academic engagement proposed in Reschly and Christenson's (2012) model of student engagement align with the behaviors that would be necessary for demonstrating effective pathway thinking in Snyder's (2002) Hope Theory. Students who, for example, attend school regularly, actively participate in class, pass classes, and graduate are engaging in behaviors that facilitate accomplishment of their goals. In this way, there is overlap between the indicators of behavioral and academic engagement with pathway thinking. Unlike cognitive, behavioral, and academic indicators of engagement, there is a less clear link between this model of student engagement and Hope Theory as it relates to affective engagement. Perhaps affective student engagement is an artifact of experiencing high hope or students who experience high hope feel a greater sense of belonging and connectedness to school. This is an area for further investigation.

Finally, both Reschly and Christenson's (2012) model of student engagement and Snyder's (2002) Hope Theory overlap with the construct of motivation. Agency thinking involved in the development of high hope reflects an individual's motivation to accomplish a goal. The individual must make a plan, feel self-efficacious, and adjust their plan when obstacles are encountered. Similarly, students who are highly engaged in school demonstrate motivation to do well. They engage in class, complete their work, are on-task, and place a high value on learning.

Defining Hope and Hope Theory

Snyder (1995) defined hope as, "the process of thinking about one's goals, along with the motivation to move toward (agency) and the ways to achieve (pathways) those goals" (p. 355).

Snyder (2002) discussed the three components of hope (i.e., agency thinking, pathway thinking, and goals) which comprise Hope Theory. Hope Theory was first proposed by Snyder and colleagues in 1991. The original theory was then expanded upon by Snyder and colleagues in 1994 and 2002, respectively, to better define and explain the theoretical components. The three previously mentioned components have been studied and empirically validated in past research in terms of their relevance and contribution to Hope Theory (Cheavens & Ritschel, 2014). The following sections discuss goals, agency, and pathways as they apply to Hope Theory, as well

as point out any overlap with our conceptualization of student engagement.

Goals

Goals are defined in Hope Theory as anything a student wishes to experience, make, attain, or become (Snyder et al., 2003). It is also important to note that an underlying assumption of goals is that all human behavior is goal-oriented, meaning that humans behave in a manner that helps them reach their goals (Snyder, 1994). Students who experience high hope have goals which serve as mental targets for promoting desired outcomes or preventing negative outcomes. To attain these goals, students with high hope are able to engage in pathway and agency thinking. That is, students who experience high hope are able to create a plausible plan to achieve their goals (i.e., they can visualize a clear pathway between their current and desired states) and believe they have the capacity to reach their goals and overcome obstacles (i.e., they feel a sense of agency).

Students with high levels of hope also tend to have more well-specified goals (Cheavens & Ritschel, 2014). Well-specified goals foster more effective pathway and agency thinking. That is, well-specified goals serve as a catalyst to guide student behavior in a manner which carries out their plausible plan. In this way, it is possible that hope, like motivation, self-efficacy, and study skills, may serve as an important academic enabler to promote student success (see DiPerna, 2006). Namely, scholars suggest that students who endorse high levels of hope and well-specified goals may be more likely to engage in behaviors that promote success in school like attending in class, completing required assignments, and engaging as active learners (Dixson, 2019). Goals set by the student and each of the correlated behaviors are reflective of the indicators of the cognitive (goal-setting), behavioral (class attendance and active participation), and academic (work completion) domains of student engagement.

Pathway Thinking

Pathway thinking is the plausible planning and thinking that a student engages in in order to attain their goals (Snyder, 1994). Ultimately, students with high levels of hope are engaging in pathway thinking when they visualize the steps necessary to progress toward achieving their well-specified goals. Referring to the previously used example, if your goal was to compete in a 5 K run, you might engage in pathway thinking by creating a plausible training plan to prepare for the race. This may involve setting a schedule to train, beginning with shorter increments, and progressively working your way up to a 5 K distance. This planning and following a path toward a goal demonstrates pathway thinking.

It is important to note that hope theorists agree that students with high hope tend to have at least one primary pathway developed to help propel them toward their goals as well as the belief that they can engage in this pathway (i.e., agency thinking; Snyder et al., 1991). However, students with high hope also tend to have flexibility in their pathways and are able to generate multiple pathways toward their goal. These students understand that obstacles and barriers may occur as they engage in goal-oriented behaviors. They are then able to appropriately assess and overcome barriers, disengage from their current pathway, and begin a new route to goal attainment (Cheavens & Ritschel, 2014; Snyder et al., 1991). Students with low hope may struggle to generate pathways toward goals or flexibility in pathways. For example, if a student with high hope has the goal of maintaining an A-average in their classes, but they are also a student athlete and practices begin to take place during their normal study times, they will have flexibility to adjust their study and practice schedule to continue working toward their goals.

Referring back to hope as it relates to student engagement, behavioral engagement is demonstrated via attendance, behavior incidents, class participation, and how well prepared a student is for school, whereas academic engagement is measured by a student's on-task behaviors, work completion, grades, and credits accrued (Reschly & Christenson, 2012). Students with high hope engage in these behaviors as they coincide with their pathway thinking to achieve educational goals, further demonstrating the relationship between Hope Theory and student engagement (Reschly & Christenson, 2012; Snyder, 2002).

Agency Thinking

Within Hope Theory, agency thinking is the motivation behind engaging in pathway-related behaviors, as well as the belief in oneself and one's ability to successfully engage in these behaviors in order to achieve goals (Snyder et al., 1998). This is perhaps the most important component of Hope Theory because if students do not believe they can engage in the pathway to their desired goals, they simply will not and thus will not achieve important goals. Agency thinking is related to student engagement because it reflects an individual's motivation to accomplish a goal. As mentioned previously, students who are highly engaged in school demonstrate motivation to do well. They engage in class, complete their work, are on-task, and place a high value on learning. They also demonstrate high self-efficacy in their ability to achieve their academic goals, aligning with the other facet of agency thinking (Reschly & Christenson, 2012; Snyder, 2002).

An example of agency thinking as it relates to student engagement is illustrated in a student with low levels of academically engaged behaviors, who still maintains the goal of passing their math class. Despite having this goal, lack of motivation and low self-efficacy are barriers to goal attainment and agency thinking (Snyder, 2002). If the student does not engage in agency thinking, they will not have the motivation, nor belief in their ability, to take the necessary steps (i.e., pathways), such as studying, getting a tutor, or paying attention in class, to attain the goal of passing math. These behaviors are also all related to academic engagement, and thus, this student's lack of agency thinking indicates both low levels of hope and low levels of academic engagement.

Measuring Student Hope

To date, few assessments have been developed and studied for the purpose of measuring hope in children and adolescents. The two most popular assessments are both trait-based measures of hope (Snyder et al., 1991, 1997). Specifically, the Child Hope Scale (CHS) was developed for use with children ages 7–14 years and the Hope Scale (HS) was created for use with adolescents who are of 15 years or older and adults. The HS is comprised of 12 items, 4 that aim to measure pathways (e.g., "I can think of many ways to get out of a jam"), 4 that aim to measure agency (e.g., "I energetically pursue my goals"), and 4 which are meant to serve as distractors (e.g., "I feel tired most of the time"), whereas the CHS consists of 3 items that aim to measure pathways (e.g., "When I have a problem, I can come up with a lot of ways to solve it") and 3 that aim to measure agency (e.g., "I am doing just as well as other kids my age"; Snyder et al., 1991, 1997). Each item on the HS is rated with a 4-point Likert scale, though more recent developments of the scale include an 8-point Likert scale to encourage diverse responses, with ratings ranging from "definitely false" to "definitely true." Each item on the CHS is rated with a 6-point Likert scale, with ratings ranging from "none of the time" to "all of the time." Scores are then calculated by adding up the numbers associated with the Likert-scale ratings and omitting the distractor items for the HS, yielding an overall score for hope. Agency and pathways scores can also be derived by only summing the Likert ratings for the items which correspond to each. Ultimately, higher scores on the HS or CHS indicate higher levels of hope in students (Snyder et al., 1991, 1997, 2002, 2003).

Both the CHS and HS have been studied across populations to validate their use as a measurement of hope among children and adolescents, respectively. Confirmatory factor analyses (CFA) have indicated that the agency and pathways items on the HS intercorrelate, and successfully confirmed these as the two components of hope measured by these tools (Babyak et al., 1993). They are dissimilar enough that the CFA reveals them as individual components of hope, but also intercorrelated to reveal that they are related. Reliability evidence has also been reported in past studies for the HS and CHS (Snyder et al., 1991, 1997, 2002, 2003). Test-retest reliability has been conducted in intervals of 3 to 10 weeks and yielded high correlations (alpha levels ranging from 0.85 for 3 weeks to 0.82 for 10 weeks; Snyder et al., 2003), indicating that hope, as a construct, may have temporal consistency. Additionally, in its applications across various populations, there was no indication that gender, race, age, or ethnicity impacted internal consistency of HS. It should be noted that across ethnic groups, it appears that individuals who identify as Caucasian tend to experience fewer obstacles (e.g., oppression and prejudice) across the lifespan and in goal attainment than individuals that identify with ethnic minority groups. However, these obstacles do not impact levels of hope for individuals belonging to ethnic minorities, and they sometimes even report higher scores on the HS than Caucasian individuals (McDermott et al., 1997; Snyder et al., 2003). Similar results were yielded in tests of reliability with the CHS (Snyder et al., 1997, 2003).

Validity evidence of the HS and CHS is also extensively available in the existing literature (Snyder et al., 1991, 1997, 2002, 2003). Past research indicates evidence of concurrent validity for the HS, with several other construct measures, including those which measure self-esteem, optimism, self-efficacy, problem-solving abilities, positive outcome expectancy, academic engagement, persistence, and student affect (Dixson, 2017; Feldman & Kubota, 2015; McDermott et al., 1997). The high level of agreement between the HS and other well-established measures indicates that hope, as a construct, may overlap with these other constructs. Similarly, evidence of concurrent validity between the CHS and measures of depression and academic outcomes exists (Dixson, 2017; Snyder et al., 2003). In addition, construct validity has been explored for both the HS and CHS, where individuals who demonstrated high levels of hope and individuals who demonstrated low levels of hope were asked to set a goal and work toward it. Those with higher levels of hope reported having more energy and demonstrated more pathways toward attaining their goals. While these differences could be explained by several factors (e.g., discrepancies in intelligence, access to resources, and individual differences in temperament), these findings suggest that the HS and CHS likely measure hope, which serves as evidence for construct validity (Snyder et al., 1991, 1997, 2002, 2003).

Along with the HS and CHS, Snyder and colleagues also developed another version of the Hope Scale, with the goal of measuring hope-related behaviors for a given moment in time. This scale was known as the State Hope Scale (SHS; Snyder et al., 1996). The SHS is a 6-item scale that, like the CHS and HS, contains subscale items for both agency thinking (i.e., "at this time, I am meeting the goals I have set for myself") and pathway thinking (i.e., "I can think of many ways to reach my current goals"). Three items comprise each subscale with the total, 6-item score indicating the level of hope an individual person is experiencing in that moment. Responses fall on a 1 to 8 Likert scale rating, ranging from "definitely false" to "definitely true." The main difference of the SHS is that the items all include words which stress the present beliefs and goals a person is working toward, indicating their current level of hope rather than their overall sense of hope. An individual's present level of hope can be different, depending upon the goals or activities that an individual is engaging in (Gallagher et al., 2019; Snyder et al., 1996).

Like the HS and the CHS, the SHS has also been tested for reliability and validity in past research. Internal reliability was demonstrated in four studies using the SHS on college students (alpha levels ranged from 0.79 to 0.95; Snyder et al., 1996). Test-retest reliability across 2 days to 4 weeks also yielded acceptable correlation coefficients (alpha levels ranging from 0.48 to 0.93; Snyder et al., 1996). In addition to reliability measures, there is also an extensive literature base which reveals the discriminant and convergent validity of the SHS with several other measures. For example, the SHS has been compared with measures of self-esteem, positive and negative affect, anxiety, depression, athletic performance, and depression and all were shown to be correlated or related to SHS measures of hope (Cheavens et al., 2006; Curry & Snyder, 2000; Curry et al., 1997; Gallagher et al., 2019; Ong et al., 2006; Snyder et al., 1996). The SHS has also been shown to reveal changes in an individual's hope over time (Cheavens et al., 2006). This means, it can be more sensitive to changes that occur with hope over time or through intervention. And finally, the SHS did not reveal differences in state hope across participant's gender or age (Martin-Krumm et al., 2015), meaning scores on it are not higher or lower as a result of any influence of these variables.

Finally, another method to measure hope in students is through the Gallup Student Poll (GSP; Lopez, 2009). The GSP is a school-wide screener or data collection tool with 20 survey items that measure students' levels of hope, engagement, and well-being. The aim of the GSP is to provide schools with data to identify which area they need to target to improve overall outcomes for students (Lopez, 2009; Lopez & Calderon, 2016). Hope, engagement, and well-being were chosen by Gallup researchers, because they have been linked to grades, academic achievement, retention rates, and employment in the future (Lopez, 2009). The poll was derived from sampling questions with over 70,000 students in grades 5 through 12. There are six items in the GSP which make up the subscale measuring hope. These include statements such as "I know I will graduate from high school" and "I can find lots of ways around a problem." Students rank their level of agreement with each on a Likert-scale, with five levels ranging from "strongly disagree" to "strongly agree." There are also seven items that measure engagement (i.e., "I feel safe in this school" and "My teachers make me feel my schoolwork is important"), and seven items that measure well-being (i.e., "Were you treated with respect all day yesterday?" and "Did you smile or laugh a lot yesterday?"). Internal consistency estimates for the hope items of the GSP are acceptable (alpha levels 0.76; Lopez & Calderon, 2011), but very little other data are available on how the scale has been validated empirically. Overall, it is a method of data collection to solve large-scale problems that schools may encounter with their students, as they relate to student hope, engagement, and well-being.

Educational Outcomes Associated with Hope

High levels of hope in students have been associated with several positive outcomes, particularly positive academic outcomes (for a summary see TeramotoPedrotti, 2018). For example, when controlling for cognitive ability in students, hope has been shown to have a positive correlation with academic achievement for elementary, secondary, and even postsecondary students (Curry et al., 1997; Snyder et al., 2002). Hope was also shown to be the greatest predictor of grade point average (GPA) in college students (Feldman & Kubota, 2015), indicating that hope may be a facilitator for achievement. In another study examining the relationship between hope and GPA, it was revealed that hope had a mediating relationship between student socioeconomic status (SES) and GPA. In initial models, Dixson and colleagues, 2017) found that SES predicted GPA, with students belonging to a lower SES group tending to have lower GPAs, whereas students belonging to higher SES groups tending to have higher GPAs. However, after adding hope to the model, the significant influence of SES was no longer observed. Instead, hope partially mediated the relationship between SES and GPA. Dixson and colleagues, (2017) concluded that "being from a low-SES background may in part have an effect on academic achievement through limiting the possibilities that the low-SES individuals perceive as reason-ably likely" (p. 512). That is, students who are from lower SES backgrounds may begin with lower levels of hope which contributes to lower achievement. It was noted that

increasing student hope among students who live in low-income households may bolster hope, and thus, result in improved achievement (Dixson and colleagues, 2017).

Students with higher levels of hope also tend to exhibit higher levels of motivation and a greater sense of belonging at school (Dixson, 2019; Dixson et al., 2017). Executive functioning has also been linked with hope in previous research. Some studies have indicated that students who experience difficulty in their executive functioning tend to have better academic outcomes when they feel a sense of belonging and hope related to their school and academic work (Dixson & Scalcucci, 2021; Kruger, 2011). Finally, higher levels of hope in students have also been associated with higher levels of academic self-efficacy and academic self-regulation (Dixson, 2020). Because the components of hope include agency and pathways, it makes sense that students with high hope, and therefore the capacity to develop plausible plans to attain goals and believe in themselves, tend to have high levels of self-efficacy and self-regulation, as these constructs appear to be related to hope.

Hope and Student Engagement

Past studies provide evidence of a relationship between hope and student engagement. Specifically, three connections between hope and engagement emerged from the extant literature. First, several studies suggest that a student's level of hope is associated with cognitive, behavioral, affective, and academic indicators of student engagement (e.g., Bryce et al., 2020; Dixson, 2019; Dixson & Stevens, 2018; Marques et al., 2017). Collectively, hope and student engagement have been associated with educational outcomes, including grade point average (GPA), grades, executive functioning skills, motivation, achievement, academic self-efficacy, and educational expectations (e.g., Dixson, 2019, 2020; Dixson & Scalcucci, 2021). Finally, some research has suggested that a mediation effect is present between hope, student engagement, and achievement. These studies, however, have not consistently identified the directionality of the relationship between these variables; that is, some research suggests hope mediates the relationship between student engagement and achievement while other findings indicate that student engagement mediates the relationship between hope and achievement (see Chen et al., 2020; Lin et al., 2021). An integrative synthesis of selected studies addressing these associations between hope and student engagement is outlined below. Table 1 summarizes the findings from the extant literature.

Is Hope Associated with Student Engagement?

According to the Gallup Student Poll which includes over 915,000 United States fifth through eighth grade respondents, students who endorsed high levels of engagement were 4.5 times more likely to endorse high levels of hope (Gallup, 2017). Supporting this notable finding, past research suggests that student hope may influence academic (i.e., GPA, task completion, and graduation rates; Marques et al., 2017; Rubens et al., 2020), cognitive (i.e., engaging in self-

Table 1 Summary of studies investigating hope and student engagement

Study	Sample characteristics	Findings
Bryce et al. (2019)	643 middle and high school students	Higher levels of cognitive (goal-oriented thinking) and behavioral (goal-oriented actions) hope were predictive of increased school engagement. High cognitive hope was also predictive of higher achievement and lower stress and anxiety.
Chen et al. (2020)	949 third—Chinese fifth grade students	Behavioral engagement mediated the relationship between hope and academic achievement.
Demirci (2020)	322 Turkish secondary students	Hope mediated the relationship between student engagement and well-being.
Dixson (2019)	447 high school students and 375 college students	Students were clustered into high, moderate, and low hope groups. Membership in the high hope cluster was associated with moderate to large effects on behavioral and affective engagement.
Dixson (2020)	447 high school students	Hope predicted academic achievement and self-efficacy after controlling for growth mindset and affective engagement.
Dixson &Scalcucci (2021)	216 high school students	Level of hope and school belongingness predicted executive functioning at school.
Dixson and Stevens (2018)	117 African American high school students	Higher levels of hope were related to greater school belonging, goal valuation, and academic motivation and self-regulation.
Lin et al. (2021)	562 Italian kindergarten-3rd grade students	Hope mediated the relationship between externalizing behaviors and student–teacher closeness, with higher hope facilitating more adaptive behaviors.
Marques (2016)	592 Portuguese sixth grade students	Students with lower levels of hope experienced diminished mental health outcomes and difficulties with school engagement.
Marques et al. (2017)	Meta-analysis of 45 studies ($N = 9250$)	12% of students with high hope demonstrated better academic outcomes than those who were low in hope with 14% having higher grades and 7% showing improved graduation rates.
Rubens et al. (2020)	41 Latinx middle school students	Agency thinking had a significant, positive effect on GPA, school support, and school engagement, while pathway thinking significantly predicted GPA and school engagement.
Tomas et al. (2020)	614 Dominican middle school students	Hope and self-efficacy were positively associated with higher behavioral, cognitive, and emotional engagement. Engagement mediated the relationship between hope and academic achievement.

regulatory behaviors and persistence toward goals; Bryce et al., 2020; Dixson & Stevens, 2018), behavioral (i.e., class participation and attendance; Dixson, 2019), and affective (i.e., belongingness, connectedness, and increased motivation; Dixson, 2019; Dixson & Stevens, 2018; Rubens et al., 2020) engagement. Study participants ranged in age from elementary school students through graduate students; most participants were in middle or high school. Across the studies reviewed, high hope was associated with higher levels of student engagement. That is, students who actively engaged in pathway and agency thinking were more likely to have higher grades and graduation rates, feel more connected to school, and engage in self-regulatory behaviors that facilitated goal achievement (see Dixson & Stevens, 2018; Marques et al., 2017).

For example, two studies were identified linking student hope to academic engagement (Marques et al., 2017; Rubens et al., 2020). Findings suggested that higher levels of hope were correlated with more positive indicators of academic engagement (e.g., higher GPA, greater work completion, and improved graduation rates). In a meta-analysis of 45 studies ($N = 9250$) examining the relationship between hope and academic outcomes (i.e., GPA, task performance, and graduation rates among elementary, secondary, undergraduate, and graduate students), findings indicated that hope had small to approaching moderate positive effects on academic indicators of engagement ($ES = 0.13–0.27$; Marques et al., 2017). Students classified as "high hope" demonstrated better indicators of academic engagement than their peers classified in the "low hope" group. Namely, when compared to students in the "low hope" group, 14% of the "high hope" group earned better grades, and 7% of the "high hope" group had higher graduation rates (Marques et al., 2017). Notably, these effects were strongest among elementary, middle, and high school students, suggesting that school level may moderate the relationship between hope and indicators of academic engagement. Similarly, Rubens et al. (2020) reported that agency and pathway

thinking were significant predictors of students' GPA and overall engagement among a sample of 41 low income, Latinx middle school students who attended a private parochial school. The relationship between agency thinking (i.e., the motivational component of hope theory) and GPA (i.e., an indicator of academic engagement) was influenced by the students' level of daytime sleepiness, with the association between hope and engagement being more robust when students demonstrated less daytime sleepiness. The authors · hypothesized that perhaps students who were more tired were less capable of engaging in agency thinking or perhaps those with greater agency were more likely to engage in healthy sleep hygiene habits (Rubens et al., 2020).

As with academic engagement, past studies have demonstrated a relationship between hope and indicators of cognitive engagement (see Bryce et al., 2020; Dixson & Stevens, 2018). Specifically, research suggests higher levels of hope are positively associated with higher cognitive engagement as measured by the Student Engagement Instrument ([SEI]; see Appleton et al., 2006 for information about the SEI) and more goal-directed thinking (Bryce et al., 2020), as well as higher levels of academic motivation and self-regulatory classroom behaviors (Dixson & Stevens, 2018) among middle and high school students. For instance, Bryce and colleagues (2020) found that students who demonstrated higher levels of cognitive (i.e., thoughts that facilitate goal attainment) and behavioral (i.e., actions that are needed to attain a goal) hope were more cognitively engaged than their peers who demonstrated lower levels of hope. Among the 634 middle school students included in their study, students with higher hope tended to show greater persistence toward their academic goals and endorsed feelingless stress and anxiety at school. Higher levels of hope were also associated with increased academic motivation and self-regulation among 117 African American high school students (Dixson & Stevens, 2018). Here, hope accounted for a significant amount of variance in academic motivation and self-regulation after controlling for sociodemographic variables and previous achievement, with the final model explaining 34.4% of the variation in these indicators of cognitive engagement. In particular, higher levels of agency thinking (i.e., the motivational component of Hope Theory) were associated with significantly higher student self-reported academic motivation and self-regulation. Hope was also a significant predictor of goal valuation, accounting for 41.9% of the variance in goal valuation among participants. Both agency and pathway thinking were unique predictors of students' goal valuation (Dixson & Stevens, 2018). These results may not be surprising given goal-directed thinking and behaviors are central to both cognitive engagement and hope. Therefore, a positive association between these constructs is to be expected.

Four studies were identified which show a significant, positive link between hope and affective engagement (i.e., belongingness, connectedness, and relationships with peers and adults). Findings from two studies indicate that agency thinking is a significant predictor of connectedness and belongingness among middle and high school students (Dixson & Stevens, 2018; Rubens et al., 2020), while one study suggested pathway thinking (i.e., goal-oriented thinking and behaviors) was positively associated with higher affective engagement in secondary students (Bryce et al., 2020). A final study investigated how the level of a student's hope (low, moderate, or high) predicted feelings of belongingness and connection at school (Dixson, 2019), finding a moderate to strong effect of high hope on affective engagement ($ES = 0.49; 1.06$) when compared to moderate and low hope membership, respectively. Dixon and Stevens (2018) examined the relationship between hope and several school-based outcomes, concluding that agency thinking explained 20.3% of the variance in belongingness in a sample of 117 African American high school students. Subsequent research supported this finding, with agency thinking being a significant predictor of school connectedness among 41 low income, Latinx middle school students ($B = 0.27$ [$SE = 0.10$], $p = <0.02$; Rubens et al., 2020).

While little evidence was identified linking hope with behavioral engagement, one study investigated this relationship with promising results. Dixson (2019) studied how low, moderate, and high hope related to behavioral engagement among high school and college students. Indicators of behavioral engagement included participation in class and regular class attendance. Membership in the high hope cluster was associated with moderate to large effects on behavioral engagement ($ES = 0.57; 1.23$) when compared to moderate and low hope membership, respectively. Students who demonstrated high hope were also significantly less likely to skip class and demonstrate academically disengaged behaviors during class.

Together, past studies provide emerging evidence that hope and academic, cognitive, behavioral, and affective engagement are related. The directionality of these relationships has not yet been established. Thus, we do not know whether higher hope contributes to greater student engagement or if student engagement contributes directly to a student's level of hope. This should be further investigated in future studies to better understand the relationship between cognitive, academic, behavioral, and affective engagement with hope.

Do Hope and Student Engagement Predict Educational Outcomes?

Past studies have also focused on the extent to which hope and student engagement predict educational outcomes (Dixson, 2020; Dixson & Scalcucci, 2021). Collectively, findings suggest that both hope and indicators of student affective engagement (i.e., belongingness) predicted positive educational outcomes and may be important targets for intervention. Dixson (2020) studied the extent to which a student's level of hope, growth mindset, and sense of belongingness (i.e., affective engagement) predicted several academic outcomes, including academic achievement, academic self-efficacy, and educational expectations. Interestingly, growth mindset and belongingness accounted for a significant amount of variance in academic self-efficacy among students after controlling for demographic variables, but they did not explain a significant amount of variance in academic achievement and educational expectations. Level of hope, however, explained a significant amount of variance in academic achievement (14.8%) and academic self-efficacy (15.9%) after controlling for demographic variables, growth mindset, and belongingness. Dixson argued that this may indicate that hope interventions are a better investment than interventions targeting mindsets or affective engagement.

Similarly, Dixson and Scalcucci (2021) examined whether hope and school belongingness and connectedness (i.e., affective engagement) predicted students' executive functioning skills in school (i.e., self-regulation, motivation, problem-solving, inhibition, and time management). They found that both hope and school belongingness positively predicted executive functioning in high school students. Pathway thinking (i.e., goal-directed thinking and planning) was a significant predictor of time management, problem-solving, and self-regulation, while belongingness significantly predicted self-regulation, motivation, and inhibition among students. Executive functioning skills are essential for positive behavioral and academic school outcomes (e.g., Masten et al., 2012; Samuels et al., 2016); therefore, the impact of hope and affective engagement on these skills has important implications for improving both behavioral and academic student outcomes.

Hope and Student Engagement: Which Is the Mediator?

Finally, previous research examining the relationship between hope and student engagement has attempted to explain the process through which hope and student engagement are related to educational outcomes (see Chen et al., 2020; Lin et al., 2021). Both studies proposed mediation models to explain variation in student outcomes; however, each utilized a different mediator (i.e., hope or student engagement) and outcome measure (i.e., student behavioral versus

achievement outcomes). First, Lin et al. (2021) studied the potential mediating effect of hope between student–teacher closeness (i.e., an indicator of affective engagement) and behavior incidents (e.g., office discipline referrals, detentions, and suspensions) among 562 Italian kindergarten through third grade students. They found that hope mediated the relationship between student–teacher closeness and externalizing behaviors (estimated indirect effect = −0.03[CI = −0.05 to −0.01]. Lin and colleagues write, "Hope is therefore likely to channel more adaptive and functional methods of dealing with situations by reducing distress" (p. 6). In this way, hope may mediate the relationship between student–teacher closeness and behavioral outcomes and may be an important factor to study to better understand how to reduce undesired behaviors in schools and increase positive affective engagement.

Conversely, Chen and colleagues (2020) investigated the relationship between hope and academic achievement (i.e., final exam scores on tests of Chinese, math and English) among a sample of 949 third through fifth grade Chinese students. They found that the relationship between hope and achievement was mediated by behavioral engagement (i.e., the student's level of participation or involvement in the classroom) as measured by the Student Engagement Questionnaire. Chen and colleagues reported, "...elementary school students with higher levels of hope reported more willingness to invest energy and behave appropriately in school activities, such as engaging with course materials, devoting time to school tasks, and asking questions, which in turn predicted successful academic outcomes" (p.7). They argued, however, that the relationship between hope, achievement, and engagement needs further investigation, highlighting that the three constructs are related and may have reciprocal influences on each other. Chen and colleagues noted students who demonstrate higher achievement probably exhibited greater effort toward earning higher grades, which in turn may have bolstered their level of hope. In this way, levels of engagement (i.e., academic engagement as measured by grades and behavioral engagement as measured by effort) may bolster hope which may influence achievement. Still, there exists the possibility that students who enter school with more hope may be more engaged which enables access to instruction and future achievement. The directionality of these relationships should be explored further in future research.

Fostering Student Hope

Given the positive association between hope and student educational outcomes as well as the evidence linking hope with student engagement, it is important to understand how high hope can be fostered among children and adolescents. This knowledge may inform intervention planning in schools, contributing to improved student outcomes. Below, three approaches to fostering hope identified from the extant literature are summarized. Notably, each is grounded in the principles of positive psychology (see Seligman, 2003).

Life Coaching Interventions

One approach to fostering hope that has been studied is solution-focused life coaching with a cognitive-behavioral orientation. Researchers implemented a life coaching intervention to examine the efficacy of this approach on fostering hope and cognitive hardiness (i.e., resilience; Green et al., 2007). The life coaching intervention was implemented with 56 female high school students with a mean age of 16 years. A randomized controlled experimental design was utilized, with participants randomly assigned to the life coaching group or control group. Participants assigned to the life coaching group met individually with a Teacher-Coach trained in life coaching psychology for ten sessions over two academic terms (Green et al., 2007).

Findings from this study indicated that the applied positive psychology approach of life coaching may be an effective intervention for the cultivation of hope and resilience with high school students. According to Green et al. (2007), participants reported significant reductions in levels of depression and increases in hope and cognitive

hardiness as measured by the Satisfaction with Life Scale (SWLS), the Positive and Negative Affect Scale (PANAS), and the Hope Scale (HS). This study provides emerging evidence that articulation of goals and interventions designed to cultivate agency with the assistance of a more skilled individual (i.e., Teacher-Coach) may lead to increased hope in students.

Single Session Hope Interventions

Another approach to bolstering hope was investigated by researchers who sought to understand how single session hope interventions might impact hopeful goal-directed thinking and grades among college students (Davidson et al., 2012; Feldman & Dreher, 2012). In these investigations, the researchers administered single session positive psychology interventions to increase student hope. Both studies focused on fostering students' strengths (e.g., sense of coherence, goal-directed thinking, and hope) and agency (i.e., self-efficacy) to achieve personal goals through the implementation of a brief intervention.

Feldman and Dreher (2012) investigated the implementation of a 90-minute, single session intervention implementing "hope visualization," where participants in the intervention condition received psychoeducation about the components of hope (i.e., goals, pathways, and agency; Feldman & Dreher, 2012). Participants included 96 college students who were assigned to either the hope intervention or one of two comparison/control conditions (i.e., progressive muscle relaxation or no intervention). Participant data regarding hope, goals, and sense of agency were assessed prior to intervention (pre-test), following intervention (post-test), and at a one-month follow-up interval. Findings suggested participants in the intervention group showed increased scores on measures of vocational calling, life purpose, and hope as measured by the Goal Specific Hope Scale, the Purpose in Life Test, and the Vocation Identity Questionnaire. Further, they observed that the hope intervention was found to increase goal progress in the college student participants when surveyed at the one-month follow-up.

Similarly, Davidson et al. (2012) investigated the impact of a brief workshop aimed at improving first year college students' hope, self-efficacy, and grades. Participants included 43 first year college students who were assigned to one of three intervention conditions, including two intervention conditions with varying components (i.e., Groups 1, 2, and 3). Participants in all three groups engaged in psychoeducation about the components of hope. Then, the Group 1 and 2 participants completed a goal-mapping activity aimed at increasing their pathway thinking. In addition to the goal-mapping activity, the Group 2 participants engaged in a "verbal persuasion" activity to bolster self-efficacy (i.e., agency thinking). Notably, Group 3 did not complete the goal-mapping or "verbal persuasion" activities; instead, Group 3 participants observed a lecture about sense of coherence and completed a cognitive-mapping worksheet focused on lessons they learned from the past and future expectations. Davidson et al. (2012) reported scores on the State Hope School and the New General Self-efficacy Scale increased across all study groups following intervention, with the increased self-efficacy scores being retained at a 1-month follow-up interval. Within each study group, results suggested that high hope and low hope subgroups emerged. Study results indicated that only members of the high hope subgroups demonstrated improved grades when compared to pre-intervention. Since there was no control group, Davidson et al. (2012) noted that the findings reported in this study may be due to maturation effects or other factors; they also were unable to distinguish variables that were correlated with membership in the high versus low hope subgroups, concluding that additional research should be conducted to identify these factors. Collectively, the findings from these studies provide limited emerging evidence that brief interventions, focused on psychoeducation and grounded in the principles of positive psychology, may increase student hope and positively impact outcomes such as

goal-directed behavior. These interventions should be a focus of future investigations.

Multiple Session Hope Interventions

Finally, other researchers have implemented manualized interventions over longer periods of time to understand how they enhance hope and correlated outcomes (Houston et al., 2017; Marques et al., 2011; Platt et al., 2020). Each multiple session hope intervention focused on improving participants' hopefulness, mental health, and well-being. Participants across the studies included middle school, high school, and undergraduate students who participated in three to eight intervention sessions. Overall, findings indicated that the multiple session hope interventions were associated with small, but significant, increases in student hope as measured by the Trait Hope Scale (Houston et al., 2017) and the Child Hope Scale (Marques et al., 2011; Platt et al., 2020).

For instance, Marques and colleagues conducted a study of the five-session *Building Hope for the Future* intervention, consisting of weekly 60-minute lessons focused on improving student hope, mental health, life satisfaction, and self-worth. Participants included 62 middle school students who were assigned to either a treatment or matched comparison group. Findings suggested that while a student's level of hope as measured by the Child Hope Scale was correlated with life satisfaction, mental health, self-worth, and academic achievement for both groups prior to intervention, only students in the intervention group benefited from increased levels of hope and subsequent improved outcomes overtime. Namely, intervention group participants "… showed a significant increase in hope from pre- to post-assessment $t(60) = -4.29, p < 0.001$ (two-tailed) and to 6-month $t(52) = -4.03, p = 0.001$ (two-tailed) and 18-month follow-up $t(49) = -3.38, p = 0.003$ (two-tailed). The comparison group showed no significant change over time" (Marques et al., 2011, p. 148). The increase in hope among those students who received the intervention was correlated with increase life satisfaction and self-worth that were not observed among comparison group peers. This study suggests that secondary students may benefit from multiple session hope interventions by experiencing not only greater levels of hope but also other positive psychological outcomes (e.g., improved self-worth).

Similar findings were reported by Platt and colleagues (2020) who examined the impact of the *Hummingbird Project*, an 8-session positive psychology intervention aimed at increasing high school students' hope, gratitude, happiness, well-being, mental health, grit, and resilience. Study participants included 90 British high school students whose baseline scores (i.e., pre-intervention) were compared to their post-intervention scores to assess changes in hope, academic tenacity, grit, and well-being. After participating in one orientation session, six psychoeducational intervention sessions, and a review session, participants reported small, but significant, increases in well-being as measured by the World Health Organization-Five Well-Being Index, academic tenacity as measured by the Bolton Uni-Stride Scale, and hope as measured by the Children's Hope Scale. Notably, the largest intervention effect was increased hope ($d = 0.24$).

Finally, in a randomized control trial study, researchers investigated the efficacy of a multiple session group intervention (Houston et al., 2017). The *Resilience and Coping Intervention,* which included three 45-minute sessions, was administered to the treatment group with the goal of bolstering hope, resilience, and coping skills and decreasing stress, anxiety, and depression. The intervention utilizes cognitive behavioral strategies to engage participants in group problem-solving, normalize stressful experiences, and teach healthy coping skills. Participants included 129 undergraduate students attending a large university in the United States. Results indicated that when compared to the control group, treatment group participants reported increases in feelings of hope, resilience, and coping skills and decreases in stress symptoms such as depression and anxiety. Each of these changes following intervention were small but significant with the

impact on hope showing a small effect (i.e., Cohen's $f^2 = 0.04$). Taken together, the results of these studies provide evidence that multiple session interventions grounded in positive psychology and using cognitive behavioral approaches may have small, yet positive, impacts on individual's experience of hope.

Directions for Future Research

While there are clear overlaps between the constructs of student engagement and hope (e.g., importance of goal-setting and engaging in behaviors that facilitate goal attainment), only emerging empirical support exists for the relationship between these two important facilitators of positive educational outcomes, and the directionality of their relationship remains unknown. There is strong evidence that both high hope and higher levels of engagement serve as enablers of academic achievement, educational attainment, and positive school-based emotional and behavioral outcomes (see Lei et al., 2018; O'Farrell & Morrison, 2003; TeramotoPedrotti, 2018). Perhaps, like motivation and self-efficacy, hope should be considered an academic enabler (DiPerna, 2006) or "psychological capital" (Luthans et al., 2007) that facilitates learning, student engagement, and subsequent positive student outcomes (e.g., life satisfaction). Future studies should explicitly explore the relationship between hope, student engagement, and student educational outcomes conceptualized broadly.

Specifically, researchers should investigate the extent to which hope mediates or moderates the relationship between student engagement and educational outcomes such as school completion, credit accrual, attendance, achievement, and behavior. Understanding the role of a student's level of hope may serve as another mechanism for increasing engagement which is positively correlated with successful educational outcomes (Lei et al., 2018). An important area of investigation would be to understand whether a student's level of hope mediates the relationship between student engagement and the proximal and distal outcomes articulated by Reschly and Christenson

(2012) or whether student engagement mediates the relationship between hope and these outcomes. An investigation fitting data to both mediation models and determining which best fits the data may help inform whether hope or student engagement has the most significant impact on student outcomes. It is essential to understand the directionality and magnitude of these relationships as this knowledge will inform intervention selection, planning, and implementation and lead to the more efficient use of resources to promote positive educational outcomes. Further, researchers may consider whether hope predicts engagement or vice versa whether engagement predicts hope. Given the alignment of cognitive, behavioral, affective, and academic engagement with hope, it would also be important to determine if there are different magnitudes of associations between the domains of engagement and student hope to determine how to intervene with students low in either competency.

In addition to investigating the relationship between student engagement and hope, future research should focus on individual differences in hope and how these differences impact student engagement and educational outcomes. Scholars should conduct research that illuminates for whom and under what conditions experiencing high hope is associated with higher levels of engagement and better school and life outcomes. Studies utilizing latent class analysis, for example, may help educators understand how students experiencing low, moderate, and high hope function differently at school and what conditions foster increased student engagement and more positive outcomes for students in each group. These types of group analyses, as well as qualitative research and single-case design studies, may help educators create school climates and programs that more effectively increase student hope and other correlated positive outcomes. Findings from these studies may also inform future research regarding the extent to which interventions and supports aimed at fostering student hope impact students' engagement and educational outcomes.

A third area for further investigation relates to unpacking the overlapping constructs of hope, student engagement, and motivation (among other related constructs; e.g., goal attainment theory and self-efficacy). Specifically, is each of these constructs unique? Are they interrelated or are they confounded? When we measure the impact of motivation, hope, or student engagement on educational outcomes, are we in actuality measuring different influences or overlapping mechanisms of success? Studies should focus on how these constructs are unique contributors to educational outcomes as well as areas of overlap, helping to inform greater clarity in our operationalization of terms and variables used in educational research.

Finally, perhaps the most practically significant future research should focus on the impact of interventions and supports that foster high hope in students. Given the strong association between high hope and more positive educational outcomes, including a positive association with student engagement (e.g., Bryce et al., 2020; Dixson & Stevens, 2018; Marques et al., 2017), it is prudent to understand how increasing student levels of hope may increase positive outcomes, such as graduation rates, work completion, academic achievement, and active participation in learning. Researchers should examine whether existing interventions that target setting and working toward realistic goals and bolstering self-efficacy and student agency influence hope, student engagement, and academic outcomes. Unveiling strategies and multi-tiered supports for fostering hope among students may have a significant effect on student outcomes.

References

Appleton, J. J., Christenson, S. L., Kim, D., & Reschly, A. L. (2006). Measuring cognitive and psychological engagement: Validation of the student engagement instrument. *Journal of School Psychology, 44*, 427–455. https://doi.org/10.1016/j.jsp.2006.04.002

Appleton, J. J., Christenson, S. L., & Furlong, M. J. (2008). Student engagement with school: Critical, conceptual and methodological issues of the construct. *Psychology in the Schools, 45*(5), 369–386. https://doi.org/10.1002/pits.20303

Babyak, M. A., Snyder, C. R., & Yoshinobu, L. (1993). Psychometric properties of the Hope Scale: A confirmatory factor analysis. *Journal of Research in Personality, 27*(2), 154–169. https://doi.org/10.1006/jrpe.1993.1011

Bryce, C. I., Alexander, B. L., Fraser, A. M., & Fabes, R. A. (2020). Dimensions of hope in adolescence:

Relations to academic functioning and well-being. *Psychology in the Schools, 57*(2), 171–190.

Cheavens, J. S., & Ritschel, L. A. (2014). Hope theory. In M. M. Tugade, M. N. Shiota, & L. D. Kirby (Eds.), *Handbook of positive emotions* (pp. 396–410). The Guilford Press.

Cheavens, J. S., Feldman, D. B., Gum, A., Michael, S. T., & Snyder, C. R. (2006). Hope therapy in a community sample: A pilot investigation. *Social Indicators Research, 77*, 61–78. https://doi.org/10.1007/s11205-005-5553-0

Chen, J., Huebner, E. S., & Tian, L. (2020). Longitudinal relations between hope and academic achievement in elementary school students: Behavioral engagement as a mediator. *Learning and Individual Differences, 78*, 101824.

Christenson, S. L., Reschly, A. L., Appleton, J. J., Berman-Young, S., Spanjers, D. M., & Varro, P. (2008). Best practices in fostering student engagement. In A. Thomas & J. Grimes (Eds.), *Best practices in school psychology V* (pp. 1099–1119). National Association of School Psychologists.

Crosnoe, R. (2002). High school curriculum track and adolescent association with delinquent friends. *Journal of Adolescent Research, 17*, 144–168. https://doi.org/10.1177/0743558402172003

Curry, L. A., & Snyder, C. R. (2000). Hope takes the field: Mind matters in athletic performances. In C. R. Snyder (Ed.), *Handbook of hope: Theory, measures, and applications* (pp. 243–259). Academic Press. http://dx.doi.org.ezproxy.mnsu.edu/10.1016/B978-012654050-5/50015-4

Curry, L. A., Snyder, C. R., Cook, D. L., Ruby, B. C., & Rehm, M. (1997). Role of hope in academic and sport achievement. *Journal of Personality and Social Psychology, 73*(6), 1257–1267. https://doi.org/10.1037/0022-3514.73.6.1257

Davidson, O. B., Feldman, D. B., & Margalit, M. (2012). A focused intervention for 1st-year college students: Promoting hope, sense of coherence, and self-efficacy. *The Journal of Psychology, 146*, 333–352. https://doi.org/10.1080/00223980.2011.634862

Demirci, İ. (2020). School engagement and well-being in adolescents: Mediating roles of hope and social competence. *Child Indicators Research, 13*(5), 1573–1595.

DiPerna, J. C. (2006). Academic enablers and student achievement: Implications for assessment and intervention services in the schools. *Psychology in the Schools, 43*(1), 7–17.

Dixson, D. D. (2017). Hope across achievement: Examining psychometric properties of the Children's Hope Scale across the range of achievement. *SAGE Open, 7*(3). https://doi.org/10.1177/2158244017717304

Dixson, D. D. (2019). Hope into action: How clusters of hope relate to success-oriented behavior in school. *Psychology in the Schools, 56*(9), 1493–1511. https://doi.org/10.1002/pits.22299

Dixson, D. D. (2020). How hope measures up: Hope predicts school variables beyond growth mindset and school belonging. *Current Psychology.* https://doi.org/10.1007/s12144-020-00975-y

Dixson, D. D., & Scalcucci, S. G. (2021). Psychosocial perceptions and executive functioning: Hope and school belonging predict students' executive functioning. *Psychology in the Schools, 58*(5), 853–872. https://doi.org/10.1002/pits.22475

Dixson, D. D., & Stevens, D. (2018). A potential avenue for academic success: Hope predicts an achievement-oriented psychosocial profile in African American adolescents. *Journal of Black Psychology, 44*(6), 532–561. https://doi.org/10.1177/0095798418805644

Dixson, D. D., Worrell, F. C., & Mello, Z. (2017). Profiles of hope: How clusters of hope relate to school variables. *Learning and Individual Differences, 59*, 55–64. https://doi.org/10.1016/j.lindif.2017.08.011

Dixson, D. D., Keltner, D., Worrell, F. C., & Mello, Z. (2018). The magic of hope: Hope mediates the relationship between socioeconomic status and academic achievement. *The Journal of Educational Research, 111*(4), 507–515. https://doi.org/10.1080/00220671.2017.1302915

Feldman, D. B., & Dreher, D. E. (2012). Can hope be changed in 90 minutes? Testing the efficacy of a single-session goal-pursuit intervention for college students. *Journal of Happiness Studies: An Interdisciplinary Forum on Subjective Well-Being, 13*(4), 745–759. https://doi.org/10.1007/s10902-011-9292-4

Feldman, D. B., & Kubota, M. (2015). Hope, self-efficacy, optimism, and academic achievement: Distinguishing constructs and levels of specificity in predicting college grade-point average. *Learning and Individual Differences, 37*, 210–216. https://doi.org/10.1016/j.lindif.2014.11.022

Finn, J. D., & Zimmer, K. S. (2012). Student engagement: What is it? Why does it matter?. In Handbook of research on student engagement (pp. 97-131). Springer, Boston, MA.

Gallagher, M. W., Long, L. J., Richardson, A., D'Souza, J., Boswell, J. F., Farchione, T. J., & Barlow, D. H. (2019). Examining hope as a transdiagnostic mechanism of change across anxiety disorders and CBT treatment protocols. *Behavior Therapy, 51*(1), 190–202. https://doi.org/10.1016/j.beth.2019.06.001

Gallup. (2017). 2016 GallupStudent poll: A snapshot of results and findings. Retrieved from: https://www.gallup.com/topic/gallup_student_poll.aspx

Green, S., Grant, A., & Rynsaardt, J. (2007). Evidence-based life coaching for senior high school students: Building hardiness and hope. *International Coaching Psychology Review, 2*(1), 24–32.

Houston, J. B., First, J., Spialek, M. L., Sorenson, M. E., Mills-Sandoval, T., Lockett, M., First, N. L., Nitiéma, P., Allen, S. F., & Pfefferbaum, B. (2017). Randomized controlled trial of the Resilience and Coping Intervention (RCI) with undergraduate university students. *Journal of American College Health, 65*, 1–9. https://doi.org/10.1080/07448481.2016.1227826

Kruger, G. H. J. (2011). Executive functioning and positive psychological characteristics: A replication and extension. *Psychological Reports, 108*(2), 477–486. https://doi.org/10.2466/04.09.21.PR0.108.2.477-486

Lei, H., Cui, Y., & Zhou, W. (2018). Relationships between student engagement and academic achievement: A meta-analysis. *Social Behavior and Personality: An International Journal, 46*(3), 517–528.

Lin, S., Fabris, M. A., & Longobardi, C. (2021). Closeness in student–teacher relationships and students' psychological well-being: The mediating role of hope. *Journal of Emotional and Behavioral Disorders.* https://doi.org/10.1177/10634266211013756

Lopez, S. J. (2009). Gallup student poll national report. America's Promise Alliance. https://www.americaspromise.org/sites/default/files/d8/legacy/bodyfiles/GSP%20National%20Report.pdf

Lopez, S. J., & Calderon, V. (2011). Gallup student poll: measuring and promoting what is right with students. Applied positive psychology: Improving everyday life, schools, work, health, and society, 117–134.

Lopez, S. J., & Calderon, V. J. (2016). Students have the will to succeed, but many lack the ways. Gallup News Brief. https://news.gallup.com/opinion/gallup/189947/students-succeed-lack-ways.aspx

Luthans, F., Avolio, B. J., Avey, J. B., & Norman, S. M. (2007). Positive psychological capital: Measurement and relationship with performance and satisfaction. *Personnel Psychology, 60,* 541–572.

Marques, S. C., Lopez, S. J., & Pais-Ribeiro, J. L. (2011). "Building hope for the future": A program to foster strengths in middle-school students. *Journal of Happiness Studies, 12,* 139–152. https://doi.org/10.1007/s10902-009-9180-3

Marques, S. C. (2016). Psychological strengths in childhood as predictors of longitudinal outcomes. *School Mental Health, 8*(3), 377–385.

Marques, S. C., Gallagher, M. W., & Lopez, S. J. (2017). Hope and academic-related outcomes: A meta-analysis. *School Mental Health, 9,* 250–262. https://doi.org/10.1007/s12310-017-9212-9

Martin-Krumm, C., Kern, L., Fontayne, P., Romo, L., Boudoukha, A. H., & Boniwell, I. (2015). French adaptation of the Orientation to Happiness scale and its relationship to quality of life in French students. *Social Indicators Research, 124*(1), 259–281. https://doi.org/10.1007/s11205-014-0774-8

Masten, A. S., Herbers, J. E., Desjardins, C. D., Cutuli, J. J., McCormick, C. M., Sapienza, J. K., ... & Zelazo, P. D. (2012). Executive function skills and school success in young children experiencing homelessness. *Educational Researcher, 41*(9), 375–384.

McDermott, D., Hastings, S., Gariglietti, K., Callahan, B., Gingerich, K., & Diamond, K. (1997). A cross-cultural investigation of hope in children and adolescents. [S.l.]: Distributed by ERIC Clearinghouse. https://eric.ed.gov/?id=ED412450

O'Farrell, S. L., & Morrison, G. M. (2003). A factor analysis exploring school bonding and related constructs among upper elementary students. *The California School Psychologist, 8,* 53–72. https://doi.org/10.1007/BF03340896

Ong, A. D., Bergeman, C. S., Bisconti, T. L., & Wallace, K. A. (2006). Psychological resilience, positive emotions, and successful adaptation to stress in later life. *Journal of Personality and Social Psychology, 91*(4), 730–749. https://doi.org/10.1037/0022-3514.91.4.730

Platt, I. A., Kannangara, C., Tytherleigh, M., & Carson, J. (2020). The hummingbird project: a positive psychology intervention for secondary school students. *Frontiers in Psychology, 11,* 2012.

Reschly, A. L., & Christenson, S. L. (2012). Jingle, jangle, and conceptual haziness: Evolution and future directions of the engagement construct. In S. L. Christenson, A. L. Reschly, & C. Wylie (Eds.), *Handbook of research on student engagement* (pp. 3–19). Springer. https://doi.org/10.1007/978-1-4614-2018-7_1

Rubens, S. L., Feldman, D. B., Soliemannjad, R. R., Sung, A., & Gudiño, O. G. (2020). Hope, daytime sleepiness, and academic outcomes in low-income, Latinx youth. *Child & Youth Care Forum, 49,* 743–757. https://doi.org/10.1007/s10566-020-09553-6

Samuels, W. E., Tournaki, N., Blackman, S., & Zilinski, C. (2016). Executive functioning predicts academic achievement in middle school: A four-year longitudinal study. *The Journal of Educational Research, 109*(5), 478–490.

Seligman, M. E. P. (2003). Positive psychology: Fundamental assumptions. *Psychologist, 126,* 127.

Snyder, C. R. (1994). *The psychology of hope: You can get there from here.* Free Press.

Snyder, C. R. (1995). Conceptualizing, measuring and nurturing hope. *Journal of Counseling and Development, 73*(3), 355–360. https://doi.org/10.1002/j.1556-6676.1995.tb01764.x

Snyder, C. R. (2002). Hope theory: Rainbows in the mind. *Psychological Inquiry, 13*(4), 249–275. https://doi-org.ezproxy.mnsu.edu/10.1207/S15327965PLI1304_01

Snyder, C. R., Harris, C., Anderson, J. R., Holleran, S. A., Irving, L. M., Sigmon, S. T., Yoshinobu, L., Gibb, J., Langelle, C., & Harney, P. (1991). The will and the ways: Development and validation of an individual-differences measure of hope. *Journal of Personality and Social Psychology, 60,* 570–585. https://doi-org.ezproxy.mnsu.edu/10.1037/0022-3514.60.4.570

Snyder, C. R., Sympson, S. C., Ybasco, F. C., Borders, T. F., Babyak, M. A., & Higgins, R. L. (1996). Development and validation of the State Hope Scale. *Journal of Personality and Social Psychology, 70*(2), 321–335. https://doi.org/10.1037/0022-3514.70.2.321

Snyder, C. R., Hoza, B., Pelham, W. E., Rapoff, M., Ware, L., Danovsky, M., Highberger, L., Ribinstein, H., & Stahl, K. J. (1997). The development and validation of the children's hope scale. *Journal of Pediatric Psychology, 22,* 399–421. https://doi-org.ezproxy.mnsu.edu/10.1093/jpepsy/22.3.399

Snyder, C. R., Lapointe, A. B., Crowson, J. J., & Early, S. (1998). Preferences of high- and low-hope people for self-referential input. *Cognition and Emotion,*

12, 807–823. http://dx.doi.org.ezproxy.mnsu.edu/10.1080/026999398379448

Snyder, C. R., Michael, S. T., & Cheavens, J. S. (1999). Hope as a psychotherapeutic foundation of common factors, placebos, and expectancies. In M. A. Hubble, B. L. Duncan, & S. D. Miller (Eds.), *The heart and soul of change: What works in therapy* (pp. 179–200). American Psychological Association. https://doi.org/10.1037/11132-005

Snyder, C. R., Shorey, H. S., Cheavens, J., Pulvers, K. M., Adams, V. H., III, & Wiklund, C. (2002). Hope and academic success in college. *Journal of Educational Psychology, 94*(4), 820–826. https://doi.org/10.1037/0022-0663.94.4.820

Snyder, C. R., Lopez, S. J., Shorey, H. S., Rand, K. L., & Feldman, D. B. (2003). Hope theory, measurements, and applications to school psychology. *School Psychology Quarterly, 18*(2), 122–139. https://doi.org/10.1521/scpq.18.2.122.21854

Snyder, C. R., Rand, K. L., & Sigmon, D. R. (2018). Hope theory: A member of the positive psychology family. In M. W. Gallagher & S. J. Lopez (Eds.), *The Oxford handbook of hope* (pp. 27–43). Oxford University Press.

TeramotoPedrotti, J. (2018). The will and the ways in school: Hope as a factor in academic success. In M. W. Gallagher & S. J. Lopez (Eds.), *The Oxford handbook of hope* (pp. 27–43). Oxford University Press.

Tomas, J. M., Gutiérrez, M., Georgieva, S., & Hernández, M. (2020). The effects of self-efficacy, hope, and engagement on the academic achievement of secondary education in the Dominican Republic. *Psychology in the Schools, 57*(2), 191–203.

Wang, M., & Fredericks, J. A. (2014). The reciprocal links between school engagement, youth problem behaviors, and school dropout during adolescence. *Child Development, 85*(2), 722–737. https://doi.org/10.1111/cdev.12138

Wurster, K. G., Kivlighan, D. M., III, & Foley-Nicpon, M. (2021). Does person-group fit matter? A further examination of hope and belongingness in academic enhancement groups. *Journal of Counseling Psychology, 68*(1), 67–76. https://doi.org/10.1037/cou0000437

Part II

Student Engagement: Positive Development and Outcomes

Relationships Between Student Engagement and Mental Health as Conceptualized from a Dual-Factor Model

Shannon M. Suldo and Janise Parker

Abstract

This chapter reviews empirical links between youth mental health and behavioral, emotional/affective, cognitive engagement among school-aged youths. Youth mental health is defined in a dual-factor model, as comprised of positive indicators of well-being (e.g., subjective well-being) and negative indicators of ill-being (e.g., internalizing and externalizing symptoms of mental health problems). After establishing the associations between student engagement and mental health as indicated from observational studies, we describe how interventions that target engagement have impacted youth mental health, and vice versa how addressing mental health problems that pose barriers to student engagement actually impact aspects of engagement. The chapter concludes with a discussion of considerations for marginalized or underrepresented groups of students, implications for practice, and directions for future research.

S. M. Suldo (✉)
Department of Educational and Psychological Studies, University of South Florida, Tampa, FL, USA
e-mail: suldo@usf.edu

J. Parker
School of Education, William & Mary, Williamsburg, VA, USA
e-mail: jparker@wm.edu

Defining Student Engagement and Mental Health

Within a larger text that examines how student engagement drives positive development for youths, in this chapter we focus on positive *emotional* development (i.e., emotional well-being) with the view that optimal mental *health* reflects a complete state of being. This view is aligned with a dual-factor model of mental health, in which a complete state of mental health is defined as (a) minimal symptoms of internalizing and externalizing forms of psychopathology (the ill-being factor), coupled with (b) the presence of positive factors such as high subjective well-being (the well-being factor; Suldo & Doll, 2021; Suldo & Shaffer, 2008). Subjective well-being is the construct scholars have used most commonly to operationalize happiness, and includes both cognitive and affective dimensions. A youth with high subjective well-being judges their life to be going well on the whole (i.e., high global life satisfaction) and on a daily basis experiences positive feelings more frequently than negative feelings. In contrast to traditional psychological research and practice that focuses on emotional and behavioral problems (i.e., the ill-being factor), a modern positive psychology lens attends to facilitating well-being beyond the mere absence of psychopathology, as reflected in high levels of indicators of eudemonic and hedonic well-being (e.g., subjective well-being).

Leaders within positive psychology purport that *flourishing* is predicted by Positive emotions, Engagement, Relationships, Meaning, and Accomplishment (PERMA; Morrish et al., 2018; Seligman, 2011). The first element—positive emotions—includes pleasant feelings such as pride, cheer, joy, enthusiasm—the positive affective dimension of subjective well-being. Kern et al. (2016) advanced the EPOCH Measure of Adolescent Well-Being to measure characteristics in youth that are believed to influence the PERMA domains later in life, specifically: Engagement, Perseverance, Optimism, Connectedness, and Happiness. In this chapter, we examine associations between student engagement and a flourishing emotional state, as conceptualized within a PERMA framework and its variants such as EPOCH. Of note, the term "engagement" within PERMA refers to complete absorption in one's activity/task—sometimes called a "flow" state (i.e., Csikszentmihalyi, 2014) where time passes differently due to focus and immersion in the task at hand. There is some overlap between engagement as conceptualized in PERMA and cognitive student engagement (as defined in the next paragraph). For instance, a youth who is totally focused on an academic task that is challenging yet doable may demonstrate both the engagement element of psychological flourishing and cognitive engagement at school. Regardless, within the positive psychology literature, use of the term engagement is generally context-free; a youth can be engaged in leisure pursuits, in community activities, in sports, at school, or in other settings.

The construct of *student engagement* pertains to "how students think, act, and feel in school" and is often conceptualized as having affective, behavioral, and cognitive dimensions (Fredricks et al., 2019, p. 1). These dimensions are interrelated but cover distinct aspects of student engagement. Affective engagement includes students' emotional reactions toward school and class, as well as their feelings of belonging to school and connectedness to adults and peers within. Behavioral engagement includes students' school attendance, conduct in class, and participation in school-based activities outside of class time such

as involvement in extracurricular activities. Cognitive engagement refers to students' deliberate investment in learning, including beliefs about the value of education, as well as use of self-regulated learning and metacognitive strategies to facilitate learning (Fredricks et al., 2019). Of note, researchers sometimes use terms such as *school engagement* and, less commonly, *study engagement* (i.e., Kwok & Fang, 2021; Ouweneel et al., 2011), but a review of items used to assess those constructs reveals conceptual alignment with one or more dimensions of student engagement as defined earlier in this paragraph. For instance, publications that reference *study engagement* provide an operational definition analogous to cognitive engagement (i.e., student experiences of vigor, dedication, and absorption in relation to academic tasks). In this chapter, we conceptualize student engagement as comprised of the three aforementioned subtypes—affective, behavioral, and cognitive engagement—and review studies that examined one or more of these subtypes of student engagement even if it was not termed such in the publication.

With these definitions of mental health and student engagement in mind, in the next sections we examine links between the two constructs as given by theory and then examined in empirical research. After summarizing the associations between student engagement and mental health as indicated from observational studies, we describe how interventions that target engagement have impacted youth mental health, and vice versa how addressing mental health problems that pose barriers to student engagement actually impact aspects of engagement. We then conclude with a summary of implications for future research.

Theoretical Associations Between Mental Health and Student Engagement

A convincing part of the argument for locating, expanding, and integrating mental health services in schools rests on the salience of youth mental health to academic success. Adelman and Taylor

(2010) delineated numerous social, economic, and health problems, including forms of psychopathology that if left unaddressed pose barriers to learning thereby making prevention and treatment of emotional and behavioral problems integral considerations in school reform efforts. By definition, youths who meet criteria for various mental health problems experience cognitive and behavioral symptoms that reduce opportunities for student engagement. Primary features of anxiety and depression such as frequent worries, lethargy, social avoidance, and somatic symptoms logically translate to increased likelihood of absences from school, challenges concentrating on academic material, and withdrawal from potential social supports. With respect to common symptoms of externalizing disorders, noncompliance, impulsivity, and affiliation with deviant peers translate to teacher and peer rejection, deficits in organizational and study skills, and truancy. Central features of thought disorders such as paranoia, hallucinations and delusions, and sleep disruptions logically pose barriers to full cognitive, behavioral, and affective engagement in and out of the classroom during episodes of psychosis. Taken together, children and adolescents without clinically impairing levels of emotional or behavioral symptoms are simply more likely to enter the classroom able to take advantage of opportunity for full student engagement, whereas students with and without diagnosed forms of psychopathology must mitigate an additional set of barriers to learning.

Is reducing and managing the aforementioned forms of *negative* emotionality sufficient to enable student engagement, or are students' positive emotions important in and of themselves? Fredrickson's (2001) Broaden-and-Build theory would suggest that positive emotions are highly salient to student learning and engagement, and essential to optimal functioning across contexts as well (see Pekrun & Linnenbrink-Garcia, chapter "Academic Emotions and Student Engagement", this volume). In particular, positive emotions create an upward spiral, marked *broadening* of one's cognitive capacity and behavioral flexibility (i.e., momentary thought–action repertoires) that, over time, allows one to

build lasting personal social, psychological, and physical resources (Fredrickson, 2001). Extensive empirical support for this "broaden-and-build" theory shows that positive emotions open up our minds to creative and flexible thinking, broaden the scope of our attentional field, and create new opportunities for positive experiences. Positive emotions foster personal knowledge and social connections, whereas negative emotions lead to impulsive, rigid, and narrow thoughts and behavioral responses. In a test of this theory to the educational context, Stiglbauer et al. (2013) found strong support for reciprocal relationships between high school students' positive affect and schooling experiences when both constructs were assessed five times during one school year. In particular, students who experienced frequent positive affect also reported the highest levels of relatedness, competency, and autonomy at school concurrently and later in the year, and such positive school experiences also predicted increases in affective well-being, illustrating the upward spiral at the core of the broaden-and-build theory.

The personal, social, and cognitive resources built by positive emotions can lead to student engagement and achievement. Case in point, Reschly et al. (2008) examined 7th–10th grade students' self-reports of frequency of emotional experiences at school, coping responses, and cognitive and affective engagement. They found that higher positive affect predicted greater use of adaptive coping strategies (a psychological and social resource), specifically responding to stress by using problem-solving strategies and/or seeking support. In contrast, frequency of negative affect at school was unrelated to coping. Such ties between positive emotional experiences and broadened psychological and social resources (i.e., problem-solving and turning to others, respectively) are in line with the broaden-and-build theory with respect to the adaptive functions served by positive emotions which, in turn, lead to better outcomes such as cognitive and affective engagement (Reschly et al., 2008).

The heightened academic success engendered by engagement likely strengthens opportunities for elements of PERMA such as accomplishment and relationships, which co-occur with and beget additional positive affect. Such pathways are illustrated in studies in which more frequent positive emotions in the academic context predicted higher levels of *psychological capital* (i.e., academic self-efficacy, optimism, hope, and resilience) among students in high school (Carmona–Halty et al., 2019) and college (Ouweneel et al., 2011), with psychological capital in turn predicting greater cognitive engagement (i.e., vigor, dedication, and absorption during academic tasks; Ouweneel et al., 2011) and better grades in math and language (Carmona–Halty et al., 2019). Further, longitudinal studies with adolescents support the existence of positive reciprocal relations between subjective well-being and student engagement (Datu & King, 2018) and achievement (e.g., 9-week grade point average; Ng et al., 2015). Recent longitudinal research with elementary school age children (grades 4–6; *M* age 10 years) examined *strengths use* as a personal resource that may mediate associations between positive emotions and cognitive engagement (i.e., perserverance and motivation in academic tasks; Kwok & Fang, 2021). Strengths use includes the identification and deployment of one's strengths, which are the "characteristics that allow a person to perform well or at their personal best" (p. 1036). Children who experienced more frequent positive emotions at the start of the study were more likely to use their strengths concurrently and later; use of strengths, in turn, predicted higher levels of cognitive engagement across time. Kwok and Fang (2021) concluded that "positive emotions may trigger the use of strengths both in school and in daily life, a kind of 'personal resource' in general" which makes students more likely to experience greater initiative, confidence, positive feedback, and mastery, which engender student engagement (p. 1047). Taken together, findings from a growing number of studies with children and adolescents indicate that attending to negative emotionality is important but insufficient, as the presence of positive emotions is critical to building resources that produce optimal outcomes.

Empirical Relationships Between Student Engagement and Youth Mental Health

Indicators of mental health (both psychopathology and subjective well-being) have been found to be associated with the various dimensions of student engagement, particularly among adolescent students. Adolescents are an appropriate focal population given the decline in student engagement that often characterizes transitions to middle and high school (Marks, 2000), and the increase in mental health problems (rising rates of mental illness; declines in average levels of subjective well-being; Casas & Gonzalez-Carrasco, 2019; Merikangas et al., 2010) seen during the adolescent years. In this section we highlight evidence of empirical relationships between mental health and engagement from observational studies assessing positive and negative indicators of youth mental health.

Subjective Well-Being

Findings from correlational studies have provided support for connections between each affective and cognitive component of subjective well-being and co-occurring student engagement. Even in regression analyses that control for the shared variance between affect and life satisfaction, Heffner and Antaramian (2016) found that higher levels of positive affect and life satisfaction in middle school students significantly predicted higher levels of cognitive engagement (academic aspirations), behavioral engagement (on-task behavior in class), and affective engagement (closeness to teachers), whereas higher levels of negative affect uniquely predicted lower affective and behavioral engagement.

Positive affect is one of multiple elements in the expanded PERMA/EPOCH framework reflecting flourishing mental health. Kern et al.'s (2016) examination of EPOCH elements in relation to youth outcomes found significant, positive correlations between participant scores on each EPOCH dimension and indicators of student engagement. The magnitude of the bivariate correlations was small for teacher-rated behavioral engagement and moderate-to-large for student-reported affective engagement. Specifically, higher levels of engagement (i.e., flow—absorption in activity, losing track of time), perseverance (i.e., task completion, determination), optimism (i.e., positive beliefs about the future), connectedness (i.e., perceived social support, caring relationships), and happiness (i.e., feeling cheerful, loving life, having fun), co-occurred with greater affective engagement (i.e., feeling excited and interest in class, and eager to go to school; r = 0.40, 0.58, 0.50, 0.37, and 0.44, respectively) and more teacher-reported effort in class (r = 0.09, 0.36, 0.16, 0.16, and 0.15, respectively). Further, Datu (2018) found that high school students who scored higher on a measure of global flourishing that taps purpose and meaning, rich social relationships, engagement, and optimism had higher levels of emotional and behavioral engagement, even after accounting for variance in student engagement explained by positive affect and other dimensions of subjective well-being.

Regarding the affective component of subjective well-being, King et al.'s (2015) observational research with postsecondary students (predominantly college freshmen) indicated that more frequent experiences of positive emotions at the start of the year co-occurred with and predicted higher levels of behavioral engagement (on-task behavior in class) and emotional engagement (e.g., perceiving class as fun, feeling interested in class), whereas higher levels of negative affect co-occurred with and predicted "disaffection" (i.e., less behavioral and emotional engagement). In an experimental follow-up study, these researchers found that students randomized to a condition designed to evoke positive emotions (specifically, through writing about a personal life event that made them feel happy) indeed then reported greater behavioral and emotional engagement (evidenced by the same indicators used in the first study) than students randomized to recall sad memories. Since the measurement of engagement occurred soon

after the induction of positive or negative emotions, it is difficult to verify from this study if positive affect translates to actual, observable heightened student engagement or simply student perception of such. In reflecting on this limitation of self-report indicators of engagement, King et al. noted that "it is possible that those in a positive affective state were more likely to sample memories wherein they were in an engaged state (vs. disengaged state) in school compared to those in a negative affective state" (pp. 70). Experimental studies reviewed in a subsequent section of this chapter on school-based interventions shed more light on this matter, and provide evidence that interventions developed to foster PERMA in children and adolescents have positive effects on *teacher-rated* indicators of engagement, in addition to *student reports of engagement* and their own subjective well-being (Shoshani & Slone, 2017; Shoshani et al., 2016).

Internalizing Problems

Internalizing forms of psychopathology may manifest when students withdraw from social interactions, avoid various tasks, and express feelings of excessive worry (anxiety), sadness, hopelessness, and depression. In relation to student engagement, researchers have found significant inverse relationships between the affective, behavioral, and cognitive aspects of student engagement and adolescent students reports of feeling sad, hopeless, depressed, or excessive worry (Conner & Pope, 2013; Wang & Peck, 2013). In fact, Wang and Peck (2013) showed that 9th and 11th grade students who reported low levels of affective (e.g., feeling happy, safe, and interested at school), behavioral (e.g., school-work completion), and cognitive engagement (e.g., using self-regulating learning strategies such as connecting learning material to other known information) reported higher rates of depression compared to their peers who reported higher levels of affective, behavioral, and cognitive engagement.

Externalizing Problems

Students' engagement in school can also be impacted by their experience of externalizing difficulties, including substance use, risky/ early sexual activity, and conduct problems/ delinquent behaviors (see Griffiths et al., chapter "Using Positive Student Engagement to Create Opportunities for Students with Troubling and High-Risk Behaviors", this volume). Case in point, studies conducted with adolescent students showed that youths who reported higher levels of one or more indicators of student engagement were significantly less likely to report high rates of substance use and sexual activity (Carter et al., 2007; Li & Lerner, 2011; Simons-Morton & Chen, 2009). Likewise, secondary students who reported being more engaged in school indicated that they were less likely partake in problematic behaviors such as fighting, bullying, stealing, cheating on assignments, and carrying a weapon (Carter et al., 2007; Conner & Pope, 2013; Li & Lerner, 2011; Simons-Morton & Chen, 2009).

Subjective Well-Being and Psychopathology Considered in Tandem

The literature summarized in the preceding paragraphs establishes that higher levels of student engagement are typically seen in students with better mental health, defined by *either* higher levels of indicators or PERMA/subjective well-being or fewer symptoms of internalizing or externalizing behavior problems. A handful of studies have examined student engagement from a dual-factor model of mental health lens, and thus used measures of both well-being and ill-being to assess mental health. Findings from studies of students in elementary school (Smith et al., 2020), middle school (Suldo & Shaffer, 2008), and high school (Rose et al., 2017; Suldo et al., 2016) indicate that the highest levels of student engagement co-occur with the experience of *complete mental health* as reflected in few symptoms of internalizing and externalizing forms of psychopathology, coupled with high subjective well-being.

Case in point, Rose et al. (2017) examined the mental health of Black teenagers using latent class analysis and identified four mental health groups characterized by high or low levels of subjective well-being (i.e., life satisfaction, self-esteem, and social integration) and psychopathology (e.g., depressive symptoms). The group with *complete mental health* (high subjective well-being, low psychopathology) reported higher affective engagement (i.e., school bonding) than the *vulnerable* group (low psychopathology but low subjective well-being) or the *symptomatic but content* group (high subjective well-being but high psychopathology), supporting advantages of high well-being coupled with low ill-being with respect to student engagement. In recent research with students in grades 4 and 5, Smith et al. (2020) found that children with complete mental health had higher levels of behavioral engagement (on-task classroom behavior) and emotional engagement (positive affect such as interest, enjoyment, and enthusiasm in class; per teacher and student report) than their peers in the *troubled* group (low subjective well-being and high psychopathology). The groups of students characterized by high subjective well-being (complete mental health, symptomatic but content) reported more emotional engagement than students with low subjective well-being (vulnerable, troubled), whereas students with low psychopathology (complete mental health, vulnerable) had higher levels of teacher-rated behavioral and emotional engagement than students with more symptoms of psychopathology (symptomatic but content, troubled). In follow-up regression analyses that controlled for internalizing and externalizing behavior problems, subjective well-being predicted greater behavioral and emotional engagement across rater, illustrating benefits associated with high subjective well-being above and beyond low psychopathology.

With respect to cognitive engagement, secondary students with complete mental health reported more positive beliefs about the value of school, and use greater use of self-regulated learning behaviors in pursuit of academic goals, in relation to their vulnerable peers (Suldo & Shaffer, 2008; Suldo et al., 2016). There were no differences in these indicators of cognitive engagement between symptomatic but content and troubled students. In sum, these studies uncovered a critical association between high subjective well-being and cognitive engagement among students without elevated psychopathology, supporting the need to foster students' positive mental health.

Mental Health Interventions and Student Engagement

Theory backed by research demonstrates undeniable links between youth mental health and student engagement, but directionality is less clear and in need of further research. Accordingly, promising school-based interventions might cultivate student engagement either directly through practices intended to increase a dimension of engagement, or indirectly by using psychological or behavioral strategies intended to improve a mental health indicator associated with student engagement. Next, we provide examples of how mental health interventions can result in improvements in student engagement and increases in engagement can lead to improvement in mental health. The following illustrations delineate exemplars of school-based mental health services within a multi-tiered preventative framework, consistent with a public health approach (Macklem, 2011; World Health Organization, 2004). We acknowledge that variables outside of the school setting (e.g., family and community) are also influential in promoting student engagement and youth mental health; however, school-based interventions have been deemed as a viable means for providing relatively low cost, accessible support for youths who are disenfranchised (Suldo et al., 2014). Therefore, our intent is to highlight how school-based practitioners could position themselves to employ interventions that are useful for promoting youth mental health and student engagement among all youths. We end this section with considerations for addressing the needs of students who have been

historically oppressed, marginalized, or forgotten, a discussion that is critical for approaching this work from a culturally responsive, social justice orientation.

Tier 1: Universal Prevention Strategies that Target Mental Health and Engagement

In a multi-tier framework, Tier 1 includes programs offered to all students regardless of current risk level. As discussed by Suldo et al. (Suldo et al., 2019a), these interventions may occur through schoolwide initiatives or through selected classrooms. Furthermore, classroom-based social and emotional learning (SEL) curricula are likely to be facilitated by teachers or interventionists with specialized training, such as school mental health providers. Relevant to this chapter, universal programs that have been found to positively impact at least one aspect of student engagement during efficacy studies may prevent or reduce psychopathology or aim to increase subjective well-being. Furthermore, we highlight examples of universal programs that are intended to target student engagement directly, as a means of fostering students' mental health.

Promoting Subjective Well-Being Through Positive Psychology Interventions

Universal interventions under this category of support—promoting subjective well-being—are typically designed to target empirically identified correlates of high subjective well-being, including ways of thinking (e.g., gratitude and optimism), behaving (e.g., using one's signature strengths in daily activities, pursuing goals), striving (e.g., hope), and relating to other people at home and school.[1] The ultimate goal, then, is to

[1]The positive psychology interventions discussed in this section focus on up-regulating positive emotions. In contrast, most traditional social-emotional learning (SEL) interventions focus on developing children and adolescents' skills in down-regulating negative emotions such as anger, sadness, and worry (Morrish et al., 2018). There are a few exceptions, as some commercially available SEL

equip students with opportunities to develop thoughts and behaviors that one would typically expect to see among happy people. For example, *Awesome Us* is a classwide program that focuses on students' understanding and use of character strengths in their daily lives (Quinlan et al., 2015). In this particular program, students participate in six weekly sessions (lasting for about 1.5 hours each) that are led by a content expert with support from the classroom teacher. Quinlan et al. (2015) found that students in grades 5 and 6 who participated in the program experienced gains in the intervention target (strengths use) and proximal outcome (positive affect), alongside increases in behavioral (on-task behavior in class) and emotional engagement (e.g., viewing class as fun and learning as enjoyable). In contrast, students in the control group experienced significant drops in engagement throughout the duration of the intervention.

Two additional examples of programs targeting correlates of subjective well-being include a 4-week classwide positive psychology intervention intended to promote gratitude among elementary students (Diebel et al., 2016) and the *Maytiv School Program* (implemented schoolwide and classwide) designed to foster multiple aspects of PERMA including positive emotions, gratitude, goal fulfillment, hope, optimism, perseverance, flow experiences, character strengths, and positive relationships (Shoshani et al., 2016). Studies of program outcomes revealed that elementary and middle school student participants reported increased aspects of emotional well-being (e.g., higher gratitude and positive affect,

and reductions in negative affect) and multiple aspects of student engagement (Diebel et al., 2016; Shoshani et al., 2016). Students in the Diebel et al. (2016) study, for example, reported increased school belongingness, an indicator of affective engagement.

Recent experimental studies examining the effects of the Maytiv program when implemented with classes of preschool and middle school students detected positive effects on *teacher*-rated indicators of engagement, in addition to student reports of engagement and their own subjective well-being (Shoshani & Slone, 2017; Shoshani et al., 2016). The Maytiv program developed by Shoshani and colleagues is a universal curriculum with lessons intended to foster youth positive emotions, flow, positive relationships, character strengths, and goal-directed behavior, in alignment with the PERMA framework. Teachers are trained in the curriculum through a series of 15 bimonthly workshops, and deliver the curricular content in their classroom during the week between workshops. In a randomized control trial with 70 teachers/classrooms with over 2500 students in grades 7, 8, and 9, over a 2-year examination period students in the intervention condition experienced significant growth in positive affect as intended, and also significant growth in teacher-rated as well as self-reported emotional engagement and cognitive engagement, in relation to the no-treatment control group (Shoshani et al., 2016). Such findings support a causal impact of positive activities intended to evoke position emotions on multiple dimensions of student engagement, as assessed by multiple methods. Similar findings were yielded from a study of a preschool version of the Maytiv program, examined with 315 children ages 3–6 served in 12 preschools randomly assigned to intervention or control (Shoshani & Slone, 2017). Compared to children in control preschools, children in the intervention condition increased significantly more in proximal mental health outcomes, namely self-reported life satisfaction and child and parent ratings of positive affect. Moreover, children in the intervention group experienced significantly larger increases in cog-

---

programs such as MindUP (The Hawn Foundation, 2011) contain comprehensive emotion regulation strategies in deliberate attempts to do both—up-regulate positive emotions and down-regulate negative emotions. However, since the emphasis or exclusive focus of most SEL programs is on prevention of mental health problems through managing negative emotions, we tend to distinguish between SEL and positive psychology interventions and recommend educational leaders integrate positive psychology interventions with their existing SEL program in accordance with a dual factor model of mental health that provides a framework for addressing both ill-being and well-being.

nitive and behavioral engagement as indicated by teacher ratings of learning behaviors displayed at the beginning and end of the school year. This study provides further support for the notion that mental health and student engagement are linked, and that deliberate efforts to evoke children's positive emotions—in addition to fostering the other PERMA elements—increase youth subjective well-being as expected and also cause concomitant improvements in student engagement that are not limited to personal perceptions of engagement.

Preventing Psychopathology at the Universal Level

A core objective of programs targeting psychopathology at the universal level is to mitigate psychological problems that will likely lead to emotional distress. To this end, programs may help students develop skills for identifying and managing emotions, coping with stress, utilizing problem-solving, and restructuring negative thoughts, while simultaneously improving student engagement and reducing mental health symptoms that pose barriers to student learning. As cited in Suldo et al. (2019a), two examples of such include the *Transformative Life Skills* program (Frank et al., 2017) and the *FRIENDS for Life* program (Ruttledge et al., 2016). Program components entail but are not limited to teaching students mindfulness strategies and relaxation techniques for managing emotions and cognitive restructuring to address worry and anxiety (*FRIENDS for Life* program).

Regarding the *Transformative Life Skills* program, Frank et al. (2017) found that middle school student participants experienced improvement in their use of adaptive coping styles to manage stressors, alongside increased behavioral and affective engagement compared to peers who were randomly assigned to a business-as-usual control group. Indicators of increased behavioral engagement included fewer unexcused absences and problem behaviors resulting in detention. Indicators of affective engagement included a greater sense of belongingness and attachment to school. Similarly, Ruttledge et al. (2016) demon-strated that elementary school children who participated in the *FRIENDS for Life* program experienced a reduction in anxiety symptoms and sustained increases in affective engagement (school connectedness) compared to students in a delayed-intervention control condition. Taken together, educators who adopt promising or evidence-based Tier 1 school mental health programs developed to either increase well-being or prevent/reduce ill-being might expect to see positive effects on student engagement in addition to enhanced mental health outcomes.

Targeting Engagement to Improve Mental Health

In this section, we draw attention to universal interventions that are intended to directly foster student engagement in conjunction with youth mental health or that improve mental health outcomes as a byproduct of program implementation. Case in point, the *Bridges to High School* program aims to prevent mental health difficulties and academic problems that Mexican American youths may encounter (Gonzalez et al., 2014). Because it is a family-focused intervention, the program targets four core areas: (1) effective parenting, (2) youth coping efficacy, (3) youth engagement with learning and at school, and (4) family cohesion. At the parent level, practices to increase student engagement include helping parents understand school expectations, cultivating parents' capacity to engage in home-school communication, and sharing strategies for strengthening parents' use of parenting practices associated with academic success. Direct work with youth included visualization of positive futures, skills training in self-regulated learning and coping strategies, and encouragement to turn to family and school resources that support personal goals. Gonzalez et al. (2014) found that seventh grade students whose families participated in the program experienced greater affective and cognitive engagement, evidenced by their reports of increased bonding to and valuing of school, compared to peers assigned to a minimal dose control condition (i.e., a single-family workshop). Follow-up research further revealed that student participation in the full program predicted better grades and lower levels of internalizing psychopathology a year later, with a sustained effect on reduced internalizing symptoms 5 years later due to the positive impact of intervention on student engagement (Gonzalez et al., 2014).

In another example of an intervention tailored to a specific population—in this case, high school freshmen entering accelerated curricula, the authors of this chapter and colleagues at the first author's institution developed the *Advancing Coping and Engagement (ACE)* program. ACE is a universal program designed to equip students taking Advanced Placement (AP) and International Baccalaureate (IB) classes with competencies in responding to academic stressors, in particular by utilizing effective coping strategies and deliberately increasing behavioral and affective engagement at school (Shaunessy-Dedrick et al., 2022). The classwide curriculum, delivered to 9th grade students in Pre-IB and AP classes consists of 12 modules with companion sessions for caregivers and AP/IB teachers. Three of the student modules focus on student engagement in response to earlier research with AP/IB students ($N = 2379$) indicating that affective and behavioral engagement are critical for promoting desired academic and mental health outcomes among this population (Suldo et al., 2018). The three engagement modules are centered on students' affective connections with the school, their AP or IB program, and class; students' relationships with teachers and classmates; and students' involvement with extracurricular activities. As reported in Suldo et al. (2019a) and Shaunessy-Dedrick et al. (2022), an initial examination of intervention acceptability as viewed by the intended users of the ACE program indicated that students, teachers, and parents who took part in a pilot of ACE at two high schools perceive skill development in these areas as salient to student success in AP/IB, and in general had a positive response to the modules that target engagement. An evaluation of the outcomes associated with student participation in ACE is underway.

Tier 2: Selective Interventions that Target Mental Health and Engagement

Tier 2 interventions focus on youths who are at-risk for academic, emotional, or behavioral difficulties and range from pairing at-risk students with adult mentors to offering time-limited small group or individual counseling to a limited number of students. The latter is typically implemented by school counselors or psychologists. Nevertheless, Doll et al. (2014) asserted that "school-based support staff are not the only resources for supporting students' healthy development" (p. 156). In this sense, mentors, or individuals without a background in professional mental health service delivery "are as essential to child mental health as the services of the school mental health professionals…[and] a comprehensive mental health plan for school mental health services will incorporate scores of adult caretakers who are not traditionally considered to be mental health providers" (Doll et al., 2014; p. 157).

There are several well-researched selective interventions that address student engagement through supplementary support offered by adult mentors. Most of these interventions focus on students who are at-risk for dropping out of school (see research on *Check & Connect*; Christenson et al., 2012; Christenson & Pohl, 2020), students who have displayed problematic externalizing behaviors (see research on Check-in/Check-out; e.g., Miller et al., 2015), or youths who are targets of peer victimization or bullying (Espelage & Swearer, 2004). There is less guidance available on evidence-based interventions with a dual focus of promotion of student engagement and improved mental health outcomes, especially for students who are experiencing internalizing difficulties. Next, we describe a promising selective intervention our team created for use by school mental health professionals to help students develop healthy coping skills and promote student engagement practices that are linked to emotional and academic success.

Grounded in motivational interviewing (Miller & Rollnick, 2012), *Motivation, Assessment, and Planning (MAP) meetings* serve as a supplemental component to the aforementioned *ACE* program. The MAP meetings are intended to help students reflect on and further develop healthy coping skills and student engagement practices that are linked to emotional and academic success in AP/IB courses. School mental health providers deliver the MAP intervention through three core steps. First, after delivery of the ACE program in the fall semester, a multimethod, multisource approach is used to identify students with signs of academic and/or emotional challenges (see Suldo et al., 2019b for a description of the screening process). Second, the interventionist administers a standard battery of surveys to assess the identified student's current coping strategies, levels of student engagement, and perceived parenting practices. Engagement indicators include (a) behavioral engagement (extent of involvement in extracurricular activities), (b) affective engagement/school connectedness (perceived relationships with AP/IB teachers, satisfaction with AP/IB classes, and pride in school); and (c) cognitive engagement (interest in AP/IB classes, persistence, and performance standards). The questionnaire also assesses the students' motivation to engage in their coursework, with specific attention to self-efficacy and flow experiences in the classroom. Third, the interventionist meets with the student individually for approximately 50 minutes to discuss their level of coping and engagement based on the assessment results, and support the student in creating a self-directed change plan. In line with motivational interviewing standards (Miller & Rollnick, 2012), the four stages in the counseling meeting include Engage, Focus, Evoke, and Plan. Following review of the student's current coping and engagement in relation to a normative database of other AP/IB students, students select a target to address (e.g., behavioral engagement: join one after-school club) and the MAP coach and student work in a collaborative manner to develop an action plan for improving the selected target.

We developed the *MAP* meetings during the 2016–17 year and field tested the MAP interven-

tion in the spring semester with 49 students who completed the ACE program during the fall semester (O'Brennan et al., 2020) and further evaluated the usability and acceptability with a different sample of 121 students during the 2017–18 year (Suldo et al., 2021). Findings from survey and interview data from participating students and coaches as well as intended end users (school mental health staff) indicate that MAP is perceived by all stakeholder groups as useful to support student progress toward goals relevant to student success. For instance, school mental health staff who listened to de-identified MAP meetings conveyed that MAP would be an appropriate brief support for students taking AP/IB courses at their school. Suldo et al. (2021) found that only 15% of the at-risk freshmen warranted a referral for more intense supports after a second MAP meeting, suggesting the intervention is an effective early support for students who might otherwise fly under the radar and develop more severe academic or emotional challenges.

Tier 3: Addressing Mental Health Problems that Pose Barriers to Student Engagement

In theory, universal and targeted supports should meet the needs of most students in the school context. Still, a smaller number of students (approximately 5% of the student body) are likely to need support that is more comprehensive and therapeutic in nature, including the provision of outpatient, community-based treatment (Doll et al., 2017). Intensive interventions provided in a school setting affords mental health specialists an opportunity to address and track the impact of students' psychological and behavioral functioning on key academic outcomes, including their engagement in school. The following section summarizes structured mechanisms for attending to students' mental health and engagement needs at this level of intense support. Of note, in contrast to the scores of professional guidance available regarding evidence-based interventions for youths with internalizing or externalizing forms of mental illness, including programs and practices evaluated in schools rather than community settings, promising practices for improving subjective well-being have been advanced only in the last 15 years and are therefore discussed after presentation of cognitive-behavioral therapy.

Counseling and Therapeutic Approaches

A natural question for the school mental health provider is: What is the best therapeutic approach for supporting youth mental health? The answer to this question may be influenced by a number of factors such as (a) one's clinical competence in relation to various approaches to psychotherapy (e.g., psychoanalysis and psychodynamic therapies, behavior therapy, cognitive therapy, and humanistic therapy); (b) the availability of time to provide school-based counseling; and (c) a review of empirical evidence relative to school-based counseling outcomes. We do not intend to be prescriptive in our discussion of cognitive-behavioral therapy (CBT) by suggesting that it is the only treatment approach for serving youths in school settings. Notwithstanding, it is important to acknowledge that the provision of school-based mental health support for individual students is often limited by time constraints due to the structure and duration of the school day. As such, therapeutic approaches that are less likely to be time limited may be less feasible in school settings. Furthermore, a great deal of research has been published demonstrating improvement in students' mental health outcomes upon the completion of counseling interventions guided by CBT techniques (Cullen, 2013; Hilt-Panahon et al., 2008). In recent years, an alternative time-limited therapeutic approach—positive psychotherapy (PPT)—has been advanced as an alternative treatment for depression, with preliminary research finding reductions in depressive symptoms as strong as those seen in adults randomized to CBT (Furchtlehner et al., 2020).

Next, we review key components and features of CBT and PPT and provide evidence of treatment efficacy based on empirical studies. We end this section with a brief review of progress monitoring techniques that interventionists can utilize, including those that may directly assess student engagement in response to individualized, long-term counseling.

Cognitive-Behavioral Therapy Components

CBT is an evidence-based intervention for treating internalizing and externalizing problems experienced by youths and adults (Hofmann et al., 2012). CBT includes a combination of cognitive and behavioral strategies that are integrated to improve client functioning (see Joyce-Beaulieu & Sulkowsi, 2020 or Kendall, 2012 for a comprehensive review). The two main cognitive components of CBT are psychoeducation and cognitive restructuring. Psychoeducation is intended to enhance one's understanding of the nature of their challenges, whereas cognitive restructuring is intended to help the client identify, challenge, and reframe negative and distorted thought patterns that are contributing to the identified concern.

Behavioral strategies typically include relaxation training, problem-solving and social skills training, exposure and response prevention, and behavioral activation. Relaxation training involves teaching clients multiple ways to reduce high levels of internal arousal associated with intense feelings of anxiety or anger (e.g., deep breathing, visual imaginary). Problem-solving and social skills training involve teaching youths to learn and apply skills for responding to challenging situations by engaging in adaptive actions (hence the behavioral nature of these two strategies) guided by a systematic process. Exposure coupled with response prevention aims to help individuals overcome intense fears by exposing them to anxiety-provoking experiences and encouraging them to employ coping strategies during such encounters—as opposed to avoiding or escaping the experience. Finally, behavioral activation is typically utilized to help clients cope with depressed feelings by encouraging them to engage in fun, distracting or productive activities to lift their mood. In addition to the aforementioned techniques, parent training can be employed as well to help caregivers learn how to support their child, especially those who display aggressive behaviors. In this regard, counselors may teach parents how to appropriately reinforce desired behaviors, deliver effective consequences for problematic behaviors, communicate effectively, set boundaries and rules, and use stress management strategies.

Evidence of CBT Effectiveness

Hilt-Panahon et al.'s (2008) review of school-based interventions for children and adolescents with and at-risk of depression concluded that CBT demonstrated moderate-to-large effect sizes, particularly when intervention activities included cognitive restructuring, pleasant activity scheduling (behavioral activation), and problem-solving training. Likewise, Cullen's (2013) meta-analysis indicated that school-based CBT is effective for treating anxiety disorders and related symptoms. Overall, Cullen found that several of the studies demonstrated moderate-to-strong evidence of treatment efficacy; and CBT interventions were especially effective when they included multiple techniques such as psychoeducation, cognitive restructuring, exposure, and social skills training.

School-based CBT can be an effective intervention for treating externalizing problems as well, such as aggression among children and adolescents. For example, Feindler and Engel's (2011) review of intervention approaches for supporting school age-youths who display physical and verbal aggression toward other people highlights the benefits of using CBT for anger management support. Feindler and Engel found that CBT-based interventions yielded significant reductions in aggressive behaviors and improvement in student coping, social skills, and self-esteem, with interventions demonstrating moderate effect sizes. Furthermore, Feindler and Engel identified psychoeducation (e.g., teaching students to identify their triggers and emotional response), arousal management (e.g., deep breathing), social skills and problem-solving training, and cognitive restructuring as critical elements of CBT for addressing aggression, all of which can be implemented in individual or group settings. By way of example of impact on an individual student, Parker et al. (2016) reported the results of a non-controlled case study illustrating the effects of a school-based selective intervention for a middle school student with aggressive behaviors. Using a treatment approach that included cognitive restructuring, psychoeducation, relaxation training, and a parent component in the form of a home-school daily report card plan, Parker and colleagues reported a reduction in the student's aggressive behaviors upon the end of the 6-month intervention period and at a 1-year follow-up.

Positive Psychotherapy Components

Positive Psychotherapy (PPT) is a clinical treatment approach that is grounded in the principles of positive psychology (in particular, the PERMA conceptualization of well-being and emphasis on character strengths) along with recognition of the critical role of a positive therapeutic alliance in improving clients' mental health (Rashid & Seligman, 2018). Regarding alliance, Rashid and Seligman contend that "effective therapeutic relationships can be built on exploration and analysis of positive personal characteristics and experiences (e.g., positive emotions, strengths, and virtues), and not just talking about troubles" (p. 21). PPT was created to balance empathic attention to the negative experiences that led to and maintain an individual's psychological distress with deliberate focus on one's resources and strengths that facilitate resilience and well-being.

The intervention manual presents a 15-session protocol (Rashid & Seligman, 2018), which has been evaluated in individual counseling and small group counseling modalities. The exercises within the sessions came from intervention research conducted to identify discrete positive activities that have empirical support for causing increases in indicators of happiness or subjective well-being. In a recent meta-analysis of the effectiveness of positive psychology interventions, Carr et al. (2020) analyzed findings from 347 studies with over 72,000 participants from 41 countries and identified ten types of positive activities that had significant effects on improving well-being or reducing ill-being (depression, anxiety), specifically: gratitude, savoring, optimism and hope, using signature strengths, humor, kindness, positive writing, meaning making, forgiveness, and goal-setting.

Positive activities included in PPT involve (a) behavioral exercises intended to increase gratitude, kindness, and forgiveness, (b) cognitive/visualization exercises intended to direct one's attention to positive aspects of one's past, present, and future, and (c) communication exercises intended to improve relationships. Communication exercises, for example, include: strengths spotting (identifying and appreciating character strengths demonstrated in family members) and using an active-constructive response style to extend positive emotions when loved ones share good news (Rashid, 2015). The counselor provides psychoeducation about the role of negative, bitter thoughts and memories in perpetuating psychological distress, alongside information about how positive cognitions lead to positive emotions, build resources, and propel psychological growth. The counselor presents one or two positive activities in a session, and assigns practice assignments for the client to complete between sessions to either rehearse or complete the specific positive psychology tool.

Evidence of PPT Effectiveness

Initial studies of PPT with diverse samples using individual and group delivery formats with varying numbers of sessions reported reductions in depressive symptoms and increases in subjective well-being (Rashid, 2015). To date, positive psychotherapy has been evaluated in at least a dozen studies with adults, and a few with youths. Walsh et al. (2017) identified nine studies published in peer-reviewed journals that used PPT in clinical treatment of adults with depression, psychosis, or suicidal ideation. This synthesis of the available research drew attention to the fact that there was considerable variability in clinical use of PPT, with some but not all activities in the PPT protocol used and treatment often supplemented with additional exercises from CBT or positive psychology. Seshadri et al.'s (2021) meta-analysis of effects of novel treatments for adult depression concluded that PPT ($N = 4$ studies) has not yet

been examined in enough well-designed studies to afford definitive conclusions, but so far appears to be comparable to CBT in terms of effectiveness in reducing depression, with the most promising outcomes among adults with moderate depression (vs. mild or severe depression).

Rashid et al. (2013) reported mixed effects of PPT in initial use with a non-clinical sample of 22 middle school students randomly assigned to intervention (8 90-min group sessions of PPT) or no-treatment control. PPT was associated with increases in self-reported well-being and parent-rated social skills, but no effects on life satisfaction or depressive symptoms. Further modification and evaluation is needed to understand optimal levels of teacher and parent involvement in the youth-focused work in order to achieve positive results of PPT across academic, social, and mental health outcomes (Rashid et al., 2013). Mahmoudi and Khoshakhlagh (2017) evaluated positive psychotherapy relative to a delayed-intervention control with 30 high school students in Iran who were referred by school counselors and diagnosed with depression. The PPT condition involved 10 large group sessions with activities that addressed identification of personal strengths, forgiveness, gratitude, hope and optimism, relationship enhancement, and evocation of positive emotions. Analysis of self-report measures from pre- to post-intervention to 2-month follow-up indicated significant, lasting improvements in self-esteem and eudemonic well-being among the intervention group in relation to the control group. Examination of indicators of psychopathology was not reported. Taken together, initial evaluation of PPT when used with youths in school settings provides preliminary support for increases in hedonic and eudemonic well-being (Mahmoudi & Khoshakhlagh, 2017; Rashid et al., 2013), with evidence of a beneficial impact on ill-being restricted to studies with adults in clinical treatment (Furchtlehner et al., 2020; Seshadri et al., 2021).

Progress Monitoring in School Settings

Examining the outcomes of efficacy studies that feature experiments and comparison conditions (as described in the preceding sections) is useful for identifying engagement and mental health interventions that are generally effective for K-12 students. However, evaluative data collected within the context of field-based support can help practitioners determine whether a given intervention is appropriate for their targeted population. When examining students' outcomes in everyday practice, educators and clinicians can utilize a variety of progress monitoring tools to assess a student's response to therapeutic interventions (see Renshaw et al., this volume). School mental health interventions should be evaluated using indicators of both well-being and ill-being, in accordance with a dual-factor model of mental health (Doll et al., 2021). Given the focus of this chapter, we highlight how the identified approaches can afford examination of indicators of student engagement as a critical aspect of treatment goals.

First, school mental health providers can examine naturally occurring school data such as office discipline referrals, incidents of in- and out-of-school suspensions, work completion status/rate, and student participation in social activities. Observational data may include (a) recording the extent to which students display on-task behaviors in the classroom and (b) noting how and to what extent students interact with peers and adults in the classroom or larger school setting. Finally, interventionists may utilize daily behavioral report cards and behavior rating scales as a mechanism to assess other adults' perceptions of the degree in which the student is displaying problematic or desired behaviors (Joyce-Beaulieu & Sulkowski, 2020).

These methods of data collection are consistent with assessing indicators of student engagement, as evidenced by students' display of problematic or adaptive behaviors, attendance patterns, and work completion rate (behavioral engagement) and social connections with peers and adults (affective engagement) (see Reschly et al., 2020). Joyce-Beaulieu and Sulkowski (2020) further explained that anecdotal accounts of students' growth are useful for determining their response to CBT interventions. Thus, inquiring about students' perceptions of the classroom and school environment may be another approach

to examining their affective and cognitive engagement. An example of such may include a student who views school and studying (an indicator of cognitive engagement) as meaningless at the beginning of treatment and later grows to appreciate school due to the implementation of cognitive restructuring, visualizing of one's best possible self in the future, or other CBT or PPT techniques.

Considerations for Supporting Marginalized and Overlooked Pupils

When supporting marginalized populations, it is important that educators take a culturally responsive approach. To this end, school mental health providers may use culturally relevant material, build upon students' cultural strengths, or help students cope with cultural-related challenges (Parker et al., 2021). For example, *Jóvenes Fuertes* is a validated version of the *Strong Teens* program that was designed for use with Latin* (Latinx) adolescents. The content includes lessons on ethnic pride (a cultural strength), in addition to using traditional CBT skills, such as cognitive reframing and problem-solving skills, to cope with acculturative stress. When delivered in a school setting, Castro-Olivo (2014) found that the intervention yielded significant effects on the students' social-emotional learning knowledge and social-emotional resiliency.

Still, this example and others we have provided thus far reflect mental health and student engagement interventions that support students directly. In recent years, more discussion has been accentuated in the professional literature about the limitations of addressing mental needs among marginalized populations at the client level alone. Scholars contend that restricting treatment to individual (and perhaps group-based) intervention does not fully address social determinants of mental health, such as systemic policies, practices, and social norms of discrimination that perpetuate ongoing disparate outcomes among people who are disenfranchised (Compton & Shim, 2015; Singh et al., 2017). Instead, individual approaches imply that clients (or students) who are marginalized are solely responsible for the outcomes of their hegemonized treatment (see Galindo et al., chapter "Expanding an Equity Understanding of Student Engagement: The Macro (Social) and Micro (School) Contexts", this volume, for a discussion of structural barriers to student engagement).

Case in point, LGBTQ+ youths are at a high risk of experiencing negative emotions and diminished mental health compared to their non-LGBTQ+ peers due to experiences of discrimination, victimization, isolation, and rejection (Russell & Fish, 2016; White et al., 2018). Consequently, LGBTQ+ youths reported higher levels of student engagement when they were surrounded by supportive, safe adults in their school setting (Seelman et al., 2012). Seelman et al. (2012) also found that indicators of affective (belonging and valuing of class content) and behavioral (being productive in school) engagement were significant predictors of decreased fear-based truancy for sexual minority youth with higher levels of subjective fear at school, providing additional evidence for the importance of fostering a positive school climate for this population.

Racial/ethnic minoritized youths represent another vulnerable population due to their encounter with racial discrimination in and out of school, and for some youths of color, exposure to neighborhood violence and inequitable access to mental health support (Alegria et al., 2010; Quirk, 2020; Rosenbloom & Way, 2004; Thomas et al., 2011; Tobler et al., 2013). It is then unsurprising that researchers have found significant, negative links between student engagement (e.g., school bonding, commitment in the school process) and discrimination, and positive associations between student engagement and social support in school settings among racial/ethnic minoritized students (Dotterer et al., 2009; Garcia-Reid et al., 2005). Taken together, it is incumbent upon school mental health providers to respond to their professional charge to advocate for antiracist and anti-discriminatory policies and practices in school settings.

As a final example of a subgroup potentially in need of additional attention, students who are enrolled in rigorous, accelerated courses will likely be overlooked for mental health interventions due to the assumption that they require little support, particularly when they excel in academic courses (Suldo et al., 2014). On the contrary, high achieving students can very well experience mental health-related challenges, which may be exacerbated by high levels of academic-related stress associated with rigorous coursework or striving toward perfectionism due to their high academic ability (e.g., Mofield et al., 2016; Shaunessy et al., 2011; Stornelli et al., 2009). These students can be impacted by self-prescribed perfectionism, wherein students may set high personal standards for themselves, as well as socially prescribed perfectionism stemming from the perception that others (e.g., parents) demand perfectionism among the students (Fletcher & Speirs Neumeister, 2012; Hewitt & Flett, 1991). Like other groups of students, school mental health providers can use systematic screening to identify students enrolled in advanced coursework who may need additional support (Suldo et al., 2019b) mental health support, including by facilitating student engagement, may be especially critical for underrepresented students who may experience increased stress due to the workload in accelerated courses *and* due to the previous mentioned factors linked to racial discrimination.

Implications for Intervention Implementation

Overall, the aforementioned examples of Tier 1 approaches underscore the benefits of universal programs for addressing student engagement directly and indirectly through structured, mental health preventative efforts. Because lower levels of student engagement and diminished youth mental health are particularly pronounced during middle and high school, programs demonstrating positive outcomes across several age groups, especially at the elementary level, support the rationale for investing in youth mental health initiatives in the early stages of their education. Mental health approaches at the Tier 2 level are generally intended to be preventative as well, with the goal of minimizing the severity of initial signs of psychopathology and academic challenges. Nevertheless, students receiving Tier 2 interventions may experience early indicators of significant mental health concerns, which warrants the use of more human capital, that is, adults from various occupational backgrounds providing short-term individual or small group support. As illustrated in the description of the *MAP* intervention, supplemental/targeted support can target student engagement and mental health indicators simultaneously to promote optimal student functioning. Some Tier 2 approaches can be provided by mentors/caregivers without a professional mental health background depending on the student's need.

This, then, reserves resources for the use of trained school mental health providers to address the needs of students who are particularly vulnerable to experiencing significant mental health challenges. As such, school-based mental health support at the Tier 3 level is more intensive due to the duration and highly individualized approach to treatment (Doll et al., 2014; Macklem, 2011; NASP, 2015). For example, positive psychotherapy requires 8–15 weekly sessions. Parker and colleagues (2016) provided a 6-month CBT intervention coupled with a 9-week behavioral intervention plan; and the intervention they executed was intended to meet the individual student's needs, as opposed to utilizing a standard treatment protocol that may have failed to address the specific challenges the student experienced.

Across all levels of interventions, student engagement can be targeted directly or indirectly through the use of empirically supported psychological strategies such as motivational interviewing, CBT, and positive psychology interventions that broaden-and-build resources that lead to student engagement and achievement. Finally, mental health support must reflect culturally sensitive practices that are responsive to marginalized youths' lived experiences. As impressed upon the readers in this chapter, responding to the needs of disenfranchised students must include the combination of student-based interventions and efforts to advocate for systemic changes to promote socially-just, equitable practices for all.

Directions for Future Research

We opened this chapter by describing and distinguishing modern conceptualizations of student engagement (i.e., behavioral, cognitive, and affective subtypes) and flourishing mental health (i.e., PERMA), and proceeded to summarize studies linking mental health to engagement and academic achievement. However, the separability of these multidimensional constructs is unclear, as is the directionality of the associations between them. Measurement studies are needed to determine if the general engagement aspect of PERMA is distinct from cognitive engagement for students, a developmental group for whom schooling is a primary focus of daily activity. Longitudinal research that tracks children and adolescents' levels of student engagement, mental well-being and ill-being, and academic achievement over time is needed to illustrate if associations are primarily reciprocal (e.g., Datu & King, 2018; Ng et al., 2015) or if instead deteriorations or improvements in one area (e.g., mental health) drive changes in another area such as student engagement, a pathway inferred by this chapter's emphasis on mental health interventions.

Experimental studies that evaluate the impact of school mental health interventions on student outcomes should include indicators of multiple student engagement subtypes, in part to permit determination of how the different foci of mental health interventions (e.g., treatment of psychopathology through CBT, fostering subjective well-being through positive psychology interventions) may impact different aspects of engagement. In addition to comprehensive assessment of student engagement and mental health (well-being and ill-being), data on distal academic outcomes via indicators of achievement (e.g., test scores, course grades, on-time graduation) should be collected to permit examination of intervention impact on those outcomes particularly relevant to administrative stakeholders who are responsible for decisions about resource allocation. Such efficacy studies should include sizeable representation of students from different gender, race/ethnicity, and socioeconomic groups to permit crucial examinations of how subgroups of students based on their intersectional identities respond to interventions targeting mental health and engagement, including systemic and culturally adapted interventions. In addition to such large-scale efficacy studies, we need more case and field-based research examining links between mental health interventions and student engagement in real-world applications of evidence-based interventions to local contexts.

Summary

Student engagement is a multidimensional construct reflected in behavioral engagement (active participation in the learning environment), affective engagement (feelings during class and learning, perceptions of belongingness and connectedness at school), and cognitive engagement (valuing of education, use of self-regulated learning strategies; Fredricks et al., 2019). In this chapter, we present literature that documents associations between student engagement and optimal mental health defined in part by subjective well-being in line with a dual-factor model (Suldo & Doll, 2021). In accordance with Fredrickson's (2001) Broaden-and-Build theory, we establish the salience of positive emotions to student learning and engagement; positive emotions create an upward spiral marked by *broadening* of cognitive capacity and behavioral flexibility that in turn *builds* lasting personal social, psychological, and physical resources (Fredrickson, 2001). In short, positive emotions serve adaptive functions that lead to better outcomes including student engagement (Reschly et al., 2008). We maintain that the superior academic outcomes that stem from student engagement foster opportunities for students' positive experiences reflective of numerous elements of PERMA (e.g., accomplishment and relationships) that foster flourishing mental health (Carmona–Halty et al., 2019; Kwok & Fang, 2021; Ouweneel et al., 2011). In sum, positive emotions and student engagement foster competencies related to coping, strengths use, and social connections that are critical to healthy emotional development as well

as academic achievement. For such reasons, universal and targeted applications of the promising or evidence-based school-based interventions that are described in this chapter as created to improve student well-being or ameliorate ill-being might conceptualize student engagement as among the proximal outcomes, and expect positive effects on student engagement in addition to enhanced mental health outcomes.

References

Adelman, H. S., & Taylor, L. (2010). *Mental health in schools: Engaging learners, preventing problems, and improving schools*. Corwin Press.

Alegria, M., Vallas, M., & Pumariega, A. J. (2010). Racial and ethnic disparities in pediatric mental health. *Child and Adolescent Psychiatric Clinics, 19*, 759–774. https://doi.org/10.1016/j.chc.2010.07.001

Carmona–Halty, M., Salanova, M., Llorens, S., & Schaufeli, W. B. (2019). How psychological capital mediates between study–related positive emotions and academic performance. *Journal of Happiness Studies, 20*, 605–617. https://doi.org/10.1007/s10902-018-9963-5

Carr, A., Cullen, K., Keeney, C., Canning, C., Mooney, O., Chinseallaigh, E., & O'Dowd, A. (2020). Effectiveness of positive psychology interventions: A systematic review and meta-analysis. *The Journal of Positive Psychology.* https://doi.org/10.1080/17439760.2020.1818807

Carter, M., McGee, R., Taylor, B., & Williams, S. (2007). Health outcomes in adolescence: Associations with family, friends and school engagement. *Journal of Adolescence, 30*(1), 51–62. https://doi.org/10.1016/j.adolescence.2005.04.002

Casas, F., & Gonzalez-Carrasco, M. (2019). Subjective well-being decreasing with age: New research on children over 8. *Child Development, 90*, 375–394. https://doi.org/10.1111/cdev.13133

Castro-Olivo, S. M. (2014). Promoting social-emotional learning in adolescent Latino ELLs: A study of the culturally adapted Strong Teens program. *School Psychology Quarterly, 29*(4), 567–577. https://doi.org/10.1037/spq0000055

Christenson, S. L., & Pohl, A. J. (2020). The relevance of student engagement: The impact of and lessons learned implementing check & connect. In A. L. Reschly, A. J. Pohl, & S. L. Christenson (Eds.), *Student engagement: Effective academic, behavioral, cognitive, and affective interventions at school* (pp. 3–30). Switzerland.

Christenson, S., Stout, K., & Pohl, A. (2012). *Check & connect: A comprehensive student engagement intervention, implementing with fidelity manual*. Institute on Community Integration, University of Minnesota.

Compton, M. T., & Shim, R. S. (2015). The social determinants of mental health. *FOCUS, 13*(4), 419–425. https://doi.org/10.1176/appi.focus.20150017

Conner, J. O., & Pope, D. C. (2013). Not just robo-students: Why full engagement matters and how schools can promote it. *Journal of Youth and Adolescence, 42*(9), 1426–1442. https://doi.org/10.1007/s10964-013-9948-y

Csikszentmihalyi, M. (2014). *Applications of flow in human development and education: The collected works of Mihaly Csikszentmihalyi*. Springer.

Cullen, R. (2013). School-based intervention for adolescent anxiety. *New Zealand Journal of Teachers' Work, 10*(1), 104–124. http://search.ebscohost.com/login.aspx?direct=true&AuthType=cookie,ip,url,shib&db=ehh&AN=93550387&site=ehost-live&scope=site

Datu, J. A. D. (2018). Flourishing is associated with higher academic achievement and engagement in Filipino undergraduate and high school students. *Journal of Happiness Studies, 19*, 27–39. https://doi.org/10.1007/s10902-016-9805-2

Datu, J. A. D., & King, R. B. (2018). Subjective well-being is reciprocally associated with academic engagement: A two-wave longitudinal study. *Journal of School Psychology, 69*, 100–110. https://doi.org/10.1016/j.jsp.2018.05.007

Diebel, T., Woodcock, C., Cooper, C., & Brignell, C. (2016). Establishing the effectiveness of a gratitude diary intervention on children's sense of school belonging. *Educational and Child Psychology, 33*, 117–129. https://psycnet.apa.org/record/2016-40016-009

Doll, B., Cummings, J. A., & Chapla, B. A. (2014). Best practices in population-based school mental health services. In P. Harrison & A. Thomas (Eds.), *Best practices in school psychology* (pp. 149–163). The National Association of School Psychologists.

Doll, B., Nastasi, B. K., Cornell, L., & Song, S. Y. (2017). School-based mental health services: Definitions and models of effective practice. *Journal of Applied School Psychology, 33*(3), 179–194. https://doi.org/10.1080/15377903.2017.1317143

Doll, B., Dart, E. H., Arora, P. G., & Collins, T. A. (2021). Framing school mental health services within a dual-factor model of mental health. In P. J. Lazarus, S. M. Suldo, & B. Doll (Eds.), *Fostering the emotional well-being of youth: A school-based approach* (pp. 40–60). Oxford University Press.

Dotterer, A. M., McHale, S. M., & Crouter, A. C. (2009). Sociocultural factors and school engagement among African American youth: The roles of racial discrimination, racial socialization, and ethnic identity. *Applied Developmental Science, 13*(2), 61–73.

Espelage, D. L., & Swearer, S. M. (2004). *Bullying in American schools: A social-ecological perspective on prevention and intervention*. Erlbaum.

Feindler, E. L., & Engel, E. C. (2011). Assessment and intervention for adolescents with anger and aggression difficulties in school settings. *Psychology in the Schools, 48*(3), 243–253. https://doi.org/10.1002/pits.20550

Fletcher, K. L., & Speirs Neumeister, K. L. (2012). Research on perfectionism and achievement motivation: Implications for gifted students. *Psychology in the Schools, 49*, 668–677. https://doi.org/10.1002/pits.21623

Frank, J. L., Kohler, K., Peal, A., & Bose, B. (2017). Effectiveness of a school-based yoga program on adolescent mental health and school performance: Findings from a randomized controlled trial. *Mindfulness, 8*, 544–553. https://doi.org/10.1080/15377903.2013.863259

Fredricks, J. A., Reschly, A. L., & Christenson, S. L. (2019). Interventions for student engagement: Overview and state of the field. In J. A. Fredricks, A. L. Reschly, & S. L. Christenson (Eds.), *Handbook of student engagement interventions: Working with disengaged youth* (pp. 1–11). Elsevier Press.

Fredrickson, B. L. (2001). The role of positive emotions in positive psychology: The broaden-and-build theory of positive emotions. *American Psychologist, 56*, 218–226. https://doi.org/10.1037/0003-066X.56.3.218

Furchtlehner, L. M., Schuster, R., & Laireiter, A. (2020). A comparative study of the efficacy of group positive psychotherapy and group cognitive behavioral therapy in the treatment of depressive disorders: A randomized controlled trial. *The Journal of Positive Psychology, 15*(6), 832–845. https://doi.org/10.1080/17439760.2019.1663250

Garcia-Reid, P., Reid, R. J., & Peterson, N. A. (2005). School engagement among Latino youth in an urban middle school context: Valuing the role of social support. *Education and Urban Society, 37*(3), 257–275. https://doi.org/10.1177/0013124505275534

Gonzalez, N. A., Wong, J. J., Toomey, R. B., Millsap, R., Dumka, L. E., & Mauricio, A. M. (2014). School engagement mediates long-term prevention effects for Mexican American adolescents. *Prevention Science, 15*, 929–939. https://link.springer.com/article/10.1007%2Fs11121-013-0454-y

Heffner, A. L., & Antaramian, S. P. (2016). The role of life satisfaction in predicting student engagement and achievement. *Journal of Happiness Studies, 17*(4), 1681–1701. https://doi.org/10.1007/s10902-015-9665-1

Hewitt, P. L., & Flett, G. L. (1991). Perfectionism in the self and social contexts: Conceptualization, assessment, and association with psychopathology. *Journal of Personality and Social Psychology, 60*, 456–470. https://doi.org/10.1037/0022-3514.60.3.456

Hilt-Panahon, A., Kern, L., Divatia, A., & Gresham, F. (2008). School-based interventions for students with or at risk for depression: A review of the literature. *Advances in School Mental Health Promotion, 1*(suppl 1), 32–41. https://doi.org/10.1080/1754730X.2008.9715743

Hofmann, S. G., Asnaani, A., Vonk, I. J., Sawyer, A. T., & Fang, A. (2012). The efficacy of cognitive behavioral therapy: A review of meta-analyses. *Cognitive Therapy and Research, 36*(5), 427–440. https://link.springer.com/article/10.1007/s10608-012-9476-1

Joyce-Beaulieu, D., & Sulkowski, M. (2020). *Cognitive behavioral therapy in K-12 school settings (2nd ed.): A practitioner's toolkit*. Springer.

Kendall, P. C. (Ed.). (2012). *Child and adolescent therapy: Cognitive-behavioral procedures* (4th ed.). Guilford.

Kern, M. L., Benson, L., Steinberg, E. A., & Steinberg, L. (2016). The EPOCH measure of adolescent Well-being. *Psychological Assessment, 28*, 586–597. https://doi.org/10.1037/pas0000201

King, R. B., McInerney, D. M., Ganotice, F. A., & Villarosa, J. B. (2015). Positive affect catalyzes academic engagement: Cross-sectional, longitudinal, and experimental evidence. *Learning and Individual Differences, 39*, 64–72. https://doi.org/10.1016/j.lindif.2015.03.005

Kwok, S. Y. C. L., & Fang, S. (2021). A cross-lagged panel study examining the reciprocal relationships between positive emotions, meaning, strengths use and study engagement in primary school students. *Journal of Happiness Studies, 22*, 1033–1053. https://doi.org/10.1007/s10902-020-00262-4

Li, Y., & Lerner, R. M. (2011). Trajectories of school engagement during adolescence: Implications for grades, depression, delinquency, and substance use. *Developmental Psychology, 47*(1), 233. https://doi.org/10.1037/a0021307

Macklem, G. L. (2011). Evidenced-based tier 1, tier 2, and tier 2 mental health interventions in schools. In G. Macklem (Ed.), *Evidenced-based school mental health services: Affect education, emotion regulation training, and cognitive behavioral therapy* (pp. 19–37). Springer Science and Business Media.

Mahmoudi, H., & Khoshakhlagh, H. (2017). The effectiveness of positive psychotherapy on psychological well-being and self-esteem among adolescents with depression disorder. *Social Behavior Research and Health, 2*(1), 153–163.

Marks, H. M. (2000). Student engagement in instructional activity: Patterns in the elementary, middle, and high school years. *American Educational Research Journal, 37*(1), 153–184. https://doi.org/10.3102/00028312037001153

Merikangas, K. R., He, J., Burstein, M., Swanson, S. A., Avenevoli, S., Cui, L., et al. (2010). Lifetime prevalence of mental disorders in US adolescents: Results from the National Comorbidity Study-Adolescent Supplement (NCS-A). *Journal of the American Academy of Child and Adolescent Psychiatry, 49*(10), 980–989. https://doi.org/10.1016/j.jaac.2010.05.017

Miller, L. M., Dufrene, B. A., Sterling, H. E., Olmi, D. J., & Bachmayer, E. (2015). The effects of check-in/check-out on problem behavior and academic engagement in elementary school students. *Journal of Positive Behavior Interventions, 17*(1), 28–38. https://doi.org/10.1177/1098300713517141.

Miller, W. R., & Rollnick, S. (2012). *Motivational interviewing: Helping people change* (3rd ed.). Guilford.

Mofield, E., Parker Peters, M., & Chakraborti-Ghosh, S. (2016). Perfectionism, coping, and underachievement in gifted adolescents: Avoidance vs. approach orientations. *Education Sciences, 6*(3), 1–22. https://doi.org/10.3390/educsci6030021

Morrish, L., Rickard, N., Chin, T. C., & Vella-Brodrick, D. A. (2018). Emotion regulation in adolescent well-being and positive education. *Journal of Happiness Studies, 19*, 1543–1564. https://doi.org/10.1007/s10902-017-9881-y

National Association of School Psychologists (NASP). (2015). *School psychologists: Qualified health professionals providing child and adolescent mental and behavioral health services* [White paper]. Author.

Ng, Z. J., Huebner, E. S., & Hills, K. J. (2015). Life satisfaction and academic performance in early adolescents: Evidence for reciprocal association. *Journal of School Psychology, 53*, 479–491. https://doi.org/10.1016/j.jsp.2015.09.004

O'Brennan, L. M., Suldo, S. M., Shaunessy-Dedrick, E., Dedrick, R. F., Parker, J. S., Lee, J., Ferron, J., & Hanks, C. (2020). Supports for youth in accelerated high school curricula: A first study of applicability and acceptability of a motivational interviewing intervention. *Gifted Child Quarterly, 64*(1), 19–40. https://doi.org/10.1177/0016986219889933

Ouweneel, E., Le Blanc, P. M., & Schaufeli, W. B. (2011). Flourishing students: A longitudinal study on positive emotions, personal resources, and study engagement. *The Journal of Positive Psychology, 6*, 142–153. https://doi.org/10.1080/17439760.2011.558847

Parker, J. S., Joyce-Beaulieu, D., & Zaboski, B. (2021). Culturally responsive mental health services. In D. Joyce-Beaulieu & B. A. Zaboski (Eds.)., *Applied cognitive behavioral therapy in schools* (pp. 100–127). Oxford University Press.

Parker, J., Zaboski, B., & Joyce-Beaulieu, D. (2016). School-based cognitive-behavioral therapy for an adolescent presenting with ADHD and explosive anger: A case study. *Contemporary School Psychology, 20*, 356–369. https://doi.org/10.1007/s40688-016-0093-y

Quinlan, D. M., Swain, N., Cameron, C., & Vella-Brodrick, D. A. (2015). How 'other people matter' in a classroom-based strengths intervention: Exploring interpersonal strategies and classroom outcomes. Journal of Positive Psychology, 10(1), 77–89. https://doi.org/10.1080/17439760.2014.920407.

Quirk, A. (2020). *Mental health support for students of color during and after the coronavirus pandemic*. https://www.americanprogress.org/issues/education-k-12/news/2020/07/28/488044/mental-health-support-students-color-coronavirus-pandemic/

Rashid, T. (2015). Positive psychotherapy: A strength-based approach. *The Journal of Positive Psychology, 10*, 25–40. https://doi.org/10.1080/17439760.2014.920411

Rashid, T., & Seligman, M. (2018). *Positive psychotherapy: Clinician manual*. Oxford University Press.

Rashid, T., Anjum, A., Lennox, C., Quinlan, D., Niemiec, R. M., Mayerson, D., & Kazemi, F. (2013). Assessment of character strengths in children and adolescents. In C. Proctor, P. A. Linley, C. Proctor, & P. A. Linley (Eds.), *Research, applications, and interventions for children and adolescents: A positive psychology perspective* (pp. 81–115). Springer Science + Business Media. https://doi.org/10.1007/978-94-007-6398-2_6

Reschly, A. L., Huebner, E. S., Appleton, J. J., & Antaramian, S. (2008). Engagement as flourishing: The role of positive emotions and coping in student engagement at school and with learning. *Psychology in the Schools, 45*(5), 419–431. https://doi.org/10.1002/pits.20306

Reschly, A. L., Pohl, A. J., & Christenson, S. L. (Eds.). (2020). Student engagement: Effective academic, behavioral, cognitive, and affective interventions at school. Springer Nature.

Rose, T., Lindsey, M. A., Xiao, Y., Finigan-Carr, N. M., & Joe, S. (2017). Mental health and educational experiences among black youth: A latent class analysis. *Journal of Youth and Adolescence, 46*, 2321–2340. https://doi.org/10.1007/s10964-017-0723-3

Rosenbloom, S. R., & Way, N. (2004). Experiences of discrimination among African American, Asian American, and Latino adolescents in an urban high school. *Youth & Society, 35*, 420–451.

Russell, S. T., & Fish, J. N. (2016). Mental health in lesbian, gay, bisexual, and transgender (LGBT) youth. *Annual Review of Clinical Psychology, 12*, 465–487. https://doi.org/10.1146/annurev-clinpsy-021815-093153

Ruttledge, R., Devitt, E., Greene, G., Mullany, M., Charles, E., Frehill, J., & Moriarty, M. (2016). A randomised controlled trial of the FRIENDS for life emotional resilience programme delivered by teachers in Irish primary schools. *Educational and Child Psychology, 33*, 69–89. https://doi.org/10.1111/camh.12030

Seelman, K. L., Walls, N. E., Hazel, C., & Wisneski, H. (2012). Student school engagement among sexual minority students: Understanding the contributors to predicting academic outcomes. *Journal of Social Service Research, 38*(1), 3–17. https://doi.org/10.1080/01488376.2011.583829

Seligman, M. E. P. (2011). *Flourish: A visionary new understanding of happiness and well-being.* Free Press.

Seshadri, A., Orth, S. S., Adaji, A., Singh, B., Clark, M. M., Frye, M. A., McGillivray, J., & Fuller-Tyszkiewicz, M. (2021). Mindfulness-based cognitive therapy, acceptance and commitment therapy, and positive psychotherapy for major depression. *American Journal of Psychotherapy, 74*, 4–12.

Shaunessy, E., Suldo, S. M., & Friedrich, A. (2011). Mean levels and correlates of perfectionism in international baccalaureate and general education students. *High Ability Studies, 22*, 61–77. https://doi.org/10.1080/13598139.2011.576088

Shaunessy-Dedrick, E., Suldo, S. M., O'Brennan, L. M., DiLeo, L., Dedrick, R. F., Ferron, J., M., & Parker, J. (2022). Acceptability of a preventative coping and connectedness curriculum for high school students entering accelerated courses. *Journal for the Education of the Gifted.* https://doi.org/10.1177/01623532221105307

Shoshani, A., & Slone, M. (2017). Positive education for young children: Effects of a positive psychology intervention for preschool children on subjective well being and learning behaviors. *Frontiers in Psychology, 8*, 1866. https://doi.org/10.3389/fpsyg.2017.01866

Shoshani, A., Steinmetz, S., & Kanat-Maymon, Y. (2016). Effects of the Maytiv positive psychology school program on early adolescents' well-being, engagement, and achievement. *Journal of School Psychology, 57*, 73–92. https://doi.org/10.1016/j.jsp.2016.05.003

Simons-Morton, B., & Chen, R. (2009). Peer and parent influences on school engagement among early adolescents. *Youth & Society, 41*(1), 3–25. https://doi.org/10.1177/0044118X09334861

Singh, G. K., Daus, G. P., Allender, M., Ramey, C. T., Martin, E. K., Perry, C.,... & Vedamuthu, I. P. (2017). Social determinants of health in the United States: Addressing major health inequality trends for the nation, 1935–2016. *International Journal of MCH and AIDS, 6*(2),139–164. https://doi.org/10.21106/ijma.236

Smith, N. D. W., Suldo, S. M., Hearon, B. V., & Ferron, J. M. (2020). An application of the dual-factor model of mental health in elementary school students: Examining academic engagement and social outcomes. *Journal of Positive School Psychology, 4*(1), 49–68.

Stiglbauer, B., Gnambs, T., Gamsjäger, M., & Batinic, B. (2013). The upward spiral of adolescents' positive school experiences and happiness: Investigating reciprocal effects over time. *Journal of School Psychology, 51*, 231–242. https://doi.org/10.1016/j.jsp.2012.12.002

Stornelli, D., Flett, G. L., & Hewitt, P. L. (2009). Perfectionism, achievement, and affect in children: A comparison of students from gifted, arts, and regular programs. *Canadian Journal of School Psychology, 24*, 267–283. https://doi.org/10.1177/0829573509342392

Suldo, S. M., & Doll, B. (2021). Conceptualizing youth mental health through a dual-factor model. In P. J. Lazarus, S. M. Suldo, & B. Doll (Eds.), *Fostering the emotional well-being of youth: A school-based approach* (pp. 20–39). Oxford University Press. https://doi.org/10.1093/med-psych/9780190918873.001.00001

Suldo, S. M., Gormley, M. J., DuPaul, G. J., & Anderson-Butcher, D. (2014). The impact of school mental health on student and school-level academic outcomes: Current status of the research and future directions. *School Mental Health, 6*, 84–98. https://doi.org/10.1007/s12310-013-9116-2

Suldo, S. M., & Shaffer, E. J. (2008). Looking beyond psychopathology: The dual-factor model of mental health in youth. *School Psychology Review, 37*(1), 52–68. https://doi.org/10.1080/0279015.2008.12087908

Suldo, S. M., Shaunessy-Dedrick, E., Ferron, J., & Dedrick, R. F. (2018). Predictors of success among high school students in advanced placement and international baccalaureate programs. *Gifted Child Quarterly, 62*(4), 350–373. https://doi.org/10.1177/0016986218758443

Suldo, S. M., Thalji-Raitano, A., Kiefer, S. M., & Ferron, J. M. (2016). Conceptualizing high school students' mental health through a dual-factor model. *School Psychology Review, 45*(4), 434–457. https://doi.org/10.17105/SPR45-4.434-457

Suldo, S., Parker, J. S., Shaunessy-Dedrick, E., & O'Brennan, L. (2019a). Mental health interventions. In J. Fredricks, A. Reschly, & S. Christenson (Eds.), *Handbook of student engagement interventions* (pp. 199–215). Academic Press.

Suldo, S. M., Storey, E., O'Brennan, L. M., Shaunessy-Dedrick, E., Ferron, J. M., Dedrick, R. F., & Parker, J. S. (2019b). Identifying high school freshmen with signs of emotional or academic risk: Screening methods appropriate for students in accelerated courses. *School Mental Health, 11*(2), 210–227. https://doi.org/10.1007/s12310-018-9297-9

Suldo, S. M., Wang, J. H., O'Brennan, L. M., Shaunessy-Dedrick, E., Dedrick, R., DiLeo, L., Ferron, J. M., & Lee, J. (2021). A motivational interviewing intervention for adolescents in accelerated high school curricula: Applicability and acceptability in a second sample. *Prevention Science.* https://doi.org/10.1007/s11121-021-01204-z

The Hawn Foundation. (2011). *The MindUP curriculum: Brain-focused strategies for learning and living.* Scholastic.

Thomas, J. F., Temple, J. R., Perez, N., & Rupp, R. (2011). Ethnic and gender disparities in needed adolescent mental health care. *Journal of Health Care for the Poor and Underserved, 22*, 101–110. https://doi.org/10.1353/hpu.2011.0029

Tobler, A. L., Maldonado-Molina, M. M., Staras, S. A., O'Mara, R. J., Livingston, M. D., & Komro, K. A. (2013). Perceived racial/ethnic discrimination, problem behaviors, and mental health among minority urban youth. *Ethnicity & Health, 18*, 337–349.

Walsh, S., Cassidy, M., & Priebe, S. (2017). The application of positive psychotherapy in mental health care: A systemic review. *Journal of Clinical Psychology, 73*, 638–651. https://doi.org/10.1002/jclp.22368

Wang, M. T., & Peck, S. C. (2013). Adolescent educational success and mental health vary across school engagement profiles. *Developmental Psychology, 49*(7), 1266. https://doi.org/10.1037/a0030028

White, A. E., Moeller, J., Ivcevic, Z., Brackett, M. A., & Stern, R. (2018). LGBTQ adolescents' positive and negative emotions and experiences in US high schools. *Sex Roles, 79*(9), 594–608. https://doi.org/10.1007/s11199-017-0885-1

World Health Organization Department of Mental Health and Substance Abuse. (2004). *Prevention of mental disorders: Effective interventions and policy options.* http://www.who.int/mental_health/evidence/en/prevention_of_mental_disorders_sr.pdf

Resilience and Student Engagement: Promotive and Protective Processes in Schools

Ann S. Masten, Kayla M. Nelson, and Sarah Gillespie

Abstract

Effective schools buffer students against the effects of adversity on learning and positive adjustment in the present and prepare them for future resilience. This chapter draws on the developmental literature about resilience in children and the educational psychology literature on student engagement to highlight the multifaceted role of schools in resilience. We adopt a scalable and multidisciplinary systems definition of resilience as the capacity of a dynamic system to adapt successfully to challenges that threaten the function, survival, or development of the system. We consider the multifaceted roles in promoting and nurturing resilience of student engagement, broadly defined to include behavioral, emotional, and cognitive processes that connect students to learning and their school communities. Student engagement affords greater access to resources and resilience capacity that can protect children at risk due to acute and chronic adverse childhood experiences while also facilitating the development of resilience factors widely implicated as the building blocks of future competence and resilience. Student engagement processes mediate, moderate, and reflect the processes by which school systems can support and nurture student resilience through multisystem interactions. A "short list" of resilience factors consistently associated with student resilience is delineated along with multiple ways that schools support and nurture these influential factors. Schools can mitigate risk, provide an array of resources and opportunities, and simultaneously nurture powerful adaptive systems that build future resilience for individuals and thereby their communities and societies.

Studies of resilience suggest that effective schools buffer children against the effects of adversity on learning and positive adjustment in the present while also nurturing their future competence and resilience (Doll, 2013; Masten, 2014b, 2021; Theron, 2021; Ungar et al., 2019). Research suggests that student engagement plays key roles in the processes by which schools contribute to this dual mobilization and development of adaptive systems that serve to protect children at risk due to acute and chronic adverse childhood experiences, while also facilitating the development of resilience factors widely implicated as foundational to future competence and resilience capacity. This chapter draws from developmental science on resilience in children

A. S. Masten (✉) · K. M. Nelson · S. Gillespie
University of Minnesota Twin Cities, Minneapolis, MN, USA
e-mail: amasten@umn.edu; nels8814@umn.edu; gille597@umn.edu

and educational science on student engagement to highlight the multiple ways that schools foster resilience in the short and long term, with a focus on the roles of student engagement in the adaptive success of students confronted with significant adversities and disadvantages.

For the purposes of this discussion, we adopt a multidimensional perspective on student engagement, encompassing indicators and processes associated with psychosocial connections of students with school that facilitate learning and academic success (Appleton et al., 2008; Christenson & Pohl, 2020; Wang & Hofkens, 2020). Broad definitions of student engagement encompass behavioral, emotional, and intellectual processes that reflect a multitude of potential interactions with curricular material; relationships with other students, staff, and teachers; participation in the norms and expectations of the school community; and active roles of students in decision making or feedback to shape their learning environments (Coates, 2007; Kuh, 2009). From this perspective, student engagement is multifaceted, including emotional, cognitive, motivational, behavioral, and relational dimensions long associated with positive outcomes in school and in life, ranging from attendance and academic achievement to later work success (Reschly et al., 2020). In addition, student engagement comprises a multisystem, multidirectional set of processes by which schools, students, families, and communities influence each other. Student engagement can be influenced by families and peers outside of school as well as by staff and students inside a school community. Moreover, the engagement of individual students as well as their families can influence the overall school climate and quality of education, with the potential for enhancing the overall quality of the school for all of its students. Consequently, there is long-standing interest in promoting student engagement in various ways in order to enhance developmental outcomes in children and youth, particularly for young children at risk of academic and psychological problems (Appleton et al., 2008; Reschly et al., 2020). Similarly, schools also may promote the resilience of the broader communities in which they are embed-

ded, fostering a sense of collective identity, building social capital among local residents, and cultivating economic growth (Good, 2019; Milofsky, 2018).

Interventions to promote student engagement and school success have historical connections to the developmental science on competence and resilience (Christenson & Pohl 2020; Masten, 2003; Masten & Motti-Stefanidi, 2009; Reynolds et al., 2007; Wang & Gordon, 1994). The importance of schools, for example, in the success of immigrant youth and in recovery from mass-casualty disasters and conflict is widely recognized by humanitarian agencies as well as researchers (Masten & Narayan, 2012; Masten et al., 2019; Motti-Stefanidi & Masten, 2013). One of the most efficacious and well-established interventions to promote student engagement and avert student dropout, Check & Connect, was explicitly designed to build protective and reduce risk factors identified in the resilience literature, along with other research evidence and theory relevant to student engagement (Christenson & Pohl, 2020).

With the goal of linking current efforts to promote student engagement with advancements in resilience science, this chapter includes the following sections. The first section provides a contemporary definition of resilience from a multisystem developmental perspective, emphasizing the salience of schools for resilience, particularly in the context of overcoming situations of high cumulative risk, including homelessness, poverty, disaster, political conflicts, migration, discrimination, maltreatment, and related adversities. The second section elaborates on parallels in the "short list" of resilience factors consistently observed in theory and empirical studies of resilience broadly defined and the more specific literature on protective influences of schools. Section three examines the evidence on mediating and moderating roles of student engagement in resilience processes. The fourth section highlights the multifaceted roles of schools in nurturing resilience and preventing adversity for their students and societies. Conclusions highlight the alignment of research on resilience and student engagement, the dual roles of schools in resilience processes present and future, the vital role schools are expected to play in pandemic recovery, and the need for resilience studies focused on adaptive processes afforded by schools that are particularly important for diverse students.

Resilience Defined from a Developmental Multisystem Perspective

Resilience can be defined from many perspectives, ranging from engineering or ecology to psychology or urban planning, referring broadly to the qualities or processes involved in withstanding or adapting to disturbances or adversities that threaten different kinds of natural or built systems (Folke, 2016; Masten, 2014b; Ungar, 2021). For the purposes of this discussion, which is focused on students in the context of schools, we adopt a multisystem view that is scalable and multidisciplinary, reflecting the growing dominance of systems thinking in developmental science and the call for integrating knowledge on resilience from different disciplines to meet challenges posed by disasters, epidemics, political conflicts, and related global challenges (Masten, 2018a; Masten & Motti-Stefanidi, 2020).

We define resilience as the capacity of a dynamic system to adapt successfully through multiple processes to challenges that threaten that system's function, survival, or development (Masten, 2014b; Masten et al., 2021). We view students as living systems, whose development (and resilience at any given time) is continually influenced by many interacting systems within their bodies and minds as well as between the whole person and their environments. Individuals are embedded in other systems, including families and schools, that in turn are connected to other systems, and they also are influenced by many processes related to culture and environments. These views are consistent with developmental systems theory (Gottlieb, 2007; Griffiths & Taber, 2013; Lerner, 2006, Overton, 2013), Bronfenbrenner's socioecological theory (Bronfenbrenner & Morris, 2006), developmental psychopathology (Masten & Cicchetti, 2016),

family resilience theory (Walsh, 2016), social-ecological theory (Folke, 2016), studies of student engagement in the education literature (Wang & Hofkens, 2020), and multisystem views of resilience emerging in many other disciplines (Ungar, 2021).

Schools also can be viewed as complex dynamic systems (Hawkins & James, 2018), influenced by individuals who attend or work in the school and by many systems outside of the school with influence on school staff, students, and curriculum, ranging from families of their students to teacher unions and policy makers. The quality of schools in terms of education and the well-being of their students and staff will depend on support from their students, families of students, their communities, and many other organizations. The quality and resilience of schools are shaped by many interactions, including the complex array of processes encompassed by the concept of student engagement, as well as excellent leadership (Hawkins & James 2018; Masten & Motti-Stefanidi, 2009; Wang & Hofkens, 2020). High-quality student engagement supports the overall effectiveness of a school as well as the individual experiences of its students.

Recognizing that many interactions shape the course of development across intersecting system levels carries with it the idea that changes at one level or in one domain of functioning in a system are likely to spread to affect other areas of function and, potentially, other system levels. The potential of multisystem interactions to change the course of development in a system is captured by the concept of *developmental cascades* (Masten & Cicchetti, 2010). Exposure to chronic, severe trauma in childhood, for example, can influence lifelong health through biological changes in stress-regulation and other neurobiological systems central to health (Boyce et al., 2021; McEwen, 2019). Early success at school, facilitated by first rate early childhood education before school entry and effective teaching and school leadership after school begins, can promote success among children who experience many forms of deprivation and adversity in childhood (Bellis et al., 2018; Masten, 2014b; Huebner et al., 2016; Reynolds et al., 2018).

From the point of view of students, schools are contexts where many learning and social interactions take place. In Bronfenbrenner's social ecological theory (Bronfenbrenner & Morris, 2006), schools represent a key microsystem for individual development. Through many interactions with staff, teachers, other students, instructional material, and the extracurricular context, students change and develop in many ways, ideally learning academic skills, such as reading and math, as well as social-emotional skills of getting along with other people, following the behavioral rules of their community and society, and understanding the values and ways of succeeding in their environment. Interactions in schools can socialize immigrant youth to the norms, expectations, and values of a new host culture, while interactions in the home promote protective connections to their heritage culture; the development of bicultural competence is linked to the success and well-being of immigrant youth (Motti-Stefanidi et al., 2020). Societies charge schools with educating and socializing their children for competence in the society, in parallel but different ways than their families. Families and societies alike expect schools to keep their children safe from harm while also preparing them for future learning, work, and civic engagement.

Going to school, getting along with other people there, and learning the skills essential for making one's way in society are some of the *developmental tasks* expected of children in most modern societies (Masten, 2014b). Developmental tasks are the physical or psychosocial milestones or accomplishments by which progress in development is typically evaluated by society, parents, and eventually by young people themselves. These are the criteria by which we often judge how well development is going, based on many generations of observation as well as research that these accomplishments indicate not only current competence but also the likelihood of future competence (Heckman, 2006; Masten et al., 2006). Such criteria have played a central role in education (Havighurst, 1974) and in resilience research as indicators of positive adaptation to adversity or risk (Masten, 2014b; Masten & Coatsworth, 1998).

The study of resilience in developmental research required the operationalization of two core components: the adversity or risk posing a threat to development and the criteria for evaluating how well the young person was doing (Masten et al., 2021). Although there are many other criteria to consider, both positive (e.g., psychological well-being) and negative (e.g., trauma symptoms) developmental tasks were popular among developmental scientists, perhaps because parents, teachers, communities, and societies agree on their importance. The thesis that "competence begets competence" was widely believed before data began to back up this idea and economist James Heckman and others documented the high return on investment in early childhood competence (Huebner et al., 2016).

Developmental tasks change, of course, as development proceeds and as the context changes. Infants and toddlers are expected to form attachment bonds and learn the language of the family, whereas students of school age are expected to attend school, follow classroom rules, and learn numerous academic and social skills. When migration occurs and young people enter school in a new culture and/or context, routine developmental tasks are often compounded by acculturation and adapting to the new context (Motti-Stefanidi & Masten, 2013, 2020). For immigrant youth, schools often serve as a primary acculturative context for learning about their new homeland, exploring their cultural identities and potential conflicts between the developmental tasks of their native culture and host culture, making friends among host-culture peers, gaining a sense of belonging, and future opportunities. Success in school also offers a gateway to success in higher education, work, and status in the new society. For receiving societies, success among immigrant youth offers enhanced human capital and a more diverse workforce.

As evidence accrued on the success of children in terms of developmental tasks in the school context, it became clear that student engagement indexed in multiple ways was generally related to competence or success in school-related developmental tasks (such as academic achievement, peer acceptance, and prosocial conduct), both for native and immigrant youth. Concomitantly, evidence grew that student engagement also was a key mediator and moderator of school success for young people at risk of school failure and developmental problems due to adverse childhood experiences, socioeconomic risks, or migration (Appleton et al., 2008; Durlak, 2009; Masten, 2014b; Masten & Motti-Stefanidi, 2009; Motti-Stefanidi & Masten, 2013). The varied processes represented by the construct of "student engagement" in this body of work included relationships with teachers and peers, attendance and participation in school activities, a sense of belonging or school spirit, and family involvement in school activities. These processes reflect behavioral, emotional, and cognitive aspects of engagement (Appleton et al., 2008).

From the perspective of the schools, student engagement can be viewed as a mediator and moderator of overall school effectiveness, with schools as systems striving to educate and promote competence of their students (Eccles & Roeser, 2011). For schools educating students at risk of learning or behavioral problems related to disadvantage, adversity, or migration, bolstering student engagement can be conceptualized as a strategy for improving the competence of all students and the resilience of their high-risk students (Reschly et al., 2020; Wang & Gordon, 1994). As a result, student engagement has been the target of interventions to bolster school effectiveness in general and promote resilience specifically among high-risk students. In their edited volume, Reschly et al. (2020) provide multiple chapters illustrating different strategies of intervention aimed at boosting emotional, cognitive, motivational, and relational engagement of students with school. Similarly, many of the preventive interventions intended to promote school achievement and adjustment among children at risk due to trauma, discrimination, migration, or poverty have focused on engaging students as foundational to facilitating the opportunities and interactions that are essential to learning and building relationships that support these students (Masten,

2014b). More specifically, in the resilience literature, student engagement processes were conceptualized as a means to build resilience capacity.

In resilience theory, general predictors of better outcomes are known as *promotive factors*, whereas influences that play an additional or exclusive role in the context of high exposure to adverse experiences are known as *protective factors* (Masten & Cicchetti, 2016). This difference reflects "main effects" versus moderating or "interactional effects" (interacting with a risk factor) of a variable on desired outcomes. Effective schools can be generally better for learning and also specifically helpful for children at risk due to disadvantages or adversities, acting as both a promotive and protective factor. Similarly, individual or family attributes, such as self-control or parenting skills, can be good for development at all risk levels but especially important for children in high-risk circumstances.

Over the years, research on children who overcame adversity or succeeded in school despite a history of risk circumstances consistently pointed to a set of individual, family, and school qualities often identified as promotive and protective factors (Masten, 2014b; Masten et al., 2021; Ungar & Theron, 2020). Striking parallels in the qualities of individual youth, families, and schools associated with resilience in children and in each of these contexts suggested that there may be multisystem processes connecting these fundamental human adaptive systems that fostered resilience, particularly when networks of these systems were aligned. In the next section, we discuss these apparent drivers of resilience and the role of student engagement in engaging and enhancing them.

Converging Research on Resilience Linking Students, Families, and Schools

Research on children at risk consistently implicated a set of recurring resilience factors associated with better outcomes in the near and far term under diverse conditions of risk or adversity

(Garmezy, 1985; Masten, 2014b; Luthar, 2006; Ungar & Theron, 2020). Examples of these factors (sometimes called the "short list") implicated a set of basic human adaptive systems associated with good adaptation, particularly under adversity. The short list included individual attributes, relationships, and qualities of a child's context, such as effective/supportive caregiving, schools, and communities. Meanwhile, other lines of research on effective families and family resilience (Henry et al., 2015; Patterson, 2002; Walsh, 2016), as well as effective schools and school resilience (Anderson, 1994; Edmonds, 1979; Masten, 2014b; Theron, 2021; Ungar et al., 2019) pointed to very similar resilience factors.

In recent theory and reviews of the literature, resilience scholars have noted the striking similarities in resilience factors identified across major social systems in the lives of children and youth, suggesting that this alignment is not coincidental. Instead, the alignment may reflect the multisystem nature of resilience and the interdependent processes that afford humans the capacity to adapt, arising from many generations of natural and sociocultural selection (Masten, 2018a; Masten et al., 2021; Ungar, 2018). Resilience factors associated with better adjustment among children at risk of various reasons also tend to co-occur, although situated in different systems, consistent with the idea that protective processes interact across systems in ways that afford synergy and thereby greater resilience capacity (Fritz et al., 2018; Höltge et al., 2021; Masten, 2011). Social networks of adaptive systems may have co-evolved, drawing on the fundamental adaptive capabilities of individuals in our highly social species. These speculations have led to interest in research on network analysis of resilience and similar efforts to measure the coordinated capacity of social-contextual systems to support individual human resilience (Fritz et al., 2018; Höltge et al., 2021).

Common psychosocial resilience factors that span individual attributes, relationships, and contexts have been reported for decades in case studies, empirical studies, and reviews of the literature on young people who show positive adjustment and outcome in the context of exposure to signifi-

cant adversity (e.g., Garmezy, 1985; Masten et al., 1990; Werner & Smith, 1992). Such observations are entirely consistent with developmental systems and social-ecological theories of resilience. Ongoing research continues to add evidence of common resilience factors, despite inconsistencies in research methods and concepts of resilience (Masten et al., 2021). Persistent inconsistencies of both concepts and methods continue to limit the feasibility of systematic reviews of this literature. Nonetheless, recent efforts to conduct systematic and scoping reviews of the literature on resilience in young people support the basic conclusions from early observations and narrative reviews that there are multisystem resilience factors that appear across cultures and diverse situations of risk (Christmas & Khanlou, 2019; Fritz et al., 2018; Meng et al., 2018; Ungar & Theron, 2020).

Examples of frequently identified factors associated with resilience in students are shown in Table 1, including comparable factors from a student and school perspective (Doll, 2013; Masten, 1994, 2007, 2014b; Masten & Motti-

Table 1 Short list of resilience factors associated with student resilience

From a student perspective	From a school perspective
Close relationships, attachment bonds with family, other adults, and friends	Caring, respectful relationships among students, faculty, and staff
Sense of security, belonging	School climate of safety and inclusion
Problem-solving skills	Effective teaching
Self-regulation (cognitive, emotional)	Structure and effective leadership
Motivation to succeed, agency	Scaffolding to enhance mastery motivation
Positive views of self, identity, self-efficacy	Positive views of students and school
Positive outlook on the future, optimism	Positive outlook on student and school future
Sense of purpose and meaning	School spirit, collective purpose
Engaged with effective school and teachers	Student engagement
Family engagement	Community engagement
Parenting and family resilience	Teacher and school resilience

Table 2 How schools enhance present and future student resilience

Meeting basic student needs for nutrition, safety, healthcare, and stimulation
Sensitive interactions and teaching that convey respect, concern, commitment, and inclusion
Opportunities for relationships with caring, committed, and competent adults and mentors
Role modeling of effective self-regulation and stress management
Support for self-regulation, autonomy, and self-determination
Fostering values and maintaining a positive school climate
High expectations in the context of supportive relationships
Opportunities for friendships with prosocial peers
Opportunities to learn and develop talents
Opportunities to experience mastery
Fostering healthy habits and daily routines
Special rituals and celebrations that reinforce belonging, accomplishment, and optimism
Connections and collaboration with students' families
Reducing school-based stress and adversity (e.g., reducing conflict, bullying, racism)

Stefanidi, 2009; Ungar & Theron, 2020; Wang & Hofkens, 2020; Wright et al., 2013). These examples of resilience factors represent leading candidates in the quest to know *"What matters?"* for resilience in children and youth. These resilience factors, comprising the short list, are assumed to reflect fundamental adaptive systems and capabilities that develop in human lives resulting from the interplay of biological, social, and ecological processes (Masten, 2014b). Identifying key resilience factors was the primary goal of the first wave of resilience science focused on children and youth (Masten, 2007; Wright et al. 2013).

Later waves of research focused on *how* questions: the processes involved in *how* these factors worked to yield successful adaptation in the midst or aftermath of adversity exposure as well as the development of the capacities for resilience indicated by these factors (Masten, 2007). It was important to understand how resilience led to successful adaptation in order to develop effective interventions for children

at risk of harm from adverse experiences and risky circumstances (Masten, 2014b). Table 2 offers a potential list of "how" schools may foster resilience based on the literature cited in this article on student resilience and effective schools (e.g., Ungar et al., 2019), a list that is highly congruent with recommendations to engage students (e.g., Reschly et al., 2020). Notably, effective schools share many of the qualities of effective families with respect to protecting children in the present and nurturing their resilience for the future (Masten, 2018a, b; Theron, 2021).

In the following section we examine more closely how schools nurture and support resilience. We suggest that student engagement plays a vital role in the processes by which schools foster resilience in the short and long term.

Student Engagement as a Mediator and Moderator of Resilience

Research from diverse corners of the literature on resilience in children and youth implicates student engagement as a mediator and moderator of resilience for children at risk due to adverse life experiences, socioeconomic disadvantage, or racial-ethnic discrimination (Fredricks et al., 2019; Motti-Stefanidi & Masten, 2013; Reschly et al., 2020; Wang & Hofkens, 2020). Success in school is a central developmental task in most contemporary societies, indicating resilience in the cases of students who encounter major obstacles to school success in their lives and serving as a harbinger of future success. Theoretically, some degree of engagement is a prerequisite for most of the resilience processes afforded by effective schools. For example, positive relationships are less likely to develop with a teacher for students who rarely attend school. Growing evidence of malleability in multiple dimensions of student engagement long associated with better school outcomes has spurred considerable interest in interventions to promote student engagement (Fredricks et al., 2019).

Cumulative Risks and Adversities Threaten School Success

Many adversities and disadvantages pose risks to school readiness, learning, conduct, achievement, completion, and psychological well-being at school. These risks often co-occur with cumulative effects on multiple indicators of school adjustment (Evans et al., 2013; Masten, 2014b). Some risks have direct effects on school success and others indirectly influence behavior or psychological well-being in ways that interfere with learning. Children experiencing homelessness may not be able to attend school regularly or may change schools frequently, either of which can disrupt learning (Cowen, 2017; Fantuzzo et al., 2012; Masten et al., 2015). Exposure to violence or neglect can interfere with children developing essential social, emotional, and self-regulation skills important for learning and school success (Labella & Masten, 2018). Youth who experience racism or discrimination based on ethnicity, gender, or weight report worse psychological well-being (e.g., low self-worth, social anxiety, depressive symptoms) and lower academic achievement, particularly if school staff or teachers are the source of the discrimination (Benner & Graham, 2013; Ghavami et al., 2020). Brain development and related cognitive functions and stress-regulation systems can also be affected in lasting ways by exposure to toxic levels of stress or profound neglect in early life (Shonkoff et al., 2012). Lower school readiness, partially mediated by self-regulation skills, is related to poverty and inequality (Blair & Raver, 2015).

Resilience in the Context of Cascading Risks

Over time the effects of such risks can accrue and cascade across domains of function at school (Masten et al., 2005; Labella & Masten, 2018). Difficulties with self-regulation skills, for example, can lead to later achievement and conduct problems that contribute to peer rejection and disengagement from school (Sabol & Pianta, 2012; Zelazo, 2020). Yet, evidence also suggests

that these cumulative and cascading harms to education can be reduced or prevented by effective family and community supports, high-quality early childhood education, and efforts by schools to engage and support students at risk during the school years (Bellis et al., 2018; Plumb et al., 2016; Robles et al., 2019; Uddin et al., 2021; Ungar et al., 2019). For example, research on families experiencing homelessness indicates that parenting quality is associated with better academic, behavioral, and social adjustment of their children in school (Labella et al., 2017; Masten et al., 2015). The Head Start REDI program, which targets social-emotional and language/literacy skills in disadvantaged preschoolers, has shown lasting effects on school success among children at risk due to poverty (Bierman et al., 2008). This intervention has shown effects on academic engagement (e.g., enthusiastic about learning, attentiveness) that were sustained through elementary school (Welsh et al., 2020) and also had protective effects on school bonding in young adolescents (Sanders et al., 2020).

Check & Connect, mentioned above, was developed in the 1990s as a dropout prevention program but quickly became recognized as a successful intervention to promote student engagement (Christenson et al., 2012; Christenson & Pohl, 2020). This program was influenced by resilience theory and, from the outset, it focused on improving students' connections to school and their sense of belonging. The aims and strategies of Check & Connect continue to align very well with protective factors and processes identified in the resilience literature. In this program, mentors build sustained, trusting relationships with students and work with them to solve problems. They monitor and facilitate student engagement with school and learning in multiple ways, engaging with parents and school personnel as well as students. The program aims to reduce risk factors while also building protective factors, such as a trusted relationships with adults at school, self-efficacy, problem-solving skills, and motivation.

Positive relationships with prosocial, engaged peers may also play a key role in student engagement. Findings from the Longitudinal Studies of Child Abuse and Neglect (LONGSCAN) suggested that positive peer relationships during adolescence had promotive effects on student engagement and protective effects against the risk of adverse childhood experiences (ACEs) on school outcomes at age 16 (Moses & Vollodas, 2017). Opportunities for positive peer interactions may also play a role in the resilience of immigrant youth, discussed further below.

Efforts to engage students in school recognize that schools have multiple academic and social contexts for engaging students (Wang & Hofkens, 2020). Schools can offer diverse social, academic, and extracurricular contexts that appeal to different students. Schools as developmental contexts can offer students different pathways of engagement that fit the individual and developmental needs of students with variable motivations, talents, and past experiences.

Student Engagement in Diverse Racial/Ethnic and Cultural Contexts

Engaging students from diverse ethnic, racial, and cultural backgrounds poses particular challenges for schools (see Galindo et al., chapter "Expanding an Equity Understanding of Student Engagement: The Macro (Social) and Micro (School) Contexts", this volume), but offers great promise for promoting resilience. Students from marginalized populations have good reason to be wary in schools or communities with a history of racism or xenophobia, and many report ongoing experiences of school-based discrimination (Ghavami et al., 2020). Nonetheless, student engagement is associated with better school outcomes and future opportunities for students from racial-ethnic minorities or immigrant families (Motti-Stefanidi & Masten, 2020; Wittrup et al., 2019). Some schools with a diverse student body manage to foster student engagement through different strategies. For example, a recent review of ethnic studies courses found that these culturally grounded curricula promote identity development, well-being, and graduation rates among ethnic minority youth and improved the racial

attitudes of white students (Sleeter & Zavala, 2020). Graham (2018) argues that, as schools become increasingly diverse due to the demographic trends in the United States, ethnic minority and majority students alike benefit from protective factors that include cross-ethnic friendships, the development of complex social identities, and reduced vulnerability to bullying or discrimination. A growing literature suggests that culturally responsive teaching and positive cross-ethnic relationships within schools can support the engagement and resilience of youth from different cultural and racial backgrounds.

Research on immigrant youth also suggests there are protective influences at multiple system levels (Motti-Stefanidi, 2018; Motti-Stefanidi & Masten, 2020; Suárez-Orozco et al., 2009, 2018). These include influences at the level of communities or society (welcoming attitudes toward immigrants, cultural pluralism valued, economic and social supports for immigrant families), schools (intermingling of immigrant and native youth, intercultural friendships, inclusive school climate), and individuals (positive identity, self-efficacy). Relationships play a central mediating role in the success of immigrant youth, facilitating both social and academic engagement. Suárez-Orozco et al. (2009) summarize the evidence from the US studies indicating the mediating role of relationships with peers and adults in schools for newcomer immigrant youth success, associated with a sense of belonging, social and emotional support, and practical help. Their findings in the Longitudinal Immigrant Student Adaptation Study (LISA) of young adolescent newcomers to the United States from multiple countries found that multiple aspects of student engagement (e.g., cognitive and behavioral engagement) were facilitated by relationships with co-national peers, teachers at school, and co-national adults in the community, all of which supplemented ongoing parental support. School-based relationships provided two distinct forms of support, emotional and practical, and these caring relationships appeared to foster academic success in a variety of ways. Numerous other studies of immigrant youth underscore the role of positive relationships with peers and teachers in facilitating student engagement, their perceived sense of belonging, and their academic success (Suárez-Orozco et al., 2018).

Research on school success of Black students in countries and communities with a history of racism and discrimination also points to the key role of student engagement. School-based racial discrimination is a risk factor for student disengagement among African American youth in the United States (Neblett et al., 2006; Leath et al., 2019). Research on resilience in African American students suggests that positive relationships and positive racial identity can counter this risk. African American students who perceive that their school supports their cultural identity development have higher grades 1 and 2 years later (del Toro & Wang, 2020). In one recent study, naturally occurring mentoring relationships, particularly when characterized by relational closeness, were found to counter the risk of discrimination on academic engagement, as defined by curiosity for new material and persistence when attempting academic tasks (Wittrup et al., 2019). In another recent study, Leath et al. (2019) found that positive racial identity beliefs protected against the effects of school-based racial discrimination experiences on academic curiosity and persistence of African American adolescents.

Student Engagement in the Context of War or Disaster

Evidence on recovery from disasters and war offers another compelling perspective on the fundamental importance of student engagement for the resilience of students, families, and communities (Masten & Narayan, 2012). Research and observations by humanitarian agencies across decades and many forms of devastating trauma have highlighted the salience of resuming school as a powerful symbol of recovery and the extraordinary value placed on student engagement by parents, community members, and students themselves in countries across the world (Lai et al., 2016; Masten, 2014a). In refugee camps and shelters with children and families who have fled terror or disaster, almost immediately after basic survival needs are met, responders or families themselves begin to set up learning centers or

in longer-term settings, schools. Similarly, the COVID-19 pandemic has revealed the importance to societies around the world of children being in school (Calao et al., 2020; Masten & Motti-Stefanidi, 2020).

In the literature on mass-trauma experiences, student engagement again appears to play multiple roles as a mediator and moderator of positive adaptation in children and their families (Masten, 2021; Osofsky & Osofsky, 2021). After tornadoes and hurricanes, students have been enlisted in recovery projects sponsored by their schools, which serves the double purpose of building self-efficacy and hope in the students and helping the community recover. After Katrina, for example, a successful Youth Leadership Program was established by the St. Bernard Unified School District in collaboration with university researchers and mental health providers, based on models of resilience and self-efficacy (Osofsky & Osofsky, 2021). Many of the interventions designed to foster recovery after disasters and wars also have been implemented in school contexts, not only because this is where the students are located but also because programs in schools are more trusted, perceived as more normative, and simultaneously serve to build resilience in the students, teachers, and parents who participate (Lai et al., 2016; Masten, 2021; Nuttman-Shwartz, 2019). Student engagement in school, more broadly, has the potential to build resilience for the future as well as enhance learning and well-being in the present.

Nurturing Resilience in Schools

Schools have multiple roles in nurturing resilience in the future, as well as providing a healthy learning environment, social support, safety, and protection in the present. Schools build resilience capacity for the future through their roles in shaping cognitive, emotional, motivational, and social skills essential for learning and success in the developmental tasks of childhood and beyond (Doll, 2013; Masten, 2018b; Masten & Motti-Stefanidi, 2009; Ungar et al., 2019). Schools were designed to promote students' development of competence in domains viewed as important for their future place in society, including reading, writing, mathematics, and the history of their country or government. There also is an implicit curriculum, described as the "hidden curriculum" by Jackson (1968), whereby schools socialize students with the values and behavior expected for successful life in their community or society. The values are likely to include respecting authority, following rules or social norms, and getting along with other people. In addition to explicit and implicit instruction, contemporary schools often provide basic food, healthcare, tutoring, and after school activities, with the goal of enhancing learning or addressing unmet basic needs of disadvantaged students. Through education, societies invest in the human capital of their future citizens and socialize them in the language, culture, and history of the country (Neem, 2017). For immigrant youth, who have acculturative as well as developmental tasks, schools serve as a key context for learning the language and culture of the receiving community or nation and cultivating cross-cultural friendships (Motti-Stefanidi & Masten, 2020). At the same time, schools may also perpetuate social stratification, inequity, and racism (Ladson-Billings & Tate IV, 1995; Theron & Theron, 2014).

For students growing up in a context of high cumulative risk or adversity, effective schools can add resources and protections that compensate for missing relational and material supports in the home or neighborhood, provide a safe haven, and buffer children from the effects of adverse childhood experiences or ongoing dangers (Masten, 2014b; Ungar et al., 2019). When risk in the home or community is or has been very high, schools play an especially important role in fostering resilience and recovery and mitigating risk. Schools that provide a rich environment of safe and positive relationships, learning, structure, routines, motivational experiences, skill-building, healthy nutrition, and prosocial friendships offer pathways to opportunity for children at risk due to current and past adversity. Student engagement and school stability can mitigate the risks associated with homelessness, particularly when the school context is proactively

resilience-informed as well as trauma-informed (Masten et al., 2015; Moore et al., 2020).

There also is evidence supporting universal resilience-focused interventions in schools, although the research is limited. A systematic review of the literature on intervention studies aiming to strengthen protective factors for children in schools found support for short-term effects of interventions (particularly cognitive-behavioral interventions) on internalizing symptoms of students (Dray et al., 2017). One might expect that effect sizes of selective and targeted school-based interventions to promote mental health and resilience would be even larger (Sanchez et al., 2018), given that selective and targeted interventions leverage student engagement in schools to provide critical additional services.

The COVID-19 pandemic, which caused prolonged school closures, abrupt shifts to distance learning, and other major educational disruptions, has underscored the importance of schools for the well-being and development of children at risk due to disadvantage and adversity (Dvorsky et al., 2020; Masonbrink & Hurley, 2020; Masten, 2021; Masten & Motti-Stefanidi, 2020; Rundle et al., 2020; Ungar & Theron, 2020; Viner et al., 2021). As school closures continued, concerns increased about the myriad ways development could be negatively impacted (e.g., by food insecurity, obesity, anxiety, suicidal thinking, depressed mood, and undetected child maltreatment), along with concerns about learning losses, particularly among children already at risk of developmental or educational problems. Fortunately, there appears to be a concomitant surge of research to document effects of school closures, distance learning, and efforts to support students as they return to school. These efforts are likely to inform future education policy on school responses to similar threats and disaster preparedness of education systems. Schools may be uniquely situated to promote resilience and recovery following this pandemic and future mass-casualty threats, and such data could inform key avenues for mobilizing and reconnecting students with multisystem promotive and protective processes afforded by effective schools.

Conclusions

Research on the role of schools in resilience continues to grow, along with increasing attention to the multisystem nature of resilience in human development. Theory and evidence on resilience factors and processes identified in the developmental literature show striking alignment with the scholarship on school resilience and the multifaceted roles of student engagement in the affordance and nurturing of student competence and resilience. It is clear that schools play a vital role in supporting children and youth burdened with past and present adversity in multiple ways, ranging from mitigating risk and providing nutrition or health care, to caring, committed, and respectful relationships that support or mobilize adaptive systems critical to resilience and recovery in the context of adversity or high cumulative risk. Resilience-effective schools, much like families, offer their students important relationships and role modeling; a sense of worthiness, belonging, security, and hope; active protections against danger; daily interactions that foster learning, problem-solving, and many skills for living in society; as well as opportunities for developing their talents and self-confidence. Through many interactions and activities, schools extend the resilience capacities of their students in the present, and through many educational processes, build resilience for the future as well. Student engagement plays many mediating and moderating roles in these adaptive processes and thereby contributes to the present and future resilience of their students. As a result of their roles in supporting the development of competence and resilience, schools and student engagement also play vital roles in building human capital and resilience of communities and societies.

Nonetheless, growing attention to the challenges and opportunities afforded by multiethnic and multicultural communities and schools has underscored the need for more nuanced research on the roles of school in addressing discrimination and fostering justice as well as acculturation. Future research is needed on the roles of student and family engagement for resilience in the intersectional contexts of diverse identities, ethnicities, cultures, individual lived experiences, and histories of oppression, political conflict, or structural violence.

Finally, the cascading threats posed by the COVID-19 pandemic to children, families, schools, communities, economies, and nations around the world have underscored the multifaceted roles played by schools in the development and resilience of children and their societies. It is already clear that some societies, including the United States, have under-invested in the resilience of children and families and underestimated how essential schools are to the function and well-being of their societies. Forthcoming research on risk, resilience, and recovery in the wake of COVID-19 will undoubtedly advance our knowledge of resilience in relation to schools as well as other vital adaptive systems.

Acknowledgments Preparation of this chapter was supported by the Irving B. Harris Professorship (Masten) and a University of Minnesota Provost's Fellowship (Gillespie).

References

Anderson, L. (1994). Effectiveness and efficiency in inner-city public schools: Charting school resilience. In M. C. Wang & E. W. Gordon (Eds.), *Educational resilience in inner-city America: Challenges and prospects* (pp. 141–149). Lawrence Erlbaum Associates, Inc.

Appleton, J. J., Christenson, S. L., & Furlong, M. J. (2008). Student engagement with school: Critical conceptual and methodological issues of the construct. *Psychology in the Schools, 45*(5), 369–386. https://doi.org/10.1002/pits.20303

Bellis, M. A., Hughes, K., Ford, K., Hardcastle, K. A., Sharp, C. A., Wood, S., Homolova, L., & Davies, A. (2018). Adverse childhood experiences and sources of childhood resilience: A retrospective study of their combined relationships with child health and educational attendance. *BMC Public Health, 18*(792), 1–12. https://doi.org/10.1186/s12889-018-5699-8

Benner, A. D., & Graham, S. (2013). The antecedents and consequences of racial/ethnic discrimination during adolescence: Does the source of discrimination matter? *Developmental Psychology, 49*(8), 1602–1613. https://doi.org/10.1037/a0030557

Bierman, K. L., Domitrovich, C. E., Nix, R. L., Gest, S. D., Welsh, J. A., Greenberg, M. T., Blair, C., Nelson, K. E., & Gill, S. (2008). Promoting academic and social-emotional school readiness: The head start REDI program. *Child Development, 79*(6), 1802–1817. https://doi.org/10.1111/j.1467-8624.2008.01227.x

Blair, C., & Raver, C. C. (2015). School readiness and self-regulation: A developmental psychobiological approach. *Annual Review of Psychology, 66*(1), 711–731. https://doi.org/10.1146/annurev-psych-010814-015221

Boyce, W. T., Levitt, P., Martinez, F. D., McEwen, B. S., & Shonkoff, J. P. (2021). Genes, environments, and time: The biology of adversity and resilience. *Pediatrics, 147*(2), e20201651. https://doi.org/10.1542/peds.2020-1651

Bronfenbrenner, U., & Morris, P. A. (2006). The bioecological model of human development. In W. Damon (Series Ed.) & R. M. Lerner (Vol. Ed.), *Handbook of child psychology: Theoretical models of human development* (pp. 793–828). Wiley. https://doi.org/10.1002/9780470147658.chpsy0114

Christenson, S. L., & Pohl, A. J. (2020). The relevance of student engagement: The impact of and lessons learned implementing Check & Connect. In A. L. Reschly, A. J. Pohl, & S. L. Christenson (Eds.), *Student engagement: Effective academic, behavioral, cognitive, and affective interventions at school* (pp. 3–30). Springer International Publishing. https://doi.org/10.1007/978-3-030-37285-9_1

Christenson, S. L., Stout, K., & Pohl, A. (2012). *Check & Connect: A comprehensive student engagement intervention: Implementing with fidelity.* University of Minnesota, Institute on Community Integration.

Christmas, C. M., & Khanlou, N. (2019). Defining youth resilience: A scoping review. *International Journal of Mental Health and Addiction, 17*(3), 731–742. https://doi.org/10.1007/s11469-018-0002-x

Coates, H. (2007). A model of online and general campus-based student engagement. *Assessment & Evaluation in Higher Education, 32*(2), 121–141. https://doi.org/10.1080/02602930600801878

Colao, A., Piscitelli, P., Pulimeno, M., Colazzo, S., Miani, A., & Giannini, S. (2020). Rethinking the role of the school after COVID-19. *The Lancet Public Health, 5*(7), e370. https://doi.org/10.1016/S2468-2667(20)30124-9

Cowen, J. M. (2017). Who are the homeless? Student mobility and achievement in Michigan 2010–2013. *Educational Researcher, 46*(1), 33–43. https://doi.org/10.3102/0013189X17694165

Del Toro, J., & Wang, M. (2020). School cultural socialization and academic performance: Examining ethnic-racial identity development as a mediator among African American adolescents. *Child Development.* https://doi.org/10.1111/cdev.13467

Doll, B. (2013). Enhancing resilience in classrooms. In S. Goldstein & R. B. Brooks (Eds.), *Handbook of resilience in children* (pp. 399–409). Springer US. https://doi.org/10.1007/978-1-4614-3661-4_23

Dray, J., Bowman, J., Campbell, E., Freund, M., Wolfenden, L., Hodder, R. K., McElwaine, K., Tremain, D., Bartlem, K., Bailey, J., Small, T., Palazzi, K., Oldmeadow, C., & Wiggers, J. (2017). Systematic

review of universal resilience-focused interventions targeting child and adolescent mental health in the school setting. *Journal of the American Academy of Child & Adolescent Psychiatry, 56*(10), 813–824. https://doi.org/10.1016/j.jaac.2017.07.780

Durlak, J. A. (2009). Prevention programs. In T. B. Gutkin & C. R. Reynolds (Eds.), *The handbook of school psychology* (4th ed., pp. 905–920). Wiley.

Dvorsky, M. R., Breaux, R., & Becker, S. P. (2020). Finding ordinary magic in extraordinary times: Child and adolescent resilience during the COVID-19 pandemic. *European Child & Adolescent Psychiatry.* https://doi.org/10.1007/s00787-020-01583-8

Eccles, J. S., & Roeser, R. W. (2011). Schools as developmental contexts during adolescence: Schools as developmental contexts. *Journal of Research on Adolescence, 21*(1), 225–241. https://doi.org/10.1111/j.1532-7795.2010.00725.x

Edmonds, R. (1979). Effective schools for the urban poor. *Educational Leadership, 37*(1), 15–24.

Evans, G. W., Li, D., & Whipple, S. S. (2013). Cumulative risk and child development. *Psychological Bulletin, 139*(6), 1342–1396. https://doi.org/10.1037/a0031808

Fantuzzo, J. W., LeBoeuf, W. A., Chen, C.-C., Rouse, H. L., & Culhane, D. P. (2012). The unique and combined effects of homelessness and school mobility on the educational outcomes of young children. *Educational Researcher, 41*(9), 393–402. https://doi.org/10.3102/0013189X12468210

Folke, C. (2016). Resilience. *Ecology and Society, 21*(4), 44. https://doi.org/10.5751/ES-09088-210444

Fredricks, J. A., Reschly, A. L., & Christenson, S. L. (2019). Interventions for student engagement: Overview and state of the field. In J. A. Fredricks, A. L. Reschley, & S. L. Christenson (Eds.), *Handbook of student engagement interventions* (pp. 1–11). Elsevier.

Fritz, J., de Graaff, A. M., Caisley, H., van Harmelen, A.-L., & Wilkinson, P. O. (2018). A systematic review of amenable resilience factors that moderate and/or mediate the relationship between childhood adversity and mental health in young people. *Frontiers in Psychiatry, 9*, 230. https://doi.org/10.3389/fpsyt.2018.00230

Garmezy, N. (1985). Stress-resistant children: The search for protective factors. In J. E. Stevenson (Ed.), *Recent research in developmental psychopathology: Journal of Child Psychology and Psychiatry Book Supplement No. 4* (pp. 213–233). Pergamon Press.

Ghavami, N., Kogachi, K., & Graham, S. (2020). How racial/ethnic diversity in urban schools shapes intergroup relations and well-being: Unpacking intersectionality and multiple identities perspectives. *Frontiers in Psychology, 11*, 503846. https://doi.org/10.3389/fpsyg.2020.503846

Good, R. M. (2019). Neighborhood schools and community development: Revealing the intersections through the Philadelphia school closure debate. *Journal of Planning Education and Research.* https://doi.org/10.1177/0739456X19839769

Gottlieb, G. (2007). Probabilistic epigenesis. *Developmental Science, 10*(1), 1–11. https://doi.org/10.1111/j.1467-7687.2007.00556.x

Graham, S. (2018). Race/Ethnicity and social adjustment of adolescents: How (not if) school diversity matters. *Educational Psychologist, 53*(2), 64–77. https://doi.org/10.1080/00461520.2018.1428805

Griffiths, P. E., & Tabery, J. (2013). Developmental systems theory. In *Advances in child development and behavior* (Vol. 44, pp. 65–94). Elsevier. https://doi.org/10.1016/B978-0-12-397947-6.00003-9

Havighurst, R. J. (1974). *Developmental tasks and education* (Third edition, newly revised). McKay.

Hawkins, M., & James, C. (2018). Developing a perspective on schools as complex, evolving, loosely linking systems. *Educational Management Administration & Leadership, 46*(5), 729–748. https://doi.org/10.1177/1741143217711192

Heckman, J. J. (2006). Skill formation and the economics of investing in disadvantaged children. *Science, 312*(5782), 1900–1902. https://doi.org/10.1126/science.1128898

Henry, C. S., Sheffield Morris, A., & Harrist, A. W. (2015). Family resilience: Moving into the third wave. *Family Relations, 64*(1), 22–43. https://doi.org/10.1111/fare.12106

Höltge, J., Theron, L., Cowden, R. G., Govender, K., Maximo, S. I., Carranza, J. S., Kapoor, B., Tomar, A., van Rensburg, A., Lu, S., Hu, H., Cavioni, V., Agliati, A., Grazzani, I., Smedema, Y., Kaur, G., Hurlington, K. G., Sanders, J., Munford, R., … Ungar, M. (2021). A cross-country network analysis of adolescent resilience. *Journal of Adolescent Health, 68*(3), 580–588. https://doi.org/10.1016/j.jadohealth.2020.07.010

Huebner, G., Boothby, N., Aber, J. L., Darmstadt, G. L., Diaz, A., Masten, A. S., Yoshikawa, H., Sachs, J., Redlener, I., Emmel, A., Pitt, M., Arnold, L., Barber, B., Berman, B., Blum, R., Canavera, M., Eckerle, J., Fox, N. A., Gibbons, J., … Zeanah, C. H. (2016). Beyond survival: The case for investing in young children globally. *National Academy of Medicine Perspective Series.* https://doi.org/10.31478/201606b

Jackson, P. W. (1968). *Life in classrooms.* Holt, Rinehart and Winston. https://doi.org/10.1002/1520-6807(196807)5:3<286::AID-PITS2310050319>3.0.CO;2-P

Kuh, G. D. (2009). The national survey of student engagement: Conceptual and empirical foundations. *New Directions for Institutional Research, 2009*(141), 5–20. https://doi.org/10.1002/ir.283

Labella, M. H., & Masten, A. S. (2018). Family influences on the development of aggression and violence. *Current Opinion in Psychology, 19*, 11–16. https://doi.org/10.1016/j.copsyc.2017.03.028

Labella, M. H., Kalstabbakken, A., Johnson, J., Leppa, J., Robinson, N., Masten, A. S., & Barnes, A. J. (2017). Promoting resilience by improving children's sleep: Feasibility among families living in supportive housing. *Progress in Community Health Partnerships: Research, Education, and Action, 11*(3), 285–293. https://doi.org/10.1353/cpr.2017.0033

Ladson-Billings, G., & Tate, W. F., IV. (1995). Toward a critical race theory of education. *Teacher's College Record, 97*(1), 47–68.

Lai, B. S., Esnard, A.-M., Lowe, S. R., & Peek, L. (2016). Schools and disasters: Safety and mental health assessment and interventions for children. *Current Psychiatry Reports, 18*(12), 109. https://doi.org/10.1007/s11920-016-0743-9

Leath, S., Mathews, C., Harrison, A., & Chavous, T. (2019). Racial identity, racial discrimination, and classroom engagement outcomes among Black girls and boys in predominantly black and predominantly White school districts. *American Educational Research Journal, 56*(4), 1318–1352. https://doi.org/10.3102/0002831218816955

Lerner, R. M. (2006). Resilience as an attribute of the developmental system: Comments on the papers of professors Masten & Wachs. *Annals of the New York Academy of Sciences, 1094*(1), 40–51. https://doi.org/10.1196/annals.1376.005

Luthar, S. S. (2006). Resilience in development: A synthesis of research across five decades. In D. Cicchetti & D. J. Cohen (Eds.), *Developmental psychopathology: Risk, disorder, and adaptation* (pp. 739–795). Wiley.

Masonbrink, A. R., & Hurley, E. (2020). Advocating for children during the COVID-19 school closures. *Pediatrics, 146*(3), e20201440. https://doi.org/10.1542/peds.2020-1440

Masten, A. S. (1994). Resilience in individual development: Successful adaptation despite risk and adversity: Challenges and prospects. In *Educational resilience in inner city America: Challenges and prospects* (pp. 3–25). Lawrence Erlbaum.

Masten, A. S. (2003). Commentary: Developmental psychopathology as a unifying context for mental health and education models, research, and practice in schools. *School Psychology Review, 32*(2), 169–173. https://doi.org/10.1080/02796015.2003.12086189

Masten, A. S. (2007). Resilience in developing systems: Progress and promise as the fourth wave rises. *Development and Psychopathology, 19*(3), 921–930. https://doi.org/10.1017/S0954579407000442

Masten, A. S. (2011). Resilience in children threatened by extreme adversity: Frameworks for research, practice, and translational synergy. *Development and Psychopathology, 23*(2), 493–506. https://doi.org/10.1017/S0954579411000198

Masten, A. S. (2014a). Global perspectives on resilience in children and youth. *Child Development, 85*(1), 6–20. https://doi.org/10.1111/cdev.12205

Masten, A. S. (2014b). *Ordinary magic: Resilience in development.* Guilford Press.

Masten, A. S. (2018a). Resilience theory and research on children and families: Past, present, and promise. *Journal of Family Theory & Review, 10*(1), 12–31. https://doi.org/10.1111/jftr.12255

Masten, A. S. (2018b). Schools nurture resilience of children and societies. *Green Schools Catalyst Quarterly, V*(3), 14–19.

Masten, A. S. (2021). Resilience of children in disasters: A multisystem perspective. *International Journal of Psychology, 56*(1), 1–11. https://doi.org/10.1002/ijop.12737

Masten, A. S., & Cicchetti, D. (2010). Developmental cascades. *Development and Psychopathology, 22*(3), 491–495. https://doi.org/10.1017/S0954579410000222

Masten, A. S., & Cicchetti, D. (2016). Resilience in development: Progress and transformation. In D. Cicchetti (Ed.), *Developmental psychopathology, Vol. 4: Risk, resilience, and intervention* (3rd ed., pp. 271–333). Wiley. https://doi.org/10.1002/9781119125556.devpsy406

Masten, A. S., & Coatsworth, J. D. (1998). The development of competence in favorable and unfavorable environments. *American Psychologist, 16*. https://doi.org/10.1037/0003-066X.53.2.205

Masten, A. S., Fiat, A. E., Labella, M. H., & Strack, R. A. (2015). Educating homeless and highly mobile students: Implications of research on risk and resilience. *School Psychology Review, 44(3), 315–330*. https://doi.org/10.17105/spr-15-0068.1.

Masten, A. S., & Motti-Stefanidi, F. (2009). Understanding and promoting resilience in children: Promotive and protective processes in schools. In T. B. Gutkin & C. R. Reynolds (Eds.), *The handbook of school psychology* (4th ed., pp. 721–738). Wiley.

Masten, A. S., & Motti-Stefanidi, F. (2020). Multisystem resilience for children and youth in disaster: Reflections in the context of COVID-19. *Adversity and Resilience Science, 1*(2), 95–106. https://doi.org/10.1007/s42844-020-00010-w

Masten, A. S., & Narayan, A. J. (2012). Child development in the context of disaster, war, and terrorism: Pathways of risk and resilience. *Annual Review of Psychology, 63*(1), 227–257. https://doi.org/10.1146/annurev-psych-120710-100356

Masten, A. S., Best, K. M., & Garmezy, N. (1990). Resilience and development: Contributions from the study of children who overcome adversity. *Development and Psychopathology, 2*(4), 425–444. https://doi.org/10.1017/S0954579400005812

Masten, A. S., Roisman, G. I., Long, J. D., Burt, K. B., Obradović, J., Riley, J. R., Boelcke-Stennes, K., & Tellegen, A. (2005). Developmental cascades: Linking academic achievement and externalizing and internalizing symptoms over 20 years. *Developmental Psychology, 41*(5), 733–746. https://doi.org/10.1037/0012-1649.41.5.733

Masten, A. S., Burt, K. B., & Coatsworth, J. D. (2006). Competence and psychopathology in development. In D. Cicchetti & D. Cohen (Eds.), *Developmental psychopathology, Vol 3, Risk, disorder and psychopathology* (2nd ed., pp. 696–738). Wiley.

Masten, A. S., Motti-Stefanidi, F., & Rahl, H. A. (2019). Developmental risk and resilience in the context of devastation and forced migration. In R. D. Parke & G. H. Elder Jr. (Eds.), *Children in changing worlds: Sociocultural and temporal perspectives* (pp. 84–111). Cambridge University Press.

Masten, A. S., Lucke, C. M., Nelson, K. M., & Stallworthy, I. C. (2021). Resilience in development and psychopathology: Multisystem perspectives. *Annual Review of Clinical Psychology, 17*(1). https://doi.org/10.1146/annurev-clinpsy-081219-120307

McEwen, B. S. (2019). Resilience of the brain and body. In G. Fink (Ed.), *Handbook of stress series Vol. 3. Stress: Physiology, biochemistry, and pathology* (pp. 19–33). Academic. https://doi.org/10.1016/B978-0-12-813146-6.00002-3

Meng, X., Fleury, M.-J., Xiang, Y.-T., Li, M., & D'Arcy, C. (2018). Resilience and protective factors among people with a history of child maltreatment: A systematic review. *Social Psychiatry and Psychiatric Epidemiology, 53*(5), 453–475. https://doi.org/10.1007/s00127-018-1485-2

Milofsky, C. (2018). Schools as community institutions. In R. A. Cnaan & C. Milofsky (Eds.), *Handbook of community movements and local organizations in the 21st century* (pp. 437–446). Springer International Publishing. https://doi.org/10.1007/978-3-319-77416-9_27

Moore, H., Astor, R. A., & Benbenishty, R. (2020). Role of school-climate in school-based violence among homeless and nonhomeless students: Individual- and school-level analysis. *Child Abuse & Neglect, 102*, 104378. https://doi.org/10.1016/j.chiabu.2020.104378

Moses, J. O., & Villodas, M. T. (2017). The potential protective role of peer relationships on school engagement in at-risk adolescents. *Journal of Youth and Adolescence, 46*(11), 2255–2272. https://doi.org/10.1007/s10964-017-0644-1

Motti-Stefanidi, F. (2018). Resilience among immigrant youth: The role of culture, development and acculturation. *Developmental Review, 50*, 99–109. https://doi.org/10.1016/j.dr.2018.04.002

Motti-Stefanidi, F., & Masten, A. S. (2013). School success and school engagement of immigrant children and adolescents: A risk and resilience developmental perspective. *European Psychologist, 18*(2), 126–135. https://doi.org/10.1027/1016-9040/a000139

Motti-Stefanidi, F., & Masten, A. S. (2020). Immigrant youth resilience: Integrating developmental and cultural perspectives. In D. Güngör & D. Strohmeier (Eds.), *Contextualizing immigrant and refugee resilience: Cultural and acculturation perspectives* (pp. 11–31). Springer International Publishing. https://doi.org/10.1007/978-3-030-42303-2_2

Motti-Stefanidi, F., Pavlopoulos, V., Mastrotheodoros, S., & Asendorpf, J. B. (2020). Longitudinal interplay between peer likeability and youth's adaptation and psychological well-being: A study of immigrant and nonimmigrant adolescents in the school context. *International Journal of Behavioral Development, 44*(5), 393–403. https://doi.org/10.1177/0165025419894721

Neblett, E. W., Philip, C. L., Cogburn, C. D., & Sellers, R. M. (2006). African American adolescents' discrimination experiences and academic achievement: Racial socialization as a cultural compensatory and protective factor. *Journal of Black Psychology, 32*(2), 199–218. https://doi.org/10.1177/0095798406287072

Neem, J. N. (2017). *Democracy's schools: The rise of public education in America.* JHU Press.

Nuttman-Shwartz, O. (2019). The moderating role of resilience resources and sense of belonging to the school among children and adolescents in continuous traumatic stress situations. *The Journal of Early Adolescence, 39*(9), 1261–1285. https://doi.org/10.1177/0272431618812719

Osofsky, J. D., & Osofsky, H. J. (2021). Hurricane Katrina and the Gulf Oil Spill: Lessons learned about short-term and long-term effects. *International Journal of Psychology, 56*(1), 56–63. https://doi.org/10.1002/ijop.12729

Overton, W. F. (2013). A new paradigm for developmental science: Relationism and relational-developmental systems. *Applied Developmental Science, 17*(2), 94–107. https://doi.org/10.1080/10888691.2013.778717

Patterson, J. M. (2002). Understanding family resilience. *Journal of Clinical Psychology, 58*(3), 233–246. https://doi.org/10.1002/jclp.10019

Plumb, J. L., Bush, K. A., & Kersevich, S. E. (2016). Trauma-sensitive schools: An evidence-based approach. *School Social Work Journal, 40*(2), 37–60(24). https://doi.org/10.1007/s11256-020-00553-3

Reschly, A. L., Pohl, A. J., & Christenson, S. L. (Eds.). (2020). *Student engagement: Effective academic, behavioral, cognitive, and affective interventions at school.* Springer Nature.

Reynolds, A. J., Temple, J. A., Ou, S.-R., Robertson, D. L., Mersky, J. P., Topitzes, J. W., & Niles, M. D. (2007). Effects of a school-based, early childhood intervention on adult health and well-being: A 19-year follow-up of low-income families. *Archives of Pediatrics & Adolescent Medicine, 161*(8), 730. https://doi.org/10.1001/archpedi.161.8.730

Reynolds, A. J., Ou, S.-R., & Temple, J. A. (2018). A multicomponent, preschool to third grade preventive intervention and educational attainment at 35 years of age. *JAMA Pediatrics, 172*(3), 247. https://doi.org/10.1001/jamapediatrics.2017.4673

Robles, A., Gjelsvik, A., Hirway, P., Vivier, P. M., & High, P. (2019). Adverse childhood experiences and protective factors with school engagement. *Pediatrics, 144*(2). https://doi.org/10.1542/peds.2018-2945

Rundle, A. G., Park, Y., Herbstman, J. B., Kinsey, E. W., & Wang, Y. C. (2020). COVID-19–related school closings and risk of weight gain among children. *Obesity, 28*(6), 1008–1009. https://doi.org/10.1002/oby.22813

Sabol, T. J., & Pianta, R. C. (2012). Patterns of school readiness forecast achievement and socioemotional development at the end of elementary school: School readiness profiles. *Child Development, 83*(1), 282–299. https://doi.org/10.1111/j.1467-8624.2011.01678.x

Sanchez, A. L., Cornacchio, D., Poznanski, B., Golik, A. M., Chou, T., & Comer, J. S. (2018). The effectiveness of school-based mental health services for elementary-aged children: A meta-analysis. *Journal of the American Academy of Child & Adolescent Psychiatry, 57*(3), 153–165. https://doi.org/10.1016/j.jaac.2017.11.022

Sanders, M. T., Welsh, J. A., Bierman, K. L., & Heinrichs, B. S. (2020). Promoting resilience: A preschool intervention enhances the adolescent adjustment of children exposed to early adversity. *School Psychology (Washington, D.C.), 35*(5), 285–298. https://doi.org/10.1037/spq0000406

Shonkoff, J. P., Garner, A. S., The Committee on Psychosocial Aspects of Child and Family Health, Committee on Early Childhood, Adoption, and Dependent Care, and Section on Developmental and Behavioral Pediatrics, Siegel, B. S., Dobbins, M. I., Earls, M. F., Garner, A. S., McGuinn, L., Pascoe, J., & Wood, D. L. (2012). The lifelong effects of early childhood adversity and toxic stress. *Pediatrics, 129*(1), e232–e246. https://doi.org/10.1542/peds.2011-2663

Sleeter, C. E., & Zavala, M. (2020). *Transformative ethnic studies in schools: Curriculum, pedagogy, and research.* Teachers College Press.

Suárez-Orozco, C., Pimentel, A., & Martin, M. (2009). The significance of relationships: Academic engagement and achievement among newcomer immigrant youth. *Teachers College Record, 111*(3), 712–749.

Suárez-Orozco, C., Motti-Stefanidi, F., Marks, A., & Katsiaficas, D. (2018). An integrative risk and resilience model for understanding the adaptation of immigrant-origin children and youth. *American Psychologist, 73*(6), 781–796. https://doi.org/10.1037/amp0000265

Theron, L. (2021). Learning about systemic resilience from studies of student resilience. In M. Ungar (Ed.), *Multisystemic resilience: Adaptation and transformation in contexts of change* (pp. 232–252). Oxford University Press. https://doi.org/10.1093/oso/9780190095888.003.0014.

Theron, L. C., & Theron, A. M. C. (2014). Education services and resilience processes: Resilient Black South African students' experiences. *Children and Youth Services Review, 47*, 297–306. https://doi.org/10.1016/j.childyouth.2014.10.003

Uddin, J., Ahmmad, Z., Uddin, H., & Tatch, A. (2021). Family resilience and protective factors promote flourishing and school engagement among US children amid developmental disorder and adverse psychosocial exposure. *Sociological Spectrum*, 1–18. https://doi.org/10.1080/02732173.2021.1875089

Ungar, M. (2018). Systemic resilience: Principles and processes for a science of change in contexts of adversity. *Ecology and Society, 23*(4), art34. https://doi.org/10.5751/ES-10385-230434

Ungar, M. (2021). *Multisystemic resilience: Adaptation and transformation in contexts of change*. Oxford University Press.

Ungar, M., & Theron, L. (2020). Resilience and mental health: How multisystemic processes contribute to positive outcomes. *The Lancet Psychiatry, 7*(5), 441–448. https://doi.org/10.1016/S2215-0366(19)30434-1

Ungar, M., Connelly, G., Liebenberg, L., & Theron, L. (2019). How schools enhance the development of young people's resilience. *Social Indicators Research, 145*(2), 615–627. https://doi.org/10.1007/s11205-017-1728-8

Viner, R. M., Bonell, C., Drake, L., Jourdan, D., Davies, N., Baltag, V., Jerrim, J., Proimos, J., & Darzi, A. (2021). Reopening schools during the COVID-19 pandemic: Governments must balance the uncertainty and risks of reopening schools against the clear harms associated with prolonged closure. *Archives of Disease in Childhood, 106*(2), 111–113. https://doi.org/10.1136/archdischild-2020-319963

Walsh, F. (2016). *Strengthening family resilience* (3rd ed.). Guilford Press.

Wang, M. C., & Gordon, E. W. (Eds.). (1994). *Educational resilience in inner-city America: Challenges and prospects*. Lawrence Erlbaum Associates.

Want, M.-T., & Hofkens, T. L. (2020). Beyond classroom academics: A school-wide and multi-contextual perspective on student engagement in school. *Adolescent Research Review, 5*, 419–433. https://doi.org/10.1007/s40894-019-00115-z

Welsh, J. A., Bierman, K. L., Nix, R. L., & Heinrichs, B. N. (2020). Sustained effects of a school readiness intervention: 5th grade outcomes of the Head Start REDI program. *Early Childhood Research Quarterly, 53*, 151–160. https://doi.org/10.1016/j.ecresq.2020.03.009

Werner, E. E., & Smith, R. S. (1992). *Overcoming the odds: High risk children from birth to adulthood*. Cornell University Press.

Wittrup, A. R., Hussain, S. B., Albright, J. N., Hurd, N. M., Varner, F. A., & Mattis, J. S. (2019). Natural mentors, racial pride, and academic engagement among black adolescents: Resilience in the context of perceived discrimination. *Youth & Society, 51*(4), 463–483. https://doi.org/10.1177/0044118X16680546

Wright, M. O. D., Masten, A. S., & Narayan, A. J. (2013). Resilience processes in development: Four waves of research on positive adaptation in the context of adversity. In *Handbook of resilience in children* (pp. 15–37). Springer.

Zelazo, P. D. (2020). Executive function and psychopathology: A neurodevelopmental perspective. *Annual Review of Clinical Psychology, 16*(1), 431–454. https://doi.org/10.1146/annurev-clinpsy-072319-024242

Developmental Relationships and Student Academic Motivation: Current Research and Future Directions

Peter C. Scales, Kent Pekel,
and Benjamin J. Houltberg

Abstract

In this chapter, we describe our applied research on student-teacher relationships and motivation, which builds on extensive theoretical and measurement foundations, most especially drawing on self-determination theory, and which blends the traditional lines of motivation and engagement research in psychology (which has tended to emphasize internal, individual influences) and education (which has tended to emphasize teacher behaviors that promote engagement, such as relationship interactions). Most importantly, our work more comprehensively defines the criteria that make student-teacher relationships more developmentally influential than being merely positive connections between young people and the "caring adults" that teachers are often urged to be on social media and in professional development workshops. Our studies and the studies of other scholars show that caring is a necessary but not sufficient element of the *developmental relationships* that enable students to learn and thrive.

Drawing on multiple studies, we outline a theory of change for how student-teacher developmental relationships influence student motivation and educational outcomes, and conclude by addressing three broad themes needing robust attention in both research and practice. These include strengthening the cultural validity and responsiveness of the Developmental Relationships Framework, better understanding and activating young people themselves as drivers of developmental relationships in and outside of school settings, and leveraging in practice a deeper knowledge of not just the adult-youth dyad but how single relationships have their effects within a larger web of developmental relationships.

We start this chapter with a thought experiment: Recall your middle and high school days. When were you engaged at/with/in school? When did you care? When did it really matter to you, not just how you did in terms of grades or tests, but whether you understood the material, because you really wanted to understand, because you were that interested in it? When did you look forward to going to school, not just to see friends, but because you knew something interesting was going to happen in at least one class? When did you work hardest at your schoolwork, especially

P. C. Scales (✉) · B. J. Houltberg
Search Institute, Minneapolis, MN, USA
e-mail: scalespc@searchinstitute.org;
benh@search-institute.org

K. Pekel
Rochester Public Schools, Rochester, MN, USA

© The Author(s), under exclusive license to Springer Nature Switzerland AG 2022
A. L. Reschly, S. L. Christenson (eds.), *Handbook of Research on Student Engagement*,
https://doi.org/10.1007/978-3-031-07853-8_13

257

when it was challenging? What was going on in those moments, who were you with, what was influencing you to care and try hard?

Most likely, the scenes you recreated included images of a favorite teacher or teachers. Friends and parents may have been in the mix, too, but our guess is that it would be rare for most people to recall their times of great motivation and engagement with school without recalling their relationships with one or more teachers.

Why a Focus on Relationships?

Relationships and Motivation

That surmise is, of course, supported by a vast literature showing that young people's experience of caring, positive relationships with teachers and other adults is significantly associated with not only student motivation and engagement in educational settings but also a wide range of other positive developmental outcomes in and outside of school (e.g., Pianta et al., 2012; Roorda et al., 2011; Wentzel, 2012), even including measures of later adult health (Kim, 2021).

The field's construct terminology is sometimes unfortunate because it inadvertently minimizes the social roots of motivation. For example, belonging and social connectedness are integral components of the theory that is nevertheless called "*self-determination* theory" (Ryan & Deci, 2000). All major theories of human motivation implicate the quality of relationships as the fuel that energizes our actions, even if they do not always explicitly center on relationships. For example, Martin and Dowson (2009) conducted an extensive review of how interpersonal relationships affect students' motivation, engagement, and achievement, concluding that influential motivational theories (e.g., attribution theory, expectancy-value theory, goal theory, self-efficacy theory, self-worth theory, and especially, self-determination theory) describe motivation in relational terms. Even when relationships are not at the core of those theories, they noted that "there is often a clear relevance for interpersonal relationships" (p.332) in achievement motivation research.

In the school setting, scholars increasingly note that student-teacher relationships are foundational for motivation, and therefore deserving of primary emphasis (e.g., Lazowski & Hulleman, 2016; Wentzel & Wigfield, 2009). For example, Pianta et al. (2012) claimed that "the central problem in school reform" (p. 368) is the need for stronger student-teacher relationships, perhaps because, as they put it, "Engagement reflects relationally mediated participation in opportunity" (p. 367). The University of Chicago Consortium on Chicago Schools Research similarly situated relationships as foundational for development, learning, and opportunity: "the intentional provision of opportunities for young people to experience, interact, and make meaning of their experiences [is] the central vehicle for learning and development" (Nagaoka et al., 2015, p. 1).

Positive student-teacher relationships are fundamental, but we should note at the outset that they also are just one part of the multilayered system of teaching and learning that both students and teachers experience, where *teacher* quality and *teaching* quality interact (not to mention student variables and the larger cultural context) to affect motivation, engagement, and performance (Darling-Hammond, 2012). A knowledgeable, pedagogically-skilled teacher who is enthusiastic, fair, adaptive, committed to all students learning and to their own ongoing improvement still "may not be able to offer high-quality instruction in a context where she is asked to teach a flawed curriculum unsupported by appropriate materials or assessments. Similarly, a well-prepared teacher may perform poorly when asked to teach outside the field of his or her preparation or under poor teaching conditions—for example, without adequate teaching materials, in substandard space, with too little time, or to classes that are far too large" (Darling-Hammond, 2012, p. 4).

Likewise, effective teaching practices from classroom management skills to how teachers provide feedback are inevitably done within—and help contribute to for better or worse—the quality of the relationships teachers have with each of their students and their classes as a whole. Thus, in this chapter, what we discuss as effective *relational* practices may be read by some as just being what is meant by good teaching practice. But the studies we cite here and the student-teacher relationships literature more broadly make it abundantly clear that strong student-teacher relationships are the vehicle within which those commonly-known effective teaching practices most powerfully occur. Developmental relationships by themselves are an important source of *motivation* in the sense of a desire to exert effort toward a purpose, but not necessarily a cause of *engagement* unless other factors are present (see more below on motivation vs. engagement).

What good teaching practice does, much like what good youth development work does, is provide students with developmental *experiences* that are, as Nagaoka et al. (2015) described them, "opportunities for action and reflection that help young people build self-regulation, knowledge and skills, mindsets, and values, and develop agency, an integrated identity, and competencies" (p. 5). Whether it is within required academic subject areas at school or in voluntary participation in out-of-school time programs in students' areas of personal interests (e.g., sports, the arts, robotics, and computers), in high-quality classes or programs it is the experiences—the opportunities for action and reflection that ultimately make meaning of the experiences—that move students from being motivated to being engaged (Immordino-Yang, 2016). Further, it is within developmental *relationships* that encouragement is given to students to "reflect on their experiences and help them to interpret those experiences in ways that expand their sense of themselves and their horizons," in a continuing cycle of experiencing, interacting, and reflecting that is a "critical engine for children's development" (Nagaoka et al., 2015, p. 5).

Relationships, Motivation, and Self-Determination Theory

Connell and Wellborn (1991) put forth a general self-system process theory of motivation (see also Skinner & Belmont, 1993), not specifically about academic motivation but highly relevant for it, that itself draws heavily on self-determination theory (Ryan & Deci, 2000). Applying Connell and Wellborn's formulation to education, teachers' provision of structure (including how they communicate about expectations), support for autonomy (including how teachers connect learning with students' interests), and "involvement" (their term for relational qualities such as expressed care, enjoying time spent with students, and being attuned and responsive to their needs) are seen as direct facilitators of motivation, which in turn more proximally affect students' school adjustment and outcomes. More recently, Guay et al. (2021) similarly situated motivation within self-determination theory, finding that initial levels and increases in relatedness with teachers (and fathers) predicted better student engagement and grades, and less risk behavior and aggression over 5 years, in a sample of nearly 1000 secondary school students in Quebec. Martin and Dowson (2009) also described how *high-quality* relationships with teachers can help students meet basic human needs for autonomy, belonging, and competence, which together then promote students' effort, participation, cooperation, self-regulation skills, and academic performance.

One such relationship-based intervention, Check & Connect, for example, is explicitly grounded in mentors helping students satisfy those needs identified in self-determination theory: "Building a trusting relationship, committing to and never giving up on students, and engaging in problem solving irrespective of student behavior and response, helps the mentor fuel students' motivation-to-learn. While cautious about over-reliance on extrinsic reinforcement and rewards, the mentor attends primarily to students' psychological needs for autonomy ('I want to and value; I make choices'), belonging ('I belong; I identify'), and competence ('I can; I am willing to try and take a risk'"; Christenson & Pohl, 2020, p. 25).

The influence of relationships on more distal outcomes (e.g., school success) may sometimes be indirect, but relationships are always in the equation. In this sense, the long-standing distinction made in the field between intrinsic and extrinsic motivation is often a false dichotomy. While it is true that extrinsic incentives for student effort such as prizes and negative consequences are often misaligned with what authentically motivates young people, in a more holistic sense, extrinsic factors that really mean something to students can be powerful sources of motivation. As Reschly and Christenson (2012) pointed out, the sources of students' "internal" motivation (e.g., values, identity and other self-perceptions, sense of the future, and goals) are themselves shaped and molded by "external" factors in the proximal and distal ecology, from relationships starting with the infant's parent and caregiver attachments, to the influence of friends, teachers, coaches, and mentors, to the students' personal and ecological socio-political contexts (racial, ethnic, sex, gender, socioeconomic, religious, historical, etc.).

In her book *Multiplication is for White People: Raising Expectations for Other People's Children,* Lisa Delpit (2012) aptly captures the interplay between students' internal motivation to learn and teacher-student relationships when she notes that "many of our children of color don't learn *from* a teacher, as much as *for* a teacher. They don't want to disappoint a teacher who they feel believes in them. They may, especially if they are older, resist the teacher's pushing initially, but they are disappointed if the teacher gives up, stops pushing" (p. 86).

Motivation Versus Engagement

Reschly and Christenson (2012) described the significant confusion in the field over the meaning of motivation and engagement, and whether and how they are distinguishable. They concluded that motivation as an internal intent or desire to get involved with and put effort into schoolwork was necessary but not sufficient for engagement in the sense of student actions in the academic, affective, cognitive, and behavioral domains. We have generally followed this dis-

tinction in how we have conceptualized and measured motivation and discuss it in this chapter. We emphasize motivation as a largely internal process and a mediating influence between student-teacher relationships and educational outcomes (e.g., wanting to exert effort, being interested in schoolwork) and engagement as a more externally observable process that can be measured using a range of educational outcome variables (e.g., attendance, class participation, grades, test scores).

Measures of students' "commitment to learning" (including achievement motivation, school engagement, and bonding to school) have been prominent for decades in our research on the external and internal developmental assets youth need to succeed (Benson et al., 2006). Thus, it has been a natural evolution for academic motivation to be the central outcome studied in Search Institute's research on student-teacher developmental relationships.

In order to examine associations between developmental relationships and students' motivation, we defined motivation more as an internal construct. Our model of student motivation draws on a mixture of social-cognitive and self-determination theories embodying effort and aspirations,[1] which are influenced by teachers (and others). In contrast, for the most part our measures of *engagement* have been conceived of as outcomes distinguished from motivation. For example, we have used sense of belonging to

---

[1]Effort and aspirations reflect intra-individual strengths such as autonomy and competence, but these do not develop independent of young people's relationships, including students' relationships with teachers. In a stand-alone measure of motivation, we would have more specifically addressed the relational component, but all of our studies in schools have used student-teacher developmental relationships as a predictor of motivation, and thus, we could not include those relationships as both predictor and outcome. In an early pilot study in a diverse high school where we combined into one measure Relationships and measures of Effort, Aspirations, Cognition, and Heart (students' deep personal interests or "sparks") (REACH), we found that students with a total REACH score at least at the average level ("Meets Goal") were nearly 2 ½ times more likely to have a B+ or higher GPA (Exp(B) = 2.44, $p = 0.001$).

school as an indicator of *affective engagement*, attendance and discipline referrals as *behavioral engagement*, and grades as an indicator of *academic engagement*. Only one of the *motivation* items we use measures self-report of actual behavior ("I work hard on all assignments even if they won't affect my grade"), with the remaining items being beliefs, values, and self-perceptions more consistent with framing motivation as an internal construct (e.g., "I am certain I can master the skills taught in school this year," "It is important to me to do well compared to others in my classes," or "I like classes that really challenge me so I can learn new things"; Scales et al., 2019b).

Our model reflects Wentzel and Miele's (2016) call for a multidimensional definition of motivation in that it consists of five scales reflecting dominant theories of motivation: mastery/performance orientation (e.g., Elliot & Church, 1997), belief in malleable intelligence (Dweck, 2015), academic self-efficacy (e.g., Midgley et al., 2000), goal orientation (e.g., Wentzel & Wigfield, 2009), and internal locus of control (e.g., Shepherd et al., 2006). These constructs emerge from the extensive body of research that shows that the way students view their own intelligence, for example, whether they consider that effort can help them become smarter (growth mindset) or whether their intelligence is set from birth (fixed mindset) has a powerful influence on the effort they put into school (Dweck & Master, 2009). Aspirations include an orientation toward setting goals and an internal locus of control. These dimensions of motivation emphasize students' sense that they have control over their own future (Damon, 2004; Yeager & Dweck, 2012; Yeager et al., 2014).

In this chapter, we describe our own applied research on student-teacher relationships and motivation, which builds on these theoretical and measurement foundations and blends the traditional lines of motivation and engagement research in *psychology* (which has tended to emphasize internal, individual influences) and *education* (which has tended to emphasize teacher behaviors that promote engagement, such

as relationship interactions; Skinner & Belmont, 1993). Most importantly, our work more comprehensively defines the criteria that make student-teacher relationships more developmentally influential than being merely connections between young people and the "caring adults" that teachers are often urged to be on social media and in professional development workshops. Our studies and the studies of other scholars show that caring is a necessary but not sufficient element of the developmental relationships that enable students to learn and thrive.

What Is the Search Institute Developmental Relationships Framework?

Literature Foundations for the Framework

There is a considerable body of research on the role of student-teacher relationships in student academic motivation, with most studies focusing on one or both of two major aspects of those relationships: Teacher expressions of their caring about students (projecting warmth, and/or providing social support, or promoting feelings of trust in their students), and teachers challenging students to grow, as when they communicate high expectations for students' performance (as reviewed in, for example, Roorda et al., 2011; Wentzel, 2002). Studies focusing largely on those aspects of caring and challenge, and sometimes social support, have shown that student-teacher relationships convincingly contribute to student motivation and achievement, including grades, test scores, and reduction in dropout (Bernstein-Yamashiro & Noam, 2013; Cornelius-White, 2007; Kannapel & Clements, 2005; Lee, 2012; Wang, 1990; Wentzel, 2012). As Wentzel's (2012) extensive research review found, teacher communications and expectations, willingness to provide help, advice, and instruction, and emotional support and safety are consistently found to be related to students' motivation, engagement, and achievement, with the effects greater for low-income students, students of color, and under-achieving students.

A significant body of research that has shown that teachers who are "warm demanders" have a particularly powerful influence on the learning and the lives of African-American young people and other young people of color. As Delpit (2012) writes in the same work cited above, "Warm demanders expect a great deal of their students, convince them of their own brilliance, and help them reach their potential in a disciplined environment" (p. 77). Delpit goes on to note that warm demanders build relationships with young people that are "imbued with a sense of trust, confidence, and psychological safety that allows students to take risks, admit errors, ask for help, and experience failure along the way to higher levels of learning" (p. 83).

Building on this research (and a dozen other large streams of research from attachment studies to mentoring to juvenile delinquency research), and most specifically extending the work of Li and Julian (2012), in 2013 Search Institute launched an effort to build a framework for *developmental relationships* that would holistically capture the essential relational nutrients that young people need to thrive. The Developmental Relationships Framework grew out of Search Institute's 30 years of theory, research, and practical application of the Developmental Assets Framework for positive youth development around the world.

First introduced in 1990, the assets framework named 40 external supports (relationships and opportunities) and internal strengths (values, skills, and self-perceptions) organized into eight broad categories (e.g., Support, Empowerment, Commitment to Learning, Social Competencies) that research had shown were linked to lower levels of risk behaviors, better odds of resilience, and more thriving behaviors in youth (e.g., reviewed in Scales & Leffert, 2004). Dozens of studies with now more than six million youth and young adults worldwide consistently showed that

Table 1 Relational emphasis of the 40 developmental assets

External assets
Support
1. **Family support**—Family life provides high levels of love and support.
2. **Positive family communication**—Young person and her or his parent(s) communicate positively, and young person is willing to seek advice and counsel from parent(s).
3. **Other adult relationships**—Young person receives support from three or more nonparent adults.
4. **Caring neighborhood**—Young person experiences caring neighbors.
5. **Caring school climate**—School provides a caring, encouraging environment.
6. **Parent involvement in schooling**—Parent(s) are actively involved in helping young person succeed in school.
Empowerment
7. **Community values youth**—Young person perceives that adults in the community value youth.
8. **Youth as resources**—Young people are given useful roles in the community.
9. **Service to others**—Young person serves in the community 1 hour or more per week.
10. **Safety**—Young person feels safe at home, at school, and in the neighborhood.
Boundaries and expectations
11. **Family boundaries**—Family has clear rules and consequences and monitors the young person's whereabouts.
12. **School boundaries**—School provides clear rules and consequences.
13. **Neighborhood boundaries**—Neighbors take responsibility for monitoring young people's behavior.
14. **Adult role models**—Parent(s) and other adults model positive, responsible behavior.
15. **Positive peer influence**—Young person's best friends model responsible behavior.
16. **High expectations**—Both parent(s) and teachers encourage the young person to do well.
Constructive use of time
17. **Creative activities**—Young person spends three or more hours per week in lessons or practice in music, theater, or other arts.
18. **Youth programs**—Young person spends three or more hours per week in sports, clubs, or organizations at school and/or in the community.
19. **Religious community**—Young person spends one or more hours per week in activities in a religious institution.

(continued)

Table 1 (continued)

20. **Time at home**—Young person is out with friends "with nothing special to do" two or fewer nights per week.

Internal assets

Commitment to Learning

21. **Achievement motivation**—Young person is motivated to do well in school.

22. School engagement—Young person is actively engaged in learning.

23. Homework—Young person reports doing at least 1 hour of homework every school day.

24. **Bonding to school**—Young person cares about her or his school.

25. Reading for pleasure—Young person reads for pleasure three or more hours per week.

Positive values

26. **Caring**—Young person places high value on helping other people.

27. **Equality and social justice**—Young person places high value on promoting equality and reducing hunger and poverty.

28. **Integrity**—Young person acts on convictions and stands up for her or his beliefs.

29. **Honesty**—Young person "tells the truth even when it is not easy."

30. **Responsibility**—Young person accepts and takes personal responsibility.

31. **Restraint**—Young person believes it is important not to be sexually active or to use alcohol or other drugs.

Social competencies

32. Planning and decision making—Young person knows how to plan ahead and make choices.

33. **Interpersonal competence**—Young person has empathy, sensitivity, and friendship skills.

34. **Cultural competence**—Young person has knowledge of and comfort with people of different cultural/racial/ethnic backgrounds.

35. **Resistance skills**—Young person can resist negative peer pressure and dangerous situations.

36. **Peaceful conflict resolution**—Young person seeks to resolve conflict nonviolently.

Positive identity

37. Personal power—Young person feels he or she has control over "things that happen to me."

38. Self-esteem—Young person reports having a high self-esteem.

39. **Sense of purpose**—Young person reports that "my life has a purpose."

40. **Positive view of personal future**—Young person is optimistic about her or his personal future.

Note: Assets with an explicit or inherent relational context are **bolded**

the more assets young people experienced, the better off they were on numerous academic, psychological, social-emotional, spiritual, and behavioral outcomes (Benson et al., 2006, 2011a, b). Table 1 shows (the **bolded** assets) that *all of the external assets and the majority of the "internal" assets are rooted in and take their meaning from interactions with others, from relationships.*

The external assets in particular were centered on the positive relationships young people had in their families, schools, communities, and peer groups. In a 2019 confirmatory analysis and invariance testing (Syvertsen et al., 2019), the original categories and assets were reduced to a more parsimonious and conceptually and empirically defensible set of measures that sharpened the core emphasis on relationships. These included *Support* (support from family, other adult relationships such as teachers, and parent involvement in school); *Mattering and Belonging* (caring school climate and community valuing youth); *Boundaries* (in the family, school, and neighborhood); and *Extra-Curricular Activity Participation* (in sports, other school activities, volunteering, creative and performing arts, and religious involvement). The Developmental Relationships Framework zeroed in on and elaborated that emphasis on the quality of young people's relationships in order to create a more comprehensive theory, measurement, and practice framework around relational quality.

Developmental Relationships Defined

We heuristically defined developmental relationships as *close connections through which young people discover who they are (their identity), cultivate abilities to shape their own lives (agency), and engage with and contribute to the world around them (connections and contributions to community*; Pekel et al., 2018). Through extensive reviews across multiple strands of relationships literature, quantitative pilot tests, and focus groups with parents, students, and youth-serving

Table 2 The developmental relationships framework

Elements	Actions	Definitions
1.1.1.1.1. **Express care** *Show me that I matter to you.*	Be dependable	Be someone I can trust.
	Listen	Really pay attention when we are together
	Believe in me	Make me feel known and valued
	Be warm	Show me you enjoy being with me
	Encourage	Praise me for my efforts and achievements
1.1.1.2. **Challenge growth** *Push me to keep getting better.*	Expect my best	Expect me to live up to my potential
	Stretch	Push me to go further
	Hold me accountable	Insist I take responsibility for my actions
	Reflect on failures	Help me learn from mistakes and setbacks
1.1.1.3. Provide support *Help me complete tasks and achieve goals.*	Navigate	Guide me through hard situations and systems
	Empower	Build my confidence to take charge of my life
	Advocate	Stand up for me when I need it
	Set boundaries	Put in place limits that keep me on track
1.1.1.4. Share power *Treat me with respect and give me a say.*	Respect me	Take me seriously and treat me fairly
	Include me	Involve me in decisions that affect me
	Collaborate	Work with me to solve problems and reach goals
	Let me lead	Give me chances to take action and lead
1.1.5. Expand possibilities *Connect me with people that broaden my world.*	Inspire	Enable me to see possibilities for my future
	Broaden horizons	Expose me to new ideas and experiences
	Connect	Introduce me to people who can help me grow

practitioners in school and community settings, we created the Developmental Relationships Framework (details in Pekel et al., 2018), which names five interconnected elements that define a developmental relationship (see Table 2). The goal was to create a framework that could be applied across contexts (families, schools, out of school time) because young people experience life across all those contexts. We also sought to create a framework that could inform both research and practice and bring the two together. Thus, we intentionally articulated the specific *actions*, 20 in all, that promote each of five broad relational elements, in order to inform and motivate their use in practice.

In this framework, *expressing care* involves actions through which teachers show students that they matter. *Challenging growth* involves the teachers' actions that push their students to keep improving. When a teacher helps their students complete tasks and achieve goals, they are *providing support*. When a teacher treats their students with respect and gives them a say in the classroom, they are *sharing power*. And finally, to *expand possibilities*, teachers connect their students with people, places, and ideas that broaden their worlds.

The Tension Between Factor Independence and Framework Holism

Although rhetorically distinguishable for the sake of clearly identifying key features of developmentally-influential relationships, the five elements of developmental relationships are best understood as connected and overlapping to varying degrees, in both conceptualization and in teacher practice. Thus, for example, even though these five elements emerged in part from factor analyses, they are not entirely orthogonal. For example, we have found in quantitative studies that the five elements are moderately to strongly correlated with each other (.50s–.80s; Scales et al., 2019b, 2020b).[2] Qualitative methods (focus groups with students and interviews with teachers) also have surfaced that it is the overall relationship that youth experience, with these features of the relationship being namable and describable, but not perceived by students and teachers as separate from each other (Sethi & Scales, 2020).

Our studies have encompassed more than the school setting, and we have reached similar conclusions across the ecological contexts of families and out-of-school-time programs. Consistently, the research has shown that when young people experience relationships with adults that are characterized by these five elements in families, schools, and out-of-school time programs, their social-emotional competencies, psychological, and academic outcomes such as grades are significantly stronger (Pekel et al., 2018; Scales et al., 2019a, b, 2020a, b; Sethi & Scales, 2020; Syvertsen et al., 2020). For example, in a study of

nearly 13,000 middle and high school students and 1200 staff in schools, out-of-school time programs, and school-based student support programs (Search Institute, 2020b), young people who reported having strong developmental relationships also perceived their own socioemotional competencies (i.e., self-awareness, self-management, responsible decision-making, social awareness, and relationship skill) to be at significantly higher levels compared to youth who reported weak and moderate levels: 22% reported strong social-emotional skills if they had weak relationships, 38% did with moderate relationships, and 68% did with strong developmental relationships in those settings.

Beyond Frequency of Interactions: Relationships as Planting Seeds of Trust

When we share the Developmental Relationships Framework with teachers, out-of-school time (OST) program staff, and other practitioners in workshops and applied research projects, their first reaction is often one of enthusiasm. They remark that the framework both validates and better informs their efforts to build relationships with all young people. Shortly after that initial wave of enthusiasm, however, someone in the session often asks, "Does this mean I need to do all twenty of these things all the time with all students?"

Practitioners are often relieved when we tell them that the answer to that question is *no*. Our studies and the studies of other scholars suggest that while the frequency with which young people experience the elements of developmental relationships matters, it is the authenticity and the timing of the action that matters even more. As Rhodes et al. (2006) noted in a study of mentoring relationships: Not "every moment in the... relationship need be packed with profundity and personal growth" (p. 697). Rhodes et al. (2006) observe that what differentiates a developmental relationship "from a series of casual contacts is the meaning attributed to those interactions" (p. 697).

---

[2]Unpublished factor analysis showed a complex factor structure, in which oblique rotation yielded either a 3- or 5-factor model (CF-Equamax and CF-Facparsim yielded the same results) that substantially but not fully reflected the a priori five elements. Although both of these models also had good CFA indices, they still did not fully fit the a priori elements conceptually and still had high cross-loadings, although the 3-factor model reflected the five elements in a more parsimonious way. The 3-factor results reflected relatively higher levels of distinctions across the following of the 20 actions named in Table 1 and can be seen as roughly representing the three motivational needs articulated in self-determination theory, namely, a Care/Warmth Factor (i.e., belonging; Listen, Value me, Be warm), an Expectations/Demandingness Factor (competence; Expect my best, Set Boundaries, Hold me Accountable), and an Empower/Motivate/Connect Factor (autonomy; Include me, Inspire, Broaden, Connect). At the same time, however, a unidimensional CFA provided the best fit to the data ($x^2 = 11,061$, $df = 140$, $p < 0.001$; RMSEA = 0.073; CFI = 0.915; TLI = 0.905; SRMR = 0.04, and meeting the criteria for metric (weak factorial) and scalar (strong factorial) invariance by school level, gender, and race/ethnicity based on ΔCFI guidelines). Thus, the five elements are best seen not as separate dimensions of developmental relationships, but as identifiable themes or descriptors of interaction that together complexly contribute to a developmental relationships construct best currently represented analytically as unidimensional (with the 3 factor model still being investigated) but that in practice is best seen as including varying degrees of the five elements.

This does not suggest that frequency is unimportant. The regularity with which an adult relates with a young people in these ways whenever interaction happens may itself be evidence to a young person of dependability and enduring affirmation from that adult. In a quite ordinary way (Masten, 2001), this kind of consistently "being there" for a young person, even if the moments are infrequent, may help fill the young person's basic psychological needs for autonomy, belonging, and competence. The 20 actions in the Developmental Relationships Framework matter because they create a sense of mutual bonding and concern, within which each person senses that the other person will "be there" for them if needed. As we noted in one of our studies of the effectiveness of social capital-building programs with and for opportunity youth, this sense of being there when it counts plants much-needed "seeds of trust" (Syvertsen et al., 2021). In that sense, a developmental relationship serves as both a current nutrient for youth today, and perhaps as or even more important, a promise and a commitment for the future (Duncan-Andrade, 2009).

Developmental relationships, whether among youth workers and youth, students and teachers, or parents and children, have ups and downs in intensity and relevance over time. Not every one of the 20 actions in Table 2 occurs with great frequency, or necessarily needs to; their importance is because those actions occur when the young person wants and needs them to, in a relationship that matters to them and meets their needs for autonomy, belonging, and competence. Over time (but not every moment), and from their web of relationships (not necessarily just from one dyadic relationship) young people need to experience all five of the relationship elements as expressed in a number (not necessarily all 20) of these actions. For example, the Express Care element is made up of actions that can and should be frequently experienced, and that are generally easy for adults in a young person's life to do. Challenge Growth is also a fairly frequent and easy to implement relational element, especially common at school. But Provide Support, Share Power, and Expand Possibilities are less common and more complex (see Scales, Roehlkepartain

et al., 2022 for a more extended treatment). The opportunities adults have to do these things in a specific way occur more situationally, not on a regular, much less a daily basis.

This much seems clear from our qualitative research work with schools and youth-serving organizations across the United States: young people notice and remember the degree to which adults create a space that feels supportive overall, and help them when they need it, where they are free to express opinions and have voice, and where they are exposed to ideas or people or things they didn't know or appreciate before. When viewed that way, the several developmental relationships elements are reflected in an overall feel for the milieu adults and young people create, a general relational repertoire that reflects a good person (stage)-environment fit (Eccles et al., 1993; Hunt, 1975) rather than being necessarily reflected in a specific number of times an action can be observed and counted.

Research Results: Developmental Relationships Predicting Motivation and School Success

Across the Search Institute student-teacher relationship studies cited in this chapter, whether using person-centered approaches (e.g., Latent Transition Analysis) or variable-centered approaches (e.g., ANCOVAs, regressions, Structural Equation Modeling), our quantitative studies have found several clear patterns. The studies have included reasonably-large and demographically diverse samples, as Table 3 shows. The measures used for student-teacher developmental relationships, academic motivation, and outcomes including sense of belonging to school, school climate, and perceptions of instructional quality have had good-to-excellent alpha reliabilities (0.70–.90s), and acceptable fit indices (i.e., CFI, TLI, SRMR, RMSEA), as presented in the associated papers listed in the table and included in the References.

The most salient conclusions we have reached about developmental relationships and academic motivation through these studies include:

Table 3 Demographic composition of search institute's student-teacher relationships samples

Scales et al. (2019a, b)	1274 middle and high school students from first-ring suburb of a large metropolitan area in the Midwest	82% grades 6–8 50% female, 1% transgender 15% African American, 9% Asian/Pacific Islander, 2% Native American/Alaska Native; 39% white; 17% mixed race; 18% other 26% Latinx 52% eligible for free and reduced-price lunch
Scales et al. (2020a, b)	534 grades 6–8 students from a middle school in the same district as above	35% grade 6, 30% grade 7, 35% grade 8 51% female, <1% transgender 12% African American, 7% Asian/Pacific Islander, 1% Native American/Alaska Native, 56% white, 13% mixed race, 11% other 13% Latinx 35% eligible for free and reduced-price lunch; 25% of total sample (not just of FRL-eligible) reported high family financial strain
Sethi and Scales (2020)	623 middle school students and 672 high school students from two of the three schools in the Scales et al., (2019a, b) study	Grade 6–12% ranged from 11% in grade 12 to 18% in grade 10 49% female, 1% transgender 17% African American, 9% Asian/Pacific Islander, 3% Native American/Alaska Native, 29% white, 20% mixed race, 23% other 35% Latinx 58% eligible for free and reduced-price lunch
Scales et al. (2021)	786 grades 6–8 students from one of the middle schools in Scales et al. (2019a, b)	35% grade 6, 35% grade 7, 30% grade 8 48% female, <1% transgender 30% African American, 8% Asian/Pacific Islander, 3% Native American/Alaska Native, 22% white, 23% mixed race, 27% other 37% Latinx 68% eligible for free and reduced-price lunch

- Only a minority of children and youth experience good/high levels of developmental relationships with their teachers.
- Share power and expand possibilities are the least-often reported relational elements.
- Levels of student-teacher developmental relationships stay flat or decline over the course of a school year.
- Middle school students report having better relationships with teachers than do high school students.
- Student-teacher developmental relationships in some studies are lower for lower-SES students (FRL eligible).
- Student-teacher developmental relationships decline over time for all socioeconomic groups of students but even more so for lower-SES students (FRL eligible and financially strained students).
- Higher levels of student-teacher developmental relationships are strongly linked to better academic motivation, perceptions of school climate, belongingness at school, and perceived quality of instruction, and indirectly to Grae-Point-Average (GPA), at both the middle and high school levels.
- Improvement in student-teacher developmental relationships over the school year is linked to higher motivation, more positive perceptions of school climate, stronger sense of belongingness, better perceptions of quality of instruction, and higher GPA.
- Only a minority of students report that student-teacher developmental relationships naturally improve by a meaningful amount over the school year when there is no specific intervention in place to strengthen them.

In addition to cross-sectional research, two recent studies (see Table 3 for sample details) have used the developmental relationship framework to track student-teacher relationships across one academic year. One study measured the quality of middle school students' relationships with their teachers (20 items measuring the 20 developmental relationships actions in Table 2) at the beginning and end of one academic year, and the other followed both middle- and high-school students across the year. In the latter study, students' academic motivation (15 items measuring mastery/performance orientation, belief in malleable intelligence, academic self-efficacy, achievement v social goal orientation, and internal locus of control) had a downward trajectory (Scales et al., 2019b), which is consistent with previous studies (Gillet et al., 2012; Wang & Eccles, 2012). However, when students reported an *increase* in the quality of their relationships with their teachers, they also reported higher year-end academic motivation, perceptions of school climate (2 items measuring whether students think teachers care about them, and feel they are disciplined fairly) and instructional quality (3 items measuring how much teachers make learning interesting, and give students specific suggestions for improvement), and had higher GPAs at year end. It was rare for student-teacher relationship quality to improve across the academic year, and so most students could not benefit from this meaningful potential influence on motivation.

In the second study, student-teacher relationships were strongly related to middle-school students' academic motivation at both the beginning and end of the year, and directly predicted students' perceptions of school climate (measured as above) and belonging (2 items measuring how much students feel like a part of their school, and feel part of a community at school; Scales et al., 2020b). Relationships indirectly predicted students' GPA, through relationships' strong effect on motivation. Student-teacher relationships declined more for students with high levels of self-reported family financial strain than they did for students reporting their families didn't face financial strain (a single item from 1 ["We have enough money to buy almost anything we want"] to 4 ["We can't buy the things we need sometimes"]).

These results take on additional salience in view of the relative importance of relationships with teachers over other relational supports for motivation. For example, in another study, we found that student-teacher developmental rela-

tionships are more important for predicting students' motivation (as well as school climate and GPA) than are relationships with parents or peers (Sethi & Scales, 2020). For middle school students, developmental relationships with both teachers and parents predicted motivation, but relationships with teachers was the far stronger influence. For high school students, only developmental relationships with teachers predicted motivation.

Student-Teacher Relationships as Social Capital

A person-centered approach in another study of a large and diverse sample of middle-school students (see demographics in Table 3; Scales et al., 2021) confirmed and extended these results about the importance of developmental relationships to students' motivation. In that research, we constructed a measure of *relational social capital* by combining the measures of the five developmental relationships elements (Express Care, Challenge Growth, Provide Support, Share Power, and Expand Possibilities) with two other aspects of student-teacher relationships: students' reports of how much teachers connected learning to student interests (3 items measuring teacher efforts to find out about students' interests and talents, and show them how their classwork relates to those interests and talents) and the degree to which students found the classroom to be culturally affirming (3 items measuring how much teachers talk positively about contributions people of the student's culture or race have made, and how much they encourage students to share about their cultural background in class).

Using Latent Transition Analysis, we found that most students (60%) were in a group characterized by low to moderate scores on all seven of these aspects of student-teacher relationships. Students in the low-scoring group reported that their relationships with their teachers were not good, their deep personal interests were not getting connected to their learning, and they were not experiencing cultural affirmation in their classrooms. Another 24% were low to moderate on six of the social capital measures but reported high levels of being challenged to grow by their teachers. Just 16% had high levels of all seven aspects of relational social capital. As found in variable-centered analyses, those with high levels of developmental relationships, feeling their interests were getting connected to learning at school, and feeling culturally affirmed at school, had higher motivation than the other two groups, and the relationally strong group as well as those high only on Challenge Growth had better GPAs than the low group on all seven dimensions of student-teacher relationships.

How Do Developmental Relationships Foster School Success? Toward a Developmental Relationships Theory of Change

This body of Search Institute work over the last decade, along with the research of numerous other scholars, suggests that one possible mechanism through which a young person's experience of developmental relationships influences positive youth development broadly (and for this chapter, school success outcomes in particular), might be through the more proximal association of developmental relationships with the three core motivational needs articulated in self-determination theory, that we have described earlier: Autonomy, belonging (relatedness), and competence. Our early findings that support this theory of change are described below and are a continuing focus of our research agenda. Specifically, it is possible, and perhaps likely, that student experience of the five elements of developmental relationships contributes to development of one of more of those three "catalytic outcomes" (Scales, Boat, & Pekel, 2020a), which in turn lay the groundwork for development of other self-perceptions and skills (e.g., motivation, social-emotional skills) that are more proximal influences on ultimate outcomes indicative of thriving (Benson & Scales, 2009), ranging from school success to work readiness to civic engagement.

Teachers build developmental relationships with students through such actions as being caring and fair (friendly, respectful, helpful, equitable), maintaining classroom order, having positive communication with parents, ensuring student safety, soliciting student "voice" and participation, having high expectations of students, providing authentic instruction (e.g., service-learning and giving students opportunities to help solve real-world issues), connecting students' interests to what they're learning at school, and respecting and honoring the cultural diversity of their students, among numerous other actions explicitly stated and implied in Table 2. All of this may be why we have found that students who experience strong developmental relationships with their teachers also rate the quality of their instruction higher (Scales et al., 2019b). All of those teacher actions are then likely to strengthen students' sense of personal and social identity, feeling that they belong and are part of the school community, sense that they are being given the tools to achieve (e.g., getting high-quality instruction), and belief that they are skilled and capable of growing even more in the competencies valued in the school environment.

Theoretical Link of the Relational Actions to Autonomy, Belonging, and Competence

We have some evidence for this theoretical connection of developmental relationships, the ABCs of self-determination theory, and positive youth development, and our strategic research agenda includes more systematic exploration of this theory of change. The 20 developmental relationships actions displayed in Table 2 were derived from a wide-ranging literature search described above (see Pekel et al., 2018 for more), but can generally be seen as encompassing and promoting the three self-determination motivational needs of autonomy (i.e., their sense of choice and self-determination; Deci & Moller, 2005), belonging, and competence, as follows:

Actions Theoretically Promoting Autonomy

- "insist I take responsibility for my actions," "help me learn from mistakes and setbacks" (both in the element of Challenge Growth)
- "build my confidence to take charge of my life" (in Provide Support)
- "involve me in decisions that affect me," "give me chances to take action and lead" (both in Share Power)
- "enable me to see possibilities for my future," and "expose me to new ideas and experiences" (both in Expand Possibilities).

Actions Theoretically Promoting Belonging

- "be someone I can trust," "really pay attention when we are together," "make me feel known and valued," "show me that you enjoy being with me," and "praise me for my efforts and achievements" (all in Express Care)
- "guide me through hard situations and systems," "stand up for me when I need it," and "put in place limits that keep me on track" (all in Provide Support)
- "take me seriously and treat me fairly,", "involve me in decisions that affect me," and "work with me to solve problems and reach goals" (all in Share Power)
- "introduce me to people who can help me grow" (in Expand Possibilities).

Actions Theoretically Promoting Competence

- "praise me for my efforts and achievements" (in Express Care)
- "expect me to live up to my potential," "push me to go further," and "help me learn from mistakes and setbacks" (all in Challenge Growth)
- "guide me through hard situations and systems," "build my confidence to take charge of my life," and "put in place limits to keep me on track" (all in Provide Support)
- "take me seriously and treat me fairly," and "work with me to solve problems and reach goals" (both in Share Power)
- "introduce me to people who can help me grow" (in Expand Possibilities).

Evidence of the Relational Actions Predicting Autonomy, Belonging, and Competence

Each of the 20 relational actions thus can be seen as theoretically promoting one or more of the three basic motivational needs. In turn, our studies have shown that students' experience of developmental relationships as defined by those relational actions directly or indirectly predict several indicators of the catalytic outcomes of autonomy, belonging, and competence based on self-determination theory. For example, developmental relationships (i.e., the 20 relational actions) predict:

- *Autonomy* (measured by students' reporting that their opinions are respected and that they are disciplined fairly; Scales et al., 2019b), and by several social-emotional competencies that reflect the need for autonomy (e.g., self-awareness, self-management, responsible decision making; Search Institute, 2020b),
- *Belonging* (measured by how much students feel cared for and connected to a community; Scales et al., 2020a, b), and
- *Competence* (measured by three indicators: students' reports of quality of instruction, that is, that teachers go out of their ways to make learning interesting, ensure students understand the material, and show students specific things they can do to improve (Scales et al., 2019b); GPA (indirectly, through motivation-Scales et al., 2019b; Scales et al., 2020b), and by greater self-report of social-emotional competencies, that is, relationships skills, social awareness; Search Institute, 2020b).

Similarly, higher levels of the 20 developmental relationships actions predict academic motivation (as measured by 15 items such as "my main reason for working hard in school is to learn new knowledge and skills," "I can get smarter by working hard," "I am confident in my ability to complete my schoolwork," "it motivates me to outperform other students in my classes," "I want to master the material presented in my classes," "I like classes that arouse my curiosity, even if they are hard," and "I am good at working toward the goals I set"; Scales et al., 2019b, 2020b; Sethi & Scales, 2020).

Further, research shows that these motivated students may then attract more teacher attentiveness (e.g., Furrer et al., 2006). As Wang et al. (2019) reported, students who are engaged at school attract more teacher investment in them, which enhances engagement and achievement, which attracts still more positive teacher response in an ongoing virtuous cycle. Positive impact anywhere in the chain thus has an increased chance of activating positive developmental cascades.

As those catalytic outcomes of autonomy, belonging, and competence are strengthened, the ground is made more fertile for the growth of students' desire to learn, willingness to focus and exert effort on schoolwork, intention to set life-enhancing educational career goals, and capacity for persevering toward those goals in the face of adversity and challenge. That motivation then more proximally affects indicators of performance and achievement, including attendance, grades, test scores, and post-secondary education and/or career plans.

Most critically from the standpoint of practice, we have found that students who report *increases* in developmental relationships with teachers over the school year have significantly better perceptions of school climate, quality of instruction, and motivation than other students at year end, as well as better GPAs, depending on whether we use the full developmental relationship measure or measures of the individual five elements (Scales et al., 2019b).

Among the five individual elements of developmental relationships, Provide Support is important for predicting multiple outcomes at both middle and high school levels, but especially at the high school level. The items tap several aspects of support, including advocating for students if they have been treated unfairly, helping students learn to advocate for themselves, and connecting students to others who can help if they have a problem. Focus group comments

gathered in the same study reflected these as well as other ways of providing both support and care, such as when teachers are flexible with deadlines and understanding when students are under stress. At the middle school level, Challenge Growth and *improvement in challenge growth* are also important in predicting multiple outcomes, including GPA. At the high school level, Share Power is particularly important in predicting multiple outcomes, including GPA.

So, there are both a reasonable theory of change and a growing body of empirical results consistent with other scholars' research that link student-teacher developmental relationships to indicators of students' senses of autonomy, belonging, and competence, and their academic motivation and performance. The developmental relationships research has, however, also revealed consistent challenges.

Challenges in Students' Experience of Developmental Relationships with Teachers

Most Students Do Not Experience High-Quality Relationships with Teachers First, on average, students reflected in Table 3 report just "okay" levels of developmental relationships with teachers, running between 3.0 and 3.4 on a 5-point scale of agreement or "like my teachers" (Scales et al., 2019b, 2020b). In the study in which we employed Latent Transition Analysis to identify classes of students based on reports of those relationships, 84% were in the low (60%) or only moderate (24%) groups (Scales et al., 2021).

Student-Teacher Relationships Do Not Get Better Over Time Second, although improvement in student-teacher relationships is linked to better school adjustment and performance, only a distinct minority of students report that their relationships with teachers improve over a school year, between 12% and 40% depending on the school studied (Scales et al., 2019b, 2020b). Those studies did not include interventions to strengthen relationships, suggesting that student-teacher relationships do not naturally become more developmental as the school year progresses. Search Institute has not yet implemented and examined an intervention to boost student-teacher developmental relationships as defined here, but other studies cited below, including through a U.S. Institute of Education Sciences grant to Search Institute to develop the Building Assets Reducing Risk program (https://ies.ed.gov/ncee/wwc/Study/132) have shown that student-teacher relationships can be positively affected through such interventions.

The Experience of Student-Teacher Developmental Relationships Is Inequitable
Third, student-teacher developmental relationships are not experienced equitably by differing groups of students. We have not found much difference across racial and ethnic groups of students in the quality of their teacher relationships. But students eligible for free- and reduced-price lunch in two of our studies were less likely to experience Challenge Growth (e.g., high expectations from teachers; Scales et al., 2021), and more likely to see their relationships with teachers get worse by the end of the school year (Scales et al., 2019b), than more affluent students, especially if they also perceived their families to be under financial strain. In addition, high-school students report significantly lower levels of developmental relationships with teachers than do middle-school students (Scales et al., 2019b).

Finally, The Individual Elements of Developmental relationships Are Not Experienced Equally Share Power and Expand Possibilities are the least often reported, both by parents (Pekel et al., 2015) and students (Scales et al., 2019b).[3] Share Power may be an especially problematic element in the school setting.

---

[3]In our unpublished data from middle- and high-school teachers in the studies cited here, teachers also report that they are least likely to Share Power and Expand Possibilities with their students. Thus, parents, students, and teachers so far all agree these are the least-commonly done or experienced elements of developmental relationships.

Another of our studies used qualitative methods including discourse analysis to conclude that when students and teachers have challenging relationships, much of the interaction seems to be around implicit negotiations of power, with it being rare for the teachers we studied to work together with students to share power or build students' agency through joint conflict resolution (Chamberlain et al., 2020). When students experience Share Power or Expand Possibilities they can accrue social capital that enables social class leverage, mobility, and contribution back to their communities (Scales et al., 2020a). Thus, engaging young people from historically marginalized communities in developmental relationships that feature high levels of Share Power and Expand Possibilities may be a particularly promising lever for advancing equity in the lives of those young people and in society as a whole.

Applications of the Developmental Relationships Research to Practice

There is great potential of developmental relationships as a contributor to student academic motivation, engagement, and performance, and even more broadly, to positive youth development and greater educational and occupational equity over time. Moreover, that positive influence and the gaps in how much students experience them, who experiences them, and which elements of student-teacher developmental relationships they experience most and least, suggest the urgent need to develop policies and practices that increase students' experience of developmental relationships with their teachers, especially among older students (i.e., high school age) and students from low-income backgrounds (whether measured with FRL eligibility or perceived financial strain).

The 20 specific actions shown in Table 2 are not intended to be exhaustive, but they describe a robust set of concrete behaviors that can inform practice: things that adults across ecological settings can do in order to deepen their developmental interaction and influence with young people. In addition, we have conducted extensive qualitative research with students and teachers, along with the quantitative research discussed here. The qualitative research in particular has illuminated specific teacher practices that build the kinds of relationships that motivate students to do their best in the classroom. It also has provided a deeper examination of the ways in which teachers' behaviors and practices can either nurture developmental relationships to flourish, or inhibit them from growing. Examples of all five of the elements of developmental relationships were evident in the comments students have made in focus groups and teachers in interviews, although stories about teachers sharing power with students were less common (a theme we examine in detail in Chamberlain et al., 2020). This is consistent with the survey methodology work that has shown that students report Share Power and Expand Possibilities as the least-experienced of the five elements (Pekel et al., 2018; Scales et al., 2019b).

The overall sense communicated by the strategies teachers use is that the most relationally-skilled teachers consistently convey to students: "I will not give up on you, and I will give you the respect of being real with you." There are powerful *meta*-messages students perceived from teachers in those fundamental teacher practices:

- You can trust me to be here through your good and bad days, and for the long haul;
- I will share some of my self with you as a person so we get to know each other, even maybe make each other laugh once in a while;
- I will be fair and honest with you;
- I will be flexible with you when I can be but I will still expect a lot from you;
- I will give you the support you need to succeed.

At a time when students are navigating significant developmental demands, opportunities, and challenges, those kinds of *meta*-messages may help to bolster students' mindsets and self-perceptions of self-efficacy, their ability to grow through self-regulated effort (Yeager et al., 2014), and the sense that they have people who care about them and will advocate for them and help

them when they need it. It is no wonder then, that students who said they experienced such teacher practices also reported feeling more confident academically and wanting to work harder for those teachers.

Experimental Studies on Educational Effects of Strengthening Relationships

Search Institute's applied research has not yet encompassed experimental studies of the impact of strengthening developmental relationships. A U.S. Department of Education grant to Search Institute enabled an early experimental evaluation of a program to combat student failure (Building Assets Reducing Risks) that was based in part on the institute's research on developmental assets, with student-teacher relationships among the emphasized intervention areas (Costello & Sharma, 2015). Results for the experimental students showed improved teacher perceptions of relationships with students, and in a subsequent study, small to modest improvements in student perceptions about feeling supported (effect size = 0.29), challenged (ES = 0.25) and engaged (ES = 0.11), as well as improvements in grades and decreases in course failures, and mixed results on standardized test scores (Bos et al., 2019). Although the results were promising, the number of teachers was relatively small, the measures of relationships quite limited, and the researchers did not tease out the effect of improved relationships from the effect of other aspects of the intervention (e.g., staff risk-review meetings and family engagement strategies), so further investigation of that model still is needed.

An inherent dilemma in this type of research is trying to produce an authentic student-teacher relationship if teachers in an experimental group are asked to perform a series of prescribed behaviors with each of their students. The danger is that the recommended actions become a constraining influence that reduces dynamic, bidirectional connectedness to a checklist that must be implemented with fidelity. Real relationships, of course, are far messier, personal, unpredictable, and idiosyncratic. One of the most prominent themes in our qualitative research, for example, has been how crucial it is, if genuine trust is to be built, for teachers to be skilled at balancing rules, accountability, and deadlines with flexibility, attunement, and responsiveness to individual needs, themes repeated both in school settings (e.g., Sethi & Scales, 2020) and in workforce readiness programs for youth who are out of the workforce and out of school (Syvertsen et al., 2021). The actions presented in Table 2 and the behaviors that students in our qualitative research have told us exemplary relationship-building teachers use (e.g., Scales et al., 2019b; Sethi & Scales, 2020) represent a research and practice-based framework of operating principles that we plan to offer as systematic suggestions for teachers to use in an eventual experimental study, while still ensuring teachers have sufficient degrees of freedom for genuine responsiveness with their students.

In the meantime, evidence from both our own longitudinal studies cited here, and other scholars' studies, points to the causal impact of making relationships more developmental. For example, Reschly and Christenson (2012) described the Check & Connect program as mentoring designed to "promote student engagement through relationship building, problem solving, and persistence for marginalized students" (p. 7). The approach "checks" on student progress through frequent data collection and analysis, and "connects" students to school through mini-interventions and support for families facilitated by the mentors over a minimum mentor commitment period of 2 years. Experimental design research, and other longitudinal pre-post studies, showed that Check & Connect students attended school more, participated more, were more eager to learn, persisted more through challenge, failed fewer classes, and were more likely to graduate from high school than other students, or in the longitudinal studies, were more likely to have those outcomes post-program than before, with some substantial effect sizes in the .50s. It should be noted, too, that this is not a brief intervention of weeks or even a few months. It requires at least

a school-year commitment to realize those impacts (Christenson & Pohl, 2020). This underscores the importance not just of intervening with adults who work with young people, but with the organizations in which they work, to ensure that visions, missions, resources, policies, and procedures are firmly supporting and prioritizing the strengthening of youth-adult (student-teacher) relationships (see Scales et al., 2022).

Similarly, Pianta and colleagues' MyTeachingPartner (MTP) aims to improve teacher-student interactions through coaching teachers how to observe their students' more accurately and be more responsive to them in their instructional strategies and classroom management (Pianta, 2016). The coaching is provided through analysis of videos of the teachers' interactions with students, and consultation from exemplar teacher colleagues. Experimental design studies from preschool through secondary levels showed that MTP significantly improved teachers' "sensitivity toward students,…[and] understanding and awareness of student perspectives" (p. 101), as well as the use of more engaging instructional strategies focusing on concepts, analysis, and other higher-order thinking than on memorization and drills. Students whose teachers received the relationship-improving coaching showed significantly better language development, self-regulation, motivation and engagement, fewer disciplinary referrals (especially among African-American students), and higher standardized test scores, with effect sizes ranging from the .50s–.90s. The effects on student-teacher relationships were also more pronounced in high-poverty classrooms.

Another relationship-targeted intervention is Establish-Maintain-Restore. It provides suggested teacher actions (such as providing 5 positive interactions for every negative interaction with a student, and spending 2 minutes/day connecting with students for 10 days) for each of those three phases of a student-teacher relationship in an effort to ensure that students "feel a sense of trust, belonging, and understanding toward those who are in charge of the setting…" (Cook et al., 2020, p. 214). Small studies (*n* from 133 to 220 students and 10 to 20 teachers) have been done with 4th–5th grade and 9th grade students and teachers. Results have shown improved student-teacher relationships and time academically engaged, and decreases in disruptive behavior (Cook et al., 2018; Duong et al., 2019) and some evidence that, when an equity focus was explicit in the teacher training, 9th grade students of color improved more than white students did on belongingness, classroom behavior, motivation and GPA (Gaias et al., 2020). One drawback to the studies so far has been that student-teacher relationships have been measured only by teacher report; our own studies show significant differences in student and teacher reports of developmental relationships, with teachers painting a far rosier picture than students (e.g., Scales et al., 2019b; Search Institute, 2020b). Those relationship improvements may thus be over-stated. However, a significant promising note for the Establish-Maintain-Restore approach is that these effects were seen following a relatively brief teacher training of just 3 hours, suggesting relative ease of implementation of the training.

A large meta-analysis of 70 youth mentoring programs and more than 25,000 participating youth (Raposa et al., 2019) provides additional evidence of the causal link between high-quality adult-youth relationships and positive youth development. The researchers used study selection criteria differing from past meta-analyses, ensuring that only programs that had a focus on improving youth outcomes through a one-on-one intergenerational relationship with a nonparent adult were included. Additionally, studies had to have a control group. The average effect size was 0.21 across all programs and all outcomes, which the authors noted (p. 437) is "well within the medium/moderate range of empirical guidelines for the average effect sizes of universal youth prevention programs." There were no significant differences in effect sizes found across school, cognitive, health, psychological, and social outcomes. Improved perception of social support among mentees appeared to be a key mechanism in producing the findings. The authors concluded that "improved perceptions of support, in turn, may lead to improvements in a wide range of developmentally-relevant outcomes, including

academic engagement and performance, self-esteem, assertiveness, and substance use" (p. 438). In a different meta-analysis study of 14 programs and more than 3500 youth that examined the effects of more informal youth-initiated mentoring (when the mentor is largely selected by youth themselves), effect sizes were slightly higher (0.30) across four domains including academic and vocational outcomes (as well as social-emotional, physical, and psychosocial outcomes; van Dam et al., 2020).

Future Directions for Research and Practice

Despite thousands of studies that have been conducted on "positive" and "caring" relationships across numerous niches of developmental, social, and educational psychology, a concluding chapter section on future directions for research and practice on developmental relationships and their connection to youth motivation could be a full chapter of its own, given how much there is still to be known. But we conclude here by addressing just three broad themes needing robust attention in both research and practice. These include: Strengthening the cultural validity and responsiveness of the Developmental Relationships Framework; better understanding and activating young people themselves as drivers of developmental relationships in and outside of school settings; and leveraging in practice a deeper knowledge of not just the adult-youth dyad but how single relationships have their effects within a larger web of developmental relationships. All three of these themes are the subject of current studies being conducted at Search Institute and elsewhere.

Cultural Validity/Responsiveness of the Developmental Relationships Framework

The extensive literature reviews, focus groups, cognitive interviews, and pilot studies we did to create and shape the Developmental Relationships

Framework suggested and then provided empirical support for the validity of the framework across sex, middle and high school levels, multiple race group designations, Latinx and non-Latinx ethnicity, and socioeconomic groups (generally designated on the basis of eligibility for free and reduced-price lunch). Our analytic samples (see Table 3) have been reasonably to extremely large (ranging from hundreds in a sample to more than 25,000) and diverse as well, ranging from 30% to 60% students of color, and similar proportions of students eligible for free and reduced-price lunch and/or feeling financial strain. The finding that higher levels of developmental relationships are correlated with and predict (in longitudinal studies) a variety of key positive youth outcomes, including academic motivation and better GPAs, has been replicated across all those sample diversities.

Nevertheless, despite the attentiveness to racial, cultural and other forms of demographic diversity, the Developmental Relationships Framework was created by a group of researchers who have been (mostly) white, non-Latinx, relatively affluent, and cis-gender. Much deeper examination of how each of the five elements and 20 actions is manifested in young people and communities of color and who face other forms of marginalization in society is needed, initially at a descriptive level. In addition, more study is needed of how experiencing different accents among the five relational elements may have differing effects on motivation and other outcomes for youth from differing racial, ethnic, and socioeconomic backgrounds, among other forms of difference.

For example, our work to date suggests that young people growing up in poverty, young people of color, and youth that face discrimination in our society may particularly benefit from relationships with teachers that feature high levels of the elements of Sharing Power and Expanding Possibilities because those elements are associated with important components of social capital (Scales et al., 2020a). That possibility is reinforced by studies that show positive and supportive relationships with teachers seem to have an even greater impact for low-income students

(e.g., Pianta, 2016; Wentzel & Wigfield, 2009). Future studies should investigate associations between elements of developmental relationships, accumulation of social capital, and outcomes in school and in the workplace with sufficiently large samples to have the power to detect possible differing paths of influence across varied demographic groups.

Thus, more research is needed, and attention in practice, to ensure that building developmental relationships does not inadvertently ignore or contribute to the perpetuation of long-standing racial, ethnic, socioeconomic, and other forms of systemic discrimination, and that, instead, a focus on building developmental relationships, in research and practice, serves as a force for promoting equity. In this light, it is encouraging that a study we did of an aggregate sample of nearly 13,000 middle and high school students and more than 1200 staff in schools, out-of-school time programs, and school-based student support programs (Search Institute, 2020a) found that settings that were high in reported developmental relationships also were high on an index of diversity, equity, and inclusion indicators (DEI), such as all people being treated fairly in the setting, no matter who they are, or students being encouraged to share their culture or background, and being encouraged to get to know others with differing cultural backgrounds. Specifically, only 6% of students with weak developmental relationships said those DEI indicators were mostly or completely true in their school or program, versus 30% who had moderate developmental relationships, and a whopping 77% of those who had strong developmental relationships also reporting that their schools and programs support diversity, equity, and inclusion.

In seeking to study and strengthen the cultural responsiveness of the Developmental Relationships Framework in the years ahead, Search Institute will build upon the decades of research on Search Institute's Developmental Assets framework. Those studies found that although the assets framework had substantial cross-cultural validity around the world, the meaning and salience of some of the constructs varied across differing cultures (Scales,

2011; Scales et al., 2017). For example, we found that notions of self, other, and identity, as well as how parents and other adults promote culturally-appropriate agency and autonomy in youth, and even what constitutes "positive youth development" were quite variable. The original Western wording and connotations of several developmental assets measures had to be adapted to be adequately valid in a number of non-Western countries. The Developmental Relationships Framework has as yet only been studied, in a very limited way, in one other country than the United States (Scales et al., 2019a). The results for youth in Guatemala did show that developmental relationships in the family were linked to better youth well-being, but considerable work in research and practice remains to be done to establish that the associations discussed in this chapter have a comparable cross-cultural reach (if not universality) as the earlier developmental assets framework.[4]

Young People as Drivers of Developmental Relationships

Relational and developmental systems theory, not to mention family systems theories, have long held that developmentally meaningful relationships are bidirectional, with each party influencing the other (Lerner, 1998). Both the literature on student-teacher relationships and our own studies have acknowledged as much, but research is less well represented in which the central question is about students' effects on the relationship with teachers. Children's reciprocal effects on their caregivers have been a core topic in the early childhood and parenting literature for many decades, such as classic studies showing that "fussy" infants elicit less warm responses from

caregivers. Emmy Werner and colleagues, for example, showed that longitudinally, infants on Kaua'i who smiled more had more extensive relationships with nonkin in the middle childhood years and were more engaged in and did better at school as adolescents, among other positive long-term patterns (Werner & Smith, 1982, 1992). The analogue in studies of student-teacher relationships may be the research showing that students who are well-behaved in the classroom are perceived as more capable by teachers, and given both more challenging work and more support to succeed at it (Reeve, 2009). Similarly, several studies in German schools found that students' motivation to engage with specific learning content was the strongest predictor of differences in student-rated teaching quality as measured by classroom management and emotional support. That is, teaching quality was not a feature of the teacher alone but of the teacher being affected by their students (Fauth et al., 2020). Likewise, the long-standing inequities in school discipline of African-American students as compared to white students, even for comparable infractions (Skiba et al., 2002), is another example of how not only students' behavior, but nonmalleable characteristics such as skin color clearly have an impact on teachers' relational and instructional behaviors.

Nevertheless, the bulk of research on student-teacher relationships prioritizes what teachers do, not what students do, to make a positive relationship "happen." This even extends to the nomenclature used: We have not counted this systematically yet, but our strong impression from deep analysis of the literature is that the term "*teacher*-student relationships" is more often used than the term we intentionally use, "*student*-teacher relationships." This emphasis on the teacher side of the relationship has meant that most of the lessons from the research are about what teachers can do to promote better relationships with their students. Our own research is guilty of the same unequal emphasis on teachers and teacher behaviors, despite our good intentions to begin rectifying this imbalance by putting "student" first in the term. How all this research gets translated into practice thus

[4]In secondary analysis of an international dataset of 30 countries, examining the frequency of relationship-centered developmental assets as proxies for developmental relationships (Scales & Roehlkepartain, 2017) reported that 48% of youth internationally had inadequate relationships with nonfamily adults in the school or learning setting and 75% had less than adequate relationships in the community setting outside of schools.

has often overlooked a critical lever: the role of students themselves as drivers of developmental relationships.

An important intervention question, for example, is that if young people are introduced to the concept of developmental relationships in schools and OST programs, can and will they take action to build relationship-based social capital that helps them achieve their goals for education, work, and life? Lessons from studies of Youth-Initiated Mentoring (e.g., Schwartz et al., 2013), as well as service-learning and youth civic engagement more broadly (e.g., Wray-Lake et al., 2016), show that young people can indeed be trained to raise their skills in seeking out people who can mentor and guide them, and that their interest and engagement in authentic, community problem-solving activities is not only substantial, but can have equity-promoting effects. In one of our studies, for example, we found that low-income students who engaged in school or community service-learning opportunities had levels of broader engagement with school that were significantly better than the school engagement (and grades) of their low-income peers without service-learning, and that were statistically indistinguishable from the engagement of affluent students without service-learning (Scales et al., 2006).

Effects of the Adult-Youth Dyad Within a Web of Developmental Relationships

Current systems and ecological theories of development are most proximally the descendants of Bronfenbrenner's seminal work on the influence of the ecology in human development, although the scholarly origins of systems thinking more broadly go back to the 1920s in physics and biology, and expansion over the decades to philosophy, economics, and computer science, all of which influenced the ecological ideas of Bronfenbrenner and the evolution of systems thinking in applied developmental science (Laszlo & Krippner, 1998; Lerner & Schmid, 2013). More specifically within the boundaries of this chapter, the study of student-teacher developmental relationships and student motivation has for the most part proceeded with an emphasis on examining the dyadic relationship between students and their teachers, and the attendant effects on various youth outcomes.

But that dyadic relationship, of course, unfolds within a much broader web of relationships in students' lives—with other teachers, friends and classmates, family, adults and other children in the neighborhood, youth programs, religious congregations, part-time workplaces, and other community settings. No matter how developmental a given student-teacher relationship might be, that single relationship is not all that young people need, and it is unlikely by itself to shape a flourishing, thriving life for a young person both now and in the future, even though it can make a considerable difference in developmental outcomes in the near-term. Each relationship offers something different, in different circumstances, and with differing effects at different times in development. A relationship with a staff person in an out-of-school time (OST) program may be just as developmental for a given young person as one with a teacher in a public school, for example, but the nonacademic context of the OST setting allows and encourages a differing basis of connection and activities than the school environment.

Similarly, the accents among the five elements that are most developmental and the impact of who provides them are probably going to be different for a seven-year-old boy trying to deal with a squabble among his friends from the elements that are relationally most helpful for a 17-year-old girl trying to decide which colleges to apply to. Moreover, a long-term developmental relationship with a teacher or coach may evolve over time from being focused on, for example, Challenge Growth and Expand Possibilities to emphasizing Provide Support and Share Power to ultimately including "only" Express Care as the young person grows up and leaves behind intense and frequent contact. The relationship may still be developmental, in the sense of its effects on identity, agency, and connection and contribution to community, still promoting growth, but it now has a different shape and features.

It is this activation not just of one dyadic relationship but a multitude of them of varying intensities and durations (in social capital theory, both the "strong" ties of bonding with people like oneself and the "weak" ties with others of differing status and power who can link one to a greater variety of opportunities; Scales et al., 2020a) that is needed to put young people on the path to becoming thriving young adults. Each young person needs this web of developmental relationships, available at different times, emphasizing different relational elements, in the service of differing youth needs and goals as they change over time. Collectively, such dynamic networks of relationships can produce the most enduring positive outcomes for young people, through helping them construct a strong autonomous identity that is integrated across time and the spaces of their lives, a sense of agency and competencies to shape their life's direction, and a firm belief that they are truly connected to communities of others who both care for them and for whom the young person desires to make meaningful contributions.

Teachers and other staff in schools are a critical strand of the broader web of relationships that young people need to thrive, but that web can and should include adults in other settings as well. In fact, a study that we conducted in 2019 (just before the start of the coronavirus pandemic) found that 70% of youth in out-of-school time programs and 62% of young people who participate in student support programs that work within schools report strong levels of developmental relationships with program staff, whereas only 40% of students report having strong developmental relationships with their teachers (Search Institute, 2020b). That finding underscores the valuable role that a wide array of youth-serving organizations can play in supplementing the developmental relationships students experience with their teachers. A participant in a qualitative study that we conducted of six career pathways programs captured this multiplying effect well when she noted that participating in the program means that, "You don't just have a hundred people in your network, you have one hundred people's networks" (Boat et al., 2020, p. 24).

Conclusion

None of these three themes for future directions are new ideas. Previous theorists, researchers, and practitioners have been writing about them for as long as there has been a scholarly tradition. The newness and relevance for today is in the greater emphasis that deserves to be placed on them.

We have described in this chapter how developmental relationships can help promote greater academic motivation, and a wealth of other youth outcomes. But schools and other institutions cannot help students enjoy the greatest benefits of those relationships without explicit commitment to do so. Our research has consistently found that less than half of middle and high school students have high-quality developmental relationships with their teachers. Those relationships don't seem to get better over time, on their own. Older students and low-income students seem to have worse relationships with their teachers, and they have fewer quality relationships with teachers over time.

For all of these reasons, more intentional effort needs to be spent in both research and practice to study and strengthen developmental relationships. We need to evaluate and, as necessary, enhance the cultural responsiveness of the Developmental Relationships Framework. We need to help more young people activate their own agency as builders of developmental relationships with teachers and other adults. And we need to facilitate not just more high-quality dyadic relationships between students and teachers, but more expansive and diverse networks and webs of developmental relationships in and out of school for all our students. Attending to all those issues in research and practice will promote not just student motivation in the near-term, but also broader and longer-term well-being and thriving in the society that today's students soon will lead.

At the outset of this chapter, we asked you to recall a teacher who motivated you to learn during your own years as a student. We hope and assume that you were able to remember more than one. It is likely that the educator who came to your mind built strong relationships with you and other students based upon their personal passions and commitments and trial-and-error experience over years in the classroom. It is also likely that you had other teachers who were *not* as successful at motivating you to learn, and if we had asked you to remember those teachers at the outset of this chapter, it would have begun our discussion at a very different place in your own education and development. Fortunately, the findings from our studies and other research are making it possible to ensure that *all* teachers have the knowledge, skills, and tools to build powerful developmental relationships with all of the students they serve.

References

Benson, P. L., & Scales, P. C. (2009). The definition and preliminary measurement of thriving in adolescence. *Journal of Positive Psychology, 4*, 85–104. https://doi.org/10.1080/17439760802399240

Benson, P. L., Scales, P. C., Hamilton, S. F., & Sesma, A., Jr. (2006). Positive youth development: Theory, research, and applications. In W. Damon & R. M. Lerner (Eds.), *Handbook of child psychology: Human development theory* (Vol. 1, 6th ed., pp. 894–941). Wiley.

Benson, P. L., Scales, P., Roehlkepartain, E. C., & Leffert, N. (2011a). *The fragile foundation: The state of developmental assets among American youth* (2nd ed.). Search Institute.

Benson, P. L., Scales, P. C., & Syvertsen, A. K. (2011b). The contribution of the developmental assets framework to positive youth development theory and practice. In R. M. Lerner, J. V. Lerner, & J. B. Benson (Eds.), *Advances in child development and behavior: Positive youth development research and applications for promoting thriving in adolescence* (pp. 195–228). Elsevier.

Bernstein-Yamashiro, B., & Noam, G. (2013). Teacher-student relationships: A growing field of study. *New Directions for Youth Development, 137*, 15–26. https://doi.org/10.1002/yd.20045

Boat, A., Sethi, J., Eisenberg, C., & Chamberlain, R. (2020). *"It was a support network system that made me believe in myself:" Understanding youth and young adults' experiences of social capital in six innovative programs.* (Report to the Bill and Melinda Gates Foundation). Minneapolis, MN: Search Institute.

Bos, J. M., Dhillon, S., Borman, T., with O'Brien, B., Graczewski, C., Park, S. J., Liu, F., Adelman-Sil, E., & Hu, L. (2019). *Building Assets and Reducing Risks (BARR) validation study final report.* American Institutes for Research.

Chamberlain, R., Scales, P. C., & Sethi, J. (2020). Competing discourses of power in teachers' stories of challenging relationships with students. *Power and Education.* https://doi.org/10.1177/1757743820931118

Christenson, S. L., & Pohl, A. J. (2020). The relevance of student engagement: The impact of and lessons learned implementing Check & Connect. In A. L. Reschly, A. J. Pohl, & S. L. Christenson (Eds.), *Student engagement: Effective academic, behavioral, cognitive, and affective interventions at school* (pp. 3–30).

Connell, J. P., & Wellborn, J. G. (1991). Competence, autonomy, and relatedness: A motivational analysis of self-system processes. In M. R. Gunnar & L. A. Sroufe (Eds.), *Self processes in development: Minnesota symposia on child psychology* (Vol. 23, pp. 43–77). Erlbaum.

Cook, C. R., Coco, S., Zhang, Y., Fiat, A. E., Duong, M. T., Renshaw, T. L., Long, A. C., & Frank, S. (2018). Cultivating positive teacher-student relationships: Preliminary evaluation of the Establish-Maintain-Restore (EMR) method. *School Psychology Review, 47*(3), 226–243. https://doi.org/10.17105/SPR-2017-0025.V47-3

Cook, C. R., Thayer, A. J., Fiat, A., & Sullivan, M. (2020). Interventions to enhance affective engagement. In A. L. Reschly, A. J. Pohl, & S. L. Christenson (Eds.), *Student engagement: Effective academic, behavioral, cognitive, and affective interventions at school* (pp. 203–237). Springer Nature.

Cornelius-White, J. (2007). Learner-centered teacher-student relationships are effective: A meta-analysis. *Review of Educational Research, 77*, 113–143. https://doi.org/10.3102/003465430298563

Costello, M., & Sharma, A. (2015). *The Building Assets-Reducing Risks Program: Replication and expansion of an effective strategy to turn around low-achieving schools.* Corsello Consulting, and S & S Consulting. Final Report on i3 Development Grant to Search Institute. https://files.eric.ed.gov/fulltext/ED560804.pdf

Darling-Hammond, L. with Cook, C., Jaquith, A., & Hamilton, M. (2012). *Creating a comprehensive system for evaluating and supporting effective teaching.* Stanford Center for Opportunity Policy in Education.

Damon, W. (2004). What is positive youth development? Annals of the American Academy of Political and Social Science, 591, 13–24. https://doi.org/10.1177/0002716203260092

Deci, E. L., & Moller, A. C. (2005). The concept of competence: A starting point for understanding intrinsic motivation and self-determined extrinsic motivation. In A. J. Eliot & C. S. Dweck (Eds.), *Handbook of competence and motivation* (pp. 579–597). The Guilford Press.

Delpit, L. (2012). *"Multiplication is for white people": Raising expectations for other people's children.* New Press.

Duncan-Andrade, J. M. R. (2009). Note to educators: Hope required when growing roses in concrete.

Harvard Educational Review, 79(2), 181–194. https://doi.org/10.17763/haer.79.2.nu3436017730384w

Duong, M. T., Pullmann, M. D., Buntain-Ricklefs, J., Lee, K., Benjamin, K. S., Nguyen, L., & Cook, C. R. (2019). Brief teacher training improves student behavior and student-teacher relationships in middle school. *School Psychology, 34*(2), 212–221. https://psycnet.apa.org/doi/10.1037/spq0000296

Dweck, C. S. (2015, September 23). Growth mindset, revisited. *Education Week, 35*(5), 20, 24.

Dweck, C., & Master, A. (2009). Self-theories and motivation: Students' beliefs about intelligence. In K. R. Wentzel & A. Wigfield (Eds.), *Handbook of motivation at school* (pp. 123–140). Routledge.

Eccles, J. S., Midgely, C., Wigfield, A., Buchanan, C. M., Reumann, D., Flanagan, C., & Mac Iver, D. (1993). Development during adolescence: The impact of stage-environment fit on young adolescents' experiences in schools and families. *American Psychologist, 48*(2), 90–101.

Elliot, A. J., & Church, M. A. (1997). A hierarchical model of approach and avoidance achievement motivation. *Journal of Personality and Social Psychology, 72*, 218–232. https://doi.org/10.1037/0022-3514.72.1.218

Fauth, B., Wagner, W., Bertram, C., Gollner, R., Roloff, J., Ludtke, O., Policoff, M. S., Klusman, U., & Trautwein, U. (2020). Don't blame the teacher? The need to account for classroom characteristics in evaluations of teaching quality. *Journal of Educational Psychology, 112*(6), 1284–1302. https://doi.org/10.1037/edu0000416

Furrer, C. J., Skinner, E., Marchand, G., & Kindermann, T. A. (2006, March). *Engagement vs. disaffection as central constructs in the dynamics of motivational development.* Paper presented at the annual meeting of the Society for Research on Adolescence, San Francisco.

Gaias, L. M., Cook, C. R., Nguyen, L., Brewer, S. K., Brown, E. C., Kiche, S., Shi, J., Buntain-Ricklefs, J., & Duong, M. T. (2020). A mixed methods pilot study of an equity-explicit student-teacher relationship intervention for ninth-grade transition. *Journal of School Health, 90*(12), 1004–1018. https://doi.org/10.1111/josh.12968

Gillet, N., Vallerand, R. J., & Lafreniere, M.-A. K. (2012). Intrinsic and extrinsic school motivation as a function of age: The mediating role of autonomy support. *Social Psychology of Education, 15*(1), 77–95. https://doi.org/10.1007/s11218-011-9170-2

Guay, F., Morin, A. J. S., Litalien, D., Howard, J. L., & Gilbert, W. (2021). Trajectories of self-determined motivation during the secondary school: A growth mixture analysis. *Journal of Educational Psychology, 113*(2), 390410. https://doi.org/10.1037/edu0000482

Hunt, D. E. (1975). Person-environment interaction: A challenge found wanting before it was tried. *Review of Educational Research, 45*, 209–230.

Immordino-Yang, M. H. (2016, invited submission) Emotion, sociality, and the brain's default mode network: Insights for educational practice and policy. *Policy Insights from the Behavioral and Brain Sciences, 3*(2), 211–219. http://journals.sagepub.com/doi/abs/10.1177/2372732216656869

Kannapel, P. J., & Clements, S. K. (2005). *Inside the black box of high-performing high-poverty schools.* Prichard Committee for Academic Excellence.

Kim, J. (2021). The quality of social relationships in schools and adult health: Differential effect of student-student versus student-teacher relationships. *School Psychology Quarterly, 36*, 6–16. https://doi.org/10.1037/spq0000373

Laszlo, A., & Krippner, S. (1998). Systems theories: Their origins, foundations, and development. In J. S. Jordan (Ed.), *Systems theories and a priori aspects of perception* (pp. 47–74). Elsevier Science.

Lazowski, R., & Hulleman, C. (2016). Motivation interventions in education: A metaanalytic review. *Review of Educational Research, 86*(2), 602–640. https://doi.org/10.3102/0034654315617832

Lee, S. J. (2012). The effects of the teacher-student relationship and academic press on student engagement and academic performance. *International Journal of Educational Research, 53*, 330–340. https://doi.org/10.1016/j.ijer.2012.04.006

Lerner, R. M. (1998). Theories of human development: Contemporary perspectives. In W. Damon (Editor-in-Chief) & R. M. Lerner (Vol. Ed.), *Handbook of child psychology: Vol. 1. Theoretical models of human development* (5th ed., pp. 1–24). Wiley.

Lerner, R. M., & Schmid, C. K. (2013). Relational developmental systems theories and the ecological validity of experimental designs. *Human Development, 56*, 372–380. https://doi.org/10.1159/000357179

Li, J., & Julian, M. M. (2012). Developmental relationships as the active ingredient: A unifying working hypothesis of "what works" across intervention settings. *American Journal of Orthopsychiatry, 82*(2), 157–166. https://doi.org/10.1111/j.1939-0025.2012.01151.x

Martin, A. J., & Dowson, M. (2009). Interpersonal relationships, motivation, engagement, and achievement: Yields for theory, current issues, and educational practice. *Review of Educational Research, 79*(1), 327–365. https://doi.org/10.3102/0034654308325583

Masten, A. S. (2001). Ordinary magic: Resilience processes in development. *American Psychologist, 56*, 227–238. https://psycnet.apa.org/doi/10.1037/0003-066X.56.3.227

Midgley, C., Maehr, M. L., Hruda, L. Z., Anderman, E., Anderman, L., Freeman, K. E., … Urdan, T. (2000). *Manual for the patterns of adaptive learning scales.* University of Michigan.

Nagaoka, J., Farrington, C. A., Ehrlich, S. B., Heath, R. D., Johnson, D. W., Dickson, S., Turner, A. C., Mayo, A., & Hayes, K. (2015). *Foundations for young adult success: A developmental framework.* University of Chicago Consortium on Chicago Schools Research.

Pekel, K., Roehlkepartain, E. C., Syvertsen, A. K., & Scales, P. C. (2015). *Don't forget the families: The missing piece in America's effort to help all children succeed.* Search Institute.

Pekel, K., Roehlkepartain, E. C., Syvertsen, A. K., Scales, P. C., Sullivan, T. K., & Sethi, J. (2018). Finding the fluoride: Examining how and why developmental relationships are the active ingredient in interventions that work. *American Journal of Orthopsychiatry, 5,* 493–502. https://doi.org/10.1037/ort0000333

Pianta, R. C. (2016). Teacher-student interactions: Measurement, impacts, improvement, and policy. *Policy Insights from the Behavioral and Brain Sciences, 3,* 98–105. https://doi.org/10.1177/2372732215622457

Pianta, R. C., Hamre, B. K., & Allen, J. P. (2012). Teacher-student relationships and engagement: Conceptualizing, measuring, and improving the capacity of classroom interactions. In S. L. Christenson, A. L. Reschly, & C. Wylie (Eds.), *Handbook of research on student engagement* (pp. 365–386). Springer.

Raposa, E. B., Rhodes, J., Stams, G. J. J. M., Card, N., Burton, S., Schwartz, S., Sykes, L. A. Y., Kanchewa, S., Kupersmidt, J., & Hussain, S. (2019). The effects of youth mentoring programs: A meta-analysis of outcome studies. *Journal of Youth and Adolescence, 48*(3), 423–443. https://doi.org/10.1007/s10964-019-00982-8

Reeve, J. (2009). Why teachers adopt a controlling motivating style toward students and how they can become more autonomy supportive. *Educational Psychologist, 44*(3), 159–175. https://doi.org/10.1080/00461520903028990

Reschly, A. L., & Christenson, S. L. (2012). Jingle, jangle, and conceptual haziness: Evolution and future directions of the engagement construct. In S. L. Christenson, A. L. Reschly, & C. Wylie (Eds.), *Handbook of research on student engagement* (pp. 3–20). Springer Science.

Rhodes, J. E., Spencer, R., Keller, T. E., Liang, B., & Noam, G. (2006). A model for the influence of mentoring relationships on youth development. *Journal of Community Psychology, 34*(6), 691–707. https://psycnet.apa.org/doi/10.1002/jcop.20124

Roorda, D. L., Koomen, H. M. Y., Spilt, J. L., & Oort, F. J. (2011). The influence of affective teacher-student relationships on students' school engagement and achievement: A meta-analytic approach. *Review of Educational Research, 81*(4), 493–529. https://doi.org/10.3102/0034654311421793

Ryan, R. M., & Deci, E. L. (2000). Self-determination theory and the facilitation of intrinsic motivation, social development, and well-being. *American Psychologist, 55*(1), 68. https://doi.org/10.1037/0003-066x.55.1.68

Scales, P. C., & Leffert, N. (2004). *Developmental assets: A synthesis of the scientific research on adolescence* (2nd ed.). Search Institute.

Scales, P. C., Roehlkepartain, E. C., Neal, M., Kielsmeier, J. C., & Benson, P. L. (2006). Reducing Academic Achievement Gaps: The Role of Community Service and Service-Learning. *Journal of Experiential Education, 29,* 38-60. https://doi.org/10.1177%2F105382590602900105

Scales, P. C., & Roehlkepartain, E. C. (2017). The contribution of nonfamily adults to adolescent well-being: A global research and policy perspective. In J. E. Lansford & P. Banati (Eds.), *The Oxford handbook of adolescent development research and its impact on global policy* (pp. 150–179). Oxford University Press.

Scales, P. C., Roehlkepartain, E. C., & Houltberg, B. J. (2022). *The elements of Developmental Relationships: A review of selected research underlying the framework.* Minneapolis: Search Institute Research Review.

Scales, P. C., Benson, P. L., & Roehlkepartain, E. C. (2011). Adolescent thriving: The role of sparks, relationships, and empowerment. *Journal of Youth and Adolescence, 40*(3), 263–277. https://doi.org/10.1007/s10964-010-9578-6

Scales, P. C., Roehlkepartain, E. C., & Shramko, M. (2017). Aligning youth development theory, measurement, and practice across cultures and contexts: Lessons from use of the Developmental Assets Profile. *Child Indicators Research, 10*(4), 1145–1178. https://doi.org/10.1007/s12187-016-9395-x

Scales, P. C., Gebru, E., & Shramko, M. (2019a). *Developmental relationships in Guatemala: A first step toward exploring the framework beyond the United States.* Search Institute. Blog available at https://www.search-institute.org/category/international-research

Scales, P. C., Pekel, K., Sethi, J., Chamberlain, R., & Van Boekel, M. (2019b). Academic year changes in student-teacher developmental relationships and their links to change in middle and high school students' motivation, engagement, and performance. *Journal of Early Adolescence, 40*(4), 499–536. https://doi.org/10.1177/0272431619858414

Scales, P. C., Boat, A., & Pekel, K. (2020a). *Defining and measuring social capital for young people: A practical review of the literature on resource-full relationships.* Search Institute. Report for the Bill & Melinda Gates Foundation.

Scales, P. C., Van Boekel, M., Pekel, K., Syvertsen, A. K., & Roehlkepartain, E. C. (2020b). Effects of developmental relationships with teachers on middle school students' motivation and performance. *Psychology in the Schools.* https://doi.org/10.1002/pits.22350

Scales, P. C., Shramko, M., Syvertsen, A. K., & Boat, A. (2021). Relational social capital and educational equity among middle-school students: A person-centered analysis. *Applied Developmental Science.* (in press).

Scales, P. C., Houltberg, B. J., & Pekel, K. (2022). *Rooted in relationships: Growing inclusive opportunity for all youth through nurturing developmental relationships.* Minneapolis: Search Institute Position Paper.

Schwartz, S. E. O., Rhodes, J. E., Spencer, R., & Grossman, J. B. (2013). Youth initiated mentoring: Investigating a new approach to working with vulnerable adolescents. *American Journal of Community Psychology, 52,* 155–159. https://doi.org/10.1007/s10464-013-9585-3

Search Institute. (2020a). *Relationships and equity: Early insights on the association to SEL.* Author.

Search Institute. (2020b). *The intersection of developmental relationships, equitable environments, and SEL [Insights & Evidence Series]*. Author. https://www.search-institute.org/wp-content/uploads/2020/10/Insights-Evidence-DRs-DEI.SEL-FINAL.pdf

Sethi, J., & Scales, P. C. (2020). Developmental relationships and school success: How teachers, parents, and friends affect educational outcomes and what actions students say matter most. *Contemporary Educational Psychology*. https://doi.org/10.1016/j.cedpsych.2020.101904

Shepherd, S., Owen, D., Fitch, T. J., & Marshall, J. L. (2006). Locus of control and academic achievement in high school students. *Psychological Reports, 98*(2), 318–322. https://doi.org/10.2466/pr0.98.2.318-322

Skiba, R. J., Michael, R. S., Nardo, A. C., & Peterson, R. L. (2002). The color of discipline: Sources of racial and gender disproportionality in school punishment. *The Urban Review, 34*, 317–342. https://doi.org/10.1023/A:1021320817372

Skinner, E. A., & Belmont, M. J. (1993). Motivation in the classroom: Reciprocal effects of teacher behavior and student engagement across the school year. *Journal of Educational Psychology, 85*(4), 571–581.

Syvertsen, A. K., Scales, P. C., & Toomey, R. B. (2019). Developmental assets framework revisited: Confirmatory analysis and invariance testing to create a new generation of assets measures for applied research. *Applied Developmental Science*, advance online publication, 1–21. https://doi.org/10.1080/10888691.2019.1613155

Syvertsen, A. K., Roskopf, J., Wu, C-Y., Sethi, J., & Chamberlain, R. (2020). *Positive disruption: The promise of the Opportunity Reboot Model* (Report to the Corporation for National and Community Service Social Innovation Fund). Search Institute.

Syvertsen, A. K., Sullivan, T. K., & Scales, P. C. (2021). *Seeds of trust: How developmental relationships in programs for opportunity youth build social capital and promote positive youth development*. Search Institute. Paper in preparation.

Van Dam, L., Blom, D., Kara, E., Assink, M., Stams, G.-J., Schwartz, S., & Rhodes, J. (2020). Youth initiated mentoring: A meta-analytic study of a hybrid approach to youth mentoring. *Journal of Youth and Adolescence*. https://doi.org/10.1007/s10964-020-01336-5

Wang, M. C. (1990). *Variables important in learning: A meta-review of reviews of the research literature (ERIC #405691)*. Center for Research in Human Development and Education, Temple University.

Wang, M.-T., & Eccles, J. S. (2012). Social support matters: Longitudinal effects of social support on three dimensions of school engagement from middle to high school. *Child Development, 83*(3), 877–895. https://doi.org/10.1111/j.1467-8624.2012.01745.x

Wang, M.-T., Degol, J. L., & Henry, D. A. (2019). An integrative development-in-sociocultural-context model for children's engagement in learning. *American Psychologist, 74*(9), 1086–1102. https://doi.org/10.1037/amp0000522

Wentzel, K. R. (2002). Are effective teachers like good parents? Teaching styles and student adjustment in early adolescence. *Child Development, 73*(1), 287–301. https://doi.org/10.1111/1467-8624.00406

Wentzel, K. R. (2012). Teacher–student relationships and adolescent competence at school. In T. Wubbels, P. den Brok, J. van Tartwijk, & J. Levy (Eds.), *Advances in learning environments research (Vol 3): Interpersonal relationships in education* (pp. 19–35). Sense Publishers. https://doi.org/10.1007/978-94-6091-939-8

Wentzel, K. R., & Miele, D. B. (2016). Introduction. In K. R. Wentzel & D. B. Miele (Eds.), *Handbook of motivation at school* (2nd ed., pp. 1–8). Routledge.

Wentzel, K. R., & Wigfield, A. (Eds.). (2009). *Handbook of motivation at school*. Routledge.

Werner, E., & Smith, R. (1982). *Vulnerable but invincible: A longitudinal study of resilient children and youth*. McGraw-Hill.

Werner, E., & Smith, R. (1992). *Overcoming the odds: High risk children from birth to adulthood*. Cornell University Press.

Wray-Lake, L., Syvertsen, A. K., & Flanagan, C. A. (2016). Developmental change in social responsibility during adolescence: An ecological perspective. *Developmental Psychology, 52*(1), 130–142. https://doi.org/10.1037/dev0000067

Yeager, D. S., & Dweck, C. S. (2012). Mindsets that promote resilience: When students believe that personal characteristics can be developed. *Educational Psychologist, 47*, 302–314. https://doi.org/10.1080/00461520.2012.722805

Yeager, D. S., Henderson, M. D., D'Mello, S., Paunesku, D., Walton, G. M., Spitzer, B. J., & Duckworth, A. L. (2014). Boring but important: A self-transcendent purpose for learning fosters academic self-regulation. *Journal of Personality and Social Psychology, 107*(4), 559–580. https://doi.org/10.1037/a0037637

Early Childhood Engagement

Stacey Neuharth-Pritchett and Kristen L. Bub

Abstract

Children's experiences with formal group early learning experiences serve as an introduction to schooling and provide foundational experiences with cognitive, language, social, emotional, behavioral, and relational skills that start the trajectory to a successful transition to elementary school and beyond. Despite evidence supporting the benefits of early childhood engagement for learning and development, there is very little consistency in how early childhood engagement is defined and measured. This chapter summarizes the evidence on early childhood engagement, describes the myriad ways early childhood engagement has been defined, and highlights some potential options for measuring early childhood engagement.

High-quality experiences with early childhood education prompt positive and enduring outcomes for children, particularly for those children from households with economic disadvantage (García et al., 2016; McCoy et al.,

2017; Ramey & Ramey, 2004; Weiland & Yoshikawa, 2013). Such experiences serve as a formal introduction to schooling for young children and provide foundational experiences with cognitive, language, social, emotional, behavioral, and relational skills that start the trajectory to a successful transition to elementary school and beyond (Ansari, 2018; Barnett, 1995; Han & Neuharth-Pritchett, 2021; Ledford et al., 2020). Longitudinal studies document the impact of early childhood experiences on the development of positive attitudes toward school and attendance patterns (Schweinhart et al., 2005; van Huizen & Plantenga, 2018; Wylie & Hodgen, 2012). Indeed, positive early childhood engagement might be a protective factor for children placed at risk by reducing problem behaviors and augmenting social skills that facilitate adjustment to the learning settings (Dominguez & Greenfield, 2009; McWayne & Cheung, 2009). Despite evidence supporting the benefits of early childhood engagement for learning and development, there is very little consistency in how early childhood engagement is defined and measured. Although a majority of studies on early childhood engagement has focused on the behavioral aspects of the construct, others have considered early childhood engagement to be multidimensional, including emotional, relational, and cognitive aspects. This chapter will summarize the evidence on early childhood engagement, describe the myriad ways early childhood engagement has been defined,

S. Neuharth-Pritchett (✉) · K. L. Bub
Department of Educational Psychology, University of Georgia, Athens, GA, USA
e-mail: sneuhart@uga.edu; Kristen.bub@uga.edu

© The Author(s), under exclusive license to Springer Nature Switzerland AG 2022
A. L. Reschly, S. L. Christenson (eds.), *Handbook of Research on Student Engagement*,
https://doi.org/10.1007/978-3-031-07853-8_14

and highlight some potential options for measuring early childhood engagement.

Longitudinal evidence of the impact of early childhood programs on students' use of special education services, retention, and graduation rates suggests that these settings are essential for setting children on a positive academic trajectory. For example, the High/Scope Perry Preschool Project suggests that children who were randomly assigned to the program spent significantly fewer years in special education programs and services compared with the control children (~1 year compared with 2.8 years, respectively). Additionally, program females completed more years of education than did nonprogram females (12.2 vs. 10.5, respectively); high school graduation or equivalence completion was also significantly higher for program females than nonprogram females. There were no differences in retention or graduation rates for program and nonprogram males (Schweinhart et al., 2005). Similarly, the Carolina Abecedarian early childhood program was associated with significantly higher education levels compared with the control group (e.g., 13.46 vs. 12.31 years, respectively), with women again benefiting more than men (Campbell et al., 2002; Campbell et al., 2012). Using follow-up data from studies examining the impact of infant and preschool programs on child development, Lazar et al. (1982) reported that children from low-income families were significantly more likely to meet basic school requirements, less likely to be retained a grade, and less likely to be referred to special education services than were children who did not attend early childhood programs. These studies provide clear evidence of the long-term benefits of early childhood education experiences for educational outcomes.

In 2021, conversations about the efficacy of early intervention, support for the early care and education workforce, and specific interventions such as universal prekindergarten for children have stimulated conversations about the quality of early childhood experiences and who accesses them (Austin et al., 2021; Eden, 2021; OECD, 2021; Shapiro, 2021). Disparities in early care and education experiences (Bernstein et al.,

2014) and variations in the individual experiences that children have within these settings trigger questions about early childhood engagement experiences and their resultant impact on long-term schooling outcomes (Williford et al., 2013). In comparison to the robust evidence base on student engagement in the elementary through high school (Finn & Zimmer, 2012; Lindstrom et al., 2021) years, literature about early childhood engagement is more limited and often focused on readiness variables (e.g., literacy, language, and mathematics) and not specifically the construct of engagement (Aydogan, 2012; Ramey & Ramey, 2004).

Engagement Foundations

Many different perspectives on the development and developmental trajectories of young children have guided the work of scholars in early childhood education. For example, Bronfenbrenner's bioecological model (Bronfenbrenner, 2005) and the Process-Person-Context-Time (PPCT) framework have been modeled in numerous studies examining the interrelations among proximal processes, personal characteristics, contexts, and time to understand how children learn and in what contexts. By examining proximal processes which Bronfenbrenner (2005) noted as primary engines of development, scholars have been able to examine children's engagement in activities and interactions that occur on a relatively regular basis along with the resources, teachers, and peers in those settings (Downer et al., 2007). Other scholars have employed dynamic systems theories to help describe how the role of context including relationships, environment, and experience drives youth learning and development (Immordino-Yang et al., 2019; Lerner, 2018). Child agency and teacher and child beliefs also have been examined to assess how young children engage to develop their identities as learners and members of the learning community (Dweck, 2016). Still other scholars advocate for understanding what early learning experiences work for which children in which contexts (Finn, 1993; Shonkoff, 2017). For example, how might the quality of a child's engagement with learning be directly related to pathways for learning (Lawson & Lawson, 2013)? Scholars have noted that children who engage in classrooms with positive and proactive involvement in learning reach higher academic outcomes than children who do not develop a proactive stance to engagement (Fredricks et al., 2004).

An emerging body of research in early childhood special education has also helped frame the way that student engagement might be operationalized in settings for young learners. For example, Finn's (1989) Participation-Identification Model suggests that both behaviors (i.e., participation) and emotions (i.e., feelings of belonging) are important for students' participation and long-term educational outcomes. He suggests it is the value of belonging which engages young children and that entry into school offers an opportunity to connect children to that feeling of belonging ultimately affecting successful participation, achievement, and identification with schooling. That is, long-term student engagement in schooling over time, combined with some level of academic success, can facilitate students' identification with school and subsequently their participation inside and outside of the classroom. This process likely begins with the earliest formative experiences with schooling (McCabe & Altamura, 2011; Mirkhil, 2010). Greenwood (1996) empirically tested a theoretical model in which the effects of instruction (e.g., exposure to materials or task quality) on student outcomes were indirect *through* student engagement. In other words, he tested whether the effects of instruction on student outcomes were not direct but instead mediated by student engagement; he found evidence to support this mediation, suggesting that the effects of instruction on student outcomes are indirect through student engagement. Ferholt and Rainio (2016) examined the role of play in children's engagement and concluded that play can serve as an important context for engaging young children. McWilliam and Bailey (1992) documented that higher levels of student engagement are strongly associated with improvements in learning across a number of developmental domains.

In engagement work with older learners, one model of student engagement is operationalized as multidimensional and encompassing activities that are malleable, responsive to contextual features of the learning environment, and amenable to environmental change (Fredricks et al., 2004). This engagement model is divided into domains of behavioral engagement, emotional engagement, and cognitive engagement. Skinner and Pitzer (2012) define school engagement as students' involvement and interactions in school as measured both by quality and quantity of such engagement. Other scholars describe student engagement as a function of dynamic and joint processes in which the environment is a primary contributor in the students' lives within the classroom (Booren et al., 2012; Carto & Greenwood, 1985; Kontos & Keyes, 1999; Wang & Degol, 2014). Although the field is in general agreement about engagement as a meta-construct, what is clear from this literature is that engagement declines as students' progress across their P-12 academic careers (Ladd & Dinella, 2009; Marks, 2000; Wang & Eccles, 2012), although the patterns of decline are not the same across youth (Wylie & Hodgen, 2012). For example, Wang and Peck (2013) identified five patterns of behavioral (e.g., how often have you gotten schoolwork done on time?), emotional (e.g., I feel happy and safe in this school), and cognitive (e.g., how often do you try to relate what you are studying to other things you know about?) engagement, including highly engaged, moderately engaged, minimally engaged, emotionally disengaged, and cognitively disengaged. Importantly, there are differences in patterns of engagement across racial/ethnic backgrounds (Johnson et al., 2001; Wang & Eccles, 2013). Thus, understanding engagement's crucial role during the early years can guide future scholarship in establishing conditions that enhance children's connections to schooling, consistency of engagement, and the subsequent success over time for an array of developmental tasks that follow (Finn, 1989; Greenwood et al., 2002; Hojnoski & Missall, 2010; Mahatmya et al., 2012; Reschly & Christenson, 2012; Skinner et al., 2008a, 2008b).

Early Childhood Engagement

McWilliam and Casey (2008) employ a broad definition of early childhood engagement to encompass the amount of time children spend in developmentally appropriate interactions in various contexts in learning settings. Copple and Bredekamp (2006) characterized early childhood classrooms as spaces where child can explore and take advantage of learning opportunities that allow them to strengthen their connections with learning. Active participation in classroom routines and appropriate interactions also have been advanced as child engagement in early learning contexts (Bennett et al., 2011; Castro et al., 2017; McWIlliam & Bailey, 1992; Odom & Bailey, 2001). Ladd and Dinella (2009) found that children who develop stable patterns of behavioral (e.g., cooperative-resistant classroom participation) and emotional (e.g., relating to school) engagement at a young age acquire skills that allow them to weather more challenging engagement tasks (e.g., embracing the student role, responding to teacher's requests, and undertaking more complex school tasks) as they make the transition to elementary and secondary schools.

Studies have documented child engagement with classroom activities and routines and their relationship to later school achievement, school completion, social and emotional outcomes, motivation, and self-regulation (Bryan & Gast, 2000; Fredricks et al., 2004; Hamre & Pianta, 2001; Hojnoski & Missall, 2010; Mashburn et al., 2008; Noltemeyer et al., 2015; Vitiello & Williford, 2016; Williford et al., 2013; Zimmerman et al., 2020). For example, Ladd et al. (1999) found that children's cooperation and self-direction in kindergarten and first grade predicted school performance (where antisocial behavior influenced peer rejection which contributed to classroom participation which influenced achievement which accounted for 53% of the total indirect effect of antisocial behavior on achievement). Young learners' positive engagement with classroom activities and processes, observed by active play, motivation, persistence (i.e., more time on a task), and comfort with

autonomy resulted in subsequent higher academic achievement and appropriate behaviors than children who did not exhibit those aspects of engagement (Fantuzzo et al., 2004; McClelland et al., 2000; McWayne & Cheung, 2009).

In addition to individual child variables, researchers have also focused on the role of various aspects of the settings in which learning and development take place (both inside and outside the classroom) in helping explain young children's engagement in school (Chien et al., 2010; Roper & Hinde, 1978; Prykanowski et al., 2018). For example, using the *Individualized Classroom Assessment Scoring System* (inCLASS; Downer et al., 2010), Vitiello et al. (2012) rated children on 10 dimensions of positive and negative engagement with teachers, peers, and tasks using (i.e., positive engagement the teacher, teacher communication, peer sociability, peer assertiveness, peer communication, engagement with tasks, self-reliance, conflict with teachers, conflict with peers, and behavioral control). Children were observed for 10 min and then rated using a seven-point Likert scale, with higher scores indicating more positive engagement on all but the conflict scales (higher scores indicated more negative engagement on these scales). Factor analyses revealed four broad dimensions: Positive engagement with teachers, which reflected positive, affectionate and confident interactions; positive engagement with peers, which reflected lower levels of rejection and higher levels of social acceptance; positive engagement with tasks, which reflected active engagement, sustained attention, motivation, persistence, and independence; and negative engagement, which was described as tense or conflictual interactions with teachers, peers, and tasks. With 283 preschool children (34–63 months; $M = 50.8$ months; $SD = 6.5$) drawn from 84 classrooms, the researchers observed children's engagement with teachers, peers, and tasks across the preschool program day. The authors found that engagement was a function of the type of activity and the learning partners with whom the children engaged. When children were engaged in free choice or outdoor time activity settings, engagement was found to be positive with both the tasks and the peers with whom the children were learning. More teacher-directed or structured activities were positively related to engagement with teachers. The authors also noted that transitions during the program day were coupled with less positive engagement with teachers (e.g., more conflict and more tension). These findings provide important insight into the contextual variables that support student engagement. The age of the child was also connected with developmental markers such as a more advanced vocabulary, which enabled older preschoolers to have more positive engagement experiences with teachers during structured activities. The authors also found children with more developed self-regulation skills, marked by better behavioral control (e.g., patience, activity level and physical awareness), also had more positive engagement. Children in the study with a language other than English spoken at home had less engagement than those dual language learners whose parents reported speaking English at home. This study is one of few studies cautioning the field to consider the language barrier or other individual variables that might prohibit full engagement in early learning settings.

A recent review and meta-analysis conducted by Lindstrom et al. (2021) examined early childhood engagement with school and subsequent achievement. Beginning with an initial screening of 13,521 studies, the authors identified a final sample of studies ($n = 21$) and calculated 199 effects sizes from those data representing 9749 children on which engagement data had been collected. Measures of the quantity and type of engagement varied considerably across studies but most commonly included the *inCLASS* (Downer et al., 2010), the *Preschool Learning Behaviors Scale* (McDermott et al., 2002), the *Learning to Learn Scale* (McDermott et al., 2011), or the *Teacher Rating Scale of School Adjustment* (Ladd, 1992). The authors found that engagement, broadly described as orientation to and interaction with instructional materials and activities, peers, and teachers, was positively and significantly associated with achievement ($r = 0.24$). The authors found a small, positive relationship between children's early childhood engagement and their subsequent achievement where higher scores on academic engagement were related to higher scores on measures of achievement. Lindstrom and colleagues then explored potential moderators to examine variability across the 21 studies and noted that across the 21 studies that individual study-level factors (e.g., demographic variables, type of engagement measure, achievement content area) did not significantly predict the correlation between engagement and achievement. Thus, the authors suggested a critical need for studies that examine the causal relationship between young children's academic engagement and achievement, including studies that examine these constructs for young children with disabilities.

Behavioral Engagement

The majority of studies on early childhood engagement have focused on the behavioral aspects of the construct. Within the construct, behavior is typically defined as compliance by following the rules in the early learning setting (Finn, 1993; Finn & Rock, 1997). Another component of the construct is participating in the learning activity by devoting attention to the work and persisting with the task even when the task is challenging (Finn et al., 1995; McWilliam et al., 2003). Early childhood studies have relied primarily on observation of these behaviors given the developmental constraints of collecting data, such as surveys, which would be developmentally inappropriate for young children in most cases. Further, the behavioral aspects of engagement are important to measure given that poor engagement is predictive of poor attention, poor impulse control, lack of persistence, navigating transitions, challenges in school readiness, and overall poorer long-term academic success (Bierman et al., 2008; Bierman et al., 2009; Bohlmann & Downer, 2016; Raver, 2002). Examining positive aspects of behavior, such as task engagement, persistence, and interest, has been shown to be related to children's regulation and overall engagement in activity settings (e.g., classrooms, schools, and out of school contexts) and positive peer acceptance (Downer et al., 2010; Hughes & Kwok, 2006; Raver et al., 2011).

Emotional Engagement

Fredricks et al. (2004) describe emotional engagement as reactions, both positive and negative, to teachers, peers, academics, and school that facilitate connectedness and belonging in a learning environment and a child's willingness to participate in that environment. By focusing on measuring social and emotional competencies, Bierman et al. (2008) supported Head Start teachers in the use of evidence-based practices in fostering social and emotional competencies and early language and literacy skills for the four-year-olds within their Head Start REDI study. Designed to help children increase participation, attention, emotional understanding, and social problem-solving, the authors implemented the Preschool PATHS Curriculum (Domitrovich et al., 2007), which encouraged friendship skills, emotional understanding and emotional expression skills, self-control, and problem-solving skills like conflict resolution and negotiation skills. Results from this intervention study supported the direct intervention of teaching social-emotional competencies and language skills with young children ultimately influencing their level of learning engagement at school, marked by self-regulation, learning motivation and involvement, and compliance. Studies documenting these types of interventions promote opportunities for teachers to support young children in forming a positive perception and liking for school as well as a sense of belonging. Such connections also support fewer concerns with behavior and increased activity engagement (Raver, 2002).

Another influential study on early childhood student engagement was conducted by Williford et al. (2013) and examined emotional engagement within a sample that included a high number of Hispanic children. The authors noted that in environments where children could engage positively with teachers and peers, outcomes included increases in compliance with classroom activities, gains in executive function (e.g., tapping a pencil once when the research assistant tapped twice (Pencil Tap task) or sorting toys into bins without playing with them (Toy Sort task; Smith-Donald et al., 2007), and gains in emotion regulation (e.g., is a cheerful child; displays appropriate negative affect in response to hostile, aggressive, or intrusive play using the Emotion Regulation Checklist; Shields & Cicchetti, 1997). The authors also found that positive peer and teacher/child engagement supported children's task orientation (e.g., completes work; functions well event with distraction) and decreased dysregulation. Another finding from the study centered on benefits for children who engaged more negatively in the classroom. For those children, higher positive engagement with teachers was related to greater reductions in dysregulation. A similar effect was found for children when they were less negatively engaged in classroom activities and more positively engaged with peers. The authors highlighted the importance of the children's positive interactions with peers and teachers and those interactions promote emotional engagement in preschool classrooms.

Other work on emotional engagement with young learners has centered on the role of helping children to establish an orientation to formal learning settings and engagement with social partners such as peers and teachers (Buhs & Ladd, 2001; Buhs et al., 2006; Ledford et al., 2020). For example, Early et al. (2010) note that Latino and African American children experience less time in free choice activity settings than their White peers. Studies have also focused on development of a mindset and other emotional connections that foster identification with and engagement in school (Finn, 1989; Ladd et al., 2000; Stipek, 2002; Trentacosta & Izard, 2007; Voelkl, 1997). Finally, studies have also focused on the role of the teacher and their interpersonal connections to children as variables that influence children's emotional engagement (Ladd et al., 1999; Skinner & Belmont, 1993; Valeski & Stipek, 2001).

Relationships

A solid body of evidence supports relationship connections between young children and their teachers and engagement with school (Fuhs et al., 2013; Hamre & Pianta, 2001; Ladd & Dinella, 2009) with engagement operationalized as classroom participation, school liking, peer relationships, and affective and cognitive processes. Young children's orientation to and interactions with teachers and peers directly influence engagement (Ledford et al., 2020; McWilliam & Bailey, 1992). In a study examining 1364 children from birth to sixth grade, O'Connor and McCartney (2007) found that children who had higher-quality relationships with their teachers demonstrated higher levels of classroom engagement (i.e., engagement in learning and engagement in the classroom) than their peers who had lower-quality relationships with their teachers; in turn, engagement predicted achievement (Sobel's $z = 2.88$, $p < 0.01$).

Searle et al. (2013) conducted a study that demonstrated the influence of adult-child relationships on hyperactivity and inattention in preschool and subsequently how the quality and strength of these relationships might improve child behavioral (e.g., effort, attention, and persistence) and cognitive (e.g., preference for challenge, flexible problem solving) engagement. In particular, more positive adult–child relationships (marked by high levels of closeness and low levels of conflict) were associated with lower levels of hyperactivity and inattention ($R^2 = 0.21$ for parent-child relations and $R^2 = 0.37$ for teacher-child relations); in turn, lower hyperactivity and inattention was associated with higher classroom behavioral and cognitive engagement ($R^2 = 0.23$). These findings prompt internal working models of success and thus facilitate a connection of belonging and eagerness to learn. Other scholars have noted the importance of healthy relationships and the impact of conflictual relationships on long-term engagement in school (Birch & Ladd, 1997; Hamre & Pianta, 2001; Hughes et al., 2006; Ladd et al., 1999; Mantzicopoulos & Neuharth-Pritchett, 2003; Roorda et al., 2011). For example, Hughes et al.

(2006) predicted first graders' peer acceptance, classroom engagement, and school belonging as a function of teacher support. The authors found that teacher-student support predicted peer acceptance and classroom engagement. Pianta et al. (1997) found similar outcomes when examining the transition from preschool to kindergarten on the engagement attributes of frustration tolerance and work habits. Within the special education literature, recent work has highlighted concerns in assessing and identifying opportunities and barriers in engagement (Adolfsson et al., 2018).

Early Childhood Engagement Measurement

Although scholars and practitioners have robust data from older students on engagement, measurement of engagement within the early childhood years and in the transition to the primary grades of school can be challenging (Fredricks & McColskey, 2012). As Janosz (2012) notes, longitudinal studies beginning in early childhood are needed to "disentangle the relations between engagement, motivation, and other biopsychosocial aspects of the child and adolescent development (p. 700)." Lam et al. (2012) note the importance of examining both indicators and facilitators of engagement that provide insight into the features and contextual factors that influence student engagement. Mahatmya et al. (2012) advocate for an ecological approach to the study of early childhood engagement which would allow for an examination of person-environment fit, the inclusion of context in engagement examinations, and an opportunity to assess contextual synchrony across transition to elementary school. Although high-quality measures for direct observation such as the BOSS-EE, inCLASS and CLASS (Downer et al., 2010; Gettinger & Walter, 2012; Pianta et al., 2008) have been developed and are incorporated in engagement studies, challenges arise in accessing engagement perceptions from children themselves (Lynch & Cicchetti, 1991; Lynch & Cicchetti, 1992). As Pianta, Hamre, and Allen (2012) note "relationships between teachers and students reflect a classroom's capacity to promote development, and it is precisely in this way that relationships and interactions are the key to understanding engagement (p. 366)." Thus, it is important to consider opportunities to collect child feedback to further examine context for engagement. As cited in other work that centers on belongingness (Finn, 1989), young children's formative experiences in early childhood settings facilitate competence and connection with others. Two measures have been developed which provide a mechanism for young children to share the relationships and engagement with teachers in classrooms, thus adding a dimension to measurement of engagement that can provide unique insights into the starts of developmental trajectories that lead to successful school completion.

Young Children's Appraisals of Teacher Support (Y-CATS). Developed with a sample of children who attended the Head Start program, the Young Children's Appraisals of Teacher Support (Y-CATS) assessment (Mantzicopoulos & Neuharth-Pritchett, 2003) examines children's perceptions of their relationships with their teachers on the constructs of warmth, conflict, and autonomy. Based in attachment theory, Y-CATS taps into children's internal working models of their interactions with their teachers that set the stage for relationship schemas from children's earliest of experiences with schooling and which might influence their perceptions as they make the transitions throughout elementary and secondary school (Howes, Phillipsen, & Peisner-Feinberg, 2000; Pianta, 1999; Pianta et al., 1995).

Y-CATS employs a developmentally appropriate assessment strategy, item formats, and concrete materials that remove concerns associated with verbal expression and information processing abilities (Martin, 1986; Measelle et al., 1998). The measure allowed children to respond to dichotomous items using concrete materials (postcards, a mailbox, and a trashcan). The original scale was developed with data from 364 children enrolled in Head Start with a sample of 187 females and 177 males with a racial/ethnic distribution of 78% White, 18.5% African American,

and 2.2% Latino. Three subscales comprised the overall measure and included: (a) 14 items on children's perceptions of their teachers' acceptance, support, and encouragement [e.g., *My teacher tells me I am smart. My teacher answers my questions.*]; (b) 9 items on the children's perceptions of their teachers' support for choice and autonomy in the activity settings [e.g., *My teacher lets me do activities that I want to do. My teacher lets me play with the kids I choose.*]; and (c) 8 items assessing children's perceived conflict and negativity in the relationship with their teacher [e.g., *My teacher tells me I do not try hard enough. My teacher gets angry with me.*]. Children place postcards for the items on which they agree in a mailbox and items on which they disagree in a trash can. Examiners assure the children that the responses they share would not be relayed to their teachers.

Concurrent validity for the Y-CATS was established along with measures of achievement (Kaufman Assessment Battery for Children-Achievement Battery [Kaufman & Kaufman, 1983] & Woodcock-Johnson-Revised [Woodcock & Johnson, 1990]), problem behaviors and social skills (Conners' Teacher Rating Scale [Conners, 1990], Social Skills Rating System [Gresham & Elliott, 1990]), and student–teacher relationships (Student Teacher Relationship Scale [Pianta & Nimetz, 1991]). Results from an exploratory factor analysis indicated that a three-factor solution best reflected the data, with subscales that included Warmth, Conflict, and Autonomy. Negatively worded autonomy items loaded on the conflict subscale instead of the autonomy subscale suggesting that teachers who discourage autonomy and choice might be perceived by children as negative and as conflict-provoking. In agreement with other early childhood studies (Birch & Ladd, 1997), analyses based on gender also revealed that males reported more conflictual relationships with their teachers than did females.

This tool presents an interesting opportunity to gather data from young children as engagement is measured. Coupled with observational data and measures of relationship quality provided by teachers, the tool can add to a more complete picture of a core feature of engagement. Further, Y-CATS can help with a more robust picture of some of the earliest experiences in school for young children.

Student Engagement Instrument-Elementary Version 2 (SEI-E2). The Student Engagement Instrument (SEI; Appleton et al., 2006) is a well-established student self-report measure examining cognitive and affective engagement of students in secondary (grades 6–12) schooling contexts. The SEI is comprised of five factors that include Control and Relevance of Schoolwork, Future Goals and Aspirations, Teacher-Student Relationships, Peer Support for Learning, and Family Support for Learning. The tool has been used in numerous student engagement studies including those that measure academic achievement, school attendance, suspensions, high school completion, and college attendance and persistence (Appleton et al., 2006; Fraysier et al., 2020; Lovelace et al., 2014; Waldrop et al., 2019). An adaptation of the scale was validated with 1943 elementary school students in 2012 who were in third through fifth grade and consisted of 36 items assessing cognitive (19 items) and affective engagement (14 items) (SEI-Elementary Version; Carter et al., 2012). A confirmatory factor analysis revealed a four-factor solution, differing from the original SEI, and included the scales of Teacher-Student Relationships, Peer Support for Learning, Future Goals and Aspirations, and Family Support for Learning. Items from the Control and Relevance of Schoolwork scale were omitted from the SEI-E.

A recent study further examined the SEI-Elementary Version by extending the collection of data on a modified tool with 1416 first and second-grade children (Wright et al., 2019). The Student Engagement Instrument-Elementary Version 2 (SEI-E2) is another potentially viable assessment tool that allows early childhood educators and researchers to assess engagement from children's perspectives. With data gathered from children who qualified for free- or reduced-price lunch meals (50%) and who were racially and ethnically diverse, a three-point scale was used with response choices of no, maybe, yes, for first

graders and both the three-point and five-point scale for second graders. Of the second graders, 391 completed the three-point scale and 336 completed the five-point scale. The SEI-E2 tool again provided a more developmentally appropriate way to gather children's perceptions by using facial expressions to pictorially guide children to complete the 24 response choices. Survey items were read aloud to the children during administration. Although preliminary in its continued downward extension of the original SEI measure, confirmatory factor analysis suggested that the items on the SEI-E2 for first-grade ratings and the second-grade five-point ratings had the same factor structure as the SEI-Elementary Version but some concerns with reliability in the first-grade responses. This preliminary work also suggests continuity in the SEI as a measure that can capture engagement of students from a young age through transition to college.

Future Directions

Evidence suggests that early childhood education and high-quality experiences that children have during preschool can be very influential for a host of subsequent academic, social, behavioral, and school completion outcomes (Camilli et al., 2010; Jimerson et al., 2000; McCoy et al., 2017). Despite this evidence, there remain areas of inquiry that should be expanded to provide a richer understanding of early childhood engagement. First, there is a need for better measurement of student engagement during early childhood. For example, tools that allow us to account for children's own perceptions of their engagement experiences in early childhood settings might place the field in a better place to document engagement at the earliest point in a student's academic trajectory (Mantzicopoulos & Neuharth-Pritchett, 2003). Recent work on tools that can include children's perceptions will allow us to better document school transitions and provide potential opportunities for both supporting children and their teachers through interventions designed to facilitate positive engagement. Second, longitudinal studies examining not just the etiology of student engagement from early childhood through adolescence (and into adulthood) but also whether and how student engagement evolves over time and across settings are essential for developing effective programs and practices that enhance student engagement. Cognizant that engagement is a process that occurs over time, understanding the initial experiences that children have in early childhood can help the field understand the role of the context, activity settings, and connections with peers and teachers that facilitate students' sense of belonging across the school years. Finally, as is evident by the many definitions of student engagement described in the preceding pages, engagement is a multidimensional construct, commonly comprised of emotional, behavioral, relational, and cognitive aspects (not to mention the instructional activities that facilitate these aspects of student engagement). As such, additional research that simultaneously considers the multiple domains of engagement in early childhood should be carried out. This work would help inform effective practices both inside and outside of the classroom and could serve to provide the field with a more coherent or consistent definition of student engagement.

References

Adolfsson, M., Sjoman, M., & Bjorck-Akesson, E. (2018). ICF-CY as a framework for understanding child engagement in preschool. *Frontiers in Education, 3*, 36. https://doi.org/10.3389/feduc.2018.00036

Ansari, A. (2018). The persistence of preschool effects from early childhood through adolescence. *Journal of Educational Psychology, 110*(7), 952–973.

Appleton, J. J., Christenson, S. L., Kim, D., & Reschly, A. L. (2006). Measuring cognitive and psychological engagement: Validation of the student engagement instrument. *Journal of School Psychology, 44*, 427–445. https://doi.org/10.1016/j.jsp.2006.04.002

Austin, L. J. E., Whitebook, W., & Williams, A. (2021). *Early care and education is in crisis: Biden can intervene.* Center for the Study of Child Care Employment, University of California, Berkeley. https://cscce.berkeley.edu/underfunded-and-broken-the-u-s-child-care-system

Aydogan, C. (2012). *Influences of instructional and emotional classroom environments and learning engagement on low-income children's achievement in the prekindergarten year.* Doctoral thesis, Vanderbilt University.

Barnett, W. S. (1995). Long-term effects of early childhood programs on cognitive and school outcomes. *The Future of Children, 5*, 25–50. https://doi.org/10.2307/1602366

Bennett, K., Reichow, B., & Wolery, M. (2011). Effects of structured teaching on the behavior of young children with disabilities. *Focus on Autism and Other Developmental Disabilities, 26*(3), 143–152. https://doi.org/cnqh4x

Bernstein, S., West, J., Newsham, R., & Reid, M. (2014). *Kindergarteners' skills at school entry: An analysis of the ECLS-K.* Mathematica Policy Research.

Bierman, K. L., Domitrovich, C. E., Nix, R. L., Gest, S. D., Welsh, J. A., Greenberg, M. T., & Gill, S. (2008). Promoting academic and social-emotional school readiness: The head start REDI program. *Child Development, 79*, 1802–1817.

Bierman, K. L., Torres, M. M., Domitrovich, C. E., Welsh, J. A., & Gest, S. D. (2009). Behavioral and cognitive readiness for school: Cross-domain associations for children attending Head Start. *Social Development, 18*, 305–323.

Birch, S. H., & Ladd, G. W. (1997). The teacher-child relationship and children's early school adjustment. *Journal of School Psychology, 35*, 61–79. https://doi.org/10.1016/S0022-4405(96)00029-5

Bohlmann, N. L., & Downer, J. T. (2016). Self-regulation and task engagement as predictors of emergent language and literacy skills. *Early Education and Development, 27*(1), 18–37. https://doi.org/frsc

Booren, L. M., Downer, J. T., & Vitiello, V. E. (2012). Observations of children's interactions with teachers, peers, and tasks across preschool classroom activity settings. *Early Education and Development, 23*(4), 517–538.

Bronfenbrenner, U. (2005). *Making human beings human: Bioecological perspectives on human development.* Sage Publications.

Bryan, L. C., & Gast, D. L. (2000). Teaching on-task and on-schedule behaviors to high-functioning children with autism via picture activity schedules. *Journal of Autism and Developmental Disorders, 30*, 553–567. https://doi.org/dngxqp

Buhs, E. S., & Ladd, G. W. (2001). Peer rejection as an antecedent of young children's school adjustment: An examination of mediating processes. *Developmental Psychology, 37*, 550–560. [PubMed: 11444490].

Buhs, E. S., Ladd, G. W., & Herald, S. L. (2006). Peer exclusion and victimization: Processes that mediate the relation between peer group rejection and children's classroom engagement and achievement? *Journal of Educational Psychology, 98*, 1–13. https://doi.org/fm2ndt

Camilli, G., Vargas, S., Ryan, S., & Barnett, W. S. (2010). Meta-analysis of the effects of early education interventions on cognitive and social development. *Teachers College Record, 112*(3), 579–620.

Campbell, F. A., Pungello, E. P., Burchinal, M., Kainz, K., Pan, Y., Wasik, B. H., … Ramey, C. T. (2012). Adult outcomes as a function of an early childhood educational program: An abecedarian project follow-up. *Developmental Psychology, 48*(4), 1033.

Campbell, F. A., Ramey, C. T., Pungello, E., Sparling, J., & Miller-Johnson, S. (2002). Early childhood education: Young adult outcomes from the abecedarian project. *Applied Developmental Science, 6*(1), 42–57.

Carter, C., Reschly, A. L., Lovelace, M. D., Appleton, J. J., & Thompson, D. (2012). Measuring student engagement among elementary students: Pilot of the elementary student engagement instrument. *School Psychology Quarterly, 27*, 61–73.

Carto, J. J., & Greenwood, C. R. (1985). Eco-behavioral assessment: A methodology for expanding the evaluation of early intervention programs. *Topics in Early Childhood Special Education, 5*(2), 88–104.

Castro, S., Granlund, M., & Almqvist, L. (2017). The relationship between classroom quality-related variables and engagement levels in Swedish preschool classrooms: A longitudinal study. *European Early Childhood Education Research Journal, 25*(1), 122–135. https://doi.org/10.1080/1350293X.2015.1102413

Chien, N. C., Howes, C., Burchinal, M., Pianta, R. C., Ritchie, S., Bryant, D. M., et al. (2010). Children's classroom engagement and school readiness gains in prekindergarten. *Child Development, 81*, 1534–1549. https://doi.org/10.1111/j.1467-8624.2010.01490.x

Conners, C. K. (1990). *Conners' rating scales: Manual.* Multi-Health Systems.

Copple, C., & Bredekamp, S. (2006). *The basics of developmentally appropriate practices in early childhood programs.* National Association for the Education of Young Children.

Dominguez, X., & Greenfield, D. (2009). Learning behaviors mediating the effects of behavior problems on academic outcomes. *NHSA Dialog, 12*, 1–17.

Domitrovich, C. E., Cortes, R., & Greenberg, M. T. (2007). Improving young children's social and emotional competence: A randomized trial of the preschool PATHS curriculum. *Journal of Primary Prevention, 28*, 67–91.

Downer, J. T., Booren, L. M., Lima, O. K., Luckner, A. E., & Pianta, R. C. (2010). The Individualized Classroom Assessment Scoring System (inCLASS): Preliminary reliability and validity of a system for observing preschoolers' competence in classroom interactions. *Early Childhood Research Quarterly, 25*(1), 1–16.

Downer, J. T., Rimm-Kaufman, S. E., & Pianta, R. C. (2007). How do classroom conditions and children's risk for school problems contribute to children's behavioral engagement in learning? *School Psychology Review, 36*(3), 413–432.

Dweck, C. (2016). *Mindset: The new psychology of success.* Ballantine.

Early, D. M., Iruka, I. U., Ritchie, S., Barbarin, O. A., Winn, D. C., et al. (2010). How do pre-kindergarteners spend their time? Gender, ethnicity, and income as predictors of experiences in pre-kindergarten classrooms. *Early Childhood Research Quarterly, 25*, 177–193.

Eden, M. (2021, February). *The drawbacks of universal pre-k: A review of the evidence.* Manhattan Institute for Policy Research.

Fantuzzo, J., Perry, M., & McDermott, P. (2004). Preschool approaches to learning and their relationship to other relevant classroom competencies for low-income children. *School Psychology Quarterly, 19*(3), 212–230.

Ferholt, B., & Rainio, A. P. (2016). Teacher support of student engagement in early childhood: Embracing ambivalence through playworlds. *Early Years, 36*(4), 413–425. https://doi.org/10.1080/09575146.2016.1141395

Finn, J. D. (1989). Withdrawing from school. *Review of Educational Research, 59*, 117–142.

Finn, J. D. (1993). *School engagement and students at risk.* National Center for Education Statistics.

Finn, J. D., Pannozzo, G. M., & Voelkl, K. E. (1995). Disruptive and inattentive withdrawn behavior and achievement among fourth graders. *Elementary School Journal, 95*, 421–454.

Finn, J. D., & Rock, D. A. (1997). Academic success among students at risk for school failure. *Journal of Applied Psychology, 82*, 221–234.

Finn, J. D., & Zimmer, K. S. (2012). Student engagement: What is it? Why does it matter? In S. Christenson, A. Reschly, & C. Wylie (Eds.), *Handbook of research on student engagement.* Springer. https://doi.org/10.1007/978-1-4614-2018-7_5

Fraysier, K., Reschly, A. L., & Appleton, J. J. (2020). Predicting postsecondary enrollment and persistence with secondary student engagement data. *Journal of Psychoeducational Assessment, 38*, 882–899. https://doi.org/10.1177/0734282920903168

Fredricks, J. A., Blumenfeld, P. C., & Paris, A. H. (2004). School engagement: Potential of the concept, state of the evidence. *Review of Educational Research, 74*, 59–109.

Fredricks, J. A., & McColskey, W. (2012). The measurement of student engagement: A comparative analysis of various methods and student self-report instruments. In S. L. Christenson, A. L. Reschly, & C. Wylie (Eds.), *Handbook of research on student engagement* (pp. 763–782). Springer.

Fuhs, M. W., Farran, D. C., & Nesbitt, K. T. (2013). Preschool classroom processes as predictors of children's cognitive self-regulation skills development. *School Psychology Quarterly, 28*, 347–359. https://doi.org/10.1037/spq0000031

García, L., Heckman, J. J., Leaf, D. E., & Prados, M. J. (2016). *The life-cycle benefits of an influential early childhood program.* NBER Working Paper No. 22993 December 2016 JEL No. C93,I28,J13

Gettinger, M., & Walter, M. J. (2012). Classroom strategies to enhance academic engagement time. In S. L. Christenson, A. L. Reschly, & C. Wylie (Eds.), *Handbook of research on student engagement* (pp. 653–674). Springer.

Greenwood, C. R. (1996). The case for performance-based instructional models. *School Psychology Quarterly, 11*(4), 283–296. https://doi.org/b4hqzz

Greenwood, C. R., Horton, B. T., & Utley, C. A. (2002). Academic engagement: Current perspectives on research and practice. *School Psychology Review, 31,* 328–349.

Gresham, F. M., & Elliott, S. N. (1990). *Social skills rating system: Manual.* American Guidance Service.

Hamre, B. K., & Pianta, R. C. (2001). Early teacher–child relationships and the trajectory of children's school outcomes through eighth grade. *Child Development, 72*(2), 625–638. https://doi.org/fcr7xg

Han, J., & Neuharth-Pritchett, S. (2021). Predicting students' mathematics achievement through elementary and middle school: The contribution of state-funded pre-kindergarten program participation. *Child & Youth Care Forum, 50*(4), 587–610. https://doi.org/10.1007/s10566-020-09595-w

Hojnoski, R. L., & Missall, K. N. (2010). Social development in preschool classrooms: Promoting engagement, competence, and school readiness. In M. R. Shinn & H. M. Walker (Eds.), *Interventions for achievement and behavior problems in a three-tier model including RTI* (pp. 703–728). National Association of School Psychologists.

Howes, C., Phillipsen, L. C., & Peisner-Feinberg, E. (2000). The consistency of perceived teacher–child relationships between preschool and kindergarten. *Journal of School Psychology, 38*(2), 113–132. https://doi.org/10.1016/S0022-4405(99)00044-8

Hughes, J. N., & Kwok, O. (2006). Classroom engagement mediates the effect of teacher–student support on elementary students' peer acceptance: A prospective analysis. *Journal of School Psychology, 43,* 465–480. https://doi.org/10.1016/j.jsp.2005.10.001

Hughes, J. N., Zhang, D., & Hill, C. R. (2006). Peer assessments of normative and individual teacher–student support predict social acceptance and engagement among low-achieving children. *Journal of School Psychology, 43,* 447–463.

Immordino-Yang, M. H., Darling-Hammond, L., & Krone, C. R. (2019). Nurturing nature: How brain development is inherently social and emotional, and what this means for education. *Educational Psychologist, 54*(3), 185–204. https://doi.org/10.1080/00461520.2019.1633924

Janosz, M. (2012). Part IV commentary: Outcomes of engagement and engages as an outcome: Some consensus, divergences, and unanswered questions. In S. L. Christenson, A. L. Reschly, & C. Wylie (Eds.), *Handbook of research on student engagement* (pp. 695–706). Springer.

Jimerson, S., Egeland, B., Sroufe, L. A., & Carlson, B. (2000). A prospective longitudinal study of high school dropouts examining multiple predictors across development. *Journal of School Psychology, 38,* 525–549. https://doi.org/10.1016/S0022-4405(00)00051-0

Johnson, M. K., Crosnoe, R., & Elder, G. H., Jr. (2001). Students' attachment and academic engagement: The role of race and ethnicity. *Sociology of Education, 2001,* 318–340.

Kaufman, A. S., & Kaufman, N. L. (1983). *The Kaufman assessment battery for children.* American Guidance System.

Kontos, S., & Keyes, L. (1999). An ecobehavioral analysis of early childhood classrooms. *Early Child Research Quarterly, 14,* 35–50. https://doi.org/10.1016/S0885-2006(99)80003-9

Ladd, G., & Dinella, L. M. (2009). Continuity and change in early school engagement: Predictive of children's achievement trajectories from first to eighth grade? *Journal of Educational Psychology, 101*(1), 190–206. https://doi.org/10.1037/a0013153

Ladd, G. W. (1992). *The teacher rating scale of school adjustment.* University of Illinois.

Ladd, G. W., Birch, S. H., & Buhs, E. S. (1999). Children's social and scholastic lives in kindergarten: Related spheres of influence. *Child Development, 70,* 1373–1400.

Ladd, G. W., Buhs, E. S., & Seid, M. (2000). Children's initial sentiments about kindergarten: Is school liking an antecedent of early classroom participation and achievement? *Merrill-Palmer Quarterly, 46,* 255–279.

Lam, S., Wong, B. P. H., Yang, H., & Liu, Y. (2012). Understanding student engagement with a contextual model. In S. L. Christenson, A. L. Reschly, & C. Wylie (Eds.), *Handbook of research on student engagement* (pp. 403–420). Springer.

Lawson, M., & Lawson, H. (2013). New conceptual frameworks for student engagement research, policy, and practice. *Review of Educational Research, 83,* 432–479. https://doi.org/10.3102/0034654313480891

Lazar, I., Darlington, R., Murray, H., Royce, J., Snipper, A., & Ramey, C. T. (1982). Lasting effects of early education: A report from the Consortium for Longitudinal Studies. *Monographs of the Society for Research in Child Development, 47,* i–151.

Ledford, J. R., Zimmerman, K. N., Severini, K. E., Gast, H., Osborne, K., & Harbin, E. R. (2020). Brief report: Evaluation of the noncontingent provision of fidget toys during group activities. *Focus on Autism and Other Developmental Disabilities, 35,* 101–107. https://doi.org/ggxg86

Lerner, R. M. (2018). *Concepts and theories of human development* (4th ed.). Routledge. https://doi.org/10.4324/9780203581629

Lindstrom, E. R., Chow, J. C., Zimmerman, K. N., Zhao, H., Settanni, E., & Ellison, A. (2021). A systematic review and meta-analysis of the relation between engagement and achievement in early childhood research. *Topics in Early Childhood Special Education, 41*(3), 221–235. https://doi.org/10.1177/02711214211032720

Lovelace, M. D., Reschly, A. L., Appleton, J. J., & Lutz, M. E. (2014). Concurrent and predictive validity of the student engagement instrument. *Journal of Psychoeducational Assessment, 32*(6), 509–520. https://doi.org/10.1177/0734282914527548

Lynch, M., & Cicchetti, D. (1991). Patterns of relatedness in maltreated and non-maltreated children:

Connections among multiple representational models. *Development and Psychopathology, 3*(2), 207–226.

Lynch, M., & Cicchetti, D. (1992). Maltreated children's reports of relatedness to their teachers. *New Directions for Child Development, 57*, 81–107.

Mahatmya, D., Lohman, B. J., Matjasko, J. L., & Farb, A. F. (2012). Engagement across developmental periods. In S. L. Christenson, A. L. Reschly, & C. Wylie (Eds.), *Handbook of research on student engagement* (pp. 45–63). Springer.

Mantzicopoulos, P., & Neuharth-Pritchett, S. (2003). Development and validation of a measure to assess head start children's appraisals of teacher support. *Journal of School Psychology, 41*, 431–451. https://doi.org/10.1016/j.jsp.2003.08.002

Marks, H. M. (2000). Student engagement in instructional activity: Patterns in elementary, middle, and high school years. *American Educational Research Journal, 37*, 153–184.

Martin, R. P. (1986). Assessment of the social and emotional functioning of preschool children. *School Psychology Review, 15*(2), 216–232.

Mashburn, A. J., Pianta, R. C., Hamre, B. K., Downer, J. T., Barbarin, O. A., Bryant, D., … Howes, C. (2008). Measures of classroom quality in prekindergarten and children's development of academic, language, and social skills. *Child Development, 79*(3), 732–749. https://doi.org/10.1111/brbr9f

McCabe, P. C., & Altamura, M. (2011). Empirically valid strategies to improve social and emotional competence of preschool children. *Psychology in the Schools, 48*(5), 513–540.

McClelland, M. M., Morrison, F. J., & Holmes, D. H. (2000). Children at-risk for early academic problems: The role of learning-related social skills. *Early Childhood Research Quarterly, 15*, 307–329.

McCoy, D. C., Yoshikawa, H., Ziol-Guest, K. M., et al. (2017). Impacts of Early childhood education on medium- and long-term educational outcomes. *Educational Researcher, 46*(8), 474–487. https://doi.org/10.3102/0013189X17737739

McDermott, P. A., Fantuzzo, J. W., Warley, H. P., Waterman, C., Angelo, L. E., Gadsden, V. L., & Sekino, Y. (2011). Multidimensionality of teachers' graded responses for preschoolers' stylistic learning behavior: The Learning-To-Learn Scales. *Educational and Psychological Measurement, 71*(1), 148–169.

McDermott, P. A., Leigh, N. M., & Perry, M. A. (2002). Development and validation of the preschool learning behaviors scale. *Psychology in the Schools, 39*(4), 353–365.

McWayne, C., & Cheung, K. (2009). A picture of strength: Preschool competencies mediate the effects of behavior problems on later academic and social adjustment for head start children. *Journal of Applied Developmental Psychology, 30*, 273–285.

McWilliam, R. A., & Bailey, D. B. (1992). Promoting engagement and mastery. In D. B. Bailey & M. Wolery (Eds.), *Teaching infants and preschoolers with disabilities* (2nd ed., pp. 229–256). Merrill.

McWilliam, R. A., & Casey, A. M. (2008). *Engagement of every child in the preschool classroom*. Brookes Publishing.

McWilliam, R. A., Scarborough, A. A., & Kim, H. (2003). Adult interactions and child engagement. *Early Education and Development, 14*, 7–27.

Measelle, J. R., Ablow, J. C., Cowan, P. A., & Cowan, C. P. (1998). Assessing young children's views of their academic, social, and emotional lives: An evaluation of the self-perceptions scales of the Berkeley Puppet Interview. *Child Development, 69*(6), 1556–1576.

Mirkhil, M. (2010). 'I want to play when I go to school': Children's views on the transition to school from kindergarten. *Australasian Journal of Early Childhood, 35*(3), 134–139.

Noltemeyer, A. L., Ward, R. M., & Mcloughlin, C. (2015). Relationship between school suspension and student outcomes: A meta-analysis. *School Psychology Review, 44*(2), 224–240. https://doi.org/f8ctv6

O'Connor, E., & McCartney, K. (2007). Examining teacher–child relationships and achievement as part of an ecological model of development. *American Education Research Journal, 44*(2), 340–369. https://doi.org/dnw96h

Odom, S. L., & Bailey, D. B. (2001). Inclusive preschool programs: Classroom ecology and child outcomes. In M. J. Guralnick (Ed.), *Early childhood inclusion: Focus on change* (pp. 253–276). Brooks.

OECD. (2021). *Family database*. https://www.oecd.org/els/family/database.htm

Pianta, R. C. (1999). *Enhancing relationships between children and teachers*. American Psychological Association.

Pianta, R. C., Hamre, B. K., & Allen, J. P. (2012). Teacher-student relationships and engagement: Conceptualizing, measuring, and improving the capacity of classroom interactions. In S. L. Christenson, A. L. Reschly, & C. Wylie (Eds.), *Handbook of research on student engagement* (pp. 365–386). Springer Science + Business Media. https://doi.org/10.1007/978-1-4614-2018-7_17

Pianta, R. C., LaParo, K. M., & Hamre, B. K. (2008). *Classroom assessment scoring system manual: Pre-K*. Brookes.

Pianta, R. C., & Nimetz, S. L. (1991). Relationship between children and teachers: Associations with classroom and home behavior. *Journal of Applied Developmental Psychology, 12*, 379–393.

Pianta, R. C., Nimetz, S. L., & Bennett, E. (1997). Mother-child relationships, teacher-child relationships, and school outcomes in preschool and kindergarten. *Early Childhood Research Quarterly, 12*, 263-280–280.

Pianta, R. C., Steinberg, M. S., & Rollins, K. B. (1995). The first two years of school: Teacher-child relationships and deflections in children's classroom adjustment. *Development and Psychopathology, 7*, 295–312.

Prykanowski, D. A., Martinez, J. R., Reichow, B., Conroy, M. A., & Huang, K. (2018). Brief report: Measurement of young children's engagement and problem behavior in early childhood settings.

Behavioral Disorders, 44(1), 53–62. https://doi.org/10.1177/0198742918779793

Ramey, C. T., & Ramey, S. L. (2004). Early learning and school readiness: Can early intervention make a difference? *Merrill-Palmer Quarterly, 50*(4), 471–491. https://doi.org/10.1353/mpq.2004.0034

Raver, C. C. (2002). Emotions matter: Making the case for the role of young children's emotional development for early school readiness. *Social Policy Report, 16*, 3–18.

Raver, C. C., Jones, S. M., Li-Grining, C., Zhai, F., Bub, K., & Pressler, E. (2011). CSRP's impact on low-income preschoolers' preacademic skills: Self-regulation as a mediating mechanism. *Child Development, 82*, 362–378.

Reschly, A. L., & Christenson, S. L. (2012). Jingle, jangle, and conceptual haziness: Evolution and future directions of the engagement construct. In S. L. Christenson, A. L. Reschly, & C. Wylie (Eds.), *Handbook of research on student engagement* (pp. 3–19). Springer.

Roorda, D. L., Koomen, H. M. Y., Spilt, J. L., & Oort, F. J. (2011). The influence of affective teacher-student relationships on students' school engagement and achievement: A meta-analytic approach. *Review of Educational Research, 81*(4), 493–529.

Roper, R., & Hinde, R. A. (1978). Social behavior in a play group: Consistency and complexity. *Child Development., 49*, 570–579.

Schweinhart, L. J., Montie, J., Xiang, Z., Barnett, S. W., Belfield, C. R., & Nores, M. (2005). *Lifetime effects: The high/scope perry preschool study through age 40.* High/Scope Press.

Searle, A. K., Miller-Lewis, L. R., Sawyer, M. G., & Baghurst, P. A. (2013). Predictors of children's kindergarten classroom engagement: Preschool adult-child relationships, self-concept, and hyperactivity/inattention. *Early Education & Development, 24*(8), 1112–1136.

Shapiro, A. (2021). The benefits of prekindergarten programs: Strong findings and open questions. *Phi Delta Kappan, 103*(2), 8–13.

Shields, A., & Cicchetti, D. (1997). Emotion regulation among school-age children: The development and validation of a new criterion Q-sort scale. *Developmental Psychology, 33*, 909–916.

Shonkoff, J. P. (2017). *Building a system for science-based R&D that achieves breakthrough outcomes at scale for young children facing adversity.* Center on the Developing Child, Harvard University.

Skinner, E. A., & Belmont, M. J. (1993). Motivation in the classroom: Reciprocal effect of teacher behavior and student engagement across the school year. *Journal of Educational Psychology, 85*, 571–581.

Skinner, E. A., Furrer, C., Marchand, G., & Kindermann, T. (2008a). Engagement and disaffection in the classroom: Part of a larger motivational dynamic? *Journal of Educational Psychology, 100*, 765–781. https://doi.org/10.1037/a0012840

Skinner, E. A., Kindermann, T. A., & Furrer, C. J. (2008b). A motivational perspective on engagement and disaffection: Conceptualization and assessment of children's behavioral and emotional participation in academic activities in the classroom. *Educational and Psychological Measurement, 69*, 493–525. https://doi.org/10.1177/0013164408323233

Skinner, E. A., & Pitzer, J. R. (2012). Developmental dynamics of student engagement, coping, and everyday resilience. In S. L. Christenson, A. L. Reschly, & C. Wylie (Eds.), *Handbook of research on student engagement* (pp. 21–44). Springer.

Smith-Donald, R., Raver, C. C., Hayes, T., & Richardson, B. (2007). Preliminary construct and concurrent validity of the Preschool Self-Regulation Assessment (PSRA) for field-based research. *Early Childhood Research Quarterly, 22*, 173–187.

Stipek, D. (2002). Good instruction is motivating. In A. Wigfield & J. Eccles (Eds.), *Development of achievement motivation.* Academic Press.

Trentacosta, C. J., & Izard, C. E. (2007). Kindergarten children's emotion competence as a predictor of their academic competence in first grade. *Emotion, 7*(1), 77–88.

Valeski, T. N., & Stipek, D. (2001). Young children's feelings about school. *Child Development, 73*, 1198–2013.

van Huizen, T., & Plantenga, J. (2018). Do children benefit from universal early childhood education and care? A meta-analysis of evidence from natural experiments. *Economics of Education Review, 66*, 206–222. https://doi.org/10.1016/j.econedurev.2018.08.001

Vitiello, V., & Williford, A. P. (2016). Relations between social skills and language and literacy outcomes among disruptive preschoolers: Task engagement as a mediator. *Early Childhood Research Quarterly, 36*, 136–144. https://doi.org/f8ssgv

Vitiello, V. E., Booren, L. M., Downer, J. T., & Williford, A. (2012). Variation in children's classroom engagement throughout a day in preschool: Relations to classroom and child factors. *Early Childhood Research Quarterly, 27*(2), 210–220. https://doi.org/10.1016/j.ecresq.2011.08.005

Voelkl, K. E. (1997). Identification with school. *American Journal of Education, 105*, 204–319.

Waldrop, D., Reschly, A. L., Fraysier, K., & Appleton, J. J. (2019). Measuring the engagement of college students: Administration format, structure, and validity of the Student Engagement Instrument-College. *Measurement and Evaluation in Counseling and Development, 52*, 90–107. https://doi.org/10.1080/07481756.2018.1497429

Wang, M. T., & Degol, J. (2014). Stay engaged: Current knowledge and future directions of student engagement research. *Child Development Perspectives, 17*, 24–29.

Wang, M. T., & Eccles, J. S. (2013). School context, achievement motivation, and academic engagement: A longitudinal study of school engagement using a multidimensional perspective. *Learning and Instruction, 28*, 12–23.

Wang, M., & Peck, S.C. (2013). Adolescent educational success and mental health vary across school engagement profiles. *Developmental Psychology, 49*(7), 1266–1276. https://doi.org/10.1037/a0030028

Wang, M.-T., & Eccles, J. S. (2012). Adolescent behavioral, emotional, and cognitive engagement trajectories in school and their differential relations to educational success. *Journal of Research on Adolescence, 22,* 31–39.

Weiland, C., & Yoshikawa, H. (2013). Impacts of a pre-kindergarten program on children's mathematics, language, literacy, executive function, and emotional skills. *Child Development, 84*(6), 2112–2130.

Williford, A. P., Whittaker, J. E., Vitiello, V. E., & Downer, J. T. (2013). Children's engagement within the preschool classroom and their development of self-regulation. *Early Education & Development, 24*(2), 162–187. https://doi.org/10.1080/10409289.2011.628270

Woodcock, R. W., & Johnson, M. B. (1990). *Woodcock – Johnson psycho-educational battery-revised.* DLM Teaching Resources.

Wright, A. G., Reschly, A. L., Hyson, D., & Appleton, J. J. (2019). *Measuring student engagement in early elementary school.* Manuscript under review.

Wylie, C., & Hodgen, E. (2012). Trajectories and patterns of student engagement: Evidence from a longitudinal study. In S. L. Christenson, A. L. Reschly, & C. Wylie (Eds.), *Handbook of research on student engagement* (pp. 585–599). Springer.

Zimmerman, K. N., Ledford, J. R., Gagnon, K. L., & Martin, J. L. (2020). Social stories and visual supports interventions for students at risk for emotional and behavioral disorders. *Behavioral Disorders, 45*(4), 207–223. https://doi.org/fjbr

Using Positive Student Engagement to Create Opportunities for Students with Troubling and High-Risk Behaviors

Amy Jane Griffiths, Rachel Wiegand, and Christopher Tran

Abstract

Only half of adolescents feel engaged in school, with almost a quarter being actively disengaged. Engagement drops as students age because older students report feeling less cared for by adults and see less value in their work. Many of the students experiencing disengagement are those who exhibit high-risk and troubling behaviors. When considering the emotional or psychological aspects of engagement, which are routinely associated with high-risk behaviors, a student must somehow conclude that, at a minimum, at least one specific person at their school truly cares about them. Be it a teacher, coach, administrator, or counselor, when this caring individual expresses respect, concern, and trust in the student, these actions often contribute to a student's belief that another person sees intrinsic value in them as a human being. In this chapter, we underscore the association between student engagement and high-risk behaviors in adolescence. Although all aspects of student engagement are essential to youth's full development, the salience of student engagement when considering troubling and high-risk behaviors in schools warrants educators' attention. We summarize research in this area and provide an overview of system-level interventions and strategies to build bonding and connectedness, specifically for those students who engage in high-risk behaviors.

Introduction

We approach the topic of adolescent student engagement, particularly considering high-risk behaviors, from the perspective that engagement research is incomplete if it only considers students' academic behaviors or personal scholastic incentives. In our view, the student and their personal beliefs and perceptions about school and the schooling process are central to engagement considerations. When examining the emotional or psychological aspects of engagement, which are routinely associated with high-risk behaviors, a student must somehow conclude that, at a minimum, at least one specific person at their school truly cares about them not only as a student but as a person (Gallagher et al., 2019; Lavy & Naama-Ghanayim, 2020; Murray & Malmgren, 2005). When this caring school staff, a teacher, coach, administrator, or counselor, expresses respect, concern, and trust in the student as part of their

A. J. Griffiths (✉) · R. Wiegand · C. Tran
Attallah College of Educational Studies, Chapman University, Orange, CA, USA
e-mail: agriffit@chapman.edu

job (Johnson, 2009), the student may begin to perceive that this person sees intrinsic value in them as a human being (Allen et al., 2018).

The literature reviewed in this chapter underscores the association between student engagement and high-risk behaviors in adolescence. To examine this topic, we first define relevant engagement terms, as well as clarify behaviors that researchers and practitioners would categorize as "troubling" or "high-risk." Next, we describe the framework and theory we use to study and explain engagement. We then summarize research describing the relationships between student engagement and significant outcomes. Finally, we discuss systems-level change, including prevention and intervention strategies to reduce adverse outcomes and build bonding and connectedness, particularly for those students who engage in high-risk behaviors. The importance and urgency of these issues are undeniable as their impacts are particularly pervasive and potentially very harmful. Nearly one-third of secondary school students report decreased engagement during their teen years (Archambault et al., 2009; Ladd et al., 2017). According to a recent study, more than half of 1047 young adults reported school engagement and environment as the primary reasons they did not graduate (McDermott et al., 2019). When looking at the nuances within engagement, most students generally involved in their schooling experience had lower levels of affective engagement than behavioral and cognitive engagement. These results suggest that academics and student behavior, rather than their reported or observed emotional disposition, are often useful indicators of the overall extent of a student's engagement (Archambault et al., 2009). Before examining these critical issues, we define the key terms used throughout this chapter.

Definition of Terms

Engagement

Researchers have studied various aspects of student engagement under a range of terms, including school connectedness, teacher support, school bonding, school climate, school engagement, and more recently, student engagement (Blum & Libbey, 2004; O'Farrell & Morrison, 2003). According to investigators, the term represents a multifaceted construct that involves student thoughts, beliefs, emotions, and behaviors related to school. Prominent voices in this field have organized the conceptualization of engagement into three subtypes: behavioral, cognitive, and emotional or affective (Fredricks et al., 2004; Jimerson et al., 2003; Reschly & Christenson, 2012; Wang & Degol, 2014). However, Appleton et al. (2008) made a convincing argument for four components of student engagement: academic, behavioral, cognitive, and affective. These four components are based on a comprehensive review of literature related to student engagement and particularly the work of Finn (1989), Connell (Connell et al., 1995; Connell & Wellborn, 1991), and McPartland (1994). Academic engagement includes variables such as points earned, homework completion, and time on task. Behavioral engagement may refer to factors such as attendance, the absence of disruptive behaviors, adhering to school rules, participation in extracurricular activities, and student participation in learning and academic assignments (Fredricks et al., 2004). Emotional engagement is the student's emotional reactions at school, including interest, boredom, happiness, sadness, and anxiety (Fredricks et al., 2004). Affective engagement consists of relationships with teachers and peers, as well as feelings of belonging. Cognitive engagement may include indicators such as personal goal development, self-regulation, the relevance of schoolwork to future goals, and the value of learning. Fredricks et al. (2004) described cognitive engagement as a student's investment in learning, self-regulation, and the use of strategies to gain knowledge and skills. This chapter will focus on the affective elements of engagement, utilizing various terms seen in the literature, such as school engagement, student engagement, school connectedness, and school bonding (See also Allen & Boyle, chapter "School Belonging and Student Engagement: The Critical Overlaps, Similarities, and Implications for

Student Outcomes", this volume). School bonding is the oldest term that connotes the personal and relational links associated with reduced participation in risky behaviors.

High-Risk Behaviors

To adequately address youths' participation in high-risk or troubling behaviors, we must define these terms to eliminate subjectivity and, in turn, personal and systemic biases as much as possible. With clear definitions, we can develop targeted and effective prevention and intervention supports. While the manifestations, severity, and circumstances of high-risk or troubling behaviors vary significantly with each individual, these behaviors often fall within one or more of the categories: injurious and/or violent behaviors, sexual behaviors associated with unplanned pregnancy, or exposure to sexually transmitted infections, substance use (e.g., alcohol, tobacco, and other drugs), unhealthy dietary habits, and insufficient physical activity (Centers for Disease Control and Prevention, 2020). This list is by no means exhaustive, but for this text, it does capture the key features of what we mean when we use the terms "high-risk" or "troubling" behaviors.

Framework for Understanding Engagement

The Engagement Process

Social development researchers (e.g., Hawkins et al., 2001) have suggested that student engagement develops in the individual through opportunities for behavioral involvement, social skills training, and rewards for using these social skills in interpersonal situations. Extending this model to include the various terms used in the student engagement literature, Furlong et al. (2003) offered the PACM model. Participation (behavioral involvement) contributes to the formation of interpersonal attachments (social bonding), which in turn results in a student's developing a

sense of personal commitment (valuing of education), ultimately incorporating school Membership (identification as a school community citizen) as part of their self-identity (P → A → C → M). Such a model is relevant to all students, particularly those engaging in high-risk behaviors. If used as the basis for educational practice, this model can guide overall school improvement efforts.

Understanding Varying Levels of Student Engagement

There is a clear distinction between active and positive engagement in school and active and negative disengagement—disengagement is not merely the absence of engagement. Cognitive engagement focuses on how intently the student participates in being a student and uses academic tasks for broader skill development and enhancing self-efficacy. However, researchers (Abbott et al., 1998; Hirschi, 1969) have long recognized that some students do not participate in such personally facilitative ways in the academic context. Drawing from resilience research (Catalano et al., 2001), models show that youth with multiple challenges (e.g., poverty, unstable housing, and racism) are at an increased risk of adverse developmental outcomes. According to current trauma research, more than half of all students report Adverse Childhood Experiences (ACEs), and almost 8% experienced four or more. Exposure to ACEs (e.g., parental separation/divorce, economic hardship, exposure to violence, racial/ethnic mistreatment, parental death, living in a disrupted household) can significantly impact a student's attendance, the likelihood of retention, school engagement, and long-term educational outcomes (Crouch et al., 2019). Demanding life experiences may make it difficult for a student to focus and be behaviorally engaged in school, further exacerbating academic issues. In other words, these vulnerable students are more likely to be disengaged in school and, in turn, continue to be more susceptible to experiencing further challenges throughout adolescence and adulthood in and outside of the school setting.

Investigators have linked disengagement to various undesirable outcomes, including problematic substance use, increased risk of dropping out, and high rates of depression (Henry et al., 2012; Li & Lerner, 2011; Wang & Peck, 2013). Long-term outcomes associated with a higher number of reported ACEs include an increased likelihood of becoming either the perpetrator or victim of violence, incarceration, juvenile arrest, felony charges, reduced life satisfaction and overall mental well-being, poor physical health, and unplanned pregnancy (Bellis et al., 2013; Giovaneli et al., 2016). Individuals with higher ACE scores are also disproportionately at risk of exposing their children to ACEs (Bellis et al., 2013), highlighting the intergenerational effects of trauma on students and families. Again, schools are uniquely positioned to disrupt the cyclical relationship between the accruement of adverse experiences, their impact on school engagement (e.g., academic, behavioral, affective, and cognitive), and overall student outcomes. While those affected by ACEs represent a wide range of demographics, according to national survey data, individuals from ethnically and racially minoritized backgrounds and lower socioeconomic status experience ACEs at higher rates (Crouch et al., 2019; Strompolis et al., 2019).

Often, school community members see these youth as more likely to be "disengaged," "disconnected," or at best inconsistently committed to the school's educational values and mission. Such students are likely to be less motivated by task mastery or performance goals (Eccles & Wigfield, 2002; Finn, 1989, 1993). They are more likely to be suspended from school (Balfanz et al., 2014) and more likely to be suspended for behaviors such as defiance, disobedience, or disrespect directed toward a teacher (Morrison & Skiba, 2001). These experiences can strain the formation of a caring, supportive relationship and undermine a teacher's authority (Gregory & Ripski, 2008). Disengaged students may not just ignore or disregard teachers and other school authority figures. Rather, if they conclude that school is not an accepting and inclusive place, they can actively resist teacher directives

(Solorzarno & Delgado Bernal, 2001). It is not just that disengaged students may believe that their teachers and others at school do not have positive regard for them. They perceive that the school context actively rejects them and does not promote or offer a supportive, caring climate (Noddings, 1995). To prevent and address these common trends among students experiencing disengagement, practitioners must consider various individual and community assets, the presence or absence of which can potentially reinforce or diminish student engagement.

Individual and Community Assets Impacting Engagement

Several organizations and measures focus on student and community assets. The Search Institute uses its framework of 40 developmental assets and their relationship to negative outcomes to inform asset building in communities. Partnering with cities and schools, The Search Institute utilizes these data to develop programs that target student engagement (see also Scales et al., chapter "Developmental Relationships and Student Academic Motivation: Current Research and Future Directions", this volume). These research efforts have led to a multiyear study of developmental assessment among school-aged youth and linked asset profiles to individual school records. The results of this research show that low assets are associated with increased participation in high-risk behaviors such as substance use and aggressive behavior (Roehlkepartain et al., 2003; Search Institute, 2021).

Our work with the California Healthy Kids Survey (CHKS) data further illustrates the association between student engagement and high-risk behaviors and the impact of protective assets on behavioral trends within a school community. The CHKS includes sections about violence, perceptions of safety, harassment, bullying, and the use of alcohol and other drugs. The CHKS also has a Resilience Youth Development Module (RYDM) to measure external resources (protective factors). RYDM external assets items measure students' perceptions of caring relationships, high expectations, and meaningful participation opportunities in school. Hanson and Kim (2007) conducted several factor analyses. They found that the six items from the Caring Relationship and High Expectation subscales combined to form one factor called "school support" with the three meaningful participation items holding together in a different factor.

We examined the CHKS surveys collected during the 2017–2018 ($N = 107,125$) school year in grades 7–12. Students were placed into one of three groups, as shown in Table 1. The first group included youth whose z-scores on the school supports and meaningful participation scales were more than one standard deviation above the entire sample's mean. These students perceived their relationships with teachers to be very positive and caring, and they believed they had ample opportunities to participate in meaningful activities at school. In brief, these students reported being highly connected and engaged with school. At the other end of the connectedness continuum, a second group included youth whose school supports and meaningful participation z-score were more than one standard deviation below the mean for the entire sample. These students were generally disengaged. The remaining students were somewhere in between these two extreme exemplar groups. As shown in Table 1, about one in five students who reported low levels of connectedness and engagement also consistently reported higher rates of involvement in substance use and aggression-related behaviors.

The students who reported school disengagement typically reported engaging in risky behaviors about twice as often as highly engaged students. It is inaccurate to conclude that these behaviors are typical for most students. However, they illustrate that when students can form positive relationships with adults at school, they are less likely to report engaging in troubling and risky behaviors. Next, focusing on high-risk behaviors, we summarize the research literature on the relations of student engagement and disengagement and key student outcomes.

Table 1 Percentage of California students in grades 7 and 12 reporting troubling and high-risk behaviors by perceptions of school support (caring adult relations and high expectations) and opportunities for meaningful participation in school activities ($N = 107,125$)

Troubling and high-risk behaviors	High[a] level of meaningful participation and school supports	All other students	Low[b] level of meaningful participation and school supports
Any past 30-day cigarettes use	1%	1%	3%
Any past 30-day marijuana use	8%	11%	18%
In past 30-days had at least 1 alcoholic drink	10%	12%	12%
Any past 30-day binge drinking	5%	5%	9%
Any past 12-month fighting at school	5%	7%	11%
Any past 12-month skipped school or cut class	20%	26%	34%
Self-report gang member	6%	3%	3%

Note. **School Support** is the total of the following six items: *At my school, there is a teacher or some other adult … (1 = Not at All True, 2 = A Little True, 3 = Pretty Much True, 4 = Very Much True)* who really cares about me; who tells me when I do a good job; who notices when I'm not there; who always wants me to do my best; who listens to me when I have something to say; who believes that I will be a success. **Meaningful participation** is the total of the following three items: *At school… (1 = Not at All True, 2 = A Little True, 3 = Pretty Much True, 4 = Very Much True)* I do interesting activities; I help decide things like class activities or rules; I do things that make a difference. (see Furlong et al., 2009; Hanson & Kim, 2007 for more information on the CHKS survey and these scales). Missing responses for each item ranged from 0.5% to 1.0%

[a] z-scores >1.0

(continued)

Table 1 (continued)

[b] *z*-scores <1.0
Data were provided by Michael Furlong at the University of California, Santa Barbara. The research reported here was supported in part by the Institute of Education Sciences, U.S. Department of Education, through Grant #R305A160157 to the University of California, Santa Barbara. The opinions expressed are those of the authors and do not represent views of the Institute of Education Sciences or the U.S. Department of Education

Student Engagement and Key Student Outcomes

Student Engagement and High-Risk Behaviors

When youth consider engaging in risky and troubling behaviors (i.e., if they are not acting on impulse), various factors can influence their choices. These factors include the behavior's danger, excitement, legality, morality, and, of relevance to this chapter's topic, the opinions of peers and adults (Moses & Villodas, 2017; Wang et al., 2019). With these factors in mind, which aspects of engagement are most salient when considering students who might otherwise be unmotivated or disengaged from school? Most research on adolescents and their involvement in troubling and high-risk behaviors has identified engagement level as particularly important. This research has multidisciplinary origins (public health, education, development, psychopathology). However, it has coalesced to encompass the core notion that adolescents' perceptions of the commitment and care of adults at school are associated with reduced involvement in troubling and high-risk behaviors. Research has established positive relationships between student engagement and student developmental outcomes, including academic achievement (Fredricks et al., 2004; Konold et al., 2018; Lee, 2014), substance use, physical and mental health problems (Carter et al., 2007; Moon et al., 2020), suicidal behavior (Moon et al., 2020), school dropout (McDermott et al., 2019; National Research Council and Institute of Medicine, 2004; Perry, 2008), as well as to conduct problems and violence (De Laet et al., 2016). This section reviews both the short-term and long-term benefits of student engagement and the negative outcomes associated with student disengagement.

Academic Achievement

Historically and presently, empirical studies indicate a distinct and impactful connection between student engagement and academic achievement (Fredricks et al., 2016; Konold et al., 2018). Finn (1989) described the long-term effects of student engagement on academic achievement through a participation-identification model. This model suggests that early disengagement from school (e.g., lack of behavioral participation) leads to unsuccessful academic outcomes. These poor school outcomes lead to student withdrawal and lack of identification with the school. This lack of identification results in nonparticipation in school-related activities, which, in turn, results in unfavorable academic outcomes. The participation-identification model is a cyclical process, meaning that school participation and school identification reciprocally influence each other over time.

Studies have found a strong positive relationship between student engagement and student academic achievement, meaning students who are more engaged tend to perform better on standardized academic assessment (e.g., Lee, 2014; Roeser et al., 1996). These results hold true across demographic variables, including gender, race/ethnicity, and socioeconomic status. Researchers have also identified academic achievement as a positive correlate to student engagement among students engaging in high-risk behaviors (Finn, 1993; Finn & Rock, 1997; Korobova & Starobin, 2015; Olivier et al., 2018). Student engagement has been identified as a critical mediator of academic achievement through academic performance, grade promotion, and grade retention (Perry et al., 2010).

Research has long revealed that students who engage with various aspects of their schooling at higher rates show increased academic achievement when compared to students who are disengaged (Fredricks et al., 2004; Konold et al., 2018). Other school-based factors such as school climate can also mitigate the relationship between engagement and educational achievement. A recent study identified links among school climate, school engagement (e.g., affective and cognitive), and academic achievement. Konold et al. (2018) analyzed survey data from the Virginia Secondary School Climate Survey, which included 60,441 students and 11,442 teachers. They found that schools where participants perceived more structure ($\beta = 0.41$, $p < 0.001$) and higher levels of support ($\beta = 0.52$, $p < 0.001$) fostered more affective (e.g., liking their school, feeling like they belong) and cognitive (e.g., finishing homework, learning as much as possible, valuing earning good grades) student engagement. Specifically, a school's adoption of a more authoritative school climate through high staff expectations of students and strong adult–student relationships correlated with higher student engagement rates. Researchers also found a positive association between academic outcomes ($\beta = 0.77$, $p < 0.001$) and student engagement and noted that implementation of an authoritative school climate framework accounted for 77% of the variance in school academics ($R^2 = 0.77$).

Gillen-O'Neel and Fuligni (2013) surveyed 572 secondary students over four years and found positive associations between students' sense of school belonging, an indicator of affective engagement, and their academic motivation, their level of enjoyment, and belief in the utility of school. Throughout the three-year study, these results sustained even after controlling for Grade Point Average (GPA). These results suggest that when students face academic difficulty, it is likely that they will still enjoy school and find it helpful if they feel a sense of belonging. Similarly, disengaged students who attend school irregularly and do not complete coursework subsequently learn less than their academically engaged peers. This disengaged behavior pattern results in lower levels of overall academic achievement (National Research Council and Institute of Medicine, 2004) and reduced opportunities for positive relationships with adults at school. The relationship between a student's level of school engagement and academic achievement is evident in primary grades (Galla et al., 2014). However, stakeholders may not observe disengagement consequences until later years in middle school and high school (Roscigno & Ainsworth-Darnell, 1999) or adulthood (Abbott-Chapman et al., 2014). Early achievement researchers have found that teacher- and parent-reported engagement (i.e., school liking and avoidance, cooperative and resistant classroom participation, and scholastic achievement) in early primary grades predicts long-term scholastic growth (Ladd & Dinella, 2009) and occupational outcomes in adulthood (Abbott-Chapman et al., 2014).

Galla et al. (2014) found that teachers' ratings of student engagement based on student effortful control (i.e., ability to focus, level of sensitivity of one's perception, exercising inhibitions, taking pleasure in low-intensity activities) and behavioral engagement (i.e., attention, persistence, and effort) in the classroom for 135 elementary-aged children were related to later achievement, as observed through academic test scores. Across this three-year study, individual levels of effortful engagement predicted students' reading scores ($B = 2.71$, $t = 2.03$, $p = 0.043$, Pseudo-$R^2 = 0.02$). In addition, when comparing students' initial levels of engagement to one another, reported effortful engagement (e.g., self-regulatory behavioral engagement and effortful control) significantly predicted both reading ($B = 10.03$, $t = 3.27$, $p = 0.001$, Pseudo-$R^2 = 0.09$) and math ($B = 11.20$, $t = 4.60$, $p < 0.001$, Pseudo-$R^2 = 0.15$) performance on standardized assessments. Early problems with school engagement, or school disengagement, have long-term effects and put students at risk for academic achievement difficulties. Research findings suggest that student engagement continues to parallel achievement patterns through high school (Roscigno & Ainsworth-Darnell, 1999). Overall, the literature suggests that engagement with the school community and academic schoolwork is a proximate determinant of current and future student academic achievement.

School Completion

School dropout is one of the most visible outcomes of pervasive student disengagement (Alliance for Excellent Education, 2009; see also Archambault et al., chapter "Student Engagement and School Dropout: Theories, Evidence, and Future Directions", this volume). In a review of research on outcomes associated with student engagement, Fredricks et al. (2004) found that student disengagement from school, including low academic participation, poor attendance, minimal work involvement, and displays of negative conduct, is a precursor of school dropout (Fredricks et al., 2004). Practices that contribute to students dropping out have been referred to as school pushout. Some of the issues relevant to student engagement include unwelcoming and uncaring school environments, lack of adult support, lack of physical and emotional safety at school, attendance policies, and zero-tolerance and attendance school policies that impact grades and push students out of school. Research demonstrates that dropping out of school (a product of pushout) has significant and lasting consequences for students, schools, and communities (Contractor & Staats, 2014).

Students commonly cite lack of school engagement and an unsupportive environment as their primary catalyst for dropping out of high school before graduation (McDermott et al., 2019). Among a sample of 1047 participants who left high school before graduating, McDermott et al. (2019) found that 52.3% of respondents reported school disengagement as the main reason for deciding to drop out. Prominent subcategories that participants reported within disengagement included, "I was bored," ($n = 104$), "I was failing too many classes," ($n = 141$), and "School wasn't relevant to my life" ($n = 80$). These results indicate that experiencing academic difficulty, consistently feeling disinterested in school, and struggling to understand the applicability of coursework to the real world can all play a part in whether or not students persist in earning their high school diploma.

Students who are not engaged in school are at a greater risk for low academic achievement and school failure and subsequently exhibit higher dropout rates than high achieving students (Janosz et al., 2008; Perry, 2008). Janosz et al. (2008) found that out of a sample of 13,300 students between the ages of 12 and 16, those students with negative or inconsistent school engagement patterns were between 10 and 80 times more likely to drop out of school than peers who exhibited typical school engagement patterns. The consequences of being disengaged from school are serious for youth with high-risk behaviors, who may not have other resources available to help counterbalance the effects of school failure. Disengaged students from impoverished backgrounds in urban school settings are more likely to drop out than disengaged students who are not from disadvantaged backgrounds (Perry, 2008). Historically, punitive practices (e.g., suspension, expulsion, zero-tolerance policies) that result in school pushout have disproportionately impacted minoritized students, including students from low-income families, LGBT students, and students in juvenile justice and alternative education settings. Students who are pushed out typically have fewer academic opportunities and reduced social networks-impacting their long-term success (Pushout, n.d.).

However, just as student disengagement can lead to student dropout, student engagement can be a protective factor against academic failure (Fredricks et al., 2004). Students with high engagement levels are more likely to exhibit high academic achievement and are less likely to drop out of school (Crosnoe et al., 2002). A student's perception of his or her connection to the school, teachers, and peers can act as a protective factor that keeps children in school (Finn & Rock, 1997; Fredricks et al., 2004; Moses & Villodas, 2017). As a product of pushout, we can address school dropout if students, families, teachers, administrators, and communities create welcoming and inclusive schools through systemic change, focusing on long-term outcomes. Prioritizing efforts to increase student engagement on a whole-school level has the potential to serve as preventative, universal support to address the needs of students at increased risk of high school pushout/dropout.

Attendance and Truancy

Student attendance and truancy issues negatively affect overall school performance (Chang & Romero, 2008; Gottfried, 2014). Not only are the impacts on academic outcomes, but overall social and psychological well-being (Gottfried, 2019). Studies have shown that students who maintain more consistent class attendance tend to achieve higher grades and perform better on exams compared to chronically absent students (Moore et al., 2003). Not only do student engagement and attendance have bidirectional impacts on one another, in some models, but attendance is also considered an indicator of student engagement. Thayer-Smith (2007) examined student engagement as measured with on-task (writing, reading, and hands-on activity) and off-task (inattentive, distracted or daydreaming, doing other work, conversing with peers, disturbing others, and playing) behaviors in primary classrooms concerning classroom attendance. Findings indicated that classrooms where student attendance was 96% or more saw higher instances of on-task behavior, while classrooms with 94% attendance or less had more students with off-task behaviors. Implications suggest that nonattendance in elementary students is worthy of greater attention.

Additionally, Miranda-Zapata et al. (2018) examined children ages 12–17 and found that student engagement, particularly affective engagement, has a positive and moderating effect on student attendance and overall academic performance. When examining the relationship between class attendance and students' exam performance, Büchele (2021) found that behavioral engagement (i.e., classroom participation, attendance, and extracurricular participation) served as a mediating factor in promoting better test scores. This finding suggests that it is not enough for students to attend class, but that meaningful engagement, particularly behavioral engagement, is encouraged to improve academic outcomes.

Many factors can contribute to student attendance issues, and in turn, student engagement that we must understand in order to appropriately plan for interventions. Maynard et al. (2017) examined students who were considered truant and used latent class analysis to investigate differences in school engagement, participation in school activities, grades, parental academic involvement, and the number of days missed. Regarding high-risk behaviors and student engagement, the researchers noted that students categorized as chronically truant were more likely to use marijuana and engage in theft, drug sales, and fighting than other groups. Youth who exhibit excessive absences, or what professionals more recently referred to as school refusal behavior, often present with complex symptoms and social-emotional profiles that often contribute to their inability to attend school consistently. Environmental circumstances both in and outside of school can also impact a student's attendance. Common factors contributing to SRB include, but are not limited to, issues related to mental health (e.g., depression, anxiety, oppositional defiant disorder) (Kearney & Albano, 2004), medical and health factors (e.g., sleep problems, chronic pain symptoms, medical symptoms that can result from co-occurring physical or neurodevelopmental conditions) (Arvans & LeBlanc, 2009; Hochadel et al., 2014; Lee et al., 2018), familial influences (Bernstein & Borchardt, 1996), and functional behavior issues (i.e., positive and negative reinforcers that contribute to SRB) (Kearney & Albano, 2004; Kearney & Silverman, 1990). These factors can not only impose barriers to consistent attendance, but when these students are in school, if stakeholders do not address underlying factors, these issues could lead to significantly diminished engagement. As multifaceted and nuanced as these cases are, it is essential to engage these students by looking at the function and causes for poor school attendance. With this information school staff can develop appropriate approaches to enhance student well-being and overall engagement in the school process.

Conduct Problems/Violence

Students who perpetrate various forms of community and school violence often have a history of social alienation and detachment at school (Henry et al., 2012). Experts have also found that students with high levels of behavioral, cognitive, and emotional (i.e., affective) engagement exhibit lower levels of problem behaviors (Finn & Rock, 1997; Olivier et al., 2020a, 2020b). Conversely, students with low engagement are more likely than engaged peers to display negative behaviors or conduct problems such as fighting, which leads to compounding ramifications, including school suspension and further disengagement from school (Carter et al., 2007; Fredricks et al., 2004; Stevenson et al., 2021). School violence and victimization pose similar repercussions for individuals on the receiving end of such behavior. Students experiencing peer victimization through the form of physical, verbal, interpersonal, or general altercations report significantly lower rates of school engagement that continue to decline over time (Ladd et al., 2017). This negative association between engagement and bullying exists among elementary and high school students across various demographics (i.e., gender, race/ethnicity, and socioeconomic status).

In many cases, these circumstances lead to school avoidance, a decline in academic achievement, and negative self-perception of one's academic competence (Ladd et al., 2017). Research shows a correlation between high levels of student engagement and a lower likelihood of being involved in violent behaviors, particularly for ethnically and socioeconomically diverse male and female adolescents in grades 7–12 (Khubchandani & Price, 2018). In addition, recent studies suggest student engagement (e.g., how much a student feels happy at school, how much a student helps keep the school clean, and how much a student feels interested in what is going on at school) can potentially mediate adverse impacts of exposure to community violence on academic achievement (Borofsky et al., 2013; Elsaesser et al., 2020). Investigators have identified student engagement (i.e., regularly attending school) as a protective factor against weapon carrying for ethnically diverse males and Black females (Khubchandani & Price, 2018). Ultimately, students who feel more engaged in school, empowered by their teachers,

and supported by their teachers and peers are less likely to bully others or be victimized by peers (Di Stasio et al., 2016). These findings hold true for both urban and suburban, ethnically diverse adolescents.

Gang Involvement

Research indicates that gang-affiliated youth and those involved in the juvenile justice system, for example, benefit from increased school engagement in many ways. Although there are various risk factors associated with why youth join gangs, student disengagement has played a part in this phenomenon. Sharkey et al. (2010) found that students are less likely to join a gang if they felt good about their academic skills, felt bonded to school, felt that education leads to a successful career, and had positive relationships with peers and mentors. In general, youth who reported a greater sense of belonging in school are more likely to resist gang membership. In the school setting, antisocial behaviors can take the form of anything that breaks school rules or harms others. Gebo and Sullivan (2014) found that youth who reported partaking in violence (i.e., carrying a weapon, physical fighting, hurting someone physically) had a higher likelihood of reported gang affiliation. This study also highlighted the fluidity and variability of gang membership—participation fluctuates both across time for members and between different members and groups making the term difficult to uniformly define and measure (Curry et al., 2002; Thornberry et al., 2003). For this study, Gebo and Sullivan relied on self-reported survey data and asked participants to identify if they were affiliated with a gang in the past year.

Similarly, Barnes et al. (2010) found that youth who reported more delinquent involvement and lower self-control levels were more likely to be in a gang. Hence, the importance of being committed and behaviorally engaged in school serve as protective factors against antisocial behavior and youth gang membership (Ang et al., 2015). Youth with multiple risk factors who have more opportunities to engage in prosocial activities will ultimately shape positive beliefs and values—decreasing the prospects of joining a gang (Bishop et al., 2017). A supportive school environment, gang-aware staff, and academic and social programs are essential aspects of school-based gang prevention and intervention efforts.

Substance Use and Physical and Mental Health Correlates

Empirical sources have also identified student engagement as impacting substance use and physical and mental health outcomes among adolescents. Student disengagement during teenage years may hinder one's ability to acquire the basic proficiencies needed to navigate life. A lack of these skill sets puts individuals at risk for poor overall health outcomes (National Research Council and Institute of Medicine, 2004). Unhealthy behaviors that begin during adolescence are more often found among students with low engagement levels than students with high engagement levels. These behaviors can have negative lifelong consequences. Over the past two decades, research has highlighted the potential protective role of school connectedness and its influence on adolescents' engagement in high-risk behaviors (Resnick et al., 1997). Seeking to strengthen educators' and researchers' understanding of this relationship, Weatherson et al. (2018) reviewed 4 years of extant survey data from a national longitudinal study (i.e., the COMPASS study) yielded from 33,313 Canadian high school participants, intending to identify whether or not a connection existed between students' feelings of school connectedness and their engagement in four health-related behaviors: smoking cigarettes, using marijuana, binge drinking, and engaging in physical activity. According to study results, researchers found lower rates of cigarette smoking was most associated with higher levels of school connectedness (OR = 1.30, $p < 0.0001$), followed by marijuana use (OR = 1.17; $p < 0.0001$) and then binge drinking (OR = 1.10, $p < 0.0001$). In other words, school connectedness may have a potential protective effect against engaging in these health-risk behaviors as students who feel more connected at school are less likely to use cigarettes, marijuana, or alcohol (Weatherson et al., 2018). Researchers have also found increased rates of school connectedness are associated with lower rates of suicidal thoughts and behaviors, particularly among populations that are more vulnerable to experiencing suicidality (e.g., sexual minority youth, youth in the welfare system, youth who engage in sexual activity, and those who report experiencing disconnectedness and bullying) (Maraccini & Brier, 2017).

Additionally, student engagement is associated with student mental health and well-being. Students with high engagement levels have a reduced risk of depression and suicidal ideation than students with low engagement (Carter et al., 2007; Moon et al., 2020; see Suldo et al., in press). These students tend to report better overall mental health and well-being outcomes than disengaged youth (Holdsworth & Blanchard, 2006). Additionally, high levels of student engagement influence healthy behaviors such as higher frequencies of physical activity, better eating habits and nutrition, safer sex, and bicycle helmet use (Carter et al., 2007).

Transition Outcomes: College and Career Readiness

In addition to considering school completion, professionals must consider the impact of engagement in future college and career prospects for students with high-risk behaviors. These impacts are long-lasting and persist well into adulthood. To better understand student engagement's long-term educational and occupational impacts, Abbott-Chapman et al. (2014) analyzed longitudinal survey data. They used data from an original cohort of 6559 respondents ages 9–15, who initially participated in the national Childhood Determinants of Adult Health study in Australia (Menzies Institute for Medical Research, 2015) in 1985. Of this sample, a subsample of 1622 participants provided follow-up responses in 2004–2006. Researchers found that individuals with high rates of school engagement in childhood and adolescence were more likely to obtain a paid position at a higher level of employment (i.e., manager or administrator) compared to those who reported lower rates of school engagement. Similarly, those who stated they completed secondary schooling and/or enrolled in higher education were also more likely to have reported higher school engagement levels during childhood or adolescence. Researchers found these linkages independent of teacher rating of childhood academic achievement, a learner's self-concept, and sociodemographic variables. This study and others indicate that student engagement can be a potential protective factor for student trajectories towards various educational and vocational opportunities accessed in adulthood (Fraysier et al., 2019).

Some studies point to the positive impacts of career and technical education (CTE) programs. For example, Furstenberg and Neumark (2007) studied a school-to-work program in Philadelphia, noting that students in the program were less likely to drop out and more likely to graduate than their peers. Castellano et al. (2014) followed more than 6600 students in three urban districts across three states. They determined that higher graduation rates were associated with earning more CTE credits. Many students, particularly those at risk, lack employability skills, appropriate work habits, and knowledge about career development pos- high school (Ivzori et al., 2020). Educators and community stakeholders should develop specialized support programs to help these youth transition successfully into adult life, particularly as many experience difficulties socially, educationally, and when entering the labor market.

Systems Change: What Can We Do?

Although all aspects of student engagement are important to youth's full development, a vast body of research recognizes the salience of student connectedness when considering troubling and high-risk behaviors in schools. Substantial evidence through randomized control trials (Langberg et al., 2008; Molina et al., 2008;

Murray & Malmgren, 2005; Sinclair et al., 2005), quasi-experimental studies (Gottfredson et al., 2004), and single-case studies (Hawken & Horner, 2003; Moore et al., 1995) strongly support the recommendation to promote positive and caring relationships among students, parents, and staff. Researchers specifically designed most of these studies to improve the school relationships of students who were at risk or had already exhibited behavior problems. Although contexts outside the school setting contribute to student engagement, school staff still need to consider ways to engage students, avoid disengaging students, and reconstruct and repair relationships with students who have disengaged. Fortunately, research indicates that alterable school-based assets influence student engagement for youth at all family risk levels, even when individual traits are considered (Sharkey et al., 2008).

With these findings in mind, it is helpful to assess the extent to which students are engaged in the multiple systems within a school community. O'Farrell et al. (2006) reviewed five levels of engagement supported within the school environment. First, schools can conduct school-wide activities (e.g., clubs, events) that reaffirm relationships with most students who are not at-risk. Second, schools can reach out and reconnect with students who are marginally involved with school and may not respond to universal strategies. Third, schools may need to reconstruct relationships with students who demonstrate emotional and behavioral difficulties through intensive interventions such as individual counseling, family support, comprehensive assessments, and targeted interventions. Fourth, for a small group of individuals, schools will need to repair the relationships of students who may have experienced marginalization or severe or chronic violence on campus and who require interventions to renew a sense of school safety and membership. For marginalized students, opportunities to repair bonds across various social contexts may be of particular importance. Suppose a student is significantly disengaged from school and possibly other environments (home and community). In that case, it may be necessary to use multiple agencies to intervene and create opportunities for attachment and self-efficacy development. We will focus on identifying student support needs and the reconstruction and rehabilitation of relationships for youth engaging in high-risk behavior.

Identifying Student Support Needs

Students spend extensive time in school, making it an optimal setting to receive resources and support, particularly for those experiencing social-emotional and behavioral difficulties (See also Masten et al., chapter "Resilience and Student Engagement: Promotive and Protective Processes in Schools", this volume). To build engaging and connected school environments for students to learn and thrive, school professionals should implement a process to monitor and screen for students' mental health, sense of safety, and engagement. However, well-being remains a narrowly defined term in education, complicating efforts to monitor it effectively in schools (Ereaut & Whiting, 2008). Generally, evaluations of student well-being in schools often include grades, attendance, or discipline incidents frequency (Soutter et al., 2014).

Emerging research and practice conceptualize student well-being in broader terms and place increased attention on physical and mental wellness, risk prevention, and resilience, as well as social-ecological contexts that facilitate safe and supportive schooling (Soutter et al., 2014). An example school-based approach that takes a more holistic view of students is the Student Well-being Model (SWBM). Developed and implemented in New Zealand schools, SWBM offers a framework for developing well-being indicators among students (Soutter et al., 2014). The developers of the SWBM identified critical domains through an extensive review of the well-being literature (Soutter et al., 2014). The seven domains—having (i.e., resources, tools, and opportunities), being (i.e., who one has been, will be and is), relating (i.e., felt and aspired influential relationships), feeling (i.e., one's spectrum of emotions), thinking (i.e., cognitive appraisals and strategies), functioning (i.e., activities, behaviors and involvements), and striving (i.e., content and outcomes of future goals)—are worthy of consideration as schools promote student well-being. The SWBM also draws from Bronfenbrenner's (1979) ecological framework because the seven domains are embedded in the ecological systems of students' lives, such as school, family, and community. In such models, school communities can consider themselves an essential part of each student's ecological system that plays a meaningful role in overall well-being.

Only 12.6% of school/district-level administrators across the nation report conducting school-wide mental health screening with their students (Bruhn et al., 2014), indicating that very few schools put this broader definition of well-being into practice. Many schools take a traditional one-sided approach to mental health by searching for evidence of mental distress concerns among students, but not their psychological strengths and resources. Kim et al. (2014) found that when practitioners use a strength-based instrument and a symptom-based instrument in combination, prediction of students' subjective well-being was significantly better than using only one of the instruments. Understanding both distress and well-being symptoms can help educators support students' psychological strengths and minimize their mental health concerns. Thus, frequently and widely used general surveillance tools of risky behavior, such as the Youth Risk Behavior Surveillance Survey (YRBSS, Kaan et al., 2016), are limited. These tools do offer meaningful information regarding current risky behaviors. However, they do not identify students' psychological strengths, positive relationships, and resources, which may reduce students' risky behaviors and create opportunities for engagement and belonging.

The Social Emotional Health Survey-Secondary (SEHS-S; Furlong et al., 2014) is an example strength-based tool that measures positive psychological traits such as self-awareness, gratitude, and optimism. It also measures social-ecological strengths and resources such as family, peer, and teacher support. These factors are closely tied to student engagement at school and related to long-term academic and well-being outcomes (Kiuru et al., 2019; Moore et al., 2018). In addition to using a measure identifying psychological distress, school professionals could implement a strength-based instrument that examines students' socioemotional strengths and resources. Professionals can use these data to construct relevant and meaningful interventions to improve engagement across the school system.

Intervention and Engaging Protective Mechanisms

Those students involved in the juvenile justice system or who have exhibited significant behavioral concerns represent a unique population at a greater risk of school and lifelong problems. High-risk behavior is related to numerous contextual influences ranging from individual factors to social/community factors. We must consider these factors when understanding how to intervene, engage protective mechanisms in their school environment, and provide these children with an ability to attain positive outcomes. An effective strategy may be to evaluate current practices and their impact, then using this information, eliminate harmful practices, as well as organize and create positive institutions or systems that promote healthy development and potentially alter a child's negative trajectory.

Dismantling Harmful Practices

Given the importance of activating protective mechanisms across multiple settings, schools may begin to intervene with high-risk and troubling behaviors from a systems perspective. To do this, stakeholders and school community members must use data to reflect on whether they are implementing practices to promote engagement in an equitable and culturally responsive way. This reflective practice can assist educators in better understanding how they might be perpetuating those systems and related ideologies that are oppressive, unjust, and harmful, as well as how they are promoting equity in their school communities. It can also shed light on how to improve our practices to make meaningful change. One school-based system historically

and currently shown to have lasting impacts on student engagement outcomes, particularly those from racially and ethnically minoritized backgrounds is school discipline.

Because youth spend much of their time at school, school staff can assist in promoting positive development. Unfortunately, when addressing behavioral problems, schools have historically relied on punitive practices to discipline students, which can lead to disengagement from school and increased involvement in the prison system. The utilization of practices that ultimately funnel students out of the schools and into prisons is a phenomenon known as the School-to-Prison Pipeline (American Civil Liberties Union, 2021). Students who faced more out-of-school suspensions and school referrals were less likely to graduate high school and more likely to engage in delinquent felonies (Teske, 2011). Researchers have identified academic failure, exclusionary discipline practices, and dropout as crucial components of the School-to-Prison Pipeline (Christle et al., 2005).

A common exclusionary practice in schools is zero-tolerance, where students are expelled or suspended from school after a single offense. Originally intended to respond to severe offenses such as gun possession, school administration often uses zero-tolerance policies to address behavioral misconduct, with most using them to curb discipline problems with students (Martinez, 2009). However, research indicates zero-tolerance policies are ineffective and most often harmful. For example, students who face school suspensions, often those from minoritized backgrounds, are at increased risk of experiencing other harmful consequences. These consequences include diminished academic performance, involvement in the juvenile justice system, incarceration, and not finishing high school (Mizel et al., 2016; Pyne, 2019). A literature review indicates that the available data on zero-tolerance contradicts the assumption that these policies reduce misbehavior while concomitantly harming adolescent development (Reynolds et al., 2008).

The existence of exclusionary practices and zero-tolerance policies in schools has raised questions about equity in education. The application of these practices has led to disproportionate and detrimental impacts on minoritized and vulnerable student populations. While the creators of these policies sought to enhance security measures, safety, and engagement in schools, research indicates that students with emotional, behavioral, and learning disabilities are more likely to receive suspensions and expulsions than their general education peers (Henson, 2012).

To understand these disproportionate and detrimental impacts, Alnaim (2018) examined litigation cases involving students in special education and school discipline. While these cases included students who exhibited aggressive behaviors towards staff and possession of weapons at school, the disciplinary actions taken failed to consider the students' disabilities concerning the offenses. Because students in special education have higher frequencies of disruptive behaviors, they are subjected excessively to the disciplinary actions proposed (Henson, 2012).

Students receiving special education services are not the only population disproportionately impacted by zero-tolerance and exclusionary discipline models. Rigid school policies that perpetuate the School-to-Prison Pipeline also affect sexual minority youth and students from racially and ethnically minoritized backgrounds. For instance, LGB (Lesbian, Gay, Bisexual) youth, specifically gender-nonconforming girls, are three times more likely to receive harsh disciplinary treatment from school administrators than their non-LGB peers (Himmelstein & Brückner, 2011). Despite LGB youth making up 5–7% of the student population, they are overrepresented in the juvenile justice system at 15% (Irvine, 2010). Moreover, these youth tend to report higher distrust towards school administrators and believe that schools do not do enough to foster safe school climates (Kosciw et al., 2012).

Recent research has also identified the adverse impacts of applying exclusionary practices and zero-tolerance policies on racially and ethnically minoritized individuals. When considering the disproportionate impact of disciplinary practices on diverse populations, we must also acknowledge the ever-present concept of intersectionality. Multiple components of a student's identity might contribute to the degree of systemic privilege or discrimination they experience with the school system and society as a whole (Azmitia & Mansfield, 2021). For example, students of color are more likely than white students to be suspended from school, particularly Black male students (Huang & Cornell, 2017; Verdugo, 2002). When examining the reasons for disciplinary action, White students tend to receive suspensions for clear violations (possession of guns, weapons, and drugs). In contrast, minoritized students, especially Black male students, are suspended for more subjective reasons such as appearing threatening or disrespectful (Bradshaw et al., 2010; Skiba, 2000; Skiba et al., 2014; Wood et al., 2018a, 2018b; Wood et al., 2021).

Through these models, students are systematically being disconnected and disengaged from their school communities. At an individual level, these marginalized students are likely to experience these practices as a form of rejection from the various systems involved and will likely need multiple opportunities to reconstruct and repair bonds across system contexts. Generally, zero-tolerance practices are blanket policies that may cover unfair and unjust disciplinary decisions because they do not always consider the various contexts in which the problem behaviors occurred, ultimately impacting engagement and infringing on educational equity.

Schools must be committed to equity and continuous improvement to address disparities in engagement and achievement for all students. School leaders can train their staff to use data to make fair decisions and effectively intervene using clear policies. Also, stakeholders must commit to consistently evaluating the school's discipline policies and practices to address fairness and equity (Contractor & Staats, 2014). The use of system-wide proactive approaches to prevent further problems will be essential to decrease problem behavior and increase student achievement, although information to support these strategies' effectiveness with high-risk populations is limited. School teams can prevent some problematic behaviors and improve the learning of all students by capturing an understanding of students' school experiences, eliminating reactive, harmful practices, and fostering positive school climates through proactive school-wide approaches.

Proactive School-Wide Interventions

When addressing student problem behaviors and academic difficulties, school efforts should focus on early prevention by implementing proactive interventions using a Multi-Tiered Systems of Support (MTSS) framework. Many schools have turned to MTSS as it addresses academic, social-emotional, and behavioral concerns. MTSS pulls from the three-tiered public health model, including early identification and prevention (universal intervention), targeted intervention (secondary), and intensive intervention (tertiary) to ensure all individuals are receiving the indicated level of support. For most students, universal interventions (e.g., school-wide positive behavioral interventions; social-emotional learning) provide sufficient support to foster appropriate development. However, some students require more intensive intervention (e.g., individual counseling, check-in check-out, special education services; Lane et al., 2013).

When addressing social-emotional and behavioral concerns, a common approach is Positive Behavioral Interventions and Supports (PBIS). PBIS organizes evidence-based support and intervention programs within three tiers, based on student responses to the intervention and the intensity of support (Horner & Sugai, 2015). PBIS requires ongoing data collection for schools to make informed decisions on student responsiveness. School staff members implement Tier 1 supports universally for all students in a school. At the universal intervention level, PBIS helps foster a safe school environment by developing clear expectations, explicitly teaching the expectations to staff and students, rewarding students when they meet school-wide expectations, and establishing a continuum of logical consequences for student misbehavior (Burke et al., 2014; Kincaid et al., 2016). Schools implementing PBIS use various sources to make data-based decisions regarding implementation fidelity, the effectiveness of interventions, and level of support for individual students. If students are not responsive to Tier 1 supports, they may require more individual or small-group interventions (Tier 2). More intensive individualized interventions (Tier 3) are warranted for students with more complex behavior problems who do not respond to Tier 1 and 2 supports. Student success requires schools to implement PBIS with fidelity: a recent two-year longitudinal study in 31 Ohio school districts found that fidelity to Tier 1 implementation was tied to decreases in suspension rates and reduced problem behaviors (James et al., 2019).

School districts interested in school-wide PBIS will need informed staff with adequate training to implement the various supports and interventions. Bradshaw et al. (2018) examined a teacher coaching program, Double Check, and its impact on student engagement and outcomes. Double Check is a preventive intervention that includes five-hour-long professional development trainings that address culturally responsive practices (i.e., connection to the curriculum, building authentic relationships, reflective thinking, effective communication, and awareness of students' culture). Additionally, individual classroom coaching was used to promote problem-solving skills to facilitate changes in teacher practices. The study took place in 12 racially and ethnically schools, six middle and six elementary schools, with approximately 56.83% of students receiving free and reduced meals. In a teacher-level randomized controlled trial (RCT) design, 100 of the eligible 158 teachers were randomly assigned to receive coaching. Results indicated lower rates of office discipline referrals for students in the classrooms of teachers who received the coaching relative to those who did not. Non-coached teachers had a predicted value of 1.99 disciplinary referrals of black students on average, versus the predicted value for coached teachers of 1.49. Additionally, in comparison to the control group, coached teachers used more proactive behavior management strategies and were more likely to anticipate student needs. Students in those classrooms were observed to be more engaged, cooperative, and displayed less disruptive behaviors (Bradshaw et al., 2018). The findings suggest the value of teacher coaching as a promising component of school-wide PBIS and reducing overall problem student behaviors.

As part of the larger school-wide PBIS, Thorne and Kamps (2008) examined the efficacy of a more targeted group contingency intervention on improving academic engagement for elementary students with behavioral risks. The intervention, which instituted a lottery system and independent group contingency, was incorporated within a previously established school-wide PBIS. Additionally, there was a self-management component to decrease further the time and costs associated with the intervention. At the six-month follow-up, data indicated a decrease in disruptive behavior and increased time engaged with reading. Trevino-Maack et al. (2015) conducted a similar study focused on high school students in remedial reading classes. The intervention had a more pronounced focus on self-monitoring: teachers explicitly taught students target behaviors to demonstrate during class. These target behaviors were displayed on the classroom wall. The teachers verified self-monitoring behaviors by reviewing permanent products (students' writing in their planners, notes taken during class, and completed reading logs). The intervention also included supports in the form of visualization notes and silent timers. While students read for 20 min, they would set timers for every 6 min, and following the timer vibration, students would write in their reading logs. Students who demonstrated the self-monitoring behavior would receive tickets that they could use to earn prizes as part of the independent group contingency intervention. Results indicated that students receiving the intervention showed increases in written work completed in independent reading logs (i.e., mean of 24.19 total words written [TWW] at baseline increased to a mean of 55.34 TWW after intervention implementation) and an overall increase in active engagement (reading aloud, taking notes, independent silent reading) (Trevino-Maack et al., 2015).

School-wide PBIS is not limited to traditional school settings but can be implemented in alternative settings, especially for youth with high-risk problem behaviors. Griffiths et al. (2019a) investigated the application of school-wide positive behavior support (SW-PBIS) in an alternative school setting. This one-year evaluation case study's main purpose was to evaluate the impact of a high school PBIS model on school-wide discipline outcomes (i.e., incident reports, teacher reports of student behavior). The overall level of implementation of PBIS during the first year of implementation reached 69%, as measured by the School-Wide Evaluation Tool. The results indicated that the overall number of incident reports did not significantly differ between the baseline and implementation years. However, there were some significant reductions in defiance-related behaviors ($z = 2.46$, $p < 0.05$) and increased on-task behavior. Process data from this case study revealed the importance of stakeholder buy-in, training opportunities, and suggested adaptations to the PBIS framework for youth in alternative school settings.

In a related study, Griffiths et al. (2019b) divided students at the alternative school based on their PBIS program engagement. Researchers divided students into two groups: "responders" and "nonresponders." Between these groups, they compared students' responses to several measures (obtained before intervention) assessing student perception of individual, school, social/community, and home systems. Results indicated that the individual system model (i.e., variables within the individual—hostility, destructive expression, depression, sense of inadequacy, hope, and life satisfaction) and the school system model (i.e., variables within the school system—academic self-concept, attitude towards teachers, and attitude towards school) could distinguish between responders and nonresponders. A one-way between-groups multivariate analysis of variance (MANOVA) was performed to explore the difference between groups (responders and nonresponders) on hostility, destructive expression of anger, hope, life satisfaction, depression, and sense of inadequacy, there was a statistically significant difference between responders and nonresponders on these combined variables ($F(1, 38) = 3.28$, $p = 0.012$; Wilks' lambda = 0.63; partial eta squared = 0.374).

When the variables were considered separately, the univariate differences to reach statistical significance were hostility, destructive expression of anger, and depression. An inspection of the mean scores indicated increased scores on all of these variables for nonresponders. Within the school system model, there was a statistically significant difference between responders and nonresponders on the combined variables ($F(1, 38) = 3.20$, $p = 0.035$; Wilks' lambda = 0.794; partial eta squared = 0.206). When the univariate analyses were considered, the differences to reach statistical significance were academic self-concept, attitude to teachers, and attitude to school. An inspection of the mean scores indicated increased scores (indicating a problem) on the attitude to teachers and attitude to school subtests for nonresponders. Responders had higher mean scores on academic self-concept. Logistic regression revealed that hostility, destructive expression of anger, depression, academic self-concept, attitude to school, and attitude to teachers, as a group, were able to distinguish responders from nonresponders (c2 (6, $N = 40$) = 12.58, $p = 0.05$).

These studies' findings indicate that PBIS had some impact on improving outcomes for specific behavior types (defiance) for some students in alternative school settings. However, given the students' path to enrollment in an alternative school, these students have likely developed an ingrained distrust and negative attitude toward school and teachers that may require more intensive intervention. These students, particularly those classified as "nonresponders," tend to experience numerous mental health concerns and contextual risk factors and require more intensive support in conjunction with universal interventions.

Targeted Interventions: Classroom-Based Interventions and Student–Teacher Relationships

In addition to considering school-wide approaches, practitioners can manipulate various classroom variables to increase a student's sense of belonging to a positive learning community which may lead to an increase in student engagement (Furlong et al., 2003). These factors include social-emotional learning curriculum, cooperative learning instructional strategies, and positive student–teacher–family relationships.

Social-emotional learning (SEL) can be employed to facilitate academic engagement, work ethic, commitment, and overall school success through explicitly teaching social-emotional skills. SEL has become a prominent prevention strategy in teaching students' key skills: recognizing and managing emotions, setting and achieving goals, appreciating others and their perspectives, and developing and maintaining healthy relationships (Durlak et al., 2011). Often part of a school-wide effort, SEL is commonly implemented at the classroom level to support students and open up communication pathways between students, parents, and school professionals. SEL programs generally aim to increase positive social behaviors and decrease conduct problems and emotional distress (Durlak et al., 2011). Schools across the United States have implemented resources and notable programming from the Collaborative for Academic, Social, and Emotional Learning (CASEL), reporting positive results in outcomes related to behavior, academics, and school environment. The graduation rate in Chicago Public Schools, for example, increased from 59.3% in 2012 to 77.5% in 2017 after integrating CASEL's SEL curriculum and policies and other initiatives to improve school climate and student well-being (Collaborative for Academic, Social, and Emotional Learning [CASEL], 2021).

There are several well-established instructional approaches that may improve students' engagement. For example, Morgan (2006) reviewed studies that examined preference and choice-making as classroom interventions for increasing behavioral task engagement. These 15 studies supported the hypothesis that preference assessment and choice-making improve students' behavior and academic performance. Morgan concluded that teachers who use preference assessment, in addition to choice making, are more likely to improve students' engagement than those using choice-making procedures alone.

Concerning student–teacher relationships, Gregory and Ripski (2008) found that student trust mediated the relationship between teacher relational (personal) discipline approaches and student and teacher-reported defiant behavior. The teachers purposefully sought to make a personal emotional connection with students in this study, and their students reciprocated. In other words, even at the classroom level, the development of a positive, trusting student–teacher relationship is associated with decreases in troubling behaviors (Gregory & Ripski, 2008). In a related study, Suldo et al. (2009) found that middle school students' perceptions of teacher emotional support were related to their global subjective well-being. On the other hand, behaviors such as noncompliance may damage student–teacher relationships and result in missed learning opportunities (Walker & Walker, 1991).

More recently, Roorda et al. (2017) conducted a meta-analysis to evaluate whether student engagement serves as a mediator between affective teacher–student relationships and academic achievement and the impact of these relationships on students' academics (see also Hoefkens & Pianta, chapter "Teacher–Student Relationships, Engagement in School, and Student Outcomes", this volume). Upon reviewing 189 studies, including 249,198 students, researchers found that affective teacher–student relationships (e.g., relationships demonstrating positive attributes—closeness, emotional support, warmth, involvement, acceptance, relatedness) directly impacted academic achievement among primary and secondary students. They also noted indirect associations between student–teacher relationships and student engagement. In longitudinal subsamples, these associations sustained over time.

Many students who engage in high-risk behaviors have had multiple experiences of failure in the school setting and a series of negative interactions with adults at school, at home, and in the community. When further examining relationships between students and their teachers, Hughes and Kwok (2007) investigated the influence of student–teacher and parent–teacher relationships on engagement and achievement. Their model suggests that the quality of the teacher's relationships with students and their parents explained the relationship between students' background and student engagement. Engagement, in turn, mediated the relationships between student-teacher and parent-teacher relatedness and student achievement the following year. Results indicated that Black children and their parents had less supportive relationships with teachers when compared with Latino and White children and their parents. In a recent study, researchers developed the GREET-STOP-PROMPT (GSP) strategy to address discipline disparities among Black male students and strengthen teacher–student relationships (Cook et al., 2018). The GSP approach focused on three components: preventative classroom management strategies to decrease occurrences of problem behavior, identifying and addressing situations in which teachers might engage in implicit bias, and techniques to respond to real or perceived misbehavior effectively and in an empathetic and consistent manner. After implementing the GSP strategy with 40 teachers across three schools, the risk of Black male students receiving an office disciplinary referral decreased by two-thirds. Black male students also reported increased school belonging and connection when comparing pre- and post-test data. This study further highlights the impact of teacher–student relationships and interactions on school performance and school engagement.

Although the link between adolescent students' perceptions of the quality of their relationships with teachers and classroom behavior is proximal (e.g., classroom behavior), other researchers report that it is associated with more distal high-risk behaviors of concern to educators and families. These behaviors include substance use (Rostosky et al., 2003), aggressive/conduct disorder behavior (Frey et al., 2008), and school dropout (Christenson & Thurlow, 2004). Given these relationships, educators should work on parental involvement in school and develop the relationship between parents and teachers, particularly with the families of students from low-income and minority backgrounds.

Career-Focused Interventions to Support Successful Transitions to Postsecondary Life

In addition to being concerned about student engagement in K-12 schooling, our larger goal should be to prepare students to participate in their community as meaningfully engaged adults. This goal must involve effective transition planning. Effective transition planning involves understanding the individual student's strengths and needs and the projected needs of the current and future labor market (Griffiths et al., 2021). A critical component of the United States' ability to sustain readiness for future workforce demands relies on the country's inclusion of a varying range of backgrounds and viewpoints. Students who have experienced adversity have a unique perspective to offer the marketplace. As 85% of the employment opportunities available in 2030 are for jobs that do not yet exist (Institute for the Future & Dell Technologies, 2017), it is essential to develop systemic pathways to employment that include the contributions of employees who offer unique and varied manners of approaching and completing tasks.

Ivzori et al. (2020) studied a program designed to improve students' transition readiness at risk. "Successful Pathways to Employment for youth at Risk" (SUPER) is an 18-week program focused on transitioning from school into employment and adult life. Investigators identified four key components of the program: (a) knowledge of the world of work and employability; (b) an understanding of their identity in terms of skills and occupational desires; (c) a future orientation, involving realistic career planning; and (d) a work experience with ongoing feedback. The program involved several teaching methods, including simulations, problem-solving, interactions with employers and managers, visits to businesses, observations, and work experience. Sixty students from three high schools participated in the program. Results indicated that students' engagement with responsibilities, knowledge about the world of work, and self-reported self-advocacy skills improved from pre-test to post. Also, supervisor ratings of work performance improved over the intervention period.

Typically, transition-related interventions center on employment experience opportunities that are immediately available to the student. While many educators focus on the student's strengths and areas of interest, less attention is paid to the guidance and support a student might need in choosing a sustainable career. School professionals should pay particular attention to projected labor market data. Specifically, teams should focus on three main areas that support well-aligned career and postsecondary education planning: (a) high demand skills (based on supply and demand), (b) in-demand jobs, and (c) projected job growth (Griffiths et al., 2021). Using this information will ensure that we prepare *all* students for long-term success.

Interventions Beyond the School Context

Given the multiple risk factors present in the lives of youth who engage in high-risk behaviors, it is likely that intervention should extend beyond the immediate school setting. However, valuable interventions occur in more than one environment. Multisystemic therapy has shown some promise in making changes for these youth (Timmons-Mitchell et al., 2006). This approach speaks to the importance of understanding each child within the context of the systems within which they are embedded and their individual experiences and needs. Understanding these students' needs on both a broad and in-depth level allows school professionals to measure the student's current status, set goals for the student, coordinate services, and evaluate intervention effectiveness. Rather than pouring multiple resources into an individual without a carefully considered outcome or plan, effective screening and coordination of services may prove to be effective, economical, and efficient.

Summaries of Strategies to Build Bonding and Connectedness for All Students

Positive connectedness to adults at school may serve as a barrier to high-risk or troubling behaviors. It is almost as if when faced with choices related to high-risk behaviors, a student would consider the question of "Who at this school would I disappoint if I engaged in this behavior?" This point highlights the importance of schools focusing on system-level change, evaluating student needs, and implementing interventions that provide the opportunity to reconstruct and repair bonds with marginalized students across various contexts.

One must consider that most students do not engage in troubling or risky behaviors whether or not they are bonded or connected to school. Other protective forces in youth lives include individual strengths and skills, extended family members, community organizations, mentors, extracurricular activities, and many others. As Masten (2009) suggested, youth seem to need and benefit from having life conditions that include adults' caring attention. For many youths, a natural, meaningful context for this to occur is in the school setting. Educators and school-based practitioners can promote school connectedness and healthy youth development by first clearly identifying the needs of their student body through school-wide evaluation. They should evaluate their current practices, reduce harmful reactive approaches, and focus on a proactive, systematic approach to intervention. School communities can establish an agreed-upon set of expectations and consequences. Schools with discipline policies or codes of conduct with clear, reasonable, and consistently applied expectations and consequences help students improve their behavior, increase their engagement, and enhance their academic achievement. Academic programs that successfully manage behavior adjust their programs to the student's functioning level and foster skills in areas of need. This adjustment allows the student to be successful and work in a positive environment. Implementing these strategies has been associated with decreased dropout rates and suspensions (Griffiths et al., 2007) and improved engagement overall.

In the past, we have classified these students themselves as "high-risk," promoting the idea that who they were and the high-risk behaviors that they engaged in were inseparable. This type of classification and labeling can negatively impact these students even if never presented to the students themselves. For example, if the label is present in the mind of any adults who interacts with the student, it would make it very challenging for the adult to connect authentically, view the child as a member of many systems, and celebrate and bolster their strengths (which are essential in fostering school engagement and connectedness). As we reflect on engaging students who are choosing to engage elsewhere (high-risk behaviors), we must seriously consider the systems in which they exist. Are these environments equitable and free of prejudicial thinking? Do they foster opportunities to build caring relationships and bonds that can compete and surpass the potential harmful bonds they might be building elsewhere? Often these students face many reasons not to come to school and begin to seek connections elsewhere. Have we taken all the necessary steps at each tier of prevention and intervention to convey to these students that school is a welcoming, safe and supportive place for them, with opportunities for success, with people who are committed and care?

References

Abbott, R. D., O'Donnell, J., Hawkins, J. D., Hill, K. G., Kosterman, R., & Catalano, R. F. (1998). Changing teaching practices to promote achievement and bonding to school. *The American Journal of Orthopsychiatry, 68*, 542–552. https://doi.org/10.1037/h0080363

Abbott-Chapman, J., Martin, K., Ollington, N., Venn, A., Dwyer, T., & Gall, S. (2014). The longitudinal association of childhood school engagement with adult educational and occupational achievement: Findings from an Australian national study. *British Educational Research Journal, 40*(1), 102–120. https://doi.org/10.1002/berj.3031

Allen, K., Kern, M. L., Vella-Brodrick, D., Hattie, J., & Waters, L. (2018). What schools need to know about fostering school belonging: A meta-analysis. *Educational Psychology Review, 30*, 1–34. https://doi.org/10.1007/s10648-016-9389-8

Alliance for Excellent Education. (2009). *The high cost of high school dropouts: What the nation pays for inadequate high schools.* http://www.all4ed.org/

Alnaim, M. (2018). The impact of zero tolerance policy on children with disabilities. *World Journal of Education, 8*(1), 1–5. https://doi.org/10.5430/wje.v8n1p1

American Civil Liberties Union. (2021). *School-to-prison pipeline.* https://www.aclu.org/issues/racial-justice/race-and-inequality-education/school-prison-pipeline

Ang, R. P., Huan, V. S., Chan, W. T., Cheong, S. A., & Leaw, J. N. (2015). The role of delinquency, proactive aggression, psychopathy and behavioral school engagement in reported youth gang membership. *Journal of Adolescence, 41*, 148–156. https://doi.org/10.1016/j.adolescence.2015.03.010

Appleton, J. J., Christenson, S. L., & Furlong, M. J. (2008). Student engagement with school: Critical conceptual and methodological issues of the construct. *Psychology in the Schools, 45*, 369–386. https://doi.org/10.1002/pits.20303

Archambault, I., Janosz, M., Morizot, J., & Pagani, L. (2009). Adolescent behavioral, affective, and cognitive engagement in school: Relationship to dropout. *The Journal of School Health, 79*, 408–415. https://doi.org/10.1111/j.1746-1561.2009.00428.x

Arvans, R. K., & LeBlanc, L. A. (2009). Functional assessment and treatment of migraine reports and school absences in an adolescent with Asperger's disorder. *Education & Treatment of Children, 32*(1), 151–166. https://doi.org/10.1353/etc.0.0046

Azmitia, M., & Mansfield, K. C. (2021). Editorial: Intersectionality and identity development: How do we conceptualize and research identity intersectionalities in youth meaningfully. *Frontiers in Psychology, 12*, 36. https://doi.org/10.3389/fpsyg.2021.625765

Balfanz, R., Brynes, V., & Fox, J. (2014). Sent home and put off track: The antecedents, disproportionalities, and consequences of being suspended in the ninth grade. *Journal of Applied Research on Children: Informing Policy for Children at Risk, 5*(2), 13. http://digitalcommons.library.tmc.edu/childrenatrisk/vol5/iss2/13

Barnes, J. C., Beaver, K. M., & Miller, J. M. (2010). Estimating the effect of gang membership on nonviolent and violent delinquency: A counterfactual analysis. *Aggressive Behavior, 36*(6), 437–451. https://doi.org/10.1002/ab.20359

Bellis, M. A., Lowey, H., Leckenby, N., Hughes, K., & Harrison, D. (2013). Adverse childhood experiences: Retrospective study to determine their impact on adult health behaviours and health outcomes in a UK population. *Journal of Public Health, 36*(1), 81–91. https://doi.org/10.1093/pubmed/fdt038

Bernstein, G. A., & Borchardt, C. M. (1996). School refusal: Family constellation and family functioning. *Journal of Anxiety Disorders, 10*(1), 1–19. https://doi.org/10.1016/0887-6185(95)00031-3

Bishop, A. S., Hill, K. G., Gilman, A. B., Howell, J. C., Catalano, R. F., & Hawkins, J. D. (2017). Developmental pathways of youth membership: A structural test of the Social Development Model. *Journal of Crime and Justice, 40*(3), 275–296. https://doi.org/10.1080/0735648X.2017.132978

Blum, R. W., & Libbey, H. P. (2004). School connectedness: Strengthening health and educational outcomes for teenagers. Executive summary. *The Journal of School Health, 74*, 231–232. https://doi.org/10.1111/j.1746-1561.2004.tb08278.x

Borofsky, L. A., Kellerman, I., Baucom, B., Oliver, P. H., & Margolin, G. (2013). Community violence exposure and adolescent's school engagement and academic achievement over time. *Psychology of Violence, 3*(4), 381–395. https://doi.org/10.1037/a0034121

Bradshaw, C. P., Mitchell, M. M., O'Brennan, L. M., & Leaf, P. J. (2010). Multi-level exploration of factors contributing to the overrepresentation of black students in office disciplinary referrals. *Journal of Educational Psychology, 102*(2), 508–520. https://doi.org/10.1037/a0018450

Bradshaw, C. P., Pas, E. T., Bottiani, J. H., Debnam, K. J., Reinke, W. M., Herman, K. C., & Rosenberg, M. S. (2018). Promoting cultural responsivity and student engagement through double check coaching of classroom teachers: An efficacy study. *School Psychology Review, 47*(2), 118–134. https://doi.org/10.17105/SPR-2017-0119.V47-2

Bronfenbrenner, U. (1979). *The ecology of human development.* Harvard University Press.

Bruhn, A. L., Woods-Groves, S., & Huddle, S. (2014). A preliminary investigation of emotional and behavioral screening practices in K–12 schools. *Education & Treatment of Children, 37*, 611–634. https://doi.org/10.1353/etc.2014.0039

Büchele, S. (2021). Evaluating the link between attendance and performance in higher education: The role of classroom engagement dimensions. *Assessment & Evaluation in Higher Education, 46*(1), 132–150. https://doi.org/10.1080/02602938.2020.1754330

Burke, M. D., Davis, J. L., Hagan-Burke, S., Lee, Y., & Fogarty, M. (2014). Using SWPBS expectations as a universal screening tool to predict behavioral risk in middle school. *Journal of Positive Behavioral Interventions, 16*, 3–15. https://doi.org/10.1177/1098300712461147

Carter, M., McGee, R., Taylor, B., & Williams, S. (2007). Health outcomes in adolescence: Associations with family, friends and school engagement. *Journal of Adolescence, 30*, 51–62. https://doi.org/10.1016/j.adolescence.2005.04.002

Castellano, M., Sundell, K. E., Overman, L. T., Richardson, G. B., & Stone, J. R. (2014). *Rigorous tests of student outcomes in CTE programs of study: Final Report.* National Research Center for Career and Technical Education. https://files.eric.ed.gov/fulltext/ED574506.pdf

Catalano, R. F., Hawkins, J. D., & Smith, B. H. (2001). Delinquent behavior. Pediatrics in Review, 23, 387–392. https://doi.org/10.1542/pir.23-11-387

Centers for Disease Control and Prevention. (2020, August). *Youth risk behavior surveillance system (YRBSS) overview.* https://www.cdc.gov/healthyyouth/data/yrbs/overview.htm

Chang, H. N., & Romero, M. (2008). *Present, engaged, and accounted for: The critical importance of addressing chronic absence in the early grades.* National Center for Children in Poverty. http://www.nccp.org/wp-content/uploads/2008/09/text_837.pdf

Christenson, S. L., & Thurlow, M. L. (2004). School dropouts: Prevention considerations, interventions, and challenges. *Current Directions in Psychological Science, 13,* 36–39. https://doi.org/10.1111/j.0963-7214.2004.01301010.x

Christle, C. A., Jolivette, K., & Nelson, C. M. (2005). Breaking the school to prison pipeline: Identifying school risk and protective factors for youth delinquency. *Exceptionality, 13*(2), 69–88. https://doi.org/10.1207/s15327035ex1302_2

Collaborative for Academic, Social, and Emotional Learning [CASEL]. (2021). *Key district findings: CDI impact on schools.* https://casel.org/key-findings/

Connell, J. P., Halpern-Felsher, B. L., Clifford, E., Crichlow, W., & Usinger, P. (1995). Hanging in there: Behavioral, psychological, and contextual factors affecting whether African American adolescents stay in high school. *Journal of Adolescent Research, 10,* 41–63. https://doi.org/10.1177/0743554895101004

Connell, J. P., & Wellborn, J. G. (1991). Competence, autonomy, and relatedness: A motivational analysis of self-system processes. In M. R. Gunnar & L. A. Sroufe (Eds.), *Self processes and development* (Vol. 23). Lawrence Erlbaum.

Contractor, D., & Staats, C. (2014). *Interventions to address racialized discipline disparities and school "push out.".* Kirwain Institute.

Cook, C. R., Duong, M. T., McIntosh, K., Fiat, A. E., Pullmann, M. D., & McGinnis, J. (2018). Addressing discipline disparities for black male students: Linking malleable root causes to feasible and effective practices. *School Psychology Review, 47*(2), 135–152. https://doi.org/10.17105/SPR-2017-0026.V47-2

Crosnoe, R., Mistry, R. S., & Elder, G. H., Jr. (2002). Economic disadvantage, family dynamics, and adolescent enrollment in higher education. *Journal of Marriage and the Family, 64,* 690–702. https://doi.org/10.1111/j.1741-3737.2002.00690.x

Crouch, E., Radcliff, E., Hung, P., & Hung. (2019). Challenges to school success and role of adverse childhood experiences. *Academic Pediatrics, 19*(8), 899–907. https://doi.org/10.1016/j.acap.2019.08.006

Curry, G. D., Decker, S. H., & Egley, A., Jr. (2002). Gang involvement and delinquency in a middle school population. *Justice Quarterly, 19,* 275–292. https://doi.org/10.1080/07418820200095241

De Laet, S., Colpin, H., Van Leeuwen, K., Van den Noortgate, W., Claes, S., Janssens, A., Goossens, L., &

Verschueren, K. (2016). Transactional links between teacher-student relationships and adolescent rule-breaking behavior and behavioral school engagement: Moderating role of a dopaminergic genetic profile score. *Journal of Youth & Adolescence, 45,* 1226–1244. https://doi.org/10.1007/210964-016-0466-6

Di Stasio, M. R., Savage, R., & Burgos, G. (2016). Social comparison, competition and teacher-student relationships in junior high school classrooms predicts bullying and victimization. *Journal of Adolescence, 53,* 207–216. https://doi.org/10.1016/j.adolescence.2016.10.002

Durlak, J. A., Weissberg, R. P., Dymnicki, A. B., Taylor, R. D., & Schellinger, K. B. (2011). The impact of enhancing students social and emotional learning: A meta-analysis of school-based universal interventions. *Child Development, 82,* 405–432. https://doi.org/10.1111/j.1467-8624.2010.01564.x

Eccles, J. S., & Wigfield, A. (2002). Motivational beliefs, values, and goals. *Annual Review of Psychology, 53,* 109–132. https://doi.org/10.1146/annurev.psych.53.100901.135153

Elsaesser, C., Gorman-Smith, D., Henry, D., & Schoeny, M. (2020). The longitudinal relations between community violence exposure and academic engagement during adolescence: Exploring families protective role. *Journal of Interpersonal Violence, 35*(17–18), 3264–3285. https://doi.org/10.1177/0886260517708404

Ereaut, G., & Whiting, R. (2008). What do we mean by 'wellbeing'? And why might it matter? (Research Report DCSF-RW073). *Department for Children, Schools and Families.* https://dera.ioe.ac.uk/8572/1/dcsf-rw073%20v2.pdf

Finn, J. D. (1989). Withdrawing from school. *Review of Educational Research, 29,* 141–162. https://doi.org/10.3102/00346543059002117

Finn, J. D. (1993). *School engagement and students at risk.* National Center for Education Statistics.

Finn, J. D., & Rock, D. A. (1997). Academic success among students at risk. *Journal of Applied Psychology, 82,* 221–234. https://doi.org/10.1037/0021-9010.82.2.221

Fraysier, K., Reschly, A., & Appleton, J. (2019). Predicting postsecondary enrollment with secondary student engagement data. *Journal of Psychoeducational Assessment, 38*(7), 882–899. https://doi.org/10.1177/0734282920903168

Fredricks, J. A., Blumenfeld, P. C., & Paris, A. H. (2004). School engagement: Potential of the concept, state of the evidence. *Review of Educational Research, 74,* 59–109. https://doi.org/10.3102/00346543074001059

Fredricks, J. A., Filsecker, M., & Lawson, M. A. (2016). Student engagement, context, and adjustment: Addressing definitional, measurement, and methodological issues. *Learning and Instruction, 43,* 1–4. https://doi.org/10.1016/j.learninstruc.2016.02.002

Frey, A., Ruchkin, V., Martin, A., & Schawb-Stone, M. (2008). Adolescents in transition: School and family characteristics in the development of violent behaviors entering high school. *Child Psychiatry and Human*

Development, 40, 1–13. https://doi.org/10.1007/s10578-008-0105

Furlong, M. J., Ritchey, K., & O'Brennan, L. (2009). Developing norms for the California Resilience Youth Development Module: Internal assets and school resources subscales. *The California School Psychologist, 14,* 35–46. https://doi.org/10.1007/BF03340949

Furlong, M. J., Whipple, A. D., St. Jean, G., Simental, J., Soliz, A., & Punthuna, S. (2003). Multiple contexts of school engagement: Moving toward a unifying framework for educational research and practice. *The California School Psychologist, 8,* 99–114. https://doi.org/10.1007/BF03340899

Furlong, M. J., You, S., Renshaw, T. L., Smith, D. C., & O'Malley, M. D. (2014). Preliminary development and validation of the Social and Emotional Health Survey for secondary school students. *Social Indicators Research, 117,* 1011–1032. https://doi.org/10.1007/s11205-013-0373-0

Furstenberg, F., & Neumark, D. (2007). Encouraging education in an urban school district: Evidence from the Philadelphia educational longitudinal study. *Education Economics, 15*(2), 135–157. https://doi.org/10.1080/09645290701263054

Galla, B. M., Wood, J. J., Tsukayama, E., Har, K., Chui, A. W., & Langer, D. A. (2014). A longitudinal multilevel model analysis of within-person and between-person effect of effortful engagement and academic self-efficacy on academic performance. *Journal of School Psychology, 52,* 295–308. https://doi.org/10.1016/j.jsp.2014.04.001

Gallagher, E. K., Dever, B. V., Hochbein, C., & DuPaul, G. J. (2019). Teacher caring as a protective factor: The effects of behavioral/emotional risk and teaching caring on office disciplinary referrals in middle school. *School Mental Health, 11,* 754–765. https://doi.org/10.1007/s12310-019-09318-0

Gebo, E., & Sullivan, C. J. (2014). A statewide comparison of gang and non-gang youth in public high schools. *Youth Violence and Juvenile Justice, 12*(3), 191–208. https://doi.org/10.1177/1541204013495900

Gillen-O'Neel, C., & Fuligni, A. (2013). Longitudinal study of school belongingness and academic motivation across high school. *Child Development, 84*(2), 678–692. https://doi.org/10.1111/j.1467-8624.2012.01862.x

Giovaneli, A., Reynolds, A. J., Mondi, C. F., & Ou, S. R. (2016). Adverse childhood experiences and adult well-being in a low-income, urban cohort. *Pediatrics, 137*(4), 10. https://doi.org/10.1542/peds.2015-4016

Gottfredson, D. C., Gerstenblith, S. A., Soule, D. A., Womer, S. C., & Lu, S. (2004). Do after school programs reduce delinquency? *Prevention Science: The Official Journal of the Society for Prevention Research, 5,* 253–266. https://doi.org/10.1023/B:PREV.0000045359.41696.02

Gottfried, M. A. (2014). Chronic absenteeism and its effects on students' academic and socioemotional outcomes. *Journal of Education for Students Placed at Risk (JESPAR), 19*(2), 53–75. https://doi.org/10.1080/10824669.2014.962696

Gottfried, M. A. (2019). Chronic absenteeism in the classroom context: Effects on achievement. *Urban Education, 54*(1), 3–34. https://doi.org/10.1177/0042085915618709

Gregory, A., & Ripski, M. B. (2008). Adolescent trust in teachers: Implications for behavior in the high school classroom. *School Psychology Review, 37,* 337–353. https://doi.org/10.1080/02796015.2008.12087881

Griffiths, A. J., Cosier, M., Wiegand, R., Mathur, S. K., & Morgan, S. (2021). Developing strong transition-focused IEPS using labor market data. *Support for Learning, 36*(3), 608–629.

Griffiths, A. J., Diamond, E. M., Alsip, J., Furlong, M., Morrison, G., & Do, B. (2019a). School-wide implementation of positive behavior intervention and supports in an alternative school setting: A case study. *Journal of Community Psychology, 47*(6), 1493–1513. https://doi.org/10.1002/jcop.22203

Griffiths, A. J., Izumi, J., Alsip, J., Furlong, M., & Morrison, G. (2019b). Positive behavior supports in the alternative education setting: Examining the risk and protective factors of responders and non-responders. *Preventing School Failure: Alternative Education for Children and Youth, 63*(2), 149–161. https://doi.org/10.1080/1045988X.2018.1534224

Griffiths, A. J., Parson, L. B., Burns, M. K., & VanDerHeyden, A. M. (2007). *Response to intervention: Research for practice.* National Association of State Directors of Special Education.

Hanson, T. L., & Kim, J. O. (2007). *Measuring resilience and youth development: The psychometric properties of the Healthy Kids Survey* (Issues & Answers Report, REL 2007–No. 034). U.S. Department of Education, Institute of Education Sciences, National Center for Education Evaluation and Regional Assistance, Regional Educational Laboratory West.

Hawken, L. S., & Horner, R. H. (2003). Implementing a targeted intervention within a school-wide system of behavior support. *Journal of Behavioral Education, 12,* 225–240. https://doi.org/10.1023/A:1025512411930

Hawkins, J. D., Guo, J., Hill, K. G., Battin-Pearson, S., & Abbott, R. D. (2001). Long-term effects of the Seattle Social Development intervention on school bonding trajectories. In J. Maggs & J. Schulenberg (Eds.), *Applied developmental science: Special issue: Prevention as altering the course of development* (Vol. 5, pp. 225–236). https://doi.org/10.1207/S1532480XADS0504_04

Henry, K. L., Knight, K. E., & Thornberry, T. P. (2012). School disengagement as a predictor of dropout, delinquency, and problem substance use during adolescence and early adulthood. *Journal of Youth and Adolescence, 41*(2), 156–166. https://doi.org/10.1007/s10964-011-9665-3

Henson, M. (2012). *Issues of crime and school safety: Zero tolerance policies and children with disabilities* (2454) [Master's thesis, University of Central Florida]. Electronic Theses and Dissertations, 2004-2019.

Himmelstein, K. E. W., & Brückner, H. (2011). Criminal-justice and school sanctions against non-heterosexual youth: A national longitudinal study. *Pediatrics, 127*(1), 49–57. https://doi.org/10.1542/peds.2009-2306

Hirschi, T. (1969). *Causes of delinquency*. University of California Press.

Hochadel, J., Frölich, J., Wiater, A., Lehmkuhl, G., & Fricke-Oerkermann, L. (2014). Prevalence of sleep problems and relationship between sleep problems and school refusal behavior in school-aged children in children's and parents' ratings. *Psychopathology, 47*(2), 119–126. https://doi.org/10.1159/000345403

Holdsworth, R., & Blanchard, M. (2006). Unheard voices: Themes emerging from studies of the views about school engagement of young people with high support needs in the area of mental health. *Australian Journal of Guidance and Counselling, 16*, 14–28. https://doi.org/10.1375/ajgc.16.1.14

Horner, R., & Sugai, G. (2015). School-wide PBIS: An example of applied behavior analysis implemented at a scale of social importance. *Behavior Analysis in Practice, 8*, 80–85. https://doi.org/10.1007/s40617-015-0045-4

Huang, F. L., & Cornell, D. G. (2017). Student attitudes and behaviors as explanations for the Black-White suspension gap. *Children and Youth Services Review, 73*, 298–308. https://doi.org/10.1016/j.childyouth.2017.01.002

Hughes, J., & Kwok, O. (2007). Influence of student teacher and parent-teacher relationships on lower achieving readers' engagement and achievement in the primary grades. *Journal of Educational Psychology, 99*, 39–51. https://doi.org/10.1037/0022-0663.99.1.39

Institute for the Future & Dell Technologies. (2017). *The next era of human machine partnerships report*. https://www.delltechnologies.com/content/dam/delltechnologies/assets/perspectives/2030/pdf/SR1940_IFTFforDellTechnologies_Human-Machine_070517_readerhigh-res.pdf

Irvine, A. (2010). "We've had three of them": Addressing the invisibility of lesbian, gay, bisexual, and gender nonconforming youths in the juvenile justice system. *Columbia Journal of Gender and Law, 19*(3), 675. https://doi.org/10.7916/cjgl.v19i3.2603

Ivzori, Y., Sachs, D., Reiter, S., & Schreuer, N. (2020). A transition to employment program (SUPER) for youth at risk: A conceptual and practical model. *International Journal of Environmental Research and Public Health, 17*(11), 3904. https://doi.org/10.3390/ijerph17113904

James, A. G., Noltemeyer, A., Ritchie, R., & Palmer, K. (2019). Longitudinal disciplinary and achievement outcomes associated with school-wide PBIS implementation level. *Psychology in the Schools, 56*, 1512–1521. https://doi.org/10.1002/pits.22282

Janosz, M., Archambault, I., Morizot, J., & Pagani, L. (2008). School engagement trajectories and their differential predictive relations to dropout. *Journal of Social Issues, 64*, 21–40. https://doi.org/10.1111/j.1540-4560.2008.00546.x

Jimerson, S. R., Campos, E., & Greif, J. L. (2003). Toward an understanding of definitions and measures of school engagement and related terms. *California School Psychologist, 8*, 7–27. https://doi.org/10.1007/BF03340893

Johnson, L. S. (2009). School contexts and student belonging: A mixed methods study of an innovative high school. *The School Community Journal, 19*, 99–118.

Kaan, L., McManus, T., Harris, W. A., Shankin, S. L., Flint, K. H., Hawkins, J., Queen, B., Lowry, R., O'Malley Olsen, E., Chyen, D., Whittle, L., Thornton, J., Lim, C., Yamakawa, Y., Brener, N., & Zaza, S. (2016). Youth risk behavior surveillance—United States, 2015. *MMWR Surveillance Summary, 65*(6), 1–174. https://doi.org/10.15585/mmwr.ss6506a1

Kearney, C. A., & Albano, A. M. (2004). The functional profiles of school refusal behavior: Diagnostic aspects. *Behavior Modification, 28*(1), 147–161. https://doi.org/10.1177/0145445503259263

Kearney, C. A., & Silverman, W. K. (1990). A preliminary analysis of a functional model of assessment and treatment for school refusal behavior. *Behavior Modification, 14*(3), 340–366. https://doi.org/10.1177/01454455900143007

Khubchandani, J., & Price, J. H. (2018). Violent behaviors, weapon carrying, and firearm homicide trends in African American adolescents, 2001-2015. *Journal of Community Health, 43*, 947–955. https://doi.org/10.1007/s10900-018-0510-4

Kim, E. K., Furlong, M. J., Dowdy, E., & Felix, E. D. (2014). Exploring the relative contributions of the strength and distress components of dual-factor complete mental health screening. *Canadian Journal of School Psychology, 29*, 127–140. https://doi.org/10.1177/0829573514529567

Kincaid, D., Dunlap, G., Kern, L., Lane, K. L., Bambara, L. M., Brown, F., Fox, L., & Knoster, T. P. (2016). Positive behavior support: A proposal for updating and refining the definition. *Journal of Positive Behavior Interventions, 18*, 69–73. https://doi.org/10.1177/1098300715604826

Kiuru, N., Wang, M. T., Salmela-Aro, K., Kannas, L., Ahonen, T., & Rikka, H. (2019). Associations between adolescents' interpersonal relationships, school Well-being, and academic achievement during educational transitions. *Journal of Youth and Adolescence, 49*, 1057–1072. https://doi.org/10.1007/s10964-019-01184-y

Konold, T., Cornell, D., Jia, Y., & Malone, M. (2018). School climate, student engagement, and academic achievement: A latent variable, multilevel multi-informant examination. *AERA Open, 4*(4), 1–7. https://doi.org/10.1177/2332858418815661

Korobova, N., & Starobin, S. S. (2015). A comparative study of student engagement, satisfaction, and academic success among international and american students. *Journal of International Students, 5*(1), 72–85. https://doi.org/10.32674/jis.v5i1.444

Kosciw, J. G., Greytak, E. A., Bartkiewicz, M. J., Boeson, M. J., & Palmer, N. A. (2012). *The 2011 National School Climate Survey: The experiences of lesbian, gay, bisexual, and transgender youth in our nation's schools.* Gay, Lesbian and Straight Education Network (GLSEN). http://glsen.org/sites/default/files/2011%20National%20School%20Climate%20Survey%20Full%20Report.pdf

Ladd, G. W., & Dinella, L. M. (2009). Continuity and change in early school engagement: Predictive of children's achievement trajectories from first to eighth grade. *Journal of Educational Psychology, 101*, 190–206. https://doi.org/10.1037/a0013153

Ladd, G. W., Ettekal, I., & Kochenderfer-Ladd, B. (2017). Peer victimization trajectories from kindergarten through high school: Differential pathways for children's school engagement and achievement? *Journal of Educational Psychology, 109*(6), 826–841. https://doi.org/10.1037/edu0000177

Lane, L. L., Menzies, H. M., Parks Ennis, R., & Bezdek, J. (2013). School-wide systems to promote positive behaviors and facilitate instruction. *Journal of Curriculum and Instruction, 7*, 6–31. https://doi.org/10.3776/joci.2013.v7n1pp6-31

Langberg, J. M., Epstein, J. N., Urbanowicz, C. M., Simon, J. O., & Graham, A. J. (2008). Efficacy of an organization skills intervention to improve the academic functioning of students with attention-deficit/hyperactivity disorder. *School Psychology Quarterly, 23*, 407–417. https://doi.org/10.1037/1045-3830.23.3.407

Lavy, S., & Naama-Ghanayim, E. (2020). Why care about caring? Linking teachers' caring and sense of meaning at work with students' self-esteem, well-being, and school engagement. *Teaching and Teacher Education, 91*, 103046. https://doi.org/10.1016/j.tate.2020.103046

Lee, J. (2014). The relationship between student engagement and academic performance: Is it a myth or reality? *The Journal of Educational Research, 107*(3), 177–185. https://doi.org/10.1080/00220671.2013.807491

Lee, K. K. S., Chong, J. Q., & Abu Bakar, A. K. (2018). School refusal in adolescents with systemic lupus erythematosus (SLE): A case series. *Asian Journal of Psychiatry, 34*, 59–60. https://doi.org/10.1016/j.ajp.2018.04.021

Li, Y., & Lerner, R. M. (2011). Trajectories of school engagement during adolescence: Implications for grades, depression, delinquency, and substance use. *Developmental Psychology, 47*(1), 233–247. https://doi.org/10.1037/a0021307

Maraccini, M. E., & Brier, Z. M. F. (2017). School connectedness and suicidal thoughts and behaviors: A systematic meta-analysis. *School Psychology Quarterly, 32*(1), 5–21. https://doi.org/10.1037/spq0000192

Martinez, S. (2009). A system gone berserk: How are zero-tolerance policies really affecting schools? *Preventing School Failure Alternative Education for Children and Youth, 53*(3), 153–158. https://doi.org/10.3200/PSFL.53.3.153-158

Masten, A. S. (2009). Ordinary magic: Lessons from research on resilience in human development. *Education Canada, 49*, 28–32. http://www.cea-ace.ca/education-canada/article/ordinary-magic-lessons-research-or-resilience-human-development

Maynard, B. R., Vaughn, M. G., Nelson, E. J., Salas-Wright, C. P., Heyne, D. A., & Kremer, K. P. (2017). Truancy in the United States: Examining temporal trends and correlates by race, age, and gender. *Children & Youth Services Review, 81*, 188–196. https://doi.org/10.1016/j.childyouth.2017.08.008

McDermott, E. R., Donlan, A. E., & Zaff, J. F. (2019). Why do students drop out? Turning points and long-term experiences. *The Journal of Educational Research, 112*(2), 270–282. https://doi.org/10.1080/00220671.2018.1517296

McPartland, J. M. (1994). Dropout prevention in theory and practice. In R. J. Rossi (Ed.), *Schools and students at risk: Context and framework for positive change* (pp. 255–276). Teachers College.

Menzies Institute for Medical Research. (2015). *Childhood determinants of adult health (CDAH) – Phase 3.* University of Tasmania. https://www.menzies.utas.edu.au/research/diseases-and-health-issues/research-projects/childhood-determinants-of-adult-health-cdah-study/childhood-determinants-of-adult-health-cdah-phase-3

Miranda-Zapata, E. D., Lara, L., Navarro, J., & Saracostti, M. (2018). Modeling the effect of school engagement on attendance to classes and school performance. *Revista de Psicodidáctica, 23*(2). https://doi.org/10.1016/j.psicoe.2018.03.001

Mizel, M. L., Miles, J. N. V., Pedersen, E. R., Tucker, J. S., Ewing, B. A., & D'Amico, E. J. D. (2016). To educate or to incarcerate: Factors in disproportionality in school discipline. *Children and Youth Services Review, 70*, 102–111. https://doi.org/10.1016/j.childyouth.2016.09.009

Molina, B. S. G., Flory, K., Bukstein, O. G., Greiner, A. R., Baker, J. L., Krug, V., et al. (2008). Feasibility and preliminary efficacy of an after school program for middle schoolers with ADHD: A randomized trial in a large public middle school. *Journal of Attention Disorders, 12*, 207–217. https://doi.org/10.1177/1087054707311666

Moon, S. S., Kim, Y. J., & Parrish, D. (2020). Understanding the linkages between parental monitoring, school academic engagement, substance use, and suicide among adolescent in U.S. *Child & Youth Care Forum, 49*, 953–968. https://doi.org/10.1007/s10566-020-09570-5

Moore, G. F., Cox, R., Evans, R. E., Hallingberg, B., Hawkins, J., Littlecott, H. J., Long, S. J., & Murphy, S. (2018). School, peer and family relationships and adolescent substance use, subjective wellbeing and mental health symptoms in Wales: A cross sectional study.

Child Indicators Research, 11, 1951–1965. https://doi.org/10.1007/s12187-017-9524-1

Moore, R., Jensen, M., Hatch, J., Duranczyk, I., Staats, S., & Koch, L. (2003). Showing up: The importance of class attendance for academic success in introductory science courses. *The American Biology Teacher, 65*(5), 325–329. https://doi.org/10.1662/0002-7685(2003)065[0325:SUTIOC]2.0.CO;2

Moore, R. J., Cartledge, G., & Heckaman, K. (1995). The effects of social skill instruction and self-monitoring on game-related behaviors of adolescents with emotional or behavioral disorders. *Behavioral Disorders, 20*, 253–266. https://doi.org/10.1177/019874299502000406

Morgan, P. L. (2006). Increasing task engagement using preference or choice making: Some behavioral and methodological factors affecting their efficacy as classroom interventions. *Remedial and Special Education, 27*, 176–187. https://doi.org/10.1177/07419325060270030601

Morrison, G., & Skiba, R. (2001). Predicting violence from school misbehavior: Promises and perils. *Psychology in the Schools, 38*, 173–184. https://doi.org/10.1002/pits.1008

Moses, J. O., & Villodas, M. T. (2017). The potential protective role of peer relationships on school engagement in at-risk adolescents. *Journal of Youth & Adolescence, 46*, 2255–2272. https://doi.org/10.1007/s10964-017-0644-1

Murray, C., & Malmgren, K. (2005). Implementing a teacher-student relationship program in a high poverty urban school: Effects on social, emotional, and academic adjustment and lessons learned. *Journal of School Psychology, 43*, 137–152. https://doi.org/10.1016/j.jsp.2005.01.003

National Research Council and Institute of Medicine. (2004). *Engaging schools: Fostering high school students' motivation to learn. Committee on increasing high school students' engagement and motivation to learn.* The National Academies Press. https://doi.org/10.17226/10421

Noddings, N. (1995). Teaching themes of care. *Phi Delta Kappa, 76*, 675–679.

O'Farrell, S., Morrison, G. M., & Furlong, M. J. (2006). School engagement. In G. Bear & K. Minke (Eds.), *Children's needs III* (pp. 45–58). National Association of School Psychologists.

O'Farrell, S. L., & Morrison, G. M. (2003). A factor analysis exploring school bonding and related constructs among upper elementary students. *The California School Psychologist, 8*, 53–72. https://doi.org/10.1007/BF03340896

Olivier, E., Archambault, I., & Dupéré, V. (2018). Boys' and girls' latent profiles of behavior and social adjustment in school: Longitudinal links with later student behavior engagement and academic achievement? *Journal of School Psychology, 69*, 28–44. https://doi.org/10.1016/j.jsp.2018.05.006

Olivier, E., Archambault, I., & Dupéré, V. (2020b). Do needs for competence and relatedness mediate the risk of low engagement of students with behavior and social problem profiles? *Learning and Individual Differences, 78*, 101842. https://doi.org/10.1016/j.lindif.2020.101842

Olivier, E., Morin, A. J. S., Langlois, J., Tardif-Grenier, K., & Archambault, I. (2020a). Internalizing and externalizing behavior problems and student engagement in elementary and secondary school students. *Journal of Youth and Adolescence, 49*, 2327–2346. https://doi.org/10.1007/s10964-020-01295-x

Perry, J. C. (2008). School engagement among urban youth of color. *Journal of Career Development, 34*, 397–422. https://doi.org/10.1177/0894845308316293

Perry, J. C., Liu, X., & Pabian, Y. (2010). School engagement as a mediator of academic performance among urban youth: The role of career preparation, parental career support, and teacher support. *The Counseling Psychologist, 38*, 269–295. https://doi.org/10.1177/0011000009349272

Pushout. (n.d.). *Supportive school discipline.* https://supportiveschooldiscipline.org/push-out

Pyne, J. (2019). Suspended attitudes: Exclusion and emotional disengagement from school. *Sociology of Education, 92*(1), 59–82. https://doi.org/10.1177/0038040718816684

Resnick, M. D., Bearman, P. S., Blum, R. W., Bauman, K. E., Harris, K. M., Jones, J., Tabor, J., Beuhring, T., Sieving, R. E., Shew, M., Ireland, M., Bearinger, L. H., & Udry, J. R. (1997). Protecting adolescents from harm: Findings from the National Longitudinal Study on Adolescent Health. *Journal of the American Medical Association, 278*, 823–832. https://doi.org/10.1001/jama.278.10.823

Reschly, A. L., & Christenson, S. L. (2012). Jingle, jangle, and conceptual haziness: Evolution and future directions of the engagement construct. In Christenson, S. L., Reschly, A. L., Wylie, C. (Eds.), *Handbook of research on student engagement* (pp. 3–20). Springer.

Reynolds, C. R., Skiba, R. J., Graham, S., Sheras, P., Conoley, J. C., & Garcia-Vasquez, E. (2008). Are zero tolerance policies effective in the schools?: An evidentiary review and recommendations. *The American Psychologist, 63*(9), 852–862. https://doi.org/10.1037/0003-066X.63.9.852

Roehlkepartain, E. C., Benson, P. L., & Sesma, A. (2003). *Signs of progress in putting children first: Developmental assets among youth in St. Louis Park, 1997–2001.* Search Institute.

Roeser, R., Midgley, C., & Urdan, T. C. (1996). Perception of the school environment and early adolescents' psychological and behavioral functioning in school: The mediating role of goals and belonging. *Journal of Educational Psychology, 88*, 408–422. https://doi.org/10.1037/0022-0663.88.3.408

Roorda, D., Zee, M., & Koomen, H. M. Y. (2017). Affective teacher–student relationships and students' engagement and achievement: A meta-analytic update and test of the mediating role of engagement.

School Psychology Review, 46(3), 1–23. https://doi.org/10.17105/SPR-2017-0035.V46-3

Roscigno, V. J., & Ainsworth-Darnell, J. W. (1999). Race and cultural/educational resources: Inequality, micropolitical processes, and achievement returns. *Sociology of Education, 72,* 158–178. https://doi.org/10.2307/2673227

Rostosky, S. S., Owens, G. P., Zimmerman, R. S., & Riggle, E. D. B. (2003). Associations among sexual attraction status, school belonging, and alcohol and marijuana use in rural high school students. *Journal of Adolescence, 26,* 741–751. https://doi.org/10.1016/j.adolescence.2003.09.002

Search Institute. (2021). *Current research on developmental assets.* https://www.search-institute.org/our-research/development-assets/current-research-developmental-assets/

Sharkey, J. D., Shekhtmeyster, Z., Chavez-Lopez, L., Norris, E., & Sass, L. (2010). The protective influence of gangs: Can schools compensate? *Aggression and Violent Behavior, 16*(1), 45–54. https://doi.org/10.1016/j.avb.2010.11.001

Sharkey, J. D., You, S., & Schnoebelen, K. J. (2008). The relationship of school assets, individual resilience, and student engagement for youth grouped by level of family functioning. *Psychology in the Schools, 45,* 402–418. https://doi.org/10.1002/pits.20305

Sinclair, M. F., Christenson, S. L., & Thurlow, M. L. (2005). Promoting school completion of urban secondary youth with emotional or behavioral disabilities. *Exceptional Children, 71,* 465–482. https://doi.org/10.1177/001440290507100405

Skiba, R. (2000). *Zero tolerance, zero evidence: A critical analysis of school disciplinary practice.* Indiana University Press.. https://doi.org/10.1002/yd.23320019204

Skiba, R. J., Chung, C., Trachok, M., Baker, T. L., Sheya, A., & Hughes, R. L. (2014). Parsing disciplinary disproportionality: Contributions of infraction, student, and school characteristics to out-of-school suspension and expulsion. *American Educational Research Journal, 51*(4), 640–670. https://doi.org/10.3102/0002831214541670

Solorzano, D. G., & Delgado Bernal, D. (2001). Examining transformational resistance through a critical race and Latcrit Theory Framework: Chicana and Chicano students in an urban context. *Equity in Urban Education, 36*(1). https://doi.org/10.1177%2F0042085901363002

Soutter, A. K., O'Steen, B., & Gilmore, A. (2014). The student well-being model: A conceptual framework for the development of student well-being indicators. *International Journal of Adolescence and Youth, 19,* 496–520. https://doi.org/10.1080/02673843.2012.754362

Stevenson, N. A., Swain-Bradway, J., & LeBeau, B. C. (2021). Examining high school student engagement and critical factors in dropout prevention. *Assessment for Effective Intervention, 46*(2), 155–164. https://doi.org/10.1177/1534508419859655

Strompolis, M., Tucker, W., Crouch, E., & Radcliff, E. (2019). The intersectionality of adverse childhood experiences, race/ethnicity, and income: Implications for policy. *Journal of Prevention & Intervention in the Community, 47*(4), 310–324. https://doi.org/10.1080/10852352.2019.1617387

Suldo, S. M., Friedrich, A. A., White, T., Farmer, J., Minch, D., & Michalowski, J. (2009). Teacher support and adolescents' subjective well-being: A mixed methods investigation. *School Psychology Review, 38,* 67–85. https://doi.org/10.1080/02796015.2009.12087850

Suldo, S. M., Parker, J., Shaunessy-Dedrick, E., & O'Brennan, L. (in press). Mental health interventions. In J. Fredricks, A. Reschly, & S. Christenson (Eds.), *Handbook of student engagement interventions: Working with disengaged youth.* Elsevier Press.

Teske, S. C. (2011). A study of zero tolerance policies in schools: A multi-integrated systems approach to improve outcomes for adolescents. *Journal of Child and Adolescent Psychiatric Nursing, 24*(2), 88–97. https://doi.org/10.1111/j.1744-6171.2011.00273.x

Thayer-Smith, R. A. (2007). *Student attendance and its relationship to achievement and student engagement in primary classrooms* (Publication No. 1539618718) [Doctoral dissertation, College of William and Mary]. Dissertations, Theses, and Masters Projects.

Thornberry, T. P., Krohn, M. D., Lizotte, A. J., Smith, C. A., & Tobin, K. (2003). *Gangs and delinquency in developmental perspective.* Cambridge University Press.

Thorne, S., & Kamps, D. (2008). The effects of a group contingency intervention on academic engagement and problem behavior of at-risk students. *Behavior Analysis in Practice, 1*(2), 12–18. https://doi.org/10.1007/BF03391723

Timmons-Mitchell, J., Bender, M. B., Kishna, M. A., & Mitchell, C. C. (2006). An independent effectiveness trial of multisystemic therapy with juvenile justice youth. *Journal of Clinical Child and Adolescent Psychology, 35,* 227–236. https://doi.org/10.1207/s15374424jccp3502_6

Trevino-Maack, S. I., Kamps, D., & Wills, H. (2015). A group contingency plus self-management intervention targeting at-risk secondary students' class-work and active engagement. *Remedial and Special Education, 36*(6), 347–360. https://doi.org/10.1177/0741932514561865

Verdugo, R. R. (2002). Race-ethnicity, social class, and zero-tolerance policies: The cultural and structural wars. *Education and Urban Society, 35*(1), 50–75. https://doi.org/10.1177/001312402237214

Walker, H. M., & Walker, J. T. (1991). *Coping with non-compliance in the classroom: A positive approach for teachers*. Pro-Ed.

Wang, M., & Degol, J. (2014). Staying engaged: Knowledge and research needs in student engagement. *Child Development Perspectives, 8*(3), 137–143. https://doi.org/10.1111/cdep.12073

Wang, M.-T., & Peck, S. C. (2013). Adolescent educational success and mental health vary across school engagement profiles. *Developmental Psychology, 49*(7), 1266–1276. https://doi.org/10.1037/a0030028

Wang, Y., Chen, M., & Lee, J. H. (2019). Adolescents' social norms across family, peer, and school settings: Linking social norm profiles to adolescent risky health behaviors. *Journal of Youth and Adolescence, 48*, 935–948. https://doi.org/10.1007/s10964-019-00984-6

Weatherson, K. A., O'Neill, M., Lau, E. Y., Qian, W., Leatherdale, S. T., & Faulkner, G. (2018). The protective effects of school connectedness on substance use and physical activity. *Journal of Adolescent Health, 63*(6), 724–731. https://doi.org/10.1016/j.jadohealth.2018.07.002

Wood, J. L., Harris, F., & Howard, T. C. (2018a). *Get out! Black male suspensions in California public schools*. Community College Equity Assessment Lab and the UCLA Black Male Institute.

Wood, J. L., Harris, F., Howard, T. C., Qas, M., Essien, I., King, T., & Escañuela, V. (2018b). Suspending our future: How inequitable disciplinary practices disenfranchise black kids in California public schools. Community College Equity Assessment Lab and the UCLA Black Male Institute.

Wood, J. L., Harris III, F., Howard, T. C., Qas, M., Essien, I., King, T. M., & Escanuela, V. (2021). Suspending our future: How inequitable disciplinary practices disenfranchise black kids in California's public schools. *The Black Minds Project*. http://bmmcoalition.com/wp-content/uploads/2021/02/SuspendingOurFuture-6-1.pdf

Student Engagement and School Dropout: Theories, Evidence, and Future Directions

Isabelle Archambault, Michel Janosz,
Elizabeth Olivier, and Véronique Dupéré

Abstract

School dropout is a major preoccupation in all countries. Several factors contribute to this outcome, but research suggests that dropouts mostly have gone through a process of disengaging from school. This chapter aims to present a synthesis of this process according to the major theories in the field and review empirical research linking student disengagement and school dropout. This chapter also presents the common risk and protective factors associated with these two issues, the profiles of students who drop out as well as the disengagement trajectories they follow and leading to their decision to quit school. Finally, it highlights the main challenges as well as the future directions that research should prioritize in the study of student engagement and school dropout.

I. Archambault (✉) · M. Janosz · E. Olivier ·
V. Dupéré
University of Montreal, Montreal, QC, Canada
e-mail: isabelle.archambault@umontreal.ca;
michel.janosz@umontreal.ca;
elizabeth.olivier@umontreal.ca;
veronique.dupere@umontreal.ca

Introduction

School dropout is a major concern in many societies. In Western countries in particular, a large proportion of youth quit school before obtaining a high school diploma (Eurostat, 2017; Statistics Canada, 2017; U.S. Department of Commerce, 2017). Many youth who drop out face important setbacks upon entering adulthood: compared to high school graduates, they rely more on social assistance services, are more likely to be involved with the justice system, present more physical and mental health problems, and have a harder time finding jobs, especially stable, well-paid ones with benefits (Tyler & Lofstrom, 2009). While it is profitable for societies to invest in education, contributing to positive development, socio-professional integration and success for youth, school dropout, and other difficulties carry a high cost. The lost income for each cohort of dropouts is estimated to be in the billions of dollars (Alliance for Excellent Education, 2013). Research suggests that many youth who drop out of school had gone through a short- or long-term process of disengagement from school (Dupéré et al., 2015; Rumberger, 2011). This process is increasingly recognized as central to understanding dropout, both in theoretical and empirical work.

This chapter aims to provide some background information regarding the disengagement process related to high school dropout. First, we define the engagement construct and its association with positive youth development. Next, we present the role of the student engagement/disengagement process in school dropout according to the main theories in the field and based on a review of empirical work. We then present the state of the evidence regarding the links between student engagement and dropout by focusing on common risk and protective factors and on student profiles and trajectories of dropout-related disengagement. Finally, we provide an overview of the main challenges and future directions regarding the study of student engagement as a means of understanding and preventing school dropout.

Student Engagement and Positive Development Outcomes

Defining Behavioral, Affective, and Cognitive Engagement

Student engagement is a multidimensional construct generally defined through three distinct components: behavioral, affective, and cognitive engagement (Fredricks et al., 2004). Behavioral engagement refers to observable actions in the classroom. Students who are behaviorally engaged participate in classroom activities, collaborate with peers, and follow their teachers' instructions. They also consistently attend school and refrain from skipping classes without valid reasons (Appleton et al., 2006; Jimerson et al., 2003; Reschly & Christenson, 2012). The affective engagement of students refers to their emotional state and reaction to school and classroom contexts and activities. Students who present high affective engagement feel interested and enthusiastic in class and develop a sense of belonging and well-being in their classroom and school (Archambault & Dupéré, 2017; Skinner et al., 2008; Wang et al., 2016). Finally, students who are cognitively engaged use appropriate self-regulation and deep-processing strategies while learning. They attentively plan their work and draw on available resources, such as grammars or worksheets, to complete their assignments. Cognitively engaged students are

proactive in preventing, correcting, and learning from their mistakes. They review their work and try to understand their errors. While more easily observable than affective engagement, student cognitive engagement also refers to an internal process and therefore remains more difficult to detect than behavioral engagement for teachers (Appleton et al., 2006; Finn & Zimmer, 2012).

The three dimensions of student engagement not only describe youth's holistic functioning demonstrating investment and attachment to school but also retain a part of specificity related to distinct underlying mechanisms, i.e., behaviors, emotions, and thoughts (Dierendonck et al., 2020; Wang et al., 2019). As such, they are interconnected across the developmental process: A change in one dimension can affect the other dimensions over time (Li & Lerner, 2011, 2013; Skinner et al., 2009), as it can promote or undermine positive youth development. Finally, while researchers have typically conceptualized disengagement as the absence of engagement, some defined engagement and disengagement as distinct constructs (Skinner & Belmont, 1993; Martin, 2007). In fact, according to Fredricks et al. (2016), both perspectives may be valid. Some indicators, like not participating in school activities, reflect a low level of engagement, while others, like guessing or forgetting answers during school-related activities, are very specific to disengagement.

Benefits of Student Engagement

Student engagement contributes to positive youth development. Across their academic journey, highly engaged students present fewer behavioral and emotional difficulties and better mental health (Fredricks et al., 2019; Henry et al., 2012; Li & Lerner, 2011; Wang & Fredricks, 2014). They also tend to show greater school and life satisfaction, feel more academically competent, connected, and attached to school, and present signs of more positive adjustment in class (Lewis et al., 2011; Skinner & Pitzer, 2012). Students with a high level of engagement are also more likely to share positive and closer interactions with teachers and peers, to be more socially competent, and to befriend more engaged peers (Hosan & Hoglund, 2017; Ladd et al., 1997). In the long run, students interest and participation in school-related activities and homework, and their use of appropriate tools while learning, promote the development of effective coping skills helping them to handle new challenges, and to feel more academically competent (Li et al., 2010; Skinner & Pitzer, 2012). This level of school investment also helps students to be more successful in school, as highly engaged youths report higher grade point averages and achievement gains, show greater perseverance, and are more likely to obtain their high school diploma (Janosz, Archambault, Morizot, & Pagani, 2008; Ladd & Dinella, 2009; Wang & Eccles, 2012). Finally, students with optimal profiles of engagement are more likely to persevere beyond high school and continue their academic journey in postsecondary education, which can ease their transition into adulthood and the labor market (Fraysier et al., 2020; Tuominen-Soini & Salmela-Aro, 2014).

Student Engagement as a Predictor of School Dropout

Student disengagement is recognized as a process associated with school dropout (Christenson & Thurlow, 2004; Rumberger, 1987). Students who present signs of behavioral, affective, and cognitive disengagement or who are following such a pathway are more likely to quit school before obtaining a high school diploma (Archambault, Janosz, Fallu, & Pagani, 2009; Wang & Fredricks, 2014). Dropout risk is also closely related to unstable pathways of engagement (Janosz, Archambault, Morizot, & Pagani, 2008). For some, this disengagement process may begin very early, even before school entry (Jimerson et al., 2000), an idea that is central to many theories of school dropout (Finn, 1989; Rumberger & Larson, 1998). However, according to recent perspectives, the disengagement process leading to school withdrawal may also occur much later, even in late adolescence (Bowers & Sprott, 2012; Dupéré et al., 2015).

The next section presents how the disengagement process unfolds according to different theories of dropout. All of these theories recognize that students' exposure to different risk and protective factors contribute to the engagement/disengagement process; as these factors are fairly consistent across theories, they will be described in a subsequent integrative section.

Engagement in Theories of School Dropout

Student disengagement is a key component of the major theories of school dropout (Dupéré et al., 2015; Finn, 1989; Rumberger & Larson, 1998; Tinto, 1975; Wehlage et al., 1989). In most of these theories, dropout is presented as the consequence of a long-term trajectory of student disengagement. Tinto's Mediation Model of College Dropout (Tinto, 1975; see also "Tinto, chapter "Exploring the Character of Student Persistence in Higher Education: The Impact of Perception, Motivation, and Engagement", this volume") was one of the first to underline the central role of this trajectory in college withdrawal. This model recognized that challenging situations may lead to an abrupt dropout, but essentially emphasized that school withdrawal typically follows a lengthy disengagement process resulting from students' interactions with the academic and social systems encountered across their academic journey. Thus, the model holds that individual and family background characteristics drive students' commitment to academic goals and their involvement in academic tasks. In turn, students' commitment informs their time investment in school, which sets the course of their engagement. Ultimately, this model proposed that student goals and involvement (corresponding in this model to behavioral engagement) contribute to their academic and social experiences (corresponding to affective engagement) in school, and may contribute to their decision to drop out of school under unfavorable conditions.

One of the most influential theories of school dropout is Finn's (1989) Participation-Identification Model. This model also relies on disengagement patterns to explain students' decision to drop out. In the model, student engagement is conceptualized through their identification with and participation in school. Student identification, an affective component, refers to their strong sense of belonging and appreciation of schooling as a way to achieve their goals. Meanwhile, student participation, a component of behavioral engagement, includes four gradated indicators: student responsiveness to requirements, participation in class-related initiatives, involvement in extracurricular activities, and involvement in decision-making. These indicators are along a continuum ranging from a minimum to a maximum level of engagement. According to Finn's model, students who strongly identify with their school are more likely to participate in school-related activities, while those showing low participation are more likely to disengage from school, and eventually quit before obtaining a diploma.

Proposed around the same time as Finn's theory, Wehlage et al.'s (1989) School Dropout Prevention model also positions engagement as central to understanding dropout. This model defined engagement through two central and distinct components: educational engagement and school membership. These components are intermediate steps associated with students' individual and social development in the school environment. For Wehlage and colleagues, student educational engagement emphasize students' efforts. In the engagement literature, effort sometimes refer to a cognitive process as it underscores student volition to consciously undertake or persist in an academic task (Lawson & Lawson, 2013). However, Wehlage et al.'s conceptualization of efforts resembles more the current definition of behavioral engagement and is associated with academic achievement and success. Similar to affective engagement, school membership is optimized when students successfully create social bonds with adults in school, including their teachers, school professionals, or authorities. Creating positive bonds with peers is another indicator of school membership. As such, students who fail to engage in school make little

academic effort and fail to develop strong social bonds, which raises their likelihood of dropping out before obtaining their high school diploma.

In their highly impactful model of school dropout, Rumberger and Larson (1998) also highlighted on the role of student engagement, which they defined through two facets: social and academic engagement. Social engagement refers to student behavioral engagement, including class attendance, rule compliance, and active participation in school-related tasks and activities. Rumberger and Larson's definition of academic engagement echoes the affective component, as it incorporates student attitudes toward school and their propensity to meet school expectations and demands. As in previous theories, Rumberger and Larson proposed that engagement is at the root of student dropout and that school withdrawal is the consequence of a long-term trajectory of student disengagement, which may start in early development.

Finally, more recently, Dupéré et al. (2015) proposed a theory of school dropout that offers a rather distinct, but complementary, perspective on student disengagement's contribution on the decision to drop out. This model's main contribution is to emphasize that the disengagement process is not always an incremental process operating over the long term. Rather, for some students, engagement can decline abruptly and unexpectedly in the wake of significant disruptions to their lives in late adolescence, not long before dropout occurs. In this theory, disengagement essentially refers to the behavioral component; other affective (i.e., relationships with others) and cognitive (i.e., self-regulation) indicators of engagement are considered, but not to the same extent.

In sum, there is a consensus among most theories regarding the central role of student disengagement in school dropout. Most models underscore the importance of behavioral and affective engagement as processes leading students to drop out. Across the theories, these processes are anchored, fully or partially, in a life course perspective, suggesting that developmental outcomes are shaped by experiences occurring throughout youth development and the academic journey (Alexander et al., 2001). These factors are potentially part of a larger context in which precipitating factors and stressful life events might lead those already at risk to disengage unexpectedly (Dupéré et al., 2015). Together, these theories suggest that student disengagement is a fundamental predictor of school dropout, an assumption that is well supported by empirical research.

Associations Between Student Engagement and Dropout from an Empirical Perspective

The association between student engagement and school dropout is well established in quantitative and qualitative research. In addition to student achievement, different indicators of student engagement such as participation, attendance, or attachment to school have repeatedly been shown to be among the strongest predictors of school dropout (Janosz et al., 1997; Rumberger, 2011). However, it is more recently that research has focused on the associations between school dropout and specific behavioral, affective, and cognitive dimensions of engagement. Even today, few studies have examined the additive or complementary role of each dimension of engagement to explain actual student dropout, rather than merely their dropout risk. Still, existing studies underline the great importance of considering all three facets of engagement, as students are more likely to drop out when reporting signs of disengagement in more than one dimension (Wang & Fredricks, 2014). Accumulating evidence also suggests that student behavioral, affective, and cognitive engagement may not have the same weight to predict school dropout. There is still no consensus regarding the specific contribution of each dimension. On the one hand, we have found that when all three dimensions of engagement are considered simultaneously, the behavioral dimension is most strongly related to school dropout (Archambault, Janosz, Morizot, &

Pagani, 2009). We further posited that student emotions and cognitions regarding school-related activities precede and affect their behaviors, which in turn lead to the decision to drop out. On the other hand, different authors have found that both the behavioral and affective dimensions of student engagement coalesce in predicting student dropout (Wang & Fredricks, 2014). Along the same lines, qualitative and ethnographic research suggests that student affective engagement represents an important protective factor against school withdrawal (Farrell, 1990).

In sum, for most dropouts, disengagement may not be a linear process. Students in general present stable levels of engagement over time, yet it seems that those who report developmental discontinuity in their engagement trajectories are more likely to drop out (Janosz, Archambault, Morizot, & Pagani, 2008). More longitudinal research is necessary to better understand the developmental nature of disengagement and the specific contribution of each dimension to school non-completion, especially the behavioral and affective dimensions, which are central to theories of school dropout. The state of the evidence regarding the cognitive component is more ambiguous; however, its definition does not reach consensus in the field and it is not clear at which specific point of the school withdrawal process that this dimension operates. For some authors, goal setting behaviors and efforts are behavioral (Duckworth, 2015; Wang et al., 2016; Wehlage et al., 1989), while for others, these indicators of student engagement underscore cognitive processes wherein students must be willful, set their objectives, and make decisions to consciously undertake a task (Lawson & Lawson, 2013; Pintrich, 2004). Some have also hypothesized that, as an internal component, cognitive engagement could be a distal predictor of student dropout and its effect mediated either by student achievement or by behavioral engagement (Wang & Fredricks, 2014). More work thus has to be achieved to get a clearer understanding of this dimension and its contribution to the disengagement process associated with student dropout.

Student Engagement as a Mediation Process

An increasing number of studies across different countries have assessed the indirect effects of student engagement dimensions, especially the behavioral and affective dimensions. These studies focused on engagement as a mediation process through which student attitudes, emotions, and beliefs, or the characteristics of their school environment (e.g., teacher discrimination or support) may impact diverse achievement and psychosocial outcomes (e.g., Buhs, 2005; Carmona-Halty et al., 2019; Chen et al., 2020; Jiang & Dong, 2020). In parallel, other studies have focused on various mechanisms, such as teacher–student relationships, potentially explaining the links between student characteristics and school dropout (Fan & Wolters, 2014; Holen et al., 2018). However, despite the fact that all school dropout theories recognize the role of the student disengagement process, there are few studies that look at the mediating role of disengagement—either in general or in terms of its specific dimensions—in predicting school non-completion. For example, a study conducted in Iceland (Blondal & Adalbjarnardottir, 2014) among a sample of adolescents showed that parents' authoritative style (i.e., parents' providing acceptance, supervision, and granting autonomy) led to a decrease in their child's behavioral (i.e., absenteeism) and affective (i.e., boredom) disengagement, which in turn was associated with lower school dropout rates after controlling for past level of achievement and student background characteristics. Similarly, a study in the United States showed that Mexican-American adolescents who participated in a family-focused intervention were less likely to drop out of school because they had increased their affective engagement (i.e., school liking and utility value) (Gonzales et al., 2014). Overall, research regarding the mediation role of each dimension of engagement on student dropout remains limited. However, consistent with the theories, the few existing studies suggests that the student disengagement process is central to school withdrawal, especially given that the two issues have common risk and protective factors.

Factors Associated with Student Engagement and Dropout

The strong connection between student engagement and dropout is also illustrated by risk and protective factors that overlap on an individual level (i.e., sociodemographic and developmental factors), a micro-level (i.e., family, peer, social, and school factors), and a macro-level (i.e., rural/urban environment and neighborhood SES; See Fig. 1). This section presents a selection of the most important predictors of student engagement/disengagement and dropout that has also been summarized in past literature reviews (see De Witte et al., 2013; Fredricks et al., 2004; Gubbels et al., 2019; Reschly & Christenson, 2012; Rosenthal, 1998; Rumberger, 2011). These predictors have generally been studied separately; however, the two fields of research converge on common factors that are generally grouped into five main categories relating to the individual, the family, the social/peer contexts, the classroom and teachers' practices, and the school and community environments (see Table 1 for summary).

Individual Factors

Among the individual determinants of disengagement and dropout, gender retains its importance. In most industrialized countries, boys are generally more likely than girls to disengage and withdraw from school before obtaining their high school diploma (Eurydice Network, 2010; U.S. Depart. Of Education, 2016). This gender gap appears early in students' academic journey and persists over time (Alexander et al., 2001). It also exists in different contexts and industrialized countries and, most importantly, persists from one socioeconomic environment to another. However, the gender gap does tend to be particularly large in disadvantaged areas (Strand, 2014). Concurrently, student temperament, effortful control, cognitive and social skills, and self-efficacy are also among the individual factors with a documented association with student disengagement and dropout (Caraway et al., 2003;

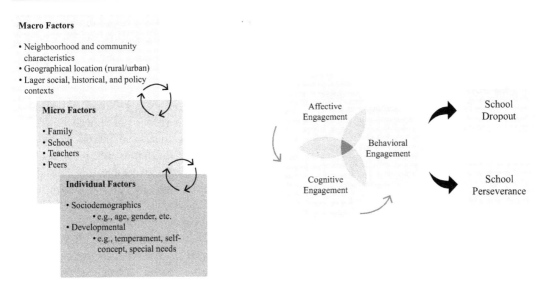

Fig. 1 Individual, micro-, and macro-level factors associated with student engagement, perseverance, or dropout

Zhou et al., 2010). In the early school years, school readiness is also a strong predictor of disengagement and dropout; children who display age-appropriate behavioral and cognitive skills upon kindergarten entry are more likely to be engaged, task focused, and perseverant in elementary school and beyond, which reduces their likelihood of school dropout (Pagani et al., 2012). Toward the end of the elementary, middle, and high school years, students' life satisfaction and well-being, use of self-regulation skills, and mastery goal orientation also contribute to engagement (Cleary et al., 2021; Datu & King, 2018). In contrast, many students who disengage from school and eventually drop out present an academic path marked by numerous school-related difficulties, such as past experiences of academic failure, delays in learning various subjects, low self-concept of abilities, and low levels of motivation (Janosz et al., 1997; Fredricks et al., 2004). Finally, from the middle to the end of adolescence, long working hours outside school or work that interferes with schooling tend to prevent optimal engagement and increase the risk of dropout (Marsh & Kleitman, 2005; Taylor et al., 2012).

Youth with behavioral problems or psychopathologies are at greater risk of schooling difficulties. In elementary school, lower behavioral engagement is reported among students presenting clinical or subclinical behavioral problems, such as opposition, deviance, hyperactivity, impulsivity, and aggressiveness (Cappella et al., 2013; Olivier, Morin, et al., 2020). In adolescence and even through college, substance use, delinquent and antisocial behaviors, or a diagnosis of conduct disorder also affect engagement and perseverance in school (Hunt et al., 2010; Mojtabai et al., 2015). Wang and Fredricks (2014) further showed that changes in adolescents' delinquency and substance use were reciprocally linked to their levels of behavioral and affective engagement and dropout. Finally, according to a recent meta-analysis (Gubbels et al., 2019), most of the aforementioned individual difficulties are associated not only with student dropout but also with student absenteeism, which is an indicator of behavioral disengagement. Yet, this meta-analysis showed that the factors most strongly linked with these outcomes were grade retention, learning difficulties, low academic achievement, negative attitudes toward school, poor well-being, major psychiatric problems, antisocial behaviors, and heavy drug abuse.

In terms of internalizing or emotional difficulties, studies that used samples of children and adolescents showed that those presenting significant levels of anxiety and depressive symptoms

Table 1 Risk and protective factors associated with student engagement and dropout

Protective factors	Risk factors
Individual factors	
Gender	Gender
Effortful control	Difficult temperament
Cognitive skills	Academic failure
Social skills	Academic delays
Self-regulation skills	Low ability self-concept
Self-efficacy	Lack of motivation
School readiness	Working hours outside
Life satisfaction	school
Well-being	Behavior problems
Mastery goal	Emotional problems
orientations	Psychopathologies
Family factors	
Family cohesion	Poverty
Effective parental	Low SES
monitoring	Teenage mother
Parent academic	Large families
aspirations and support	Parents/siblings who
	dropped out
	Blended or single-parent
	family
	Permissive parenting
Social and peer context factors	
Social acceptance	Peer rejection
Quality friendships	Social isolation
	Victimization
	Friends/romantic partners
	who dropped out
Classroom and teacher practices factors	
Student–teacher close	Student–teacher conflictual
relationship	relationships
Autonomy support	Unfair or harsh discipline
Structure	
School and community environment factors	
Positive school climate	Large school size
Fair disciplinary	Low-SES inner-city schools
policies	Rural or remote areas
Immigration and	
integration policies	

were less likely to show optimal behavioral and affective engagement (Curhan et al., 2020; Kurdi & Archambault, 2020). Yet, such as those that look at students' externalizing difficulties, studies have not reached a consensus on the risk that internalizing behaviors represent for student cognitive engagement (Olivier et al., 2018). Finally, the contribution of students' internalizing difficulties to school dropout is increasingly recognized (Brière et al., 2017; Melkevik et al., 2016),

although research on the topic remains limited compared to externalizing difficulties.

Family Factors

Several family characteristics contribute to early student disengagement and intentions to drop out. First, family hardship is well recognized for its association with student educational disadvantage (Duncan & Murnane, 2011). Students who present significant signs of disengagement are more likely to come from low-SES families, experience poverty, and attend large public schools located in populous, socioeconomically disadvantaged, central urban neighborhoods (Leventhal & Dupéré, 2019). In parallel, already disengaged youth living in low-SES neighborhoods have a higher risk of quitting school, even compared to students who are also highly disengaged but hail from privileged backgrounds or attend schools in privileged areas (Perry, 2008). However, authors suggest that links between family socioeconomic status and student success or dropout are not necessarily direct and could be affected by many other context-, school-, and community-based factors (Brooks-Gunn & Duncan, 1997).

Disengagement and dropout are also more frequent among adolescents who come from large families and have parents and siblings who do not have a high school diploma (Björklund & Salvanes, 2011; Dupéré et al., 2020), who were born to teenage mothers, or who grew up in blended or single-parent families (Gubbels et al., 2019). These outcomes are also relatively more common among youth from disorganized families characterized by chaos, ambiguous rules, permissive parenting styles, and a lack of parental supervision, support, and academic aspirations for their children (Afia et al., 2019; Gubbels et al., 2019). Household disorganization during early childhood also decreases parents' tendency to engage in responsive interactions with their children, which, in turn, undermines the development of self-regulatory skills and global engagement in children throughout elementary school

(Garrett-Peters et al., 2019). On the other hand, youth with authoritative parents, i.e., who help their adolescent in case of problems, explain the rational for rules and expectations, set limits, and provide monitoring and supervision, are generally less likely to disengage and drop out of school compared to their peers with permissive parents (Blondal & Adalbjarnardottir, 2014). Similarly, family cohesion and effective parental monitoring promote student affective (i.e., school belonging) and cognitive (i.e., school relevance for achieving ones' goals) engagement in school (Krauss et al., 2017) and potentially prevent dropout.

In parallel, a growing body of literature has examined the links between families' ethnocultural or migratory characteristics and student engagement and disengagement or dropout. This scientific literature is complex, as these links vary considerably not only between different ethnic groups and contexts but also from one country to another. For example, several studies conducted in the United States raise important concerns regarding the socioeconomic conditions that undermine the engagement and perseverance of some groups of Black and Hispanic American students compared to their Caucasian or Asian-American peers (e.g., Bingham & Okagaki, 2012; Crosnoe & Turley, 2011; "Galindo et al., chapter "Expanding an Equity Understanding of Student Engagement: The Macro (Social) and Micro (School) Contexts", this volume"). However, in other countries with separate histories of migration and different ethnocultural composition, concerns relate to other populations (OECD, 2015). Moreover, the distinct realities of immigrant students compared to those of ethnic minorities established in the country for generations also raise different questions and concerns. For both groups, discrimination, racism, and poverty might undermine student experience in school (Hoff et al., 2002; Suárez-Orozco et al., 2009). Nonetheless, the engagement and perseverance of immigrant students are also likely to be influenced by their family's migration status when entering the country (e.g., economic immigrant versus refugee), by the host country's immigration and integration policies, as well as by the national social safety nets (Archambault et al., 2017; Suárez-Orozco et al., 2009). Therefore, these diverse contexts may, in part, explain the great disparities observed between immigrant-based studies at the international scale. For instance, some suggest that youth from immigrant families present lower engagement and higher dropout rates compared to their native-born peers (Crul & Mollenkopf, 2012; OECD, 2015). Yet others indicate that students from immigrant families generally perform better regarding these outcomes than their non-immigrant counterparts (Archambault et al., 2017; García Coll & Marks, 2012; Georgiades et al., 2007). It is well beyond the scope of this chapter to disentangle the factors contributing to these important discrepancies between studies and countries, but this overview underscores the need for extreme vigilance and care when interpreting studies linking student ethnocultural or migratory characteristics with student disengagement or dropout.

Social and Peer Factors

Relationships with classmates represent a micro-level context that can nurture or hinder youth development and engagement in school. For example, Wang et al. (2018) showed that youth tend to become similar to their peers over time in terms of behavioral, affective, and cognitive engagement, but that they select their new friends essentially according to similarity in terms of behavioral engagement only (Wang et al., 2018). According to a recent meta-analysis, peer characteristics or student social status within the peer group may also have a weak association with student disengagement indicators, such as school absenteeism (Gubbels et al., 2019). The impact of peers is also reported to vary based on the stage of schooling. In childhood, peer group social acceptance and friendship quality contribute to student emotional (i.e., interest) and behavioral engagement (i.e., autonomous participation, cooperation, efforts) (e.g., Buhs, 2005; Hosan & Hoglund, 2017). In their meta-analysis, Wentzel et al. (2020) further suggested that children who are socially accepted by their peers tend to be behaviorally engaged (i.e., cooperation, effort, persistence) in school, which, in turn, supports their achievement. Peers may even strengthen student participation in school by providing social approval, acceptance, and a sense of security. Conversely, peer dissatisfaction (i.e., loneliness and lack of support) might explain why children with a difficult temperament report weak affective engagement (i.e., school bonding) (Buhs et al., 2018). Throughout schooling, peer rejection, social isolation, and victimization also diminish behavioral and affective engagement (Buhs, 2005; Cornell et al., 2013).

At the beginning of adolescence, social experiences and friendship may start to have an enhanced, but different effect, not only on student disengagement but also on their decision to drop out of school (Danneel et al., 2019; Dupéré et al., 2020; Véronneau et al., 2008). More specifically, while students' peer group status at this stage is not necessarily associated with dropout (French & Conrad, 2001; Lansford et al., 2016; Véronneau et al., 2008), having friends or romantic partners who have dropped out themselves represents an important risk factor (Dupéré et al., 2020; Staffs & Kreager, 2008; Véronneau et al., 2008). According to Dupéré et al. (2020), through social contagion, youth who have more than one same-age intimate who has dropped out are at greater risk of school withdrawal. Moreover, membership in a deviant peer group could also interfere with student engagement and contribute to dropout, once again through social contagion but also through modeling (Janosz et al., 1997). Finally, isolation and social rejection by peers in school are alienating experiences for adolescents, for whom leaving school could become an inevitable outcome (Hymel et al., 1996).

Classroom and Teachers Practices

Teachers' attitudes toward students as well as the practices they promote in class are determinants for student engagement (Reeve, 2009; Skinner & Belmont, 1993). Teachers who share close and involved relationships with students and who provide them with autonomy support and struc-

ture are recognized as promoting the three dimensions of engagement and preventing school dropout, an assertion established in different contexts and countries and across the whole academic journey (Archambault et al., 2021; Hospel & Galand, 2016; Liu et al., 2018; van Uden et al., 2016). Seeking help from teachers and teachers' autonomy support are even recognized as counteracting the negative effects of youth characteristics, such as difficult temperament, low engagement (i.e., on the behavioral, affective, and cognitive dimensions), academic difficulties, or poor mastery goal orientation (Buhs et al., 2018; Duchesne et al., 2019; Jang et al., 2012). Conversely, poor teacher–student relationships characterized by a high level of conflict, ineffective instruction, unfair or harsh disciplinary practices, conditional provision of affection and attention, or low sense of self-efficacy are likely to undermine students' interest and involvement in school, in turn increasing their disengagement and risk of dropping out (Gubbels et al., 2019; Olivier, Galand, et al., 2020).

Community Factors and School Factors

Although no communities are immune to high school dropout, studies indicate that this issue is more highly concentrated in specific contexts, like low-SES inner-city schools, those in rural or remote areas, and, notably, in Indigenous communities (DePaoli et al., 2015; Leventhal & Dupéré, 2019). In many of these schools, students are also more likely to present negative self-perceptions, worsening their disengagement (Agirdag et al., 2013). For instance, in underprivileged neighborhoods, a much lower proportion of students present high attendance, participation, enthusiasm, and self-regulation and successfully obtain their high school diploma, with graduation gaps up to 40% compared with schools in advantaged environments (CAE, 2012). Such "concentration effects" reflect larger historical, social, economic, and political drivers of inequality and geographical sorting (Leventhal & Dupéré, 2019).

Schools' structural characteristics, such as school size and student demographic composition, also contribute to student engagement and graduation rates (Brault et al., 2014; Christle et al., 2007). In small schools with a lower proportion of students with difficulties, disengagement and dropout rates are lower (Gubbels et al., 2019). In opposition, a negative school climate, marked by safety problems and a lack of control from school staff, increases student behavioral disengagement (i.e., absenteeism, lack of compliance) and dropout risk (Gubbels et al., 2019; Janosz, Archambault, Morizot, & Pagani, 2008; Janosz, Archambault, Pagani, et al., 2008). Also, school disciplinary policies can influence schooling outcomes, including engagement and dropout, notably through the so-called "push-out policies," which particularly affect minority students attending the most socioeconomically disadvantaged schools (Jordan et al., 1999; Rocque & Snellings, 2018).

Overall, student disengagement and dropout share a great number of risk factors. However, student engagement is not a status. It is rather an alterable outcome that may be affected by many favorable characteristics relating to students, their family, social network, or school environment (Reschly & Christenson, 2006a; Christenson & Thurlow, 2004). Research nonetheless remains relatively silent on the role of these factors in the short- and long-term trajectories of engagement.

Profiles and Trajectories of Student Engagement Associated with Student Dropout

An increasing number of studies have highlighted the presence of diverse profiles or trajectories characterizing student engagement. A few studies have first identified, within specific developmental periods, different cross-sectional patterns of engagement by incorporating some or all dimensions. For example, Luo et al. (2009) found that, during childhood, academically at-risk first graders presented four profiles of behavioral (i.e., cooperation and antisocial behaviors) and affective (i.e., bonding with peers) engagement: (1) a

highly engaged group labeled the "cooperative group," in which children presented high behavioral and psychological engagement; (2) an enthusiastic group, wherein children presented a high level of affective engagement, but a low level of behavioral engagement; (3) a disaffected group in which children were behaviorally but not emotionally engaged; and (4) a resistive group, in which children presented low behavioral and psychological engagement. Among adolescents, a greater number of studies have identified behavioral (i.e., energy, dedication, and absorption in school work vs non-compliance), affective (i.e., interest vs disinterest), and cognitive (i.e., self-regulation vs lack of efforts) engagement or disengagement patterns (Fredricks et al., 2019; Tuominen-Soini & Salmela-Aro, 2014; Wang & Peck, 2013). In certain identified profiles, students presented low, moderate, or high levels of behavioral, affective, and cognitive engagement. There were also profiles in which adolescents presented a low level of engagement, but only on one or two dimensions. The low engagement profiles were more likely to be associated with lower school completion and/or postsecondary school enrollment.

In addition to studies focusing solely on engagement indicators, others have identified different profiles of students who dropped out of high school by combining several indicators of self-assessed educational and psychosocial factors (see Table 2 for summary). These studies suggest that students having dropped out are a more heterogeneous group than anticipated by theories. For instance, 20 years ago, Janosz et al. (2000) identified four different groups of dropouts in a longitudinal study. Students from the first group, labeled the "Quiet Dropouts," represented 40% of students and had the most positive profile. They reported a high level of combined affective (i.e., school interest) and cognitive engagement (i.e., achievement goals), and showed well-adjusted patterns of behavioral engagement and psychological functioning. These students even presented better patterns of adaptation compared to their average peers having graduated. In addition, this typology identified another 40% of dropouts who experienced severe difficulties in school, presenting a very low level of engagement accompanied by significant behavioral and psychosocial problems and by academic underachievement. Finally, these authors identified two groups, each comprising 10% of students: a disengaged group, characterized by low levels of behavioral and affective engagement, and a low-achieving group mainly presenting academic difficulties. This study was one of the first to empirically demonstrate that student disengagement, combined with other facets of youth psychosocial adjustment, is a key factor for some dropouts.

In subsequent years, these results were partly replicated by others. Table 2 presents some of studies conducted among actual dropouts or students at risk of dropout, or assessing links between typologies and student dropout. These studies all use indicators of disengagement (e.g., absenteeism, misbehavior, disinterest, etc.) and converge on three to four groups of dropouts somewhat akin to those of Janosz et al.: (1) profiles in which students present disruptive behaviors and high levels of behavioral disengagement; (2) profiles in which youth mostly exhibit academic difficulties in terms of achievement or engagement, (3) profiles in which youth present psychosocial problems, and (4) profiles for which youths' difficulties are less observable, whether because they were covert or internalizing or because they were related to external factors (e.g., residential or school mobility, instability in friends or family relationships). Students in types 2 (academic problems; see Table 2) and 4 (mixed problems) showed the lowest levels of engagement, which was associated with higher school dropout.

Beyond cross-sectional profiles of student engagement and disengagement, longitudinal studies among children and adolescents have also highlighted heterogeneous trajectories of student engagement that range across all dimensions or are specific to behavioral (i.e., participation, cooperation), affective (i.e., subject-specific interest), or cognitive (i.e., self-regulation) engagement. In elementary school, various large-scale studies (Archambault & Dupéré, 2017; Pagani et al., 2012) have iden-

tified subgroups of children presenting longitudinal patterns of classroom engagement, either starting at early schooling or later on in the elementary school years. These studies have identified specific groups of children with high, moderate, or low levels of engagement in terms of behaviors or across the three dimensions, and still other groups who present irregular (transitory declining or inclining) or declining trajectories of engagement. Among adolescents, a study by Wang and Eccles (2012) showed that the average developmental trajectories of behavioral (i.e., participation), affective (i.e., school belonging), and cognitive (i.e., self-regulated learning) engagement in school decreased at different rates, with the affective dimension presenting the steepest decline over time. Other studies (Archambault, Janosz, Morizot, & Pagani, 2009; Janosz, Archambault, Morizot, & Pagani, 2008) conducted among adolescents have identified normative groups, including students presenting relatively high and stable engagement levels, either globally or specifically in terms of the behavioral (i.e., school compliance), affective (i.e., school belonging) or cognitive (i.e., efforts) dimensions. These studies have also identified different non-normative groups composed of students mostly presenting downward, but also upward, trajectories whether in terms of global engagement or for each specific dimension. Interestingly, Archambault, Janosz, Morizot, and Pagani (2009b) showed that student affective engagement, measured in terms of school belonging, was lower than the other dimensions in all subgroups of students, even among the highly engaged who were the most likely to graduate from high school. This study also identified a particularly interesting developmental pattern: Although some students report low affective and cognitive engagement but high levels of behavioral engagement, the reverse pattern has not been found. When students presented positive emotions and thoughts in school throughout their secondary school years, they were also more behaviorally engaged and less likely to drop out. These findings suggest that students' negative emotions and thoughts could precede

Table 2 Profiles of dropouts combining student engagement, educational, and psychosocial factors

Typology indicators	Link with Dropout	Typologies				
		Normative or not at risk	Type 1 Quiets (low apparent risk)	Type 2 Academic Problems (achievement or engagement)	Type 3 Psychosocial Problems (intern., extern., or peer)	Type 4 Mixed Problems (high all)
Bowers & Sprott (2012; USA) GPA Reading at home Extracurricular Academic delay Absenteeism and suspensions Misbehavior Teaching quality School safety	Conducted among actual dropouts	NA	Quiets (52.7%) Involved (9.3%)			Jaded (38.0%)
Fortin et al. (Fortin et al., 2004; Canada) Math grades **Dropout risk score (includes indicators similar to low aff. eng.)** Externalizing and delinquency Depression Teacher attitude Classroom order and organization Family cohesion and organization	Conducted among students at risk of dropout	NA		Uninterested in school (39.8%)	Antisocial covert behavior (18.9%) Depressive (10.7%)	School and social adjustment difficulties (30.6%)
Goulet et al. (2020; Canada) **Behavior problems in school (includes low behav. and aff. eng.)** Academic problems in school (i.e., low achievement) Externalizing and internalizing Social withdrawal Peer victimization Coercive parenting Parental distress	Profiles predicting risk of dropout	Normative (57.9%) Family risk (4.9%)			Social risk (9.6%; internalizing, social withdrawal, peer victimization)	Global risk (4.9%) Individual risk (22.7%; externalizing and school problems)
Janosz et al. (2000; Canada) Achievement **Commitment to education (similar to aff. eng.)** Grade retention School misbehavior	Conducted among actual dropouts	NA	Quiets (38%)	Disengaged (11%) Low achievers (13%)		Maladjusted (39%)

(continued)

Table 2 (continued)

	Typology indicators	Link with Dropout	Typologies		Type 1 Quiets (low apparent risk)	Type 2 Academic Problems (achievement or engagement)	Type 3 Psychosocial Problems (intern., extern., or peer)	Type 4 Mixed Problems (high all)
				Normative or not at risk				
Korhonen et al. (2014; Finland)	Reading, spelling, and math performance **Academic self-concept (includes indicators similar to aff. eng.)** Perceived learning difficulties **School burnout (includes indicators similar to aff. diseng.)**	Profiles predicting actual dropout	Average performing (41%) High performing (34%)			Low performing (18%) Negative academic well-being (7%; learning diff., burnout, and low self-concept)		
McDermott et al. (2017; USA)	Failing classes Extracurricular Expelled from school Delinquency Teacher attitude Parent supervision Family adversity Moving/changing schools Foster care/homeless/jail	Conducted among actual dropouts	NA		Quiets (57.6%)			Instability (39.1%; moderate on all indicators) High adversity (3.3%; high on all indicators)

Note. *Abbreviations*: *Aff. Eng.* affective engagement, *Behav. Eng.* behavioral engagement their behavioral disengagement. This downward spiral from emotions to thoughts to actions (Li & Lerner, 2011, 2013) might also play a leading role in the dynamics between declining behavioral disengagement and student dropout (Reschly & Christenson, 2012). Youth engage in school because they enjoy and are interested in the proposed tasks and to the extent that they feel able to accomplish them. In an effort to nurture students' behavioral engagement, research suggests that school figures should promote the development of students' positive feelings and cognitions while in school.

Student Engagement and School Dropout: What Is Next?

In recent decades, researchers have developed definitions of student engagement as a multidimensional construct. They generally agree on three dimensions pertaining to student behaviors, emotions, and thoughts, all contributing to positive youth development. Theories also acknowledge that student disengagement can lead to school dropout. Empirical research supports this claim by showing that (1) there are various disengagement trajectories relating to student dropout; and (2) student engagement is a mechanism linking individual, family, social, classroom, teachers, school, and community characteristics to student achievement and perseverance-related outcomes. In addition, not only do student disengagement and school dropout share common risk factors but they are also intertwined within different profiles of dropouts, highlighting the key role of student behavioral and affective engagement. Nonetheless, although this field of research has been thriving for several years, more work is yet to be accomplished to address the remaining challenges in understanding the nexus between disengagement and dropout. The first challenge relates to existing gaps between school dropout theories and student engagement research. The second challenge involves the universality and specificity of student engagement and the processes associated with dropout.

Theory-Research Gaps

From a theoretical perspective, three important gaps emerge between the state of empirical evidence and theoretical proposals. They pertain to (1) the trajectories of student engagement associated with student dropout, (2) the short- and long-term processes of student disengagement leading to school dropout, and (3) the role of the three dimensions of student engagement in theories of school withdrawal. The first gaps relate to the absence of empirical validations of existing school dropout theories. All theories postulate the presence of factors shaping trajectories of engagement that concern the family (e.g., structure, income), the social context (i.e., social integration), the classroom and teachers (i.e., support, teaching practices), the school (i.e., composition, quality of instruction, extracurricular activities), and the community (i.e., resources). Nonetheless, although several studies tested some of these models' assumptions, there is no research that fully tests these theories. Moreover, while all theories suggest that these factors may interact with student trajectories of engagement to predict school dropout, studies having examined their contribution as moderators of engagement remain limited. We have learned more in recent years on stressors leading some students to drop out unexpectedly (Dupéré et al., 2015), but more research is needed to understand how these stressors interact to influence the understanding of the heterotypic continuity of the disengagement process associated with dropout (Archambault, Janosz, Morizot, & Pagani, 2009). With that said, not all students presenting signs of disengagement have the same likelihood of dropping out (Janosz et al., 2000). As such, a number of protective factors probably explain the multifinality of student disengagement trajectories (Cicchetti & Rogosch, 1996). Many of these protective factors (e.g., support from and relationships with a significant adult, academic, and family support) are already put forward in effective multimodal interventions promoting student engagement (see Fredricks et al., 2019 for an exhaustive review). Nonetheless, research needs to further identify the specific protective factors preventing highly disengaged students from dropping out of school, in order to assess whether and how the contribution of these factors varies over time as to understand which of them are more relevant at different stages of schooling.

A second aspect that should be further developed in school dropout theories is the conceptualization of engagement as a short versus long-term process. Although research indicates that this process often begins at school entry or even earlier (Alexander et al., 2001; Jimerson et al., 2000), long-term longitudinal and person-centered approaches are still insufficient to properly uncover the heterogeneous disengagement trajectories leading to dropout. Moreover, beyond the hypothesized long-term processes of disengagement, the life course framework argues that students may also face discontinuity, points of rupture, or shifts in their trajectories, which can lead to an abrupt decision to drop out of school (Crosnoe & Johnson, 2011; Janosz, Archambault, Morizot, & Pagani, 2008). Other than Dupéré et al.'s Stress Process–Life Course Model of High School Dropout, the possibility that student disengagement results from a short-term precipitating process has received scant attention in theories; nevertheless, it is increasingly supported by empirical research (see Dupéré et al., 2018; McDermott et al., 2019; Samuel & Burger, 2020). Documenting these abrupt changes in student behavioral, affective, and cognitive engagement is thus critical to further understanding its theoretical and empirical role in school dropout.

Finally, there is a clear empirical consensus regarding the multidimensionality of student engagement, which most authors have defined through at least three components: behavioral, affective, and cognitive (e.g., Fredricks et al., 2004; Wang et al., 2019). Yet, despite the central role of engagement in all theories of school dropout, no theory is clearly based on this three-dimensional conceptualization of the construct. All theoretical models refer to the behavioral dimension, presented in terms of student participation, efforts, involvement, or the absence of problematic behaviors, such as indiscipline and truancy displayed in the classroom or school. In addition, all theories discuss student affective engagement, whether in terms of school identification, social experiences, academic engagement, or school membership. Nonetheless, other than Finn's Participation-Identification Model, the affective facet of engagement is not as central in school dropout theories compared to its behavioral counterpart. Surprisingly, student cognitive engagement is also very neglected by school dropout theories. Tinto's mention of commitment to academic goals, Finn's decision-making component of the participation process, and Dupéré's reference to self-regulation abilities are vague allusions to cognitive engagement. Still, these studies take only a superficial look at these indicators of cognitive engagement. This virtual absence of the cognitive dimension might stem from the fact that empirical studies have mainly focused on its association with classroom-related learning processes (e.g., Lovelace et al., 2018). Given that school dropout theories focus on more macro-level processes, the little attention paid to cognitive engagement is thus unsurprising. However, since students' actions, emotions, and thoughts are dynamically interrelated across the development of engagement (Hong et al., 2020; Li & Lerner, 2013), and are sometimes even considered to be part of a global indicator of engagement (Dierendonck et al., 2020; Wang et al., 2019), the place of cognitive engagement in the decision process leading students to drop out of school deserves to be better understood. Greater balance between the three recognized dimensions of engagement and the theoretical proposals linking them to school dropout is needed to improve our response to students' needs regarding the most central facets of their development.

Universality and Specificity of Student Engagement and School Dropout

An overview of literature suggests that students are not at equal risk of not obtaining a high school diploma: Important gaps in dropout rates are found between different populations of students sharing stable characteristics. Disparities in upper secondary school completion rates are estimated at 7% between boys and girls, 20% between students of different immigrant or ethnic backgrounds, 7% between rural and urban regions, 20% between students from different SES backgrounds, 30% between youth with and without special needs, and up to 40% between students who live in Indigenous communities and those who do not (Mahuteau et al., 2015; UNESCO, 2020). The OECD (2018) qualifies equity in education as an international concern, which is why one of the biggest upcoming challenges in research focusing on the links between disengagement and dropout relates to the universality and specificity of disengagement across different populations of students.

First, boys are overrepresented among youth who drop out of school compared to females (Lavoie et al., 2019). These discrepancies sometimes, but not always, apply to student engagement (Archambault, Janosz, Fallu, & Pagani, 2009), especially in subjects, such as language in which girls are typically more engaged (Brozo et al., 2014). In STEM-related subjects, this gender gap is either found to be absent or in favor of boys, who are more engaged (Fredricks et al., 2018; Wang & Degol, 2014). Beyond these differences of prevalence, a question that has been scarcely addressed is whether the processes through which each dimension of engagement leads to dropout might differ between genders. There are some indications that for the purposes of maintaining proper engagement, boys may be more sensitive to some aspects of the learning environment, whereas that girls are more sensitive to their social surroundings (Lavoie et al., 2019). As such, the gender gap in high school dropout and the behavioral, affective, and cognitive processes leading to it raise key questions for future research.

Second, a growing body of research indicates that student engagement differs across groups of students from different immigration or ethnic backgrounds (Suárez-Orozco et al., 2009). For instance, in the United States, Wang et al. (2011) found that, compared to European American students, African American students reported higher affective engagement, but lower behavioral engagement. In a Canadian study, Archambault

et al. (2017) further showed that a number of factors generally associated with student dropout had a weak or non-existent correlation with school withdrawal for immigrant students, including academic achievement, school aspirations, competency beliefs in language classes, and family economic resources. However, others found that parental practices had a similar effect on school dropout among immigrant and non-immigrant students (Afia et al., 2019). The current state of the evidence thus suggests that well-known factors associated with student dropout do not have the same amount of influence on the academic journey of immigrant students and ethnic minorities, possibly because these students experience challenges related to their migration history and adjustment to a new school and country, or are more often the target of discrimination. Nonetheless, much remains to be explored in order to fully understand all the complex issues affecting disengagement and dropout for immigrants and racialized youth in different countries and across different cultures.

Third, youth with special needs, whether they are gifted or present clinical or subclinical mental health or academic problems, may have a modified or greater risk of disengagement and school dropout compared to students without such characteristics (Landis & Reschly, 2013; Olivier, Morin, et al., 2020). For example, a literature review showed that for gifted students presenting a potential for high academic achievement, absenteeism, academic failure and underachievement, substance use, learning disabilities, family conflicts, and behavioral disengagement were all associated with school dropout, as they are for students from the general population (Landis & Reschly, 2013). However, for gifted students, school dropout was surprisingly less associated with the affective dimension of engagement and more associated with the cognitive dimension. In parallel, research suggests that students with various emotional and behavioral problems (e.g., internalizing, externalizing, hyperactivity–inattention, delinquency, substance use, learning disabilities) seem to display suboptimal patterns of engagement (for review, see Olivier, Morin, et al., 2020). However, studies have rarely assessed whether the role of behavioral, affective, and cognitive engagement is more or less salient in explaining these students' risk of dropping out. Finally, one study suggests that although youth with learning disabilities presented less favorable engagement than youth without disabilities, they nonetheless presented a similar association between engagement and dropout similarly (Reschly & Christenson, 2006b). Considering that the disparity in dropout rates between youth with and without special needs is one of the largest (30%) in Western countries, it is surprising that little attention has been devoted in research to understanding the processes and moderating factors contributing to the disengagement of these students and their eventual decision to quit school.

Finally, the contribution of acute and chronic stressors to students' disengagement and decision to drop out has also been under-addressed (Dupéré et al., 2015; Samuel & Burger, 2020), especially in light of the macro-level or systemic contexts in which they unfold. This represents a worthy area for further inquiry, as recent results suggest that a certain kind of stressor—for example, those related to social relationships and delinquency or interactions with the legal system and the police—is differentially associated with school withdrawal in socioeconomically disadvantaged rural communities vs. their urban counterparts (Dupéré et al., 2019). Along similar lines, school mobility is also more strongly associated with dropout among adolescents living in disadvantaged communities (Crowder & South, 2003). Lastly, beyond school factors such as size, climate, or support for students, educational systems do not perform at the same level in terms of promoting youth educational success. School systems' organization and characteristics (private vs. public sector; composition, etc.) are also associated with gaps in student engagement and dropout (Teese et al., 2007). However, this field of research remain acutely under-investigated. Better understanding how these macro-level factors act on these outcomes would allow practitioners and decision makers to find more effective ways to improve based on factors they can control and that constitute important levers for intervention.

In sum, more work is to be done to further the understanding of how student engagement relates to school dropout for specific groups of students, such as boys and girls, ethnic minorities, immigrants, students from low-SES families and rural communities, gifted students, and youth presenting academic or mental health challenges or who are exposed to chronic stressors. Addressing these discrepancies in coming years should inform equitable practices to be implemented in schools as a way to promote engagement and success for all (Basharpoor et al., 2013; Landis & Reschly, 2013)

Conclusion

Although a disengagement process preceding school dropout is recognized by theories and research in the field, more empirical research is needed to identify the mechanisms linking student behavioral, affective, and cognitive engagement to school dropout. While student behavioral and affective engagement have increasingly been identified as mediators connecting student or school characteristics to student achievement and well-being, these mechanisms have rarely been studied in the context of predicting school dropout. Research focusing on trajectories or dropout typologies mostly considers two out of the three critical dimensions of engagement, generally the behavioral and affective component, leaving questions surrounding the role of student cognitive engagement in the decision process to quit school. Moreover, despite the growing consensus regarding the multidimensionality of engagement and the existence of heterogeneous profiles of students having dropped out of school, we have worryingly limited knowledge on the larger context within which school dropout is salient, especially for some populations of students as boys, immigrants or ethnic minorities, students with special needs, and those from low-SES or rural backgrounds or who are exposed to major stressors. This chapter aims to raise awareness of the need to better understand the interconnected nature of all dimensions of student engagement in the short- and long-term process leading to school dropout, especially among students who are most at risk.

References

Afia, K., Dion, E., Dupéré, V., Archambault, I., & Toste, J. (2019). Parenting practices during middle adolescence and high school dropout. *Journal of Adolescence, 76,* 55–64. https://doi.org/10.1016/j.adolescence.2019.08.012

Agirdag, O., Van Houtte, M., & Van Avermaet, P. (2013). School segregation and self-fulfilling prophecies as determinants of academic achievement in Flanders. In S. De Groof & M. Elchardus (Eds.), *Early school leaving and youth unemployment (pp. 46e74).* Amsterdam University Press.

Alexander, K. L., Entwisle, D. R., & Kabbani, N. S. (2001). The dropout process in life course perspective: Early risk factors at home and school. *Teachers College Record, 103*(5), 760–822. https://doi.org/10.1111/0161-4681.00134

Alliance for Excellent Education. (2013). *Saving futures, saving dollars: The impact of education on crime reduction and earnings.* Retrived from https://mk0all4edorgjxiy8xf9.kinstacdn.com/wp-content/uploads/2013/09/SavingFutures.pdf.

Appleton, J. J., Christenson, S. L., Kim, D., & Reschly, A. L. (2006). Measuring cognitive and psychological engagement: Validation of the student engagement instrument. *Journal of School Psychology, 44*(5), 427–445. https://doi.org/10.1016/j.jsp.2006.04.002

Archambault, I., Pascal, S., Tardif-Grenier, K., Dupéré, V., Janosz, M., Parent, S., & Pagani, L. (2021). The contribution of teacher structure, involvement, and autonomy support on student engagement in low-income elementary schools. *Teachers and Teaching, 26*(5–6), 428–445. https://doi.org/10.1080/13540602.2020.1863208

Archambault, I., & Dupéré, V. (2017). Joint trajectories of behavioral, affective, and cognitive engagement in elementary school. *The Journal of Educational Research, 110*(2), 188–198. https://doi.org/10.1080/00220671.2015.1060931

Archambault, I., Janosz, M., Dupéré, V., Brault, M.-C., & Andrew, M. M. (2017). Individual, social, and family factors associated with high school dropout among low- SES youth: Differential effects as a function of immigrant status. *British Journal of Educational Psychology, 87*(3), 456–477. https://doi.org/10.1111/bjep.12159

Archambault, I., Janosz, M., Fallu, J.-S., & Pagani, L. S. (2009a). Student engagement and its relationship with early high school dropout. *Journal of Adolescence, 32*(3), 651–670. https://doi.org/10.1016/j.adolescence.2008.06.007

Archambault, I., Janosz, M., Morizot, J., & Pagani, L. (2009b). Adolescent behavioral, affective, and cogni-tive engagement in school: Relationship to dropout. *Journal of School Health, 79*(9), 408–415. https://doi.org/10.1111/j.1746-1561.2009.00428.x

Basharpoor, S., Issazadegan, A., Zahed, A., & Ahmadian, L. (2013). Comparing academic self-concept and engagement to school between students with learning disabilities and normal. *The Journal of Education and Learning Studies, 5,* 47–64.

Bingham, G. E., & Okagaki, L. (2012). Ethnicity and student engagement. In S. L. Christenson, A. L. Reschly, & C. Wylie (Eds.), *Handbook of research on student engagement* (pp. 65–95). Springer Science + Business Media). https://doi.org/10.1007/978-1-4614-2018-7_4

Björklund, A., & Salvanes, K. G. (2011). Education and family background: Mechanisms and policies. In E. A. Hanushek, S. Machin, & L. Woessmann (Eds.), *Handbook in economics of education* (Vol. 3, pp. 201–247). Elsevier.

Blondal, K. S., & Adalbjarnardottir, S. (2014). Parenting in relation to school dropout through student engagement: A longitudinal study. *Journal of Marriage and Family, 76*(4), 778–795. https://doi.org/10.1111/jomf.12125

Bowers, A. J., & Sprott, R. (2012). Why tenth graders fail to finish high school: A dropout typology latent class analysis. *Journal of Education for Students Placed at Risk, 17*(3), 129–148. https://doi.org/10.1080/10824669.2012.692071

Brault, M.-C., Janosz, M., & Archambault, I. (2014). Effects of school composition and school climate on teacher expectations of students: A multilevel analysis. *Teaching and Teacher Education, 44,* 148–159. https://doi.org/10.1016/j.tate.2014.08.008

Brière, F. N., Pascal, S., Dupéré, V., Castellanos-Ryan, N., Allard, F., Yale-Soulière, G., & Janosz, M. (2017). Depressive and anxious symptoms and the risk of secondary school non-completion. *The British Journal of Psychiatry, 211,* 163–168. https://doi.org/10.1192/bjp.bp.117.201418

Brooks-Gunn, J., & Duncan, G. J. (1997). The effects of poverty on children. *The Future of Children: Children and Poverty, 7*(2), 55–71. https://doi.org/10.2307/1602387

Brozo, W. G., Sulkunen, S., Shiel, G., Garbe, C., Pandian, A., & Valtin, R. (2014). Reading, gender, and engagement. *Journal of Adolescent & Adult Literacy, 57*(7), 584–593. https://doi.org/10.1002/jaal.291

Buhs, E. S., Koziol, N. A., Rudasill, K. M., & Crockett, L. J. (2018). Early temperament and middle school engagement: School social relationships as mediating processes. *Journal of Educational Psychology, 110*(3), 338–354. https://doi.org/10.1037/edu0000224

Buhs, E. S. (2005). Peer rejection, negative peer treatment, and school adjustment: Self-concept and classroom engagement as mediating processes. *Journal of School Psychology, 43*(5), 407–424. https://doi.org/10.1016/j.jsp.2005.09.001

Cappella, E., Kim, H. Y., Neal, J. W., & Jackson, D. R. (2013). Classroom peer relationships and behavioral engagement in elementary school: The role of social network equity. *American Journal of Community Psychology, 52*(3–4), 367–379. https://doi.org/10.1007/s10464-013-9603-5

Caraway, K., Tucker, C. M., Reinke, W. M., & Hall, C. (2003). Self-efficacy, goal orientation and fear of failure as predictors of school engagement in high school students. *Psychology in the Schools, 40*(4), 417–427. https://doi.org/10.1002/pits.10092

Carmona-Halty, M., Salanova, M., Llorens, S., & Schaufeli, W. B. (2019). Linking positive emotions and academic performance: The mediated role of academic psychological capital and academic engagement. *Current Psychology*, 1–10. https://doi.org/10.1007/s12144-019-00227-8

Chen, J., Huebner, E., & Tian, L. (2020). Longitudinal relations between hope and academic achievement in elementary school students: Behavioral engagement as a mediator. *Learning and Individual Differences, 78*, 101824. https://doi.org/10.1016/j.lindif.2020.101824

Cicchetti, D., & Rogosch, F. A. (1996). Equifinality and multifinality in developmental psychopathology. *Development and Psychopathology, 8*, 597–600. https://doi.org/10.1017/S0954579400007318

Chiefs Assembly on Education. (2012). A portrait of first nations and education. Retrived from https://www.afn.ca/uploads/files/events/fact_sheet-ccoe-3.pdf

Christenson, S. L., & Thurlow, M. L. (2004). School dropouts: Prevention considerations, interventions, and challenges. *Current Directions in Psychological Science, 13*(1), 36–39. https://doi.org/10.1111/j.0963-7214.2004.01301010.x

Christle, C. A., Jolivette, K., & Nelson, M. (2007). School characteristics related to high school dropout rates. *Remedial and Special Education, 28*(6), 325–339. https://doi.org/10.1177/07419325070280060201

Cleary, T. J., et al. (2021). Linking student self-regulated learning profiles to achievement and engagement in mathematics. *Psychology in the Schools, 58*(3), 443–457. https://doi.org/10.1002/pits.22456

Cornell, D., Gregory, A., Huang, F., & Fan, X. (2013). Perceived prevalence of teasing and bullying predicts high school dropout rates. *Journal of Educational Psychology, 105*(1), 138–149. https://doi.org/10.1037/a0030416

Crosnoe, R., & Johnson, M. K. (2011). Research on adolescence in the twenty-first century. *Annual Review of Sociology, 37*, 439–460. https://doi.org/10.1146/annurev-soc-081309-150008

Crosnoe, R., & Turley, R. N. (2011). K-12 educational outcomes of immigrant youth. *The Future of Children, 21*(1), 129–152. https://doi.org/10.1353/foc.2011.0008

Crowder, K. D., & South, S. J. (2003). Neighborhood distress and school dropout: The variable significance of community context. *Social Science Research, 32,* 659–698. https://doi.org/10.1016/S0049-089X(03)00035-8

Crul, M., & Mollenkopf, J. (2012). *The changing face of world cities: Young adult children of immigrants in Europe and the United States* (pp. 3–25).

Russell Sage Foundation. https://www.jstor.org/stable/10.7758/9781610447911

Curhan, A. L., Rabinowitz, J. A., Pas, E. T., & Bradshaw, C. P. (2020). Informant discrepancies in internalizing and externalizing symptoms in an at-risk sample: The role of parenting and school engagement. *Journal of Youth and Adolescence, 49*(1), 311–322. https://doi.org/10.1007/s10964-019-01107-x

Danneel, S., Colpin, H., Goossens, L., Engels, M., Van Leeuwen, K., Van Den Noortgate, W., & Verschueren, K. (2019). Emotional school engagement and global self-esteem in adolescents: Genetic susceptibility to peer acceptance and rejection. *Merrill-Palmer Quarterly, 65*(2), 158–182. https://doi.org/10.13110/merrpalmquar1982.65.2.0158

Datu, J. A. D., & King, R. B. (2018). Subjective Well-being is reciprocally associated with academic engagement: A short-term longitudinal study. *Journal of School Psychology, 69*, 100–110. https://doi.org/10.1016/j.jsp.2018.05.007

DePaoli, J. L., Hornig Fox, J., Ingram, E. S., Maushard, M., Bridgeland, J. M., & Balfanz, R. (2015). Building a grad nation: Progress and challenge in ending the high school dropout epidemic.

De Witte, K., Cabus, S., Thyssen, G., Groot, W., & van Den Brink, H. M. (2013). A critical review of the literature on school dropout. *Educational Research Review, 10*, 13–28. https://doi.org/10.1016/j.edurev.2013.05.002

Dierendonck, C., Milmeister, P., Kerger, S., & Poncelet, D. (2020). Examining the measure of student engagement in the classroom using the bifactor model: Increased validity when predicting misconduct at school. *International Journal of Behavioral Development, 44*(3), 279–286. https://doi.org/10.1177/0165025419876360

Dupéré, V., Dion, E., Cantin, S., Archambault, I., & Lacourse, E. (2020). Social contagion and high school dropout: The role of friends, romantic partners, and siblings. *Journal of Education Psychology, 113*(3), 572–584. https://doi.org/10.1037/edu0000484

Dupéré, V., Dion, E., Leventhal, T., Crosnoe, R., Archambault, A., & Goulet, M. (2019). Circumstances preceding dropout among rural high schoolers: A comparison with urban peers. *Journal of Research in Rural Education, 35*, 1–20. https://doi.org/10.1037/edu0000484

Dupéré, V., Dion, E., Leventhal, T., Archambault, I., Crosnoe, R., & Janosz, M. (2018). High school dropout in proximal context: The triggering role of stressful life events. *Child Development, 89*(2), e107–e122. https://doi.org/10.1111/cdev.12792

Dupéré, V., Leventhal, T., Dion, E., Crosnoe, R., Archambault, I., & Janosz, M. (2015). Stressors and turning points in high school and dropout: A stress process, life course framework. *Review of Educational Research, 859*(4), 591–629. https://doi.org/10.3102/0034654314559845

Duchesne, S., Larose, S., & Feng, B. (2019). Achievement goals and engagement with academic work in early high school: Does seeking help from teachers matter?

The Journal of Early Adolescence, 39(2), 222–252. https://doi.org/10.1177/0272431617737626

Duckworth, A. (2015). *OECD report of skills for social progress: The power of social emotional skills* (Peer Commentary on IECD report). Retrieved from https://www.oecd.org/edu/ceri/seminarandlaunchofthereportskillsforsocialprogressthepowerofsocialandemotionalskills.htm

Duncan, G. J., & Murnane, R. J. (2011). *Whither opportunity? Rising inequality, schools, and children's life chances*. Russel Sage Foundation.

Eurostats. (2017). Decrease in "early school leavers" in the EU. Retrived from https://ec.europa.eu/eurostat/en/web/products-eurostat-news/-/edn-20170908-1.

Fan, W., & Wolters, C. A. (2014). School motivation and high school dropout: The mediating role of educational expectations. *British Journal of Educational Psychology, 84*(1), 22–39. https://doi.org/10.1111/bjep.12002

Farrell, E. (1990). *Hanging in and dropping out: Voices of at-risk students*. Teachers College Press.

Finn, J. D. (1989). Withdrawing from school. *Review of Educational Research, 59*(2), 117–142. https://doi.org/10.3102/00346543059002117

Finn, J. D., & Zimmer, K. S. (2012). Student engagement: What is it? Why does it matter? In S. L. Christenson, A. L. Reschly, & C. Wylie (Eds.), *Handbook of research on student engagement* (pp. 97–131). Springer.

Fortin, L., Royer, É., Potvin, P., Marcotte, D., & Yergeau, É. (2004). La prediction du risque de decrochage scolaire au secondaire : Facteurs personnels, familiaux et scolaires [Prediction of risk for secondary school dropout: Personal, family and school factors]. *Canadian Journal of Behavioural Science, 36*(3), 219–231. https://doi.org/10.1037/h0087232

Fraysier, K., Reschly, A., & Appleton, J. (2020). Predicting postsecondary enrollment with secondary student engagement data. *Journal of Psychoeducational Assessment, 38*(7), 882–899. https://doi.org/10.1177/0734282920903168

Fredricks, J. A., Hofkens, T., Wang, M.-T., Mortenson, E., & Scott, P. (2018). Supporting girls' and boys' engagement in math and science learning: A mixed methods study. *Journal of Research in Science Teaching, 55*(2), 271–298. https://doi.org/10.1002/tea.21419

Fredricks, J. A., Ye, F., Wang, M., & Brauer, S. (2019). Profiles of school disengagement: Not all disengaged students are alike. In J. A. Fredricks, A. L. Reschly, & S. L. Christenson (Eds.), *Handbook of student engagement interventions* (pp. 31–43). Academic Press.

Fredricks, J. A., Wang, M., Schall, J., Hokfkens, T., Snug, H., Parr, A., & Allerton, J. (2016). Using qualitative methods to develop a survey of math and science engagement. *Learning and Instruction, 43*, 5–15. https://doi.org/10.1016/j.learninstruc.2016.01.009

Fredricks, J. A., Blumenfeld, P. C., & Paris, A. H. (2004). School engagement: Potential of the concept, state of the evidence. *Review of Educational Research, 74*(1), 59–109. https://doi.org/10.3102/00346543074001059

French, D. C., & Conrad, J. (2001). School dropout as predicted by peer rejection and antisocial behavior. *Journal of Research on Adolescence, 11*(3), 225–244. https://doi.org/10.1111/1532-7795.00011

García Coll, C. G., & Marks, A. K. (Eds.). (2012). *The immigrant paradox in children and adolescents: Is becoming American a developmental risk?* American Psychological Association.

Garrett-Peters, P. T., Mokrova, I. L., Carr, R. C., Vernon-Feagans, L., & Family Life Project Key Investigators. (2019). Early student (dis)engagement: Contributions of household chaos, parenting, and self-regulatory skills. *Developmental Psychology, 55*(7), 1480–1492. https://doi.org/10.1037/dev0000720

Georgiades, K., Boyle, M. H., & Duku, E. (2007). Contextual influences on children's mental health and school performance: The moderating effects of family immigrant status. *Child Development, 78*(5), 1572–1591. https://doi.org/10.1111/j.1467-8624.2007.01084.x

Gonzales, N. A., Wong, J. J., Toomey, R. B., Millsap, R., Dumka, L. E., & Mauricio, A. M. (2014). School engagement mediates long-term prevention effects for Mexican American adolescents. *Prevention Science, 15*(6), 929–939. https://doi.org/10.1007/s11121-013-0454-y

Goulet, M., Clément, M.-E., Helie, S., & Villatte, A. (2020). Longitudinal associations between risk profiles, school dropout risk, and substance abuse in adolescence. *Child & Youth Care Forum, 49*, 687–706.

Gubbels, J., van der Put, C. E., & Assink, M. (2019). Risk factors for school absenteeism and dropout: A meta-analytic review. *Journal of Youth and Adolescence, 48*(9), 1637–1667. https://doi.org/10.1007/s10964-019-01072-5

Henry, K. L., Knight, K. E., & Thornberry, T. P. (2012). School disengagement as a predictor of dropout, delinquency, and problem substance use during adolescence and early adulthood. Journal of Youth and Adolescence, 41(2), 156–166. https://doi.org/10.1007/s10964-011-9665-3.

Hoff, E., Laursen, B., & Tardiff, T. (2002). Socioeconomic status and parenting. In P. M. Greenfield & R. R. Cocking (Eds.), *Cross-cultural roots of minority children development* (pp. 285–313). Lawrence Erlbaum Associates.

Holen, S., Waaktaar, T., & Sagatun, Å. (2018). A chance lost in the prevention of school dropout? Teacher-student relationships mediate the effect of mental health problems on noncompletion of upper-secondary school. *Scandinavian Journal of Educational Research, 62*(5), 737–753. https://doi.org/10.1080/00313831.2017.1306801

Hong, W., Zhen, R., Liu, R.-D., Wang, M.-T., Ding, Y., & Wang, J. (2020). The longitudinal linkages among Chinese children's behavioral, cognitive, and emotional engagement within a mathematics context. *Educational Psychology, 40*(6), 666–680. https://doi.org/10.1080/01443410.2020.1719981

Hosan, N. E., & Hoglund, W. (2017). Do teacher–child relationship and friendship quality matter for children's school engagement and academic skills? *School Psychology Review, 46*(2), 201–218. https://doi.org/10.17105/SPR-2017-0043.V46-2

Hospel, V., & Galand, B. (2016). Are both classroom autonomy support and structure equally important for students' engagement? A multilevel analysis. *Learning and Instruction, 41,* 1–10. https://doi.org/10.1016/j.learninstruc.2015.09.001

Hunt, J., Eisenberg, D., & Kilbourne, A. M. (2010). Consequences of receipt of a psychiatric diagnosis for completion of college. *Psychiatric Services (Washington, D.C.), 61*(4), 399–404. https://doi.org/10.1176/ps.2010.61.4.399

Hymel, S., Comfort, C., Schonert-Reichl, K., & McDougall, P. (1996). Academic failure and school dropout: The influence of peers. In J. Juvonen & K. R. Wentzel (Eds.), *Cambridge studies in social and emotional development. Social motivation: Understanding children's school adjustment* (pp. 313–345). Cambridge University Press. https://doi.org/10.1017/CBO9780511571190.015

Jang, H., Kim, E. J., & Reeve, J. (2012). Longitudinal test of self-determination theory's motivation mediation model in a naturally occurring classroom context. *Journal of Educational Psychology, 104*(4), 1175–1188. https://doi.org/10.1037/a0028089

Janosz, M., Archambault, I., Morizot, J., & Pagani, L. S. (2008a). School engagement trajectories and their differential predictive relations to dropout. *Journal of Social Issues, 64*(1), 21–40. https://doi.org/10.1111/j.1540-4560.2008.00546.x

Janosz, M., Archambault, I., Pagani, L. S., Pascal, S., Morin, A. J., & Bowen, F. (2008b). Are there detrimental effects of witnessing school violence in early adolescence? *The Journal of Adolescent Health : Official Publication of the Society for Adolescent Medicine, 43*(6), 600–608. https://doi.org/10.1016/j.jadohealth.2008.04.011

Janosz, M., Le Blanc, M., Boulerice, B., & Tremblay, R. E. (2000). Predicting different types of school dropouts: A typological approach with two longitudinal samples. *Journal of Educational Psychology, 92*(1), 171–190. https://doi.org/10.1037/0022-0663.92.1.171

Janosz, M., Le Blanc, M., Boulerice, B., & Tremblay, R. E. (1997). Disentangling the weight of school dropout predictors: A test on two longitudinal samples. *Journal of Youth and Adolescence, 26*(6), 733–762. https://doi.org/10.1023/A:1022300826371

Jiang, S., & Dong, L. (2020). The effects of teacher discrimination on depression among migrant adolescents: Mediated by school engagement and moderated by poverty status. *Journal of Affective Disorders, 275,* 260–267. https://doi.org/10.1016/j.jad.2020.07.029

Jimerson, S. R., Campos, E., & Greif, J. L. (2003). Towards an understanding of definitions and measures of school engagement and related terms. *The California School Psychologist, 8,* 7e28. https://doi.org/10.1016/S0022-4405(00)00051-0

Jimerson, S. R., Egeland, B., Sroufe, L. A., & Carlson, B. (2000). A prospective longitudinal study of high school dropouts: Examining multiple predictors across development. *Journal of School Psychology, 38*(6), 525–549. https://doi.org/10.1016/S0022-4405(00)00051-0

Jordan, W. J., McPartland, J. M., & Lara, J. (1999). Rethinking the causes of high school dropout. *The Prevention Researcher, 6,* 1–4.

Krauss, S. E., Kornbluh, M., & Zeldin, S. (2017). Community predictors of school engagement: The role of families and youth-adult partnership in Malaysia. *Children and Youth Services Review, 73,* 328–337. https://doi.org/10.1016/j.childyouth.2017.01.009

Korhonen, J., Linnanmäki, K., & Aunio, P. (2014). Learning difficulties, academic well-being and educational dropout: A person-centered approach. *Learning & Individual Differences, 31,* 1–10. https://doi.org/10.1016/j.lindif.2013.12.011

Kurdi, V., & Archambault, I. (2020). Self-perceptions and engagement in low socio-economic elementary school students: The moderating effects of immigration status and anxiety. *School Mental Health, 12,* 400–416. https://doi.org/10.1007/s12310-020-09360-3

Ladd, G. W., & Dinella, L. M. (2009). Continuity and change in early school engagement: Predictive of children's achievement trajectories from first to eighth grade? *Journal of Educational Psychology, 101*(1), 190–206. https://doi.org/10.1037/a0013153

Ladd, G. W., Kochenderfer, B. J., & Coleman, C. C. (1997). Classroom peer acceptance, friendship, and victimization: Distinct relational systems that contribute uniquely to children's school adjustment? *Child Development, 68*(6), 1181–1197. https://www.jstor.org/stable/1132300

Landis, R. N., & Reschly, A. L. (2013). Reexamining gifted underachievement and dropout through the lens of student engagement. *Journal for the Education of the Gifted, 36*(2), 220–249. https://doi.org/10.1177/0162353213480864

Lansford, J. E., Dodge, K. A., Pettit, G. S., & Bates, J. E. (2016). A public health perspective on school dropout and adult outcomes: A prospective study of risk and protective factors from age 5 to 27 years. *Journal of Adolescent Health, 58*(6), 652–658. https://doi.org/10.1016/2Fj.jadohealth.2016.01.014

Lavoie, L., Dupéré, V., Dion, E., Crosnoe, R., Lacourse, É., & Archambault, I. (2019). Gender differences in adolescents' exposure to stressful life events and differential links to impaired school functioning. *Journal of Abnormal Child Psychology, 47*(6), 1053–1064. https://doi.org/10.1007/s10802-018-00511-4

Lawson, M. A., & Lawson, H. A. (2013). New conceptual frameworks for student engagement research, policy, and practice. *Review of Educational Research, 83*(3), 432–479. https://doi.org/10.3102/0034654313480891

Leventhal, T., & Dupéré, V. (2019). Neighborhood effects on youth development in experimental and nonexperimental research. *Annual Review of Developmental Psychology, 1,* 149–176. https://doi.org/10.1146/annurev-devpsych-121318-085221

Lewis, A. D., Huebner, E. S., Malone, P. S., & Valois, R. F. (2011). Life satisfaction and student engagement in adolescents. *Journal of Youth and Adolescence, 40*(3), 249–262. https://doi.org/10.1007/s10964-010-9517-6

Li, Y., & Lerner, R. M. (2013). Interrelations of behavioral, emotional, and cognitive school engagement in high school students. *Journal of Youth and Adolescence, 42*(1), 20–32. https://doi.org/10.1007/s10964-012-9857-5

Li, Y., & Lerner, R. M. (2011). Trajectories of school engagement during adolescence:Implications for grades, depression, delinquency, and substance use. *Developmental Psychology, 47*(1), 233–247. https://doi.org/10.1037/a0021307

Li, Y., Lerner, J. V., & Lerner, R. M. (2010). Personal and ecological assets and academic competence in early adolescence: The mediating role of school engagement. *Journal of Youth and Adolescence, 39*, 801–815. https://doi.org/10.1007/s10964-010-9535-4

Liu, R.-D., Zhen, R., Ding, Y., Liu, Y., Wang, J., Jiang, R., & Xu, L. (2018). Teacher support and math engagement: Roles of academic self-efficacy and positive emotions. *Educational Psychology, 38*(1), 3–16. https://doi.org/10.1080/01443410.2017.1359238

Lovelace, M. D., Reschly, M. L., & Appleton, J. J. (2018). Beyond school records: The value of cognitive and affective engagement in predicting dropout and on-time graduation. *Professional School Counseling, 21*(1), 70–84. https://doi.org/10.5330/1096-2409-21.1.70

Luo, W., Hughes, J. N., Liew, J., & Kwok, O. (2009). Classifying academically at-risk first graders into engagement types: Association with long-term achievement trajectories. *The Elementary School Journal, 109*(4), 380–405. https://doi.org/10.1086/593939

Mahuteau, S., Karmel, T., Mavromaras, K., & Zhu, R. (2015). *Educational outcomes of young Indigenous Australians*. National Centre for Student Equity in Higher Education, Curtin University, Bentley, viewed 7 February 2017. https://www.ncsehe.edu.au/educationaloutcomes-of-young-indigenous-australians/

Marsh, H. W., & Kleitman, S. (2005). Consequences of employment during high school: Character building, subversion of academic goals, or a threshold? *American Educational Research Journal, 42*(2), 331–369. https://doi.org/10.3102/00028312042002331

Martin, A. J. (2007). Examining a multidimensional model of student motivation and engagement using a construct validation approach. *British Journal of Educational Psychology, 77*, 413–440. https://doi.org/10.1348/000709906X118036

McDermott, E. R., Donlan, A. E., & Zaff, J. F. (2019). Why do students drop out? Turning points and long-term experiences. *The Journal of Educational Research, 112*, 270–282. https://doi.org/10.1080/00220671.2018.1517296

McDermott, E. R., Anderson, S., & Zaff, J. (2017). Dropout typologies: Relating profiles of risk and support to later educational re-engagement. *Applied Developmental Science, 22*, 217–232. https://doi.org/10.1080/10888691.2016.1270764

Melkevik, O., Nilsen, W., Evensen, M., Reneflot, A., & Mykletun, A. (2016). Internalizing disorders as risk factors for early school leaving: A systematic review. *Adolescent Research Review, 1*(3), 245–255. https://doi.org/10.1007/s40894-016-0024-1

Mojtabai, R., Stuart, E. A., Hwang, I., Eaton, W. W., Sampson, N., & Kessler, R. C. (2015). Long-term effects of mental disorders on educational attainment in the National Comorbidity Survey ten-year follow-up. *Social Psychiatry and Psychiatric Epidemiology, 50*(10), 1577–1591. https://doi.org/10.1007/s00127-015-1083-5

Organisation for Economic Co-operation and Development (OECD). (2018). *Equity in education: Breaking down barriers to social mobility*. PISA, OECD.

Olivier, E., Galand, B., Morin, A. J. S., & Hospel, V. (2020a). Need-supportive teaching and student engagement : Comparing the additive, synergistic, and balanced contributions. *Learning and Instruction, 71*, 1–18. https://doi.org/10.1016/j.learninstruc.2020.101389

Olivier, E., Morin, A. J. S., Langlois, J., Tardif-Grenier, K., & Archambault, I. (2020b). Internalizing and externalizing behavior problems and student engagement in elementary and secondary school. *Journal of Youth and Adolescence, 49*, 2327–2346. https://doi.org/10.1007/s10964-020-01295-x

Olivier, E., Archambault, I., & Dupéré, V. (2018). Boys' and girls' latent profiles of behavior and social adjustment in school: Longitudinal links with later student behavioral engagement and academic achievement? *Journal of School Psychology, 69*, 28–44. https://doi.org/10.1016/j.jsp.2018.05.006

Organisation for Economic Co-operation and Development (OECD). (2015). *Helping immigrant students to succeed at school – and beyond*. OECD Publishing. https://www.oecd.org/education/Helping-immigrant-students-to-succeed-at-school-and-beyond.pdf

Pagani, L. S., Fitzpatrick, C., & Parent, S. (2012). Relating kindergarten attention to subsequent developmental pathways of classroom engagement in elementary school. *Journal of Abnormal Child Psychology, 40*(5), 715–725. https://doi.org/10.1007/s10802-011-9605-4

Perry, J. C. (2008). School engagement among urban youth of color: Criterion pattern effects of vocational exploration and racial identity. *Journal of Career Development, 34*(4), 397–422. https://doi.org/10.1177/0894845308316293

Pintrich, P. R. (2004). Conceptual framework for assessing motivation and self-regulated learning in college students. *Psychological Bulletin, 16*, 385–407.

Reeve, J. (2009). Why teachers adopt a controlling motivating style toward students and how they can become more autonomy supportive. *Educational Psychologist, 44*(3), 159–175. https://doi.org/10.1080/00461520903028990

Réseau Eurydice. (2010). Différences entre les genres en matière de réussite scolaire: étude sur les mesures prises et la situation actuelle en Europe.

Reschly, A. L., & Christenson, S. L. (2012). Jingle, jangle, and conceptual haziness: Evolution and future directions of the engagement construct. In S. L. Christenson, A. L. Reschly, & C. Wylie (Eds.), *Handbook of research on student engagement* (pp. 3–19). Springer Science + Business Media). https://doi.org/10.1007/978-1-4614-2018-7_1

Reschly, A., & Christenson, S. L. (2006a). Promoting school completion. In G. Bear & K. Minke (Eds.), *Children's needs III: Understanding and addressing the developmental needs of children*. Bethesda.

Reschly, A. L., & Christenson, S. L. (2006b). Prediction of dropout among students with mild disabilities: A case for the inclusion of student engagement variables. *Remedial and Special Education, 27*(5), 276–292. https://doi.org/10.1177/07419325060270050301

Rocque, M., & Snellings, Q. (2018). The new disciplinology: Research, theory, and remaining puzzles on the school-to-prison pipeline. *Journal of Criminal Justice, 59*, 3–11.

Rosenthal, B. S. (1998). Non-school correlates of dropout: An integrative review of the literature. *Children and Youth Services Review, 20*(5), 413–433. https://doi.org/10.1016/S0190-7409(98)00015-2

Rumberger, R. W. (2011). *Dropping out: Why students drop out of high school and what can be done about it*. Harvard University Press. https://doi.org/10.4159/harvard.9780674063167

Rumberger, R. W., & Larson, K. A. (1998). Student mobility and the increased risk of high school dropout. *American Journal of Education, 107*(1), 1–35. https://doi.org/10.1086/444201

Rumberger, R. W. (1987). High school dropouts: A review of issues and evidence. *Review of Educational Research, 57*(2), 101–121. https://doi.org/10.3102/00346543057002101

Samuel, R., & Burger, K. (2020). Negative life events, self-efficacy, and social support: Risk and protective factors for school dropout intentions and dropout. *Journal of Educational Psychology, 112*(5), 973–986. https://doi.org/10.1037/edu0000406

Skinner, E. A., & Pitzer, J. R. (2012). Developmental dynamics of student engagement, coping, and everyday resilience. In S. L. Christenson, A. L. Reschly, & C. Wylie (Eds.), *Handbook of research on student engagement* (pp. 21–44). Springer Science + Business Media). https://doi.org/10.1007/978-1-4614-2018-7_2

Skinner, E. A., Kindermann, T. A., & Furrer, C. J. (2009). A motivational perspective on engagement and disaffection: Conceptualization and assessment of children's behavioral and emotional participation in academic activities in the classroom. *Educational and Psychological Measurement, 69*(3), 493–525. https://doi.org/10.1177/0013164408323233

Skinner, E., Furrer, C., Marchand, G., & Kindermann, T. (2008). Engagement and disaffection in the classroom: Part of a larger motivational dynamic? *Journal of Educational Psychology, 100*(4), 765–781. https://doi.org/10.1037/a0012840

Skinner, E. A., & Belmont, M. J. (1993). Motivation in the classroom: Reciprocal effects of teacher behavior and student engagement across the school year. *Journal of Educational Psychology, 85*(4), 571–581. https://doi.org/10.1037/0022-0663.85.4.571

Staffs, J., & Kreager, D. A. (2008). Too cool for school? Violence, peer status and high school dropout. *Social Forces, 87*(1), 445–471. https://doi.org/10.1353/sof.0.0068

Statistics Canada (2017). Insights on Canadian society young men and women without a high school diploma. Retrived from https://www150.statcan.gc.ca/n1/pub/75-006-x/2017001/article/14824-fra.htm

Suárez-Orozco, C., Rhodes, J., & Milburn, M. (2009). Unraveling the immigrant paradox: Academic engagement and disengagement among recently arrived immigrant youth. *Journal of Education for Students Placed at Risk, 6*, 7–25. https://doi.org/10.1177/0044118X09333647

Strand, S. (2014). School effects and ethnic, gender and socio-economic gaps in educational achievement at age 11. *Oxford Review of Education, 40*(2), 223–245. https://doi.org/10.1080/03054985.2014.891980

Taylor, G., Lekes, N., Gagnon, H., Kwan, L., & Koestner, R. (2012). Need satisfaction, work-school interference and school dropout: An application of self-determination theory. *The British Journal of Educational Psychology, 82*(4), 622–646. https://doi.org/10.1111/j.2044-8279.2011.02050.x

Teese, R., Lamb, S., & Duru-Bellat, M. (2007). *International studies in education inequality, theory and policy*. Springer.

Tinto, V. (1975). Dropout from higher education: A theoretical synthesis of recent research. *Review of Educational Research, 45*(1), 89–125. https://doi.org/10.2307/1170024

Tuominen-Soini, H., & Salmela-Aro, K. (2014). Schoolwork engagement and burnout among Finnish high school students and young adults: Profiles, progressions, and educational outcomes. *Developmental Psychology, 50*(3), 649–662. https://doi.org/10.1037/a0033898

Tyler, J., & Lofstrom, M. (2009). Finishing high school: Alternative pathways and dropout recovery. *The Future of Children, 19*(1), 77–103. https://doi.org/10.1353/foc.0.0019

UNESCO. (2020). *World inequality database on education*. UNESCO Institute for Statistics.

U.S. Department of Commerce. (2017). *Census bureau, current population survey (CPS), selected years, October 1977 through 2017*. Table 2.5. Retrived from https://nces.ed.gov/programs/dropout/ind_02.asp.

U.S. Department of Education. (2016). *Digest of Education Statistics 2016, table 219.70*. Retrived from https://nces.ed.gov/pubs2017/2017094.pdf

Van Uden, J. M., Ritzen, H., & Pieters, J. M. (2016). Enhancing student engagement in pre-vocational and vocational education: a learning history. *Teachers and Teaching, 22*(8), 983–999. https://doi.org/10.1080/13540602.2016.1200545

Véronneau, M.-H., Vitaro, F., Pedersen, S., & Tremblay, R. E. (2008). Do peers contribute to the likelihood of secondary school graduation among disadvantaged boys? *Journal of Educational Psychology, 100*(2), 429–442. https://doi.org/10.1037/0022-0663.100.2.429

Wang, M. T., Fredricks, J., Ye, F., Hofkens, T., & Linn, J. S. (2019). Conceptualization and assessment of adolescents' engagement and disengagement in school. *European Journal of Psychological Assessment, 35*(4), 592–606. https://doi.org/10.1027/1015-5759/a000431

Wang, M.-T., Kiuru, N., Degol, J. L., & Salmela-Aro, K. (2018). Friends, academic achievement, and school engagement during adolescence: A social network approach to peer influence and selection effects. *Learning and Instruction, 58*, 148–160. https://doi.org/10.1016/j.learninstruc.2018.06.003

Wang, M. T., Fredricks, J. A., Ye, F., Hofkens, T. L., & Linn, J. S. (2016). The math and science engagement scales: Scale development, validation, and psychometric properties. *Learning and Instruction, 43*, 16–26. https://doi.org/10.1016/j.learninstruc.2016.01.008

Wang, M. T., & Degol, J. (2014). Motivational pathways to STEM career choices: Using expectancy-value perspective to understand individual and gender differences in STEM fields. *Developmental Review, 33*, 304e340. https://doi.org/10.1016/j.dr.2013.08.001

Wang, M.-T., & Fredricks, J. A. (2014). The reciprocal links between school engagement, youth problem behaviors, and school dropout during adolescence. *Child Development, 85*(2), 722–737. https://doi.org/10.1111/2Fcdev.12138

Wang, M. T., & Peck, S. C. (2013). Adolescent educational success and mental health vary across school engagement profiles. *Developmental Psychology, 49*(7), 1266–1276. https://doi.org/10.1037/a0030028

Wang, M.-T., Willett, J. B., & Eccles, J. S. (2011). The assessment of school engagement: Examining dimensionality and measurement invariance by gender and race/ethnicity. *Journal of School Psychology, 49*(4), 465–480. https://doi.org/10.1016/j.jsp.2011.04.001

Wang, M.-T., & Eccles, J. S. (2012). Adolescent behavioral, emotional, and cognitive engagement trajectories in school and their differential relations to educational success. *Journal of Research on Adolescence, 22*(1), 31–39. https://doi.org/10.1111/j.1532-7795.2011.00753.x

Wehlage, G. G., Rutter, R. A., Smith, G. A., Lesko, N., & Fernandez, R. R. (1989). *Reducing the risk: Schools as communities of support.* The Falmer Press.

Wentzel, K. R., Jablansky, S., & Scalise, N. R. (2020). Peer social acceptance and academic achievement: A meta-analytic study. *Journal of Educational Psychology, 113*(1), 157–180. https://doi.org/10.1037/edu0000468

Zhou, Q., Main, A., & Wang, Y. (2010). The relations of temperamental effortful control and anger/frustration to Chinese children's academic achievement and social adjustment: A longitudinal study. *Journal of Educational Psychology, 102*(1), 180–196. https://doi.org/10.1037/a001590

Exploring the Character of Student Persistence in Higher Education: The Impact of Perception, Motivation, and Engagement

Vincent Tinto

Abstract

This chapter begins with an overview of what we know about rates of college persistence and completion in the United States; what they are for different types of students and types of institutions, and how they have changed over the time between two nationally representative surveys of college persistence carried out by the US Department of Education. This chapter then reviews extant models that seek to explain student persistence. It begins with models that take on the perspective of the institution that asks what it has to do to retain its students, then turns to models that take on the perspective of students who ask how they can persist. Taking on that perspective leads to a discussion of the role of student engagement and motivation in persistence and completion and in turn to the way student self-efficacy, sense of belonging, and perceptions of the relevance of their studies impact decisions to persist. This leads to a more detailed analysis of engagement and the impact of its constituent parts in shaping stu-

dent persistence and completion. This chapter concludes with a discussion of how network analysis can shed light on the impact of micro-engagements with different members of a network on student persistence and completion.

The completion of a higher educational degree matters. It does so for individuals, the institutions they attend, and our society writ large. For individuals, the attainment of a higher educational degree yields a range of benefits not the least of which is its' economic benefits. It is estimated that individuals who attain an undergraduate degree earn approximately $900,000 more in median lifetime earnings than high school graduates. They also have greater access to job opportunities, increased marketability, and greater occupational and economic stability. For institutions, gains in persistence and completion lead, among other things, to greater revenue not only from having more tuition-paying students remain in the institution but also from the resulting reduction of costs associated with recruiting

Here higher education refers to undergraduate education.

V. Tinto (✉)
School of Education, Syracuse University, Syracuse, NY, USA
e-mail: vtinto@syr.edu

fewer students to replace those who leave.[1] For our society, a more educated citizenry yields higher rates of employment, increased tax revenue, higher rates of voting, community involvement, and philanthropic contributions. In addition, it allows our industries to better meet the demands of an increasingly technological society.

Given these benefits, it is little wonder that increasing college completion has become an issue of widespread concern. Thus, the focus of this chapter is as follows. We will explore not only what we know about college completion in the United States but also what we know about what promotes persistence and completion. In doing so, we will explore what is known about the role of student motivation and student engagement and consider how our changing view of the character of student engagement influences our understanding of how it comes to influence persistence and completion.

This chapter begins with an overview of what we know about rates of college persistence and completion in the United States; how they have changed, and how they vary for students of different attributes. It follows with a review of theories that have sought to explain persistence and completion beginning with theories, often referred to as institutional theories, that view retention through the lens of the institution that asks how it can retain more students. Then it turns to social-psychological theories that look at the issue through the eyes of students who ask, not how they can be retained, but how they can persist to completion. That perspective leads to a discussion of theoretical frameworks that argue that student motivation is central to our understanding of student persistence and completion. The following section turns to a more detailed discussion of the concept of engagement and its role in motivation and, in turn, student persistence and completion. It argues that the concept of engagement as commonly understood is a

meta construct that consists of several forms of engagement that have separate impacts on motivation. A theoretical framework is proposed that seeks to explain how those forms of engagement influence motivation over time and, in turn, persistence and completion. The section closes with a discussion of several issues that require further exploration, including the role of student networks and the importance of micro-engagements to student success. This chapter concludes with comments on institutional practice and next steps in our search for a more complete understanding of how student engagement comes to influence student persistence and completion.

College Completion in the United States: What We Know

We begin by examining what we know about the overall rate of college completion in the United States. To do so, we turn to the most recent data on college persistence and completion of students 6 years after entering higher education. These come from the National Center for Education Statistics (NCES) six-year follow-up study of a nationally representative sample of first-time students who began in public and private, two- and four-year colleges in 2011–2012 (McFarland et al., 2019). As we consider these data, the reader is reminded that aggregate data are exactly that, namely, averages that unavoidably mask what may be important variations in outcomes within any one category. Furthermore, aggregate data in any one category may reflect intersections with other categories as, for instance, does race with socio-economic background.

Turning first to overall six-year persistence and attainment rates, a total of 36.8 percent of all first-time students who began in 2011 earned their Bachelor's Degree (BA) within 6 years of entry (Table 1). Another 10.9 percent earned an Associate's Degree (AA) and 8.5 percent an Undergraduate Certificate (UC). Among those who began in a four-year institution, a total of 59.1 percent earned a BA. Since 8.3 percent are still enrolled in a four-year institution, one can

---

[1]In those states that use graduation rates in their formula to fund public institutions, higher graduation rates also lead to increased funding, though the degree to which it does vary from state to state.

Table 1 Six-year persistence and attainment at any institution of first-time students who began in 2011–12

	Bachelor's degree	Associate's degree	Undergraduate certificate	Still enrolled at four-year institution	Left first institution, enrolled at less than four-year institution	Not enrolled
Four-year institutions	59.1	6.0	2.3	8.3	2.6	21.7
Public	59.4	5.8	2.4	9.3	2.8	20.3
Private nonprofit	73.6	2.9	1.4	5.4	2.1	14.7
Private for-profit	14.1	17.9	12.2	11.4	3.3	50.2
Two-year institutions	11.4	17.9	12.2	4.4	9.5	44.6
Public	12.7	18.1	8.4	4.8	9.8	46.3
Private nonprofit	10.6	21.0	20.4	*	*	38.4
Private for-profit	*	16.0	44.4	1.4	6.8	30.7

*Reporting standards not met. Too few cases for reliable estimate
Source: US Department of Education (2020). National Center for Education Statistics. *A 2017 Follow-up: Six-Year Persistence and Attainment at Any Institution for 2011–12 First-time Postsecondary Students*. NCES 2020–238. Washington, DC: 2002

reasonably expect the total completion rate among four-year college entrants to increase to at least 63.3 percent over a longer time frame if only half of those still enrolled complete their degrees. Among students who entered a two-year college, 11.4 percent earned a BA, 17.9 percent an AA, and another 12.2 percent earned an undergraduate certificate in 6 years. As with BA degree attainment, one can also expect these figures to increase somewhat over time.

Beyond the understandable differences in persistence and attainment between four and two-year institutions, it is apparent that where one goes to a four- or two-year institution matters. For instance, among students who first began in a public four-year institution in 2011, 59.4 percent completed their BA degrees in 6 years, while 73.6 percent of those who began in a private nonprofit institution did so. This is not surprising if only because of the differences, on average, of the socio-economic background of students who attend public and private nonprofit institutions.[2]

As before, if half of those still enrolled complete their degrees, one can expect those figures to increase over time to at least 64 and 76 percent, respectively. That the BA completion rate among students who entered private for-profit institutions is so much lower reflects a number of factors not the least of which is that only an estimated twenty percent of beginning students who enter those institutions enroll in a four-year degree program.[3]

Among students who began in public two-year institutions in 2011, 12.7 percent earned a BA by 2017, 18.1 percent earned an AA, and 8.4 percent earned an undergraduate certificate in 6 years. Among those who began in private nonprofit two-year colleges, 10.6 percent completed their BA degrees, 21.0 percent their AA, and 20.4 percent their undergraduate certificates. By contrast, very few students who entered private for-

[2]Brookings Institute report indicates little differences in entering ACT/SAT scores for four-year public and private institutions. See https://www.brookings.edu/research/dont-forget-private-non-profit-colleges/

[3]Four-year private for-profit institutions offer many niche or job-specific programs not requiring a four-year degree that attracts many non-traditional students who need more flexible programs. These are often funded by investors or by subsidiaries of larger corporations. It is noteworthy that their average tuition in 2017–2018 was roughly 45 percent higher than the average four-year public institution (NCES 2017–2018).

Table 2 Six-year persistence and attainment at any institution of first-time students who began in 1995–1996

	Bachelor's degree	Associate's degree	Undergraduate certificate	Still enrolled at a four-year institution	Still enrolled at less than a four-year institution	Not enrolled
Four-year institutions						
Public	53.0	4.4	2.8	14.5	2.8	22.5
Private nonprofit	68.8	2.8	1.8	7.1	2.3	17.2
Private for-profit	19.5	15.1	18.1	7.8	3.3	36.2
Two-year institutions						
Public	10.3	15.7	9.7	8.4	9.1	46.9
Private nonprofit	11.5	26.7	19.8	3.6	4.6	33.8
Private for-profit	1.9	24.4	28.2	1.2	3.0	41.4

Source: US Department of Education (2002). National Center for Education Statistics. *Descriptive Summary of 1995–96 Beginning Postsecondary Students: 6 Years Later*, NCES 2003–151. Washington, DC: 2002

profit colleges earned a BA degree, while 16 percent earned an AA degree and over 44 percent earned an undergraduate certificate. It should be noted that many students who enter public two-year colleges do so with the intent of transferring to a four-year institution and more than a few who begin in private two-year colleges, in particular for-profit ones, do so to earn work-related undergraduate certificates.[4]

Changes in College Completion

Have rates of degree completion changed? To answer this question, we turn to Table 2 that provides data from the National Center for Education Statistics (NCES) six-year follow-up study of the persistence and attainment of a representative sample of first-time students who began college in 1995–1996 (Curtin et al., 2002) and compare those data to the data presented in Table 1. For public and private nonprofit four-year institutions, rates of completion have changed. They

have increased from 53.0 to 59.4 percent for public institutions and from 68.8 to 73.6 percent for private nonprofit institutions. For private for-profit institutions, however, they have decreased from 19.5 to 14.1 percent. While BA and AA completion rates among students beginning in public two-year institutions have increased from 10.3 to 12.7 percent, they have decreased somewhat in private nonprofit institutions. Among private for-profit colleges, while the proportion who earned AA has decreased, the proportion earning Undergraduate Certificates has risen dramatically.[5]

Finally, while the total rate of attainment and continuation has increased over time for public and private nonprofit four-year institutions, from 77.5 and 82.8 percent to 79.7 and 85.3 percent respectively, it has declined for private for-profit four-year institutions from 63.8 to 49.8 percent. Among two-year colleges, though it remained steady for public colleges, it has declined for private nonprofit colleges and increased for private for-profit institutions. Much of the gain for the latter institutions results from the increased

[4]It is also important to note there are many students in two-year institutions who do not fit the profile of the traditional first-time student. In addition to the many students who transfer between institutions, others re-enroll in higher education after having left some years earlier.

[5]It is likely that this increase reflects an increasing demand among students for work-related undergraduate certificates.

percentage of students earning Undergraduate Certificates

College Completion by Student Attributes

How do rates of college completion vary by student attributes? To answer this question. We first turn to the most recent data on the persistence and attainment of students entering public four-year institutions in 2011–2012 as a function of student gender, race/ethnicity, parental educational background, and high school grade point average (Table 3). What these data tell us is that, on average, females do better than males, Asians and White students do better than Black or

Hispanic students, students from more educated families do better than students from less educated families, and students who have higher grade point averages in high school fare better than students who have lower grade point averages. Of those attributes, differences in cumulative high school grade point average are associated with the greatest differences in the completion of BA degrees followed by differences in parental educational level. To restate a point made at the outset of this section, these aggregate data unavoidably mask important intersections with other student attributes, most notably those of ethnicity, parental educational level, and high school grade point average.

The data on the six-year persistence and attainment of students entering private nonprofit

Table 3 Six-year persistence and attainment at any institution of first-time students who began public four-year institutions in 2011–2012 by student attributes

	Bachelor's degree	Associate's degree	Undergraduate certificate	Still enrolled at four-year institution	Left first institution, enrolled at less than four-year institution	Not enrolled
Gender						
Male	55.1	5.7	2.0	11.1	2.5	23.6
Female	62.7	5.9	2.7	7.8	3.0	17.7
Race/ethnicity						
White	65.2	5.9	1.6	8.0	1.8	17.5
Black	41.4	6.0	4.7	10.7	7.1	30.2
Hispanic	50.5	5.7	4.2	12.8	4.1	22.7
Asian	66.5	4.7	++	9.0	++	14.3
Highest level of education attained by either parent						
High school or less	44.2	5.6	3.6	13.5	3.9	29.2
Some postsecondary	49.2	8.8	3.4	8.2	3.6	26.8
Bachelor's degree or more	71.8	4.3	1.3	7.9	1.7	13.0
High school cumulative grade point average#						
Less than 2.50	32.8	8.6	3.6	13.8	5.3	35.9
2.5–2.99	47.4	7.4	2.0	11.9	4.5	26.8
3.0–3.49	60.8	6.3	2.7	10.3	2.4	17.6
3.5–4.0	76.3	2.2	1.5	4.9	1.7	13.4

For students under age 30
++ Insufficient data for reliable estimate
Source: US Department of Education (2020). National Center for Education Statistics. *A 2017 Follow-up: Six-Year Persistence and Attainment at Any Institution for 2011–12 First-time Postsecondary Students*. NCES 2020–238. Washington, DC: 2002

four-year institutions in 2011–2012 indicate that all groups fare better in private nonprofit institutions than in public ones. It is also the case that, as in public institutions, females do better than males, Asian and White students fare better than Hispanic and Black students, and students from more educated background and with higher grade point averages do better than students from less educated backgrounds and lower grade point averages (Table 4). Again, differences in high school grade point average are associated with the largest differences in attainment followed by differences in parental educational backgrounds. It is notable that differences in attainment between students of different parental educational background are larger in private nonprofit institutions than in public institutions, but smaller among students of different grade point averages.

Changes in College Completion by Student Attributes

Have these differences changed over time? The data for public 4-year institutions tell us that while they have not changed in the pattern of differences seen in 2011–2017, they have changed both in rates of attainment of students of different attributes and in differences in between them in attainment (Table 5). In all cases, rates of attainment have increased over time, the largest gain being for Hispanic students whose BA completion rate increased from 39.9 percent to 50.5 per-

Table 4 Six-year persistence and attainment at any institution of first-time students who began in private nonprofit four-year institutions in 2011–2012 by student attributes

	Bachelor's degree	Associate's degree	Undergraduate certificate	Still enrolled at four-year institution	Left first institution, enrolled at less than four-year institution	Not enrolled
Gender						
Male	70.3	2.5	0.5!	6.4	2.1	18.1
Female	76.1	3.1	1.8	4.6	2.1	12.3
Race/ethnicity						
White	77.6	2.2	0.9!	4.6	1.9	12.8
Black	50.1	5.9	2.7	7.3	4.5!	29.5
Hispanic	71.0	5.7!	2.4!	6.7	2.5!	11.6
Asian	86.4	++	++	7!.0	++	6.0!
Highest level of education attained by either parent						
High school or less	50.6	4.6	2.5!	7.7	4.6!	29.8
Some postsecondary	66.6	5.9!	1.7!	5.1	2.9!	17.7
Bachelor's degree or more	82.3	1.2	0.6!	4.8	1.3	9.8
High school cumulative grade point average#						
Less than 2.50	48.0	7.7	2.6!	7.9	3.8	30.0
2.50–2.99	56.5	++	++	5.1!	2.8!	27.9
3.0–3.49	73.1	2.8	1.5!	6.3	1.9	14.4
3.5–4.0	85.8	++	++	3.8	1.9	7.3

\# For students under age 30
! Interpret with caution as estimate is unstable because standard error represents more than 30 percent of estimate
++ Insufficient data for reliable estimate
Source: US Department of Education (2020). National Center for Education Statistics. *A 2017 Follow-up: Six-Year Persistence and Attainment at Any Institution for 2011–12 First-time Postsecondary Students.* NCES 2020–238. Washington, DC: 2002

Table 5 Six-year persistence and attainment at any institution of first-time students who began in public four-year institutions in 1995–1996 by student attributes

	Bachelor's degree	Associate's degree	Undergraduate certificate	Still enrolled at four-year institution	Still enrolled at less than four-year institution	Not enrolled
Gender						
Male	49.5	3,7	2.3	16.4	3.0	25.2
Female	56.0	4.9	3.3	12.9	2.8	20.1
Race/ethnicity						
White	56.1	4.4	2.9	13.3	2.3	21.0
Black	39.0	3.5	3.4	17.4	5.0	31.8
Hispanic	39.9	5.4	2.7	20.2	4.2	27.7
Asian/Pacific Islander	64.2	2.8	0.3	13.5	2,6	16.6
Highest level of education attained by either parent						
High school or less	39.0	4.7	3.9	16.5	3.3	32.7
Some postsecondary	47.7	5.3	3.5	14.4	4.3	25.0
Bachelor's degree	62.4	5.0	1.9	14.1	2.2	14.6
Advanced degree	67.3	1.3	1.7	12.8	2.1	14.6
High school cumulative grade point average						
B's or less	35.5	5.6	3.7	19.6	5.2	30.5
B+ to A-	56.6	3.8	2.8	13.9	2.4	20.6
Mostly A's	76.9	2.1	1.2	11.1	0.8	8.0

Source: US Department of Education (2002). National Center for Education Statistics. *Descriptive Summary of 1995–96 Beginning Postsecondary Students: 6 Years Later*, NCES 2003–151. Washington, DC

cent. But while rates of completion have increased for all groups, differences between the groups have, in some cases, increased. Putting aside differences in the measures in some of categories (e.g., parental education and high school grade point average), it is noteworthy that while the gap in BA completion between females and males has increased only slightly, the gap between White students and Black students has increased substantially from 17.1 percent to 23.8 percent. This is true even after one accounts for the likely increase in BA attainment over time of Black and White students. These findings are striking, indeed disturbing, given the increased emphasis on affirmative action over the span of years between the two surveys.

The data for private nonprofit four-year institutions show that BA completion increased for most groups, especially for Hispanic students whose rate of BA completion increased from 55.6 to 71 percent (Table 6). At the same time, they decreased slightly for Black students and 3.4 percent for students from least educated families. As in public institutions, the gap in completion rates between Black and White students increased over time, in this case from 21.7 to 27.5 percent.

Together with data on public four-year institutions, the 1995–1996 and 2011–2012 studies paint a picture, on one hand of improvement in attainment, but on the other of very different outcomes for Black and Hispanic students in public and private nonprofit institutions. More importantly, it is a picture that makes clear that the gap in BA completion between White and Black students has increased over time for both public and private nonprofit institutions but decreased between White and Hispanic students. The gap between them decreased from 16.8 to 14.7 percent among public institutions and from 16.2 to 6.6 percent among private nonprofit institutions.

Table 6 Six-year persistence and attainment at any institution of first-time students who began private nonprofit four-year institutions in 1995–1996 by student attributes

	Bachelor's degree	Associate's degree	Undergraduate certificate	Still enrolled at four-year institution	Left first institution, enrolled at less than four-year institution	Not enrolled
Gender						
Male	65.8	2.6	1.9	8.5	2.3	18.9
Female	71.2	3.0	1.7	6.0	2.3	15.9
Race/ethnicity						
White	72.4	2.6	1.2	5.8	1.6	16.4
Black	50.7	2.7	5.9	11.8	5.3	23.7
Hispanic	55.6	6.3	3.0	10.1	4.8	20.3
Asian	77.6	0.8	++	6.3	2.8	12.6
Highest level of education attained by either parent						
High school or less	54.0	4.1	3.4	7.0	4.5	27.1
Some postsecondary	58.0	4.9	2.4	8.9	3.2	22.6
Bachelor's degree	73.7	2.4	1.0	6.7	1.5	14.8
Advanced degree	82.7	1.3	0.2	6.1	0.9	8.9
High school cumulative grade point average						
B's or less	35.5	5.6	3.7	19.6	5.2	30.5
B+ to A−	56.6	3.8	2.8	13.9	2.4	20.6
Mostly A's	76.9	2.1	1.2	11.1	0.8	8.0

++ Insufficient data for reliable estimate

Source: US Department of Education (2002). National Center for Education Statistics. *Descriptive Summary of 1995–96 Beginning Postsecondary Students: 6 Years Later*, NCES 2003–151. Washington, DC

Institutional Completion

Now we turn to institutional completion, specifically to the persistence and attainment of students in their first institution of registration. While rates of completion anywhere are of interest, especially at the state level where state higher educational policy is set, institutional rates of completion are a special concern to institutions as much of their revenue depends not only on enrollments but also on the persistence and graduation of their students. In this case, we will focus on three questions, namely how do rates of institutional completion vary among different types of institutions, how have they changed over time, and how have they changed for students of different attributes. In each instance, we will limit our analysis to institutional completion in four-year institutions. We do so because students attending two-year colleges, especially public ones, often use them as inexpensive gateways to

entry to four-year institutions without completing an Associate's Degree.[6] As a result, aggregate data on institutional completion among two-year colleges often misrepresents their success in promoting degree attainment among their students.

How then do rates of institutional completion differ among different types of four-year institutions? Given what we already know about differences in overall persistence and attainment between public and private nonprofit and private for-profit four-year, it is not surprising that institutional persistence and attainment is higher among private nonprofit institutions than public ones (Table 7). This is the case even if one accounts for the likely increase in completion over time that results from the completion of stu-

---

[6]One of the costs of doing so is that students who do not complete their Associate's Degree before transferring to a four-year institution have, on average, lower Bachelor's Degree completion rates than students who leave after completing their degree.

Table 7 Changes in six-year persistence and attainment in first institution of first-time beginning four-year college students between 1996 and 2017

	Bachelor's degree	Associate's degree	Undergraduate certificate	Still enrolled initial institution	Transferred	No credential at any institution as of Spring 2001
NLS 1995–1996						
Public	45.5	1.9	1.0	8.3	17.1	26.3
Private nonprofit	61.0	1.0	0.6	3.2	10.9	23.3
Private for-profit	17.5	11.7	9.2	6.0	29.8	25.9
NLS 2011–2012						
Public	50.9	4.4	0.4	5.5	24.9	13.8
Private nonprofit	63.6	1.3	*	2.1	23.5	9.2
Private for-profit	11.4	12.9	1.6	6.3	24.8	42.8

*Reporting standards not met. Too few cases for reliable estimate

Source: US Department of Education (2002). National Center for Education Statistics. *Descriptive Summary of 1995–96 Beginning Postsecondary Students: 6 Years Later*, NCES 2003–151. Washington, DC: 2002

Source: US Department of Education (2020). National Center for Education Statistics. *A 2017 Follow-up: Six-Year Persistence and Attainment at Any Institution for 2011–2012 First-time Postsecondary Students*. NCES 2020–238. Washington, DC: 2002

dents still enrolled in their initial institution. But while this is the case, rates of institutional completion have increased somewhat more for public than for private nonprofit institutions (5.4 percent versus 2.6 percent). At the same time, rates of transfer to another institution have increased more for private nonprofit institutions than for public ones (i.e., 12.6 versus 7.8 percent). The net effect is that after 6 years, the total rates of degree completion and continuation (i.e., the percentage of students still enrolled in their institution or transferred to another) remains higher in private nonprofit institutions than in public ones (i.e., 90.8 versus 86.2 percent). That the total rate of six-year degree completion of all types of degrees and continuation is high in both public and private nonprofit institutions speaks not only to the increased capacity of these institutions to graduate their students but also the greater mobility of students between institutions.

Institutional Completion by Student Attributes

What then of persistence and attainment rates of first-time students of differing attributes who began a four-year institution in 2011–2021? To answer this question, we turn to the data on the persistence and attainment of students of different gender, race/ethnicity, parental educational background, and high school grade point average (Table 8). Consistent with the data on rates of persistence and attainment from any institution (Tables 3 and 4), the data for institutional persistence and attainments at the initial institution of entry also show that females fared better than males, students from more educated backgrounds did better than those from less educated backgrounds, students who had higher high school grade point average had higher rates of attainment than students with lower high school grade point average, and Asian/Pacific and White students fared better than Black and Hispanic students. As in other data, Asian and/or Asian/Pacific students outperformed all other students.

Changes in Institutional Completion: The Intersection of Gender and Race/Ethnicity

Next we consider changes between 1995–2001 and 2011–2017 in institutional completion of students of different attributes. Unfortunately, the available data do not allow us to replicate the data shown in Table 8. But they do allow for an analysis of how institutional completion rates vary over time for students of different gender and race/ethnicity who begin in public and private nonprofit four-year institutions. More importantly, they allow for an exploration of the intersection between gender and race/ethnicity that was not possible before. In this case, the available data are for first-time, full-time bachelor's degree-seeking students who began in four-year public and private nonprofit institutions. Consequently, they are not directly comparable to the data presented above that are for all first-time students, some of whom do not have that goal.

Turning to first to public institution, the data indicate that the overall total rates of six-year institutional completion have increased for all first-time, full-time students as well as for males and females generally (Table 9). But whereas rates of institutional completion increased for White, Black, Hispanic, and Asian/Pacific Island students, the increase for Black students was less than one percent, while the gain for Hispanic students was nearly ten percent. In every instance, females outperformed males of similar racial/ethnic backgrounds. The same findings, with one notable exception, apply to completion in private nonprofit institutions (Table 10). That exception is for Black students. Their overall rates of completion did not increase but declined somewhat. For males they declined a little more than one percent, but increased less than one percent for female students.

Regardless, male and female students of all racial/ethnic backgrounds completed their degrees more often in a private nonprofit four-year than in four-year public institutions. That they did is, at first appearance, not surprising. But

Table 8 Six-year persistence and attainment in first institution of first-time, four-year college students who began in 2011–2012 by student attributes

NLS 2011–2017	Bachelor's degree	Associate's degree	Undergraduate certificate	Still enrolled at first institution	Left first institution, but enrolled at another institution	Left first institution and never enrolled at another institution
Gender						
Males	48.0	4.1	0.5	5.7	23.9	17.8
Females	52.2	4.5	0.6	3.7	24.9	13.5
Race/ethnicity						
White	55.3	4.2	0.4!	3.9	23.1	13.1
Black	32.7	4.1	0.8	4.5	35.0	22.9
Hispanic	43.4	6.5	0.9	7.4	24.9	16.9
Asian	64.9	2.7!	++	5.6	15.8	10.9
Parental education						
High school or less	32.1	6.4	1.0	6.2	27.2	27.1
Some postsecondary	41.9	5.8	0.6!	5.0	28.3	18.4
BA or more*	64.3	2.7	0.2	3.6	21.2	8.0
High school grade point average#						
Below 2.00	14.7	6.6!	0.2!	5.2	32.3	41.1
2.00–2.49	27.5	6.0	1.0	8.1	32.9	24.4
2.50–2.99	38.6	4.4	0.8!	6.6	30.9	18.6
3.00–3.49	52.8	4.0	0.4	4.8	25.1	12.9
3.50–4.00	67.8	2.3	++	2.3	18.6	8.8

*Estimated from BA and Advanced Degrees
For students under the age of 30
! Estimate unstable
++ Reporting standards not met
Source: US Department of Education (2019). Persistence, Retention, and Attainment of 2011–12 First-Time Beginning Postsecondary Students as of Spring 2017: First Look. NCES 2019-401. Washington, DC: 2002

Table 9 Six-year completion in first institution of first-time, full-time, bachelor's degree-seeking who began in public four-year institutions in 1996 and 2012

	Total	White	Black	Hispanic	Asian/Pacific Island
1996					
Total	55.4	58.1	38.9	45.7	63.4
Males	52.0	54.8	32.8	41.3	59.8
Females	58.2	60.9	43.0	49.1	75.3
2012					
Total	60.4	64.4	39.8	55.0	71.8
Males	57.3	61.4	34.1	50.7	68.7
Females	63.0	66.9	43.9	58.2	76.7

Source: US Department of Education (2019). National Center for Education Statistics. *Digest of Educational Statistics*. Washington, DC: 2002

much depends on the selectivity of the institutions in which students are enrolled. Since institutional selectivity and institutional completion rates are correlated, some of the differences observed in Tables 8 and 9, in particular, those for Black students, may reflect the changing average

Table 10 Six-year completion in first institution of first-time, full-time, bachelor's degree-seeking who began in private nonprofit four-year institutions in 1996 and 2011

	Total	White	Black	Hispanic	Asian/Pacific Island
1995–1996					
Total	63.1	65.7	44.6	55.7	73.5
Males	60.4	63.0	38.9	52.1	71.5
Females	65.4	67.9	48.4	58.3	75.0
2011–2012					
Total	66.5	69.7	44.0	62.8	79.1
Males	63.1	66.7	37.5	59.3	76.9
Females	69.2	72.2	49.0	65.3	80.7

Source: US Department of Education (2019). National Center for Education Statistics. *Digest of Educational Statistics*. Washington, DC: 2002

selectivity of institutions in which they enrolled in 1996 and 2012. Unfortunately we do not have such data. Be that as it may, what is striking is that the gap in the completion rates of White and Black male students and White and Black female students increased over time in both public and private nonprofit institutions. In the public institutions, they increased from 22.0 to 27.3 percent for male and 17.9 to 23.0 percent for females. In private nonprofit institutions, they increased from 24.1 to 29.2 percent for males and from 19.5 to 23.2 percent for females. Again, it is clear we still have much to do to address the many issues that shape the educational experience of students of Black students.

Models of Student Retention

Although public higher education, as we know it, has its roots in the Morrill Land Grant of 1862, it was not until the late 1930s when the first study of student retention was carried out by McNeeley (1937). Data involving 15,535 students from fourteen public and eleven private institutions who initially enrolled as freshmen in 1931–1932 were analyzed to ascertain how various student attributes were related to what was then called student mortality.

The following year, the first significant national study of retention in the United States was carried out by the US Department of Interior and the Office of Education. Like other national studies that would follow, it collected data from a

sample of institutions on a range of demographic student characteristics, social engagement, and reasons for departure (Demetriou & Schmitz-Sciborski, 2011). Other studies, such as those by Gekoski and Schwartz (1961), Astin (1964, 1975, 1984), Panos and Astin (1968), Feldman and Newcomb (1969), and Kamens (1971), followed as retention became a matter of national and institutional interest. Of these, Astin's (1984) study was particularly important for it called attention to the importance of involvement, or what is now referred to as engagement, to student retention.

While these studies looked at the correlates of student retention, it was not until my 1975 article (Tinto, 1975), which built upon and extended Spady's article (1971) article, did attention turn to the development of models to explain how retention arose in institutions.[7] Key to my model is the role of student engagement in the formal and informal academic and social systems of the institution and their impact on student integration, or what would now be called student inclu-

---

[7]It is important to note that my model and those like it do not distinguish between students who leave an institution to enroll in another institution, in other words a student transfer from those who leave higher education altogether. From the perspective of the institution, a leaver is a leaver regardless of what follows after departure. This is not the case for how states in which institutions are located view student departure. For them, transfer is a more desirable outcome than withdrawal from all forms of higher education within the state.

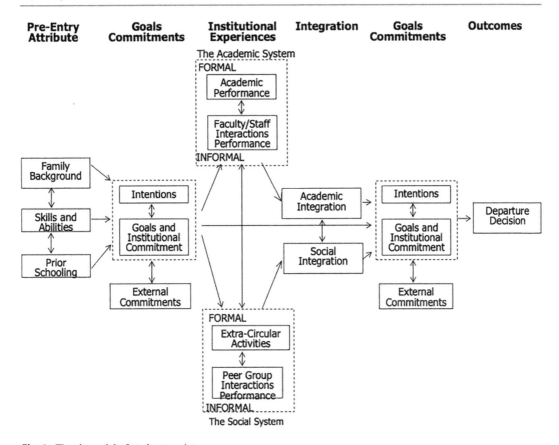

Fig. 1 Tinto's model of student persistence

sion, in the life of the institution.[8] Given student attributes, goals, and commitments, experiences that promote integration/inclusion lead to a commitment of the student to the goal of college completion and to the institution. Those commitments drive retention. But, as described in my revised model (Tinto, 1993), they do so within a context in which external events can mitigate those commitments. Indeed, those events may lead a student, who would otherwise remain in college, to withdraw.[9] Moreover, my revised

model recognizes that students bring intentions, goals, and commitments with them into college that can be strengthened or weakened depending on the way in which students are integrated into the academic and social communities of the college. That model is presented in Fig. 1.

Unlike my model of persistence, Bean's model (1980) is based upon research on worker turnover in organizations. Bean argued that student intentions to leave are similar to those of employees dissatisfied with their career or employer, that it reflected the attributes of the organization and its reward structures. Whether the process of turnover in work organizations is a suitable analog to student experiences in institutions of higher education is, however, an open question. Working with Metzner, a revised model was developed to address the retention of commuting students (Bean & Metzner, 1985). Unlike Bean's earlier model, their model stressed the particular impor-

---

[8]The term integration when used in the context of 1960s and 1970s was not meant to suggest, as some observers argue (e.g., Tierney, 1992) that students of color had to become culturally "white" to persist. Rather it was used as a bookmark to describe the opposite of segregation, a major issue of the time. In today's context the term inclusion better captures the intent of my work.

[9]As opposed to students who leave of their own accord, these students are often referred to as involuntary leavers.

tance of environmental and external forces in shaping student retention decisions. Focusing on the role of faculty, Pascarella (1980) constructed a Student-Faculty Contact Model that stressed the importance of the extent and quality of student–faculty nonclassroom interactions to student satisfaction and in turn retention.

It is important to note that one of the primary drivers that led to the development of my model and that of others was the rejection of the tendency of some earlier writers to "blame the victim" for their dropout, namely, that it reflected the attributes of students. Instead, I and others argued that light had to be shed on the role the institution plays in constructing environments that have the effect of increasing the likelihood that some of their students, in particular, those from low-income and minority backgrounds, would not persist. To improve student persistence for all students, institutions had to change. This focus on institutional change remains at the center of much of the current research on student retention.

Although my model has been critiqued (e.g., Berger & Braxton, 1998; Tierney, 1992), it has generally been supported in its application to the study of retention in different institutions and among different groups of students (e.g., Karp et al., 2009). As Pascarella and Terenzini's (1980) stated their "results generally support the predictive validity of the major dimensions of Tinto's model" (p. 70). More importantly, "it has significantly influenced how researchers and practitioners alike approach the study of undergraduate retention" (Demetriou & Schmitz-Sciborski, 2011).

This is not to say that my model is not without need of modification and improvement. It is. As Braxton et al. (1997) observed, it would be improved by exploring additional psychological, social, and organizational forces that also impact retention. Nor is it to say that there are no other ways of explaining student retention. There are. Beyond those already noted, these include economic theories (e.g., Stampen & Cabrera, 1986; Cabrera et al., 1992; Paulsen & St. John, 1997), anthropological theories (e.g., McCarty et al., 2013; Tierney, 1992), and recently social network

theory (e.g., Eckles & Stradley, 2011). Except for the latter, to which we will return later in this chapter, other theories, though useful in their own right, have, with the possible exception of Tierney (1992), done relatively little to explore the role of student engagement in persistence. Of those models that have, my model and its several derivatives (e.g., Berger & Braxton, 1998) continue to influence how practitioners view institutional retention. Furthermore, the emphasis on the importance of social and academic involvement/engagement has been integral to the development of instruments to assess student engagement in both four-year (NSSE) and two-year (CCSSE) institutions.

It is important that one understands that what are referred to in the literature as theories of student retention are not theories in the strictest sense of the word. Unlike many theories in the physical world, social science theories do not predict individual behavior. Rather they describe the association between various individual, institutional, and situational attributes and patterns of retention. As they pertain to student retention, they argue that there is an association between patterns of student engagement and patterns of student retention such that more engagement is, on average, associated with higher rates, on average, of retention. It does not follow that this will apply to each and every student, but only to students on average.[10] It is far better to use the terms, like framework or conceptual model, that do not imply prediction. The term conceptual model can be thought of as a type of middle-range theory that comprises a limited number of variables, each of limited scope, as evidence for the usefulness of particular forms of practice (Merton,

---

[10] Many argue that it is unlikely that social scientists will ever be able to predict individual behavior, not only because we will never be able to completely account for all possible events that shape an individual event but also because it is not clear what is the behavior we are trying to predict. Is it the behavior an external view observes or is it the intent of the actor of the behavior? This is but one reason why experienced student advisors are well aware that while certain attributes are associated, on average, with certain types of student behaviors, they can never assume that the average association applies to the individual student with whom they meet.

1957). The term framework, as used here, is not conceptual model as much as it is a way of thinking about how a particular outcome, in this case student retention, comes about.[11]

Models of Engagement, Motivation, and Student Persistence

For the most part, past models of student persistence have taken on the perspective of the institution that asks what it can do to improve the retention of their students. Another way, arguable a more important way, is to take on the perspective of the student. Although it is understandable that an institution would ask how it can retain its students, this is not the question students ask. Instead, they ask what they can do to persist. The two perspectives, that of the institution and that of the student, though related, are different. They speak to different issues and give rise to different actions.

Understanding what this means for the process of persistence begins with realizing that the term "to persist," or its adjective form "persistent," is but one way of speaking about student motivation. Simply put, students have to want to persist and be motivated to do so, otherwise there is little reason for them to expend the effort and sometimes considerable resources to do so.

Social-Psychological Models of Persistence and Student Motivation

This perspective, what is referred to as a social-psychological perspective, has increasingly come to mark recent research and theory. Although Summerskill (1962) first suggested that both psychological and sociological theories and concepts should be applied to the study of student retention, it was not until recently that others took up his suggestion. Doing so is not just a matter of adding psychological variables into models of student retention, as have Bean and Metzner (1985), but of building a model based on that perspective. This has happened in a number of ways.

Bean and Eaton (2001) in addressing what they saw as the shortcomings of my model of institutional retention, specifically that it gave "no explanation of the mechanisms by which activities would lead to increased academic and social integration and reduced attrition" (p. 74), proposed a model of retention in which psychological processes play a key role in students' academic and social integration. They argued that students "emotional reactions to college environments motivate students to engage in adaptive strategies" (p. 75). Of the possible emotional reactions, they stressed the role of students' self-efficacy assessments, their coping behaviors, and their locus of control (i.e., whether students believe they have control over their success or failure in college). Graham et al. (2013) proposed a different framework, one which also stresses the importance of motivation, in their case for the persistence of students in STEM. Their framework sees persistence as influenced by student learning and developing a professional identity as a scientist. More importantly, they posit a feedback loop over time such that as students learn and begin to see themselves as a scientist, they gain confidence in their abilities. That, in turn, leads to enhanced motivation to persist that furthers their willingness to learn and become scientists.

As do Bean and Eaton (2001) and Graham et al. (2013), I begin with the premise that motivation is central to persistence (Tinto, 2015, 2017).[12] Student motivation is, in turn, seen as being shaped by student perceptions of their experiences in the institution. Like Hurtado and Carter (1966), I argue that it is not engagement per se that matters, as it is students' perceptions of their engagements and the meanings they draw from them as to their self-efficacy, sense of belonging, and the relevance of their studies.

---

[11]Qualitative researchers typically do not assume a conceptual model or framework beforehand. They argue that doing so would restrict their ability to discover what explanations make sense for the data they collect. Only then they may ask what existing models or frameworks might apply to their data.

[12]Also see Rizkallah & Seitz (2017).

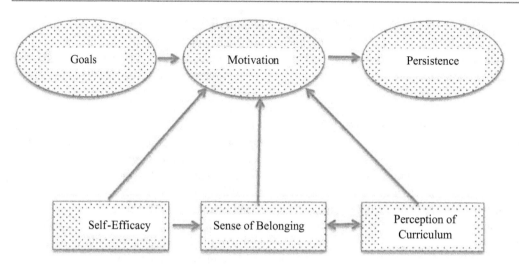

Fig. 2 A framework for the study of student motivation and persistence

Given student goals, this framework for the analysis of the impact of perceptions on motivation and persistence is shown in Fig. 2.

Self-efficacy refers to a person's belief in their ability to succeed at particular task or in a specific situation (Bandura, 1977). It is not inherited, but learned from past experiences. Moreover, it is malleable. It can change as student experiences change.[13] What matters for the present discussion is that students who believe they can succeed at a particular educational task will engage more readily in that task, spend more time on it, and expend more effort on its completion. Sense of belonging speaks to a student's perception of being an accepted member of the community of the institution whose participation is valued by others.[14] It can refer to the larger university community or to one or more smaller academic and social communities of the university. Students who perceive themselves as belonging are more likely to be motivated to persist because of the connection between students' sense of belonging and their commitment to the institution or the particular community in which they participate (Strayhorn, 2019). That commitment drives motivation to persist. Student's perceptions of the curriculum, specifically their perceptions of the relevance of their studies to matters that concern them, is also seen as influencing motivation. This is the case if only because studies that are seen as irrelevant will undermine student effort. A student can reasonably question the point of investing the time and effort and, in many cases, considerable resources needed to complete a degree program when they see little relevance of their studies.

It should be noted that studies of persistence of culturally diverse students often use the term validation as well as sense of belonging. They do so as a way of emphasizing the importance of having students' presence on campus and in the classrooms be validated by others, especially the faculty, that their voice matters (e.g., Barnett, 2011; Rendón, 1994). In stressing validation, theorists like Rendón highlight the critical role institutional culture plays in shaping students' sense of being validated and, in turn, persistence (Yi, 2008). It is one thing to have their presence on campus tolerated, it is entirely another to have their presence valued and their voices validated as contributing to the dialogue of learning.

---

[13]Dweck (2006) argues that change in a person's self-efficacy depends on their mindset, specifically that they believe that it can change.

[14]It is widely understood that sense of belonging is a fundamental human need that shapes all aspects of human development. See: https://www.psychologytoday.com/us/blog/sense-belonging/201906/the-importance-belonging-across-life

By including motivation as a driver of persistence, as do Bean and Eaton (2001), I propose a mechanism that provides the causal link, not explicitly discussed in my 1993 model of persistence, between students' academic and social engagements in the communities of the institution and their academic and social integration/inclusion. As so much depends on student perceptions of their engagements, I further argue that to effectively address student persistence, institutions must look at the issue of retention and persistence through the eyes of their students (Tinto, 2015). They need to understand how students make sense of their experiences. One of the advantages of doing so is that it not only gives voice to students, it also more clearly raises questions about the experiences of students of different racial and ethnic, socio-economic, and immigrant backgrounds and their perceptions of those experiences. To improve persistence while addressing issues of equity, institutions need to take the voices of all their students, not just some, seriously and ask not only what they need to do to help those students persist but also what they need do to lead them to want to persist.

Student Engagement: Its Components and Role in Student Persistence

Most models of student retention and persistence, whether they approach the issue from the view of the institution or that of the student, have one thing in common, namely, the centrality of engagement to student success. But exactly what researchers and theorists mean by that term is often unclear. This is the case, in part, because engagement is not a single construct but comprises different types of engagement. Fredricks et al. (2004) and Jimerson et al. (2003), for instance, argue that engagement comprises three types of engagement, namely, behavioral (e.g., attendance, participation), affective (e.g., interest, belonging, identification, attitudes), and cognitive (e.g., perceived relevance of learning).[15]

Reschly and Christenson (2006, 2012) postulate that engagement consists of not three but four subtypes, behavioral, affective, cognitive, and academic (e.g., engagement in learning, time on task, credits earned, grades). They further speculate that cognitive and affective engagement mediates academic and behavioral engagement. In other words, affective and cognitive engagement precedes students' behavioral and academic engagement. Moreover, as do Graham et al. (2013) and Reschly (2010), Reschly and Christenson (2012) draw upon Ceci and Papierno (2005) to postulate a feedback loop between student perceptions of engagement, that are shaped by the context in which engagement occurs, and future engagements. Doing so leads directly to the argument that engagement in context is a longitudinal process, one which leads to greater or lesser levels of engagement over time.

Following Hurtado and Carter (1966), it is argued here that affective engagement precedes other forms of engagement, namely, behavioral, academic, and cognitive. It does so via its impact on motivation which, in turn, impacts subsequent engagements (Ben-Eliyahua et al., 2018). Here affective engagement refers to students' perceptual responses to their academic and social environment; behavioral engagement to their social interactions with others on campus; academic engagement to their engagements in academic activities; and cognitive engagement as the degree to which students' are willing to seriously engage in learning the curriculum.

To understand this process, put yourself in the position of new student entering the university. She, like most new students, begins meeting and interacting with a range of people, instructors, administrators, staff, and other students. Her perceptions of those interactions, especially with instructors and peers, and the meanings she derives from them, that is her affective engagement, matter. They do because they begin to influence her sense of her ability to succeed, her sense of academic and social belonging, and her perceptions of the curriculum. These influence her motivation and, in turn, her willingness to engage in other ways, namely, behavioral, academic, and cognitive. Affective engagements that are positive tend to enhance other forms of

---

[15] Although these authors were speaking of engagement in high school, it is the view here that the same applies to college.

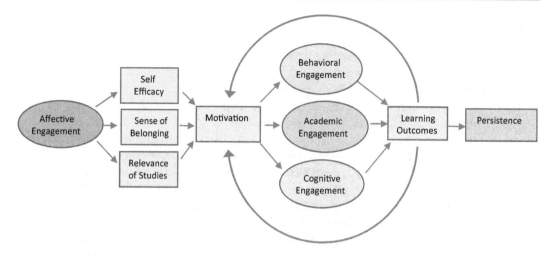

Fig. 3 A model for the study of the longitudinal process of engagement, motivation, and persistence

engagement that promote outcomes, such as learning. As students learn more, their motivation increases. In other words, there is a feedback loop between an outcome such as learning and motivation, as discussed above (Graham et al., 2013; Reschly, 2010), and subsequent engagements. Increased motivation furthers subsequent engagements that enhances learning over time. The end result of this longitudinal process is persistence and eventually completion. A model that captures this process in depicted in Fig. 3.

Of course, not all engagements are positive. Nor are student engagements and the meanings students derive from them are consistently in one direction or the other. They can and often do vary over time if only because students also vary over time in their perceptions of their experiences.[16] Nor does it follow that intensity of engagements follows a similarly uniform pattern. But how they impact any individual student's persistence is a more complex issue. Nevertheless, one would expect an especially negative affective engagement, for instance, experiencing racial bigotry, can significantly influence a student's willingness to further engage and remain at the institution despite earlier experiences. Conversely, a partic-

ularly positive experience, for instance, very positive feedback in a class, may enhance a student's willingness to become more academically and cognitively engaged even when other classes are far less engaging.

It should be noted that the process described above provides not only the causal link between motivation and persistence missing in Fig. 2 but also the causal link missing in my model of student retention between students integration/inclusion and retention (Tinto, 1975). More importantly, it provides for a feedback mechanism that helps explain how a student's decision about persistence may vary over time.

There remains another unaddressed question about engagement, namely, do the effects of engagement depend on with whom one engages. In other words, do students' micro-engagements matter. As regards student learning, specifically as it is influenced by faculty, we know that it does (e.g., Pascarella, 1980; Pascarella & Terenzini, 1991). It is also possible that positive engagements with a smaller group of students with whom one shares common values or perspectives can lead to the persistence as it does, for instance, for minority students (e.g., Simmons, 2013). The same may also be true for peer friendships.

But determining whether this is the case demands another form of analysis not yet common in studies of student persistence, namely,

---

[16]Given what we know from student development theory (Evans et al., 2010), it is also likely that traditional age students' perceptions of their environments change as they develop over the college years.

social network analysis. Social network analysis is based on the relatively simple idea that peoples' social behavior is largely brought about through social ties with other people whose behavior influences their own (Wasserman & Faust, 1994). Network of relationships defines, in effect, the social space within which individual interactions occur and influence, in differing degrees, individual behaviors, and views. To what degree it does, depends on both the density of the network, that is the number of connections divided by the number of possible connections, and the person's location in the network, that is whether they are at the center or on periphery of the network. The denser a network is, the greater the number of interactions among its members. The more central individuals are to the center of a network, the more interactions they have with other members of the network. These matter because students who are at or near the center of dense networks of affiliation with other students are more likely to find social support in those affiliations (Eggens et al., 2008), have a greater sense of community (Dawson, 2008), improved academic performance (Rizzuto et al., 2009) and greater persistence (Thomas, 2000). Presumably, having more connections leads to more social support, a greater sense of belonging, heightened performance, and, in turn, greater likelihood of persistence to completion. But much depends on the views and behavior of members of the network. Not all networks yield positive outcomes. As it pertains to persistence, Eckles and Stradley's (2011) study of second-year retention found that the retention of a student's friends in the network had a greater impact on second-year retention than any background variable. If a student's friends stay, the student is more likely to do so. Conversely if a student's friend leave, the student is more likely to leave. These and other studies (e.g., Eggens et al., 2008; Smith et al., 2013) lend support to not only the importance of students' network of affiliations in understanding student performance and persistence but also the importance of affiliations with specific individuals play in that process. They tell us that while it is evident that engagement matters, engagement with particular individuals, faculty, and peers, or what

I refer to as micro-engagements, may matter as much if not more.[17]

Two final observations are as follows. First, Smith and Vonhoff (2019) argue that conceptualizing communities as networks of interrelationships among students can reveal largely overlooked degrees of complexities in academic and social communities and patterns of engagement within them that influence student persistence. Second, as it pertains to current theories of persistence, Thomas (2000) argues that the strength and range of a student's network of affiliations provides another way of making sense of how student academic and social integration/inclusion and, in turn, student persistence are shaped by student engagements on campus.

In closing, it should be noted that our conversation about motivation and persistence should not be taken to suggest that student ability does not matter. We know that it does. That is but one reason why universities invest in academic support programs, especially in the first year of university study. They understand that while some students begin their studies insufficiently prepared for the academic demands of university study, others will struggle in that year to adjust to the heightened demands of university study. The fact is that many students struggle in the first year. It is part and parcel of the first-year experience. That being said, it is clear that the provision of academic support can improve students' academic performance. To the degree that it does, it can also improve students' perception of their ability to succeed in the university and in turn their motivation to persist.

The provision of social support, in particular that which helps new students become engaged with others can also improve students' performance and persistence. As is the case for academic adjustment, more than a few new students struggle to adjust to the social life of an institution. It is not always easy to meet new people

---

[17] The use of mentor programs, especially but not only for underrepresented students, is but one concrete example how a student's affiliation with a particular individual within a network of affiliations can enhance the likelihood of student persistence (e.g., Campbell & Campbell, 1997; Crisp & Cruz, 2009; and Ma, 2010).

and make friends. In response, institutions have developed a range of programs beginning as early as orientation that are designed to build student communities. To the degree that they do, they can also promote a sense of belonging and in turn student motivation to persist. But whether these communities are perceived by students to be inclusive depends on the value-laden environment in which students find themselves.

Closing Thoughts

Our discussion of the impact of different forms and networks of engagement on student persistence gives rise to a number of questions about institutional practice. First, it raises questions about how institutions can direct its early actions to better promote student persistence. Given the view here that students' affective engagement influences subsequent academic and behavioral as well as cognitive engagement, institutions would be advised to focus their early efforts to ensuring, as best it can, that students' affective engagements are positive and that they lead students to believe they can succeed, see themselves as belonging, and perceive the relevance of the first-year curriculum. This is not to say that efforts to enhance academic and behavioral engagement should not be pursued. Rather it is to say that to promote those engagements in ways that include all students, institutions have to address the various issues on campus that influence their affective engagement, not the least of which is the value-laden culture of the institution that gives meaning to those engagements.

Second, it raises the question of whether it is possible for institutions to intentionally construct networks of affiliation that enhance the likelihood of persistence. For instance, can carefully constructed first-year learning communities, both residential and nonresidential, serve to develop networks of affiliation that promote persistence?

Some research suggest that they can, at least in the short term (Tinto, 2003, 2015). As regards academic performance, can the same apply to carefully constructed classrooms, especially those that apply well-implemented cooperative learning and problem or project learning. Again, we have evidenced that they can, at least in the short term (Nilson, 2010). Whether those networks, in a learning community or a classroom, endure over time as students develop other affiliations is another question that has yet to be answered. But to do so, we have to better understand how micro-engagements within networks of affiliation shape different forms of engagement more broadly understood. We know that it is possible, for instance, for a student to have rewarding micro-engagements with other members of the institution, students, faculty, and administrators (e.g., smaller networks of like students or a faculty mentor), yet have negative affective engagements with the institution more broadly. Think here of underrepresented students feeling connected to and supported by faculty and students of similar backgrounds, but feel disconnected from the institution. As regards persistence, though we know that such micro-engagements can lead to persistence, what we do not yet fully understand is to what degree and in what manner the former can offset the latter. Knowing how it can may help institutions build more effective programs to promote the persistence of all students.

We have slowly begun to unravel the complex role of engagement in student persistence and only recently have considered the ways in different forms of engagement and different networks of engagement and micro-engagements within them influence persistence. But while we have learned much about engagement and persistence, it is evident there is still much more to learn. Here I am reminded of a quote of the late Daniel Boorstin of The University of Chicago who said "Education is learning what you didn't even know you didn't know."

References

Astin, A. W. (1964). Personal and environmental factors associated with college dropout among high aptitude students. *Journal of Educational Psychology, 55*(4), 219–227. https://doi.org/10.1037/h0046924

Astin, A. W. (1975). *Preventing students from dropping out.* Jossey-Bass.

Astin, A. W. (1984). Student involvement: A developmental theory for higher education. *Journal of College Student Personnel, 25,* 297–308.

Bandura, A. (1977). Self-efficacy: Toward a unifying theory of behavioral change. *Psychological Review, 84,* 191–215. https://doi.org/10.1037/0033-295X.84.2.191

Barnett, E. (2011). Validation experiences and persistence among community college students. *The Review of Higher Education, 32*(2), 193–230. https://doi.org/10.1353/rhe.2010.0019

Bean, J. (1980). Dropouts and turnover: The synthesis and test of a causal model of student attrition. *Research in Higher Education, 12*(2), 165–133. https://doi.org/10.1007/BF00-76194

Bean, J., & Eaton, S. (2001). The psychology underlying successful retention practices. *Journal of College Student Retention, 3*(1), 73–89. https://doi.org/10.2190/6R55-4B30-28XG-L8U0

Bean, J., & Metzner, B. S. (1985). A conceptual model of nontraditional undergraduate student attrition. *Review of Educational Research, 55*(4), 485–540. https://doi.org/10.3102/00346543055004485

Ben-Eliyahua, A., Moore, D., Dorph, R., & Schunn, C. D. (2018). Investigating the multidimensionality of engagement: Affective, behavioral, and cognitive engagement across science activities and contexts. *Contemporary Educational Psychology, 53*(April), 87–105. https://doi.org/10.1016/j/edpsych.2018.01.002

Berger, J. B., & Braxton, J. M. (1998). Revising Tinto's Interactionalist theory of student departure through theory elaboration. *Research in Higher Education, 39*(2), 103–119. https://doi.org/10.1023/A:1018760513769

Braxton, J. M., Sullivan, A. S., & Johnson, R. (1997). Appraising Tinto's theory of college student departure. In J. S. Smart (Ed.), *Higher education: Handbook of theory and research* (Vol. XII). Agathon.

Cabrera, A. F., Nora, A., & Castaneda, M. B. (1992). The role of finances in the persistence process: A structural model. *Research in Higher Education, 33,* 571–593. https://doi.org/10.2307/1982157

Campbell, T. A., & Campbell, E. D. (1997). Faculty/Student mentor program: Effects on academic performance and retention. *Research in Higher Education, 38*(6), 727–742. https://doi.org/10.1023/A:1024911904627

Ceci, S. J., & Papierno, P. B. (2005). The rhetoric and reality of gap closing: When the "have-nots" gain but the "haves" gain even more. *American Psychologist, 60*(2), 149–160. https://doi.org/10.1037/0003-066X.60.2.149

Crisp, G., & Cruz, I. (2009). Mentoring college students: A critical review of the literature between 1990 and 2007. *Research in Higher Education, 50*(6), 525–545. https://doi.org/10.1007/s11162-009-9130-2

Curtin, T. R., Ingels, S. J., Wu, S., & Heuer, R. E. (2002). *Base-Year to Fourth Follow-up Data File User's Manual.* National Education Longitudinal Study of 1988. NCES 2002-323. National Center for Education Statistics.

Dawson, S. (2008). A student of the relationship between student social networks and sense of community. *Educational Technology & Society, 11*(3), 224–238.

Demetriou, C., & Schmitz-Sciborski, A. (2011). Integration, motivation, strengths and optimism: Retention theories past, present and future. In R. Hayes (Ed.), *Proceedings of the 7th National Symposium on Student Retention. Charleston* (pp. 300–312). The University of Oklahoma.

Dweck, C. S. (2006). *Mindset.* Random House.

Eckles, J. E., & Stradley, E. G. (2011). A social network analysis of student retention using archival data. *Social Psychology of Education, 15*(2), 165–180. https://doi.org/10.1007/s11218-011-9173-z

Eggens, L., Van der Werf, M. P. C., & Bosker, R. J. (2008). The influence of personal networks and social support on study attainment of students in university education. *Higher Education, 55*(5), 553–573.

Evans, N. J., Forney, D. S., Guido, F. M., Patton, L. D., & Renn, K. A. (2010). *Student development in college: Theory, research, and practice* (2nd ed.). Jossey-Bass & Sons..

Feldman, K. A., & Newcomb, T. M. (1969). *The impact of college on students.* Jossey-Bass Inc.

Fredricks, J. A., Blumenfeld, P. C., & Paris, A. H. (2004). School engagement: Potential of the concept, state of the evidence. *Review of Educational Research, 74*(1), 59–109. https://doi.org/10.3102/00346543074001059

Gekoski, N., & Schwartz, S. (1961). Student mortality and related factors. *The Journal of Educational Research, 54*(5), 192–193. https://doi.org/10.1080/00220671.1961.10882710

Graham, M., Frederick, J., Byars-Winston, A., Hunter, A., & Handelsman, J. (2013). Increasing persistence of college students in STEM. *Science, 341*(6153), 1455–1456. https://doi.org/10.1126/science.1240487

Hurtado, S., & Carter, D. (1966). Latino students' sense of belonging in the college community: Rethinking the concept of integration on campus. In F. K. Stage, G. L. Anaya, J. Bean, D. Hossler, & G. Kuh (Eds.), *College students: Evolving nature of research* (pp. 123–136). Simon & Schuster Custom Publishing.

Jimerson, S. R., Campos, E., & Greif, J. L. (2003). Toward an understanding of definitions and measures of school engagement and related terms. *California School*

Psychologist, 8(1), 7–27. https://doi.org/10.1007/BF03340893

Kamens. (1971). The college "charter" and college size: Effects on occupational choice and college attrition. *Sociology of Education, 47*(3), 270–296. https://doi.org/10.2307/2111994

Karp, M. H., Hughes, K., & O'Gara, L. (2009). An exploration of Tinto's integration framework for community college students. *Journal of College Student Retention: Theory and Practice, 12*(1), 69–86. https://doi.org/10.2190/CS.15.3.b

Ma, S. Y. (2010). Mentoring and student persistence in college: A study of the Washington State Achievers program. *Innovative Higher Education, 35*(5), 329–341. https://doi.org/10.1007/s10755-010-9147-7

McCarty, T., Brayboy, B. M. J., Datnow, A., Hamann, E. T., & The Anthropology of Educational Persistence Thought Collective, "The Anthropology of Educational Persistence: What Can We Learn from Anthropology to Improve Educational Opportunities and Outcomes for Underserved Students?". (2013). *Faculty publications: Department of teaching, learning and teacher education.* 149. http://digitalcommons.unl.edu/teachlearnfacpub/149

McFarland, J., Hussar, B., Zhang, J., Wang, X., Wang, K., Hein, S., Diliberti, M. K., Cataldi, E. F., Mann, F. B., & Barmer, A. (2019). *The Condition of Education 2019.* NCES 2019-144. National Center for Education Statistics.

McNeeley, J. H. (1937). *College Student Mortality.* U.S. Department Interior Bulletin, No. 11. In National Center for Education Statistics (2003). *Descriptive Summary of 1995–96 Beginning Postsecondary Students: Six Years Later.* U.S. Department of Education.

Merton, R. (1957). *Social theory and social structure.* Free Press.

Nilson, L. B. (2010). *Teaching at its best: A research-based resources for college instructors* (2nd ed.). Jossey-Bass.

Panos, R. J., & Astin, A. W. (1968). Attrition among college students. *American Educational Research Journal, 5*(1), 57–72. https://doi.org/10.2307/1161701

Pascarella, E. T. (1980). Student-faculty informal contact and college outcomes. *Review of Educational Research, 50*(4), 545–595. https://doi.org/10.3102/00346543050004545

Pascarella, E. T., & Terenzini, P. T. (1980). Predicting freshman persistence and voluntary dropout decisions from a theoretical model. *Journal of Higher Education, 51*(1), 60–75. https://doi.org/10.1080/00221546.1980.11780030

Pascarella, E. T., & Terenzini, P. T. (1991). *How college effects students: Findings and insights from twenty years of research.* Jossey-Bass.

Paulsen, M. B., & St. John, E. P. (1997). The financial nexus between college choice and persistence. *New Directions for Institutional Research, 95*, 65–82. https://doi.org/10.1002/ir.9504

Rendón, L. I. (1994). Validating culturally diverse students: Toward a new model of learning and student development. *Innovative Higher Education, 19*(1), 33–51. https://doi.org/10.1007/BF01191156

Reschly, A. (2010). Reading and school completion: Critical connections and Matthew effects. *Reading and Writing Quarterly, 26*(1), 67–90.

Reschly, A. L., & Christenson, S. L. (2006). Prediction of dropout among students with mild disabilities: A case for the inclusion of student engagement variables. *Remedial and Special Education, 27*(5), 276–292. https://doi.org/10.1177/07419325060270050311

Reschly, A. L., & Christenson, S. L. (2012). Jingle, jangle, and conceptual haziness. Evolution and future directions of the engagement construct. In S. L. Christenson, A. M. Reschly, & C. Wylie (Eds.), *Handbook of research on student engagement.* Springer Publishing. https://doi.org/10.1007/978-1-4614-2018-7_1

Rizkallah, E. J., & Seitz, V. (2017). Understanding student motivation: A key to retention in higher education. *Scientific Annals of Economics and Business, 64*, 45–57.

Rizzuto, T. E., LeDoux, J., & Hatala, J. P. (2009). It's not just what you know, it's who you know: Testing a model of the relative importance of social networks to academic performance. *Social Psychology of Education, 12*(2), 175–189.

Simmons, L. (2013). Factors of persistence for African American men in a student support organization. *The Journal of Negro Education, 82*(1), 62–74. https://doi.org/10.7709/jnegroeducation.82.1.0062

Smith, A., & Vonhoff, C. (2019). Problematizing community: A network approach to conceptualizing campus communities. *Journal of College Student Development, 60*(3), 255–270. https://doi.org/10.1353/csd.2019.0025

Smith, J., Pender, M., & Howell, J. (2013). The full extent of student-college academic undermatch. *Economics of Education Review, 32*, 247–261. https://doi.org/10.1016/j.econedurev.2012.11.001

Spady, W. G. (1971). Dropouts from higher education: Toward an empirical model. *Interchange, 2*(3), 38–62. https://doi.org/10.1007/BF02282469

Stampen, J. O., & Cabrera, A. F. (1986). Exploring the effects of student aid on attrition. *Journal of Student Financial Aid, 16*(2), 28–40.

Strayhorn, T. (2019). *College students' sense of belonging: A key to educational success for all students* (2nd ed.). Routledge.

Summerskill, J. (1962). Dropouts from college. In Stanford (Ed.), *The American college: A psychological and social interpretation of the higher learning* (pp. 627–657). Wiley. https://doi.org/10.1037/11181-019

Thomas, S. L. (2000). Ties that bind: A social network approach to understanding student integration and persistence. *The Journal of Higher Education, 71*(5), 591–615. https://doi.org/10.2307/2649261

Tierney, W. G. (1992). An anthropological analysis of student participation in college. *Journal of Higher*

Education, 63(6), 603–618. https://doi.org/10.1080/00 221546.1992.11778391

Tinto, V. (1975). Dropout from higher education: A theoretical synthesis of recent research. *Review of Educational Research, 45*(1), 89–125. https://doi.org/10.2307/1170024

Tinto, V. (1993). *Leaving college: Rethinking the causes and cures of student attrition* (2nd ed.). The University of Chicago Press.

Tinto, V. (2003). *Learning better together: The impact of learning communities on student success (Higher education monograph series,* no 6). Syracuse University.

Tinto, V. (2015). Through the eyes of students. *Journal of College Student Retention: Research, Theory & Practice, 19*(3), 254–269. https://doi.org/10.1177/1521025621917

Tinto, V. (2017). Through the eyes of students. *Journal of College Student Retention: Research, Theory & Practice, 19*, 54–269.

U.S. Department of Education. (2002). National Center for Education Statistics. *Descriptive summary of 1995–96 beginning postsecondary students: Six years later,* NCES 2003–151. Washington, DC: 2002.

U.S. Department of Education. (2019). National Center for Education Statistics. *Integrated postsecondary education data system.* Spring 2004 through Spring 2013 and Winter 2013–2014 through Winter 2018–2019.

U.S. Department of Education. (2020). National Center for Education Statistics. *A 2017 follow-up:Six-year persistence and attainment at any institution for 2011–12 first-time postsecondary students.* NCES 2020–238. Washington, DC: 2002.

Wasserman, S., & Faust, K. (1994). *Social network analysis: Methods and applications.* Cambridge University Press.

Yi, P. (2008). Institutional climate and student departure: A multinomial multilevel modeling approach. *Review of Higher Education, 31*(2), 161–183. https://doi.org/10.1353/rhe.2007.0076

Part III

Contexts for Engagement

Expanding an Equity Understanding of Student Engagement: The Macro (Social) and Micro (School) Contexts

Claudia L. Galindo, Tara M. Brown, and Justine H. Lee

Abstract

Decades of research have positioned student engagement as a malleable factor that can help improve learning outcomes. Research also demonstrates that schools struggle to support the engagement of students coping with poverty, especially Black and Brown students, and in many cases blame them for their low engagement. In this chapter, we argue that scholars must consider the role of societal macro-level conditions and the multiple ways in which these conditions are reflected in school features to gain a nuanced understanding of student engagement. This chapter reviews conventional conceptions of student engagement and proposes a holistic framing. We discuss race and racism, and economic inequality as two macro-level conditions that affect student engagement. We examine current evidence about school funding inequity, racial and economic segregation, deficit conceptions of students and families, exclusionary disciplinary practices, and pedagogical approaches. Finally, we provide consider-

C. L. Galindo (✉) · T. M. Brown · J. H. Lee
Department of Teaching, Learning, Policy, and Leadership, University of Maryland, College Park, MD, USA
e-mail: galindo@umd.edu; tmbrown@umd.edu; jlee718@umd.edu

ations for developing school strategies to improve student engagement.

Introduction

Decades of disciplinary research have positioned student engagement as a malleable factor that can help improve students' learning outcomes. Most of this research centers on a conceptualization of engagement that emphasizes individual attributes, including cognitive, emotional, and behavioral elements (Fredricks et al., 2004). Other research has taken an ecological approach to frame engagement by considering the bidirectional influence of engagement and the multiple proximal contexts in which students are embedded (e.g., families, schools, and communities; Furlong et al., 2003; Quin et al., 2018). However, few studies have considered the direct and indirect influences of societal macro-level conditions (race and racism, and economic inequality) on student engagement.

Expanding the understanding of student engagement is an important imperative. We use the term student engagement as an integrative and broad construct to refer to conventional conceptions, including positive feelings about schooling, participating in school activities, and engagement with learning, among others. A plethora of studies demonstrate the relationships between conventional measures of engagement and learning outcomes in K-12 schools (Quin, 2017) and persistence in high school and college (Finn & Zimmer, 2012). Other researchers show the influence of student engagement on social-emotional development, social behaviors, and psychological well-being (Wang & Fredricks, 2014). In addition, research demonstrates that schools struggle to support the engagement of students coping with poverty, and Black and Brown students. Although not all minoritized students[1] have low engagement, on average, these students are less engaged in school than their higher income and White peers (Bingham & Okagaki, 2012; Fredricks et al., 2004). Engagement disparities have become more evident during the COVID-19 pandemic, as many minoritized students have had difficulty participating in online learning due to lack of resources (García & Weiss, 2020).

In this chapter, we argue that to gain a nuanced understanding of student engagement and disparities, we must consider the role of two intertwined societal macro-level conditions, race and racism, and economic inequality. We also argue that these macro-level conditions are often rendered invisible, yet they are manifested and reflected in micro-level school and classroom features, influencing students' daily experiences and their engagement in diverse ways. By paying attention to macro-level conditions and school micro-level features, we hope to inform policies and practices to support student engagement that are responsive to their multiple needs and struggles.

Two important caveats are worth mentioning at this point. First, although this chapter focuses on structural social conditions that shape students' experiences in schools, we embrace and recognize students' agency. There is ample evidence showing that students are not passive recipients, but active agents in the construction of their schooling experiences (Brown & Rodriguez, 2017). However, we acknowledge that student agency could be constrained by multiple institutional and societal barriers that are reflected in schooling practices and policies. Second, we conceptualize students' beliefs and behaviors as evolving and responsive to multiple contexts. A student could be actively engaged in their community but not in school, or with a particular content area but not another. These two caveats add complexity to the way that we conceptualize student engagement and have implications for exploring strategies to reduce disparities in engagement.

This chapter is organized in four sections. It begins by reviewing conventional conceptions of student engagement and proposing a holistic way to frame this construct. Second, we analyze two essential macro-level conditions that directly and indirectly affect students' schooling experiences and outcomes: race and racism, and economic inequality. Third, we discuss current literature on how schools are reflective of these social conditions, paying particular attention to funding inequity; racial and economic segregation; deficit conceptions of students and families; exclusionary disciplinary practices; and pedagogical approaches. Finally, we examine considerations for developing school strategies to improve student engagement.

A Holistic Conceptualization of Student Engagement

The ways in which scholars have conceptualized student engagement have evolved over time. A major difference across the disciplinary conceptualizations of engagement is the relative emphasis on individual versus structural social dimensions.

Initially, student engagement was commonly conceptualized as an individual attribute that includes cognitive, emotional, and behavioral elements (Fredricks et al., 2004). Some of these conceptualizations consider the three elements as part of a unidimensional construct, whereas others examine each element separately—and therefore acknowledge that each uniquely influences diverse student outcomes. Much of this scholar-

[1] We utilize the label minoritized students as an encompassing term to refer to students coping with poverty and Black and Brown students; the label Brown refers to Latinxs or indigenous peoples.

ship measures student engagement using student involvement in learning and in-school activities or feelings of connection to school, teachers, and peers. Also, these conceptions of engagement emphasize students' individual dispositions and behaviors and promote increasing students' resilience, grit, self-efficacy, and growth mindsets (Tang et al., 2019).

Building from Bronfenbrenner' (1992) ecological system theory, other scholars put forward conceptions of engagement that emphasize an ecological or socio-ecological approach. These definitions of student engagement emphasize the bidirectional influence of engagement and the multiple proximal contexts and social relations in which students are embedded (e.g., families, schools, and communities). In this line of work, student engagement is conceptualized as context specific because it is responsive to the organizational and cultural features of a given context (Lawson & Lawson, 2013). In other words, instead of defining student engagement as a stable trait, a student could be socio-emotionally engaged with friends outside of class, but not in class, or they can be cognitively engaged in learning at home, but not in learning their least favorite school subject. Ecological perspectives also acknowledge the importance of young people's developmental stages for understanding how their engagement is manifested and the relative influence of diverse contexts and interactions with meaningful individuals (e.g., parents, teachers, peers) (You & Sharkey, 2009).

Although previous scholarship has significantly expanded the knowledge base on student engagement, most conceptualizations of engagement are rooted in White or middle-class ideologies and experiences. Freedom of choice and meritocracy, for instance, are two ideological assumptions—rooted in the experiences of Whites or middle-class individuals, that inform the different ways that scholarship approaches educational experiences and outcomes (Hochschild & Scovronick, 2003), including student engagement. The beliefs that individuals are free to choose and that their outcomes are dependent solely on ability or effort center personal responsibility as a key determinant of student

engagement. Unfortunately, this narrow understanding does not reflect the realities of minoritized students and takes for granted their unique experiences and challenges. This understanding also perpetuates the belief that all students, regardless of race and economic status, have the same opportunities to be engaged. As Goodman and Fine (2018) point out, we argue that we must consider the role of macro-level social conditions, race and racism, and economic inequality—and the multiple school inequities to gain a holistic understanding of student engagement.

Macro-Level Conditions: Race and Racism, and Economic Inequality

This section examines two macro dimensions of society and their intersections which frame students' dispositions, behaviors, and schooling experiences. While these dimensions do not always directly influence students, they may constrain the opportunities available to them. To gain a nuanced understanding of student engagement, we need to acknowledge first the macro context in which schools and individuals are embedded.

Race and Racism

Racism has been an enduring attribute of the United States since before the country's inception. In the 345 years after European "settlers" brought 20 captive Africans to Virgina in 1619, laws and ordinances ensured the marginalization of Blacks and other racially minoritized groups (Bennett, 1980). Ideological and legal constructions of race and property ownership dispossessed Native Americans of their lands and contributed to the enslavement of African descendant people for 250 years (Harris, 1993). Further, during the 90-year period of Jim Crow in the South, many Blacks, Latinxs, Asians, and Native Americans across the country were denied full citizenship rights and barred from K-12 schools and post-secondary institutions (Haney-López, 2006). The segregationist policies observed in

Southern states were modeled after similar policies in the Northern and Mid-Western states that excluded these groups from education and political participation since the 17th century (Bell, 2004). However, decades of Black political resistance and agitation for the expansion of human and civil rights led to a shift in the mechanisms that perpetuated racial inequality, as White dominance shifted to more covert forms of structural and interpersonal racism.

After racial discrimination was legally addressed at the federal level with the passage of the Civil Rights Act of 1964, racism became "masked in unofficial practices and 'neutral' standards" (Bell, 1992, p. 7). This covert form of racism is grounded in the ideology of colorblindness, which argues that race does not influence opportunities for upward mobility and success. Proponents of this ideology posit that race is not a social marker that limits or facilitates individuals' social or economic positions in a hierarchical society. Beliefs about the inferiority of Black and Brown individuals, in comparison to Whites, are expressed through claims of individualism, meritocracy, egalitarianism, as well as cultural inferiority (Bonilla-Silva, 2014). The presumption of equal opportunity embedded in these notions permits the attribution of Black and Brown people's overall lower economic status on their perceived personal and cultural deficits while neglecting institutional responsibility. One manifestation of this ideology is resistance to affirmative action programs, which are designed to promote racial equity in employment and higher education. Claims that affirmative action programs are unfair to Whites are grounded in beliefs about "a level playing field" which deny the enduring obstacles that Black and Brown individuals face due to historical and current racism.

Racism is manifested at the individual and institutional levels. At the individual level, it shapes individuals' beliefs and behaviors in interactions with others. One form of individual racism is microaggressions, which are subtle everyday messages and actions that draw on racial stereotypes and colorblind paradigms to belittle or marginalize Black and Brown individuals (Sue, 2010). Examples of microaggressions include mispronunciation of names or comments like, "I'm not a racist. I have Black friends," or telling a Latinx or Asian student how good their English is.

At the institutional level, race and racism are considered central organizational principles of the US society and its power structure. The hierarchical racial order and its systems of subordination uphold White dominance and perpetuate the marginalization of Black and Brown individuals in our social institutions (Lawrence & Keleher, 2004). Individuals who are the top of the hierarchy are granted greater opportunities, most of their behaviors are rewarded, and their beliefs, values, and normative practices are considered frames of reference for subordinate groups (Bonilla-Silva, 1997). This racial order becomes part of all social institutions (e.g., education, health care, criminal justice) and it is reflected in many aspects of society. As an example, Blacks are grossly overrepresented and Whites are underrepresented among people incarcerated for drug use. As Alexander (2010) showed, Blacks and Whites have similar rates of illegal drug use, yet the "war on drugs" has largely targeted Black communities. For Latinxs, one way in which institutional racism is manifested is through the criminalization of immigration and its associated discourses about the prevalence of criminals among, particularly, Latinx immigrants (Ewing et al., 2015). Due to current immigration policies, undocumented Latinx students face stressors and limitations that negatively influence their school engagement because their efforts towards social and economic upward mobility are interrupted (Enriquez, 2017).

Economic Inequality

National data show that one in ten adults and one in five children live in poverty in the United States (Semega et al., 2020), which indicates that many families face difficulties in meeting their basic needs and achieving overall well-being. Institutional factors significantly contribute to these economic difficulties. For example, the current federal minimum wage, which has not increased since 2009, is $7.25, and 42% of workers in the United States make less than $15 per hour. While the *flow of money* received regularly (income) is important to support families' daily living, wealth, or the *stock* of values of one's home, retirement funds, and financial assets, is vital for upward mobility. Wealth, which can be transmitted across generations, enables families to buy a home in a high-performing school district, invest in their children's post-secondary education, and weather unforeseen financial problems.

Wealth and income inequality have significantly increased over time. Income gaps have widened since the late 1970s, especially among the middle and upper classes. In 2018, households in the top fifth of the income distribution (i.e., those who earned $130,001 or more) accumulated about half of the national income (Schaeffer, 2020). The same report showed that wealth disparities in the United States have doubled between 1989 and 2016 and those in the bottom 20th percentile of the income distribution have no wealth.

A plethora of research demonstrates the negative consequences of living with economic hardship. For example, students coping with poverty are more likely than their affluent counterparts to experience food insecurity (i.e., inconsistent food intake) and family disruption, including because of an incarcerated parent (Turney & Goodsell, 2018). Poverty is also associated with health problems (e.g., poor nutrition, vision problems, asthma, and lead poisoning) and inadequate access to health care (Voelkl, 2012). Families coping with poverty face challenges related to eviction, homelessness, residential mobility, and poor housing conditions, which negatively impacts young people's academic progress (Desmond, 2016). Other emerging evidence shows that low-income families tend to live in economically impoverished urban neighborhoods that have high levels of exposure to street crime and interpersonal violence (Brown, 2016).

Although causes of economic disparities in the United States are multifaceted (e.g., due to global economic disparities and historical events, including the Great Depression and Great Migration, deindustrialization, and residential changes), the US political economy has very few protections for families and youth who are economically disadvantaged. Therefore, in addition to race and racism, the economy is another system of subordination in US society. For example, the federal government taxes wages from work at a higher rate than income from investments, held mainly by the affluent (Saez & Zucman, 2019). In this context of economic inequality, social institutions perpetuate advantages and opportunities for families and individuals with greater income and wealth than those with fewer financial resources.

Intersections of Race and Economic Inequalities

Race and poverty often operate in tandem; racially minoritized families and youth are overrepresented among those facing economic hardships. Of note, although child poverty (poverty among individuals under 18 years old) has decreased for all racial groups since 2010, persistent racial disparities are prevalent (e.g., current poverty rates are 40% for Native Americans, 26% for Blacks, and 21% for Latinxs as compared to 8% for Whites; Thomas & Fry, 2020). Researchers anticipate that these disparities will increase as the COVID-19 pandemic has had a disproportionately negative economic impact on Black and Brown communities (Save the Children, 2021).

Further, labor market growth in the United States indicates increasingly low-quality employment opportunities for minoritized individuals (Carnevale et al., 2019). There has been an increase in the number of poor quality, low-wage, part-time, and unstable service jobs, which are largely occupied by Black and Brown workers (Ton, 2020). The number of well-paying professional jobs has also grown, albeit at a far slower pace, and these jobs require increasingly higher levels of educational attainment (Katz & Kearney, 2006), excluding many Black and Brown workers from low-income backgrounds (Brown et al., 2005). Relatedly, income inequality largely falls along racial lines with

Black and Brown individuals being overrepresented among low-wage workers and families living in poverty (Massey, 2007). As compared to the median White household income of $76,507, Black and Latinx household incomes are just $46,073 and $56,113, respectively (Wilson, 2020). Importantly, racial disparities exist at all income and education levels, reflecting the negative impact of racism on even middle-class, affluent, and college-educated Blacks and Latinxs.

In comparison to racial disparities in income, those in wealth are even greater. For example, the Federal Reserve reports "the typical White family has eight times the wealth of the typical Black family and five times the wealth of the typical Hispanic family" (Bhutta et al., 2020, p. 1). Among Black and Brown adults, starting in their twenties, half of the wealth disparities are explained by the economic disadvantages of their parents (Killewald & Bryan, 2018). For many Blacks, in particular, the history of enslavement, Jim Crow, educational disenfranchisement, as well as enduring employment discrimination (Massey, 2007) have significantly contributed to their limited wealth accumulation. For many Latinxs, their concentration in unstable jobs that do not provide benefits and their larger financial family responsibilities, which includes financially supporting family members living elsewhere (Hanks et al., 2018), are important contributors of their limited wealth.

Thus, the multiple ways in which Black and Brown individuals are disproportionately represented at the bottom of the economic distribution in the United States impede their ability to move up the economic ladder and to overcome the negative effects of systemic racism that plague our social institutions. As macro-level conditions impact nearly all aspects of US society, racism and economic inequality also shape schools in ways that pose obstacles to student engagement.

Schools as Micro-Reflections of Social Inequalities

Social inequalities at the macro-level lead to multiple in-school and classroom conditions, over which students have no control. In this section, we examine five interrelated features of schooling—school funding, racial and economic segregation, deficit conceptions of students and their families, exclusionary discipline practices, and pedagogical approaches. These conditions reflect macro social conditions and are indicative of how racism and economic inequality contribute to not only many of the challenges students face outside of schools but also the inequitable conditions they experience inside schools, which have a direct link to student engagement.

School Funding

While high-poverty schools serve many students with the greatest needs due to their families' economic marginalization, these schools are often under-resourced. A recent study by the Education Trust found that in many states, districts with a large concentration of students facing poverty receive inadequate funding, as compared to districts with lower poverty (Morgan & Amerikaner, 2018). This study also found that school funding is negatively associated with prevalence of Black and Brown students at the district level.

Inequitable school resources are attributable to how public schools are financed, largely through state funding and local property taxes. Schools that serve large numbers of students coping with poverty are located in districts where property tax revenues are lower than schools in more affluent areas. This inequity becomes even more consequential during state budget crises, which often occur. Presently, many states are experiencing significant budget shortfalls due to lost tax revenue during the COVID-19 pandemic, which has cut into K-12 public school budgets

(NCSL, 2021). In addition, Title I funding, which provides additional federal money to schools that serve a significant number of students from low-income backgrounds, in many cases, does not accomplish its redistributive purpose in ways that significantly narrow school funding disparities (Snyder et al., 2019).

Through financial neglect, many schools that serve large numbers of students coping with poverty, particularly in urban areas, have been allowed to deteriorate. For example, a Johns Hopkins report on Baltimore City Public Schools (BCPS)—a district whose student body is over 90% Black and Latinx and more than 50% low income—reports deplorable physical conditions (Sharfstein et al., 2020). Many classrooms in BCPS schools have no heat in the winter and no air conditioning in the summer, leaking pipes, water fountains contaminated with lead, and broken toilets. Unfortunately, schools in BCPS are not the exception; these conditions are also found in other high-poverty urban schools across the country (Alonso et al., 2009). The derelict conditions of schools in poor communities of Color, which would unlikely be tolerated in White middle-class neighborhoods, show how minoritized students are often relegated to physical school environments that are not conducive of academic or social engagement.

Inadequate school funding affects multiple aspects of schools' functioning and limits students' educational opportunities, including their engagement. Dilapidated schools have unstable teaching staff, affect teacher attendance, and cause periodic school closures (Sharfstein et al., 2020). Deplorable school conditions exacerbate students' medical conditions, such as asthma, depress students' morale, and make them feel uncared for. These school conditions often lead to chronic absenteeism, difficulty focusing on schoolwork, and limited feelings of belonging (Schultz, 2008). High-poverty schools also often lack high-quality teachers and learning resources (e.g., over-crowded classrooms, inadequate numbers of books, computers, and internet connections, and uncertified teachers; Alonso et al., 2009). Of course, students are more likely to academically disengage when they have neither a skilled teacher who can make learning meaningful nor the materials needed for high-quality instruction. In addition to contributing to out-of-school challenges and inequitable access to functioning schools, socio-structural racism and economic inequality also shape the sociocultural practices and interactions of schools in ways that further disadvantage these student populations. We come back to this point below.

Racial and Economic School Segregation

The separation of students by race and economic status in schools and school districts remains a stubborn reality. In 1954, *Brown v. Board of Education* and later in 1970, *Cisneros v. Corpus Christi Independent School District* spurred various school desegregation efforts for Black and Latinx students, respectively (Donato & Hanson, 2019). But, significant progress in desegregating schools through the 1970s slowed when the Court ruled, in *Milliken v. Bradley,* against between-district desegregation. This lead to the re-segregation of many schools, separating Black and Latinx students into different school districts from White and middle-class peers (Orfield et al., 2014).

Today, desegregation efforts remain stalled by related factors. Besides legal setbacks in integration efforts (Reardon et al., 2012), demographic shifts (Fuller et al., 2019), residential mobility patterns (Iceland, 2009), rand recently school-choice policies (Coughlan, 2018) limit many school desegregation efforts. Also, housing and zoning policies and real estate markets that push a disproportionate number of families coping with poverty into isolated and increasingly poor areas are other major factors influencing school segregation (Massey & Denton, 1993). These multiple factors have further enabled White middle-class families to place their children in schools where there are very few low-income Black and Brown students.

Presently, on average, Black and Latinx students attend schools that are 70% Black and Latinx, and White students attend schools that are nearly 70% White (Frankenberg et al., 2019). Similarly, Richards and Stroub (2020) found significant and rising economic segregation among K-12 schools which was "most severe at the extremes of the income distribution, with very poor and very affluent students experiencing the highest levels of segregation from students in all other income quintiles" (p. 17). Further, nearly half of Black and Latinx public school students attend high-poverty schools—those in which more than 75% of students are eligible for free and reduced price lunch—as compared to only 8% of White students (NCES, 2018). Of note, district-level segregation is more pronounced than school-level segregation (Owens et al., 2016), with limited potential for desegregation if policymakers do not implement inter-district integration practices (Fuller et al., 2021).

Segregation limits educational opportunities for many students. At the district level, segregation is associated with an unequal distribution of resources (Owens, 2018). At the school level, segregation is associated with fewer effective teachers and limited availability of advanced placement and college-preparatory courses and other instructional resources (Lewis, 2003). Some scholars believe desegregating schools will provide equitable educational opportunities for minoritized students (e.g., Frankenberg et al., 2019). However, other researchers challenge the assumption that exposure to White or middle-class students will automatically improve their schooling experiences and educational outcomes. Scholar caution about the potential loss of students' own linguistic and cultural frames and the likelihood they will be stigmatized, relative to the dominant group (Borman & Pyne, 2016; Carter, 2016). Within schools, tracking (separation of students by ability in classrooms or groups) is also a mechanism that segregates students by race and economic status even when minoritized students share schools with White students. Through tracking, schools often reproduce disparities, further structuring inequities rather than yielding learning benefits for minoritized students (DeSena & Ansalone, 2009; Oakes, 2005).

Deficit Conceptions of Students and Families

Deficit perspectives of students coping with poverty and Black and Brown students have existed in K-12 schools since the inception of public education. Through the mid-20th century, Brown and, especially, Black students were considered intellectually inferior to White students: a perception reinforced by intelligence testing and the Eugenics Movement (Tyack, 1974). With Oscar Lewis' (1966) research on Puerto Ricans coping with poverty in New York City and San Juan, genetic inferiority explanations of Black and Brown students' relative academic "underachievement" gave way to cultural interpretations, such as the culture of poverty, cultural deprivation, and cultural disadvantage. That is, students coping with poverty and Black and Brown students were not considered inherently less capable but hindered by their racial and familial cultures, which were seen as not conducive to school success.

By the early 1990s, researchers had developed a cultural difference theory to move beyond cultural deprivation perspectives (Banks, 2013). Instead of positioning minoritized students as inferior, they were considered culturally different from White students, with unique norms, beliefs, and values. The cultural difference theory encourages teachers to embrace the multiple cultural manifestations of minoritized students and utilize pedagogical practices that build from their strengths. While there has been widespread rhetorical and, in some cases, practical adoption of the principles of cultural difference theory (e.g., culturally relevant teaching), many teachers and schools take an assimilationist perspective and socialize students based on White middle-class norms, values, and expectations and, therefore, erase their cultural particularities (Dyke et al., 2020). Thus, beliefs in the cultural deprivation and intellectual inferiority of minoritized students remain a reality in schools, and many educators still hold deficit perceptions of these students and their families (Yosso, 2005).

Deficit perspectives among educators include negative assumptions, biases, and stereotypes associated with race, skin color and phenotype, English proficiency and accent, poverty, and immigration status. There is plenty of evidence indicating that many teachers hold deficit perspectives of minoritized students in preschool and across the K-12 grades (Cochran-Smith, 2004). For example, in a study where teachers were told to identify behavioral problems in a video experiment, even though there were none, Gilliam et al. (2016) found that caregivers in preschool expected more problematic behaviors from Black boys than from Black girls and White children of both sexes. Oates (2003) showed that high school teachers had negative behavioral expectations (e.g., for homework completion) of Black students when compared to White students even after controlling for student covariates including previous GPA and test scores. High school teachers have also described Black and Latinx students' classroom behaviors (e.g., homework completion, attentiveness, disruption) less favorably, especially when there was a racial mismatch between the teacher and student (Dee, 2005). Other studies indicate that mainstream teachers hold similar deficits thinking about emergent bilingual students (e.g., Pettit, 2011). Instead of acknowledging the roles that society and schools play in perpetuating educational disparities, school personnel often blame minoritized students' "underperformance" on these students' and their families' perceived deficits.

In many cases, teachers' and administrators' deficit perspectives are associated with low expectations for students (Brown & Rodriguez, 2017). Lawson and Lawson (2013) point out that "students with positive dispositions and/or expectancies toward academic work may have difficulty engaging in academic activity if their teacher has low expectations for their learning or performance" (p. 454). Also, low expectations contribute to the disproportionate number of low-income students of Color relegated to low academic tracks and special education classes where they are exposed to remedial curriculum that is neither intellectually challenging nor engaging (Payne & Brown, 2016).

Further, teachers' racial and cultural biases often lead to poor student/teacher relationships; caring relationships with school personnel are particularly important for Black and Latinx students' academic engagement (Carey, 2020; Griffin et al., 2020; Irizarry, 2011). In a study of 160 predominantly Black and Latinx high school students, Fallis and Opotow (2003) found many students "were selectively cutting [the] classes" (p. 103) in which they had poor relationships with teachers. Notably, middle-class teachers of Color can also display biases towards low-income students of Color (Lynn et al., 2010), which reflects the ubiquity of racism and classism in US society.

In addition, teachers often struggle to recognize the diverse assets of minoritized students and families. Some teachers believe minoritized families lack the competencies and dispositions for positive child-rearing (Lawrence-Lightfoot, 2004) or that they do not care about their children's education (Montoya-Ávila et al., 2018). Yet, in her community cultural wealth framework, Yosso (2005) describes cultural "assets students of Color bring with them from their homes and communities into the classroom" (p. 70), drawn from generational and personal experiences of navigating a racist and classist society. As she asserts, school personnel often do not recognize or disregard these assets rather than capitalizing on them to strengthen students' connections to school and academic learning. Research also demonstrates that Black and Latinx families are highly interested and invested in the education of their children (e.g., Cooper, 2009; Galindo et al., 2019). Empirical evidence demonstrates these parents' strong commitment to supporting learning at home and attending school events and activities, especially when they feel safe and have positive perceptions of the school climate (Jasis & Ordóñez-Jasis, 2004).

Exclusionary Discipline

Exclusionary discipline refers to a set of beliefs and practices that encourages removal of students from educational spaces (i.e., classrooms or schools) in response to school personnel's perceptions of student misbehavior. Mechanisms of exclusion include in- and out-of-school suspensions and expulsions as well as school cultures of surveillance in which security measures, such as body and bag searches, live-feed security cameras, ID card scanning, and metal detectors, are ubiquitous (Caton, 2012). Exclusionary discipline practices, in general, significantly increased from 1972 to 2012 (Losen & Skiba, 2010), but some types of discipline practices (out-of-school suspensions and in-school suspensions) have decreased in recent years (Harper et al., 2018). Yet, high rates of racial disparity in suspension, expulsion, and classroom removal have persisted across the P-12 pipeline. Teachers and administrators continue to widely use exclusionary discipline practices despite overwhelming research findings on the deleterious effects they can have on youth development (Gregory & Fergus, 2017; Perry & Morris, 2014; Skiba et al., 2014a).

Prior research indicates that exclusionary discipline practices are, in many cases, unfair and a source of institutional discrimination. This disciplinary approach is disproportionately inflicted on students coping with poverty and Black and Brown students (Verdugo, 2002). Black students are most unfairly targeted and subjected to higher rates of exclusionary discipline than other racial/ethnic groups even after controlling for socioeconomic status and severity of behavioral infraction (Huang & Cornell, 2018). In 2011–2012, for instance, while Black students accounted for 16% of students enrolled in schools, they made up 42% of students receiving multiple out-of-school suspensions, and 34% of expelled students (US Department of Education, 2014). During that year, Black male students were suspended at a rate three times higher than their White male peers, and Black female students were suspended at a rate six times higher than White female peers (Crenshaw et al., 2015). A significant racial disproportionality is also observed among students with disabilities, where Black and Brown students are also overrepresented among students who are suspended or expelled (Losen & Martinez, 2013).

Although the reasons for racial disparities in discipline practices are multifaceted, correlational evidence indicates that implicit bias (unconscious negative attitudes or stereotypes associated with a social group) among school personnel is a major determinant. Three areas of research support this claim: (1) research directly analyzing school personnel's implicit biases and associated attitudes and beliefs (e.g., principals' attitudes toward discipline, and teachers' responses to student behavior), (2) research focusing on student misbehavior, and (3) research examining schools' demographic influences on exclusionary discipline practices (e.g., race and economic composition) (Skiba et al., 2014b; Welsh & Little, 2018).

First, Gullo (2017) found that school administrators with high levels of implicit racial bias, measured by the Implicit Associations Test, chose more severe disciplinary actions for minoritized students than those with less implicit bias. Also, principals who favored zero-tolerance approaches to discipline (use of severe and exclusionary sanctions to specific misbehaviors) oversee schools with higher rates of suspension and expulsion than their counterparts who favor more inclusive approaches (Heilbrun et al., 2015). Similarly, Gregory and Mosely (2004) documented how teachers' approaches to discipline can be rooted in cultural deficit and colorblind paradigms. In this qualitative study, less than 10% of teachers considered how issues of race and racism affected their beliefs and practices.

Second, many scholars have cast doubt on student behavior as an explanatory factor in exclusionary discipline disparities by race and economic status (Anyon et al., 2014). Research demonstrates that Black students often receive discipline referrals for vaguer, more ill-defined, and more subjectively assessed than White students (Smolkowski et al., 2016). For instance, in a study on racial disparities in school discipline, Skiba et al. (2002) found Black students were more likely than White students to be sent to the principal's office for "disrespect," "excessive noise," "threat," and "loitering"—behaviors that are subjectively assessed, difficult to prove, and subject to school staff members' interpretations. In contrast, White students were more often referred for "an objective event... that leaves a permanent product" (p. 334), such as smoking, leaving school without permission, vandalism, and obscene language. Butler-Barnes and colleagues (2015) documented similarly ambiguous reasoning (e.g., "disobedience" "disruptive behavior") in referrals of Black girls for out-of-school suspensions in a state where they accounted for 16% of enrollment, but 48% of suspensions.

A third group of studies shows the prevalence of exclusionary discipline practices is associated with school attributes. Skiba et al. (2014b) found that the most significant predictor of out-of-school suspensions was the racial composition of the student body, specifically the percentage of Black students. Percentage of Black students was not only positively associated with out-of-school suspensions but also with the likelihood of school personnel using more extreme forms of exclusion. Together, the three bodies of research demonstrate that educators' biased perceptions of student behavior significantly contribute to racial disparities in school discipline.

Removing students from schools often results in academic obstacles produced by lost instructional time, a fragmented experience of curriculum, and fractured student–teacher relationships (Brown, 2007). For example, in Balfanz and colleagues' (2014) longitudinal study, suspension accounted for 40% of the total number of student absences. Accumulation of lost instructional time can lead to feeling overwhelmed by the need to catch up on missed coursework (Kennedy-Lewis & Murphy, 2016), grade retention, decreased likelihood of high school graduation (Chu & Ready, 2018; Losen, 2015), and an increased risk of involvement with the justice system (Skiba et al., 2014a). Moreover, students' perceptions of unjust and unequal treatment from their teachers and administrators can negatively impact their feelings of connectedness to school. As an example, in a qualitative study about school factors that influence Latinx students to leave high school, a participant share:

> With Latinos everything is gang related...I walked into one of my English classes and I just had a sweater and I just sat down and put my head down and the teacher actually, she called the school police thinking that I was going to shoot up the school only because I had my hoodie up and I put my hands down (p. 29, Luna & Revilla, 2013).

As evident from the previous quote, minoritized students can feel negatively judged and labeled as "troublemakers." Such feelings have detrimental implications for student engagement.

Pedagogical Approaches

Learning is conceptualized as the product of social interactions between students and teachers and among students, and it is influenced by classroom members' understandings and practices. Learning requires that students are actively involved in the creation of knowledge through exchanges with others including teachers and peers. This conceptualization of learning is in contradiction with traditional, teacher-centered, or "banking" (Freire, 1972) approaches to teaching in which young people—especially Black and Brown youth—have been seen as incapable of guiding their own learning. Thus, many scholars are calling for a commitment to move away from instruction that reflects deficit perspectives and towards student-centered pedagogical practices that promote educational equity and social justice.

There are diverse pedagogical approaches that place students at the center of instructional processes and take an asset-based approach (e.g., culturally relevant pedagogy, culturally responsive pedagogy, and humanizing pedagogies). Although there are differences across these approaches, all of them elevate the importance of enhancing students' content knowledge and higher-order critical thinking skills while at the same time strengthening their academic identity and overall well-being and prioritizing their sense of belonging to their own racial and cultural groups (Milner, 2006). These pedagogical approaches acknowledge the cultural experiences of minoritized students and their communities' ways *of being*. In the classroom, teachers reframe curricula to incorporate diverse students' cultural understandings (e.g., discourse conventions and social norms) to make academic content more meaningful, validate students' differences, and facilitate cultural competence. This pedagogical approach also empowers students to take charge of their learning and positions them as active learners in exploring, discussing, and experiencing academic content and becoming creators rather than mere consumers of knowledge (Ladson-Billings, 1995; Paris, 2012).

Unfortunately, many teachers, across K-12 schools, struggle to provide minoritized students with high-quality learning opportunities. In particular, students coping with poverty and Black and Brown students disproportionately experience low-quality teaching, remedial instruction, and poor relationships with teachers (e.g., Blanchett, 2006; Ladson-Billings, 2006; Milner, 2010). Research by Morton and Riegle-Crumb (2020) shows that teachers spend less time on algebra and advanced content, such as geometry, in predominantly Black schools (60% or more of the school is Black) than in predominantly White schools. Also, Shores, Kim, and Still (2020) showed pronounced racial inequalities in access to gifted and talented programs and advanced placement (AP) courses. Further, Umansky's (2016) longitudinal study of middle school students in California found that students classified as English Language Learners are overrepresented in lower level and remedial courses, underrepresented in upper level (e.g., honors, gifted and talented, AP courses) classes, and are excluded from core academic courses, especially English language arts.

In many classrooms, minoritized students are not exposed to teaching practices and curricula that reflect their cultures, languages, racial/ethnic group experiences, and everyday lives. In many cases the schools' curricula, normative practices, and cultures reflect White (and middle-class) preferences, perspectives, norms, and values. In her seminal book, "Other People's Children," Delpit (2006) describes this as "The clash between school culture and home culture"

(p. 167). When students perceive schooling as culturally irrelevant, dismissive, or disparaging, they are more likely to academically disengaged, which is manifested in behaviors such as irregular school attendance or limited homework completion (Paris & Alim, 2017). For Latinx students, most of whom are multilingual learners, this clash is also manifested around the use of home language in the classroom, which enhances these students' learning, academic confidence levels, and sense of belonging in school. Consequently, classroom policies and practices that prevent multilingual learners from speaking in their home languages signal that their languages are antithetical to learning (Brown et al., 2012) and deny them opportunities for diverse social and academic engagement.

The racial make-up of the K-12 educator workforce, which is predominantly White, is also related to the inadequate instruction that many students coping with poverty and Black and Brown students receive in the classroom. Presently, 79% of K-12 public school teachers are White (Taie & Goldring, 2020), while racially minoritized students make up more than half of the student population. The problem of teacher diversity is multifaceted, although it has been linked to historical and contemporary racism. When Black schools in the South were desegregated in the 1950s–1970s, the Black teaching force was decimated; few Black teachers were hired in the newly desegregated schools (Milner & Howard, 2004). At the time, de facto segregated Black and Latinx schools in non-Southern regions already had mostly White teachers (MacDonald, 2004; Oakley et al., 2009). These conditions, which foreground the predominantly White teaching force of today, were designed to maintain White dominance in the K-12 labor market and appease racist Whites who did not want teachers of Color to teach White children.

Of note, scholars do not automatically equate having Black or Brown teachers with academic success among minoritized students. However, when students and teachers have similar cultural backgrounds, it enhances the odds that Black and Brown students will be exposed to educational environments that speak to and nurture their identities and lived experiences as racialized young persons. The current racial "mismatch" between the K-12 teaching force and student body negatively impacts student engagement in a variety of ways. First, many White middle-class teachers "lack cultural competencies" (Brown & Rodriguez, 2017 p. 75) and do not practice the culturally responsive and sustaining approaches found to be successful among students most likely to become academically disengaged. Teachers of Color, who are in short supply, are more likely to employ these practices (Souto-Manning & Emdin, 2020).

Secondly, the underrepresentation of teachers of Color, who are often able to connect with and relate to minoritized students and their families (Kohli, 2018; Neason, 2014), negatively impacts student engagement. For example, research indicates that non-White students, especially boys, are less likely to be absent and suspended from school when they have a teacher from the same racial/ethnic background (Holt & Gershenson, 2019). Further, a John Hopkins study found,

> Having at least one black teacher in third through fifth grades reduced a black student's probability of dropping out of school by 29 percent... For very low-income black boys, the results are even greater – their chance of dropping out fell 39 percent (Rosen, 2017, p. 2).

These findings point to not only the positive effect of teachers of Color on student engagement among minoritized students but also how "non-White students, and particularly non-White males are disproportionately harmed" (Holt & Gershenson, 2019, p. 1087) by having White teachers due, in part, to their racial biases.

Informing Policy and Practice

Student engagement, as a malleable factor, has been the focus of interdisciplinary research in recent years. Given the positive links between conventional indicators of engagement and academic success, researchers have sought to understand the factors shaping student engagement and to evaluate interventions designed to enhance it. Many of these interventions focus on generating changes at the individual level; others focus on the immediate school context by examining students' relationships with teachers and peers. Individual-level strategies, such as strengthening teacher–student relationships and reinforcing engagement behaviors with positive rewards, are important to enhance student engagement (Irizarry & Brown, 2014; Paris & Alim, 2017). Such targeted approaches may be particularly useful for students who have adult responsibilities (e.g., are parents or have financial obligations in their families) or for those who do not see their schooling experiences as valuable to their futures.

However, these individual-level approaches alone will not generate long-term, significant improvements to or eradicate student engagement disparities. Instead, we must pay attention to inequalities at the macro-level social context and recognize the central role that race and racism, and economic inequities play in shaping student engagement (Goodman & Fine, 2018), and the multiple ways in which these inequities are reflected in school processes through funding, segregation, exclusionary disciplines, deficit conceptions, and instructional pedagogies. Each of these schooling dimensions portray the damaging ways macro social inequities impact the daily experiences of students coping with poverty and Black and Brown students.

This chapter is an invitation to reconceptualize the scope of student engagement research and a call for an equity-oriented approach to studying minoritized students' engagement. Students' forms of and potential for school engagement can be discounted and even discouraged because of the daily struggles that students face in society and schools. Without denying the commensurable role that the social and micro contexts have on student engagement, we offer considerations for developing school strategies to improve student engagement.

Equity-Oriented Approaches

As Ladson-Billings (1995) argued more than 25 years ago, social institutions, including schools, must acknowledge the cumulative and dehumanizing multiple injustices that students coping with poverty and Black and Brown students face. Educators must recognize the historical and present forms of discrimination, move beyond centering White middle-class' norms, expectations, and behaviors, and combat injustice and unequal power structures within schools. An equity-oriented approach to student engagement starts by acknowledging the need to build trust between educators and students and their families. Part of this trust-building endeavor will require attention to the racial literacy of school personnel, who must continuously reflect on their own (lack of) knowledge of race and how it functions on the interpersonal *and* institutional levels (Young, 2011), without charging minoritized students and communities with the responsibility to be *their* teachers in this regard. A true commitment to building trusting relationships—intentional and sustained practices—is necessary to diminish minoritized students' and families' apprehension of schools as mainstream institutions that perpetuate the US history of racial and economic oppression and discrimination.

Because many school practices are rooted in deficit conceptions of Black and Brown students, schools must embrace the knowledge and experiences of minoritized students and recognize that their racial and cultural backgrounds influence the ways they experience schools (Arzubiaga et al., 2008). Therefore, students' perspectives must guide the development and implementation of school-based efforts to support their engagement. Moreover, a true equity-oriented approach requires decision-making about school discipline that abides by Milner's (2020) distinction between *punishment* and *discipline*; whereas punishment excludes and isolates, discipline focuses on providing multiple opportunities for students to feel successful.

Whole School Reform Strategy

Given the diverse nature of student engagement and the ways school conditions reflect social inequities, it is important to utilize a multidimensional strategy to generate a major cultural shift in schools. Although the specific configuration of reform may vary depending on particular schools' and students' needs and struggles, equity-oriented goals and processes must be placed at the center of this effort. Also, the school leadership team must create expectations and conditions to facilitate buy-in from all school personnel and develop the structures and practices needed to monitor progress. Besides offering supportive programs and services, this cultural change should be reflected in an inclusive school climate, a commitment to affirm all students, and mutually respectful relationships among students, families, and school personnel.

Emphasis on Promoting and Protective Factors

It is important to acknowledge the many cases in which minoritized students have been academically successful in the face of multiple institutional obstacles. Researchers advocating a strengths-based approach, in contrast to deficit-oriented perceptions of students, have identified the salience of the "promoting" (e.g., benefitting student engagement directly) and "protecting" (e.g., serving as a buffer for contextual negative influences) roles that schools can play in influencing educational outcomes, including student engagement. Although scholars are in the process of developing a cohesive conceptual framework of promoting and protecting factors, research has identified key attributes that could benefit the engagement of minoritized students. These factors include a positive racial school climate (Griffin et al., 2020) and caring relations between and among teachers and students (Wittrup et al., 2019) affirming students' cultural pride and self-efficacy (Butler-Barnes et al., 2013), among others.

Elevating the Role of Teachers

Given the critical role teachers play in the successful implementation of any educational reform, it is an imperative to improve the recruitment of minoritized teachers and provide all teachers the required professional development to support improvement efforts. Given rising college costs and teachers' low salaries, as compared to other professionals, teaching is an impractical career choice for many Black and Brown people (Gold, 2020), who are overrepresented among those with low incomes. Further, racism in teacher education programs deters individuals of Color from pursuing teaching careers and, in K-12 schools, leads to attrition among teachers of Color (Kohli, 2018; Neason, 2014). Explicit efforts need to be implemented to diversify the teaching profession.

In addition, professional development can provide teachers and principals with alternative ways of understanding and addressing underlying impetuses for student engagement. Specifically, professional development initiatives need to address teacher racial literacy, or the ability to read race in its historical, structural, and interpersonal dimensions (Guinier, 2004). These initiatives need to move beyond conceptions of race as a matter of interpersonal prejudice to see how institutional racism shapes the experiences of Black and Brown students (Young, 2011). This professional development also needs to combat "raceless pedagogies" (Ladson-Billings, 2003) rooted in colorblind paradigms if they are to be truly impactful in facilitating students' opportunities to develop multiple and positive identities.

Conclusion

To gain a more robust understanding of student engagement and the multiple roles schools play in perpetuating or ameliorating disparities, research must consider the direct and indirect influences of societal macro-level conditions (race and racism, and economic inequality) on student engagement. It is also important to examine the multiple inequities—school funding, racial and economic segregation, deficit conceptions of students and their families, disciplinary practices, and pedagogical approaches—through which macro social conditions are reflected in schools. In this chapter, we propose an equity-oriented conceptualization of student engage-

ment that centers race and racism, and economic inequities as key factors. Moving away from conceptions of student engagement as an individual problem, we acknowledge its multiple social dimensions. Equally relevant, we argue that policies and practices that are responsive to students' multiple needs and struggles are the best approach to reduce student disengagement. In doing so, we hope to promote meaningful schooling experiences, positive learning outcomes, and overall well-being for all students and specifically for minoritized students.

References

Alexander, M. (2010). *The new Jim Crow: Mass incarceration in the age of colorblindness*. The New Press.

Alonso, G., Anderson, N. S., Su, C., & Theoharis, J. (2009). *Our schools suck: Students talk back to a segregated nation on the failures of urban education*. New York University Press.

Anyon, Y., Jenson, J. M., Altschul, I., Farrar, J., McQueen, J., Greer, E., ... & Simmons, J. (2014). The persistent effect of race and the promise of alternatives to suspension in school discipline outcomes. *Children and Youth Services Review, 44*, 379–386.

Arzubiaga, A. E., Artiles, A. J., King, K. A., & Harris-Murri, N. (2008). Beyond research on cultural minorities: Challenges and implications of research as situated cultural practice. *Exceptional Children, 74*(3), 309–327.

Balfanz, R., Byrnes, V., & Fox, J. (2014). Sent home and put off-track: The antecedents, disproportionalities, and consequences of being suspended in the ninth grade. *Journal of Applied Research on Children: Informing Policy for Children at Risk, 5*(2), 13.

Banks, J. A. (2013). The construction and historical development of multicultural education, 1962–2012. *Theory Into Practice, 52*(suppl 1), 73–82. https://doi.org/10.1080/00405841.2013.795444

Bell, D. A. (1992). *Faces at the bottom of the well: The permanence of racism*. Basic Books.

Bell, D. A. (2004). *Silent covenants: Brown v. Board of Education and the unfulfilled hopes for racial reform*. Oxford University Press.

Bennett, L. (1980). *Before the Mayflower: A history of the Negro in American 1619–1964*. Penguin Books.

Bhutta, N., Chang, A. C., Dettling, L. J., & Hsu, J. W. (2020). *Disparities in wealth by race and ethnicity in the 2019 survey of consumer finances*. The Federal Reserve System. https://www.federalreserve.gov

Bingham, G. E., & Okagaki, L. (2012). Ethnicity and student engagement. In S. L. Christenson, A. L. Reschly, & C. Wylie (Eds.), *Handbook of research on student engagement* (pp. 65–95). Springer. https://doi.org/10.1007/978-1-4614-2018-7

Blanchett, W. J. (2006). Disproportionate representation of African American students in special education: Acknowledging the role of white privilege and racism. *Educational Researcher, 35*(6), 24–28.

Bonilla-Silva, E. (1997). Rethinking racism: Toward a structural interpretation. *American Sociological Review, 62*(3), 465–480. https://doi.org/10.2307/2657316

Bonilla-Silva, E. (2014). *Racism without racists: Color-blind racism and the persistence of racial inequality in the United States* (4th ed.). Rowman & Littlefield Publishers, Inc.

Borman, G. D., & Pyne, J. (2016). What if Coleman had known about stereotype threat? How social-psychological theory can help mitigate educational inequality. *RSF: The Russell Sage Foundation Journal of the Social Sciences, 2*(5), 164–185. https://doi.org/10.7758/rsf.2016.2.5.08

Bronfenbrenner, U. (1992). *Ecological systems theory.* Jessica Kingsley Publishers.

Brown, M. K., Carnoy, M., Currie, E., Duster, T., & Oppenheimer, D. B. (2005). *Whitewashing race.* University of California Press.

Brown, T. M. (2007). Lost and turned out: Academic, social and emotional experiences of students excluded from school. *Urban Education, 42*(5), 432–455.

Brown, T. M. (2016). "Hitting the streets": Youth street involvement as adaptive well-being. *Harvard Educational Review, 86*(1), 48–71. https://doi.org/10.17763/0017-8055.86.1.48

Brown, T. M., Clark, S., & Bridges, T. (2012). Youth teaching teachers: Bridging racial and cultural divides between teachers and students. In S. Hughes & T. Berry. (Eds), *The evolving significance of race* (pp. 69–82). Peter Lang.

Brown, T. M., & Rodriguez, L. F. (2017). Collaborating with urban youth to address gaps in teacher education. *Teacher Education Quarterly, 44*(3), 75–92.

Butler-Barnes, S. T., Chavous, T. M., Hurd, N., & Varner, F. (2013). African American adolescents' academic persistence: A strengths-based approach. *Journal of Youth and Adolescence, 42*(9), 1443–1458. https://doi.org/10.1007/s10964-013-9962-0

Butler-Barnes, S. T., Estrada-Martinez, L., Colin, R. J., & Jones, B. D. (2015). School and peer influences on the academic outcomes of African American adolescents. *Journal of Adolescence, 44*, 168–181.

Carey, R. L. (2020). Making Black boys and young men matter: Radical relationships, future oriented imaginaries and other evolving insights for educational research and practice. *International Journal of Qualitative Studies in Education (QSE), 33*(7), 729–744. https://doi.org/10.1080/09518398.2020.1753255

Carnevale, A. P., Strohl, J., Gulish, A., Van Der Werf, M., & Peltier Campbell, K. (2019). *The unequal race for good jobs: How Whites made outsized gains in education and good jobs compared to Blacks and Latinos.* Georgetown University: Center of Education and the Work Force. https://vtechworks.lib.vt.edu/handle/10919/96132

Carter, P. L. (2016). Educational equality is a multifaceted issue: Why we must understand the school's sociocultural context for student achievement. *RSF: The Russell Sage Foundation Journal of the Social Sciences, 2*(5), 142–163.

Caton, M. T. (2012). Black male perspectives on their educational experiences in high school. *Urban Education, 47*(6), 1055–1085.

Chu, E. M., & Ready, D. D. (2018). Exclusion and urban public high schools: Short- and long term consequences of school suspensions. *American Journal of Education, 124*, 479–509.

Cochran-Smith, M. (2004). *Walking the road: Race, diversity, and social justice in teacher education.* Teachers College Press.

Cooper, C. W. (2009). Parent involvement, African American mothers, and the politics of educational care. *Equity & Excellence in Education, 42*, 379–394. https://doi.org/10.1080/10665680903228389

Coughlan, R. W. (2018). Divergent trends in neighborhood and school segregation in the age of school choice. *Peabody Journal of Education, 93*(4), 349–366. https://doi.org/10.1080/0161956X.2018.1488385

Crenshaw, K. W., Ocen, P., & Nanda, J. (2015). Black girls matter: Pushed out, overpoliced and underprotected. Columbia Law School: Scholarship Archive. https://scholarship.law.columbia.edu/faculty_scholarship/3227

Dee, T. S. (2005). A teacher like me: Does race, ethnicity, or gender matter? *American Economic Review, 95*(2), 158–165.

Delpit, L. (2006). *Other people's children: Cultural conflict in the classroom.* The New Press.

DeSena, J. N., & Ansalone, G. (2009). Gentrification, schooling, and social inequality. *Educational Research Quarterly, 33*(1), 61–76.

Desmond, M. (2016). *Evicted: Poverty and profit in the American city.* Crown Publishing Group.

Donato, R., & Hanson, J. (2019). Mexican-American resistance to school segregation. *Phi Delta Kappan, 100*(5), 39–42.

Dyke, E. L., El Sabbagh, J., & Dyke, K. (2020). "Counterstory mapping our city": Teachers reckoning with Latinx students' knowledges, cultures, and communities. *International Journal of Multicultural Education, 22*(2), 30–45.

Enriquez, L. E. (2017). A 'master status' or the 'final straw'? Assessing the role of immigration status in Latino undocumented youths' pathways out of school. *Journal of Ethnic and Migration Studies, 43*(9), 1526–1543. https://doi.org/10.1080/1369183X.2016.1235483

Ewing, W. A., Martinez, D., & Rumbaut, R. G. (2015). *The criminalization of immigration in the United States.* American Immigration Council Special Report.

Fallis, R. K., & Opotow, S. (2003). Are students failing school or are schools failing students? Class cutting in high school. *Journal of Social Issues, 59*(1), 103–119. https://doi.org/10.1111/1540-4560.00007

Finn, J. D., & Zimmer, K. S. (2012). Student engagement: What is it? Why does it matter? In S. L. Christenson, A. L. Reschly, & C. Wylie (Eds.), *Handbook of research on student engagement* (pp. 97–131). Springer. https://doi.org/10.1007/978-1-4614-2018-7

Frankenberg, E., Ee, J., Ayscue, J. B., & Orfield, G. (2019). *Harming our common future: America's segregated schools 65 years after Brown*. The Civil Rights Project/Proyecto Derechos Civiles.

Fredricks, J. A., Blumenfeld, P. C., & Paris, A. H. (2004). School engagement: Potential of the concept, state of the evidence. *Review of Educational Research, 74*(1), 59–109. https://doi.org/10.3102/00346543074001059

Freire, P. (1972). Pedagogy of the Oppressed. 1968. Trans. Myra Bergman Ramos. New York: Herder.

Fuller, B., Bathia, S., Bridges, M., Galindo, C., & Lagos, F. (2021). Local variation in the segregation of Latino children – Role of place, poverty, and culture. *American Journal of Education, 128*(2), 245–280.

Fuller, B., Kim, Y., Galindo, C., Bathia, S., Bridges, M., Duncan, G. J., & Valdivia, I. G. (2019). Worsening school segregation for Latino children? *Educational Researcher, 48*(7), 407–420. https://doi.org/10.3102/0013189X19860814

Furlong, M. J., Whipple, A. D., Jean, G. S., Simental, J., Soliz, A., & Punthuna, S. (2003). Multiple contexts of school engagement: Moving toward a unifying framework for educational research and practice. *The California School Psychologist, 8*(1), 99–113.

Galindo, C., Sonnenschein, S., & Montoya-Ávila, A. (2019). Latina mothers' engagement in children's math learning in the early school years: Conceptions of math and socialization practices. *Early Childhood Research Quarterly, 47*(2), 271–283. https://doi.org/10.1016/j.ecresq.2018.11.007

García, E., & Weiss, E. (2020). *COVID-19 and student performance, equity, and U.S. education policy*. https://www.epi.org/publication/the-consequences-of-the-covid-19-pandemic-for-education-performance-and-equity-in-the-united-states-what-can-we-learn-from-pre-pandemic-research-to-inform-relief-recovery-and-rebuilding/

Gilliam, W. S., Maupin, A. N., Reyes, C. R., Accavitti, M., & Shic, F. (2016). *Do early educators' implicit biases regarding sex and race relate to behavior expectations and recommendations of preschool expulsions and suspensions?* Yale University Child Study Center. https://charleshamiltonhouston.org/research/early-educators-implicit-biases-regarding-sex-race-relate-behavior-expectations-recommendations-preschool-expulsions-suspensions/

Gold, T. (2020). Pipeline and retention of teachers of color: Systems and structures impeding growth and sustainability in the United States.

Goodman, S. & Fine, M. (2018). *It's not about grit: Trauma, inequity, and the power of transformative teaching*. Teachers College Press.

Gregory, A., & Mosely, P. M. (2004). The discipline gap: Teachers' views on the over-representation of African American students in the discipline system. Equity & Excellence in Education, 37(1), 18–30.

Gregory, A., & Fergus, E. (2017). Social and emotional learning and equity in school discipline. *The Future of Children, 27*(1), 117–136.

Griffin, C. B., Stitt, R. L., & Henderson, D. X. (2020). Investigating school racial climate and private racial regard as risk and protector factors for black high school students' school engagement. *Journal of Black Psychology, 46*(6-7), 514–549. https://doi.org/10.1177/0095798420946895

Guinier, L. (2004). From racial liberalism to racial literacy: Brown v. Board of Education and the interest-divergence dilemma. *Journal of American History, 91*(1), 92–118.

Gullo, G. L. (2017). *Implicit bias in school disciplinary decisions* (Doctoral dissertation, Lehigh University).

Haney-López, I. (2006). *White by law: The legal construction of race* (10th ed.). New York University Press.

Hanks, A., Solomon, D., & Weller, C. E. (2018). *Systematic inequality: How America's structural racism helped create the black-white wealth gap* (p. 21). Center for American Progress. https://www.americanprogress.org/issues/race/reports/2018/02/21/447051/systematic-inequality/

Harper, K., Ryberg, R., & Temkin, D. (2018). Schools report fewer out-of-school suspension, but gaps by race and disability persist. *Child Trends*. https://www.childtrends.org/blog/schools-report-fewer-out-of-school-suspensions-but-gaps-by-race-and-disability-persist

Harris, C. I. (1993). Whiteness as a property. *Harvard Law Review, 106*(8), 1707–1791. https://doi.org/10.2307/1341787

Heilbrun, A., Cornell, D., & Lovegrove, P. (2015). Principal attitudes regarding zero tolerance and racial disparities in school suspensions. *Psychology in the Schools, 52*(5), 489–499.

Hochschild, J., & Scovronick, N. (2003). *The American dream and public schools*. Oxford University Press.

Holt, S. B., & Gershenson, S. (2019). The impact of demographic representation on absences and suspensions. *Policy Studies Journal, 47*(4), 1069–1099.

Huang, F. L., & Cornell, D. (2018). The relationship of school climate with out-of-school suspensions. Children and Youth Services Review, 94, 378–389. https://doi.org/10.1016/j.childyouth.2018.08.013

Iceland, J. (2009). *Where we live now: Immigration and race in the United States*. University of California Press.

Irizarry, J. (2011). *The Latinization of U.S. schools: Successful teaching and learning in shifting cultural contexts*. Paradigm Publishers.

Irizarry, J. G., & Brown, T. M. (2014). Humanizing research in dehumanizing spaces: The challenges and opportunities of conducting participatory action research with youth in schools. In D. Paris, & M. Winn (Eds.), *Humanizing research: Decolonizing qualitative inquiry with youth and communities* (pp. 63–80). Sage Publications.

Jasis, P., & Ordóñez-Jasis, R. (2004). Convivencia to empowerment: Latino parent organizing at La Familia. *The High School Journal, 88*(2), 32–42.

Katz, L. F., & Kearney, M. S. (2006). *The polarization of the US labor market (No. w11986)*. National Bureau of Economic Research.

Kennedy-Lewis, B. L., & Murphy, A. S. (2016). Listening to "frequent flyers": What persistently disciplined students have to say about being labeled as "bad". *Teachers College Record, 118*(1), 1–40.

Killewald, A., & Bryan, B. (2018). Falling behind: The role of inter-and intragenerational processes in widening racial and ethnic wealth gaps through early and middle adulthood. *Social Forces, 97*(2), 705–740. https://doi.org/10.1093/sf/soy060

Kohli, R. (2018). Behind school doors: The impact of hostile racial climates on urban teachers of color. *Urban Education, 53*(3), 307–333.

Ladson-Billings, G. (1995). Toward a theory of culturally relevant pedagogy. *American Educational Research Journal, 32*(3), 465–491. https://doi.org/10.3102/00028312032003465

Ladson-Billings, G. (2003). *Critical race theory perspectives on the social studies: The profession, policies, and curriculum*. IAP.

Ladson-Billings, G. (2006). From the achievement gap to the education debt: Understanding achievement in U.S. schools. *Educational Researcher, 35*(7), 3–12. https://doi.org/10.3102/0013189x035007003

Lawrence, K., & Keleher, T. (2004). *Structural racism*. Paper presented at the Race and Public Policy Conference, Berkeley, CA.

Lawson, M. A., & Lawson, H. A. (2013). New conceptual frameworks for student engagement research, policy, and practice. *Review of Educational Research, 83*(3), 432–479. https://doi.org/10.3102/0034654313480891

Lewis, A. E. (2003). *Race in the schoolyard: Negotiating the color line in classrooms and communities*. Rutgers University Press.

Lewis, O. (1966). The culture of poverty. *Scientific American, 215*(4), 19–25.

Lightfoot, S. L. (2004). *The essential conversation: What parents and teachers can learn from each other*. Ballantine Books.

Losen, D. J., & Martinez, T. E. (2013). *Out of school and off track: The overuse of suspensions in American middle and high schools*. The Civil Rights Project/Proyecto Derechos Civiles.

Losen, D. J., & Skiba, R. J. (2010). *Suspended education*. Policy report for the Southern Poverty Law Center.

Losen, D. J. E. (2015). *Closing the school discipline gap: Equitable remedies for excessive exclusion*. Teachers College Press.

Luna, N., & Revilla, A. T. (2013). Understanding Latina/o school pushout: Experiences of students who left school before graduating. *Journal of Latinos and Education, 12*(1), 22–37. https://doi.org/10.1080/15348431.2012.734247

Lynn, M., Bacon, J. N., Totten, T. L., Bridges, T. L., & Jennings, M. (2010). Examining teachers' beliefs about African American male students in a low-performing high school in an African American school district. *Teachers College Record, 112*(1), 289–330.

MacDonald, V. (Ed.). (2004). *Latino education in the United States: A narrated history from 1513–2000*. Springer.

Massey, D., & Denton, N. A. (1993). *American apartheid: Segregation and the making of the underclass*. Harvard University Press.

Massey, D. S. (2007). *Categorically unequal: The American stratification system*. Russell Sage Foundation.

Milner, H. R., IV. (2010). *Start where you are, but don't stay there: Understanding diversity, opportunity gaps, and teaching in today's classrooms*. Harvard Education Press.

Milner, R. H., IV. (2006). Preservice teachers' learning about cultural and racial diversity: Implications for urban education. *Urban Education, 41*(4), 343–375. https://doi.org/10.1177/0042085906289709

Milner IV, H. R. (2020). Fifteenth annual AERA Brown lecture in education research: Disrupting punitive practices and policies: Rac(e) ing back to teaching, teacher preparation, and Brown. *Educational Researcher, 49*(3), 147–160.

Milner, H. R., & Howard, T. C. (2004). Black teachers, Black students, Black communities, and Brown: Perspectives and insights from experts. *Journal of Negro Education*, 285–297.

Montoya-Ávila, A., Ghebreab, N., & Galindo, C. (2018). Towards improving the educational opportunities of Black and Latinx students: Strengthening partnerships between families and schools. In S. Sonnenschein & B. E. Sawyer (Eds.), *Academic socialization of young Black and Latino children: Building on family strengths* (pp. 209–231). Springer.

Morgan, I., & Amerikaner, A. (2018). *Funding gaps: An analysis of school funding equity across the U.S. and within each state*. The Education Trust. https://edtrust.org/wp-content/uploads/2014/09/FundingGapReport_2018_FINAL.pdf

Morton, K., & Riegle-Crumb, C. (2020). Is school racial/ethnic composition associated with content coverage in algebra?. *Educational Researcher, 49*(6), 441–447.

National Center for Education Statistics (NCES). (2018). *The condition of education 2018: Concentration of public school students eligible for free or reduced-price lunch*. https://nces.ed.gov/programs/coe/indicator/clb

National Conference of State Legislatures (NCSL). (2021). *State actions to close budget shortfalls in response to COVID-19*. https://www.ncsl.org/research/fiscal-policy/state-actions-to-close-budget-shortfalls-in-response-to-covid-19.aspx

Neason, A. (2014). Our teacher diversity problem is not just about recruitment. It's about retention. SLATE. https://slate.com/human-interest/2014/12/teacher-diversity-accomplishing-it-is-not-just-about-recruitment-its-aboutretention.html

Oakes, J. (2005). *Keeping track: How schools structure inequality.* Yale University Press.

Oates, G. L. S. C. (2003). Teacher-student racial congruence, teacher perceptions, and test performance. *Social Science Quarterly, 84*(3), 508–525. https://doi.org/10.1111/1540-6237.8403002

Oakley, D., Stowell, J., & Logan, J. R. (2009). The impact of desegregation on black teachers in the metropolis, 1970–2000. Ethnic and Racial Studies, 32(9), 1576–1598.

Orfield, G., Frankenberg, E. D., Ee, J., & Kuscera, J. (2014). *Brown at 60: Great progress, a long retreat and an uncertain future.* Civil Rights Project/Proyecto Derechos Civiles.

Owens, A. (2018). Income segregation between school districts and inequality in students' achievement. *Sociology of Education, 91*(1), 1–27. https://doi.org/10.1177/0038040717741180

Owens, A., Reardon, S. F., & Jencks, C. (2016). Income segregation between schools and school districts. *American Educational Research Journal, 53*(4), 1159–1197. https://doi.org/10.3102/0002831216652722

Paris, D. (2012). Culturally sustaining pedagogy: A needed change in stance, terminology, and practice. *Educational Researcher, 41*(3), 93–97.

Paris, D., & Alim, H. S. (Eds.). (2017). *Culturally sustaining pedagogies: Teaching and learning for justice in a changing world.* Teachers College Press.

Payne, Y. A., & Brown, T. M. (2016). "I'm still waiting on that golden ticket": Attitudes toward and experiences with opportunity in "The Streets" of Black America. *Journal of Social Issues, 72*(4), 789–811. https://doi.org/10.1111/josi.12194

Perry, B. L., & Morris, E. W. (2014). Suspending progress: Collateral consequences of exclusionary punishment in public schools. *American Sociological Review, 79*(6), 1067–1087. https://doi.org/10.1177/0003122414556308

Pettit, S. K. (2011). Teachers' beliefs about English language learners in the mainstream classroom: A review of the literature. *International Multilingual Research Journal, 5*(2), 123–147. https://doi.org/10.1080/19313152.2011.594357

Quin, D. (2017). Longitudinal and contextual associations between teacher–student relationships and student engagement: A systematic review. *Review of Educational Research, 87*(2), 345–387. https://doi.org/10.3102/0034654316669434

Quin, D., Heerde, J. A., & Toumbourou, J. W. (2018). Teacher support within an ecological model of adolescent development: Predictors of school engagement. *Journal of School Psychology, 69*, 1–15. https://doi.org/10.1016/j.jsp.2018.04.003

Reardon, S. F., Grewal, E. T., Kalogrides, D., & Greenberg, E. (2012). Brown fades: The end of court-ordered school desegregation and the resegregation of American public schools. *Journal of Policy Analysis and Management, 31*(4), 876–904. https://doi.org/10.1002/pam.21649

Richards, M. P., & Stroub, K. J. (2020). Metropolitan public school district segregation by race and income, 2000-2011. *Teachers College Record, 122*(5), 21–41.

Rosen, J. (2017, April 5). *With just one black teacher, black students more likely to graduate.* https://releases.jhu.edu/2017/04/05/with-just-one-black-teacher-black-students-more-likelyto-graduate/

Saez, E., & Zucman, G. (2019). *The triumph of injustice: How the rich dodge taxes and how to make them pay.* W. W. Norton & Company.

Save the Children. (2021). *Child poverty in America.* https://www.savethechildren.org/us/charity-stories/poverty-in-america

Schaeffer, K. (2020). *6 facts about economic inequality in the U.S.* Pew. https://www.pewresearch.org/fact-tank/2020/02/07/6-facts-about-economic-inequality-in-the-u-s/

Schultz, B. D. (2008). *Spectacular things happen along the way: Lessons from an urban classroom.* Teachers College Press.

Semega, J., Kollar, M., Shrider, E. A., & Creamer, J. F. (2020). *Income and poverty in the United States: 2019. Current Population Reports P60-270.* U.S. Census Bureau. https://www.census.gov/library/publications/2020/demo/p60-270.html

Sharfstein, J., Klosek, K., Thronton, R., & Lofton, R. (2020). *School conditions and educational equity in Baltimore City: Why do the physical conditions of schools matter?* https://gisanddata.maps.arcgis.com/apps/Cascade/index.html?appid=3ddf7ded140d4dc38bedc27d6c0e44f7

Shores, K., Kim, H. E., & Still, M. (2020). Categorical inequality in Black and White: Linking disproportionality across multiple educational outcomes. *American Educational Research Journal, 57*(5), 2089–2131.

Skiba, R. J., Arredondo, M. I., & Williams, N. T. (2014a). More than a metaphor: The contribution of exclusionary discipline to a school-to-prison pipeline. *Equity & Excellence in Education, 47*(4), 546–564. https://doi.org/10.1080/10665684.2014.958965

Skiba, R. J., Chung, C. G., Trachok, M., Baker, T. L., Sheya, A., & Hughes, R. L. (2014b). Parsing disciplinary disproportionality: Contributions of infraction, student, and school characteristics to out-of-school suspension and expulsion. *American Educational Research Journal, 51*(4), 640–670. https://doi.org/10.3102/0002831214541670

Skiba, R. J., Michael, R. S., Nardo, A. C., & Peterson, R. (2002). The color of discipline: Sources of racial and gender disproportionality in school punishment. *The Urban Review, 34*(4), 317–342.

Snyder, T. D., Dinkes, R., Sonnensberg, W., & Cornman, S. (2019). *Study of the Title I, part A grant program mathematical formulas (2019–2016). U.S. Department of Education.* National Center for Education Statistics. http://nces.ed.gov/pubsearch

Smolkowski, K., Girvan, E. J., McIntosh, K., Nese, R. N., & Horner, R. H. (2016). Vulnerable decision points for disproportionate office discipline referrals: Comparisons of discipline for African American and White elementary school students. *Behavioral Disorders, 41*(4), 178–195.

Souto-Manning, M., & Emdin, C. (2020). On the harm inflicted by urban teacher education programs: Learning from the historical trauma experienced by teachers of color. *Urban Education*, 0042085920926249.

Sue, D. W. (2010). *Microaggressions in everyday life: Race, gender, and sexual orientation*. Wiley.

Taie, S., & Goldring, R. (2020). Characteristics of Public and Private Elementary and Secondary School Teachers in the United States: Results from the 2017–18 National Teacher and Principal Survey. First Look. NCES 2020–142. National Center for Education Statistics.

Tang, X., Wang, M.-T., Guo, J., & Salmela-Aro, K. (2019). Building grit: The longitudinal pathways between mindset, commitment, grit, and academic outcomes. *Journal of Youth and Adolescence, 48*(5), 850–863. https://doi.org/10.1007/s10964-019-00998-0

Thomas, D., & Fry, R. (2020). *Prior to COVID-19, child poverty rates had reached record lows in U.S.* Pew Research Center. https://www.pewresearch.org/fact-tank/2020/11/30/prior-to-covid-19-child-poverty-rates-had-reached-record-lows-in-u-s/

Ton, Z. (2020). *Equality in the U.S. starts with better jobs*. Harvard Business Publishing. https://hbr.org/2020/08/equality-in-the-u-s-starts-with-better-jobs

Turney, K., & Goodsell, R. (2018). Parental incarceration and children's wellbeing. *The Future of Children, 28*(1), 147–164.

Tyack, D. B. (1974). *The one best system: A history of American urban education*. Harvard University Press.

Umansky, I. M. (2016). To be or not to be EL: An examination of the impact of classifying students as English learners. *Educational Evaluation and Policy Analysis, 38*(4), 714–737.

U.S. Department of Education. (2014). *Civil rights data collection: Data Snapshot (School discipline)*. Issue brief No. 10.

Verdugo, R. R. (2002). Race-ethnicity, social class, and zero-tolerance policies: The cultural and structural wars. *Education and Urban Society, 35*(1), 50–75.

Voelkl, K. E. (2012). School identification. In S. L. Christenson, A. L. Reschly, & C. Wylie (Eds.), *Handbook of research on student engagement* (pp. 193–218). Springer. https://doi.org/10.1007/978-1-4614-2018-7

Wang, M. T., & Fredricks, J. A. (2014). The reciprocal links between school engagement and youth problem behavior during adolescence. *Child Development, 85*, 722–737. https://doi.org/10.1111/cdev.12138

Welsh, R. O., & Little, S. (2018). The school discipline dilemma: A comprehensive review of disparities and alternative approaches. *Review of Educational Research, 88*(5), 752–794.

Wilson, V. (2020). *Racial disparities in income and poverty remain largely unchanged amid strong income growth in 2019*. Economic Policy Institute. https://www.epi.org/blog/racial-disparities-in-income-and-poverty-remain-largely-unchanged-amid-strong-income-growth-in-2019/

Wittrup, A. R., Hussain, S. B., Albright, J. N., Hurd, N. M., Varner, F. A., & Mattis, J. S. (2019). Natural mentors, racial pride, and academic engagement among black adolescents: Resilience in the context of perceived discrimination. *Youth & Society, 51*(4), 463–483. https://doi.org/10.1177/0044118X16680546

Yosso, T. J. (2005). Whose culture has capital? A critical race theory discussion of community cultural wealth. *Race Ethnicity and Education, 8*(1), 69–91. https://doi.org/10.1080/1361332052000341006

Young, E. Y. (2011). The four personae of racism: Educators'(mis) understanding of individual vs. systemic racism. *Urban Education, 46*(6), 1433–1460.

You, S., & Sharkey, J. (2009). Testing a developmental–ecological model of student engagement: A multilevel latent growth curve analysis. *Educational Psychology, 29*(6), 659–684. https://doi.org/10.1080/01443410903206815

Parental Influences on Achievement Motivation and Student Engagement

Janine Bempechat, David J. Shernoff, Shira Wolff, and Hannah J. Puttre

Abstract

Underachievement and school disengagement have serious consequences, both at an individual and societal level. In this chapter, we adopt a strength-based perspective to examine the multiple ways in which parents foster achievement motivation and student engagement. Our theoretical orientation is grounded in Bronfenbrenner's (1977) ecological systems theory, in which the child is situated at the center of increasingly distal and interconnected spheres of influence, from family and school to community and societal institutions. Given the increasingly diverse composition of our nation's schools, we place a premium on understanding how varied ethnic and cultural models of learning and socialization, particularly among low-income families, differentially influence parents' educational socialization strategies, and how these come to affect children's developing achievement-related beliefs and behaviors. We examine several theoretical models of engagement, motivation, and parental involvement and highlight some notable research efforts that seek to explain parents' roles in fostering motivation and engagement. We then share several models of innovative programs that have experienced success in creating authentic partnerships between parents, children, schools, and communities towards the goal of fostering achievement and student engagement.

J. Bempechat (✉) · H. J. Puttre
Boston University Wheelock College of Education and Human Development, Boston, MA, USA
e-mail: jbempech@bu.edu; hputtre@bu.edu

D. J. Shernoff · S. Wolff
Rutgers University, New Brunswick, NJ, USA
e-mail: david.shernoff@rutgers.edu;
shira.wolff@rutgers.edu

The Role of Parents in Student Motivation and Engagement

Student disengagement is reported to be pervasive, both nationally and internationally. The Program for International Student Assessment survey evaluated 540,000 15-year-old students from 72 countries and found that over one in every four students felt disaffected from school, and the same proportion skipped at least one class over a 2-week period [Organization for Economic Cooperation and Development (OECD), 2016]. Overall, student disengagement tends to worsen as students advance in the school system (Lam et al., 2015), a trend that can be more severe for males, students of color, and low-income students (Martin et al., 2015). *Student engagement* has been conceptualized variably by numerous researchers, but recently conceptualized as a multidimensional phenomenon with

A. L. Reschly, S. L. Christenson (eds.), *Handbook of Research on Student Engagement*,
https://doi.org/10.1007/978-3-031-07853-8_19

behavioral (e.g., participation and completion of learning activities), cognitive (e.g., cognitive and self-regulatory strategies in the learning process), and emotional (affective and reactive experience in learning activities) aspects (Fredericks et al., 2004). Prior research has demonstrated that student engagement is integral to learning and retention (Shernoff, 2013). As documented by a recent meta-analysis (Lei et al., 2018), there is clear evidence that student engagement is one of the most robust predictors of academic achievement. Furthermore, underachievement and school disengagement can have serious consequences, including school dropout and related problems, such as unemployment, underemployment, and poverty. School dropouts are more likely to be unemployed, earn low wages, suffer from health problems, face poverty and social exclusion, rely heavily on public services, and become incarcerated during their lifetime as compared to students who graduate (Lei et al., 2018; Rumberger, 2011).

Such problems are intensified for students who live in poverty. Among children under 18 years of age, approximately one in five in the United States lives in poverty, and 39% of children live in low-income households. In 2017, more than half of Black and Hispanic children lived in low-income families (Child Trends, 2019). Students from low socioeconomic communities face significant educational challenges, such as schools of lower quality and higher teacher turnover compared to students from higher socioeconomic communities (Simon & Johnson, 2015). Children in such schools are more likely to be held back one or more grades and experience higher rates of suspension and school dropout (Duncan & Murnane, 2014). Living in poverty is also negatively associated with children's cognitive, physical, and social development, which presents challenges to academic skill and social-emotional development (Aber et al., 2012). Such challenges were exacerbated by the COVID-19 pandemic, which forced the closures of schools across the U.S. in March, 2020. Vast inequality in access to remote learning resources in urban and rural communities left children with little contact with their teachers,

fueling disengagement with school over this time period (Bacher-Hicks et al., 2021). The combined effects of school closures and inequality in accessing remote learning have been projected to lead to significant learning loss (Kuhfeld et al., 2020).

Although the mechanisms underlying these challenges are not well understood, most research evidence places parents in a central role (Shonkoff, 2017). Children in poverty are more likely to live in single-parent, female-headed households (43%) than two-parent families (9%), and are more likely to have a parent with low educational attainment than children from more affluent communities (Pew Research Center, 2015). Financial and other life challenges can also lead to inconsistencies in the quality of childcare critical for the well-being of children, with parenting practices accounting for up to 50% of the variance in children's cognitive and academic abilities (Brooks-Gunn et al., 1993).

As children's first and primary guides through their schooling experiences, parents can also serve to greatly buffer risk factors for disengagement and low achievement. The achievement-related beliefs and behaviors of parents can have a profound influence on how children come to perceive their intellectual abilities and the value of learning and education (Eccles et al., 2006). There are a variety of ways in which parental socialization beliefs and practices can foster children's achievement motivation and beliefs about learning, resulting in persistence, diligence, and other educational assets. Thus, it is important to better understand how parents, in collaboration with their children and their children's teachers, schools, and communities, can work to support school achievement and engagement.

In this chapter, we adopt a strength-based perspective to examine the multiple ways in which parents foster achievement motivation and student engagement. Our theoretical orientation is grounded in Bronfenbrenner's (1977) ecological systems theory, in which the child is situated at the center of increasingly distal and interconnected spheres of influence, from family and school to community and societal institutions. Given the increasingly diverse composition of our nation's schools, we place a premium on understanding how varied ethnic and cultural models of learning and socialization, particularly among low-income families, differentially influence parents' educational socialization strategies, and how culturally informed strategies come to positively affect children's developing achievement-related beliefs and behaviors (Rogoff et al., 2017).

In this chapter, we explore similar questions to those we have investigated in our own research (Bempechat, 2000; Shernoff & Schmidt, 2008): What are the learning beliefs, dispositions, and emotions that characterize achievement motivation and student engagement among low-income and racial/ethnic minority students? What are the primary influences on the motivation and engagement of such students? Importantly, to what extent may parental involvement and other family-related variables influence students' motivation and engagement with school learning and achievement? Finally, what is the role of culture in influencing educational socialization practices, and what differences in parental influences and socialization strategies exist among students from different cultures? We will herein examine several theoretical models of engagement and motivation and highlight notable research efforts that seek to explain parents' roles in fostering motivation and engagement. We will then share several models of innovative programs that have experienced success in creating authentic partnerships between parents, children, schools, and communities towards the goal of fostering achievement and school engagement.

Theoretical Perspective on Motivation and Engagement

Referring to students' "active participation in academic or cocurricular or school-related activities, and commitment to educational goals and learning" (Christenson et al., 2012, p. 817), student engagement involves behaviors, cognitions, and emotions and encompasses effort and persistence in school work (Fredericks et al., 2004). Engagement and motivation to learn are highly

related and overlapping concepts, having many commonalities as measurable constructs (see Fig. 1). However, motivation has been traditionally viewed as a psychological construct and thus the property of an *individual*. Engagement, even in its common definition, refers to an emotional involvement, experiential intensity, or commitment to an object or goal and thus characterizes a *relationship* or *interaction* between an individual and object of engagement in the environment. It can refer to one's temporal involvement or interactions with activities and social partners in the immediate environments, as well as a more sustained relationship, as with continuing engagement in the process of schooling or a domain of interest. Engagement is increasingly recognized to be a complex, latent construct involving both overt, observable, non-psychological events (e.g., attending class), unobservable psychological events (e.g., "investment" in learning), *and* positive emotions (e.g., enjoyment and interest) (Appleton et al., 2008). It is presumed to encompass actions and behaviors, effort, as well as ambient emotional states.

Both motivation and engagement have been conceptualized as a personal trait and context-varying psychological state (Fredericks et al., 2004). We find this to be a useful distinction, and to simplify, we generally think of *engagement* as the quality of temporal interactions with the learning activity, task, social companions, and other components of the proximal environment, not dissimilar from the concept of *situational interest* (Mitchell, 1993). We characterize *motivation* as a more global set of personal orientations that influence how students approach school work, learning, and achievement.

Conceptualizing Engagement

Many studies rely on observer ratings of engagement, but as a latent and multidimensional construct, engagement may not always be an observable characteristic. In addition, behaviors rated high on engagement by observers may represent only compliance to authority figures or "going through the motions" characteristic of

Fig. 1 Conceptual
model of the interaction
between deep
engagement and
motivation, with
associated short-term
and long-term outcomes

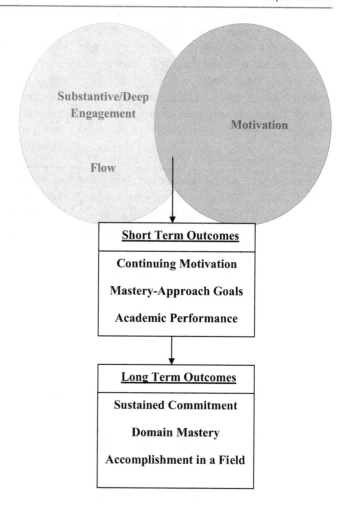

procedural engagement (i.e., superficial forms of
behavioral engagement). This contrasts with substantive engagement characterized by deep pro
cessing and intrinsic motivation (i.e., deep
cognitive engagement and activated emotional
engagement) (Nystrand & Gamoran, 1991). For
purposes of identifying students who are academically resilient, we are interested in identifying engagement that is more substantive and less
procedural, because substantive engagement is
likely to be more strongly related to motivational
orientations and educational attitudes that are
transferrable into higher levels of academic performance (See Fig. 1). We believe that when students are substantively engaged in learning, the

psychological state can be characterized as *flow
experiences,* or deep absorption in an activity that
is   intrinsically   interesting   and   enjoyable
(Csikszentmihalyi, 1990).

Based on flow theory, we have found it useful
to define and operationalize engagement in educational contexts as the simultaneous experience
of concentration, interest, and enjoyment in the
task at hand (Shernoff, 2013). In the schooling
context, student engagement conceptualized in
this manner can be promoted by *environmental
complexity,* or the simultaneous combination of
environmental challenge (e.g., instructional relevance, clear goals) and environmental support
(e.g., motivational support, performance feed-

back, positive relationships) (Shernoff et al., 2016; Shernoff et al., 2017).

Conceptualizing Motivation

In Hidi and Renninger's (2006) four-phase model of interest development, early interest in a topic is often facilitated by situational factors, but as value in the activity or topic deepens, interest becomes an enduring and sustained trait of the individual. Similarly, engagement with learning activities can have a cumulative and compounding result, developing into more general motivational orientations and proclivities. Not all instances of motivation, such as motivation to obtain a reward or other forms of extrinsic motivation, are developed this way, however. We are particularly interested in motivational orientations that support learning and school achievement, or *achievement motivation*. Broadly speaking, achievement motivation consists of a constellation of beliefs influencing patterns of school achievement, including expectations and standards for performance, value placed on learning, and competence-related beliefs (Schunk et al., 2014). Research in achievement motivation has been located within a social-cognitive framework (Schunk & DiBenedetto, 2020). That is, achievement-related beliefs are seen as influenced by the ways in which students co-construct meaning from school-related experiences with influential adults and peers. These experiences may include feedback from parents and teachers, academic-related interactions with peers, motivational and affective responses to success and failure, and placement within school structures through ability grouping and tracking. As reviewed below, evidence-based interventions have demonstrated that children and their parents can successfully learn to adopt and transmit adaptive achievement-related beliefs.

While a review of achievement motivation theories is beyond the scope of this chapter, we highlight in our review below theories that are particularly useful in helping to understand the ways in which parents can foster achievement-related beliefs and behaviors.

Goal Theory and Theories of Intelligence

Goal theory and theories of intelligence are focused on competence-related beliefs. Early goal theory research focused on two achievement goal orientations—mastery and performance— that students adopt about the nature and purpose of learning (Bardach et al., 2020). Mastery goals are conceptualized as the desire to attain knowledge and understanding, implying a positive form of motivation. As illustrated in Fig. 1, this motivational pattern can be maintained over time both in the short term and in the long term (Weiner, 1979), underscoring the quality of involvement and a continued commitment to learning (Paris & Winograd, 1990; Pelletier et al., 1995; Pintrich & De Groot, 1990). An impressive body of research has demonstrated that individuals with mastery goals perform better, have more positive affect and self-efficacy beliefs, are more persistent in the face of difficulty, prefer challenging over easy tasks, continue their interests as they make choices to enroll in college courses, and are otherwise better oriented towards learning (Ames, 1992; Brophy, 1983; Elliot et al., 2011; Hulleman et al., 2008; Meece et al., 1988; Nicholls, 1989). In contrast, performance goals represent a desire to appear competent (a performance-approach orientation), or at least to avoid appearing incompetent (a performance-avoidance orientation) (Elliot et al., 2015).

Implicit theories of intelligence, or mindsets, speak to two primary conceptions of ability as either fixed or malleable (Dweck & Molden, 2017). A variety of studies across different methods has established that a fixed mindset is associated with the view that intelligence is stable, uncontrollable, limited, and limiting. Research has shown that students who adhere to this view of ability tend to be primarily concerned with demonstrating competence or avoiding appearing incompetent; their focus is on the perceived product of school learning—grades. They view mistakes as an inherent condemnation of their abilities. In contrast, a growth mindset is associated with the belief that intelligence is malleable, unlimited, and can grow with effort. Students who endorse this view of learning are primarily concerned with increasing skills and knowledge, even at the risk of making mistakes or looking confused at times. Their focus is on the process of learning, and thus they tend to adopt mastery goals and embrace challenging tasks as opportunities for expanding their knowledge. Consistent with these tendencies, a growth mindset is associated with higher performance in school (Haimovitz & Dweck, 2017).

It is not surprising that parents play a key role in socializing their children's beliefs about intelligence. Researchers have conducted elegant studies in which they observed parents providing feedback to their children on school-related tasks. Findings have revealed differential learning belief outcomes depending on whether the preponderance of parents' feedback was person-oriented (i.e., focused on their child's ability and outcomes) or process-oriented (i.e., focused on the process of effortful learning). For example, process praise used by parents of children between 1 and 3 years of age predicted a stronger growth mindset and mastery-oriented beliefs for learning (e.g., value on effort) 4–5 years later than did person-oriented feedback (Gunderson et al., 2013).

Somewhat counterintuitively, it is not parents' own mindsets that predict children's mindsets, but rather how parents ascribe meaning to failure in general. Researchers have shown that parents who believed failure to be hurtful and an outcome to be avoided expressed anxiety and concern in the face of their children's struggles, fostering a fixed mindset in their children. In contrast, parents who viewed failure as a learning opportunity presented their children with strategies for managing their challenge, fostering a growth mindset. Importantly, varied interventions across subjects have been shown to be very successful in promoting a growth mindset both in the short term and the long term (Haimovitz & Dweck, 2017).

Situated Expectancy- Value Theory

Situated expectancy-value theory has been an especially useful framework for understanding students' interest and persistence in learning. This theory proposes that students' achievement beliefs and behaviors are jointly determined by the expectancy they have for success and the value they place on learning (Eccles & Wigfield, 2002; see also Gladstone, Wigfield, & Eccles, chapter "Situated Expectancy Value Theory, Dimensions of Engagement, and Academic Outcomes", this volume). Eccles and Wigfield (2020) recently updated their model by adding "situated" to the name of the theory, highlighting the cultural beliefs, values, and situations that influence individuals' goals and task choices (Eccles & Wigfield, 2020). Students' expectancies for success across domains are strong predictors of their performance (Guo et al., 2015; Nagengast et al., 2013). Value on learning itself is multifaceted. Students may value doing well in school for personal reasons (*attainment value*); for the inherent interest and the pure enjoyment that comes from learning or performing certain tasks (*intrinsic value*); and/or for the way it relates to current or future goals, such as wanting to please parents or completing a course prerequisite (*utility value*). Students also consider the *cost value* of engaging in a task, as when the task in question induces anxiety (emotional cost) or when time devoted to the task entails sacrificing time for more pleasurable activities (opportunity cost).

Self-Determination Theory

With roots in Robert White's (1959) concept of effectance motivation (i.e., the desire to develop personal mastery), Ryan and Deci's (2017) self-determination theory (SDT) offers a powerful lens through which we can understand motivation for learning. In this framework, motivation is undergirded by the fulfillment of three psychological needs—the need for competence, autonomy, and relatedness. Individuals' inherent need for competence leads them to seek fulfilling experiences, and to experience mastery as intrinsically rewarding. At the same time, individuals have a strong need to feel agentic—that that they are in control of their actions and not coerced by external factors, such as punishments, rewards, or social expectations. With respect to relatedness, SDT suggests that we all have an inherent need to feel connected and supported by others in learning contexts (Ryan & Deci, 2020). As we show further on, parent involvement that is warm and supportive of autonomy fosters competence beliefs and engagement. Importantly, parents can be shown how to support autonomy successfully.

In this regard, we see a strong connection between studies in which researchers have coached parents on ways to foster adaptive learning beliefs and behaviors, and studies of parent involvement that have examined how schools can strengthen the home–school connection (e.g., Epstein, 1995; Reschly & Christenson, 2009). Supporting children with their schoolwork and general academic socialization (e.g., high expectations) are two of three primary components that comprise parent involvement (school-based involvement, such as attending parent–teacher nights, is the third component; Hill & Tyson, 2009).

Considering Sociodemographic Factors in Motivation

Most research on academic motivation has been conducted on White middle-class students, and scholars are increasingly concerned that the field has not fully considered how motivational factors influence the learning of sociodemographically diverse students (Urdan & Bruchmann, 2018; Usher, 2018). As an example, Gray et al. (2018) have observed that while relatedness is an integral component of numerous theories of motivation, such as self-determination theory, research often does not take into consideration the fact that the school and its agents foster a sense of relatedness that is experienced differently by diverse groups of students (Gray et al., 2018). For

example, at an interpersonal or relationship level, racialized tracking, through which low-income students of color are held to lower achievement standards by teachers than their White peers, threatens students' sense of belonging (Francis & Darity, 2021). At an instructional level, "color-blind" pedagogy has been criticized as it perpetuates social inequities (Gray et al., 2018). Finally, at the institutional level, zero-tolerance and punitive discipline policies disproportionly target non-White students (American Psychological Association Zero Tolerance Task Force, 2008). We expect that greater awareness of this research disparity, such as that evidenced in a recent special issue of Educational Psychologist (Zusho & Kumar, 2018), will foster research agendas that are more focused on the educational experiences of sociodemographically diverse students and how these experiences exert their influence on motivation for learning.

Ecological Theory as Guidepost

In proposing his ecological model underscoring the primacy of context in child development, Bronfenbrenner (1977) observed that developmental psychology had become "…the science of the strange behavior of children in strange situations with strange adults for the briefest periods of time" (p.513). His theory of nested and reciprocal spheres of influence in child development served to highlight a widely accepted organizing principle of development: individuals do not evolve in a vacuum, but are active participants in multiple social and historical contexts that shape their emerging beliefs about the world and their place within it.

The microsystem consists of the proximal settings that contain the child—for example, what parents and families say and do in support of academic achievement. With respect to human development, Bronfenbrenner placed the greatest emphasis on proximal processes as the engines of development, including parenting. More recently, longitudinal studies have found that most important factor in promoting positive youth development is caring, competent, and committed adults—typically, parents and guardians (Lerner et al., 2011).

In Bronfenbrenner's model, the mesosystem represents interactions between the environments that contain the child, and thus theoretically situates the home–school connection in studies of how bonds between these settings can foster achievement and engagement (Sheridan & Kim, 2016) as we discuss later in this chapter. No less important for the influence of parenting on developmental outcomes are the two more distal circles of influence. Psychological anthropologists and cultural psychologists alike have argued that societal contexts (the exosystem) as well as cultural and historical contexts (the macrosystem) are critical in shaping thinking and the development of belief systems, including those that guide parental educational socialization practices (Harkness & Super, 2020; Rogoff, 2016; Vygotsky, 1978; Weisner, 2002).

Culture and context can play especially central roles in helping us to understand how parents foster their children's engagement with school. The child's role, however, is equally critical. Children actively co-construct their developing understanding of the nature and value of learning and education through their ongoing interactions with their caregivers, teachers, and mentors. As we will discuss below, ecocultural theory and bioecological models of development are critical in understanding ethnic and cultural diversity in parental influences on student engagement.

The Influence of Parental Relationship Support

The importance of parental relations for social competence and other positive developmental outcomes is rooted in the continuity view of relationships, which suggests that one's relationship style is relatively stable and strongly influenced by one's attachment to a primary caregiver as early as infancy, like relational "templates" carried forward into to adolescence and adulthood (Furrer & Skinner, 2003). A variety of studies corroborate this finding by demonstrating the significant, positive influence of warm and caring

parent or family support on student engagement and motivation (e.g., Brewster & Bowen, 2004; Furrer & Skinner, 2003; Marchant et al., 2001; Murray, 2009; Wentzel et al., 2016). The quality of parental relations may also operate in a variety of ways to influence students' motivation and engagement with school. Several studies have found an influential role of both parents and teachers on student engagement and motivation. For example, Quin, Hemphill and Heerde (Quin et al., 2017) found that both sources of social support uniquely and positively predicted Australian students' emotional engagement in school. Estell and Perdue (2013) found that parent support, but not teacher support, uniquely and positively predicted sixth graders' behavioral engagement (i.e., work habits in the classroom). Other studies have oppositely found positive effects of teachers but not parents (e.g., Duchesne & Larose, 2007; Kindermann, 2007; Wentzel, 2016).

Some studies have shown that various sources of social support may exert differential effects on various aspects of academic motivation and engagement. For example, Wang and Eccles (2012) found that parent social support was a stronger predictor of school identification, the subjective valuing of learning, and participation in extracurricular activities than peer social support. Peers, however, exerted a stronger influence on school-related behavioral outcomes than did parents and teachers. Despite the mixed nature of these findings, research on the whole suggests that students navigate complex social ecologies with the potential for multiple contexts supporting their academic engagement or motivation. Minimally, parents have been shown to be a primary source of influence on these processes, along with teachers and peers.

The Influence of Parental Involvement on Well-Being and Engagement

Research evidence suggests at least two fundamental reasons that parental involvement influences engagement and motivation. The first is the strong association between parental relations with their children and overall psychological well-being, which positions parental involvement as a primary protective factor against disengagement. The second is the more direct influence of caring and supportive relationships with parents on students' motivation and engagement with schooling.

Parental Relations and Psychological Well-Being

Our conceptualization of engagement as defined by students' self-perceptions of their level of involvement in an activity places an emphasis on the relational and emotional well-being of the student. Such an outlook is based on the premise that engagement with learning environments is situated within the larger context of psychological and relational well-being emanating from effective adaptation to the environment (Griffiths et al., 2009). Within this larger perspective, meaningful engagement that leads to sustained motivation may be seen as a key driver of positive youth development (Larson, 2006), and fostering it is a primary goal of educational approaches that emphasize strengths and well-being of students rather than deficit-driven and reactive approaches (Gilman et al., 2009).

Indeed, there appears to be a strong relationship between engagement and well-being (see Suldo & Parker, chapter "Relationships Between Student Engagement and Mental Health as Conceptualized from a Dual-Factor Model", this volume). Students who are interested and involved in skill-building and productive pursuits score higher on measures of psychological adjustment, including measures of self-esteem, responsibility, competence, and social relations, whereas students who report feeling alienated from school are more likely to have behavioral problems ranging from withdrawal to depression to aggression (Shernoff, 2013). Research has shown that the resources of families, schools, and communities may foster the positive development of youth through provisions of physical safety and security, developmentally appropriate structure and expectations for behavior, emo-

tional and moral support, and opportunities to make a contribution to one's community (Eccles & Gootman, 2002).

Because family life and parental relations are such powerful forces in overall adaptation and relational well-being, family cohesiveness and parental relations may be seen as a primary protective factor against behavioral and psychological problems, including disengagement from school, while reciprocally serving as a salient influence on resiliency and positive psychological outcomes (Barger et al., 2019). One longitudinal study in Australia found that having a strong relationship with one's parents across childhood and adolescence contributed to positive development across five domains (e.g., social competence, life satisfaction) at age 20 (O'Connor et al., 2011).

How Parents Influence Engagement and Foster Adaptive Achievement Beliefs

A considerable body of research has focused on what parents can do to foster their children's engagement and achievement in school, and how schools can support parents in their efforts. The quality of parent–child relations has been linked not only to higher engagement (Chen, 2008) but also to academic performance (Furrer & Skinner, 2003; Sirin & Rogers-Sirin, 2004) and achievement (Hughes & Kwok, 2007). These linkages suggest that supportive parental relations are important for students' engagement and attitudes about schooling beyond providing the child with templates for relating to others in the early years of life (Furrer & Skinner, 2003). For example, particular activities that parents do with their children, such as reading to them, can influence school grades and achievement test scores (Kaplan Toren, 2013). Further, parental involvement in the form of school- and home-based involvement has additionally been linked to students' academic engagement (i.e., homework completion; feelings of interest in, enjoyment, and value of school learning) and success, as well as positive mental health outcomes in high school (Jeynes, 2012; Wang & Sheikh-Khalil, 2014).

Importantly, our understanding of the benefits of parent involvement has expanded to include the motivational factors that can be transmitted through such interactions. Research at the intersection of sociocultural theory and social cognitive theory has revealed that parents' own attitudes about learning, value on education, achievement expectations, and approaches with the school and its agents have a profound influence on the development of their children's achievement-related beliefs and behaviors (Jeynes, 2010). The impact of parents' attitudes towards and approaches to learning has been extensively studied in research on children's homework and on the ways in which parents communicate and transmit their educational values to their children (Bempechat, 2019).

Parent Involvement in Homework

A large body of research on parent involvement in homework has demonstrated that parents can have a profound influence on their children's developing achievement-related beliefs and behaviors. This influence is best understood in light of the fact that students' subjective experiences while doing homework tend to be characterized by negative affect, including anxiety and low engagement (Goetz et al., 2012; Katz et al., 2014). Parents who provide assistance with homework play a critical role, not only in fostering learning, but also in scaffolding strategies for time management and problem solving (Moroni et al., 2015). Their interest in and assistance with homework also predicts their children's self-perceptions of competence (Grolnick, 2015; Hoover-Dempsey et al., 2001; Pomerantz et al., 2006).

Much recent research grounded in self-determination and goal theories provides evidence that help for the sake of help, however, tends not to foster adaptive learning beliefs or behaviors. Indeed, the quality of parental help matters (Moroni et al., 2015). For example, self-determination theory would predict that parents who support children's autonomy would provide hints and suggestions when children encounter difficulty and refrain from solving the problem in question themselves. From a goal theory perspec-

tive, parents whose focus is mastery would likely orient their children towards learning for understanding and not be concerned with the grade earned.

Against this theoretical backdrop, research has converged to show that parental autonomy support and mastery orientation predict engagement with learning, greater persistence, increased intrinsic motivation, heightened self-regulation, and academic achievement (Cheung & Pomerantz, 2015; Lerner & Grolnick, 2020; Madjar et al., 2016). For example, Doctoroff and Arnold (2017) observed caregivers (mostly mothers) of first through fourth grade students help their children with homework-like language arts worksheets. Findings showed that supportive parenting behavior that was highly encouraging of autonomy predicted reading achievement, even controlling for support for relatedness and competence. Autonomy support also predicted children's increased engagement in the task. When the relative importance of the types of parenting support were examined, autonomy support emerged as particularly salient for children's reading achievement and engagement.

In a study of the influence of parents' attitudes on children's motivation towards homework assignments, Madjar et al. (2016) surveyed fourth through sixth grade parents and their children. Children reported on their own and their parents' homework goal orientations, while parents reported on their achievement-oriented goals towards homework. Results showed that parental focus on mastery goal orientation while doing homework (e.g., focus on understanding and self-improvement) was associated with children's mastery orientations. In contrast, parent-reported emphasis on performance while doing homework (e.g., competing with peers, avoiding negative evaluation) was associated with children's performance-approach and performance-avoidance orientation, respectively. These associations were mediated by children's perceptions of their parents' goal orientations.

Much research on parental help with homework has found a negative relationship between parental homework help and student achievement. This may be because some parents step in to provide assistance when their children are struggling to succeed. However, as A. Li and Hamlin (2019) pointed out, these studies do not distinguish between parents who do help and those who do not help at all. The researchers addressed this oversight by examining the relationship between parent homework help and student achievement at the elementary school level, focusing on *only* those parents who were highly inclined to provide daily homework help. They found that low socioeconomic status (SES), minority status, and student low academic achievement were associated with a high propensity to help children with homework on a daily basis, independent of other background factors. In addition, there was a positive relationship between the propensity to provide daily homework help and academic achievement (as measured by standardized math and reading scores). As the authors suggested, many low-income parents are well aware that their children attend a low-quality school. Their propensity to help with homework may reflect their need to compensate for the academic support their children may not be receiving. The authors noted that these findings may reflect, in part, parents' decisions to support their children's learning in light of the fact that their schools are under-resourced.

Importantly, research has shown that parents can be successfully instructed to adopt an autonomy-supportive style when helping their children with homework. Froiland (2011, 2015) conducted a field-based intervention study during which he provided parents of fourth and fifth grade children with role-modeling sessions that demonstrated how to provide homework help in an autonomy-supportive fashion (e.g., warm listening, empathic feedback), and how to convey learning goals to their children as they worked on their homework. In survey responses, parents in the training group perceived an increase in intrinsic motivation and autonomy in their children, and their children reported experiencing more positive emotions while doing their homework and becoming more passionate about learning. Further, an analysis of weekly diary entries kept by parents revealed that they generalized the autonomy-supportive strategies that they learned

to foster learning in contexts other than school (e.g., music lessons).

Research has shown that, in and of itself, homework help is not a necessary factor in the promotion of academic achievement (Benner et al., 2016). Parents can also create environments for study and help their children to manage homework behavior (Epstein & Van Vooris, 2001; Xu & Corno, 1998, 2003). Grolnick, Raftery-Helmer, Flamm, Marbell, & Cardemil (2014) examined the relationship between the ways that parents provide academic structure (i.e., providing clear rules and expectations about homework completion and studying, applied consistently) and sixth graders' competence-related beliefs, motivation, and academic achievement. Interviews conducted with these middle schoolers showed that parental provision of structure in an autonomy-supportive manner was positively associated with greater feelings of competence, school engagement, and high performance in English. These and other studies (e.g., O'Sullivan et al., 2014) demonstrate the extent to which homework is partly a social experience that is co-constructed through children's interactions with their parents.

The ongoing debate about the influence of homework on academic achievement has at times pitted parents against educators, and educators against homework researchers (Bempechat, 2019). Mixed findings on the extent to which homework enhances achievement, especially at the elementary school level (where effects are more muted), have contributed to a popular view that homework should be more measured if not reconsidered (Kohn, 2006; Kralovec & Buell, 1991). The above body of research, however, makes clear that homework can be a powerful vehicle for fostering the development of adaptive motivational tendencies. When parent involvement with homework is warm and supportive, it serves to enhance both academic achievement and the development of adaptive beliefs about learning.

The Transmission of Educational Values

Parents' own educational attitudes and beliefs have been shown to be a major influence on the educational attitudes that their children gradually adopt (Halle, Kurtz-Costes, & Mahoney, 1997). Through the process of socialization, children gradually internalize their parents' beliefs and attitudes, including those regarding the value parents place on education (Vygotsky, 1978). Parent involvement is multidimensional (Boonk et al., 2018; Grolnick & Slowiaczek, 1994). When parents express interest in what their children are learning (personal involvement), attend school events (behavioral involvement), and help with homework and otherwise expose children to intellectually enriching activities (cognitive/intellectual involvement), they are conveying educational messages that have a profound impact on children's developing achievement-related beliefs, behaviors, and outcomes (Pomerantz & Grolnick, 2017). These dimensions of parent involvement have been shown to be associated with social class, such that cognitive/intellectual involvement is more characteristic of more educated parents. Importantly, however, as we stated in the previous section, parent educational level is not always predictive of behavioral involvement; and indeed, parents do not necessarily have to be actively involved in homework help in order for their children to do well in school.

Cheung and Pomerantz (2015) studied the extent to which the effect of parent involvement on their children's educational values was mediated by children's perceptions of their parents versus their direct experience with their parents. Specifically, they tested two models or pathways through which parents may transmit their educational values to their children. Following Grusec and Goodenow (1994, as cited in Cheung & Pomerantz, 2015), the *perception-acceptance* model proposes that parent involvement (e.g., attendance at school events, help with homework, provision of resources) leads children to believe that their parents value academic achievement, which leads to children adopting this value, and ultimately fosters greater school achievement. The more direct *experience-development pathway* proposes that as a consequence of being involved in their children's schooling, parents create experiences (e.g., discussing school activities) that heighten the value children place on school, regardless of their parents' own values. Cheung and Pomerantz (2015) surveyed American and Chinese seventh graders through their eighth year and reported evidence on the strength of both pathways. They found that both pathways uniquely contributed to the valuing of school achievement, greater school engagement (e.g., self-regulation), and higher grades in both populations of students.

Parents' educational messages are themselves influenced by culture, an influence that is enduring and slow to change. Indeed, children readily develop learning beliefs from the culturally informed educational messages that they receive from their parents (Bornstein, 2012). In a recent qualitative study, Bempechat, Cheung, and J. Li (2021) conducted a discourse analysis of low-income Chinese American adolescents' construction of their immigrant parents' educational messages. Using J. Li's (2012) *mind* versus *virtue* model of learning as a framework, the authors found that students constructed their parents' educational messages in ways that supported their internalization of the Confucian-influenced model of learning as a virtue, encompassing a set of qualities including diligence, perseverance, concentration, humility, endurance of hardship, respect for teachers, and knowledge as essential (J. Li, 2012). For example, one participant's constructions of her parents' educational messages coalesced around the discourses of mutual obligation and self-improvement. She constructed her parents as having sacrificed much to immigrate to the U.S. and provided her with opportunities that they did not have in China. This construction positioned her as obligated to her parents to consistently put forth her best efforts in school.

Jeynes' (2010) analysis of parent involvement research showed that parent expectations, communicated through parental sacrifice, low stress communication, and a shared value on education, were more powerful in predicating academic outcomes than even open communication in which parents and children freely expressed themselves without fear of retribution. Grolnick and Ryan (1989) also found evidence for the indirect influence of parent involvement on student achievement and the development of value on education through motivational factors. Youth whose parents were both autonomy supportive and involved in their schoolwork (i.e., talked with them about school and helped them with challenges) internalized the value of doing well in school, as demonstrated by regularly completing homework, enjoying their schoolwork, and doing their best to succeed. With greater internalization of their parents' educational values also came higher achievement and better psychological adjustment. Thus, parents who are present at school meetings or events may be communicating its importance to children, as well as modeling ways to deal with questions or concerns. As a result, children also come to view schooling as within their realm of control. Similarly, parents who are involved intellectually, by reading to their children or helping with homework, may foster beliefs that these are manageable and controllable tasks.

Studies of mentoring have likewise shown that a mentor's tacit values and practices leading towards high-quality work within a profession were found to become absorbed by multiple subsequent generations of mentees in the context of supportive relationships (Nakamura & Shernoff, 2009). Values that get transmitted from one generation to the next can be conceptualized as memes, the cultural units of intergenerational inheritance, as an analog to genes. In the case of mentoring and apprenticeship within professions, the tacit transmission of values and practices appears to be one way in which professions are maintained and evolve. Similarly, cultural values transmitted from parents to children may be an important mechanism for the evolution and maintenance of culture itself, speaking to the potential interaction of parental influences with the macrosystem.

Parental Involvement and the Building of Social Capital

Parent involvement is well illustrated through the construct of social capital, the notion that individuals have at their disposal cultural resources that they can access through their social networks (Bourdieu, 1985). Parent networks operate as a form of social capital in which individuals share tangible (books, educational videos) and intangible (knowledge about the college application process) resources to enhance their children's learning (Lareau, 2000). A body of ethnographic research has emerged to show that parents' means of creating and accessing social capital varies as a function of both social class and ethnicity (e.g., Horvat et al., 2003). Lareau's (2002, 2011) influential ethnographic work underscores the power of social class in how parents build and use social networks to enhance their children's educational experiences. Lareau (2011) identified two distinct models of parent involvement that are driven by social class and influence both how families interact with schools and how schools, in turn, interact with families. Working- and middle-class parents did not differ in the value they placed on education. However, given their own limited education and social status, working-class parents perceived a clear distinction between their roles and that of their children's teachers (Lareau, 1987). Working-class parents believed that education takes place at the school and as such invested teachers with the responsibility to guide their children's academic trajectories. In contrast, middle-class parents, who had more years of formal education and enjoyed higher social status, viewed themselves as the teachers' equals. They felt empowered to question and challenge teachers' pedagogy, including the frequency of homework assignments. As such, they initiated contact with teachers and participated in school events to a greater extent than their working-class peers.

Lareau (2002) characterized middle-class Black and White parents as engaging in what she termed "concerted cultivation" to enhance their children's intellectual and social development (e.g., enrollment in extracurricular activities, use of reasoning as a means of socialization), and in turn, their children came to view themselves as both talented and entitled (Lareau, 2002, p.748). Greater involvement in organized activities further extended middle-class parents' social networks by exposing them to similarly well-educated and connected adults, while at the same time limiting their exposure to extended family. In contrast, low-income parents in both groups socialized their children towards the "accomplishment of natural growth" by structuring their children's lives around more spontaneous events, such as family gatherings. This pattern of kinship ties clearly had its own advantages but resulted in a social network composed of few professionals and more limited understanding of how to negotiate the school system. Clearly, concerted cultivation reflects middle-class norms. Working-class parents were not uninvolved in their children's education; rather, their model of involvement privileged the expertise of teachers.

Calarco (2020) extended Lareau's findings through an extensive study of how middle-class students learn to negotiate opportunities for themselves in their classrooms. Her classroom observations and interviews with students, their parents, and their teachers revealed that middle-class parents characterized teachers as facilitators of their children's academic success. In the process, parents taught their children strategies to advocate for themselves (e.g., asking for extra time to complete a task, repeatedly requesting assistance and clarifications). As a result, these students were able to garner the support they needed to overcome challenges in the classroom. In contrast, working-class parents emphasized the importance of personal responsibility in their learning and exhorted their children not to unnecessarily encumber their teachers with questions. These children were more self-reliant in the classroom than their wealthier peers, but at a cost to their learning, understanding, and achievement.

In a recent homework-related study, Calarco (2020) showed how White middle-class parents can undermine teachers' homework policy, and how teachers themselves can privilege higher SES students in the homework process. She reported that third through fifth grade teachers valued homework as a tool to foster independence and self-regulation. Despite this, teachers yielded to higher SES parent requests for exemptions from homework-related sanctions (e.g., allowing a child to phone his mother and request that she bring his forgotten homework to school). Their children, then, were subject to far fewer disciplinary sanctions than their working-class peers. Calarco describes schools as "privilege-dependent organizations" whose reputations emanate from the families they serve (Calarco, 2020, p. 223). Thus, teachers may see incentives inherent in catering to higher SES, White families, resulting in the differential treatment of students.

Research on parents' social networks has begun to consider how culture and ethnicity, in conjunction with social class, may help to explain students' academic achievement. A variety of survey, ethnographic, and qualitative studies of Latinx students and their families have converged to show that, contrary to stereotypes (Colegrove, 2018; Landa et al., 2020), Latino parents care deeply about their children's learning (Delgado-Gaitan, 1992; Gándara, 1995; Valenzuela, 1999); they communicate their values and expectations through cultural narratives, including *consejos* (advice) and *dichos* (proverbs), that serve as guides to navigate school and life (Delgado-Gaitan, 1994; Rendón et al., 2014; Yosso, 2005). A qualitative study of 32 Mexican-origin ninth graders revealed that their parents' *consejos* were the most salient and meaningful form of involvement (Holloway et al., 2014). These students spoke, for example, about their parents' compelling messages about the value of education as a path to a better life than the ones they were experiencing.

J. Li and colleagues demonstrated the primacy of culture in the creation and use of social networks among low-income Chinese American families (Li et al., 2008). Individual interviews with ninth-graders revealed that their relatively high level of achievement (mean GPA of 3.27) was attained with little practical assistance from parents. Rather, students described parents as engaging in three strategies that supported their learning. First, they identified and designated at least one person in the home or extended family (older sibling, relative)—an *"anchor helper"*—to be charged with guiding the student's school progress and providing tutoring. Second, according to students, their parents tried to motivate them by invoking *good learning models*—an exemplary individual(s) in the home or community whom they urged their children to emulate. Finally, students reported that their parents enlisted the *long reach of kin*—family members who were invited or obliged to be involved in their schooling, but who also willingly became involved by staying current about their progress in school. This work presents a challenge, both to "deficit model" approaches to understanding achievement outcomes, and to the premium placed on higher SES in social capital explanations of achievement.

Parental Influences on STEM Learning and Programming

Increasing attention has been paid to parental influences on student achievement and engagement in STEM subjects (Science, Technology, Engineering, and Mathematics). This attention reflects a concern that, relative to their more affluent peers, lower-income students are less likely to enroll in advanced mathematics and science courses (Bozick & Ingels, 2008; Tyson et al., 2007).

Gathering reports from students and their parents about their expectations, values, and identities for STEM topics between middle school through age 20, Svoboda and colleagues (2016) found that parental education predicted mathematics and science course enrollment in high school and college. This relationship was also found to be partially mediated by students' and parents' future identity and motivational beliefs about mathematics and science. Consistent with expectancy-value theories of motivation (Wigfield & Eccles, 2000), the most influential

motivational beliefs related to the perceived expectancy for achievement in STEM disciplines and careers, and the underlying value of education in mathematics and science. Importantly, researchers have reported successful interventions focused on parents' involvement in students' STEM-related achievement and study. Specifically, Harackiewicz, Rozek, Hulleman, and Hyde (Harackiewicz et al., 2012) designed a randomized controlled study in which parents in the treatment group received materials (brochures, website) about the utility and relevance of STEM subjects for their 10th and 11th grade children. They were encouraged to share the information with their children and provided advice on how to communicate the information therein. Relative to students in the control group, whose parents did not receive the STEM-related materials, students in the intervention group enrolled on average in one additional semester STEM study. A follow-up study found that this intervention resulted in significantly improved math and science scores on the standardized ACT exam. Students' enhanced STEM preparation in high school was associated with greater STEM course enrollment in college, as well as greater STEM career aspiration and perceived value of STEM (Rozek et al., 2017).

Some of this research has focused on one STEM subject specifically, especially mathematics. For example, Ing (2014) used latent growth curve analysis to analyze nationally representative longitudinal data and found that parents' motivational practices influenced their children's mathematics achievement trajectories between 7th and 12th grade. The influencing motivational practices were conceptualized as extrinsic (e.g., use of rewards and emphasizing grades) vs. intrinsic (e.g., praise of effort, encouragement of intrinsic interest in mathematics interest). Several other studies have supported the proposition that parents' own math anxiety and attitudes influence that of their children, and ultimately their achievement in math. Maloney and colleagues (2015) found that children are more anxious and learn less mathematics when their parents are anxious, but only when those parents provided frequent help with math homework. Children's attitudes and achievement were not related to their parents' math anxiety when parents helped with math homework less often. Similarly, Soni and Kumari (2017) studied 595 students in India, along with one parent each, and found that parental math anxiety and attitudes act as precursors to that of their children, significantly influencing their mathematics achievement scores between the ages of 10 and 15.

Parental Overinvolvement

Since parental involvement is clearly an important factor influencing students' academic engagement and motivation, a good question is whether parents can be too involved in their children's schooling for the influence to remain positive. One characterization of overinvolvement has been referred to as "helicopter parenting," defined as overparenting (Schiffrin et al., 2014). As children develop into young adults, the need for autonomy increases and helicopter parenting can undermine that need. LeMoyne and Buchanan (2011) explored this issue by surveying sample of 317 college students and concluded that helicopter parenting adversely affected students' psychological well-being and increased their chance of using prescription medication for mental health. The study suggested that the net effect of "helicopter parenting" on college student motivation and well-being was negative—an effect that can be explained by undermining students' need for autonomy (Schiffrin et al., 2014).

In a study designed to examine the effects of helicopter parenting on academic motivation, Schiffrin and Liss (2017) surveyed 192 college students and their mothers ($N = 121$) and found that parents and their college-age children often had different views about parenting behaviors, and that there were frequently negative consequences associated with children's perception that their parents were "helicoptering." Overall, the results implied that helicopter parenting is related to maladaptive academic motivation (e.g., diminished sense of autonomy), which, in turn, can negatively impact academic achievement.

Not all studies, however, support the narrative that helicopter parenting is common or a barrier to student success (e.g., Howard et al., 2020).

Howard, Nicholson and Chesnut (2019) studied overparenting as it relates to *grit*, or the tolerance for adversity in the pursuit of goal achievement (Duckworth et al., 2007; Von Culin et al., 2014). The success of college students can be linked to their ability to handle common stressors during the transition to college, such as academic concerns, interpersonal relationships, and finances (Galatzer-Levy et al., 2012; Prevatt et al., 2011). An important question becomes what protective factors can help college students mitigate the risk of common stressors during the college years. Howard et al. (2019) proposed that grit could be one such factor. In surveying 226 undergraduate students, they found that parental acceptance and involvement positively predicted students' academic success, while overparenting negatively predicted it. They further found that grit mediated both relationships. That is, parental involvement had a positive effect on students' grit, which in turn positively predicted students' academic success. Grit also was found to mediate the negative relationship between helicopter parenting and academic success: helicopter parenting exerted a negative effect on grit, reducing its potential to positively influence college success.

Programs Modeling Parental Involvement and Home–School Partnerships

Since relational warmth, care, and support consistently emerge as critical factors in students' engagement in school, it may not be surprising that these qualities are essential for the development of home–school partnerships drawing on community resources in addition to parents. School-based family centers and high-quality after-school have effectively modeled the building of social capital by leveraging resources and networks in the neighborhood or community in addition to families.

Family–School Partnerships

Family–school partnership models are child-focused approaches that bring families and school professionals together to increase opportunities and accomplishments for children's well-being and development (Albright & Weissberg, 2010). A notable example of an effective family–school partnership model is the Getting Ready intervention, premised on building school readiness in children (Sheridan et al., 2008). This is accomplished by developing a partnership between early childhood professionals (ECPs) and parents through the use of a strength-based framework that promotes positive parental responses such as parental warmth, sensitivity, and participation in their children's learning to support the child's autonomy and independence. ECPs are instrumental in promoting these values through the intentional use of strategies that foster strong parent–child interactions and a positive family–school relationship, such as modeling positive behaviors, fostering open communication, and validating parent competence. A randomized study of the Getting Ready intervention, in which the interactions of 234 parents and their children were videotaped over a 16-month period, revealed that intervention participants demonstrated higher-quality interactions with their children in terms of warmth, sensitivity, and autonomy support (Knoche et al., 2012). Parents, children, teachers, and other early childhood professionals participating in the Getting Ready approach also reported positive experiences regarding parent–child and family–school relationships, demonstrating the value of the program in terms of providing a setting that enables a healthy dynamic for families to support the child's development and learning (Sheridan & Kim, 2016). More recently, a goal of the Getting Ready intervention was to strengthen parent–teacher partnerships, a model that demonstrated social validity, in part by the inclination of the various participants' (parents, teachers and early intervention coaches) to mutually value the academic and behavioral goals established for children (Kuhn et al., 2016).

Since 1989, the Mexican American Legal Defense and Education Fund (MALDEF) has sponsored a Parent School Partnership (PSP) program to educate and empower parents, and Latinx parents in particular, to be advocates for their children's educational attainment. This program is designed to foster leadership skills and knowledge of the processes associated with school-based involvement (Bolívar & Chrispeels, 2011). In a 12-week study of the program's impact, Mexican-origin parents met weekly for 2 hours in sessions led by a Spanish-speaking MALDEF instructor. Sessions included training in community advocacy and information on their rights as parents, as well as their children's rights. At the conclusion of the program, participants developed a sense of relational trust with the instructor and fellow parents, felt knowledgeable about the norms for engaging with the school and its personnel, became aware of their rights as immigrants and the roles they were expected to fulfill, and gained understanding and skills needed to work collectively to effect change. In short, MALDEF's program has been successful in supporting parents' abilities to build social and individual capital in the service of their children's education (Bolívar & Chrispeels, 2011).

Out-of-School Time Programs

Out-of-school time programs, which can be both school and community based, can also provide a model of leveraging social capital and community resources to positively influence student engagement and motivation. Developmental psychologists have taken a keen interest in out-of-school time because structured and supervised after-school and extracurricular activities can help children and adolescents to negotiate salient developmental tasks (Mahoney et al., 2005); organized after-school programs can be a unique context for supporting positive youth development in particular (Y. Li et al., 2014). Noam and Shaw (2014) argued that well-designed after-school programs for informal science activities can be supportive of youth development beyond helping youth to develop talents in skill-building activities like sports, art, music, community projects, and special-interest academic pursuits. Another important reason programs are developmentally supportive is that they can foster enhanced relations with peers and adults, and improve social competence among participants (Hoxie & DeBellis, 2014; Mahoney et al., 2007; Shernoff, 2010). For example, youth participating in organized after-school programs reported learning cooperation and teamwork critical to positive youth development (Hansen et al., 2003; Lower et al., 2017) and experiencing increased empathy and understanding essential to perspective taking (Dworkin et al., 2003). There is also evidence that participation in after-school activities is a supportive context for student engagement (Shernoff & Vandell, 2007; Vandell et al., 2005). Recently, Vandell et al. (2020) found that children who regularly participated a high-quality after-school program, often combined with extracurricular activities, were reported by their teachers to have better work habits, task persistence, and academic performance compared to students who did not.

Students join in after-school programs for both internal and external reasons. For example, students may join a program for intrinsic enjoyment of the activities provided, or to satisfy adults such as teachers and, most frequently, parents. Barry and LaVelle (2013) tested whether self-joined program participants had better socioemotional outcomes than those who joined programs for the sake of their parents and others. They found self-joined students demonstrated significantly higher autonomy, self-efficacy, and prosocial behaviors over time compared to other-joined participants. Participants whose motivation switched from self-joined to other-joined decreased in socioemotional ratings significantly compared to other participants. Although studies such as this suggest that parents can exert a negative effect on students' motivation in after-school activities, it stands to reason that, conversely, they can play a positive role in supporting good decision-making, perceived autonomy, and engagement in out-of-school time activities as well. More research in this area is needed.

Discussion

As we have seen, student engagement is a pervasive problem both nationally and internationally (OECD), 2016). The problem is intensified for students in underserved communities, and while the mechanisms are in need of further study, much research evidence places parents in a central role (Offord, 2001; Federal Interagency Forum on Child and Family Statistics, 2007). Bronfenbrenner's ecological systems theory is an especially useful lens for enhancing our understanding of parents' roles in fostering student motivation and engagement. It suggests that interactions between the proximal (micro- and mesosystems) and distal (exo- and macrosystems) spheres of influences are dynamic and continually evolving to meet the varied and changing needs of children and families. This bioecological paradigm has allowed researchers and practitioners to design family-centered and culturally sensitive research programs that operate from a strength-based perspective.

The preponderance of research evidence suggests that parents are a significant influence on student engagement, along with teachers and peers (Estell & Perdue, 2013; Quin et al., 2017; Wang & Eccles, 2012). According to some studies, parents may be the most important factor contributing to positive youth development (R. M. Lerner et al., 2011), and parents can be a stronger predictor of students' engagement than teachers (Estell & Perdue, 2013) and peers (Wang & Eccles, 2012). For example, parents' motivational beliefs have been found to influence math and science course taking in high school (Wigfield & Eccles, 2000), and several studies have suggested that parents' math anxiety can influence their children's anxiety and achievement in mathematics (Maloney et al., 2015; Soni & Kumari, 2017). At the same time, overparenting can have a negative influence on children's persistence in college (Howard et al., 2019).

Parents can influence their students' school engagement and achievement in a variety of ways. A central message underlying the considerable body of research that we have reviewed is that affective and instrumental relational support across contexts is essential for student motivation and engagement. Perceptions of general acceptance, respect for and interest in students as individuals, and expressions of warmth and care are critical to well-being and essential for students' motivation to learn and expressions of engagement with schooling. This includes pragmatic assistance (e.g., shepherding students through the college application process) that adults such as teachers and mentors can provide to enable students to meet their goals. Importantly, research has demonstrated the extent to which relational support is also vital to the individuals and entities that serve students. These elements of relational support serve as sources of guidance and represent protective factors that can help initiate, maintain, and reengage students' adaptive beliefs about learning and engagement in school.

One way that parents may model flow and engagement is by engaging in activities such as play with their children. Research suggests that engaging in activities with children during childcare is frequently a rich opportunity for both the parents' and child's optimal experiences (Delle Fave et al., 2013). Engaging in enjoyable and fulfilling activities directly with one's child is also an important way that parents demonstrate their value in parenting and their children's well-being.

A number of frameworks reviewed in this chapter place the primary responsibility for student engagement on schools. However, schools cannot be effective in providing support when they hold deficit-driven models of students, families, and communities (Posey-Maddox & Haley-Lock, 2016). Teachers, families, and schools interact in multiple spheres of a child's ecology and cannot work together in a mutually supportive fashion if they do not understand and accept each other in light of cultural influences. Our review highlights the extent to which the traditional model of parent involvement privileges White, middle-class parents, and underestimates the importance of cultural differences in how socioculturally diverse parents perceive their roles in home- and school-based involvement (Posey-Maddox & Haley-Lock, 2016). Expressing respect for diverse families may not be enough; respect must be visible in the actions that teachers take to understand their students' families and appreciate their involvement strategies.

Importantly, our review makes clear that much more attention must be paid to the ways in which culture, context, and social class bear unique influences in the development of children's learning beliefs and behaviors. The research we have presented highlights the extent to which sociocultural models of learning influence the ways in which parents socialize their children for academic achievement and how children come to make meaning of and internalize their parents' educational messages. Further, we have highlighted researchers' call for motivation research that places the educational experiences of sociodemographically diverse students at the center of future study and theory development.

The research evidence and models of effective programming that we have reviewed suggests that larger collaborative networks of schools, families, community organizations, and public institutions can provide for the nurturing and supportive socialization of youth, promoting engagement beyond what may be achieved by a single individual teacher or parent. For example, studies demonstrating the efficacy and social reliability of the Getting Ready intervention (Knoche et al., 2012; Kuhn et al., 2016) suggest that socializing agents within various systems of a child's ecology can collaborate to create greater continuity and consistency of children's care and support than when agents of a single system work in isolation (Sheridan et al., 2017). Similarly, high-quality after-school programs that can bridge school and family contexts have been shown to foster social and developmental competencies, like teamwork and perspective taking (Hoxie & DeBellis, 2014; Lower et al., 2017; Shernoff, 2010), which can lead to enhanced student engagement and academic performance (e.g., Vandell et al., 2005, 2020).

Implications and Future Directions for Research

Achievement motivation researchers have noted that an overreliance on experimental and survey methods may limit our understanding of the complex nature of students' achievement beliefs (Dowson & McInerney, 2001; Kaplan & Maehr, 2007). For example, experimental settings can bear little resemblance to the complex nature of classroom learning (Urdan & Turner, 2005). As Dowson and McInerney (2001) also pointed out, the deductive approach to studying students' achievement goal orientations involves making a priori assumptions about the presence of certain achievement goals and then using quantitative, decontextualized measures to test these assumptions. Furthermore, there may be a variety of ways children construct meaning and form goals from their everyday educational experiences (Bempechat & Boulay, 2001). In particular, students who differ in social class, culture, ethnicity and educational experiences may interpret survey or questionnaire items about their achievement beliefs differentially, further limiting our understanding.

Researchers in achievement motivation have therefore recognized the need to integrate qualitative methods in their investigations of students' and parents' learning beliefs. Ethnographic research has enhanced our understanding of meaning making among both higher- and lower-income White and culturally diverse families. The work of scholars such as Guerra and Nelson (2013) illustrates the value inherent in understanding the underlying cultural meanings of words and expressions that can encourage and motivate students.

Despite the knowledge gleaned from research that has examined ethnic groups, researchers and educators must be wary about adopting stereotypic views of Latinx, African American, or Asian immigrant/Asian descent parents' educational socialization practices. While cultural beliefs may indeed guide parenting styles, it is important to recognize that within cultures and ethnicities, there exists variation in how individuals interpret cultural beliefs.

Engaging Students, Families, and Communities

In moving away from a deficit perspective to a strength-building approach, research and theory in achievement motivation and student engagement have expanded to deepen our understanding of how some low-income or children of color may succeed in the face of fewer resources than those available to their more affluent peers. Engagement and motivation appear to be strong mediators of the resiliency to thrive in school as well as life in general. Superior engagement in skill-building tasks and an adaptive motivational orientation to succeed in school are often based on strong values for education and learning. Those values are neither created nor maintained in a vacuum, however. Parents, guardians, and teachers are perhaps the best poised to foster the motivation and engagement of children, and have the potential to make a long-lasting influence since these adults may have the most intimate understanding of their children's needs and potentialities. The most successful models converge to reveal that healthy patterns of engagement and motivation are fostered in supportive networks, including students, teachers, parents, and community members who share a mutual interest and commitment to the future welfare of youth.

References

Aber, L., Morris, P., & Raver, C. (2012). *Children, families and poverty: Definitions, trends, emerging science and implications for policy and commentaries* (2379–3988). Retrieved from https://doi.org/10.1002/j.2379-3988.2012.tb00072.x

Albright, M. I., & Weissberg, R. P. (2010). School-family partnerships to promote social and emotional learning. In S. L. Christenson & A. L. Reschly (Eds.), *Handbook of school-family partnerships for promoting student competence* (pp. 246–265). Routledge.

Ames, C. (1992). Achievement goals and the classroom motivational climate. In D. H. Schunk (Ed.), *Student perceptions in the classroom*. Erlbaum.

Appleton, J. J., Christenson, S. L., & Furlong, M. J. (2008). Student engagement with school: Critical conceptual and methodological issues of the construct. *Psychology in the Schools, 45*(5), 369–386.

Bacher-Hicks, A., Goodman, J., & Mulhern, C. (2021). Inequality in household adaptation to schooling shocks: Covid-induced online learning engagement in real time. *Journal of Public Economics, 193*, 104345.

Bardach, L., Oczlon, S., Pietschnig, J., & Lüftenegger, M. (2020). Has achievement goal theory been right? A meta-analysis of the relation between goal structures and personal achievement goals. *Journal of Educational Psychology, 112*(6), 1197.

Barger, M. M., Kim, E. M., Kuncel, N. R., & Pomerantz, E. M. (2019). The relation between parents' involvement in children's schooling and children's adjustment: A meta-analysis. *Psychological Bulletin, 145*(9), 855–890. https://doi.org/10.1037/bul0000201

Bempechat, J. (2000). *Getting our kids back on track: Educating children for the future.* Jossey-Bass.

Bempechat, J. (2019). The case for (quality) homework: Why it improves learning, and how parents can help. *Education Next, 19*(1), 36–43.

Bempechat, J., & Boulay, B. (2001). Beyond dichotomous characterizations: New directions in achievement motivation research. In D. McInerney & S. V. Etten (Eds.), *Research on sociocultural influences on motivation and learning* (Vol. 1, pp. 15–36). Information Age Publishing.

Bempechat, J., Cheung, A., & Li, J. (2021). A qualitative analysis of educational messaging: Case studies of four low income chinese american youth. *Journal of Ethnographic and Qualitative Research, 15*(3), 173–190.

Benner, A. D., Boyle, A. E., & Sadler, S. (2016). Parental involvement and adolescents' educational success: The roles of prior achievement and socioeconomic status. *Journal of Youth and Adolescence, 45*(6), 1053–1064. https://doi.org/10.1007/s10964-016-0431-4

Berry, T., & LaVelle, K. B. (2013). Comparing socioemotional outcomes for early adolescents who join after school for internal or external reasons. *The Journal of Early Adolescence, 33*(1), 77–103. https://doi.org/10.1177/0272431612466173

Bolívar, J. M., & Chrispeels, J. H. (2011). Enhancing parent leadership through building social and intellectual capital. *American Educational Research Journal, 48*(1), 4–38. https://doi.org/10.2307/27975280

Boonk, L., Gijselaers, H. J. M., Ritzen, H., & Brand-Gruwel, S. (2018). A review of the relationship between parental involvement indicators and academic achievement. *Educational Research Review, 24*, 10–30. https://doi.org/10.1016/j.edurev.2018.02.001

Bornstein, M. H. (2012). Cultural approaches to parenting. *Parenting: Science and Practice, 12*, 212–221.

Bourdieu, P. (1985). The forms of capital. In J. G. Richardson (Ed.), *Handbook of theory and research for the sociology of education* (pp. 241–258). Greenwood.

Bozick, R., & Ingels, S. J. (2008). *Mathematics coursetaking and achievement at the end of high school: Evidence from the education longitudinal study of 2002 (els: 2002) (statistical analysis report nces 2008–319).* National Center for Education Statistics.

Brewster, A. B., & Bowen, G. L. (2004). Teacher support and the school engagement of Latino middle and high school students at risk of school failure. *Child and Adolescent Social Work Journal, 21*(1).

Bronfenbrenner, U. (1977). Toward an experimental ecology of human development. *American Psychologist, 32*(7), 513–531.

Brooks-Gunn, J., Guo, G., & Furstenberg, F. F., Jr. (1993). Who drops out of and who continues beyond high school? A 20-year follow-up of black urban youth. *Journal of Research on Adolescence (Lawrence Erlbaum), 3*(3), 271–294. https://doi.org/10.1111/1532-7795.ep11301616

Brophy, J. E. (1983). Conceptualizing student motivation. *Educational Psychologist, 18*(3), 200–215.

Calarco, J. M. (2020). Avoiding us versus them: How schools' dependence on privileged "helicopter" parents influences enforcement of rules. *American Sociological Review, 85*(2), 223–246. https://doi.org/10.1177/0003122420905793

Chen, J. J.-L. (2008). Grade-level differences: Relations of parental, teacher and peer support to academic engagement and achievement among Hong Kong students. *School Psychology International, 29*(2), 183–198.

Cheung, C. S.-S., & Pomerantz, E. M. (2015). Value development underlies the benefits of parents' involvement in children's learning: A longitudinal investigation in the United States and China. *Journal of Educational Psychology, 107*(1), 309–320. https://doi.org/10.1037/a0037458

Children in poverty. (2019). Retrieved from https://www.childtrends.org/?indicators=children-in-poverty.

Christenson, S. L., Reschly, A. L., & Wylie, C. (2012). Epilogue. In S. L. Christenson, A. L. Reschly, & C. Wylie (Eds.), *Handbook of research on student engagement* (pp. 813–817). Springer.

Colegrove, K. S. S. (2018). Building bridges, not walls, between Latinx immigrant parents and schools. *Supporting Young Children of Immigrants in PreK-3, 130.* https://doi.org/10.1080/15348431.2020.1794875

Csikszentmihalyi, M. (1990). *Flow: The psychology of optimal experience.* Harper Perennial.

Delgado-Gaitan, C. (1992). School matters in the Mexican-American home: Socializing children to education. *American Educational Research Journal, 29*(3), 495–513.

Delgado-Gaitan, C. (1994). *Consejos*: The power of cultural narratives. *Anthropology and Education Quarterly, 25*, 298–316.

Delle Fave, A., Pozzo, M., Bassi, M., & Cetin, I. (2013). A longitudinal study on motherhood and well-being: Developmental and clinical implications. *Terapia Psicologica, 31*, 21–33. https://doi.org/10.4067/S0718-48082013000100003

Doctoroff, G. L., & Arnold, D. H. (2017). Doing homework together: The relation between parenting strategies, child engagement, and achievement. *Journal of Applied Developmental Psychology, 48*, 103–113. https://doi.org/10.1016/j.appdev.2017.01.001

Dowson, M., & McInerney, D. M. (2001). Psychological parameters of students' social and work avoidance goals: A qualitative investigation. *Journal of Educational Psychology, 93*(1), 35–42.

Duchesne, S., & Larose, S. (2007). Adolescent parental attachment and academic motivation and performance in early adolescence. *Journal of Applied Social Psychology, 37*(7), 1501–1521. https://doi.org/10.1111/j.1559-1816.2007.00224.x

Duckworth, A. L., Peterson, C., Matthews, M. D., & Kelly, D. R. (2007). Grit: Perseverance and passion for long-term goals. *Journal of Personality and Social Psychology, 92*(6), 1087.

Duncan, G. J., & Murnane, R. J. (2014). *Restoring opportunity: The crisis of inequality and the challenge for American education.* Harvard Education Press.

Dweck, C. S., & Molden, D. C. (2017). Mindsets: Their impact on competence motivation and acquisition. In A. J. Elliot, C. S. Dweck, & D. S. Yeager (Eds.), *Handbook of competence and motivation: Theory and application* (2nd ed., pp. 135–154). Guilford Press.

Dworkin, J. B., Larson, R., & Hansen, D. (2003). Adolescents' accounts of growth experiences in youth activities. *Journal of Youth and Adolescence, 32*(1), 17–26.

Eccles, J. S., & Gootman, J. A. (2002). *Community programs to promote youth development.* National Academy Press.

Eccles, J. S., & Wigfield, A. (2002). Motivational beliefs, values, and goals. *Annual Review of Psychology, 53*, 109–132.

Eccles, J. S., & Wigfield, A. (2020). From expectancy-value theory to situated expectancy-value theory: A developmental, social cognitive, and sociocultural perspective on motivation. *Contemporary Educational Psychology, 61*, 101859. https://doi.org/10.1016/j.cedpsych.2020.101859

Eccles, J. S., Roeser, R., Vida, M., Fredericks, J. A., & Wigfield, A. (2006). Motivational and achievement pathways through middle childhood. In L. Balter & C. S. Tamis-LeMonda (Eds.), *Child psychology: A handbook of contemporary issues* (2nd ed., pp. 325–355). Psychology Press.

Elliot, A. J., Murayama, K., & Pekrun, R. (2011). A 3 × 2 achievement goal model. *Journal of Educational Psychology, 103*(3), 632–648. https://doi.org/10.1037/a0023952

Elliot, A., Murayama, K., Kobeisy, A., & Lichtenfeld, S. (2015). Potential-based achievement goals. *British Journal of Educational Psychology, 85*(2), 192–206. https://doi.org/10.1111/bjep.12051

Epstein, J. L. (1995). School/family/community partnerships: Caring for the children we share. *Phi Delta Kappan, 76*(9), 701–712.

Epstein, J. L., & Van Vooris, F. L. (2001). More than minutes: Teachers' roles in designing homework. *Educational Psychologist, 36*(3), 181–193.

Estell, D. B., & Perdue, N. H. (2013). Social support and behavioral and affective school engagement: The effects of peers, parents, and teachers. *Psychology in the Schools, 50*(4), 325–339. https://doi.org/10.1002/pits.21681

Federal Interagency Forum on Child and Family Statistics. (2007). *America's children: Key national indicators of well-being.* U.S.: Government Printing Office.

Francis, D. V., & Darity, W. A. (2021). Separate and unequal under one roof: How the legacy of racialized tracking perpetuates within-school segregation. *RSF: The Russell Sage Foundation Journal of the Social Sciences, 7*(1), 187–202. https://doi.org/10.7758/rsf.2021.7.1.11

Fredericks, J., Blumenfeld, P. C., & Paris, A. H. (2004). School engagement: Potential of the concept, state of evidence. *Review of Educational Research, 74*(1), 59–109.

Froiland, J. M. (2011). Parental autonomy support and student learning goals: A preliminary examination of an intrinsic motivation intervention. *Child & Youth Care Forum, 40*(2), 135–149. https://doi.org/10.1007/s10566-010-9126-2

Froiland, J. M. (2015). Parents' weekly descriptions of autonomy supportive communication: Promoting children's motivation to learn and positive emotions. *Journal of Child and Family Studies, 24*(1), 117–126. https://doi.org/10.1007/s10826-013-9819-x

Furrer, C., & Skinner, E. (2003). Sense of relatedness as a factor in children's academic engagement and performance. *Journal of Educational Psychology, 95*(1), 148–162.

Galatzer-Levy, I. R., Burton, C. L., & Bonanno, G. A. (2012). Coping flexibility, potentially traumatic life events, and resilience: A prospective study of college student adjustment. *Journal of Social and Clinical Psychology, 31*(6), 542–567. https://doi.org/10.1521/jscp.2012.31.6.542

Gándara, P. (1995). *Over the ivy walls: The educational mobility of low income chicanos.* SUNY Press.

Gilman, R., Huebner, E. S., & Furlong, M. J. (Eds.). (2009). *Handbook of positive psychology in schools.* Routledge.

Goetz, T., Nett, U. E., Martiny, S. E., Hall, N. C., Pekrun, R., Dettmers, S., & Trautwein, U. (2012). Students' emotions during homework: Structures, self concept antecedents, and achievement outcomes. *Learning and Individual Differences, 22*(2), 225–234. https://doi.org/10.1016/j.lindif.2011.04.006

Gray, D. L., Hope, E. C., & Matthews, J. S. (2018). Black and belonging at school: A case for interpersonal, instructional, and institutional opportunity structures. *Educational Psychologist, 53*(2), 97–113.

Griffiths, A.-J., Sharkey, J. D., & Furlong, M. J. (2009). Student engagement and positive school adaptation. In R. Gilman, E. S. Huebner, & M. J. Furlong (Eds.), *Handbook of positive psychology in schools* (pp. 197–211) Routledge/Taylor & Francis Group.

Grolnick, W. S. (2015). Mothers' motivation for involvement in their children's schooling: Mechanisms and outcomes. *Motivation and Emotion, 39*(1), 63–73.

Grolnick, W. S., & Ryan, R. M. (1989). Parent styles associated with children's self-regulation and competence in school. *Journal of Educational Psychology, 81*(2), 143–154.

Grolnick, W. S., & Slowiaczek, M. L. (1994). Parents' involvement in children's schooling: A multidimensional conceptualization and motivational model. *Child Development, 65*(1), 237–252.

Grolnick, W. S., Raftery-Helmer, J. N., Flamm, E. S., Marbell, K. N., & Cardemil, E. V. (2014). Parental provision of academic structure and the transition to middle school. *Journal of Research on Adolescence, 25*(4), 668–684. https://doi.org/10.1111/jora.12161

Grusec, J. E., & Goodnow, J. J. (1994). Impact of parental discipline methods on the child's internalization of values: A reconceptualization of current points of view. *Developmental Psychology, 30*(1), 4–19. https://doi.org/10.1037/0012-1649.30.1.4

Gunderson, E. A., Gripshover, S. J., Romero, C., Dweck, C. S., Goldin-Meadow, S., & Levine, S. C. (2013). Parent praise to 1- to 3-year-olds predicts children's motivational frameworks 5 yearlater. *Child Development, 84*(5), 1526–1541.

Guo, J., Parker, P. D., Marsh, H. W., & Morin, A. J. (2015). Achievement motivation and educational choices: A longitudinal study of expectancy and value using a multiplicative perspective. *Developmental Psychology, 51*(8), 1163–1176.

Haimovitz, K., & Dweck, C. S. (2017). The origins of children's growth and fixed mindsets: New research and a rew proposal. *Child Development, 6*, 1849. https://doi.org/10.1111/cdev.12955

Halle, T. G., Kurtz-Costes, B., & Mahoney, J. L. (1997). Family influences on school achievement in low-income, African American children. *Journal of Educational Psychology, 89*(3), 527–537. https://doi.org/10.1037/0022-0663.89.3.527

Hansen, D. M., Larson, R. W., & Dworkin, J. B. (2003). What adolescents learn in organized youth activities: A survey of self-reported developmental experiences. *Journal of Research on Adolescence, 13*, 25–56.

Harackiewicz, J. M., Rozek, C. S., Hulleman, C. S., & Hyde, J. S. (2012). Helping parents to motivate adolescents in mathematics and science: An experimental test of a utility-value intervention. *Psychological Science, 23*(8), 899–906.

Harkness, S., & Super, C. M. (2020). Cross-cultural research on parents: Applications to the care and education of children introduction to the issue. *New Directions for Child and Adolescent Development, 2020*(170), 7–11. https://doi.org/10.1002/cad.20341

Hidi, S., & Renninger, K. A. (2006). The Four-Phase Model of Interest Development. *Educational Psychologist, 41*(2), 111–127. https://doi.org/10.1207/s15326985ep4102_4

Hill, N. E., & Tyson, D. F. (2009). Parental involvement in middle school: A meta-analytic assessment of the strategies that promote achievement. *Developmental Psychology, 45*(3), 740–763. https://doi.org/10.1037/a0015362

Holloway, S. D., Park, S., Jonas, M., Bempechat, J., & Li, J. (2014). "My mom tells me I should follow the rules, that's why they have those rules": Perceptions of parental advice giving among Mexican-heritage adolescents. *Journal of Latinos and Education, 13*(4), 262–277. https://doi.org/10.1080/15348431.2014.887468

Hoover-Dempsey, K. V., Battiato, A. C., Walker, J. M., Reed, R. P., DeLong, J. M., & Jones, K. P. (2001). Parental involvement in homework. *Educational Psychologist, 36*(3), 195–209.

Horvat, E. M., Weininger, E. B., & Lareau, A. (2003). From social ties to social capital. *American Educational Research Journal, 40*, 319–351.

Howard, A. L., Alexander, S. M., Dunn, L. C. (2020). Helicopter parenting is unrelated to student success and well-being: A latent profile analysis of perceived parenting and academic motivation during the transition to university. *Emerging Adulthood, 10*, 1–15. https://doi.org/10.1177/2167696820901626

Howard, J. M., Nicholson, B. C., & Chesnut, S. R. (2019). Relationships between positive parenting, overparenting, grit, and academic success. *Journal of College Student Development, 60*(2), 189–202. https://doi.org/10.1353/csd.2019.0018

Hoxie, A.-M. E., & DeBellis, L. M. (2014). Engagement in out-of-school time: How youth become engaged in the arts. In D. J. Shernoff & J. Bempechat (Eds.), *Engaging youth in schools: Evidence-based models to guide future innovations*. NSSE Yearbooks by Teachers College Record.

Hughes, J. N., & Kwok, O.-M. (2007). Influence of student-teacher and parent-teacher relationships on lower achieving readers' engagement and achievement in the primary grades. *Journal of Educational Psychology, 99*(1), 39–51.

Hulleman, C. S., Durik, A. M., Schweigert, S. B., & Harackiewicz, J. M. (2008). Task values, achievement goals, and interest: An integrative analysis. *Journal of Educational Psychology, 100*(2), 398–416.

Ing, M. (2014). Can parents influence children's mathematics achievement and persistence in stem careers? *Journal of Career Development, 41*(2), 87–103. https://doi.org/10.1177/0894845313481672

Jeynes, W. H. (2010). The salience of the subtle aspects of parental involvement and encouraging that involvement: Implications for school-based programs. *Teachers College Record, 112*(3), 747–774.

Jeynes, W. H. (2012). A meta-analysis of the efficacy of different types of parental involvement programs for urban students. *Urban Education, 47*(4), 706–742.

Kaplan, A., & Maehr, M. (2007). The contributions and prospects of goal orientation theory. *Educational Psychology Review, 19*, 141–184.

Kaplan Toren, N. (2013). Multiple dimensions of parental involvement and its links to young adolescent self-evaluation and academic achievement. *Psychology in the Schools, 50*(6), 634–649.

Katz, I., Eilot, K., & Nevo, N. (2014). 'I'll do it later': Type of motivation, self-efficacy and homework procrastination. *Motivation and Emotion, 1*, 111. https://doi.org/10.1007/s11031-013-9366-1

Kindermann, T. A. (2007). Effects of naturally existing peer groups on changes in academic engagement in a cohort of sixth graders. *Child Development, 78*(4), 1186–1203. https://doi.org/10.1111/j.1467-8624.2007.01060.x

Knoche, L. L., Sheridan, S. M., Clarke, B. L., Edwards, C. P., Marvin, C. A., Cline, K. D., & Kupzyk, K. A. (2012). Getting ready: Results of a randomized trial of a relationship-focused intervention on the parent-infant relationship in rural early head start. *Infant Mental Health Journal, 33*(5), 439–458. https://doi.org/10.1002/imhj.21320

Kohn, A. (2006). *The homework myth: Why our kids get too much of a bad thing*. De Capo Lifelong Books.

Kralovec, E., & Buell, J. (1991). End homework now. *Educational Leadership (April)*, 39–42. Retrieved from http://www.ascd.org/publications/educational--leadership/apr01/vol58/num07/End-Homework-Now.aspx

Kuhfeld, M., Soland, J., Tarasawa, B., Johnson, A., Ruzek, E., & Liu, J. (2020). Projecting the potential impact of COVID-19 school closures on academic achievement. *Educational Researcher, 49*(8), 549–565.

Kuhn, M., Marvin, C. A., & Knoche, L. L. (2016). In it for the long haul: Parent–teacher partnerships for addressing preschool children's challenging behaviors. *Topics in Early Childhood Special Education, 37*(2), 81–93. https://doi.org/10.1177/0271121416659053

Lam, S. F., Jimerson, S., Shin, H., Cefai, C., Veiga, F. H., Hatzichristou, C., … Zollneritsch, J. (2015). Cultural universality and specificity of student engagement in school: The results of an international study from 12 countries. *The British Journal of Educational Psychology, 86*(1), 137–153. https://doi.org/10.1111/bjep.12079

Landa, L., Snodgrass Rangel, V., & Coulson, H. (2020). Parent engagement at a primarily Latinx high school campus. *Journal of Latinos and Education*, 1–17.

Lareau, A. (1987). Social class differences in family-school relationships: The importance of cultural capital. *Sociology of Education, 60*, 73–85.

Lareau, A. (2000). *Home advantage: Social class and parental intervention in elementary education*. Rowman & Littlefield Publishers.

Lareau, A. (2002). Invisible inequality: Social class and childrearing in black families and White families. *American Sociological Review, 67*(5), 747–776.

Lareau, A. (2011). *Unequal childhoods: Class, race, and family life* (2nd ed.). University of California Press.

Larson, R. W. (2006). Positive youth development, willful adolescents, and mentoring. *Journal of Community Psychology, 34*(6), 677–689.

Lei, H., Cui, Y., & Zhou, W. (2018). Relationships between student engagement and academic achievement: A meta-analysis. *Social Behavior and Personality, 46*(3), 517–528.

LeMoyne, T., & Buchanan, T. (2011). Does "hovering" matter? Helicopter parenting and its effect on well-being. *Sociological Spectrum, 31*(4), 399–418. https://doi.org/10.1080/02732173.2011.574038

Lerner, R. E., & Grolnick, W. S. (2020). Maternal involvement and children's academic motivation and achievement: The roles of maternal autonomy support and children's affect. *Motivation and Emotion, 44*(3), 373–388. https://doi.org/10.1007/s11031-019-09813-6

Lerner, R. M., Lerner, J. V., & Colleagues. (2011). *Waves of the future – 2009: Report of the findings from the first six years of the 4-H study of positive youth development*. National 4-H Council.

Li, J. (2012). *Cultural foundations of learning: East and west*. Cambridge University Press.

Li, A., & Hamlin, D. (2019). Is daily parental help with homework helpful? Reanalyzing national data using a propensity score–based approach. *Sociology of Education, 92*(4), 367–385. https://doi.org/10.1177/0038040719867598

Li, J., Holloway, S. D., Bempechat, J., & Loh, E. (2008). Building and using a social network: Nurture for low income chinese american adolescents' learning. In Y. Hirokazu & N. Way (Eds.), *The social contexts of immigrant children and adolescents. New directions for child and adolescent development* (Vol. 121, pp. 9–25). Wiley.

Li, Y., Agans, J. P., Chase, P. A., Arbeit, M. R., Weiner, M. B., & Lerner, R. M. (2014). School engagement and positive youth development: A relational developmental systems perspective. *Teachers College Record, 116*(13), 37–57.

Lower, L. M., Newman, T. J., & Anderson-Butcher, D. (2017). Validity and reliability of the teamwork scale for youth. *Research on Social Work Practice, 27*(6), 716–725. https://doi.org/10.1177/1049731515589614

Madjar, N., Shklar, N., & Moshe, L. (2016). The role of parental attitudes in children's motivation toward homework assignments. *Psychology in the Schools, 53*(2), 173–188. https://doi.org/10.1002/pits.21890

Mahoney, J. L., Larson, R. W., & Eccles, J. S. (Eds.). (2005). *Organized activities as contexts of development: Extracurricular activities, after-school and community programs*. Lawrence Erlbaum.

Mahoney, J. L., Parente, M. E., & Lord, H. (2007). After-school program engagement: Links to child competence and program quality and content. *Elementary School Journal, 107*(4), 385–404.

Maloney, E. A., Ramirez, G., Gunderson, E. A., Levine, S. C., & Beilock, S. L. (2015). Intergenerational effects of parents' math anxiety on children's math achievement and anxiety. *Psychological Science, 26*(9), 1480–1488. https://doi.org/10.1177/0956797615592630

Marchant, G. J., Paulson, S. E., & Rothlisberg, B. A. (2001). Relations of middle school students' perceptions of family and school contexts with academic achievement. *Psychology in the Schools, 38*(6), 505–519. https://doi.org/10.1002/pits.1039

Martin, A. J., Way, J., Bobis, J., & Anderson, J. (2015). Exploring the ups and downs of mathematics engagement in the middle years of school. *The Journal of Early Adolescence, 35*(2), 199–244. https://doi.org/10.1177/0272431614529365

Meece, J. L., Blumenfeld, P. C., & Hoyle, R. H. (1988). Students' goal orientations and cognitive engagement in classroom activities. *Journal of Educational Psychology, 80*(4), 514–523.

Mitchell, M. (1993). Situational interest: Its multifaceted structure in the secondary school mathematics classroom. *Journal of Educational Psychology, 85*(3), 424–436.

Moroni, S., Dumont, H., Trautwein, U., Niggli, A., & Baeriswyl, F. (2015). The need to distinguish between quantity and quality in research on parental involvement: The example of parental help with homework. *Journal of Educational Research, 108*(5), 417–431. https://doi.org/10.1080/00220671.2014.901283

Murray, C. (2009). Parent and teacher relationships as predictors of school engagement and functioning among low-income urban youth. *The Journal of Early Adolescence, 29*(3), 376–404. https://doi.org/10.1177/0272431608322940

Nagengast, B., Trautwein, U., Kelava, A., & Lüdtke, O. (2013). Synergistic effects of expectancy and value on homework engagement: The case for a within-person perspective. *Multivariate Behavioral Research, 48*(3), 428–460.

Nakamura, J., & Shernoff, D. J. (2009). *Good mentoring: Fostering excellent practice in higher education.* Jossey-Bass.

Nicholls, J. G. (1989). *The competitive ethos and democratic education.* Harvard University Press.

Noam, G. G., & Shaw, A. M. (2014). Informal science and youth development: Creating convergence in out-of-school time. In D. J. Shernoff & J. Bempechat (Eds.), *Engaging youth in schools: Evidence-based models to guide future innovations* (pp. 199–218). NSSE Yearbooks by Teachers College Record.

Nystrand, M., & Gamoran, A. (1991). Instructional discourse, student engagement, and literature achievement. *Research in the Teaching of English, 25*(3), 261–290.

O'Connor, M., Sanson, A., Hawkins, M. T., Letcher, P., Toumbourou, J. W., Smart, D., … Olsson, C. A. (2011). Predictors of positive development in emerging adulthood. *Journal of Youth and Adolescence, 40*(7), 860–874. https://doi.org/10.1007/s10964-010-9593-7

O'Sullivan, R. H., Chen, Y.-C., & Fish, M. C. (2014). Parental mathematics homework involvement of low-income families with middle school students. *School Community Journal, 24*(2), 165–188.

Offord, D. R. (2001). Reducing the impact of poverty on children's mental health. *Current Opinion in Psychiatry, 14*(4), 299–301.

Organization for Economic Cooperation and Development (OECD). (2016). *PISA 2015 results: Policies and practices for successful schools — Vol II/students' wellbeing — Vol III.* Organization for Economic Cooperation and Development.

Paris, S. G., & Winograd, P. (1990). Promoting metacognition and motivation of exceptional children. *Rase: Remedial & Special Education, 11*(6), 7–15.

Pelletier, L. G., Tuson, K. M., Fortier, M. S., Vallerand, R. J., Briere, N. M., & Blais, M. R. (1995). Toward a new measure of intrinsic motivation, extrinsic motivation, and amotivation in sports: The sport motivation scale (sms). *Journal of Sport and Exercise Psychology, 17*(1), 35–53.

Pew Research Center. (2015). *Parenting in America: Outlook, worries, aspirations are strongly linked to financial situation.* Retrieved from Washington D.C.: https://www.pewresearch.org/social--trends/2015/12/17/1-the-american-family-today/

Pintrich, P. R., & De Groot, E. V. (1990). Motivational and self-regulated learning components of classroom academic performance. *Journal of Educational Psychology, 82*(1), 33–40.

Pomerantz, E. M., & Grolnick, W. S. (2017). The role of parenting in children's motivation and competence: What underlies effective parenting? In A. J. Elliot, C. S. Dweck, & D. S. Yeager (Eds.), *Handbook of competence and motivation* (pp. 566–585). Guilford Press.

Pomerantz, E. M., Ng, F. F., & Wang, Q. (2006). Mothers' mastery-oriented involvement in children's homework: Implications for the well-being of children with negative perceptions of competence. *Journal of Educational Psychology, 98*(1), 99–111.

Posey-Maddox, L., & Haley-Lock, A. (2016). One size does not fit all: Understanding parent engagement in the contexts of work, family, and public schooling. *Urban Education, 55*(5), 671–698.

Prevatt, F., Li, H., Welles, T., Festa-Dreher, D., Yelland, S., & Lee, J. (2011). The academic success inventory for college students: Scale development and practical implications for use with students. *Journal of College Admission, 211*, 26–31.

Psychological Association Zero Tolerance Task Force. (2008). Are zero tolerance policies effective in the schools? An evidentiary review and recommendations. *The American Psychologist, 63*, 852–862. https://doi.org/10.1037/0003-066X.63.9.852

Quin, D., Hemphill, S. A., & Heerde, J. A. (2017). Associations between teaching quality and secondary students' behavioral, emotional, and cognitive engagement in school. *Social Psychology of Education, 20*(4), 807–829. https://doi.org/10.1007/s11218-017-9401-2

Rendón, L. I., Nora, A., & Kanagala, V. (2014). *Ventajas/assets y conocimientos/knowledge: Leveraging Latin@ Strengths to foster student success.* Retrieved from https://www.utsa.edu/strategicplan/documents/2017_12%20Student%20Success%20_Ventajas_Assets_2014.pdf

Reschly, A. L., & Christenson, S. L. (2009). Parents as essential partners for fostering students' learning outcomes. In R. Gilman, E. S. Huebner, & M. J. Furlong (Eds.), *Handbook of positive psychology in schools* (pp. 257–272). Routledge.

Rogoff, B. (2016). Culture and participation: A paradigm shift. *Current Opinion in Psychology, 8*, 182–189. https://doi.org/10.1016/j.copsyc.2015.12.002

Rogoff, B., Coppens, A. D., Alcalá, L., Aceves-Azuara, I., Ruvalcaba, O., López, A., & Dayton, A. (2017). Noticing learners' strengths through cultural research. *Perspectives on Psychological Science, 12*(5), 876–888. https://doi.org/10.1177/1745691617718355

Rozek, C. S., Svoboda, R. C., Harackiewicz, J. M., Hulleman, C. S., & Hyde, J. S. (2017). Utility-value intervention with parents increases students' STEM preparation and career pursuit. *Proceedings of the National Academy of Sciences*, 201607386. https://doi.org/10.1073/pnas.1607386114

Rumberger, R. W. (2011). *Dropping out: Why students drop out of high school and what can be done about it.* Harvard University Press.

Ryan, R. M., & Deci, E. L. (2017). *Self-determination theory: Basic psychological needs in motivation, development, and wellness.* The Guilford Press.

Ryan, R. M., & Deci, E. L. (2020). Intrinsic and extrinsic motivation from a self-determination theory perspective: Definitions, theory, practices, and future directions. *Contemporary Educational Psychology, 61*, 101860. https://doi.org/10.1016/j.cedpsych.2020.101860

Schiffrin, H. H., & Liss, M. (2017). The effects of helicopter parenting on academic motivation. *Journal of Child and Family Studies, 26*(5), 1472–1480.

Schiffrin, H. H., Liss, M., Miles-McLean, H., Geary, K. A., Erchull, M. J., & Tashner, T. (2014). Helping or hovering? The effects of helicopter parenting on college students' well-being. *Journal of Child and Family Studies, 23*(3), 548–557.

Schunk, D. H., & DiBenedetto, M. K. (2020). Motivation and social cognitive theory. *Contemporary Educational Psychology, 60*, 101832. https://doi.org/10.1016/j.cedpsych.2019.101832

Schunk, D. H., Meece, J. L., & Pintrich, P. R. (Eds.). (2014). *Motivation in education: Theory, research, and applications* (4th ed.). Pearson.

Sheridan, S. M., & Kim, E. M. (Eds.). (2016). *Family-school partnerships in context.* Springer.

Sheridan, S. M., Marvin, C., Knoche, L., & Edwards, C. P. (2008). Getting ready: Promoting school readiness through a relationship-based partnership model. *Early Childhood Services, Special Issue on Young Children's Relationships, 2*(3), 149–172.

Sheridan, S. M., Moen, A. L., & Knoche, L. L. (2017). Family-school partnerships in early childhood. In E. Votruba-Drzal & E. Dearing (Eds.), *The Wiley handbook of early childhood development programs, practices, and policies* (1st ed., pp. 289–309). Wiley.

Shernoff, D. J. (2010). Engagement in after-school programs as a predictor of social competence and academic performance. *American Journal of Community Psychology, 45*, 325–337.

Shernoff, D. J. (2013). *Optimal learning environments to promote student engagement.* Springer.

Shernoff, D. J., & Schmidt, J. A. (2008). Further evidence of an engagement-achievement paradox among U.S. High school students. *Journal of Youth and Adolescence, 36*, 891–903.

Shernoff, D. J., & Vandell, D. L. (2007). Engagement in after-school program activities: Quality of experience from the perspective of participants. *Journal of Youth and Adolescence, 36*(7), 891–903. https://doi.org/10.1007/s10964-007-9183-5

Shernoff, D. J., Kelly, S., Tonks, S. M., Anderson, B., Cavanagh, R. F., Sinha, S., & Abdi, B. (2016). Student engagement as a function of environmen-

tal complexity in high school classrooms. *Learning and Instruction, 43*, 52–60. https://doi.org/10.1016/j.learninstruc.2015.12.003

Shernoff, D. J., Ruzek, E. A., & Sinha, S. (2017). The influence of the high school classroom environment on learning as mediated by student engagement. *School Psychology International, 38*(2), 201–218. https://doi.org/10.1177/0143034316666413

Shonkoff, J. P. (2017). Breakthrough impacts: What science tells us about supporting early childhood development. *YC Young Children, 72*(2), 8–16.

Simon, N. S., & Johnson, S. M. (2015). Teacher turnover in high-poverty schools: What we know and can do. *Teachers College Record, 117*(3), 1–36.

Sirin, S. R., & Rogers-Sirin, L. (2004). Exploring school engagement of middle-class African American adolescents. *Youth & Society, 35*(3), 323–340.

Soni, A., & Kumari, S. (2017). The role of parental math anxiety and math attitude in their children's math achievement. *International Journal of Science and Mathematics Education, 15*(2), 331–347. https://doi.org/10.1007/s10763-015-9687-5

Svoboda, R. C., Rozek, C. S., Hyde, J. S., Harackiewicz, J. M., & Destin, M. (2016). Understanding the relationship between parental education and STEM course taking through identity-based and expectancy-value theories of motivation. *Aera Open, 2*(3), 2332858416664875. https://doi.org/10.1177/2332858416664875

Tyson, W., Lee, R., Borman, K. M., & Hanson, M. A. (2007). Science, technology, engineering, and mathematics (STEM) pathways: High school science and math coursework and postsecondary degree attainment. *Journal of Education for Students Placed at Risk (JESPAR), 12*(3), 243–270. https://doi.org/10.1080/10824660701601266

Urdan, T. C., & Bruchmann, K. (2018). Examining the academic motivation of a diverse student population: A consideration of methodology. *Educational Psychologist, 53*(2), 114–130. https://doi.org/10.1080/00461520.2018.1440234

Urdan, T. C., & Turner, J. C. (2005). Competence motivation in the classroom. In A. J. Elliot & C. S. Dweck (Eds.), *Handbook of competence and motivation* (pp. 297–317). Guilford.

Usher, E. L. (2018). Acknowledging the whiteness of motivation research: Seeking cultural relevance. *Educational Psychologist, 53*(2), 131–144.

Valenzuela, A. (1999). *Subtractive schooling: US-Mexican youth and the politics of caring.* SUNY Press.

Vandell, D. L., Shernoff, D. J., Pierce, K. M., Bolt, D. M., Dadisman, K., & Brown, B. B. (2005). Activities, engagement, and emotion in after-school programs (and elsewhere). *New Directions for Youth Development*, (105), 121–129. https://doi.org/10.1002/yd.111

Vandell, D. L., Simpkins, S. D., Pierce, K. M., Brown, B. B., Bolt, D., & Reiser, E. (2020). Afterschool programs, extracurricular activities, and unsupervised time: Are patterns of participation linked to children's academic and social well-being? *Applied Developmental Science.* https://doi.org/10.1080/1 0888691.2020.1843460. Advance online publication. Retrieved from https://escholarship.org/uc/item/17q604gf

Von Culin, K. R., Tsukayama, E., & Duckworth, A. L. (2014). Unpacking grit: Motivational correlates of perseverance and passion for long-term goals. *The Journal of Positive Psychology, 9*(4), 306–312. https://doi.org/10.1080/17439760.2014.898320

Vygotsky, L. S. (1978). *Mind in society: The development of higher psychological processes.* Harvard University Press.

Wang, M.-T., & Eccles, J. S. (2012). Social support matters: Longitudinal effects of social support on three dimensions of school engagement from middle to high school. *Child Development, 83*(3), 877–895. https://doi.org/10.1111/j.1467-8624.2012.01745.x

Wang, M.-T., & Sheikh-Khalil, S. (2014). Does parental involvement matter for student achievement and mental health in high school? *Child Development, 85*(2), 610–625. https://doi.org/10.1111/cdev.12153

Weiner, B. (1979). A theory of motivation for some classroom experiences. *Journal of Educational Psychology, 71*(1), 3–25.

Weisner, T. (2002). Ecocultural understanding of children's developmental pathways. *Human Development, 45*(4), 375–281.

Wentzel, K. R. (2016). Teacher-student relationships. In K. R. Wentzel & D. B. Miele (Eds.), *Handbook of Motivation at School* (pp. 211–230). Routledge.

Wentzel, K. R., Russell, S., & Baker, S. (2016). Emotional support and expectations from parents, teachers, and peers predict adolescent competence at school. *Journal of Educational Psychology, 108*(2), 242–255. https://doi.org/10.1037/edu0000049

White, R. W. (1959). Motivation reconsidered: The concept of competence. *Psychological Review, 66*, 297–333.

Wigfield, A., & Eccles, J. S. (2000). Expectancy-value theory of achievement motivation. *Contemporary Educational Psychology, 25*(1), 68–81.

Xu, J., & Corno, L. (1998). Case studies of families doing third grade homework. *Teachers College Record, 100*(2), 402–436.

Xu, J., & Corno, L. (2003). Family help and homework management reported by middle school students. *The Elementary School Journal, 103*(5), 503–519.

Yosso, T. J. (2005). Whose culture has capital? A critical race theory discussion of community cultural wealth. *Race, Ethnicity, and Education, 8*(1), 69–91.

Zusho, A., & Kumar, R. (2018). Critical reflections and future directions in the study of race, ethnicity, and motivation. *Educational Psychologist, 52*(2). https://doi.org/10.1080/00461520.2018.1432362

Teacher–Student Relationships, Engagement in School, and Student Outcomes

Tara L. Hofkens and Robert C. Pianta

Abstract

Classrooms are complex relational settings, and student engagement in these settings reflects relationally mediated participation in opportunities that are structured through interactions with teachers. Specifically, we posit that relationships with teachers either produce or inhibit student engagement to the extent that interactions meaningfully challenge students in a context of consistent and effective relational and instructional supports. In this chapter, we describe the Teaching Through Interactions (TTI) framework for understanding, studying, and ultimately improving engagement. Importantly, our work reflects the view that engagement is not a characteristic of a student; rather, engagement emerges in the context of interactions with their teacher, which are fundamental to the classroom setting as a developmental context for children and adolescence. Engagement, in this view, is both a mediator of impacts and an outcome in its own right that our work shows can be improved by leveraging the capacity of relationships and interactions to nurture the quality and durability of students' involvement in classroom learning. We conclude with suggestions for future research and education policy.

Introduction

Over the past three decades, there has been an explosion of interest in student engagement. Nationally, there is a pressing need to raise academic achievement, psychological wellbeing, and civic engagement and to address gaps among low-income and underrepresented children and youth (Aud et al., 2012; Carbonaro & Gamoran, 2002). Because classrooms are the primary school context in which children and adolescents develop and learn, a significant emphasis in education research and policy has been to better understand how to support student engagement in classroom learning.

Classrooms are essentially relational settings, and the mechanisms by which the time children spend engaged in a classroom are conditioned by the quality of interactions with teachers. Students spend almost one-quarter of their waking hours in classrooms, and the quality of students' interactions with teachers, on average, is modest at best (Hamre et al., 2013; Kane et al., 2014; Pianta et al., 2007) and can vary throughout the day (Brock & Curby, in press). Adolescents describe experiences that promote disengagement, a sense that classrooms and adults are disconnected from their developmental needs (e.g., Morin et al.,

T. L. Hofkens (✉) · R. C. Pianta
University of Virginia, Charlottesville, VA, USA
e-mail: th7ub@virginia.edu; rcp4p@virginia.edu

© The Author(s), under exclusive license to Springer Nature Switzerland AG 2022
A. L. Reschly, S. L. Christenson (eds.), *Handbook of Research on Student Engagement*,
https://doi.org/10.1007/978-3-031-07853-8_20

2013) and, in urban settings, many lack easy access to supportive adults or helpful feedback from teachers (Los Angeles Unified School District, 2013). In our view, students' relationships and interactions with teachers either produce or inhibit student engagement to the extent that they meaningfully challenge students in a context of consistent and effective instructional and relational supports. From this perspective, relationships between teachers and students reflect a classroom's capacity to promote development, and it is precisely in this way that relationships and interactions are keys to understanding engagement.

In this chapter, we describe three decades of work to conceptualize, measure, and improve the quality of teacher–student interactions as a framework for understanding how engagement unfolds in classrooms and how to harness the power of teacher interactions to improve students' engagement and outcomes. In what follows, we first describe the theoretical foundations of the classroom setting as a salient developmental context for children and youth. We then explain our view on student engagement and interactions, using the TTI framework for conceptualizing interaction quality in early childhood, elementary, and secondary classrooms (Hamre et al., 2013; Hamre et al., 2014; Pianta et al., 2004, 2007). Finally, we describe efforts to improve the quality of interactions by working with and supporting teachers to deepen and leverage the power of relationships to support student engagement in classroom learning. The chapter concludes with implications for education policy and future research.

Classroom Setting as a Context for Child and Adolescent Development

Research in education and child development consistently confirms that the quality of students' experiences in the classroom setting is critical, if not necessary, to determining the value of educational opportunity (e.g., Connell & Wellborn, 1991; Pianta et al., 2007). In studies that examine

the factors in education settings that contribute to academic achievement (e.g., funding, class size, teacher qualifications, curriculum), factors at the classroom level consistently account for the greatest proportion of student learning gains over and above students' prior performance and family background. These large-scale evaluations that assess the impacts of educational investments reinforce the idea that the quality of what takes place in classrooms may be the essential educational ingredient for fostering student success (e.g., Kane et al., 2014; Pianta et al., 2007, 2008a, b). Therefore, in this section, we briefly describe the ways in which the interactions that students have with teachers relate to engagement by targeting processes that foster development, relationships, and motivation; foster student motivation to engage in learning; and serve as a resource for student persistence and resilience.

Within classrooms, children's direct and interactive experiences with others form the basis for learning and development gained from spending time in those settings. Urie Bronfenbrenner, the renowned developmental psychologist, emphasized that proximal processes—or interactions between an individual and their context over time—drive human development (e.g., Bronfenbrenner & Morris, 1998). Lev Vygotsky, the Russian psychologist, described how effective social interactions "tune" to children's developmental and learning needs. Specifically, he described the "Zone of Proximal Development" as the quality of an interaction that effectively blends support and challenge to promote learning (Vygotsky, 1978, 1991; Wood et al., 1976). These theories, along with thousands of studies in education, psychology, and human development, provide conceptual and empirical support for the simple and powerful idea that the interactions that students have in class are fundamental proximal processes that contribute to growth in broad areas of development.

Although interactions are broadly developmentally salient, interactions with teachers have an outsized impact as outcomes emerge as a consequence of interactions between the capacities and skills of the person and the opportunities and resources available to them (Bronfenbrenner &

Morris, 1998; Magnusson & Stattin, 1998; Vygotsky, 1991). In the classroom, teachers structure opportunities for students to engage, and can either produce or inhibit developmental growth in the extent to which they can provide social and relational resources while challenging students on meaningful tasks. In particular, there is evidence that teacher–student interactions that foster positive relationships and critical thinking, problem-solving and communication skills predict multiple aspects of student development (e.g., Pianta & Allen, 2008; Pianta et al., 2008a; b).

Interactions are the behavioral component of a broader classroom relational system, within which the quality of teacher–student relationships is the engine. Extensive research over the past two decades consistently confirms that teachers are important attachment figures for children and adolescents in school and, as such, are in a unique position to foster students' development through interactions as relational mechanisms that shape development (see Pianta et al., 2003; Sabol & Pianta, 2012). Teacher–student relationships are conceptualized as coordinated systems consisting of (1) teacher and student beliefs and expectations about self, other, and the relationship; (2) behavioral exchanges that shape and reflect experience and beliefs; and (3) individual characteristics (e.g., temperament) and experiences (prior attachments) that shape other components (see Pianta, 1999). For example, providing an emotionally consistent and safe classroom environment in which children experience teachers' sensitive responsiveness to their individual experiences creates a secure base for children to explore and take risks behaviorally, cognitively, and socially (e.g., Ainsworth et al., 1978; Bowlby, 1969; Hamre & Pianta, 2001; Pianta, 1999). At the same time, providing feedback and scaffolding that acknowledges student perspectives and ideas contributes to the development of their aspirations and sense of belonging and competence. In this way, relational processes are foundational to qualities of persistence, motivation, and engagement that drive positive youth development.

Teacher–student interactions are a resource that enriches the skills, attitudes, and resourcefulness in engaging in class. Students who experience positive and productive interactions with their teachers acquire skills and attitudes that can help them successfully navigate academic challenges in school (Dawes & Larson, 2011; Eccles & Roeser, 2011; Wentzel, 2009). These resources include emotional support, promotion of efficacy beliefs, and instrumental support (Martin & Dowson, 2009; Wentzel, 2012). For example, teacher interactions support behavioral and emotional functioning in school and contribute to the development of perceived competencies that support high-level engagement in academics (Farb & Matjasko, 2012; Wang & Eccles, 2012a; Wentzel, 2002). Interactions with teachers serve as a positive outlet and a resource for coping with stressors adaptively (Finn & Zimmer, 2012). Students who experience positive interactions are also more likely to report their psychological needs fulfilled, making them more motivated to persist through challenging work and re-engage after setbacks or failure (Ryan & Patrick, 2001; Wang & Eccles, 2012b). Self-determination (or self-system) theory argues that students' motivation to engage in classroom learning is fostered when adults support their need to feel connected to others and a sense of competence and autonomy (Connell & Wellborn, 1991; Ryan & Deci, 2000; Skinner & Belmont, 1993). Students who enjoy and feel competent in their interactions with teachers are more likely to enlist support on academic tasks (Patrick et al., 2007; Wang & Degol, 2016).

In summary, relationships between teachers and students are foundational to a classroom's capacity to foster learning and development and, in this formulation, relationships and interactions are the key to understanding engagement.

Engagement in Classroom Settings

Engagement as a Relational Process

We define student engagement as a relational process in which the quantity and quality of students' behavioral, cognitive, and emotional involvement in the classroom setting (Skinner,

2016) emerge in the context of interactions with teachers, who activate and organize student engagement in the service of a developmental task or aim (Pianta et al., 2012). From this perspective, engagement is not a characteristic of a student. A student is not engaged or disengaged *as a person*. Instead, a student is engaged *in* or disengaged *from* activities or people within the classroom context (Hofkens & Ruzek, 2019). Student engagement emerges within this relational context; it reflects relationally mediated participation in opportunities that are structured through interactions with teachers.

Conceptually, this relational view of engagement acknowledges the multidimensional nature of student involvement in classroom learning, while highlighting the critical importance of teacher–student interactions. Both interactions and engagement have been described as separate mechanisms by which time spent in classrooms shapes student outcomes. In our view, interactions and engagement are inextricably linked: teacher relationships and interactions shape the relational environment in the classroom within which engagement emerges as a property of students' experience of that environment (Allen et al., 2011; Pianta et al., 2012). In other words, while student engagement can be described in terms of behavioral, cognitive, and emotional components, engagement is a dynamic process that unfolds within the social milieu of the classroom environment, the fabric of which is overdetermined by the quality of students' relationships and interactions with teachers.

At the same time, it should be recognized that engagement is an outcome in its own right. Initiating and sustaining involvement in classroom interactions and activities is, itself, a developmental task and skill. For the student, it reflects successfully coordinating their own ability and skill with motivation and attitudes toward learning in a rich and complex social setting (Wang & Hofkens, 2019). Under circumstances in which students are enabled to apply their skills to meaningfully challenging work, they can attain a deep state of absorption referred to as flow (Csikszentmihalyi, 1996). Flow is a state of high engagement, characterized by the simultaneous experience of concentration, interest, and enjoyment (Csikszentmihalyi & Csikzentmihaly, 1990), the experience of which is its own outcome or reward (DeCharms, 1968; Deci, 1975). The balance of challenge and skill required to achieve a flow state is fragile, and interactions with teachers play a determining role in ensuring that students' skills are neither overmatched nor underutilized during classroom work (Shernoff et al., 2014).

Trajectories of Engagement

Unfortunately, an abundance of evidence indicates that student engagement declines throughout children's and adolescents' education, with particularly steep and consequential declines after the transition from elementary to secondary school (e.g., Eccles & Roeser, 2011; Wang & Eccles, 2012a). Although some of these declines are attributed to system- or school-level factors (e.g., larger schools, a more bureaucratic education system), research consistently links these declines with changes in the relational, organizational, and instructional context of secondary classrooms (e.g., Eccles & Roeser, 2011; Wang, Chow, Hofkens, & Salmela-Aro, 2015). To start, the nature and quality of teacher–student relationships shifts dramatically from elementary to middle school. Adolescents spend less time with more teachers throughout each school day and, in class, secondary school teachers tend to be less emotionally supportive than elementary teachers (Zimmer-Gembeck et al., 2006). Lacking positive relationships with teachers is a missed opportunity for adolescents, since close teacher–student relationships is positively associated with engagement among secondary school students (Roorda et al., 2011; Roorda et al., 2017). Secondary teachers also tend to focus more on academic performance, with a particular emphasis on evaluative and social comparison-based feedback (Wang & Degol, 2016). At the same time, academic work in secondary school tends to be more passive and less cognitively demanding (Juvonen, 2007), and the content is often not presented in ways that is relevant or useful to adolescents (Eccles, 2009). Presenting and having students grapple over personally relevant, real-world information is conspicuously absent in the vast majority of classrooms (see Pianta et al., 2008a, b). Furthermore, ability grouping becomes more common in secondary school, which restricts the types and range of interactions that students experience and are exposed to in class (Crosnoe et al., 2004).

These contextual changes foster competition and undermine a sense of belonging at a time when adolescents experience a significant need for successful peer and adult relationships (Ryan & Patrick, 2001). Developmentally, adolescents are attuned to the nature and quality of social interactions, and they strive to form meaningful connections with adults and peers (Wang & Eccles, 2012a, b). Adolescents who have interactions with their teachers that meet their developmental capacities and needs and that leverage the importance of relationships maintain their motivation and achievement after the transition into secondary school (Eccles & Roeser, 2011). Conversely, young students who lack developmentally supportive interactions or, worse, have negative interactions with teachers in class, avoid or struggle to engage in classroom learning (Morrison et al., 2005). This puts students at a dual disadvantage: they fail to develop the skills and resources that support learning while withdrawing from interactions that could foster productive engagement in academics (Wang & Hofkens, 2019).

In both cases, as a mediator or as an outcome of classroom effects, supporting student engagement requires understanding relationships and their behavioral expression as embedded in interpersonal interactions in the classroom—through observation of exchanges and interpretation of their value and meaning with regard to fostering opportunity to learn and develop.

Teaching Through Interactions

Theory of Teacher–Student Interactions

Over the past three decades, our team has worked to conceptualize, measure, and improve the quality of teacher–student interactions across grade levels. A major part of that work is framed by a series of theoretical and empirical papers (Hamre et al., 2013; Hamre et al., 2014; Pianta et al., 2004, 2007) in which we describe the resulting TTI framework of effective teaching. In a very real sense, this framework provides the conceptual basis for how we define, operationalize, and measure teacher–student interaction. Informed by theories of human development, motivation, and learning science previously described, the TTI framework provides a comprehensive framework for understanding how relationships and interactions relate to student engagement.

Drawing upon the TTI and operationalizing it for purposes of assessing teacher–student interaction, the Classroom Assessment Scoring System (CLASS; Pianta et al., 2008a, b) is an observational measure of teacher–student interaction quality that aligns to the TTI framework. Specifically, the CLASS categorizes observable behaviors that reflect various types and levels of interaction quality, which is measured in the average quality of interactions observed among the teacher and students in the classroom. In theory and design, the CLASS measure is an applied reflection of the TTI, with its reliability and validity having been examined in a wide range of educational settings across the globe. These studies provide empirical support for the TTI framework and link overall and specific elements of interaction quality to a broad spectrum of developmental and educational outcomes. In this section, we describe the foundational role of relational support, relevance, and autonomy/competence supports provided by teachers as activating aspects of interaction that are incorporated into the domains of effective teaching practice. We then describe the three domains of interactions in the TTI framework and results from studies that use the CLASS to examine how interaction quality relates to classroom engagement.

Foundational Elements of Classrooms: Relationships, Relevance, and Autonomy/Competence

Changing the classroom's capacity for student engagement means understanding how to leverage the developmental salience of relationships and interactions in the classroom setting. We explained that in our view engagement emerges through a dynamic process mediated by relationships and interactions engagement in the classroom (Bronfenbrenner & Morris, 1998; Magnusson & Stattin, 1998). The activating components of the relational setting are the extent to which students experience positive relationships, that interactions reflect an openness to and understanding of what is relevant to them, and that students feel a sense of autonomy and competence.

For children and adolescents, it is fair to say that there is nothing more important to them than their relationships with others (Collins & Repinski, 1994). Regarding relationships with teachers, a large and growing body of research has highlighted the importance of *closeness* (i.e., high levels of warmth, positive affect, and approachability between student and teacher) and *conflict* (i.e., negativity and lack of rapport between student and teacher). The degree of closeness and conflict—also referred to as positive and negative teacher–student relationships—has been associated with achievement (e.g., Lippard et al., 2018; McCormick & O'Connor, 2015; Pianta & Stuhlman, 2004; Spilt et al., 2012); multiple indicators of social-behavioral development, such as sociability, internalizing behavior, externalizing behavior, and engagement in risky behavior (e.g., Heatly & Votruba-Drzal, 2017; Kobak et al., 2012; Pianta & Stuhlman, 2004; Spilt et al., 2012); and students' educational beliefs and aspirations (e.g., Clem et al., 2020; McFarland et al., 2016;

Verschueren et al., 2012). Altogether, the literature consistently confirms that the presence of positive and absence of negative relationships between teachers and students are foundational for students at every age and grade level (Roorda et al., 2011, 2017).

This general pattern of results across the K-12 years is evident when relationships are assessed through teacher report, observation, and student report as children reach adolescence (Pianta, 2006). Although much of the literature has focused on teacher report of relationship quality in the early years, investigations on the nature and developmental salience of students' relationships with teachers extend through adolescence (Allen et al., 2011), with particularly strong evidence for the importance of adolescents' perceptions of their relationships with their teachers. In a systematic review of 46 published studies about predictive associations between teacher–student relationships and engagement among adolescents, Quin (2017) found that student perceptions of higher-quality teacher–student relationships were associated cross-sectionally and longitudinally with multiple indicators of student engagement. Specifically, students who report higher-quality teacher–student relationships had higher grades, attendance, and a lower likelihood of dropping out of school. In contrast, declines in the quality of teacher–student relationships over 1–4 years were associated with commensurate declines in behavioral engagement, including attendance and compliance (De Wit et al., 2010; Wang & Eccles, 2012b). Indeed, research has found that even making modest efforts to connect with students can significantly increase student motivation and emotional wellbeing (Roeser et al., 2000; Skinner et al., 1998). Even with students whom teachers find challenging, spending a small amount of non-directive one-on-one time can decrease disruptive behavior and improve that student's orientation toward learning (Mashburn et al., 2008).

Relevance is important for all students but is a particularly important factor for adolescent engagement. Developmentally, adolescents are focused on making meaning of their lives. Research consistently shows that youth are more engaged in classes where they perceive what they are learning as relevant to their lives; and that the lack of relevance can contribute to withdraw and disengagement from learning (e.g., Assor et al., 2002; Fredricks et al., 2016). Connecting what students are learning to their personal lives can draw them in and keep them engaged in classroom learning. Tying the curriculum with real-world applications in ways that are perceived as meaningful to the student can improve classroom behavior (Allen et al., 1997) and contributes to a sense of autonomy that feeds students, intrinsic motivation to learn (Assor et al., 2002; Deci, 1975).

The importance of autonomy and competence is reflected in several theories of human development and learning. All of these perspectives agree that engagement is maximized when students are presented with meaningful challenges that stretch their knowledge and skills to just within reach in ways that maintain their sense of efficacy and control (Bandura et al., 1996; Vygotsky, 1991). In particular, adolescents feel competent and autonomous when they can express their views and make meaningful choices regarding their academic work (Niemiec & Ryan, 2009) and when the structures and scaffolds provided by teachers is not overly controlling (Wang & Holcombe, 2010). Contrary to the perception of some secondary teachers that the desire for autonomy or competence is a hindrance or burden, these developmental needs are a source of energy that teachers can channel into productive and sustained engagement in learning. Ideally, teachers interact with students in ways that provide a balance of following students lead meaningfully challenging work while using scaffolds to channel their engagement toward attaining the developmental or learning goal.

In summary, relational supports, relevance, and autonomy/competence supports are how teachers, through relationships and interactions, establish a classroom environment with a high capacity to engage students. These supports produce cycles of student engagement that effectively contribute to student performance and are reflected throughout our view of the domains of effective, high-quality interactions.

Interaction Domains

The TTI framework organizes interactions into three major domains based on the salience of specific types of interactions for student social and emotional development, self-regulation and attention, and achievement: emotional supports, classroom organization, and instructional support (Hamre et al., 2013). Together, the domains represent a latent structure of teacher–child interaction quality that can be reliably observed and is applicable from preschool through secondary school. The framework is unique in that the latent structure of teacher–student interactions is grade invariant while also allowing for developmentally relevant variation in the indicators of positive and negative interactions across grade levels and corresponding stages of children's development. In this section we briefly describe each of the domains of the TTI and their association with student engagement.

Emotional Support Interactions in the Emotional Support domain promote the sense of security necessary for students to explore novel experiences and develop connectedness to others (Pianta & Hamre, 2009). This domain builds on research of teachers as a secure base that can support risk-taking and persistence when they develop relationships with students are characterized by warmth, consistency, and structure (e.g., Ainsworth et al., 1978; Bowlby, 1969; Hamre & Pianta, 2001; Pianta, 1999). Emotionally supportive interactions also foster motivation by meeting children and adolescents' psychological needs to feel connected to others and a sense of competence and autonomy (Connell & Wellborn, 1991; Ryan & Deci, 2000; Skinner & Belmont, 1993). Students who are emotionally connected to teachers and peers demonstrate positive trajectories of social development and academic achievement (Hamre & Pianta, 2001; Harter, 1996; Ladd et al., 1999; Roeser et al., 2000; Silver et al., 2005; Wentzel, 1998).

In the TTI framework, emotional support consists of interactions that establish a positive emotional climate and are indicative of teacher sensitivity to students' emotional needs and regard for student perspectives. Emotional climate refers to the overall affective quality of the classroom social environment, specifically the presence of warm and caring interactions that establish a positive climate and the absence of punitive, agitated, or humiliating interactions that contribute to a negative climate. Teacher sensitivity refers to the timing and responsiveness to cues about student's individual emotional needs. Teacher sensitivity is critical to student engagement as it reflects the extent to which teachers elicit and sustain student involvement in classroom learning. When children and adolescents experience that their teachers are tuned in to, understand, and support their individual needs, they feel freer to explore and learn in class (Pianta et al., 2004). Students in classrooms with teachers who notice and respond to how they feel are more engaged and self-reliant in class and have lower parent-reported internalizing problems than children with less sensitive teachers (NICHD ECCRN, 2003; Rimm-Kaufman et al., 2002). Finally, regard for students' perspectives captures the extent to which the teacher orients classroom learning and interactions to the interests and motivations of their students. Interactions that elicit and incorporate student feedback and follow students' lead invite students to work with one another to take an active role in their classroom engagement (Pianta et al., 2004). While some research suggests that the optimal level of teacher control may vary depending on the learning objectives (Brophy & Good, 1986; Soar & Soar, 1979) or grade level (Valeski & Stipek, 2001), overall children and adolescents are more motivated and engaged when they experience more autonomy-supportive instruction (de Kruif et al., 2000; Gutman & Sulzby, 2000; NRC, 2004; Pianta et al., 2002).

Teachers vary in the extent to which they develop positive relationships among the students in their class (Hamre et al., 2005; Mashburn et al., 2007). Research shows that children and youth in classrooms with teachers who offer higher levels of support are more engaged in class than peers in less-supportive classrooms,

even after controlling for individual levels of teacher support (Hughes et al., 2006). In the United States, teacher support (e.g., teacher caring, involvement, and encouragement) is predictive of behavioral, emotional, and cognitive engagement (Pianta et al., 2012; Roorda et al., 2011; Wang & Eccles, 2012b; Wang & Holcombe, 2010). Among Finnish adolescents, emotionally supportive interactions with teachers are associated with students' own report of their situational engagement (Pöysä et al., 2019). Finally, in a sample of Swiss fifth graders, high levels of emotional support protected students who reported feeling emotionally disengaged from academics (i.e., reported feeling overwhelmed by schoolwork and that it was not meaningful) from developing perceptions of their teacher as unjust (Gasser et al., 2018). Furthermore, in Swedish preschools, teachers' emotional support predicted observed indicators of students' behavioral engagement over time (e.g., student focus on and participation in class; Castro et al., 2017) and a combination of positive climate, instructional learning formats, and language modeling predicted children's engagement in literacy learning (Norling et al., 2015). This research contributes to evidence that, together, relationships and the interactions that develop and reflect them serve a fundamental role in supporting student engagement.

Instructional Support Instructional support refers to the ways that teachers orchestrate and facilitate learning opportunities, including how they deliver curriculum and provide responsive, constructive feedback that emphasizes conceptual understanding and relevant knowledge or skills (Pianta & Hamre, 2009). Reflecting research in cognitive development, language development, and learning science (e.g., Carver & Klahr, 2001), the instructional support domain is a broad, cognitively focused definition of instruction. The domain includes several dimensions that describe the types of interactions that scaffold student engagement in tasks that build students' critical thinking and metacognitive skills and deep conceptual understanding of what they are learning (Bransford et al., 1999; Mayer, 2002; Veenman et al., 2005; Williams et al., 2002; Vygotsky, 1991). For example, teachers support students' concept development with activities, conversations, and behaviors that foster higher-order thinking skills and knowledge acquisition and transfer (Mayer, 2002; Pianta et al., 2004). Teachers further nurture and cement deep understanding through feedback that provides students with specific information about the content or process of learning. In the TTI framework, high-quality feedback goes beyond offering praise or evaluation. To provide high-quality feedback, teacher provides frequent information and back and forth exchanges to direct or sustain student engagement in ways deepen their understanding, improve their performance, or how their performance relates to their larger goals (Pianta et al., 2004).

The instructional support domain is reflected in the education policies that aim to raise learning standards and reform instruction to position and support students to actively engage in challenging academic work (e.g., Achieve, 2006). The development of Common Core and other State standards of learning (e.g., Common Core State Standards, 2015), increase in pedagogy focused on dialogue and meta-cognitive skills (see Cohen & Ball, 1999), and rise in teacher evaluation policies (Danielson, 2012; Cohen & Ball, 1999; Resnick & Resnick, 1992) all reflect student-centered approaches to learning and instruction. The difference in the TTI framework is that these interactions are situated in a broader view of interaction quality, such that they are considered alongside the relational and organizational factors that shape students' willingness and ability to engage in the opportunities provided to them.

Interactions described in the instructional support domain play a multi-purpose role in supporting student engagement. While cognitively focused, when delivered effectively, instructional support does more than support cognitive engagement in learning tasks. It also targets intrinsic motivation by providing scaffolds needed to support a sense of competence and structured dialogue and feedback in ways that support autonomy by following students lead. Instructional support also invites and sustains student engagement. In a sample of Finnish kindergarten students, for example, the quality of instructional support was positively associated with empathy and negatively associated with disruptive behavior in class (Siekkinen et al., 2013) and less task-avoidant behavior in class (Pakarinen et al., 2011). Directing the efforts of students who are already engaged contributes to learning—and interacting with students in ways that get and keep them engaged—is also crucial to their success in class.

Classroom Organization Among the interactions that establish a high-quality classroom environment, there is a particularly strong emphasis on classroom organization and management. In the TTI framework, the classroom organization domain includes interactions that promote engagement by organizing students' behavior, time, and attention (Downer et al., 2010; Emmer & Stough, 2001). The domain includes organizing interactions that research has linked with student engagement and academic achievement, including effective behavior management (Arnold et al., 1998; Emmer & Stough, 2001; Evertson & Harris, 1999), routines and management structures that maximize productivity (Bohn et al., 2004; Cameron et al., 2008), and instructional learning formats that support students active participants in classroom activities (Bowman & Stott, 1994; Bruner, 1996; Rogoff, 1990; Vygotsky, 1978). Behavior management refers specifically to interactions that promote positive behavior and prevent or stop misbehavior, including providing clear and consistent expectations and proactively monitoring student behavior to reinforce positive behavior and prevent misbehavior (Emmer & Stough, 2001; Pianta et al., 2004). Productivity includes teacher preparation, organization, and timely facilitation of activities and transitions. Instructional learning formats refer to teachers providing and facilitating active engagement in interesting activities and materials (Bowman & Stott, 1994; Bruner, 1996; Rogoff, 1990; Vygotsky, 1978).

The classroom organization domain reflects the ways in which the engagement of individual students is nested in how activities and productivity are facilitated and unfold at the classroom level. Teachers high in this dimension effectively use instruction and materials to support behavioral engagement among all of the students in their class (Rimm-Kaufman et al., 2005). In these classrooms, everyone in the class seems to know what is expected and how to go about doing it (Pianta et al., 2004). Teachers low in this dimension fail to format activities and instruction in ways that provide timely opportunities for interactions that foster engagement. They may focus on lecture or being underprepared or unorganized to support engagement in more complex activities. In these classrooms, student engagement in learning can be derailed by boredom or wasted time and energy as students search for materials, inundate the teacher for logistical support, or simply sit around. In Finland, for example, the quality of teachers' classroom organization predicted learning motivation among Finnish kindergartners (Pakarinen et al., 2011) and self-reports of behavioral and cognitive engagement among Finnish secondary students (Pöysä et al., 2019).

In summary, there is substantial support for the conceptualization of overall interaction quality and corresponding evidence of the theorized components as being impactful for student engagement.

Levels of Interaction Quality

Research from across the globe confirms that interactions are a powerful lever for supporting educational reform and excellence through improving engagement in classroom learning. In the United States and in international studies, each domain of interaction quality is associated with student engagement in classroom learning from early education through secondary school.

The potential for interactions to drive engagement is dampened, however, by the state of interaction quality across the globe. Observational studies reveal that the quality of teacher–student interactions vary widely. For example, from early education to elementary to secondary settings,

the proportion of students in classrooms that offer low levels of emotional, instructional, and organizational support far exceeds those in classrooms with high-quality interactions in those domains. In a large study of early education settings, children in only 15 percent of classrooms experienced high emotional and instructional support (NCES), and poor and African American children are more likely to experience lower-quality interactions. At the elementary level, a national study of American classrooms revealed that the quality of instructional and social support offered to young elementary school students is generally low, and even lower for less-advantaged students (NICHD ECCRN, 2003; Pianta et al., 2007; Kane & Staiger, 2012). Similarly, in a study of adolescents' experiences in more than 3000 4th–10th grade classrooms in 4 large school districts, the Measures of Effective Teaching (MET) Study (Kane et al., 2014; Kane & Staiger, 2012) found that classroom learning experiences were largely rote in nature and rarely called for reasoning, problem solving, or analytic skills; instruction was delivered primarily in large groups; content was discrete and isolated rather than made relevant and connected to other knowledge (Kane et al., 2014; Kane & Staiger, 2012).

Observational studies also suggest that variability in the quality of interactions that students experience could undermine their engagement. The quality of teacher–student interactions varies throughout the school day (Brock & Curby, in press). In middle school variation in interaction quality across teachers and within days is related to their levels of problem behavior (LoCasale-Crouch et al., 2018). While the research on consistency of interaction quality is still growing, studies on the cumulative effects of closeness or conflict with teachers over time suggest that both the level of quality and the consistency with which student experience high-quality interactions meaningfully contribute to engagement and associated outcomes over time.

In summary, in many ways the evidence on interaction quality reflects what we know about engagement: interaction quality is not as high as desired nor as high as it could be. Similarly, like student engagement, to improve interactions, teachers need targeted training and relational supports. As just a matter of context, in a national Gallup Poll (Gallup., 2014), teachers report of daily stress exceeded all other occupations surveyed (Gallup., 2014) and predictably results in higher levels of burnout (Betoret, 2009), reduced teacher self-efficacy (Klassen et al., 2012), and increased teacher attrition (Skaalvik & Skaalvik, 2011). Given these concerns, it should not be surprising that the quality of teachers' interactions with students may suffer.

Improving Teacher–Student Interactions

Evidence from our and others' efforts clearly demonstrates that interaction quality can be improved with a system of relational and learning supports for teachers and that increasing the quality of interactions contributes to subsequent improvements in student outcomes. Our team has developed and evaluated in experiments a set of interventions, that includes coaching, courses (in-person and online) and a range of video analysis and knowledge-focused activities to increase teachers' knowledge of and observation skills for identifying effective and ineffective interactions.

For example, one of these techniques uses coaches to guide the development of teachers' observation skills as they learn how to analyze video of their own or others' interactions. The My Teaching Partner (MTP) coaching model (Allen et al., 2011; Pianta, Mashburn, et al., 2008b) is a systematic professional development program designed specifically to use a supportive consulting relationship to support teachers' study of CLASS exemplars and analysis of moment-to-moment cycles of other's and their own interactions with students.

MTP coaching has been shown to produce positive growth across several features of teacher–child interaction (with a large effect size, $d = 0.77 - 0.97$; Pianta, Mashburn, et al., 2008b), particularly for teachers in high-poverty classrooms. Children whose teachers received coaching showed greater gains in literacy skills and lower levels of problem behavior (e.g., Hamre et al., 2010). In a larger-scale experimental evaluation with nearly 500 teachers in preschool programs from 10 sites, there was evidence of positive impacts on teachers' instructionally focused interactions (Downer et al., 2010), such as support for higher-order thinking skills, more intensive and frequent feedback, and support for language development (with moderately large effects, $d = 0.51–0.69$), while also improving children's multi-word language behavior and inhibitory control.

In the secondary grades, MTP was adapted (My Teaching Partner-Secondary, MTP-S) to emphasize interactions that enable autonomy, increase relevance, and integrate peers as resources (My Teaching Partner-Secondary, MTP-S) (Allen et al., 2011). In a randomized controlled evaluation, MTP-S yielded 9 percentile point gains in year-end standardized achievement tests, mediated in part by higher levels of student motivation and observed behavioral engagement (Gregory et al., 2014). Coaching significantly improved teachers' sensitivity toward students, behavioral indications of their understanding and awareness of students' perspectives, and greater use of instructional strategies focused on concepts and analysis. A modified version of MTP-S also demonstrated clear and significant benefits, this time during the first year of treatment, on students' state standardized test scores, as well as a range of observed and student-reported engagement (Allen et al., 2011). In these two controlled evaluations of interactions-focused coaching, not only were the improved quality of teacher–student interactions and a nearly 10 percentile point benefit attributed to coaching but also achievement gains were equal in magnitude across content areas (i.e., math, language arts, science, history).

The MTP interventions are also effective at addressing the racial discipline gap. MTP-S increased teachers' use of clear routines, fair implementation of rules, and proactive monitoring of behavior, which fostered respectful relationships that recognized students' needs for autonomy, leadership, relevancy, and peer interactions (Gregory et al., 2014). MTP-S coaching reduced levels of disciplinary referrals for all students and lowered the odds that African American students were referred for disciplinary reasons. In a post-MTP year with new students, African American students in the control teacher classrooms were over twice more likely to be issued a discipline referral, compared to non-African American students, a disparity that was significantly reduced for teachers who received MTP-S the prior year.

The coursework interventions are equally effective at producing improvements in teacher–student interaction. These courses (both the online and in-person versions) provide structured, didactic material to teachers that describes the TTI framework, with a large number of accompanying video clips demonstrating exemplars of effective and ineffective interactions across the TTI domains. They also include skills training that involves tagging videos to identify effective exemplars and activities that involve analysis of teachers' impacts on student engagement (Hamre et al., 2013). As evaluated in a series of experimental studies, these courses, online or in-person, have significant and large effects on improving teacher–student interactions.

In summary, there is clear evidence that interactions can be improved in ways that effectively increase the capacity of the classroom for student engagement. We hypothesize—and have heard in focus groups of participating teachers—that the relational, observational, and learning supports provided in the intervention seem to influence the behavioral, psychological, and emotional systems that shape how teachers self-regulate around their interactions with students. The CLASS observational tool serves as a "roadmap," providing a common language and landscape for teachers to improve their interactions with students.[1]

Conclusion and Future Directions

The discussion above informed the following suggestions and directions for further research in the area of teacher–student interaction and student engagement. First, it continues to be important for research to specify how engagement is positioned in their conceptual models and empirical work. It is also important to clarify what are considered indicators of engagement and to distinguish indicators of engagement from antecedents (e.g., facilitators, like teacher–student relationships or interactions) and outcomes (e.g., academic achievement) in how engagement is operationalized and measured (Lam et al., 2012; Skinner & Pitzer, 2012). In our work, engagement is situated as a mediator of classroom inputs and as a potential outcome in classrooms. In this view, relationships and interactions are not considered antecedents to engagement in the traditional temporal, linear, and causal sense. The TTI framework describes relationships and interactions as establishing the *capacity* of a classroom for student engagement; engagement emerges through the dynamic relationship between the students' capacities and skills and the relational, instructional, and organizational resources available to them (Bronfenbrenner & Morris, 1998; Magnusson & Stattin, 1998). Thus, engagement *emerges* in classrooms, with the nature and quality of engagement conditioned on the quality of interactions between teachers and students in that setting. By extension, interventions and policies that improve the quality of relationships and interactions enrich the conditions for student engagement.

An important area for future research is to examine how relationships and interactions support the emergence and coordination of subtypes of engagement. Research differs in terms of focusing on overall engagement or specifically on behavioral, cognitive, and emotional subtypes of engagement (Lam et al., 2012; Skinner & Pitzer, 2012). In light of evidence of differential associations between subtypes and specific outcomes, it is important to systematically study how we might leverage relationships and interactions in interventions targeting different types of outcomes

---

[1]Please see the Teachstone website for more information about the CLASS measures and coaching (https://teachstone.com/). Note that co-author Pianta has a financial interest in Teachstone as the distributor of CLASS-related observation and professional development materials.

(e.g., behavioral and cognitive engagement consistently predicts achievement in secondary math and science, while emotional engagement predicts with career aspirations, e.g., Wang et al., 2017). Importantly, this also means attending to how engagement is measured and from whose perspective (e.g., student report of emotional engagement in secondary math and science coursework predicts their career aspirations in these fields, but teacher report does not; Wang et al., 2016). Furthermore, subtypes of involvement in classroom learning are part of a self-system of engagement in school (Wang & Hofkens, 2019). Future research could help us understand how teacher relationships and interactions relate to students' coordinating their engagement across different components of school (Mikami et al., 2017; Wang & Hofkens, 2019).

Future research could also help us better support and understand engagement by examining how the quality of teacher–student relationships and interactions relate to student *disengagement*. Some research suggests that disengagement may represent more than the absence of engagement; that disengagement may be a distinct process that includes both the absence of positive engagement and the presence of negative engagement in class (Skinner et al., 2009; Wang et al., 2015, 2017, 2020). In this view, students who are disengaged lack sustained involvement in class and engage in maladaptive behavior (Skinner et al., 2009), which has negative consequences for outcomes that are independent from the effects of engagement (Jimerson, Campos, & Greif, 2003). Studying how relationships and interactions relate to disengagement is necessary for addressing the process by which students become alienated, disconnected, and/or withdrawn from classroom relationships and learning (Schussler, 2009; Fredricks, 2014) and can help us leverage the power of teacher interactions in classrooms to address disengagement from school (Anderson et al., 2004).

Regarding implications for policy, education policy could recognize and leverage teacher–child interactions as a powerful resource for student learning and achievement. Instead of policies that intend to improve educational opportunity by focusing on distal factors, like teachers' degrees or outcomes, such as student test scores, policies aimed at improving teacher effectiveness could focus on classroom processes that are proximal to teaching and student learning, which would increase the capacity for student engagement. For example, school reform efforts that have focused on increasing academic demands and standardized tests have strained an already overloaded education workforce. In the context of increased economic stressors placed on students, families, teachers, and communities over the past decade (Kena et al., 2014), one might characterize the rising rates of teachers' use of exclusionary discipline practices (e.g., suspension) as reflecting notable misalignment between demands on students and educators and resources that are relevant for their success (Sullivan & Bal, 2013). With 50 percent of the teaching workforce leaving the profession after 5 years, the vast majority report feeling inadequately trained to respond effectively to students' social needs and behaviors, and more than 10% of schools in America are chronically failing to engage students in productive learning opportunities (Kena et al., 2014), it is abundantly clear that policies are needed that direct investments in teachers' wellbeing and relational capacity.

In sum, we recognize the tremendous value of a focus on student engagement as a lever for improving educational opportunity and student outcomes. In the framing and analysis presented in this chapter, engagement is viewed as an emergent property of effective and supportive teacher–student interactions and relationships. Using that conceptualization for engagement and interaction, the evidence for impacts on students of improving the qualities of teacher–student interaction reinforces the value of these interactions for enhancing the capacity of classroom settings to support engaged, involved students. This framing of engagement as central to learning and as embedded in relationships and interactions forces us to understand classrooms as social systems, with consequent implications for research and policy.

References

Achieve, Inc. (2006). *Closing the expectations gap: An annual 50-state progress report on the alignment of high school policies with the demands of college and work*. Achieve. https://www.achieve.org/publications/closing-expectations-gap-2014.

Ainsworth, M. D., Blehar, M. C., Waters, E., & Wall, D. (1978). *Patterns of attachment: A psychological study of the strange situation*. Erlbaum.

Allen, J. P., Philliber, S., Herrling, S., & Kuperminc, G. P. (1997). Preventing teen pregnancy and academic failure: Experimental evaluation of a developmentally based approach. *Child Development*, 729–742. https://doi.org/10.2307/1132122

Allen, J. P., Pianta, R. C., Gregory, A., Mikami, A. Y., & Lun, J. (2011). An interaction-based approach to enhancing secondary school instruction and student achievement. *Science, 333*(6045), 1034–1037. https://doi.org/10.1126/science.1207998

Anderson, A. R., Christenson, S. L., Sinclair, M. F., & Lehr, C. A. (2004). Check & connect: The importance of relationships for promoting engagement with school. *Journal of School Psychology, 42*(2), 95–113. https://doi.org/10.1016/j.jsp.2004.01.002

Arnold, D. H., McWilliams, L., & Arnold, E. H. (1998). Teacher discipline and child misbehavior in day care: Untangling causality with correlational data. *Developmental Psychology, 34*(2), 276. https://doi.org/10.1037/0012-1649.34.2.276

Assor, A., Kaplan, H., & Roth, G. (2002). Choice is good, but relevance is excellent: Autonomy-enhancing and suppressing teacher behaviours predicting students' engagement in schoolwork. *British Journal of Educational Psychology, 72*(2), 261–278. https://doi.org/10.1348/000709902158883

Aud, S., Hussar, W., Johnson, F., Kena, G., Roth, E., Manning, E., Wang, X., & Zhang, J. (2012). *The condition of education 2012 (NCES 2012–045)*. National Center for Education Statistics.

Bandura, A., Barbaranelli, C., Caprara, G. V., & Pastorelli, C. (1996). Multifaceted impact of self-efficacy beliefs on academic functioning. *Child Development, 67*(3), 1206–1222. https://doi.org/10.1111/j.1467-8624.1996.tb01791.x

Betoret, F. D. (2009). Self-efficacy, school resources, job stressors and burnout among Spanish primary and secondary school teachers: A structural equation approach. *Educational Psychology, 29*(1), 45–68. https://doi.org/10.1080/01443410802459234

Bohn, C. M., Roehrig, A. D., & Pressley, M. (2004). The first days of school in the classrooms of two more effective and four less effective primary-grades teachers. *The Elementary School Journal, 104*(4), 269–287. https://doi.org/10.1086/499753

Bowlby, J. (1969). *Attachment and loss (Attachment, Vol. 1)*. Basic Books.

Bowman, B., & Stott, F. (1994). Understanding development in a cultural context: The challenge for teachers.

In B. Mallory & R. New (Eds.), *Diversity and developmentally appropriate practices: Challenges for early childhood education* (pp. 19–34). Teachers College Press.

Bransford, J., Brown, A. L., & Cocking, R. R. (Eds.). (1999). *How people learn: Brain, mind, experience, and school*. National Academy Press.

Brock, L. B., & Curby, T. W. (in press). Emotional support consistency and teacher-child relationships forecast social competence and problem behaviors in pre-kindergarten and kindergarten. *Early Education and Development*. 10.1080/10409289.2014.866020.

Bronfenbrenner, U., & Morris, P. A. (1998). The ecology of developmental processes. In W. Damon & R. M. Lerner (Eds.), *Handbook of child psychology (theoretical models of human development)* (Vol. 1, 5th ed., pp. 993–1029). Wiley.

Brophy, J. E., & Good, T. L. (1986). Teacher behavior and student achievement. In M. C. Wittrock (Ed.), *Handbook of research on teaching* (3rd ed., pp. 328–375). Macmillan.

Bruner, J. (1996). *The culture of education*. Harvard University Press.

Cameron, C. E., Connor, C. M., Morrison, F. J., & Jewkes, A. M. (2008). Effects of classroom organization on letter–word reading in first grade. *Journal of School Psychology, 46*(2), 173–192. https://doi.org/10.1016/j.jsp.2007.03.002

Carbonaro, W. J., & Gamoran, A. (2002). The production of achievement inequality in high school English. *American Educational Research Journal, 39*, 801–827. https://doi.org/10.3102/00028312039004801

Carver, S. M., & Klahr, D. (Eds.). (2001). *Cognition and instruction: 25 years of progress*. Erlbaum.

Castro, S., Granlund, M., & Almqvist, L. (2017). The relationship between classroom quality-related variables and engagement levels in Swedish preschool classrooms: A longitudinal study. *European Early Childhood Education Research Journal, 25*(1), 122–135. https://doi.org/10.1080/1350293X.2015.1102413

Clem, A. L., Rudasill, K. M., Hirvonen, R., Aunola, K., & Kiuru, N. (2020). The roles of teacher–student relationship quality and self-concept of ability in adolescents' achievement emotions: Temperament as a moderator. *European Journal of Psychology of Education*, 1–24. https://doi.org/10.1007/s10212-020-00473-6

Cohen, D. K., Ball, D. L., & Educational Resources Information Center (U.S.). (1999). *Instruction, capacity, and improvement*. Consortium for Policy Research in Education, University of Pennsylvania, Graduate School of Education. http://files.eric.ed.gov/fulltext/ED431749.pdf

Collins, W. A., & Repinski, D. J. (1994). Relationships during adolescence: Continuity and change in interpersonal perspective. In R. Montemayor, G. Adams, & T. P. Gullotta (Eds.), *Personal relationships during adolescence* (pp. 7–36). Sage Publications.

Common Core State Standards Initiative. (2015). *Mathematics Standards*. Retrieved from http://www.corestandards.org/

Connell, J. P., & Wellborn, J. G. (1991). Competence, autonomy, and relatedness: A motivational analysis of self-system processes. In M. Gunnar & L. A. Sroufe (Eds.), *Self-processes in development: Minnesota symposium on child psychology* (Vol. 23, pp. 43–77). Erlbaum.

Crosnoe, R., Johnson, M. K., & Elder, G. H., Jr. (2004). Intergenerational bonding in school: The behavioral and contextual correlates of student-teacher relationships. *Sociology of Education, 77*(1), 60–81. https://doi.org/10.1177/003804070407700103

Csikszentmihalyi, M. (1996). *Flow: The psychology of engagement in everyday life. The masterminds series.* Basic Books.

Csikszentmihalyi, M., & Csikzentmihaly, M. (1990). *Flow: The psychology of optimal experience (Vol. 1990).* Harper & Row.

Danielson, C. (2012). Observing classroom practice. *Educational Leadership, 70*(3), 32–37.

Dawes, N. P., & Larson, R. (2011). How youth get engaged: Grounded-theory research on motivational development in organized youth programs. *Developmental Psychology, 47*(1), 259. https://doi.org/10.1037/a0020729

de Kruif, R. E. L., McWilliam, R. A., Ridley, S. M., & Wakely, M. B. (2000). Classification of teachers' interaction behaviors in early childhood classrooms. *Early Childhood Research Quarterly, 15*, 247–268. https://doi.org/10.1016/S0885-2006(00)00051-X

De Wit, D. J., Karioja, K., & Rye, B. J. (2010). Student perceptions of diminished teacher and classmate support following the transition to high school: Are they related to declining attendance? *School Effectiveness and School Improvement, 21*(4), 451–472. https://doi.org/10.1080/09243453.2010.532010

DeCharms, R. (1968). *Personal causation: The internal effective determinants of behavior.* Academic Press.

Deci, E. L. (1975). *Intrinsic motivation.* Plenum Press.

Downer, J., Sabol, T. J., & Hamre, B. K. (2010). Teacher-child interactions in the classroom: Toward a theory of within- and cross-domain links to children's developmental outcomes. *Early Education and Development, 21*, 699–723. https://doi.org/10.1080/10409289.2010.497453

Eccles, J. (2009). Who am I and what am I going to do with my life? Personal and collective identities as motivators of action. *Educational Psychologist, 44*(2), 78–89. https://doi.org/10.1080/00461520902832368

Eccles, J. S., & Roeser, R. W. (2011). Schools as developmental contexts during adolescence. *Journal of Research on Adolescence, 21*, 225–241. https://doi.org/10.1111/j.1532-7795.2010.00725.x

Emmer, E. T., & Stough, L. M. (2001). Classroom management: A critical part of educational psychology, with implications for teacher education. *Educational Psychologist, 36*(2), 103–112. https://doi.org/10.1207/S15326985EP3602_5

Evertson, C., & Harris, A. (1999). Support for managing learning-centered classrooms: The classroom organization and management program. In H. J. Freiberg (Ed.), *Beyond behaviorism: Changing the classroom management paradigm* (pp. 59–74). Allyn & Bacon.

Farb, A. F., & Matjasko, J. L. (2012). Recent advances in research on school-based extracurricular activities and adolescent development. *Developmental Review, 32*(1), 1–48. https://doi.org/10.1016/j.dr.2011.10.001

Finn, J. D., & Zimmer, K. (2012). Student engagement: What is it? Why does it matter? In S. L. Christenson, A. L. Reschly, & C. Wylie (Eds.), *Handbook of research on student engagement* (pp. 97–132). Springer.

Fredricks, J. A. (2014). *Eight myths of student disengagement: Creating classrooms of deep learning.* Corwin Press.

Fredricks, J. A., Wang, M. T., Linn, J. S., Hofkens, T. L., Sung, H., Parr, A., & Allerton, J. (2016). Using qualitative methods to develop a survey measure of math and science engagement. *Learning and Instruction, 43*, 5–15. https://doi.org/10.1016/j.learninstruc.2016.01.009

Gallup. (2014). *State of America's schools: The path to winning again in education.* Gallup.

Gasser, L., Grütter, J., Buholzer, A., & Wettstein, A. (2018). Emotionally supportive classroom interactions and students' perceptions of their teachers as caring and just. *Learning and Instruction, 54*, 82–92.

Gregory, A., Allen, J. P., Mikami, A. Y., Hafen, C. A., & Pianta, R. C. (2014). Effects of a professional development program on behavioral engagement of students in middle and high school. *Psychology in the Schools, 51*(2), 143–163. https://doi.org/10.1002/pits.21741

Gutman, L. M., & Sulzby, E. (2000). The role of autonomy-support versus control in the emergent writing behaviors of African American kindergarten children. *Reading Research and Instruction, 39*, 170–184. https://doi.org/10.1080/19388070009558319

Hamre, B. K., & Pianta, R. C. (2001). Early teacher-child relationships and the trajectory of children's school outcomes through eighth grade. *Child Development, 72*(2), 625–638. https://doi.org/10.1111/1467-8624.00301

Hamre, B. K., & Pianta, R. C. (2010). Classroom environments and developmental processes: Conceptualization and measurement. In Handbook of research on schools, schooling, and human development (pp. 25-41). Routledge.

Hamre, B. K., Pianta, R. C., Downer, J. T., & Mashburn, A. J. (2005). Teachers' perceptions of conflict with young students: Looking beyond problem behaviors. *Social Development, 17*(1), 115–136. https://doi.org/10.1111/j.1467-9507.2007.00418.x

Hamre, B. K., Pianta, R. C., Downer, J. T., DeCoster, J., Mashburn, A. J., Jones, S. M., … Hamagami, A. (2013). Teaching through interactions: Testing a developmental framework of teacher effectiveness in over 4,000 classrooms. *The Elementary School Journal, 113*(4), 461–487. https://doi.org/10.1086/669616

Hamre, B., Hatfield, B., Pianta, R., & Jamil, F. (2014). Evidence for general and domain-specific elements of teacher–child interactions: Associations with preschool children's development. *Child Development, 85*(3), 1257–1274. https://doi.org/10.1111/cdev.12184

Harter, S. (1996). Teacher and classmate influences on scholastic motivation, self-esteem, and level of voice in adolescents. In J. Juvonen & K. Wentzel (Eds.), *Social motivation: Understanding children's school adjustment* (pp. 11–42). Cambridge University Press.

Heatly, M. C., & Votruba-Drzal, E. (2017). Parent-and teacher-child relationships and engagement at school entry: Mediating, interactive, and transactional associations across contexts. *Developmental Psychology, 53*, 1042–1062. https://doi.org/10.1037/dev0000310

Hofkens, T. L., & Ruzek, E. (2019). Measuring student engagement to inform effective interventions in schools. In *Handbook of student engagement interventions* (pp. 309–324). Academic Press.

Hughes, J. W., Zhang, D., & Hill, C. R. (2006). Peer assessment of normative and individual teacher-student support predict social acceptance and engagement among low-achieving children. *Journal of School Psychology, 43*, 447–463. https://doi.org/10.1016/j.jsp.2005.10.002

Jimerson, S. R., Campos, E., & Greif, J. L. (2003). Toward an understanding of definitions and measures of school engagement and related terms. *The California School Psychologist, 8*(1), 7–27.

Juvonen, J. (2007). Reforming middle schools: Focus on continuity, social connectedness, and engagement. *Educational Psychologist, 42*(4), 197–208. https://doi.org/10.1080/00461520701621046

Kane, T. J., & Staiger, D. O. (2012). Gathering feedback for teaching: Combining high-quality observations with student surveys and achievement gains. Research Paper. MET Project. *Bill & Melinda Gates Foundation*.

Kane, T. J., Kerr, K. A., & Pianta, R. C. (Eds.). (2014). *Designing teaching evaluation systems*. Wiley & Sons.

Kena, G., Aud, S., Johnson, F., Wang, X., Zhang, J., Rathbun, A., & Kristapovich, P. (2014). The Condition of Education 2014. NCES 2014–083. *National Center for Education Statistics*. http://files.eric.ed.gov/fulltext/ED545122.pdf

Klassen, R. M., Perry, N. E., & Frenzel, A. C. (2012). Teachers' relatedness with students: An underemphasized component of teachers' basic psychological needs. *Journal of Educational Psychology, 104*(1), 150–165. https://doi.org/10.1037/a0026253

Kobak, R., Herres, J., Gaskins, C., & Laurenceau, J. P. (2012). Teacher–student interactions and attachment states of mind as predictors of early romantic involvement and risky sexual behaviors. *Attachment & Human Development, 14*(3), 289–303. https://doi.org/10.1080/14616734.2012.672282

Ladd, G. W., Birch, S. H., & Buhs, E. S. (1999). Children's social and scholastic lives in kindergarten: Related spheres of influence? *Child Development, 70*, 1373–1400. https://doi.org/10.1111/1467-8624.00101

Lam, S., Wong, B. P. H., Yang, H., & Liu, Y. (2012). Understanding student engagement with a contextual model. In S. L. Christenson, A. L. Reschly, & C. Wylie (Eds.), *Handbook of research on student engagement* (pp. 403–419). Springer.

Lippard, C. N., La Paro, K. M., Rouse, H. L., & Crosby, D. A. (2018). A closer look at teacher-child relationships and classroom emotional context in preschool. *Child & Youth Care Forum, 47*, 1–21. https://doi.org/10.1007/s10566-017-9414-1

LoCasale-Crouch, J., Jamil, F., Pianta, R. C., Rudasill, K. M., & DeCoster, J. (2018). Observed quality and consistency of fifth graders' teacher–student interactions: Associations with feelings, engagement, and performance in school. *SAGE Open, 8*(3), 2158244018794774. https://doi.org/10.1177/2158244018794774

Los Angeles Unified School District (LAUSD). (2013). *LAUSD school experience survey*. http://home.lausd.net/apps/news/article/299935

Magnusson, D., & Stattin, H. (1998). Person-context interaction theory. In W. Damon & R. M. Learner (Eds.), *Handbook of child psychology (theoretical models of human development)* (Vol. 1, 5th ed., pp. 685–760). Wiley.

Martin, A. J., & Dowson, M. (2009). Interpersonal relationships, motivation, engagement, and achievement: Yields for theory, current issues, and educational practice. *Review of Educational Research, 79*(1), 327–365. https://doi.org/10.3102/0034654308325583

Mashburn, A. J., Hamre, B. K., Downer, J. T., & Pianta, R. C. (2007). Teacher and classroom characteristics associated with teachers' ratings of prekindergartners' relationships and behavior. *Journal of Psychoeducational Assessment, 24*, 367–380. https://doi.org/10.1177/0734282906290594

Mashburn, A. J., Pianta, R. C., Hamre, B. K., Downer, J. T., Barbarin, O., Bryant, D., Burchinal, M., Early, D., & Howes, C. (2008). Measures of classroom quality in prekindergarten and children's development of academic, language, and social skills. *Child Development, 79*, 732–749. https://doi.org/10.1111/j.1467-8624.2008.01154.x

Mayer, R. E. (2002). Rote versus meaningful learning. *Theory Into Practice, 41*, 226–233.

McCormick, M. P., & O'Connor, E. E. (2015). Teacher-child relationship quality and academic achievement in elementary school: Does gender matter? *Journal of Educational Psychology, 107*, 502. https://doi.org/10.1037/a0037457

McFarland, L., Murray, E., & Phillipson, S. (2016). Student–teacher relationships and student self-concept: Relations with teacher and student gender. *Australian Journal of Education, 60*(1), 5–25. https://doi.org/10.1177/0004944115626426

Mikami, A. Y., Ruzek, E. A., Hafen, C. A., Gregory, A., & Allen, J. P. (2017). Perceptions of relatedness with classroom peers promote adolescents' behavioral engagement and achievement in secondary school. *Journal of Youth and Adolescence, 46*(11), 2341–2354. https://doi.org/10.1007/s10964-017-0724-2

Morin, A. J., Maïano, C., Marsh, H. W., Nagengast, B., & Janosz, M. (2013). School life and adolescents' self-esteem trajectories. *Child Development, 84*(6), 1967–1988. https://doi.org/10.1111/cdev.12089

Morrison, F. J., Connor, C. M., & Bachman, H. J. (2005). The transition to school. In *Handbook of early literacy*, Dickinson, D. K. and Neuman, S. B. Guilford. Vol. 2 National Center for Education Statistics. (2003). The condition of education 2003. : U.S. Department of Education, Institute of Education Sciences.

National Research Council. (2004). *Engaging schools: Fostering high school students' motivation to learn.* National Academies Press.

NICHD Early Child Care Research Network. (2003). Social functioning in first grade: Prediction from home, childcare and concurrent school experience. *Child Development, 74*, 1639–1662. https://doi.org/10.1046/j.1467-8624.2003.00629.x

Niemiec, C. P., & Ryan, R. M. (2009). Autonomy, competence, and relatedness in the classroom: Applying self-determination theory to educational practice. *Theory and Research in Education, 7*(2), 133–144. https://doi.org/10.1177/1477878509104318

Norling, M., Sandberg, A., & Almqvist, L. (2015). Engagement and emergent literacy practices in Swedish preschools. *European Early Childhood Education Research Journal, 23*(5), 619–634. https://doi.org/10.1080/1350293X.2014.996423

Pakarinen, E., Kiurua, N., Lerkkanenb, M. K., Poikkeusb, A. M., Ahonena, T., et al. (2011). Instructional support predicts children's task avoidance in kindergarten. *Early Childhood Research Quarterly, 26*, 376–386. https://doi.org/10.1016/j.ecresq.2010.11.003

Patrick, H., Ryan, A. M., & Kaplan, A. (2007). Early adolescents' perceptions of the classroom social environment, motivational beliefs, and engagement. *Journal of Educational Psychology, 99*, 83–98. https://doi.org/10.1037/0022-0663.99.1.83

Pianta, R. C. (1999). *Enhancing relationships between children and teachers.* Washington, DC: American Psychological Association. In M. B. Shinn & H. Yoshikawa (Eds.), *Toward positive youth development: Transforming schools and community programs* (pp. 21–40). Oxford University Press.

Pianta, R. B. (2006). Teacher–child relationships and early literacy. In D. K. Dickinson & S. B. Neuman (Eds.), *Handbook of early literacy research* (pp. 149–162). Guilford Press.

Pianta, R. C., & Allen, J. P. (2008). Building capacity for positive youth development in secondary school classrooms: Changing teachers' interactions with students. In M. Shinn & H. Yoshikawa (Eds.), *Toward positive youth development: Transforming schools and community programs* (pp. 21–39). Oxford University Press. https://doi.org/10.1093/acprof:oso/9780195327892.003.0002

Pianta, R. C., & Hamre, B. K. (2009). Conceptualization, measurement, and improvement of classroom processes: Standardized observation can leverage capacity. *Educational Researcher, 38*(2), 109–119. https://doi.org/10.3102/0013189X09332374

Pianta, R. C., & Stuhlman, M. W. (2004). Teacher-child relationships and children's success in the first years of school. *School Psychology Review, 33*(3), 444–458. https://doi.org/10.1080/02796015.2004.12086261

Pianta, R. C., Hamre, B., & Stuhlman, M. (2003). Relationships between teachers and children. In W. M. Reynolds & G. E. Miller (Eds.), Handbook of psychology: Educational psychology, Vol. 7, pp. 199–234). John Wiley & Sons Inc.

Pianta, R. C., La Paro, K. M., Payne, C., Cox, M., & Bradley, R. (2002). The relation of kindergarten classroom environment to teacher, family, and school characteristics and child outcomes. *The Elementary School Journal, 102*(3), 225–238. https://doi.org/10.1086/499701

Pianta, R. C., La Paro, K. M., & Hamre, B. K. (2004). *Classroom assessment scoring system [CLASS].* Unpublished measure, University of Virginia, Charlottesville, VA.

Pianta, R. C., Belsky, J., Houts, R., & Morrison, F. (2007). Opportunities to learn in America's elementary classrooms. *Science, 315*(5820), 1795–1796. https://doi.org/10.1126/science.1139719

Pianta, R. C., Belsky, J., Vandergrift, N., Houts, R., Morrison, F., & The NICHD Early Child Care Research Network. (2008a). Classroom effects on children's achievement trajectories in elementary school. *American Educational Research Journal, 45*(2), 365–397. https://doi.org/10.3102/0002831207308230

Pianta, R. C., Mashburn, A. J., Downer, J. T., Hamre, B. K., & Justice, L. (2008b). Effects of web-mediated professional development resources on teacher–child interactions in pre-kindergarten classrooms. *Early Childhood Research Quarterly, 23*(4), 431–451. https://doi.org/10.1016/j.ecresq.2008.02.001

Pianta, R. C., Hamre, B. K., & Allen, J. P. (2012). Teacher-student relationships and engagement: Conceptualizing, measuring, and improving the capacity of classroom interactions. In *Handbook of research on student engagement* (pp. 365–386). Springer.

Pöysä, S., Vasalampi, K., Muotka, J., Lerkkanen, M. K., Poikkeus, A. M., & Nurmi, J. E. (2019). Teacher–student interaction and lower secondary school students' situational engagement. *British Journal of Educational Psychology, 89*(2), 374–392. https://doi.org/10.1111/bjep.12244

Quin, D. (2017). Longitudinal and contextual associations between teacher–student relationships and student engagement: A systematic review. *Review of Educational Research, 87*(2), 345–387. https://doi.org/10.3102/0034654316669434

Resnick, L. B., & Resnick, D. P. (1992). Assessing the thinking curriculum: New tools for educational reform. In *Changing assessments* (pp. 37–75). Springer.

Rimm-Kaufman, S. E., Early, D. M., & Cox, M. J. (2002). Early behavioral attributes and teachers' sensitivity as predictors of competent behavior in the kindergarten classroom. *Journal of Applied Developmental Psychology, 23*(4), 451–470. https://doi.org/10.1016/S0193-3973(02)00128-4

Rimm-Kaufman, S. E., La Paro, K. M., Downer, J. T., & Pianta, R. C. (2005). The contribution of classroom setting and quality of instruction to children's behavior in kindergarten classrooms. *The Elementary School Journal, 105*(4), 377–394. https://doi.org/10.1086/429948

Roeser, R. W., Eccles, J. S., & Sameroff, A. J. (2000). School as a context of early adolescents' academic and social-emotional development: A summary of research findings. *The Elementary School Journal, 100*, 443–471. https://doi.org/10.1086/499650

Rogoff, B. (1990). *Apprenticeship in thinking: Cognitive development in social context.* Oxford University Press.

Roorda, D. L., Koomen, H. M., Spilt, J. L., & Oort, F. J. (2011). The influence of affective teacher–student relationships on students' school engagement and achievement: A meta-analytic approach. *Review of Educational Research, 81*(4), 493–529. https://doi.org/10.3102/0034654311421793

Roorda, D. L., Jak, S., Zee, M., Oort, F. J., & Koomen, H. M. (2017). Affective teacher–student relationships and students' engagement and achievement: A meta-analytic update and test of the mediating role of engagement. *School Psychology Review, 46*(3), 239–261. https://doi.org/10.17105/SPR-2017-0035.V46-3

Ryan, R. M., & Deci, E. L. (2000). Self-determination theory and the facilitation of intrinsic motivation, social development, and well-being. *American Psychologist, 55*(1), 68–78. https://doi.org/10.1037/0003-066X.55.1.68

Ryan, A. M., & Patrick, H. (2001). The classroom social environment and changes in adolescents' motivation and engagement during middle school. *American Educational Research Journal, 38*(2), 437–460. https://doi.org/10.3102/00028312038002437

Sabol, T. J., & Pianta, R. C. (2012). Patterns of school readiness forecast achievement and socioemotional development at the end of elementary school. *Child Development, 83*(1), 282–299. https://doi.org/10.1111/j.1467-8624.2011.01678.x

Salmela-Aro, K. (2015). Toward a new science of academic engagement. *Research in Human Development, 12*(3-4), 304–311. https://doi.org/10.1080/15427609.2015.1068038

Schussler, D. L. (2009). Beyond content: How teachers manage classrooms to facilitate intellectual engagement for disengaged students. *Theory Into Practice, 48*(2), 114–121.

Shernoff, D. J., Csikszentmihalyi, M., Schneider, B., & Shernoff, E. S. (2014). Student engagement in high school classrooms from the perspective of flow theory. In *Applications of flow in human development and education* (pp. 475–494). Springer. https://doi.org/10.1080/00405840902776376

Siekkinen, M., Pakarinen, E., Lerkkanen, M. K., Poikkeus, A. M., Salminen, J., Poskiparta, E., & Nurmi, J. E. (2013). Social competence among 6-year-old children and classroom instructional support and teacher stress.

Early Education & Development, 24(6), 877–897. https://doi.org/10.1080/10409289.2013.745183

Silver, R. B., Measelle, J., Essex, M., & Armstrong, J. M. (2005). Trajectories of externalizing behavior problems in the classroom: Contributions of child characteristics, family characteristics, and the teacher-child relationship during the school transition. *Journal of School Psychology, 43*, 39–60. https://doi.org/10.1016/j.jsp.2004.11.003

Skaalvik, E. M., & Skaalvik, S. (2011). Teacher job satisfaction and motivation to leave the teaching profession: Relations with school context, feeling of belonging, and emotional exhaustion. *Teaching and Teacher Education, 27*(6), 1029–1038. https://doi.org/10.1016/j.tate.2011.04.001

Skinner, E. A. (2016). Engagement and disaffection as central to processes of motivational resilience development. In K. Wentzel & D. Miele (Eds.), *Handbook of motivation at school* (2nd ed., pp. 145–168). Erlbaum.

Skinner, E. A., & Belmont, M. J. (1993). Motivation in the classroom: Reciprocal effects of teacher behavior and student engagement across the school year. *Journal of Educational Psychology, 85*, 571–581. https://doi.org/10.1037/0022-0663.85.4.571

Skinner, E. A., & Pitzer, J. R. (2012). Developmental dynamics of student engagement, coping, and everyday resilience. In *Handbook of research on student engagement* (pp. 21–44). Springer.

Skinner, E. A., Zimmer-Gembeck, M. J., & Connell, J. P. (1998). Individual differences in the development of perceived control. In *Monographs of the Society for Research in Child Development, Serial No. 254, Vol. 63*. The University of Chicago Press.

Skinner, E. A., Kindermann, T. A., & Furrer, C. J. (2009). A motivational perspective on engagement and disaffection: Conceptualization and assessment of children's behavioral and emotional participation in academic activities in the classroom. *Educational and Psychological Measurement, 69*(3), 493–525. https://doi.org/10.1177/0013164408323233

Soar, R., & Soar, R. (1979). Emotional climate and management. In P. Peterson & H. Walberg (Eds.), *Research on teaching: Concepts, findings, and implications* (pp. 97–119). McCutchan.

Spilt, J. L., Hughes, J. N., Wu, J. Y., & Kwok, O. M. (2012). Dynamics of teacher–student relationships: Stability and change across elementary school and the influence on children's academic success. *Child Development, 83*, 1180–1195. https://doi.org/10.1111/j.1467-8624.2012.01761.x

Sullivan, A. L., & Bal, A. (2013). Disproportionality in special education: Effects of individual and school variables on disability risk. *Exceptional Children, 79*(4), 475–494. https://doi.org/10.1177/001440291307900406

Valeski, T., & Stipek, D. (2001). Young children's feelings about school. *Child Development, 72*, 1198–1213. https://doi.org/10.1111/1467-8624.00342

Veenman, M. V., Kok, R., & Blöte, A. W. (2005). The relation between intellectual and metacognitive skills in early adolescence. *Instructional Science, 33*(3), 193–211. https://doi.org/10.1007/s11251-004-2274-8

Verschueren, K., Doumen, S., & Buyse, E. (2012). Relationships with mother, teacher, and peers: Unique and joint effects on young children's self-concept. *Attachment & Human Development, 14*(3), 233–248. https://doi.org/10.1080/14616734.2012.672263

Vygotsky, L. S. (1978). *Mind and society: The development of higher mental processes.* Harvard University Press.

Vygotsky, L. S. (1991). Genesis of the higher mental functions. In P. Light, S. Sheldon, & M. Woodhead (Eds.), *Learning to think* (pp. 32–41). Taylor & Frances/ Routledge.

Wang, M. T., & Degol, J. L. (2016). School climate: A review of the construct, measurement, and impact on student outcomes. *Educational Psychology Review, 28*(2), 315–352. 10.1007/s10648-015-9319-1.

Wang, M. T., & Eccles, J. S. (2012a). Adolescent behavioral, emotional, and cognitive engagement trajectories in school and their differential relations to educational success. *Journal of Research on Adolescence, 22*(1), 31–39. https://doi. org/10.1016/10.1111/j.1532-7795.2011.00753.x

Wang, M. T., & Eccles, J. S. (2012b). Social support matters: Longitudinal effects of social support on three dimensions of school engagement from middle to high school. *Child Development, 83*(3), 877–895. https:// doi.org/10.1111/j.1467-8624.2012.01745.x

Wang, M. T., & Hofkens, T. L. (2019). Beyond classroom academics: A school-wide and multi-contextual perspective on student engagement in school. *Adolescent Research Review, 1–15.* https://doi.org/10.1007/ s40894-019-00115-z

Wang, M. T., & Holcombe, R. (2010). Adolescents' perceptions of school environment, engagement, and academic achievement in middle school. *American Educational Research Journal, 47*(3), 633–662. https://doi.org/10.3102/0002831209361209

Wang, M. T., Chow, A., Hofkens, T., & Salmela-Aro, K. (2015). The trajectories of student emotional engagement and school burnout with academic and psychological development: Findings from Finnish adolescents. *Learning and Instruction, 36*, 57–65. https://doi.org/10.1016/j.learninstruc.2014.11.004

Wang, M. T., Fredricks, J. A., Ye, F., Hofkens, T. L., & Linn, J. S. (2016). The math and science engagement scales: Scale development, validation, and psychometric properties. *Learning and Instruction, 43*, 16–26.

Wang, M. T., Fredricks, J., Ye, F., Hofkens, T., & Linn, J. S. (2017). Conceptualization and assessment of adolescents' engagement and disengagement in school: A multidimensional school engagement scale. *European Journal of Psychological Assessment, 35*(4), 592. https://doi.org/10.1027/1015-5759/a000431

Wang, M. T., Hofkens, T., & Ye, F. (2020). Classroom quality and adolescent student engagement and performance in mathematics: A multi-method and multi-informant approach. *Journal of Youth and Adolescence, 49*(10), 1987–2002. https://doi. org/10.1007/s10964-020-01195-0

Wentzel, K. (1998). Social relationships and motivation in middle school: The role of parents, teachers, and peers. *Journal of Educational Psychology, 90*(2), 202–209. https://doi.org/10.1037/0022-0663.90.2.202

Wentzel, K. R. (2002). Are effective teachers like good parents? Teaching styles and student adjustment in early adolescence. *Child Development, 73*(1), 287–301. https://doi.org/10.1111/1467-8624.00406

Wentzel, K. R. (2009). Students' relationships with teachers as motivational contexts. In K. Wentzel & A. Wigfield (Eds.), *Handbook of motivation in school* (pp. 301–322). Erlbaum.

Wentzel, K. R. (2012). Teacher-student relationships and adolescent competence at school. In *Interpersonal relationships in education* (pp. 17–36). Brill Sense.

Williams, W. M., Blythe, T., White, N., Li, J., Gardner, H., & Sternberg, R. J. (2002). Practical intelligence for school: Developing metacognitive sources of achievement in adolescence. *Developmental Review, 22*(2), 162–210. https://doi.org/10.1006/drev.2002.0544

Wood, D., Bruner, J. S., & Ross, G. (1976). The role of tutoring in problem solving. *Journal of Child Psychology and Psychiatry, 17*(2), 89–100. https://doi. org/10.1111/j.1469-7610.1976.tb00381.x

Zimmer-Gembeck, M. J., Chipuer, H. M., Hanisch, M., Creed, P. A., & McGregor, L. (2006). Relationships at school and stage-environment fit as resources for adolescent engagement and achievement. *Journal of Adolescence, 29*(6), 911–933. https://doi. org/10.1016/j.adolescence.2006.04.008

The Role of Peer Relationships on Academic and Extracurricular Engagement in School

Casey A. Knifsend, Guadalupe Espinoza, and Jaana Juvonen

Abstract

Peer relationships are a major part of youths' experiences at school. Moreover, both close friendships and peer group affiliations are related to student engagement in school. This chapter reviews research on school belonging, friendships, and negative social experiences (e.g., rejection or bullying) as related to engagement, with discussion of effects of peer relationships for youth from historically underrepresented backgrounds. Across these sections, research on both academic and extracurricular engagement is reviewed to understand if peer relationships operate in similar ways across these two domains. The chapter concludes with a discussion of areas for future research and implications for policy and practice, with consideration of existing policies that can restrict peer relationships (e.g., academic tracking or selection of participants in extracurricular activities).

C. A. Knifsend (✉)
Department of Psychology, California State University, Sacramento, CA, USA
e-mail: casey.knifsend@csus.edu

G. Espinoza
Department of Child and Adolescent Studies, California State University, Fullerton, CA, USA

J. Juvonen
Department of Psychology, University of California, Los Angeles, CA, USA

Introduction

Peers are a major part of schooling, and most students say they like school because that is where they get to affiliate with their friends (Erath et al., 2008). Given the amount of time students spend with their classmates and friends in school, they are also likely to be influenced by them. Moreover, when students have friends and feel socially connected and supported at school, one would expect these factors to predispose them to feel positively towards academic work and other school activities. The assumption guiding this review is that friends and other peer relationships can motivate students to engage in schoolwork as well as in extracurricular activities. However, we recognize that some peers and social experiences in school can also discourage engagement. To be able to understand when and how peers matter, we review research on the positive and negative engagement "effects" of friendships, peer support, and socially marginalizing experiences, such as peer rejection and bullying.

Our review is largely based on the assumption that positive relationships with schoolmates facilitate a sense of belonging to school (Juvonen, 2006). Consistent with the path diagram below (Fig. 1), we presume that both peer rela-

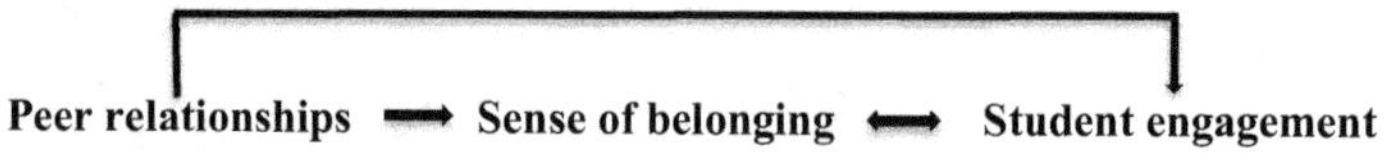

Peer relationships ➡ Sense of belonging ⬌ Student engagement

Fig. 1 Conceptual framework guiding the review of the current chapter

tionships, as well as school belonging, are related to student engagement (e.g., Kindermann et al., 1996; Voelkl, 1997). The primary focus of the current chapter is to review research that enables us to understand how different peer relationship experiences may or may not be associated with student engagement. Terms referring to school belonging and peer relationships are used broadly. For example, we use belongingness and connectedness interchangeably. The term peer relationships is used as a superordinate construct to refer to close friendships (i.e., relationships characterized by mutual liking) as well as to peer group affiliations (i.e., less tight relationships united by common interests and activities). Social status, in turn, refers to position or rank within a classroom.

We also rely on a broad and inclusive definition of engagement. Research on both academic engagement and extracurricular involvement is reviewed. Our definition of academic engagement entails a range of observable indicators, including emotional (e.g., interest, boredom), behavioral (e.g., effort, following classroom rules), and cognitive (e.g., investment in learning, preference for challenging tasks) dimensions (Fredricks et al., 2004), more so than self-reported expectations, values, and aspirations that are typically used to assess academic motivation. School-based extracurricular involvement in sports, arts, and other clubs is included for two reasons. First, by assessing both academic and non-academic engagement in school activities, we are able to determine whether peer relationships operate in similar ways across these two domains. Second, although extracurricular participation mostly involves non-academic activities, such involvement is related to academic engagement (e.g., Mahoney & Cairns, 1997). Thus, we review how peer relationships affect and are affected by extracurricular involvement in ways that can facilitate academic engagement.

Both academic and extracurricular engagement are of interest given links with adaptive academic outcomes. For instance, dimensions of behavioral, cognitive, and emotional engagement are associated with grade point average among teens (Chase et al., 2014), as well as adaptive coping (e.g., strategizing how to solve problems or seeking help from teachers or other adults) among young children (Skinner et al., 2016). Similarly, extracurricular engagement (measured by the type of activity, or duration of involvement) is linked with outcomes including higher competence, achievement, and perceived value of education (Hughes et al., 2016; Im et al., 2016).

We start the chapter with some illustrative examples of research demonstrating the links between school belonging and academic engagement as well as extracurricular involvement. We then proceed to review the ways in which the selection of friends and the influence of friends is related to students' engagement. Thereafter, the quality of the friendships and the type of support (academic vs. emotional) are discussed. Studies examining whether the size of the peer network and friendship stability are related to student engagement are also reviewed. Research on students who are rejected or bullied by their peers, in turn, captures the ways in which negative social experiences may alienate students from school and possibly increase the chances of dropping out. We also discuss whether peers are particularly salient for some youth, compared to others. The chapter ends with a discussion about future research needs and implications for school policies (e.g., academic tracking, grade retention, extracurricular practices).

This second edition chapter follows the structure of our first edition with several key revisions and additions. Our goal was to include robust findings from studies relying on larger, more diverse, and/or longitudinal samples that employ newer and sophisticated analytic techniques (e.g., social network analysis). Additions include an overview of peer influence processes including youth from historically underrepresented ethnic-racial groups and youth who have experienced adverse childhood experiences.

School Belonging

Research on school belonging presumes that environments characterized by caring and supportive relationships facilitate student engagement (e.g., Felner & Felner, 1989; Goodenow & Grady, 1993; Voelkl, 1997). Consequently, engagement can be undermined when students feel unsupported and disconnected from others (e.g., Becker & Luthar, 2002; Finn, 1989). Although both relationships with teachers and peers matter (Furrer & Skinner, 2003), the need to "fit in" with one's peers is especially pronounced during adolescence (LaFontana & Cillessen, 2010). Hence, it is not surprising that much of the existing research on school belonging has focused on middle and high school students. The following section examines evidence across development from elementary, middle, and high school, and we note where studies rely on longitudinal data.

Does Sense of Belonging Promote Academic Engagement?

Capitalizing on a large sample of over 4000 students and across 24 elementary schools, Battistich et al. (1995) investigated the association between students' sense of school community (e.g., perceptions of caring and supportive interpersonal relationships) and a range of measures tapping attitudes, motivation, and achievement. By relying on hierarchical linear modeling techniques that allow examination of students nested within schools, the findings revealed that a greater sense of community was associated with higher levels of class enjoyment and lower levels of work avoidance. Generally, stronger associations were documented in schools serving the most economically disadvantaged families, suggesting that

sense of belonging might be particularly important for students from educationally and financially disadvantaged homes.

Similarly, a sense of belonging is linked with engagement among adolescents. In one of the earliest studies on sense of belonging in middle school, a strong sense of belonging was associated with increased academic engagement (i.e., measured as the importance of schoolwork and persistence) among an ethnically diverse sample of students (Goodenow & Grady, 1993). The link between a sense of belonging at school and student engagement has been studied most extensively among high school students. Focusing on a predominantly Latino sample of urban high school seniors, school belonging was associated with more frequent classroom participation, homework completion, exam preparation, and better school attendance (Sánchez et al., 2005). Similarly, in a diverse sample assessed in the fall and spring of ninth grade, school climate (which consisted of belonging, fairness, and interracial climate as dimensions) was linked with student- (i.e., perceptions of own engagement, like paying attention in class) and teacher-rated (i.e., ratings of the student as engaged vs. disaffected from schoolwork) engagement concurrently, with a stronger link for student-rated engagement. Fall engagement, in turn, was linked with subsequent grade point average (Benner et al., 2008). Thus, a sense of belonging may facilitate the social conditions that help youth do better academically.

It is important to recognize that sense of belonging and engagement vary across individuals and also over time in complex ways. On one hand, there is evidence that year-to-year changes in engagement (i.e., perceived usefulness and intrinsic value of school) across high school are related to corresponding levels of belonging (Gillen-O'Neel & Fuligni, 2013). But research on school transitions suggests that changes in sense of belonging can affect changes in engagement in different ways. In a study of predominately Latino and African American teens, Benner et al. (2017) found that students reporting decreased belonging across the transition from middle school to high school were less engaged (e.g., perceived to pay less attention in class), compared to those reporting increased or relatively stable sense of school belonging across the transition. Thus, while a lack of sense of belonging is generally related to lower student engagement, high or stable levels of belonging across school transitions may also buffer against a declining engagement.

In sum, these findings suggest that students' sense of belonging is an important factor associated with academic involvement and engagement, especially in secondary school. Although most research in this area does not allow us to conclude that sense of belonging *causes* students to engage, there is strong support that declines in sense of belonging are related to lack of engagement. Moreover, it appears that a sense of connectedness may be particularly important for some groups of students and during normative school transitions. We now turn to examine the connections between a sense of belonging and students' levels of engagement outside of the classroom in extracurricular activities.

Is Extracurricular Participation a Way to Strengthen Sense of Belonging?

A handful of survey and qualitative studies have examined the association between belonging and students' engagement in extracurricular activities. Students with a stronger sense of school belonging are more likely to engage in activities such as after-school sports or extracurricular programs. In a study relying on daily phone interviews of African American students in sixth to ninth grade, the more time students spent on extracurricular activities, the more strongly they bonded with school (e.g., felt close to others, happy, safe, and that teachers treated students fairly; Dotterer et al., 2007).

Qualitative research provides some insights into the mechanisms through which extracurricular involvement is linked with a sense of belonging. High school girls were surveyed before and interviewed after they received notification of whether they had been selected to the cheer or dance team following competitive tryouts (Barnett, 2006). The girls who made the

team maintained their high levels of school liking (which is partly tapping school belonging), whereas school liking significantly decreased among the unsuccessful aspirants. When interviewed, one of the non-selected girls explained that one of the main reasons why she wanted to be on the dance team was "to find a way to be connected with my school", showing how success and failure can each affect connection to school. Another qualitative study conducted focus groups among Chilean teens participating in a range of mostly school-based extracurricular activities, including sports, music, and academics (Berger et al., 2020). Teens discussed themes related to a positive social climate within the activity and development of social-emotional skills. Particularly, they noted instances where lessons learned through activities transferred to the school setting, including the value of collaboration and teamwork. These studies suggest that experiences within activities are likely associated, whether directly or indirectly, with belonging.

Taken together, a sense of belonging appears to be related to a wide range of student engagement in school activities. Research on extracurricular activities provides some important insights into how engagement in turn promotes a sense of belonging, reinforcing the notion of bidirectional effects. We now turn to examine how positive peer relationships facilitate engagement. This analysis also shows why social bonds – and a corresponding sense of belonging – are not always associated with increased levels of student engagement.

Peer Selection and Socialization

To understand when socially connected youth may not engage, it is critical to understand peer selection and socialization processes. Children and youth tend to have relationships and affiliate with similar others (Laursen, 2017). That is, academically motivated students form friendships with engaged classmates, whereas unmotivated students are friends with disengaged peers. Given the similarities between friends, it is not surprising that such peer relationships amplify students' school-related behaviors, whether positive or negative (Dishion et al., 1996; Mounts & Steinberg, 1995). Whether these peer "effects" also reflect the influence of friends is at times difficult to discern based on correlational data, although more recent studies tend to rely on longitudinal data that can help address this question.

Characteristics of Peers and Academic Engagement

Earlier research in this area tested effects of selection or influence on engagement in separate investigations. Evidence for peer influence on academic engagement is seen in studies on peer networks (Cairns et al., 1989; Kindermann, 1993). For instance, when students were members of groups with high average academic engagement, their own academic engagement improved over time (Kindermann et al., 1996). Analyses of groups and group members suggest that students select peer groups, and groups welcome members based on similarities. Moreover, a range of characteristics of friends is related to academic engagement. Students with all-around adjusted friends (based on academic, social, and mental health attributes) spent more time doing homework and in extracurricular activities, and were absent less frequently, than students with friends who obtained lower grades and engaged in drug use or other misbehaviors (Cook et al., 2007).

More recently, large-scale longitudinal investigations have tested the effects of selection and influence simultaneously. A longitudinal study of Finnish 10th graders employed a social network approach to examine selection and influence effects on emotional (e.g., the perceived value of school), cognitive (i.e., effort in school), and behavioral (i.e., truancy) engagement (Wang et al., 2018). Youth nominated up to three peers with whom they most liked to spend time in the 10th and 11th grade, and together, these data were used to compare effects of selection (e.g., does similarity in engagement in 10th grade pre-

dict peer nomination in 11th grade?) and influence (e.g., do youth become more similar to those they nominated in 10th grade?). Both selection and influence effects were shown for behavioral engagement, but only influence effects were present for emotional and cognitive engagement. These results highlight both selection and influence effects operating, but these effects depend on the type of engagement under investigation.

Extracurricular Engagement: Are Friends a Reason to Get and Stay Involved?

Consistent with findings regarding academic engagement, students with friends who are involved in extracurricular activities are more likely to participate in activities themselves. An investigation in the National Longitudinal Study of Adolescent Health (Add Health) dataset surveyed seventh to 12th grade youth across an eight-month span with reciprocated nominations of their closest friends as well as participation in school-based clubs, organizations, or sports activities (Schaefer et al., 2011). Analyses employed a social network approach, accounting for multiple friendship processes (e.g., homophily or triadic closure) simultaneously. Those who were in the same activities were more likely to be friends than those who did not share a common activity, and this effect was strongest for high school students compared to middle school students. Moreover, analyses of these effects over time showed that those in the same activity at the first time point had a greater likelihood of becoming friends 8 months later, controlling for friendships at the first time point. Although this study did not test relative contributions of selection and influence per se, these findings support the idea of the selection of friends who share common activities. Given that no other studies to our knowledge test selection and influence within extracurricular activities, additional research is needed in this area to test whether effects operate similarly to academic engagement.

In sum, friends' behaviors and overall adjustment, as well as perceived behaviors and values of friends and peers, are related to student engagement. Research on the mechanisms of peer influence and selection suggests roles of each in affecting academic engagement. Similarly, those with friends involved in extracurricular activities are more likely to become friends with those sharing the same activity. What is not clear from these studies is whether the quality of friendships and type of peer support might also be linked with engagement.

Quality of Friendships and Type of Peer Support

High-quality friendships typically involve positive features such as support, companionship, and commitment, as well as low levels of conflict (Berndt, 2002). It is easy to see why these types of relationships in school would also facilitate a sense of belonging. Below, we review evidence on the connection between high-quality friendships and student engagement in schoolwork, as well as in extracurricular activities.

How Does Quality of Friendships Affect Academic Engagement?

In an ethnically diverse sample of Canadian children in kindergarten to 3rd grade assessed three times over one school year, Hosan and Hoglund (2017) measured friendship quality (i.e., closeness and conflict) and emotional and behavioral dimensions of engagement, among other variables. Cross-lagged models showed that friendship closeness was associated with higher emotional (e.g., enjoying learning new things) and behavioral (e.g., working hard) engagement over time, and friendship conflict was associated with lower emotional and behavioral engagement. Earlier behavioral engagement, in turn, predicted greater friendship closeness, as well as lower friendship conflict. Similar findings have been shown in studies of seventh and eighth graders (Berndt & Keefe, 1995), where the perceived quality of the friendship predicted changes in

self-reported behaviors (involvement and disruptiveness) across the school year. Students with a supportive, intimate, and validating closest friend became more involved in class across the school year. In contrast, students whose closest friendship involved frequent conflict and rivalry or competition increased in disruptive behavior during the school year. These results highlight that it is not only the behaviors of friends but also the relationship qualities of the friendships that matter.

In addition to individual-level friendships, school-level friendship quality and academic engagement may also affect one's own academic engagement. A large-scale, longitudinal study assessed how individual- and school-level characteristics in the fifth grade, including perceived friendship quality (e.g., trust and caring) and self-reported engagement behaviors, were associated with academic engagement in the sixth grade (Lynch et al., 2013). Individual-level friendship quality and academic engagement in fifth grade predicted sixth grade academic engagement. Over and above individual effects, school-level average friendship quality and academic engagement among all survey participants in the fifth grade were also associated with engagement. Thus, a school climate where youth experience positive peer relations and high levels of engagement is likely to bolster academic engagement, independent of the quality of individuals' specific friendships.

The *type* of peer support received might also matter, whether it is academic support or social-emotional support more broadly. Focusing on seventh grade students, Murdock (1999) demonstrated that students who reported high levels of academic support from peers were rated by their teachers as attending classes, participating in class, and completing assignments more frequently than those who did not feel academically supported by their peers. Perceived academic support from peers was also related to lower rates of discipline problems (e.g., detention, in-school suspension). While academic support might be particularly critical in allowing students to work together on homework or projects, emotional or social support might be especially critical at times of heightened distress. In concurrent and short-term longitudinal analyses (i.e., start and end of kindergarten), Ladd et al. (1996) found that when young elementary school students considered their friends as sources of aid and validation, they were particularly likely to develop positive attitudes toward school as the year progressed.

Positive Youth Development and Peer Support in Extracurricular Activities

Although relatively little is known about the relation between extracurricular involvement and peer support, it is possible that at least some types of extracurricular activities foster skills that allow students to be more supportive of one another. Activities can provide a setting for positive youth development (PYD), including competence in specific domains (e.g., social, academic), confidence, connection, character, and caring (Lerner et al., 2005). Activities may also support other skills, like empathy and stress management (e.g., Dworkin et al., 2003). Thus, the effects of extracurricular activities on academic engagement may be indirect: the personal skills and competencies to understand and support peers in distress gained in the context of extracurricular activities likely help them also to provide academic support.

Taken together, the quality of student friendships and peer support are each related to academic engagement. Students with stable, non-conflictive friendships, and who attend schools with high-quality friendships on average, are likely to engage in academic tasks. While close friends can encourage engagement, students are also likely to seek friends who can help them with academic work. Although friends are in the position to provide various types of support, not surprisingly, academic support is consistently related to academic engagement. Extracurricular involvement, in turn, may aid the ability to support others.

Does the Number of Friends and Ability to Make and Keep Friends Matter?

As shown above, school-based friendships often serve as sources of instrumental and social support. Does this mean then that students with larger friendship networks are more engaged in school?

Size of Friendship Networks and Academic Engagement

Focusing on initial school entry in a short-term longitudinal study conducted over the course of kindergarten, Ladd (1990) found that children with multiple existing friendships during school entrance developed more favorable school attitudes during the first 2 months of kindergarten, accounting for preschool experience, mental age, and gender. Those maintaining these friendships also liked school more over time. Ladd (1990) also found that children who formed new friendships during kindergarten performed better academically (as measured by teacher reports and student performance on school readiness and achievement tests) than children who did not establish friendships. New friendships accounted for a significant proportion of the variance in academic performance even when controlling for existing friendships.

In a study of students transitioning from fifth to sixth grade, Kingery and Erdley (2007) examined the role of schoolmates as students acclimate to their new middle school. Correlation analysis showed that greater peer acceptance and number of friends prior to the transition to middle school was related to greater involvement (e.g., participating in class and other school activities) at the start of the sixth grade. Hence, the ability to have friends even before the transition seems to help students when transitioning to a new school. In a longitudinal study spanning the middle school years, Lessard and Juvonen (2018) found that not only was friendship network size related to more student academic engagement, but also that friendship instability (i.e., proportion of friend losses and gains) was linked to lower academic engagement and academic performance (i.e., student GPA). Specifically, greater friendship instability in the first year of middle school was predictive of lower engagement, and this in turn was predictive of lower academic performance by the last year of middle school. Thus, the most socially skilled students (who are likely to have lots of friends and also have friendship stability) may have the easiest time navigating a new environment, and therefore, they remain highly engaged throughout the middle school years.

Although a greater number of friends might help, having one friend may be sufficient to help adjust to a new school environment. The power of one friend is highlighted in research on school transitions when students frequently experience a disruption in peer networks and loss of friends (Kenny, 1987). Linking early middle school friendships with school outcomes in a longitudinal survey study over the course of middle school, Wentzel et al. (2004) found that students with no reciprocated friends in the first year of middle school were initially more distressed and received lower grades in their school record than students with at least one friend. A significant difference in distress, but not grades, was also found in the eighth grade for those with no friends, compared to those with at least one friend. Although it is possible that a lack of friends caused distress which interfered with achievement, it is also possible that stress caused by low grades from elementary school made it hard for students to make friends. Nevertheless, this study demonstrates that an absence of even just one friend is related with compromised academic performance.

While one good friendship may be enough to get students more engaged in school, friends are not the only way to improve academic outcomes. Wentzel et al. (2004) also found that the students with no friends in the first year of middle school improved their academic performance over the course of middle school, despite initially having lower grades in sixth grade than those with friendships. It is possible that friendless students

obtain support for academic engagement from other sources (e.g., adults at school, parents). Alternatively, if it is perceived as "cool" among classmates to be disengaged (Galván et al., 2011), academically engaged students may simply not "fit in" with their classmates. In that case, it could be that lack of connections with classmates behaving in accordance with peer group norms protects engagement for some youth.

Number of Friends and Extracurricular Engagement

Research on extracurricular activities suggests that indeed one friend may be sufficient to get students engaged in non-academic activities. Huebner and Mancini (2003) showed that high school students with just one friend whom they could "count on" were more likely to report that they participate in after-school extracurricular activities (e.g., sports, clubs), regardless of whether that friend participated in that activity or not. Additionally, one study found that there may be an added benefit to participating in extracurricular activities with friends. In a study of eighth grade students, Poulin and Denault (2013) found that over 70% of students reported having friends in their activities (on average, students had about four friends participating in extracurricular activities with them), and those students with co-participating friends reported better grades (Poulin & Denault, 2013). In a study examining extracurricular activity involvement, Knifsend et al. (2018) found that middle school students with more friends engaged in extracurricular activities reported a greater sense of belongingness at school (as measured by feelings of connectedness to others at school). Moreover, school belonging mediated the link between friends' involvement in activities and student engagement (Knifsend et al., 2018). The findings highlight the importance of adolescent friendships within extracurricular engagement and how this may promote student engagement and achievement. Thus, it is possible that close friendships provide enough support and confidence for students to explore and become involved in school, much like secure attachment to a caregiver is related to exploration early in life.

Taken together, lack of close friendships is typically associated with lower student engagement (especially at times of school transitions), while the ability to develop and maintain friendships is related with academic engagement. Although a larger number of friends might increase the probability of receiving positive support for academic performance, the size of the peer network may simply reflect social skills that are particularly helpful to students during school transitions. Yet, having just one friend is enough to help students become involved in both academic and extracurricular activities. But what happens when a student is rejected or bullied in school? We now turn to research on negative social experiences with peers.

Negative Social Experiences: Rejected and Bullied Students

Given the literature covered thus far, it appears that having high quality, supportive friendships can promote school engagement behaviors possibly because such relationships help facilitate school belonging. Conversely, students who are friendless are less engaged perhaps because they feel they do not belong in school. In this section, we go beyond the lack of friends to examine how negative peer experiences (rejection and bullying) are related to academic disengagement, and potentially to alienation from school.

Peer Rejection and Engagement

Peer rejection is commonly defined as peers' social avoidance of, dislike of, or reluctance to affiliate with a student. Therefore, rejection by classmates may threaten a sense of belonging in school even more than lack of friends inasmuch as rejection affects group membership at the classroom level (cf. Furman & Robbins, 1985). Indeed, peer rejection is associated with avoidance of school, less positive perceptions about school, and lower academic performance in kin-

dergarten (Ladd, 1990), as well as lower grades in the first and second grade (O'Neil et al., 1997). In secondary school, peer rejection is related to increased absenteeism and truancy (DeRosier et al., 1994; Kupersmidt & Coie, 1990), decreased emotional school engagement (Danneel et al., 2019), and subsequent grade retention (Coie et al., 1992). It is important to note that even temporary or one-time rejection (Greenman et al., 2009) is associated with negative academic outcomes, and that negative experiences with schoolmates can also be associated with lasting disengagement (Buhs et al., 2006).

Given that aggressive students are at high risk for being rejected by classmates at least in elementary school (Asher & Coie, 1990), it is important to understand whether peer rejection (i.e., peer nomination of disliking) independently contributes to subsequent problems, or whether it functions merely as a marker of problem behaviors (Parker & Asher, 1987). Following a large sample of African American children from elementary school to middle school, Coie et al. (1992) demonstrated that childhood peer rejection (based on social preference scores calculated from peer nominations) contributed to behavior problems 3 years later, over and above earlier levels of aggression. Subsequent analyses of data from the same sample revealed that the combination of childhood aggression and peer rejection significantly increased the risk of committing assaults by the second year in high school (Coie et al., 1995). Because aggression is associated with school disengagement, independent of rejection (e.g., Lessard et al., 2008), it is, therefore, likely that rejection amplifies the risk for subsequent school disengagement.

Peer Victimization and Engagement

Consistent with the findings on rejected students, victims of bullying in elementary school are less likely to feel that they belong in school and are more likely to disengage by avoiding school (e.g., Kochenderfer & Ladd, 1996). Examining the association between bullying experiences and teacher-rated academic engagement as well as grade point average in middle school, Juvonen et al. (2011) discovered that bullied students were less engaged and obtained lower academic grades across 3 years of middle school. Although the study did not test the directionality of the associations (i.e., whether bullying experiences preceded disengagement or vice versa), the robust association between bullying experiences (regardless of whether they were assessed based on self-reports or peer nominations) and the academic indicators among an ethnically diverse sample of about 1500 students suggests that bullying cannot be ignored when trying to improve academic engagement and performance. In addition, daily diary studies have shown that Latino high school students who are bullied at school report more daily academic problems (i.e., poor performance on a test, quiz or homework; Espinoza et al., 2013) and Latino youth who are bullied online report more school attendance problems (Espinoza, 2015). Thus, increasingly longitudinal and daily methodology research has highlighted the ways in which bullying experiences may be linked to student engagement.

Evidence for both direct and mediated effects of bullying on school functioning has also been documented (e.g., Totura et al., 2013). For example, by focusing on close to 2000 ethnically diverse students in the first year of middle school, Nishina et al. (2005) found that bullying experiences at the start of the sixth grade were linked with subsequent psychological maladjustment as well as health complaints, which were related to end of the year absences and grades. At the same time, symptoms of psychological distress at the start of the sixth grade also increased the chances of students being bullied by the end of the year, which was associated with higher absences and lower grades. Hence, negative peer experiences and distress are interrelated in a cyclical manner (see also Egan & Perry, 1998) and therefore especially likely to compromise academic engagement (see also Juvonen et al., 2000).

Research has also examined the complex ways in which bullying and school climate impact student engagement. Yang et al. (2018) found that peer victimization among elementary, middle and high school students was related to multiple forms of student engagement (i.e., cognitive-behavioral engagement, emotional engagement). School climate, which included students' perceptions related to teacher relationships, fairness of rules, respect for diversity and school safety, moderated the relationship between victimization and engagement such that a positive school climate intensified the negative link between victimization and engagement. That is, if a student attends a school that is perceived as safe and positive, their experiences with bullying may be rarer, and particularly damaging to their engagement (Yang et al., 2018). A similar set of school climate moderation findings were found between adolescents' experiences with cyberbullying and engagement (Yang et al., 2020). Thus, there are likely structural and climate-specific aspects of students' school that play an important role in how these negative peer experiences relate to their engagement levels.

In sum, both peer rejection and bullying experiences are associated with lower levels of academic engagement and academic performance. It is likely that negative social experiences cause students to disengage. However, it is also possible that low performing students are bullied and rejected by their classmates. In the latter case, the odds against these students accumulate. Their distress and concerns about being ridiculed or excluded can propel students into avoiding school altogether. Thus, the associations are likely to be cyclical. Moreover, even mere concerns about rejection are related to decreased academic engagement in middle and high school. Although additional longitudinal research on this topic is warranted, there is important evidence illustrating that a sense of social alienation precedes an ultimate form of disengagement, namely dropping out of school, as summarized below.

Social Alienation and Dropping Out

Approximately one in five youth report that they dropped out of school because they felt that they did not belong at school (Doll et al., 2013). Finn (1989, 1993) proposed that the association between students not participating in school and dropping out is explained by a lack of sense of belonging and of identification with school. Consistent with this idea, an early study (Dillon & Grout, 1976) reported that students become alienated from school when they feel they are denied meaningful participation in both classroom and other school activities. A meta-analytic review of 82 correlational studies concluded that school belonging was negatively related to dropout rates (Korpershoek et al., 2020), further providing evidence that students' sense of school belonging facilitates their engagement and their commitment to school.

Extracurricular involvement may also protect youth from dropping out of school. Focusing on Mexican-American and White non-Hispanic students who were either in good academic standing or had dropped out of school, Davalos et al. (1999) found that students who had been involved in any extracurricular activity were more than twice as likely to be enrolled in school. In a prospective longitudinal study, Mahoney and Cairns (1997), in turn, demonstrated that students who participated in extracurricular activities in middle or high school were less likely to drop out of school, and effects were strongest for those at highest risk of dropping out. Similarly, Neely and Vaquera (2017) extended this research examining the impact of extracurricular participation on the likelihood of school dropout by accounting for the impact of antecedents of dropout and potential selection biases. The results from this rigorous, large nationally representative study showed that engagement in extracurricular activities was associated with a reduced likelihood of dropout, with the largest associations shown among African American students who participate in athletic activities. These findings suggest that opportunities to engage in school-related activities together with peers are critical, especially for youth who might otherwise be at risk of leaving school prematurely (Hymel et al., 1996).

Consistent with the idea about the importance of sense of belonging with one's peers, Kaplan et al. (1997) showed that in addition to low grades and lack of motivation, social alienation from school-based peer networks and relationships with deviant schoolmates during eighth

and ninth grade independently contributed to the risk of dropping out. Ties to friends in school may provide students with the connection and sense of belonging they need to continue in school. A large study with over 10,000 secondary students found that students who eventually dropped out of high school nominated fewer friends compared to students who completed school, suggesting that students who drop out experience more social isolation in school (Carbonaro & Workman, 2013). Similarly, a longitudinal study among Canadian high school students showed that reciprocal friendships were a predictor of school dropout, over and above the impact of academic motivation and teacher support (Ricard & Pelletier, 2016). Also, students who were held back during middle school were seven times more likely to drop out of school than their peers with similar academic performance who were not held back (Alexander et al., 2001). The authors concluded that this independent effect of grade retention partly reflects a lack of social integration. Hence, feeling that one does not socially "fit in" or belong is an important risk factor for dropping out.

In sum, socially alienated youth who feel that they do not belong at school are at risk of dropping out. Although both grade retention and behavior problems may in part alienate youth from their peers as well as their teachers (Juvonen, 2006), students who are bullied and rejected are a particular risk group. In addition to not retaining students, encouraging socially vulnerable youth to participate in extracurricular activities might help keep these students engaged in the schooling process.

Do Peer Effects Vary Across Groups?

Increasingly, research is demonstrating the ways in which peers may be particularly important in promoting school engagement among historically underrepresented students. Earlier, we referred to a large study of elementary school students where a greater sense of community was associated with greater enjoyment and lower work avoidance, particularly in schools serving the most economically disadvantaged students (Battistich et al., 1995). More recent findings highlight differences across ethnic-racial groups. For example, Wang and Eccles (2012) examined the impact of social support on various dimensions of school engagement across the middle and high school years and found that peer support was more strongly associated with both school identification (i.e., sense of school belonging and valuing of education) and the subjective valuing of learning among African American youth compared to European American youth. Also, in a study comprised of 527 academically at-risk adolescents, Hughes et al. (2015) found that increases in school belonging from fifth to eighth grade predicted achievement for African American students, but not for Euro-American students. The authors noted that it may be especially important to maintain a sense of school belonging (i.e., perceived acceptance at school, feelings of respect and encouragement from teachers) for students who typically face more challenges within the school context. Also, Moses and Villodas (2017) found that positive peer factors such as peer companionship were protective against the negative impact of adverse childhood experiences on perceptions of school importance (measured by adolescents' response to how important it is for them to do well in school). Conversely, negative peer factors such as peer conflict exacerbated the impact of adverse childhood experiences on school dropout contemplation. Taken together, these studies point to the potential value of identifying strategies that boost school belonging via peer connections to reduce engagement and school completion disparities. More research is needed to better understand group variations in how peer factors and belongingness relate to engagement.

Final Conclusions

We have reviewed evidence suggesting that the way students feel about "fitting in" or belonging with their schoolmates is associated with their level of engagement in school. Let us now summarize some of our main conclusions and point out questions that need to be further examined.

Summary of Positive Peer "Effects"

Relationships with friends who are academically engaged in school are associated with higher academic motivation and achievement. Even mere perceptions of friends' values and their academic behaviors are related to more active class participation. Friends' overall social adjustment (e.g., lack of behavior problems) is also associated with involvement in both academics and extracurricular activities. In addition to these individual-level effects, there is also evidence of school-level factors, such as average friendship quality within a grade level, that affect engagement. Although having a greater number of friends may help students get engaged in school, having just one friend helps alleviate the stress related to transitioning to a new school. Friends are typically good sources of emotional and social support; however, it is academic support that is most clearly associated with engagement behaviors, like attendance and participating in class. Extracurricular activities, in turn, provide students with opportunities to form new friendships, just as those with friends are more likely to explore new extracurricular options and stay involved. In turn, engagement in extracurricular activities is likely to feed into academic engagement. Based on the research reviewed, we conclude that friendships and peer affiliations with engaged classmates generally facilitate belonging with school that in turn promotes engagement, as suggested by the pathway depicted in the beginning of the chapter.

Summary of Negative Peer "Effects"

Not all friendships are beneficial, however. Not only do critical qualities (e.g., supportiveness, validation) of friendships vary, but also the level of support and collaboration on school assignments varies depending on the abilities and aspirations of friends. Students who have disengaged friends are unlikely to excel academically. Additionally, negative social experiences with classmates may make rejected youth seek the company of other students who misbehave and encourage bullied students to avoid school. Feelings of social alienation from school and repeated absences, in turn, increase the risk of dropping out of school. Similar to the positive "effects" noted above, there is support for school-level factors, like its climate, that are linked with engagement. Thus, particular types of friendships, lack of any friendships, as well as bullying and rejection experiences, are all related to school disengagement.

Are Peers Necessary to Maintain Engagement?

Although many students are motivated to attend school to spend time with their friends, it should be clear from the research reviewed that peers are not the only source of enhanced engagement and achievement. There is evidence that parent support and teacher support may be more important than peer support (Chen, 2005; Garcia-Reid, 2007; Wentzel, 1998). When and how these other sources of support can compensate for the support that friends provide in relation to academic engagement, or whether other sources of support can counter negative social experiences (such as bullying), are critical questions to further investigate.

The studies reviewed in this chapter also convey that not all peer relationships promote academic engagement. Clearly, there are peer groups of disengaged students whose effects are more harmful than productive. Also, while a lack of friends might be a sign of social isolation or alienation, there are students with no friends in school who do well. For some, it may be to their benefit not to form close ties with classmates who are not engaged. Moreover, youth can form valuable peer relationships outside of school. That is, neighborhood friends or friends from out-of-school activities may compensate for the lack of close ties in school. These are questions that remain to be investigated.

Implications for Future Research and School Policies

A few key longitudinal studies suggest that both selection of friends and their influence play a part in whether students engage in class or get involved in extracurricular activities. It is therefore important to consider the opportunities that schools provide for students to seek and find friends who are in the position to provide support. This is particularly critical when considering how certain educational policies and practices may restrict students' opportunities to establish and maintain positive peer relationships. Based on the current review, it seems that academic tracking is particularly problematic. In low track classrooms that often have an overrepresentation of disengaged students, youth lack opportunities to form positive peer relationships supporting academic involvement. Similar problems can arise in classrooms that segregate students with disabilities. That is, the range of potential friends is limited (Juvonen, 2018).

For extracurricular activities, in turn, selection procedures are problematic. Exclusion based on tryouts can disengage and alienate students from school. When non-selected students are the ones who need most support, an opportunity to make them feel part of the school is lost. Therefore, schools should consider offering meaningful alternative activities for students who are not among the top performers within their extracurricular activities.

The benefits of having at least one friend through the transition to a new school are consistent across studies of kindergartners to middle school students. Similarly, research on bullying suggests that one friend is enough to both decrease the risk of getting bullied and buffer the emotional distress associated with peer harassment (Hodges et al., 1999; Hodges et al., 1997). Whether one friend or *any* friend is enough in other stressful situations as well is less clear. It is therefore important to examine the potential power of one friend when youth experience academic difficulties, or when they get cut from a team. Equally important is research examining the ways in which some extracurricular involvement (e.g., team sports) might help students provide support to one another. Unless group work and other cooperative methods are used in classrooms, certain extracurricular activities may be one of the only ways to learn support giving.

Because the bodies of research on academic and extracurricular activities are largely separate, it is valuable to compare the two domains of engagement. It is interesting not only to note differences in assumptions and research traditions for each but also to learn about the generalizability of the findings across the two domains. For example, it appears that rejection by peers and exclusion from a sports team may have similarly alienating effects that are related to disengagement. Whether course selections, much like extracurricular choices, might be influenced in part by whether friends or high status (i.e., popular) peers are involved in the class is also needed to understand fully whether peers have similar effects on academic as well as extracurricular engagement. Particularly intriguing is the idea that extracurricular activities or peer relations fostered by those activities might help us explain academic engagement.

References

Alexander, K. L., Entwisle, D. R., & Kabbani, N. (2001). The dropout process in life course perspective: Early risk factors at home and school. *Teachers College Record, 103*, 760–822. https://doi.org/10.1111/0161-4681.00134

Asher, S. R., & Coie, J. D. (1990). *Peer rejection in childhood*. (S. R. Asher & J. D. Coie (Eds.)). Cambridge University Press.

Barnett, L. A. (2006). Flying high or crashing down: Girls' accounts of trying out for cheerleading and dance. *Journal of Adolescent Research, 21*, 514–541. https://doi.org/10.1177/0743558406291687

Battistich, V., Solomon, D., Kim, D., Watson, M., & Schaps, E. (1995). Schools as communities, poverty levels of student populations, and students' attitudes, motives and performance: A multilevel analysis. *American Educational Research Journal, 32*, 627–658. https://doi.org/10.2307/1163326

Becker, B. E., & Luthar, S. S. (2002). Social-emotional factors affecting achievement outcomes among disadvantaged students: Closing the achievement gap. *Educational Psychologist, 37*(4), 197–214. https://doi.org/10.1207/S15326985EP3704_1

Benner, A. D., Graham, S., & Mistry, R. S. (2008). Discerning direct and mediated effects of ecological structures and processes on adolescents' educational outcomes. *Developmental Psychology, 44*(3), 840–854. https://doi.org/10.1037/0012-1649.44.3.840

Benner, A. D., Boyle, A. E., & Bakhtiari, F. (2017). Understanding students' transition to high school: Demographic variation and the role of supportive relationships. *Journal of Youth and Adolescence, 46*(10), 2129–2142. https://doi.org/10.1007/s10964-017-0716-2

Berger, C., Deutsch, N., Cuadros, O., Franco, E., Rojas, M., Roux, G., & Sánchez, F. (2020). Adolescent peer processes in extracurricular activities: Identifying developmental opportunities. *Children & Youth Services Review, 118*, N.PAG. https://doi.org/10.1016/j.childyouth.2020.105457

Berndt, T. J. (2002). Friendship quality and social development. *Current Directions in Psychological Science, 11*, 7–10. https://doi.org/10.1111/1467-8721.00157

Berndt, T. J., & Keefe, K. (1995). Friends' influence on adolescents' adjustment to school. *Child Development, 66*, 1312–1329. https://doi.org/10.2307/1131649

Buhs, E. S., Ladd, G. W., & Herald, S. L. (2006). Peer exclusion and victimization: Processes that mediate the relation between peer group rejection and children's classroom engagement and achievement? *Journal of Educational Psychology, 98*, 1–13. https://doi.org/10.1037/0022-0663.98.1.1

Cairns, R. B., Cairns, B. D., & Neckerman, H. J. (1989). Early school dropout: Configurations and determinants. *Child Development, 60*, 1437–1452. https://doi.org/10.2307/1130933

Carbonaro, W., & Workman, J. (2013). Dropping out of high school: Effects of close and distant friendships. *Social Science Research, 42*, 1254–1268. https://doi.org/10.1016/j.ssresearch.2013.05.003

Chase, P., Hilliard, L., John Geldhof, G., Warren, D., & Lerner, R. (2014). Academic achievement in the high school years: The changing role of school engagement. *Journal of Youth and Adolescence, 43*(6), 884–896. https://doi.org/10.1007/s10964-013-0085-4

Chen, J. J. (2005). Relation of academic support from parents, teaches, and peers to Hong Kong adolescents' academic achievement: The mediating role of academic engagement. *Genetic, Social, and General Psychology Monographs, 131*(2), 77–127. https://doi.org/10.3200/MONO.131.2.77-127

Coie, J. D., Lochman, J., Terry, R., & Hyman, C. (1992). Predicting early adolescent disorder from childhood aggression and peer rejection. *Journal of Consulting and Clinical Psychology, 60*, 783–792. https://doi.org/10.1037/0022-006X.60.5.783

Coie, J. D., Terry, R., Lenox, K., & Lochman, J. (1995). Childhood peer rejection and aggression as predictors of stable patterns of adolescent disorder. *Development and Psychopathology, 7*, 697–713. https://doi.org/10.1017/S0954579400006799

Cook, T. D., Deng, Y., & Morgano, E. (2007). Friendship influences during early adolescence: The special role of friends' grade point average. *Journal of Research on Adolescence, 17*, 325–356. https://doi.org/10.1111/j.1532-7795.2007.00525.x

Danneel, S., Colpin, H., Goossens, L., Engels, M., Van Leeuwen, K., Van Den Noortgate, W., & Verschueren, K. (2019). Emotional school engagement and global self-esteem in adolescents: Genetic susceptibility to peer acceptance and rejection. *Merrill-Palmer Quarterly, 65*, 158–182. https://doi.org/10.13110/merrpalmquar1982.65.2.0158

Davalos, D. B., Chavez, E. L., & Guardiola, R. J. (1999). The effects of extracurricular activity, ethnic identification, and perception of school on student dropout rates. *Hispanic Journal of Behavioral Sciences, 21*, 61–77. https://doi.org/10.1177/0739986399211005

DeRosier, M. E., Kupersmidt, J. B., & Patterson, C. P. (1994). Children's academic and behavioral adjustment as a function of the chronicity and proximity of peer rejection. *Child Development, 65*, 1799–1813. https://doi.org/10.2307/1131295

Dillon, S. V., & Grout, J. A. (1976). Schools and alienation. *The Elementary School Journal, 76*, 481–489. https://doi.org/10.1086/461014

Dishion, T. J., Spracklen, K. M., Andrews, D. W., & Patterson, G. R. (1996). Deviancy training in male adolescent friendships. *Behavior Therapy, 27*, 373–390. https://doi.org/10.1016/S0005-7894(96)80023-2

Doll, J. J., Eslami, Z., & Walters, L. (2013). Understanding why students drop out of high school, according to their own reports: Are they pushed or pulled, or do they fall out? A comparative analysis of seven nationally representative studies. *SAGE Open, 3*, 1–15. https://doi.org/10.1177/2158244013503834

Dotterer, A. M., McHale, S. M., & Crouter, A. C. (2007). Implications of out-of-school activities for school engagement in African American adolescents. *Journal of Youth and Adolescence, 36*, 391–401. https://doi.org/10.1007/s10964-006-9161-3

Dworkin, J. B., Larson, R., & Hansen, D. (2003). Adolescents' accounts of growth experiences in youth activities. *Journal of Youth and Adolescence, 32*, 17–26. https://doi.org/10.1023/A:1021076222321

Egan, S. K., & Perry, D. G. (1998). Does low self-regard invite peer victimization? *Developmental Psychology, 34*, 299–309. https://doi.org/10.1037/0012-1649.34.2.299

Erath, S. A., Flanagan, K. S., & Bierman, K. L. (2008). Early adolescent school adjustment: Associations with friendship and peer victimization. *Social Development, 17*(4), 853–870. https://doi.org/10.1111/j.1467-9507.2008.00458.x

Espinoza, G. (2015). Daily cybervictimization among Latino adolescents: Links with emotional, physical and school adjustment. *Journal of Applied Developmental Psychology, 38*, 39–48. https://doi.org/10.1016/j.appdev.2015.04.003

Espinoza, G., Gonzales, N. A., & Fuligni, A. J. (2013). Daily school peer victimization experiences among Mexican-American adolescents: Associations with psychosocial, physical and school adjustment. *Journal of Youth and Adolescence, 42*, 1775–1788. https://doi.org/10.1007/s10964-012-9874-4

Felner, R. D., & Felner, T. Y. (1989). Primary prevention programs in the educational context: A transactional-ecological framework and analysis. In L. A. Bond & B. E. Compas (Eds.), *Primary prevention and promotion in the schools* (pp. 13–49). Sage.

Finn, J. D. (1989). Withdrawing from school. *Review of Educational Research, 59*, 117–142. https://doi.org/10.2307/1170412

Finn, J. D. (1993). *School Engagement & Students at Risk*. Washington DC: National Center for Education Statistics. https://eric.ed.gov/?id=ED362322

Fredricks, J. A., Blumenfeld, P. C., & Paris, A. H. (2004). School engagement: Potential of the concept, state of the evidence. *Review of Educational Research, 74*(1), 59–109. https://doi.org/10.3102/00346543074001059

Furman, W., & Robbins, P. (1985). What's the point?: Selection of treatment objectives. In B. Schneider, K. H. Rubin, & J. E. Ledingham (Eds.), *Children's peer relations: Issues in assessment and intervention* (pp. 41–54). Springer.

Furrer, C., & Skinner, E. (2003). Sense of relatedness as a factor in children's academic engagement and performance. *Journal of Educational Psychology, 95*, 148–163. https://doi.org/10.1037/0022-0663.95.1.148

Galván, A., Spatzier, A., & Juvonen, J. (2011). Perceived norms and social values to capture school culture in elementary and middle school. *Journal of Applied Developmental Psychology, 32*(6), 346–353. https://doi.org/10.1016/j.appdev.2011.08.005

Garcia-Reid, P. (2007). Examining social capital as a mechanism for improving school engagement among low income Hispanic girls. *Youth and Society, 39*(2), 164–181. https://doi.org/10.1177/0044118X07303263

Gillen-O'Neel, C., & Fuligni, A. (2013). A longitudinal study of school belonging and academic motivation across high school. *Child Development, 84*(2), 678–692. https://doi.org/10.1111/j.1467-8624.2012.01862.x

Goodenow, C., & Grady, K. E. (1993). The relationship of school belonging and friends' values to academic motivation among urban adolescent students. *Journal of Experimental Education, 62*, 60–71. https://doi.org/10.1080/00220973.1993.9943831

Greenman, P. S., Schneider, B. H., & Tomada, G. (2009). Stability and change in patterns of peer rejection: Implications for children's academic performance over time. *School Psychology International, 30*, 163–183. https://doi.org/10.1177/0143034309104151

Hodges, E. V. E., Malone, M. J., & Perry, D. G. (1997). Individual risk and social risk as interacting determinants of victimization in the peer group. *Developmental Psychology, 33*, 1032–1039. https://doi.org/10.1037/0012-1649.33.6.1032

Hodges, E. V. E., Boivin, M., Vitaro, F., & Bukowski, W. M. (1999). The power of friendship: Protection against an escalating cycle of peer victimization. *Developmental Psychology, 25*, 94–101. https://doi.org/10.1037/0012-1649.35.1.94

Hosan, N. E., & Hoglund, W. (2017). Do teacher-child relationship and friendship quality matter for children's school engagement and academic skills? *School Psychology Review, 46*(2), 201–218. https://doi.org/10.17105/SPR-2017-0043.V46-2

Huebner, A. J., & Mancini, J. A. (2003). Shaping structured out-of-school time use among youth: The effects of self, family, and friend systems. *Journal of Youth and Adolescence, 32*, 453–463. https://doi.org/10.1023/A:1025990419215

Hughes, J. N., Im, M. H., & Allee, P. J. (2015). Effect of school belonging trajectories in grades 6–8 on achievement: Gender and ethnic differences. *Journal of School Psychology, 53*, 493–507. https://doi.org/10.1016/j.jsp.2015.08.001

Hughes, J., Cao, Q., & Kwok, O. (2016). Indirect effects of extracurricular participation on academic adjustment via perceived friends' prosocial norms. *Journal of Youth and Adolescence, 45*(11), 2260–2277. https://doi.org/10.1007/s10964-016-0508-0

Hymel, S., Comfort, C., Schonert-Reichl, K., & McDougall, P. (1996). Academic failure and school dropout: The influence of peers. In K. Wentzel & J. Juvonen (Eds.), *Social motivation: Understanding children's school adjustment* (pp. 313–345). Cambridge University Press.

Im, M. H., Hughes, J. N., Cao, Q., & Kwok, O. (2016). Effects of extracurricular participation during middle school on academic motivation and achievement at Grade 9. *American Educational Research Journal, 53*(5), 1343–1375. https://doi.org/10.3102/0002831216667479

Juvonen, J. (2006). Sense of belonging, social relationships, and school functioning. In P. A. Alexander & P. H. Winne (Eds.), *Handbook of educational psychology* (2nd ed., pp. 255–674). Erlbaum.

Juvonen, J. (2018). The potential of schools to facilitate and constrain peer relationships. In W. M. Bukowski, B. Laursen, & K. H. Rubin (Eds.), *Handbook of peer interactions, relationships, and groups* (2nd ed., pp. 491–509). The Guilford Press.

Juvonen, J., Nishina, A., & Graham, S. (2000). Peer harassment, psychological adjustment, and school functioning in early adolescence. *Journal of Educational Psychology, 92*, 349–359. https://doi.org/10.1037/0022-0663.92.2.349

Juvonen, J., Wang, Y., & Espinoza, G. (2011). Bullying experiences and compromised academic performance across middle school grades. *The Journal of Early Adolescence, 31*, 152–173. https://doi.org/10.1177/0272431610379415

Kaplan, D. S., Peck, B. M., & Kaplan, H. B. (1997). Decomposing the academic failure-dropout relationship: A longitudinal analysis. *The Journal of Educational Research, 90*, 331–343. https://doi.org/10.1080/00220671.1997.10544591

Kenny, M. (1987). Family ties and leaving home for college: Recent findings and implications. *Journal of College Student Personnel, 28*, 438–442.

Kindermann, T. A. (1993). Natural peer groups as contexts for individual development: The case of children's motivation in school. *Developmental Psychology, 29*, 970–977. https://doi.org/10.1037/0012-1649.29.6.970

Kindermann, T. A., McCollam, T., & Gibson, E. (1996). Peer networks and student's classroom engagement

during childhood and adolescence. In J. Juvonen & K. Wentzel (Eds.), *Social motivation: Understanding children's school adjustment* (pp. 279–312). Cambridge University Press.

Kingery, J. N., & Erdley, C. A. (2007). Peer experiences as predictors of adjustment across the middle school transition. *Education and Treatment of Children, 30*, 73–88. https://doi.org/10.1353/etc.2007.0007

Knifsend, C. A., Camacho-Thompson, D. E., Juvonen, J., & Graham, S. (2018). Friends in activities, school-related affect, and academic outcomes in diverse middle schools. *Journal of Youth and Adolescence, 47*, 1208–1220. https://doi.org/10.1007/s10964-018-0817-6

Kochenderfer, B. J., & Ladd, G. W. (1996). Peer victimization: Cause or consequence of school maladjustment? *Child Development, 67*, 1305–1317. https://doi.org/10.2307/1131701

Korpershoek, H., Canrinus, E. T., Fokkens-Bruinsma, M., & de Boer, H. (2020). The relationships between school belonging and students' motivational, social-emotional, behavioral, and academic outcomes in secondary education: A meta-analytic review. *Research Papers in Education, 35*, 641–680. https://doi.org/10.1080/02671522.2019.1615116

Kupersmidt, J. B., & Coie, J. D. (1990). Preadolescent peer status, aggression, and school adjustment as predictors of externalizing problems in adolescence. *Child Development, 61*, 1350–1362. https://doi.org/10.2307/1130747

Ladd, G. W. (1990). Having friends, keeping friends, and being liked by peers in the classroom: Predictors of children's early school adjustment? *Child Development, 61*, 1081–1100. https://doi.org/10.2307/1130877

Ladd, G. W., Kochenderfer, B. J., & Coleman, C. C. (1996). Friendship quality as a predictor of young children's early school adjustment. *Child Development, 67*, 1103–1118. https://doi.org/10.2307/1131882

LaFontana, K. M., & Cillessen, A. H. N. (2010). Developmental changes in the priority of perceived status in childhood and adolescence. *Social Development, 19*(1), 130–147. https://doi.org/10.1111/j.1467-9507.2008.00522.x

Laursen, B. (2017). Making and keeping friends: The importance of being similar. *Child Development Perspectives, 11*, 282–289. https://doi.org/10.1111/cdep.12246

Lerner, R. M., Lerner, J. V., Almerigi, J. B., Theokas, C., Phelps, E., Gestsdottir, S., Naudeau, S., Jelicic, H., Alberts, A., Ma, L., Smith, L. M., Bobek, D. L., Richman-Raphael, D., Christiansen, E. D., & von Eye, A. (2005). Positive youth development, participation in community youth development programs, and community contributions of fifth-grade adolescents: Findings from the first wave of the 4-H study of positive youth development. *Journal of Early Adolescence, 25*(1), 17–71. https://doi.org/10.1177/0272431604273211

Lessard, L., & Juvonen, J. (2018). Losing and gaining friends: Does friendship instability compromise academic functioning in middle school? *Journal of School Psychology, 69*, 143–153. https://doi.org/10.1016/j.jsp.2018.05.003

Lessard, A., Butler-Kisber, L., Fortin, L., Marcotte, D., Potvin, P., & Royer, E. (2008). Shades of disengagement: High school dropouts speak out. *Social Psychology of Education, 11*(1), 25–42. https://doi.org/10.1007/s11218-007-9033-z

Lynch, A., Lerner, R., & Leventhal, T. (2013). Adolescent academic achievement and school engagement: An examination of the role of school-wide peer culture. *Journal of Youth and Adolescence, 42*(1), 6–19. https://doi.org/10.1007/s10964-012-9833-0

Mahoney, J. L., & Cairns, R. B. (1997). Do extracurricular activities protect against early school dropout? *Developmental Psychology, 33*, 241–253. https://doi.org/10.1037/0012-1649.33.2.241

Moses, J. O., & Villodas, M. T. (2017). The potential protective role of peer relationships on school engagement in at-risk adolescents. *Journal of Youth and Adolescence, 46*, 2255–2272. https://doi.org/10.1007/s10964-017-0644-1

Mounts, N. S., & Steinberg, L. (1995). An ecological analysis of peer influence on adolescent grade point average and drug use. *Developmental Psychology, 31*, 915–922. https://doi.org/10.1037/0012-1649.31.6.915

Murdock, T. B. (1999). The social context of risk: Status and motivational predictors of alienation in middle school. *Journal of Educational Psychology, 91*, 62–75. https://doi.org/10.1037/0022-0663.91.1.62

Neely, S. R., & Vaquera, E. (2017). Making it count: Breadth and intensity of extracurricular engagement and high school dropout. *Sociological Perspectives, 60*, 1039–1062. https://doi.org/10.1177/0731121417700114

Nishina, A., Juvonen, J., & Witkow, M. R. (2005). Sticks and stones may break my bones, but names will make me feel sick: The psychosocial, somatic and scholastic consequences of peer harassment. *Journal of Clinical Child and Adolescent Psychology, 34*, 37–48. https://doi.org/10.1207/s15374424jccp3401_4

O'Neil, R., Welsh, M., Parke, R. D., Wang, S., & Strand, C. (1997). A longitudinal assessment of the academic correlates of early peer acceptance and rejection. *Journal of Clinical Child Psychology, 26*, 290–303. https://doi.org/10.1207/s15374424jccp2603_8

Parker, J. G., & Asher, S. R. (1987). Peer relations and later personal adjustment: Are low-accepted children at risk? *Psychological Bulletin, 102*, 357–389. https://doi.org/10.1037/0033-2909.102.3.357

Poulin, F., & Denault, A. S. (2013). Friendships with co-participants in organized activities: Prevalence, quality, friends' characteristics, and associations with adolescents' adjustment. In J. A. Fredricks & S. D. Simpkins (Eds.), *Organized out-of-school activities: Setting for peer relationships. New directions for child and adolescent development, 140* (pp. 19–36). Wiley Periodicals, Inc.

Ricard, N. C., & Pelletier, L. G. (2016). Dropping out of high school: The role of parent and teacher self-determination support, reciprocal friendships and academic motivation. *Contemporary Educational Psychology, 44–45*, 32–40. https://doi.org/10.1016/j.cedpsych.2015.12.003

Sánchez, B., Colón, Y., & Esparza, P. (2005). The role of sense of school belonging and gender in the academic adjustment of Latino adolescents. *Journal of Youth and Adolescence, 34*, 619–628. https://doi.org/10.1007/s10964-005-8950-4

Schaefer, D. R., Simpkins, S. D., Vest, A. E., & Price, C. D. (2011). The contribution of extracurricular activities to adolescent friendships: New insights through social network analysis. *Developmental Psychology, 47*(4), 1141–1152. https://doi.org/10.1037/a0024091

Skinner, E. A., Pitzer, J. R., & Steele, J. S. (2016). Can student engagement serve as a motivational resource for academic coping, persistence, and learning during late elementary and early middle school? *Developmental Psychology, 52*(12), 2099–2117. https://doi.org/10.1037/dev0000232

Totura, C. M. W., Karver, M. S., & Gesten, E. L. (2013). Psychological distress and student engagement as mediators of the relationship between peer victimization and achievement in middle school youth. *Journal of Youth and Adolescence, 43*, 40–52. https://doi.org/10.1007/s10964-013-9918-4

Voelkl, K. E. (1997). Identification with school. *American Journal of Education, 105*, 294–318. https://doi-org.proxy.lib.csus.edu/10.1086/444158

Wang, M.-T., & Eccles, J. S. (2012). Social support matters: Longitudinal effects of social support on three dimensions of school engagement from middle to high school. *Child Development, 83*, 877–895. https://doi.org/10.1111/j.1467-8624.2012.01745.x

Wang, M.-T., Kiuru, N., Degol, J. L., & Salmela-Aro, K. (2018). Friends, academic achievement, and school engagement during adolescence: A social network approach to peer influence and selection effects. *Learning and Instruction, 58*, 148–160. https://doi.org/10.1016/j.learninstruc.2018.06.003

Wentzel, K. R. (1998). Social relationships and motivation in middle school: The role of parents, teachers, and peers. *Journal of Educational Psychology, 90*, 202–209. https://doi.org/10.1037/0022-0663.90.2.202

Wentzel, K. R., Barry, C. M., & Caldwell, K. A. (2004). Friendships in middle school: Influences on motivation and school adjustment. *Journal of Educational Psychology, 96*, 195–203. https://doi.org/10.1037/0022-0663.96.2.195

Yang, C., Sharkey, J. D., Reed, L. A., Chen, C., & Dowdy, E. (2018). Bullying victimization and student engagement in elementary, middle, and high schools: Moderating role of school climate. *School Psychology Quarterly, 33*, 54–64. https://doi.org/10.1037/spq0000250

Yang, C., Sharkey, J. D., Reed, L. A., & Dowdy, E. (2020). Cyberbullying victimization and student engagement among adolescents: Does school climate matter? *School Psychology, 35*, 158–169. https://doi.org/10.1037/spq0000353.supp

Instruction and Student Engagement: Implications for Academic Engaged Time

Matthew K. Burns, Mallory A. Stevens, and James Ysseldyke

Abstract

Student engagement is related to various positive academic outcomes and can be facilitated by specific school structures. The current chapter hypothesizes that academic engaged time (AET) is the proportion of instructional time that students are behaviorally, cognitively, and affectively engaged, and that schools directly influence AET by facilitating engagement and determining amount of total instructional time. Several psychological theories are presented as potential foundations of AET, including Flow Theory and Instructional Level. Finally, the Planning Instruction, Managing Instruction, Delivering Instruction, and Evaluating Instruction model is presented as a framework to examine school structures and instructional practices that lead to increased AET.

M. K. Burns (✉) · M. A. Stevens
University of Missouri, Columbia, MO, USA
e-mail: burnsmk@missouri.edu;
mashx5@mail.missouri.edu

J. Ysseldyke
University of Minnesota, Minneapolis, MN, USA
e-mail: jim@umn.edu

Student Engagement, Academic Engaged Time, and Student Achievement

There is a well-established link between student engagement and academic outcomes such as school completion or dropping out (Fredricks et al., 2004). One potential reason why engagement and academic outcomes are linked is because higher levels of engagement led to increased student academic engaged time (AET), which subsequently increased achievement. The amount of instructional time has long been linked to student learning (Guida et al., 1985; Rosenshine, 1978), but more instructional time by itself did not necessarily increase student outcomes (Lopez-Agudo & Marcenaro-Gutierrez, 2020) because the relationship between the two was influenced by the nature of the classroom environment (Nomi & Allensworth, 2013; Rivkin & Schiman, 2015). The purpose of this chapter is to discuss the relationship between instructional practices and AET, and specific practices that can enhance the relationship. Next is a description of engagement and AET, theoretical underpinnings of AET, and specific school practices that facilitate AET.

Definitions of Engagement and AET

Student engagement was once a confusing and controversial term (Axelson & Flick, 2010). Research has provided some clarity, but the clarity has led to additional questions and points in need of continued research. Many have proposed engagement as a multifaceted construct (Li & Lerner, 2013) driven primarily by Fredricks et al.' (2004) classic delineation of behavioral engagement (active participation in school including academic, social, and extracurricular activities), emotional engagement (positive feelings towards teachers, classmates), and cognitive engagement (putting forth the effort needed for success). More recent engagement theorists have identified four areas of engagement that essentially kept the concepts of cognitive and behavioral engagement, reconceptualized emotional engagement as affective engagement (feelings of belonging and identification with the school), and added academic engagement (time on task, credit hours accrued, and homework completion; Reschly & Christensen, 2012). Engagement is defined for this chapter as a broad sense of an emotional connection with a school and a desire to succeed that leads to generally active participation in and completion of school activities.

A deeper understanding of student engagement has led to much clearer implications for intervening to improve engagement and subsequent student outcomes (Fredricks et al., 2019), and affective ($r = 0.22$), behavioral ($r = 0.35$), and cognitive ($r = 0.25$) engagement have been correlated to student achievement across 69 studies (Lei et al., 2018). However, a more precise understanding of student engagement has also demonstrated the need for further clarity. It was long believed, and empirically demonstrated, that student motivation led to behavior, which led to outcomes, but engagement theories have placed aspects of behavior on the motivation side of the formula and components of motivation into the behavior variable (Eccles & Wigfield, 2020).

Academic engaged time (AET; Rosenshine & Berliner, 1978) is "the proportion of instructional time during which students are cognitively and behaviorally on task or engaged in learning, as evidenced by paying attention, completing work, listening, or participating in relevant discussion" (Gettinger & Walter, 2012, p. 663). Thus, the definition of AET is the amount of time, in relation to total instructional time, that students are cognitively and behaviorally engaged. Affective engagement is also related to student achievement, but the relationship is mediated by behavioral engagement (Lee, 2014) and there is a bidirectional relationship between affective and behavioral engagement (Li & Lerner, 2013). Although related to engagement, AET is fundamentally different from student engagement because engagement is a broad or general sense of connection and AET is specific to a given task or set of tasks. Moreover, AET is also different from academic engagement because it relies on the number of instructional minutes available to the student, and academic engagement involves more general indicators than the frequency with which students are on task such as credit hours accrued and class grades (Reschly & Christensen, 2012).

Research has consistently found that AET affects positive student development. Interventions that increased AET led to immediate gains in student outcomes. For example, implementing interventions for AET with high-school and middle-school students with disabilities led to increased AET and subsequent higher long-term retention of the material learned during the instructional task (Duchaine et al., 2018), and higher ongoing classroom quiz scores (Müllerke et al., 2019). AET is also linked to long-term growth in academic achievement. A review of 38 meta-analyses found that how well a student remained on task during instruction was more closely related to student achievement than 59% of the 105 variables examined (Schneider & Preckel, 2017), perhaps because AET led to more active participation in instruction, more frequent productive teamwork in classrooms, and better self-directed learning (Rotgans & Schmidt, 2011).

In the original conceptualization of AET, it was suggested that the number of instructional minutes in which students were engaged was directly related to content covered and teacher activities (Rosenshine, 1978). As shown in Fig. 1, several environmental variables can facilitate and support cognitive and affective engagement, including school structure, teaching for relevance, and teacher support, which accounts for 46% of the variance in affective engagement, and 32% of the variance in cognitive engagement (Wang & Eccles, 2013). Affective and cognitive engagement facilitate behavioral and academic engagement, which in turn leads to AET. However, specific classroom practices (e.g., providing choice $r = 0.44$–0.59, using tasks that are challenging but provide opportunities for success $r = 0.61$, and framing goals intrinsically $\eta^2 = 0.42$–0.59) also facilitate student engagement (Guthrie et al., 2012), and school structures also directly influence the AET formula by establishing the denominator (total number of instructional minutes). Therefore, the focus of this chapter will be on school structures and instructional practices that influence AET.

Theoretical Underpinnings of AET and School Structures

There are several well-established theories that can help explain the relationship between school structures and AET including Stage Environmental Fit Theory (SEFT; Eccles & Midgley, 1989), Self-Determination Theory (SDT; Deci & Ryan, 2012), and Expectancy-Value Theory (EVT; Eccles et al., 1983). We will discuss these theories next and expand on the instructional level conceptual framework as an extension of Flow Theory (Getzels & Csikszentmihalyi, 1976). All four theories, and their implications for AET, are succinctly outlined in Table 1.

Common Theories for Student Engagement

SEFT has clear implications for emotional and cognitive engagement because it hypothesizes a varying relationship between changing school environments and evolving student psychological needs as they progress through the grades (Symonds & Hargreaves, 2016); however, the implications for behavioral engagement are less clear other than its relationship to the other aspects of engagement. SDT is more closely related to behavioral engagement because it hypothesizes that a student's desire to meet basic psychological needs (i.e., autonomy, relatedness, and competence) affects motivation, engagement, and achievement (Deci & Ryan, 2012). Moreover, EVT is more centered on student perceptions than school context because it hypothesizes that the student's expectation for success and the degree to which the student sees the task as important or interesting determine effort, but school structures can modify perceived task value and expectancy of success.

The primary theories described above tell us that student engagement is both developmental and alterable. Student engagement can change based on the environment that schools provide in relation to students' changing psychological needs as they progress through the grades (SEFT). A strong sense of self-determination can change the relationship between environmental stress and student engagement, which suggests that strengthening a student's sense of autonomy, relatedness, and competence will help facilitate school engagement (Raufelder et al., 2014). Students see intrinsic value in some tasks over others, and that value changes as the context and student experiences change (Eccles & Wigfield, 2020). Although the intrinsic value of math and science tasks predicted student behavior more than the perceived utility of the task (Galla et al., 2018), the expectancy of success was also directly linked to behavioral engagement and student achievement among elementary-aged students (Putwain et al., 2019), and environmental variables can change the expectancy of success (Magidson et al., 2014; Wigfield & Tonks, 2002).

Flow Theory and Instructional Level

Although the three theories previously described provide strong conceptual underpinnings to better understand student engagement, they have

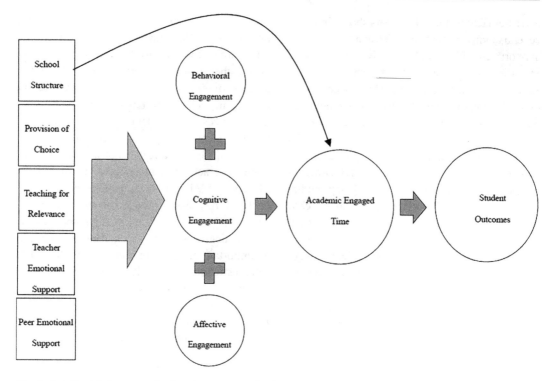

Fig. 1 Relationship between school environment, academic engaged time, and student outcomes

Table 1 Theories to explain relationship between school structures and academic engaged time (AET)

Theory	Definition	Implications for AET
Stage Environmental Fit Theory (Eccles & Midgley, 1989)	Characteristics of the individual and environment influence each other	Students have higher AET when the environment meets their developmental needs
Self-Determination Theory (Deci & Ryan, 2012)	Humans are motivated to complete tasks that are aligned with their own goals and when environmental conditions meet their basic needs	AET is influenced by student's perceptions of autonomy, competence, and relatedness
Expectancy-Value Theory (Eccles et al., 1983)	Behavior is driven by perceived probability of successfully completing the task and the value that is assigned to completing the task	AET is influenced by student interests, goals, academic self-concept, and sense of self-efficacy
Flow Theory (Getzels & Csikszentmihalyi, 1976)	People enter a mental state of complete absorption in tasks that represent optimal experiences	AET is facilitated by tasks that are challenging, but not too difficult, with clear goals and feedback

less direct implications for AET or for school practices that enhance AET. Instructional practices are linked to AET (Rosenshine, 1978). In fact, instructional practices were more closely related to AET than behavioral management practices, accounting for 12% of the variance beyond class size and lesson format, and opportunities for students to respond (OTR) was the single best predictor of AET $r = 0.30$ (Lekwa et al., 2019).

Flow Theory (FT; Getzels & Csikszentmihalyi, 1976) purports that students have an optimal experience ("deep absorption" Shernoff et al., 2014, p. 476) when they are presented with (a) "perceived challenges, or opportunities for action, that stretch but do not overmatch individual skills;" and (b) "clear proximal goals and immediate feedback about the progress being made" (Nakamura & Csikszentmihalyi, 2009, p. 195). Research with a national dataset found high levels of student engagement (self-reported interest, concentration, enjoyment, and attention throughout the school day) when the perceived challenge of the task and skill were balanced (i.e., instructional match; Treptow et al., 2007), especially for individual or group work as opposed to more passive learning activities like listening to lectures or watching videos (Shernoff et al., 2014). It seems that the idea is similar to Vygotsky's (1978) zone of proximal development, but puts less emphasis on the scaffolded support from a more knowledgeable or skilled partner. FT also focuses on task demands and how well they are matched to student skills, which is an important daily instruction task.

Instructional Level

Gickling and Armstrong (1978) attempted to operationally define Flow Theory's concept of the perceived balance between the challenge of the task and skill based on an instructional level (Betts, 1949). Their seminal research defined an instructional level as the percentage of known material within the learning task that provided the optimal balance between review and new items so that the task was not too difficult to be frustrating, but still provided an opportunity to learn. Students in the study with reading disabilities demonstrated increased AET, defined as time on task and task completion, when they accurately read 93–97% of the words correctly. Students who read less than 93% of the words correctly were reading at a frustration level and those who read more than 97% of the words correctly were reading at an independent level, both of which led to decreased AET.

The relationship between student skill and performance is curved rather than linear. The higher the student's background knowledge and skill for a specific task, then the higher the AET, but only to a point. Once the student exceeds 97% of known items within the task, AET decreases (Beck et al., 2009; Gickling & Armstrong, 1978; Treptow et al., 2007).

Gickling's definition of an instructional level provides an easily implemented framework to help facilitate increased AET. For example, the simulated data presented in Fig. 2 are from a fourth-grade male who experienced significant behavioral difficulties and who increased AET by reading at the instructional level. He was observed with a momentary time sampling with 10-second intervals and was on task approximately 60–70% of the intervals during instruction and completed less than 33% of the assigned tasks. His reading skills were assessed with a curriculum-based assessment for instructional design (CBA-ID; Burns & Parker, 2014) in which he read an average of 76% of the words correctly from the fourth-grade reading material. Next, the student was presented with three sets of passages to read. He was presented with a list of the words in each passage before reading them. Those that he read 93–97% of the words within 2 seconds of presentation were identified as instructional level passages, those in which he read less than 93% of the words correctly were identified as frustration level, and those for which he read more than 97% of the words correctly were identified as independent level passages. He was then asked to read the passages silently during instruction and was observed. The data in Fig. 2 represented the percentage of intervals that he was observed to be on task while reading the passages (top panel) and the percentage of tasks completed for each passage (bottom panel). There was clear differentiation for instructional level passages, which resulted in higher time on task and task completion than the independent and frustration level passages.

The variables described here (time on task and task completion) are likely manifestations of behavioral and cognitive engagement within AET more than they are direct measures of them. Behavioral engagement is both directly related to student achievement (Ponitz et al., 2009) and mediates the relationship between other aspects of engagement and student achievement (Lee, 2014; Li & Lerner, 2013). As hypothesized in Fig. 1, AET represents the proportion of instructional time that the students are engaged in, which can be assessed with variables such as time on task and task completion.

Acquisition Rate

The amount of information taught is also a variable to consider when establishing an instructional level with individual students. The amount of information that a student can rehearse and later recall during one intervention session is called the acquisition rate (AR; Burns, 2001) and is a critical component of providing an appropri-

ate level of challenge for individual students (Burns & Parker, 2014). Teaching the number of items that represented a student's AR, in comparison to teaching too many or too few items, resulted in increased retention (Burns et al., 2016), generalization of the information (Haegele & Burns, 2015), and AET during a specific task

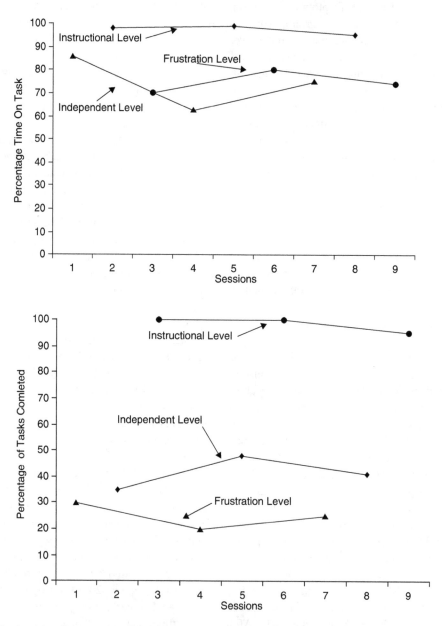

Fig. 2 Simulated data from actual student data to demonstrate time on task (top panel) and task completion (bottom panel) while reading instructional level (93–97%) passages Compared to independent level (>97%) and frustration level passages (<93%)

or instructional activity (Burns & Dean, 2005; Burns et al., 2021).

The AR construct was based on Ceraso's (1967) retroactive cognitive interference construct and seminal finding that exceeding an individual student's limits on the number of new items to be taught resulted in poor retention of new information and reduced retention of previously learned material. For example, if a student is capable of learning 5 items during instruction and is taught 10 items, the student will learn the first 5 with little difficulty, but will not remember that last 5 items taught, and attempting to teach them will result in the student forgetting the first 5 items that he had just learned.

A student's AR is measured by teaching unknown words (or math facts, letter sounds, etc.) until the student makes three errors while rehearsing one new word (Burns, 2001). An error is counted whenever the student does not provide the correct response to the stimulus within 2 seconds. The number of new words successfully rehearsed at that point at which three errors are made is considered the student's AR. The reliability of assessing AR was estimated at $r = 0.83$ for kindergarten students (Taylor et al., 2018), $r = 0.76$ among first-grade students and $r = 0.91$ for third- and fifth-grade students (Burns, 2001). AR data also correlated well with a standardized memory measure (corrected $r = 0.70$; Burns & Mosack, 2005) and with the number of words retained 1 day later ($r = 0.70$, Taylor et al., 2018).

An instructional match is an approach for teachers to directly influence AET that is both consistent with theory and well-researched. Ensuring that students can complete a high percentage of the task (e.g., read 93–97% of the words) and that the amount of new material to learn falls within a student's acquisition rate are instructional decisions for which effective account, and doing so facilitates higher AET. Next, we will discuss other decisions throughout the phases of instruction and how each can help facilitate AET.

Enhancing AET Through Phases of Instruction

Instructional practices are clearly linked to AET, or the proportion of the instructional time that students are engaged (Lekwa et al., 2019; Ponitz et al., 2009; Rosenshine, 1978). As stated previously, opportunities for students to respond (OTR) was the single best predictor of AET (Lekwa et al., 2019), and using instructional materials that represented an instructional level increased student outcomes such as time on task (Beck et al., 2009; Burns et al., 2021; Treptow et al., 2007). Thus, it makes sense to ensure an appropriate level of challenge with high OTR to increase AET.

Algozzine and Ysseldyke (1992) proposed a framework to examine instruction, which was later refined by Algozzine et al. (1997) and Ysseldyke and Christenson (2002). The model examines instruction through four phases, planning instruction, managing instruction, delivering instruction, and evaluating instruction. Although the model addresses general effective instruction, we will discuss the implications for increasing AET as summarized in Table 2.

Planning Instruction

Planning instruction involves making decisions about what to teach, how to teach, and the communication of realistic expectations. All of these decisions are driven by student data to enhance AET.

Deciding What to Teach

The primary task in deciding what to teach to enhance AET is to determine what materials and levels represent an instructional level, and then the secondary decisions such as task characteristics (e.g., sequence, cognitive demands) and classroom characteristics (e.g., instructional groupings, materials) can be made. Most teachers follow some curriculum or district instruction guide based on state standards, which is the starting point for deciding what to teach. Teachers typically first identify the standard being taught or point in the curriculum and identify the content, process, and product that would best meet each student's needs (Levy, 2008). Students who have not mastered prerequisite skills will likely be frustrated during instruction, which would reduce AET. Alternatively, students who have already mastered the new content will likely be bored, which also results in reduced AET (Treptow et al., 2007). Thus, instruction is most effective when the material represents an instructional level, or when prerequisite skills are taught. Moreover, effective teachers consider which assessment approach would best demonstrate individual student competence (e.g., writing for a student with strong writing skills, but perhaps drawing or verbally stating information for students for whom writing is a particular struggle).

Deciding How to Teach

The best way to decide how to teach is to assess the kinds of instructional practices that work best for some students and do not work for others. Previously, many teachers relied on teaching practices based on the assessment of students' learning styles, attempting to identify visual learners, auditory learners, or kinesthetic learners and match instruction to students' alleged preferred styles. Such practices are an ineffective yet persistent educational myth (Cuevas, 2015). The professional literature is filled with guidelines for effective instruction (e.g., Hattie, 2009). Stockard et al. (2018) reviewed 328 studies across 50 years of research and found significant effects for reading, math, and spelling that were maintained when information was taught through direct instruction that incorporated explicit modeling, guided practice, and teaching to mastery, which is an instructional approach that has been linked to enhanced student engagement as measured by observations of students attending to instruction (Hollingsworth & Ybarra, 2017; Lekwa et al., 2019). In fact, modeling while teaching academic tasks is one of the most effective ways for teachers to facilitate high AET (Harbour et al., 2015). However, teacher-led lessons reduced AET ($r = -0.27$; Lekwa et al., 2019). Thus, effective

Table 2 Phases of instruction and activities to support academic engaged time (AET)

Phase of instruction	Instructional decision	Tasks for AET
Plan instruction	Decide what to teach	Determine what materials represent an instructional level and identify task characteristics and classroom characteristics for optimal learning
	Decide how to teach	Model new concepts that build on previously taught material, but in an interactive way with guided practice and immediate corrective feedback. Determine the need for peer tutoring.
	Communicate realistic expectations	Set mastery goals, make them known to the students, and report progress toward the goals
Manage instruction	Prepare for instruction	Set rules early in the year, communicate them to the students, teach students the consequences of behavior. Preteach new concepts and facts to students who need support
	Use time productively	Provide procedures, organized physical space, short transitions, and minimal interruptions. Use warmup activities and watch for frequent errors with all of the students
	Establish a positive environment	Promote positive relationships, and feelings of excitement and comfort. Be sensitive toward student academic and social needs, and show regard for student perspectives

(continued)

teachers consider how to best incorporate modeling of a new concept in a sequence that builds on

Table 2 (continued)

Phase of instruction	Instructional decision	Tasks for AET
Deliver instruction	Effectively present information	Promote frequent active student participation
	Provide practice	Provide frequent opportunities to respond that incorporates a high percentage of known items
	Provide feedback	Provide information to improve student learning that takes into account the stage of the learning cycle and is positively worded at least three times more frequently than negatively
	Modify or adapt instruction	Observe student behavior for need for change. Base adaptations on the distinction between deficits in effort and skill
Evaluate instruction	Monitor AET	Observe time on task for classrooms. Assess individual student engagement with surveys or direct behavior ratings
	Monitor structures and student activities	Assess instructional environment. Monitor grades, homework completion, attendance, and participation in school activities as part of school improvement process

previously taught material, but in an interactive way that then allows for guided practice with immediate corrective feedback before providing independent practice until mastery. Previous research also found that spending more time introducing new concepts and student work time increased academic engaged time, but more time spent on closing the lessons decreased academic engaged time (Maulana et al., 2012).

Task analysis in comparison to state standards or the given curriculum is the starting point, but it is also important to take into account the ways in which classrooms are organized. Physical space, peer interactions, and instructional grouping arrangements affect a teacher's planning (Squires, 1983). A review of 20 studies found that peer tutoring had a direct effect on student learning ($d = 0.75$), but also had an effect on decreasing time off task ($d = 0.60$) and increasing academic engagement ($d = 0.38$; Bowman-Perrott et al., 2014). The effects of peer tutoring were also noted among students for whom English was not their native language (Bowman-Perrott et al., 2016). Heterogenous dyads provide scaffolding from a more expert partner, as described by Vygotsky (1978). Effective teachers arrange the room to allow for peer interaction as part of the learning process to enhance AET.

Communicating Realistic Expectations

Both EVT and Flow Theory emphasize the importance of setting and communicating goals. Making shared goals public and frequently discussing them facilitated enhanced AET with high school students (Shernoff et al., 2016). Students do better when they are expected to perform well and when their performance is monitored and reported. Mastery-oriented goals are especially important among students attending schools in high-poverty neighborhoods (Lawson & Lawson, 2013).

Managing Instruction

Effectively managing instruction directly influences AET. Observations and ratings of instructional and behavioral management strategies among 107 teachers in 11 urban elementary schools serving approximately 2000 students found larger effects for instructional practices (12% unique variance) than behavior management practices (6% unique variance) on student AET (Lekwa et al., 2019). There are three principles of effective instructional management, (a) preparing for instruction, (b) using time productively, and (c) establishing a positive classroom environment.

Preparing for Instruction

Preparing for instruction does not mean preparing materials etc. Rather, it refers to preparing students for success. Teachers set rules early in the year, communicate them to the students, and teach students the consequences of behavior and how to manage their own behavior. Corrective feedback for behavior problems is negatively correlated with AET (Lekwa et al., 2019), in that the more time spent correcting behavioral difficulties, the less time that students are spent engaged in learning. Thus, it is best to handle disruptions effectively and quickly and to follow up disruptions with reteaching as needed.

Preteaching is an effective strategy to prepare students to receive instruction that has been linked to increased achievement and AET. The process of preteaching involves the teacher or interventionist reviewing the material, identifying key concepts or facts, and providing initial instruction and practice with the content or facts before the students receive formal instruction (Burns & Parker, 2014). Burns (2007) studied the effects of preteaching words before reading instruction with 58 students identified with learning disabilities in reading. The average reading growth for students randomly assigned to the preteaching condition increased at a rate that exceeded the active control group and the national norm for growth for students in their grade. Several studies have used preteaching of academic content (e.g., words) with students with and without disabilities to facilitate increased academic achievement (Berg & Wehby, 2013; Burns et al., 2011; Watt & Therrien, 2016). Moreover, Beck et al. (2009) pretaught words and letter sounds to elementary-aged students with emotional disorders before they received reading instruction, which increased AET for each student. Spending 5–10 minutes preteaching key concepts or facts to students who struggle may be time well spent given the effects of AET.

Using Time Productively

When time is used productively, this maximizes the amount of time students spend actively engaged in learning and minimizes the time spent on activities not related to learning. It is important to allocate sufficient time to the content being taught but to also use time efficiently through well-established routines and procedures, organized physical space, short transitions between activities, and minimal interruptions that break the flow of classroom activities (Algozzine & Ysseldyke, 1992). Lessons are more effective if they begin with a practiced routine, an agenda, and warm-up activities to build interest and activate prior knowledge so that AET will be enhanced (Masci, 2008). Moreover, total instructional time can be conserved by planning activities and tasks to fit learning materials (Evertson & Harris, 1992).

Productive use of instructional time relies on high AET or ensuring that students are on task during instruction. Above we talked about deciding what to teach, but part of delivering instruction productively is monitoring student errors to determine if reteaching is needed and if students are reaching an AR. Burns et al. (2021) observed kindergarten instruction with sight words using a commonly used video that presented the words in a song. They assessed each student's AR, as described above, and found that time off task increased dramatically immediately after presenting a word that exceeded their AR. Students were on task 88.1% of the instructional time before reaching an AR, but it fell to 61% afterward. When presenting new items (e.g., letter sounds, math facts, sight words, spelling words, vocabulary), monitoring student responses and sudden increases in errors will suggest that the students are reaching an AR, and time may not be efficiently used from that point on. The teacher then stops instruction, reviews what was just taught, provides an opportunity for students to apply and discuss what was just learned, and then changes instructional focus.

Establishing a Positive Classroom Environment

Positive interactions and classroom environments are consistently linked to AET. A meta-analysis of 61 studies found a significant relationship ($r = 0.25$) between classroom environment and engagement, and all dimensions of classroom environment (instructional support, socioemotional support, and classroom organization) all equally predicted engagement (Wang et al., 2020). Classroom climates that are built on "positive relationships, enjoyment and excitement, feelings of comfort, and experiences of appropriate levels of autonomy" (p. 704), teacher sensitivity toward student academic and social needs, and regard for student perspectives led to student engagement and subsequent achievement (Reyes et al., 2012). Teachers can also notice activities for which students have intrinsic motivation and build them into instructional routines, which also is linked to increase student AET (Shernoff et al., 2017).

Delivering Instruction

Teaching is the systematic presentation of content assumed necessary for mastery of the subject matter (Burns & Ysseldyke, 2009), and it does not happen accidentally. Careful intentional planning of the delivery of instruction ensures that (a) instruction is presented in effective ways, (b) students are given relevant practice, (c) feedback is provided, (d) students are actively involved, and (e) instruction is modified based on information on pupils' performance (Algozzine & Ysseldyke, 1992). Effective teachers use a variety of strategies to deliver instruction in ways that enhance AET (Algozzine et al., 1997). They find effective and unique ways to present instruction, provide students with relevant practice, provide feedback, modify instruction based on student progress, continually evaluate their instruction, monitor engaged time, and monitor what is going on in classrooms. We briefly touch on these below.

Effectively Presenting Instruction

Almost any study on AET identified active student responding as an important instructional component (Harbour et al., 2015; Haydon et al., 2009; Lekwa et al., 2019). Active Student Responding (ASR) is defined as a method to promote frequent student participation for effective learning (Jerome & Barbetta, 2005). Student attention spans may be as short as 2–4 minutes depending on the age and stage of the lesson (Bunce et al., 2010), which suggests that students need to provide an active response at least every 2–4 minutes. Responding can be verbal, physical, or in writing, and can be whole-class or group. Some suggestions for providing ASR include providing time for students to think before responding, waiting 3–5 seconds before asking for a response, providing a clear and consistent cue when to respond, and maintain an active pace (Griffin & Ryan, 2016). Teachers can also build AET with frequent questioning, especially if the questions ask students to apply and analyze information, and to engage in reasoning while dialoguing with each other (Smart & Marshall, 2013).

Providing Relevant Practice

Much like active responding, providing high opportunities to respond (OTR) is an important component of instruction and can help build AET. Practice is how any skill moves from initial learning to generalization (Klubnik & Ardoin, 2010), but not all practice approaches lead to high AET. Research has consistently shown that incorporating a high percentage of known items within a practice task has increased retention of the newly learned material when rehearsing math facts (Burns et al., 2016), letter sounds (Peterson et al., 2014), words to be read in context (Burns, 2007), and many other academic tasks (Burns et al., 2012). However, including known items within practice sets also led to increased AET. Billington et al. (2004) asked students to practice multidigit math computation problems and found that interspersing single-digit problems with every third problem increased preference and engagement for the task. Burns and Dean (2005) compared to time on task of students with learning disabilities while rehearsing sight words with four conditions (0% known, 50% known, 83% known, and 90% known). The least challenging condition (90% known) led to the highest percentage of AET with all data points being above 90% time on task.

Providing Feedback

Feedback is one of the most effective instructional techniques available to teachers (Hattie, 2009) and has consistently been linked to high AET (Harbour et al., 2015; Shernoff et al., 2016). In fact, quality feedback was the strongest classroom predictor of behavioral engagement in 54 fifth- and sixth-grade classrooms (McKellar et al., 2020). A review of 435 studies found a moderate effect ($d = 0.55$), and 86% of the effects for engagement were positive (Wisniewski et al., 2020). However, feedback must provide information to improve student learning and consider the stage of the learning cycle (e.g., immediate feedback for initial learning and delayed feedback to build autonomy for fluency building or generalization), and be positively presented at least three times more frequently than negatively (Voerman et al., 2012). Moreover, setting goals for the students and providing feedback on progress toward those goals have been consistently linked to AET (Adams et al., 2020; Winstone et al., 2017).

Modifying or Adapting Instruction

Effective instruction involves adjusting the instructional content and techniques for individual students as a result of observations and data. Teachers can observe student behavior to determine if modifications are needed. If students are making sufficient progress and exhibiting high AET, then no modifications are needed. However, effective teachers who observe frequent behavioral difficulties or off-task behavior assessed the behavior by observing times of day and physical locations of difficulties, so to make simple modifications such as rearranging student seats, providing areas for personal space, creating separate work areas, or using teacher proximity control (Guardino & Fullerton, 2010).

Adaptations are more effective if they are also based on the distinction between deficits in effort and skill (Passyn & Sujan, 2012). VanDerHeyden and Witt (2008) differentiated between two profiles of students with low AET; a can't do profile in which students experience a mismatch between task demands and skill, and a won't do profile in which students have sufficient skill to be successful but are choosing not to engage for some unknown reason. As shown in Table 3, low AET with academic skills that fall below the aforementioned instructional level criteria indicates that the student cannot successfully complete the task (can't do) and needs an adaptation that either strengthens their skills or changes the task demands. Low AET and adequate skill suggest an effort deficit (won't do), which may be remediated with goal setting, feedback, and other AET techniques described within this chapter.

Evaluating Instruction

Evaluation is the process by which practitioners examine data to determine if their instruction is effective through both formative evaluation and summative evaluation approaches. The process of evaluating instruction has consistently been shown to improve student learning (Jung et al., 2018), and effective teachers tend to more frequently evaluate their instruction (Bolt et al., 2010). Moreover, closely monitoring student

Table 3 Interaction between student levels of skill and effort for academic engaged time (AET)

		Skill level	
		Low	High
Effort level	Low	Can't do AET is facilitated by strengthening student skill (e.g., preteach) or changing task demands (e.g., use instructional level material)	Won't do Intervene to increase AET (e.g., set goals for student, provide feedback, and provide relevant practice)
	High	Academically engaged Provide appropriately challenging tasks	

progress has also been linked to increased AET (Spicuzza et al., 2001; Ysseldyke & Bolt, 2007). There are many readily available resources on how to best evaluate instruction (see https:// intensiveintervention.org/intensive-intervention/ progress-monitor). This chapter focuses on evaluating instruction to improve AET and will next discuss monitoring engaged time and monitoring student activity.

Monitoring Engaged Time

There are several scales and assessment approaches to determine behavioral, cognitive, and affective engagement (Fredricks, chapter, "The Measurement of Student Engagement: Methodological Advances and Comparison of New Self-report Instruments", this volume; Fredricks & McColskey, 2012). AET is often assessed in research by observing student time on task on a regular interval (e.g., every minute) and recording if students are rated as on task or not (e.g., Beck et al., 2009; Treptow et al., 2007). Researchers have also recorded the data for an entire classroom by again observing behavior on a regular interval and recording the number of students who are rated as on task at the precise moment in relation to the total number of students (Taylor et al., 2000). Independent observers could collect time on task data to help identify tasks and instructional approaches associated with higher or lower rates of AET, but this approach is not practical for classroom teachers and has other limitations.

Although time on task is a frequently used and easily collected measure, it is an indirect and incomplete measure of AET and other assessments may be needed for individual students. Spanjers et al. (2008) correlated a self-rating of academic engagement to data from systematic direct observations of time on task, which suggested low correlations between the two $r = -0.15$ to $r = 0.30$. Measures of time on task were significantly correlated to direct behavior ratings of behavior (DBR), and the direct ratings were more sensitive to changes in behavior across time (Briesch et al., 2010; Riley-Tillman et al., 2008). Thus, effective teachers often informally observe AET among their students and take steps to change behavior of individual students with

consistently low AET. However, effective teachers also rate the AET of their entire classroom with DRB to get a more empirically determined sense of what activities, topics, and times of day facilitate high AET or lead to decreased AET, and rate behaviors of individual students with DBR to monitor their AET. Readers are referred to https://dbr.education.uconn.edu/ for more information on how to do so.

Monitoring Classroom Structures and Student Activities

Effective schools assess instructional environments to ensure that they are creating environments that lead to AET. The Classroom Assessment Scoring System (CLASS; Pianta et al., 2008) is an observational system that was developed from 10 years of research with over 3000 classrooms. The CLASS assesses teacher-student interaction, emotional support, classroom organization, and instructional support, all of which contribute to student engagement.

There are many surveys to assess behavioral engagement for students (Nguyen et al., 2018), but observational data may support analysis to examine the effectiveness of school systems in addressing student engagement. Schools best meet student needs by monitoring grades, homework completion, attendance, and participation in school activities including extracurricular activities, and then using those data to examine trends to inform future school improvement plans.

Implications for Future Research

AET and student engagement generally are frequently studied constructs in educational psychology in the past 15 years, but there are many unanswered questions. Additional research is needed to identify which components of engagement are most closely related to AET and other student outcomes. Second, the relationship between AET and behavioral, cognitive, and emotional engagement is not well studied, nor is the uniqueness of AET from components of engagement Thus, Fig. 1 is hypothetical because it proposes a relationship between AET and engagement, and presents school structures as both supporting engagement and providing the denominator for the AET equation. Third, additional research is needed regarding how to best measure AET and student engagement for research or in applied settings, and how to best intervene for AET. Several studies have examined AET as a dependent variable (Common et al., 2020), but relatively few studies examined the effect of AET on academic outcomes and suggested an area for additional research. Finally, the phases of instruction outlined above can be used to consult with teachers, but previous research on the model did not focus on the effects on AET, which suggests a potentially important area for future research.

Conclusion

AET is an important concept in education because it is both consistent with several major psychological theories, and is an observable and easily assessed type of student engagement. Moreover, AET is directly influenced by the school environment, which makes it malleable and an area for potential intervention, and many of the instructional approaches discussed in this chapter help foster AET. Additional research is needed to better understand the relationship between AET and student engagement, and how to measure both, but given the importance of AET for student achievement and other positive outcomes, additional research seems warranted.

References

Adams, A. M., Wilson, H., Money, J., Palmer-Conn, S., & Fearn, J. (2020). Student engagement with feedback and attainment: The role of academic self-efficacy. *Assessment & Evaluation in Higher Education, 45*(2), 317–329.

Algozzine, B., & Ysseldyke, J. (1992). *Strategies and tactics for effective instruction*. Sopris West.

Algozzine, B. S., Ysseldyke, J. E., & Elliott, J. (1997). *Strategies and tactics for effective instruction*. Sopris West.

Axelson, R. D., & Flick, A. (2010). Defining student engagement. *Change: The Magazine of Higher Learning, 43*(1), 38–43.

Beck, M., Burns, M. K., & Lau, M. (2009). The effect of preteaching reading skills on the on-task behavior of children identified with behavioral disorders. *Behavioral Disorders, 34*(2), 91–99.

Berg, J. L., & Wehby, J. (2013). Preteaching strategies to improve student learning in content area classes. *Intervention in School and Clinic, 49*(1), 14–20.

Betts, E. A. (1949). Readability: Its application to the elementary school. *The Journal of Educational Research, 42*(6), 438–459.

Billington, E. J., Skinner, C. H., & Cruchon, N. M. (2004). Improving sixth-grade students perceptions of high-effort assignments by assigning more work: Interaction of additive interspersal and assignment effort on assignment choice. *Journal of School Psychology, 42*(6), 477–490.

Bolt, D. M., Ysseldyke, J. E., & Patterson, M. J. (2010). Students, teachers, and schools as sources of variability, integrity and sustainability in implementing progress monitoring. *School Psychology Review, 39*(4), 612–630.

Bowman-Perrott, L., Burke, M. D., Zhang, N., & Zaini, S. (2014). Direct and collateral effects of peer tutoring on social and behavioral outcomes: A meta-analysis of single-case research. *School Psychology Review, 43*(3), 260–285.

Bowman-Perrott, L., de Marín, S., Mahadevan, L., & Etchells, M. (2016). Assessing the academic, social, and language production outcomes of English language learners engaged in peer tutoring: A systematic review. *Education and Treatment of Children, 39*(3), 359–388.

Briesch, A. M., Chafouleas, S. M., & Riley-Tillman, T. C. (2010). Generalizability and dependability of behavior assessment methods to estimate academic engagement: A comparison of systematic direct observation and direct behavior rating. *School Psychology Review, 39*(3), 408–421.

Bunce, D. M., Flens, E. A., & Neiles, K. Y. (2010). How long can students pay attention in class? A study of student attention decline using clickers. *Journal of Chemical Education, 87*(12), 1438–1443.

Burns, M. K. (2001). Measuring sight-word acquisition and retention rates with curriculum-based assessment. *Journal of Psychoeducational Assessment, 19*(2), 148–157. https://doi.org/10.1177/073428290101900204

Burns, M. K. (2007). Reading at the instructional level with children identified as learning disabled: Potential implications for response-to-intervention. *School Psychology Quarterly, 22*(3), 297–313. https://doi.org/10.1037/1045-3830.22.3.297

Burns, M. K., & Dean, V. J. (2005). Effect of drill ratios on recall and on-task behavior for children with learning and attention difficulties. *Journal of Instructional Psychology, 32*(2), 118–126.

Burns, M. K., & Mosack, J. L. (2005). Criterion-related validity of measuring sight-word acquisition with curriculum-based assessment. *Journal of Psychoeducational Assessment, 23*(3), 216–224.

Burns, M. K., & Parker, D. C. (2014). *Curriculum-based assessment for instructional design: Using data to individualize instruction*. Guilford Publications.

Burns, M. K., & Ysseldyke, J. E. (2009). Reported prevalence of evidence-based instructional practices in special education. *The Journal of Special Education, 43*(1), 3–11.

Burns, M. K., Hodgson, J., Parker, D. C., & Fremont, K. (2011). Comparison of the effectiveness and efficiency of text previewing and preteaching keywords as small-group reading comprehension strategies with middle-school students. *Literacy Research and Instruction, 50*(3), 241–252.

Burns, M. K., Zaslofsky, A. F., Kanive, R., & Parker, D. C. (2012). Meta-analysis of incremental rehearsal using phi coefficients to compare single-case and group designs. *Journal of Behavioral Education, 21*(3), 185–202.

Burns, M. K., Zaslofsky, A. F., Maki, K. E., & Kwong, E. (2016). Effect of modifying intervention set size with acquisition rate data while practicing single-digit multiplication facts. *Assessment for Effective Intervention, 41*(3), 131–140.

Burns, M. K., Aguilar, L. N., Warmbold-Brann, K., Preast, J. L., & Taylor, C. N. (2021). Effect of acquisition rates on off-task behavior of kindergarten students while learning sight words. *Psychology in the Schools, 58*(1), 5–17.

Ceraso, J. (1967). The interference theory of forgetting. *Scientific American, 217*(4), 117–127.

Common, E. A., Lane, K. L., Cantwell, E. D., Brunsting, N. C., Oakes, W. P., Germer, K. A., & Bross, L. A. (2020). Teacher-delivered strategies to increase students' opportunities to respond: A systematic methodological review. *Behavioral Disorders, 45*(2), 67–84. https://doi.org/10.1177/0198742919828310

Cuevas, J. (2015). Is learning styles-based instruction effective? A comprehensive analysis of recent research on learning styles. *Theory and Research in Education, 13*(3), 308–333.

Deci, E. L., & Ryan, R. M. (2012). Self-determination theory. In P. A. M. Van Lange, A. W. Kruglanski, & E. T. Higgins (Eds.), *Handbook of theories of social psychology* (pp. 416–436). Sage Publications Ltd.. https://doi.org/10.4135/9781446249215.n21

Duchaine, E. L., Jolivette, K., Fredrick, L. D., & Alberto, P. A. (2018). Increase engagement and achievement with response cards: Science and mathematics inclusion classes. *Learning Disabilities: A Contemporary Journal, 16*(2), 157–176.

Eccles, J. S., & Midgley, C. (1989). Stage– Environment fit: Developmentally appropriate classrooms for young adolescents. In C. Ames & R. Ames (Eds.), *Research on motivation in education* (Goals and cognitions) (Vol. 3, pp. 13–44). Academic.

Eccles, J. S., & Wigfield, A. (2020). From expectancy-value theory to situated expectancy-value theory: A developmental, social cognitive, and sociocultural perspective on motivation. *Contemporary Educational Psychology, 61*, 101859.

Eccles, J., Adler, T. F., Futterman, R., Goff, S. B., Kaczala, C. M., Meece, J., & Midgley, C. (1983). Expectancies, values and academic behaviors. In J. T. Spence (Ed.), *Achievement and achievement motives*. W. H. Freeman.

Evertson, C. M., & Harris, A. H. (1992). What we know about managing classrooms. *Educational Leadership, 49*(7), 74–78.

Fredricks, J. A., Blumenfeld, P. C., & Paris, A. H. (2004). School engagement: Potential of the concept, state of the evidence. *Review of Educational Research, 74*(1), 59–109.

Fredricks, J. A., Reschly, A. L., & Christenson, S. L. (2019). Interventions for student engagement: Overview and state of the field. In *Handbook of student engagement interventions* (pp. 1–11). Elsevier Science.

Fredricks, J. A., & McColskey, W. (2012). The measurement of student engagement: A comparative analysis of various methods and student self-report instruments. In S. L. Christenson, A. L. Reschly, & C. Wylie (Eds.) *Handbook of research on student engagement* (pp. 763–782). Springer.

Galla, B. M., Amemiya, J., & Wang, M. T. (2018). Using expectancy-value theory to understand academic self-control. *Learning and Instruction, 58*, 22–33.

Gettinger, M., & Walter, M. J. (2012). Classroom strategies to enhance academic engaged time. In S. L. Christenson, A. L. Reschly, & C. Wylie (Eds.), *Handbook of research on student engagement* (pp. 653–673). Springer.

Getzels, J. W., & Csikszentmihalyi, M. (1976). *The creative vision: A longitudinal study of problem finding in art*. Wiley.

Gickling, E. E., & Armstrong, D. L. (1978). Levels of instructional difficulty as related to on-task behavior, task completion, and comprehension. *Journal of Learning Disabilities, 11*(9), 559–566. https://doi.org/10.1177/002221947801100905

Griffin, C. & Ryan, M. (2016). *Active student responding: Supporting student learning and engagement*. Retrieved from https://www.into.ie/ROI/Publications/InTouch/FullLengthArticles/Fulllengtharticles2016/ActiveStudentResponding_InTouchMay2016.pdf

Guardino, C. A., & Fullerton, E. (2010). Changing behaviors by changing the classroom environment. *Teaching Exceptional Children, 42*(6), 8–13.

Guida, F. V., Ludlow, L. H., & Wilson, M. (1985). The mediating effect of time-on-task on the academic anxiety/achievement interaction: A structural model. *Journal of Research & Development in Education, 19*(1), 21–26.

Guthrie, J. T., Wigfield, A., & You, W. (2012). Instructional contexts for engagement and achievement in reading. In S. L. Christenson, A. L. Reschly, & C. Wylie (Eds.), *Handbook of research on student engagement* (pp. 601–634). Springer.

Haegele, K., & Burns, M. K. (2015). Effect of modifying intervention set size with acquisition rate data among students identified with a learning disability. *Journal of Behavioral Education, 24*(1), 33–50.

Harbour, K. E., Evanovich, L. L., Sweigart, C. A., & Hughes, L. E. (2015). A brief review of effective teaching practices that maximize student engagement. *Preventing School Failure: Alternative Education for Children and Youth, 59*(1), 5–13.

Hattie, J. A. C. (2009). *Visible learning: A synthesis of 800 meta-analyses relating to achievement.* Routledge.

Haydon, T., Mancil, G. R., & Van Loan, C. (2009). Using opportunities to respond in a general education classroom: A case study. *Education and Treatment of Children, 32*(2), 267–278.

Hollingsworth, J. R., & Ybarra, S. E. (2017). *Explicit direct instruction (EDI): The power of the well-crafted, well-taught lesson.* Corwin Press.

Jerome, A., & Barbetta, P. M. (2005). The effect of active student responding during computer-assisted instruction on social studies learning by students with learning disabilities. *Journal of Special Education Technology, 20*(3), 13–23.

Jung, P. G., McMaster, K. L., Kunkel, A. K., Shin, J., & Stecker, P. M. (2018). Effects of data-based individualization for students with intensive learning needs: A meta-analysis. *Learning Disabilities Research & Practice, 33*(3), 144–155.

Klubnik, C., & Ardoin, S. P. (2010). Examining immediate and maintenance effects of a reading intervention package on generalization materials: Individual verses group implementation. *Journal of Behavioral Education, 19*(1), 7–29.

Lawson, M. A., & Lawson, H. A. (2013). New conceptual frameworks for student engagement research, policy, and practice. *Review of Educational Research, 83*(3), 432–479.

Lee, J. S. (2014). The relationship between student engagement and academic performance: Is it a myth or reality? *The Journal of Educational Research, 107*(3), 177–185.

Lei, H., Cui, Y., & Zhou, W. (2018). Relationships between student engagement and academic achievement: A meta-analysis. *Social Behavior and Personality: An International Journal, 46*(3), 517–528.

Lekwa, A. J., Reddy, L. A., & Shernoff, E. S. (2019). Measuring teacher practices and student academic engagement: A convergent validity study. *School Psychology, 34*(1), 1091–1118.

Levy, H. M. (2008). Meeting the needs of all students through differentiated instruction: Helping every child reach and exceed standards. *The Clearing House: A Journal of Educational Strategies, Issues and Ideas, 81*(4), 161–164.

Li, Y., & Lerner, R. M. (2013). Interrelations of behavioral, emotional, and cognitive school engagement in high school students. *Journal of Youth and Adolescence, 42*(1), 20–32.

Lopez-Agudo, L. A., & Marcenaro-Gutierrez, O. D. (2020). Instruction time and students' academic achievement: A cross-country comparison. *Compare:*

A Journal of Comparative and International Education, 1–17. https://doi.org/10.1080/03057925.2020.1737919

Magidson, J. F., Roberts, B. W., Collado-Rodriguez, A., & Lejuez, C. W. (2014). Theory-driven intervention for changing personality: Expectancy value theory, behavioral activation, and conscientiousness. *Developmental Psychology, 50*(5), 1442.

Masci, F. (2008). Time for time on task and quality instruction. *Middle School Journal, 40*(2), 33–41.

Maulana, R., Opdenakker, M. C., Stroet, K., & Bosker, R. (2012). Observed lesson structure during the first year of secondary education: Exploration of change and link with academic engagement. *Teaching and Teacher Education, 28*(6), 835–850.

McKellar, S. E., Cortina, K. S., & Ryan, A. M. (2020). Teaching practices and student engagement in early adolescence: A longitudinal study using the Classroom Assessment Scoring System. *Teaching and Teacher Education, 89,* 102936.

Müllerke, N., Duchaine, E. L., Grünke, M., & Karnes, J. (2019). The effects of a response card intervention on the active participation in math lessons of five seventh graders with learning disabilities. *Insights into Learning Disabilities, 16*(2), 107–120.

Nakamura, J., & Csikszentmihalyi, M. (2009). Flow theory and research. In C. R. Snyder & S. J. Lopez (Eds.), *Handbook of positive psychology* (pp. 195–206). Oxford.

Nomi, T., & Allensworth, E. M. (2013). Sorting and supporting: Why double-dose algebra led to better test scores but more course failures. *American Educational Research Journal, 50*(4), 756–788.

Nguyen, T. D., Cannata, M., & Miller, J. (2018). Understanding student behavioral engagement: Importance of student interaction with peers and teachers. *The Journal of Educational Research, 111*(2), 163–174.

Passyn, K., & Sujan, M. (2012). Skill-based versus effort-based task difficulty: A task-analysis approach to the role of specific emotions in motivating difficult actions. *Journal of Consumer Psychology, 22*(3), 461–468.

Peterson, M., Brandes, D., Kunkel, A., Wilson, J., Rahn, N. L., Egan, A., & McComas, J. (2014). Teaching letter sounds to kindergarten English language learners using incremental rehearsal. *Journal of School Psychology, 52*(1), 97–107.

Pianta, R. C., La Paro, K. M., & Hamre, B. K. (2008). *Classroom assessment scoring system™: Manual K-3.* Paul H Brookes Publishing.

Ponitz, C. C., Rimm-Kaufman, S. E., Grimm, K. J., & Curby, T. W. (2009). Kindergarten classroom quality, behavioral engagement, and reading achievement. *School Psychology Review, 38*(1), 102–120.

Putwain, D. W., Nicholson, L. J., Pekrun, R., Becker, S., & Symes, W. (2019). Expectancy of success, attainment value, engagement, and achievement: A moderated mediation analysis. *Learning and Instruction, 60,* 117–125.

Raufelder, D., Kittler, F., Braun, S. R., Lätsch, A., Wilkinson, R. P., & Hoferichter, F. (2014). The interplay of perceived stress, self-determination and school engagement in adolescence. *School Psychology International, 35*(4), 405–420.

Reschly, A. L., & Christenson, S. L. (2012). Jingle, jangle, and conceptual haziness: Evolution and future directions of the engagement construct. In S. L. Christenson, A. L. Reschly, & C. Wylie (Eds.). *Handbook of research on student engagement (pp. 3–19). Springer.*

Reyes, M. R., Brackett, M. A., Rivers, S. E., White, M., & Salovey, P. (2012). Classroom emotional climate, student engagement, and academic achievement. *Journal of Educational Psychology, 104*(3), 700–712.

Riley-Tillman, T. C., Chafouleas, S. M., Sassu, K. A., Chanese, J. A., & Glazer, A. D. (2008). Examining the agreement of direct behavior ratings and systematic direct observation data for on-task and disruptive behavior. *Journal of Positive Behavior Interventions, 10*(2), 136–143.

Rivkin, S. G., & Schiman, J. C. (2015). Instruction time, classroom quality, and academic achievement. *The Economic Journal, 125*(588), F425–F448.

Rosenshine, B. V. (1978). Academic engaged time, content covered, and direct instruction. *Journal of Education, 160*(3), 38–66.

Rosenshine, B. V., & Berliner, D. C. (1978). Academic engaged time. *British Journal of Teacher Education, 4*(1), 3–16.

Rotgans, J. I., & Schmidt, H. G. (2011). Situational interest and academic achievement in the active-learning classroom. *Learning and Instruction, 21*(1), 58–67. https://doi.org/10.1016/j.learninstruc.2009.11.001

Schneider, M., & Preckel, F. (2017). Variables associated with achievement in higher education: A systematic review of meta-analyses. *Psychological Bulletin, 143*(6), 565–600. https://doi.org/10.1037/bul0000098

Shernoff, D. J., Csikszentmihalyi, M., Schneider, B., & Shernoff, E. S. (2014). Student engagement in high school classrooms from the perspective of flow theory. In M. Csikszentmihalyi (Ed.), *Applications of flow in human development and education* (pp. 475–494). Springer. https://doi.org/10.1007/978-94-017-9094-9_24

Shernoff, D. J., Kelly, S., Tonks, S. M., Anderson, B., Cavanagh, R. F., Sinha, S., & Abdi, B. (2016). Student engagement as a function of environmental complexity in high school classrooms. *Learning and Instruction, 43*, 52–60.

Shernoff, D. J., Ruzek, E. A., & Sinha, S. (2017). The influence of the high school classroom environment on learning as mediated by student engagement. *School Psychology International, 38*(2), 201–218.

Smart, J. B., & Marshall, J. C. (2013). Interactions between classroom discourse, teacher questioning, and student cognitive engagement in middle school science. *Journal of Science Teacher Education, 24*(2), 249–267.

Spanjers, D. M., Burns, M. K., & Wagner, A. R. (2008). Systematic direct observation of time on task as a measure of student engagement. *Assessment for Effective Intervention, 33*(2), 120–126. https://doi.org/10.1177/1534508407311407

Spicuzza, R., Ysseldyke, J., Lemkuil, A., Kosciolek, S., Boys, C., & Teelucksingh, E. (2001). Effects of using a curriculum-based monitoring system on the classroom instructional environment and math achievement. *Journal of School Psychology, 39*(6), 521–542.

Squires, D. A. (1983). *Effective schools and classrooms: A research-based perspective*. Association for Supervision and Curriculum Development.

Stockard, J., Wood, T. W., Coughlin, C., & Rasplica Khoury, C. (2018). The effectiveness of direct instruction curricula: A meta-analysis of a half century of research. *Review of Educational Research, 88*(4), 479–507.

Symonds, J., & Hargreaves, L. (2016). Emotional and motivational engagement at school transition: A qualitative stage-environment fit study. *The Journal of Early Adolescence, 36*(1), 54–85.

Taylor, B. M., Pearson, P. D., Clark, K., & Walpole, S. (2000). Effective schools and accomplished teachers: Lessons about primary-grade reading instruction in low-income schools. *The Elementary School Journal, 101*(2), 121–165.

Taylor, C. N., Aguilar, L., Burns, M. K., Preast, J. L., & Warmbold-Brann, K. (2018). Reliability and relationship to retention of assessing an acquisition rate for sight words with kindergarten students. *Journal of Psychoeducational Assessment, 36*(8), 798–807.

Treptow, M. A., Burns, M. K., & McComas, J. J. (2007). Reading at the frustration, instructional, and independent levels: The effects on students' reading comprehension and time on task. *School Psychology Review, 36*(1), 159–166.

VanDerHeyden, A. M., & Witt, J. C. (2008). Best practices in can't do/won't do assessment. In A. Thomas & J. Grimes (Eds.), *Best practices in school psychology V* (pp. 131–140). National Association of School Psychologists.

Voerman, L., Meijer, P. C., Korthagen, F. A., & Simons, R. J. (2012). Types and frequencies of feedback interventions in classroom interaction in secondary education. *Teaching and Teacher Education, 28*(8), 1107–1115.

Vygotsky, L. S. (1978). Socio-cultural theory. *Mind in Society, 6*, 52–58.

Wang, M. T., & Eccles, J. S. (2013). School context, achievement motivation, and academic engagement: A longitudinal study of school engagement using a multidimensional perspective. *Learning and Instruction, 28*, 12–23.

Wang, M. T., Degol, J. L., Amemiya, J., Parr, A., & Guo, J. (2020). Classroom climate and children's academic and psychological wellbeing: A systematic review and meta-analysis. *Developmental Review, 57*, 100912.

Watt, S. J., & Therrien, W. J. (2016). Examining a pre-teaching framework to improve fraction computation outcomes among struggling learners. *Preventing*

School Failure: Alternative Education for Children and Youth, 60(4), 311–319.

Wigfield, A., & Tonks, S. (2002). Adolescents' expectancies for success and achievement task values during the middle and high school years. *Academic Motivation of Adolescents, 2*, 53–82.

Winstone, N. E., Nash, R. A., Parker, M., & Rowntree, J. (2017). Supporting learners' agentic engagement with feedback: A systematic review and a taxonomy of recipience processes. *Educational Psychologist, 52*(1), 17–37.

Wisniewski, B., Zierer, K., & Hattie, J. (2020). The power of feedback revisited: A meta-analysis of educational feedback research. *Frontiers in Psychology, 10*, 3087.

Ysseldyke, J., & Bolt, D. M. (2007). Effect of a technology-enhanced continuous progress monitoring system on math achievement. *School Psychology Review, 36*(3), 453–467.

Ysseldyke, J., & Christenson, S. (2002). *Functional assessment of academic behavior*. Sopris West.

The Role of Academic Engagement in Students' Educational Development: Insights from Load Reduction Instruction and the 4M Academic Engagement Framework

Andrew J. Martin

Abstract

School is difficult for many students. In part, this is because there are instructional burdens that impose a significant cognitive load on students as they try to learn. As cognitive load escalates, there is the risk of declining academic engagement which then reduces students' learning and achievement. It is vital that teachers deliver instruction in a way that eases the cognitive load on students as they learn and supports students' academic engagement, learning, and achievement. Load reduction instruction (LRI) is an instructional approach aimed at managing the cognitive demands experienced by students as they learn. This discussion explores how LRI can enhance students' academic engagement and how these improvements in engagement assist academic outcomes such as achievement—thus, hypothesizing a mediating role for academic engagement. The discussion also introduces a novel engagement framework—the 4M Academic Engagement Framework—that hierarchically conceptualizes engagement in terms of students' engagement with their broad educational development (the "mega" level) through to the granular operationalization of specific engagement variables (the "micro/measured" level). The theoretical and empirical connections between LRI and the academic engagement dimensions of the 4M Framework are then described, with a particular focus on how academic engagement mediates the link between LRI and achievement. Implications of these findings for engagement assessment and practice are discussed. Taken together, it is clear that academic engagement plays an important part in young people's educational development and the instructional factors aimed at supporting that development.

A. J. Martin (✉)
School of Education, University of New South Wales, Sydney, NSW, Australia
e-mail: andrew.martin@unsw.edu.au

Introduction

The pace and nature of academic demands at school escalate as students move from one academic year to the next. These demands include escalations in subject difficulty, assessment tasks, homework frequency and complexity, etc. and impose cognitive and other burdens on students as they strive to keep up with instruction and assessment, particularly at points of significant transition such as from elementary school to middle school and then to high school (Anderman, 2013; Anderman & Mueller, 2010; Graham & Hill, 2003; Martin et al., 2015). As these demands and burdens escalate, there is also the risk of declines in students' academic engagement. In turn, declines in engagement are associated with declines in students' academic outcomes (e.g., learning, achievement) (Martin, 2016; Martin & Evans, 2018). There is thus a cycle in which the demands of school adversely impact academic engagement that adversely impacts young people's academic development (Martin et al., 2020b). This being the case, it is important for teachers to deliver instruction in a way that eases the burden on students as they learn and thereby supports students' academic engagement and subsequent academic outcomes (Evans & Martin, 2022; Martin, 2016; Martin & Evans, 2018, 2019; Moreno, 2010; Moreno & Mayer, 2007).

Cognitive load theory (CLT) has identified key elements of instruction that ease the cognitive burden on students as they learn (Sweller, 2012; Sweller et al., 2011). Recently, these elements were harnessed in a newly proposed instructional model, "load reduction instruction" (LRI; Martin, 2016; Martin & Evans, 2018, 2019, 2021; Martin et al., 2020b, 2021b). LRI is a practical instructional approach aimed at managing the cognitive demands experienced by students as they learn. LRI comprises five key principles:

1. Reducing the difficulty of instruction during initial learning, as appropriate to learners' levels of prior knowledge and skill
2. Instructional support and scaffolding
3. Ample structured practice
4. Appropriate provision of instructional feedback-feedforward (combination of corrective information and specific improvement-oriented guidance)
5. Guided independent application (Martin, 2016; see also Martin & Evans, 2018, 2019; Martin et al., 2020b, 2021b).

The present chapter examines the relationships between LRI, academic engagement, and young people's academic development (by way of their learning and achievement). Specifically, this chapter: introduces an integrative academic engagement framework; explains the role of academic engagement in this framework; describes LRI; discusses links between LRI (and related instructional approaches) and distinct dimensions of academic engagement; unpacks key connections between academic engagement and academic outcomes, and explores the role of academic engagement in mediating the link between LRI and young people's academic outcomes.

Academic Engagement: Introducing the 4M Framework

It is proposed herein that academic engagement comprises a hierarchy of general and granular engagement dimensions. Figure 1 introduces the hierarchical engagement framework that is developed to guide the present discussion.

Mega Level Construct At the apex is the "mega" construct of "academic engagement". This refers to students' commitment to, involvement with, and investment in the learning and instruction factors and processes implicated in their academic life (at school, college, university, etc.).

Meta Level Constructs Subsumed under the mega construct are the "*meta*" constructs that seek to capture engagement in the major broad modes of contemporary learning and instruction. These meta engagement constructs reflect students' commitment to, investment in, and involvement with digital learning and instruction, non-digital learning and instruction, and blended/hybrid learning and instruction—respectively, their "digital engagement", "non-digital engagement", and "blended/hybrid engagement". With substantial shifts to digital and hybrid learning and instruction in recent years, these three modes (digital, non-digital, and hybrid) represent the near-totality of students' learning and instruction experiences today (Escueta et al., 2017; Nguyen, 2015; OECD, 2015). Digital engagement refers to students' commitment to, investment in, and involvement with learning through or facilitated by technology, including synchronous or asynchronous online lessons and tasks, computer/software-based resources, electronic media, virtual reality, learning management systems, etc. Non-digital engagement refers to students' com-

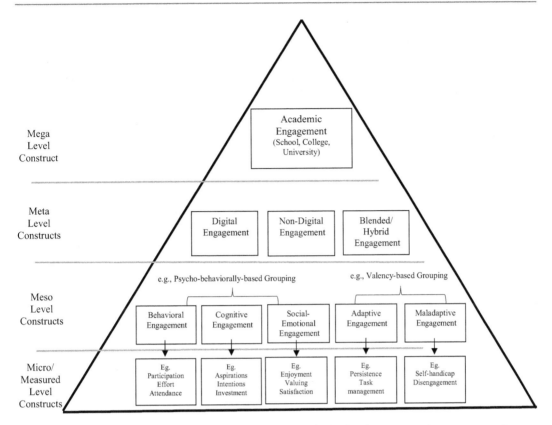

Fig. 1 The 4M Academic Engagement Framework

Note: At the meso level, other engagement groupings are plausible. For example, the present chapter has cited agentic engagement as one possibility at the meso level, comprised of micro-measured engagement elements such as asking questions, requesting clarification, offering suggestions, and expressing interests and preferences

mitment to, investment in, and involvement with learning in real-time and physical space (e.g., the physical classroom), teacher and peers in real-time and physical space, hard-copy materials, physical resources, etc. Blended/hybrid engagement refers to students' commitment to, investment in, and involvement with learning and instruction that comprises a combination of digital and non-digital modes. Importantly, blended/hybrid learning and instruction are more than the sum of digital and non-digital components; there are distinct tasks, processes, and dynamics involved in integrating digital and non-digital modes to attain an optimal balance that meets learners' needs (Bernard et al., 2014). To the extent digital, non-digital, and blended/hybrid modes comprise unique learning and instruction processes (Means et al., 2009), it is contended that students will differentially engage with and learn through each of them (e.g., Bergdahl et al., 2020; Bernard et al., 2014; Kirschner & De Bruyckere, 2017; McGuinness & Fulton, 2019).

Meso-Level Constructs Under the meta level is the "meso" level that refers to the substantive engagement groupings relevant to each mode of digital, non-digital, and blended/hybrid engagement. At this meso level, the nature of the engagement constructs is such that they substantively connect the granular (micro-measured) dimensions of engagement with the broader engagement constructs at mega and meta levels. As relevant to the present chapter, these may be considered in terms of their psycho-behavioral functions (e.g., *behavioral, cognitive, and social-emotional engagement* under tripartite perspectives; e.g., Fredricks et al., 2004; Martin et al., 2021a) or in terms of valence (e.g., *adaptive and maladaptive engagement* under the Motivation and Engagement Wheel; Martin, 2007, 2009). Or (beyond the focus of this chapter), other engagement frameworks may come into play at this meso level—such as students' agentic engagement that can be applied to each mode of digital, non-digital, and blended/hybrid engagement and which also comprises its granular micro/measured components (described below) (Patall et al., 2019; Reeve & Shin, 2020). Thus, in relation to tripartite perspectives, for example, students will differ in the extent to which they are behaviorally, cognitively, and socially-emotionally engaged (or not) in digital modes of learning and instruction, non-digital modes of learning and instruction, and blended/hybrid modes of learning and instruction.

Micro/Measured Level Constructs Finally, subsumed under the meso level is the "micro/measured" level which is the specific operationalized form for each of the meso level engagement constructs. Under focus in this chapter are examples such as *participation and attendance* (for behavioral engagement), *aspirations and intentions* (for cognitive engagement), *enjoyment and satisfaction* (for social-emotional engagement), *persistence and task management* (for adaptive engagement), and *self-handicapping and disengagement* (for maladaptive engagement). Other examples (but outside the focus of this chapter) include asking questions, requesting clarification, offering suggestions, and expressing interests and preferences (for agentic engagement; Reeve, 2013). This framing of academic engagement in terms of its mega, meta, meso, and micro/measured levels is referred to as the 4M Academic Engagement Framework (Fig. 1).

In considering major reviews of engagement, it is evident that most of the factors proposed in the 4M Academic Engagement Framework are part of the established engagement landscape (Finn & Zimmer, 2012; Fredricks et al., 2004; Fredricks & McColskey, 2012; Martin, 2007, 2009; Skinner & Pitzer, 2012). However, there

can be differences among researchers as to the precise topography of this landscape, where specific factors reside on this topography, and how they synergistically and dynamically interact (see Lawson & Lawson, 2013 for review). For example, Skinner and Pitzer (2012) also identify a hierarchy of engagement, with institutional engagement at the apex, subsumed by school engagement (comprising sport, club, classroom, and government dimensions) and then classroom engagement (comprising teacher, curriculum, and peer dimensions). Fredricks et al. (2004) and Fredricks and McColskey (2012) identify engagement as a tripartite meta-construct subsumed by behavioral, cognitive, and emotional engagement. Finn and Zimmer (2012) summarize an overarching engagement concept in terms of behavioral (academic, social, and cognitive) and emotional dimensions. Appleton et al. (2006) and Christenson et al. (2008) identify engagement as subsumed by academic, behavioral, cognitive, and affective dimensions. There are, then, alignments and distinctions among major engagement models.

The 4M Academic Engagement Framework is developed here as a means to systematically connect LRI to engagement at its different levels and to advance engagement conceptualizing in numerous ways, as follows:

1. It is aimed at formally incorporating digital, non-digital, and blended/hybrid modes of learning and instruction, and thus the digital, non-digital, and blended/hybrid modes of engagement relevant to these. Learning and instruction have been transformed in recent years, with an increasing focus on digital delivery (Escueta et al., 2017; Nguyen, 2015; OECD, 2015)—which has vastly accelerated since the onset of the COVID-19 pandemic (Australian Academy of Science, 2020). It is appropriate that contemporaneous academic engagement frameworks take these modes of engagement into account.

2. Because digital and hybrid instruction can impose a distinct cognitive burden on learners (Kirschner & De Bruyckere, 2017) and because cognitive burden has distinct implica-

tions for students' academic engagement (Martin, 2016; Martin et al., 2020b), developing a conceptual framework that integrates salient engagement dimensions of digital and hybrid modes has potentially wide application to contemporary learning.

3. It is framed to generalize across diverse educational institutions and contexts—e.g., school, college, and university.

4. It is designed to represent a parsimonious alignment of superordinate and subordinate engagement constructs—e.g., the meso dimensions of behavioral, cognitive, and social-emotional engagement can apply to each of the meta dimensions of digital, non-digital, and blended/hybrid engagement; in addition, each meso dimension has its unique micro/measured analogues.

5. There is inherent flexibility by including "placeholders" in the framework—e.g., the meta level is designed to be sufficiently flexible to allow diverse groupings of engagement themes—Figure 1 shows just two examples by way of a psycho-behaviorally based grouping (behavioral, cognitive, social-emotional engagement) and a valency-based grouping (adaptive, maladaptive engagement)—but as noted, there are others such as agentic engagement.

6. Drawing on the construct validity tradition (e.g., Campbell & Fiske, 1959; Marsh, 2002), there is explicit recognition in the 4M Framework that engagement typically involves hypothetical constructs that are conceptual or theoretical abstractions (like most psychological constructs; Marsh et al., 2006). This being the case, constructs are often inferred indirectly via concrete indicators— such as the micro/measured constructs at the base of the 4M Framework. By undergirding the 4M Framework with the micro/measured level of engagement, there is an acknowledgment (consistent with the aims of construct validation) that conceptual (upper) and operationalized (lower) levels of engagement are inextricably intertwined such that one cannot be understood without understanding the other.

This chapter attends to the meso and micro/measured levels of the 4M Academic Engagement Framework. At the meso level, it addresses the behavioral, cognitive, and social-emotional engagement dimensions of the tripartite perspective (Fredricks et al., 2004; Fredricks & McColskey, 2012; Martin et al., 2021a)—and also the adaptive and maladaptive engagement dimensions of the Motivation and Engagement Wheel (Martin, 2007, 2009). Then, at the micro level, the chapter reviews recent research into LRI and specific measured forms of engagement (e.g., participation, persistence, etc.) and provides pedagogical advice at this micro/measured level.

Where Have We Been and Where Are We Going?

The issues addressed in this chapter are in part grounded in the first edition of this handbook (Christenson et al., 2012). In that volume, leading researchers offered their perspectives on the interface between academic motivation and engagement. The researchers described the processes underlying the relationship between academic motivation and engagement and the subsequent impacts on academic outcomes. In his commentary on their chapters, Martin (2012) noted there was broad agreement that academic motivation underpins academic engagement and that academic engagement impacts academic outcomes such as achievement. For example, Reeve (2012) described how inner motivational resources allow students to academically engage in class. Anderman and Patrick (2012) identified how motivation is present before and during a task, while academic engagement is predominantly present during a task. Cleary and Zimmerman (2012) differentiated "will" (motivation) from "skill" (engagement) and suggested the former gives rise to the latter. Similarly, Schunk and Mullen (2012) described the energizing role of academic motivation for engagement. Pekrun and Linnenbrink-Garcia (2012) suggested that academic engagement mediates the relationship between emotion (motivation) and achievement. Ainley (2012) also described how motivation (by way of interest) leads to achievement via engagement.

These contributing researchers also explored the contextual factors implicated in students' academic motivation and engagement. Reeve (2012) described how good teacher-student relationships are important for motivation and engagement to flourish. Likewise, Voelkl (2012) reported how being supported by teachers, being treated fairly, and feeling safe was important for academic engagement. Anderman and Patrick (2012), as well as Pekrun and Linnenbrink-Garcia (2012), explored the role of classroom goal structures (students' subjective perceptions of the meaning and purpose of tasks within the classroom) and their impacts on student motivation and engagement. In a similar vein, Schunk and Mullen (2012) identified the role of collective agency (students' shared beliefs about what they can achieve as a class) in the development of academic motivation and engagement.

Schunk and Mullen (2012) also identified the educational influences that shape students' academic motivation and engagement—bringing into focus the role of instruction in impacting students' academic engagement and the consequent impact of engagement on academic learning and achievement. Indeed, it is at this very point where the present chapter picks up. Specifically, with a focus on LRI, CLT and related instructional frameworks, the present chapter reviews the role of academic engagement in mediating the relationship between instruction and young people's academic development (i.e., their learning, achievement, etc.). Moreover, because LRI is a highly cognitive model of instruction, it is contended there are natural alignments in the processing implicated in how learners acquire their knowledge and skill and how they are psychologically oriented to their academic life and academic subject matter, particularly when it comes to their cognitive orientations that take the form of, inter alia, cognitive dimensions of engagement. Thus, a comprehensive assessment of engagement would benefit from also assessing contexts and factors that may shape it. Instructional and cognitive burdens rep-

resent a significant source of difficulty for many students and may adversely impact student engagement if not effectively managed (Martin et al., 2020b). This being the case, researchers and practitioners would benefit from also assessing instructional practices that are relevant to ease (or not) the cognitive load on students as they learn.

It is also appropriate to note that although the focus of this chapter is on LRI and CLT, it is acknowledged there are numerous instructional frameworks that recognize the realities (and limits) of the cognitive architecture of the human memory system and formulate effective principles, strategies, and practices aimed at accommodating these realities (for examples and relevant reviews, see Adams & Engelmann, 1996; Cromley & Byrnes, 2012; Lee & Anderson, 2013; Marzano, 2003, 2011; Mayer & Moreno, 2010; Nandagopal & Ericsson, 2012; Purdie & Ellis, 2005; Rosenshine, 1995, 2009; Rosenshine & Stevens, 1986). These principles have also been present in other instructional approaches over the past five decades (e.g., Brophy & Good, 1986; Christenson et al., 1989; Slavin, 1995).

Cognitive Load Theory and Load Reduction Instruction

According to CLT, two kinds of cognitive loads can be imposed by teachers on students that are a barrier to learning: intrinsic and extraneous cognitive load (Sweller et al., 2011). Intrinsic cognitive load is the inherent difficulty of instructional material and learning activities. Teachers manage the intrinsic cognitive load by presenting instructional material and learning activities that are appropriate to students' level of knowledge and skill (Sweller et al., 2011). Extraneous cognitive load is a function of how instructional material and learning activities are structured and presented (Sweller et al., 2011). They can be presented to students in sequential, clear, and explicit ways, so the students are guided through learning in a structured and linear manner—leading to low extraneous load. Alternatively, instructional material and learning activities can be presented in a way that places a greater onus and responsibility on students to derive and determine the structure of the information and nature of the activity, navigate through a range of possible solutions, and draw on and apply the information they have relatively little prior knowledge about—all leading to higher levels of extraneous load (Sweller et al., 2011). Extraneous cognitive load is identified as an unnecessary burden on students and thus does not contribute to learning (Sweller et al., 2011).

LRI draws on these major principles of CLT. LRI comprises a suite of instructional principles that are aimed at reducing the extraneous cognitive load (as the primary yield)—and to some extent, a certain level of associated intrinsic cognitive load (as a secondary yield) (Martin, 2016; Martin et al., 2020b). It is especially important to reduce extrinsic and intrinsic cognitive load when students are in the early stages of learning—thus, when they are novices (e.g., when beginning a new subject, a new unit of a course or work, etc.). Failure to do so not only risks learners not acquiring the required knowledge or skill but also risks alienating learners from an academic engagement perspective (Martin, 2016). Then, when students have developed an adequate level of automaticity and fluidity in knowledge and skill, there is an appropriate point for engaging in guided discovery approaches (Liem & Martin, 2012; see also Kalyuga et al., 2012). In terms of broader pedagogical terrain, then, LRI is clear that explicit and constructivist perspectives are not only compatible but essentially synergistic—the success of one is intertwined with the success of the other (Liem & Martin, 2012; Martin, 2016; Martin & Evans, 2018, 2019; Martin et al., 2020b). Nonetheless, the order in which explicit and constructivist processes are enacted is key: extraneous cognitive load is likely to result if discovery approaches are carried out before students have acquired the necessary skill and knowledge, and this will impede students' learning (Martin, 2016). Thus, particularly when students are novices, LRI emphasizes that explicit and structured instructional approaches must precede guided discovery approaches.

The Human Memory System, LRI, and the Potential Role of Engagement

Human Memory

The human memory system is a major consideration when developing principles and strategies for instruction that reduce the cognitive load on learners. Particularly for learning academic subject matter, working and long-term memory are primary components of the human memory system (Kirschner et al., 2006; Sweller, 2012; Winne & Nesbit, 2010). Working memory is the component that receives and processes information (e.g., solving problems, performing tasks, etc.), including unfamiliar and new information. Learning is deemed to have occurred when information is "moved" from working memory and is encoded in long-term memory such that the student can successfully retrieve it later (Kirschner et al., 2006; Martin & Evans, 2018, 2019; Sweller, 2012; Winne & Nesbit, 2010).

A major challenge for teachers and students is that working memory is very limited. This challenge is especially present when teachers are attempting to teach new material to students (Sweller et al., 2011; Winne & Nesbit, 2010). On the other hand, long-term memory has no such limits; it has a vast capacity (Sweller, 2012). It is therefore important for instruction to take into account the reality of students' working memory limits and help them to transfer knowledge between working and long-term memory (Martin, 2015, 2016; Martin & Evans, 2018, 2019; Paas et al., 2003; Sweller, 2004; Winne & Nesbit, 2010). Instruction is a primary means by which they do this. As Kirschner and colleagues caution: "Any instructional theory that ignores the limits of working memory when dealing with novel information or ignores the disappearance of those limits when dealing with familiar information is unlikely to be effective" (2006, p. 77).

Fluency, Automaticity, and LRI

Fluency and automaticity are important concepts when considering effective means by which teachers can help move, encode, and store information in long-term memory. When teachers deliver instruction in ways that enable opportunities for developing students' fluency and automaticity in skill and knowledge they help free up working memory resources. Fluency and automaticity reduce cognitive burden and help students to transfer novel information into long-term memory (Rosenshine, 2009).

As relevant to LRI, Martin and Evans (2019; see also Martin, 2016; Martin et al., 2020b) explain how LRI develops fluency and automaticity—especially through its first four principles: (principle #1) reducing the difficulty of instruction in the initial stages of learning, as appropriate to the learner's level of prior knowledge and skill (see also Pollock et al., 2002; Mayer & Moreno, 2010); (principle #2) providing appropriate support and scaffolding to learn relevant skill and knowledge (see also Renkl, 2014; Renkl & Atkinson, 2010); (principle #3) allowing sufficient opportunity for practice (see also Nandagopal & Ericsson, 2012; Purdie & Ellis, 2005; Rosenshine, 2009); and (principle #4) providing appropriate feedback-feedforward (com-

bination of corrective information and specific improvement-oriented guidance) as needed (see also Hattie, 2009; Mayer & Moreno, 2010; Shute, 2008). Figure 2 demonstrates.

With increasing fluency and automaticity, students' working memory is freed up and they are better placed to apply their knowledge and skill to learning tasks that may have previously been too great a cognitive load on them. These learning tasks include novel or more complex tasks, activities that involve higher-order thinking, problem solving, and discovery learning (Martin, 2016; Martin & Evans, 2019). These latter learning tasks are collectively represented by principle #5 in LRI: guided independent learning. CLT research demonstrates that when expertise is developed by learners (i.e., learners have developed sufficient automaticity and fluency in skill and knowledge), their learning is not further assisted by approaches that are overly explicit and structured. In fact, when students have developed fluency and automaticity in skill and knowledge, they benefit from more open, problem-solving approaches. This has been empirically shown via the "expertise reversal effect" (e.g., Kalyuga, 2007; Kalyuga et al., 2003; Kalyuga et al., 2001).

Taken together, when the teacher provides the appropriate difficulty reduction, instructional sup-

Fig. 2 Load reduction instruction (LRI) framework. (Adapted with Permission from Martin (2016))

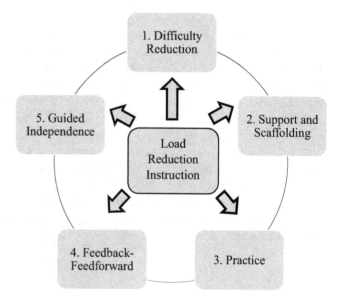

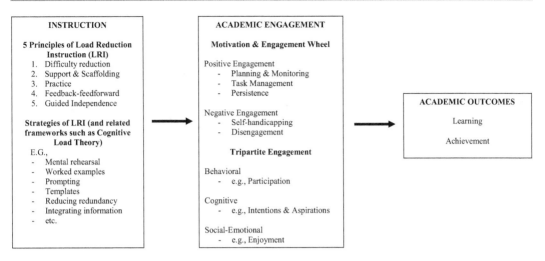

Fig. 3 Role of academic engagement in mediating the link between instruction and academic outcomes

port, guided practice, and feedback-feedforward through LRI principles #1-#4, learners are ideally placed to develop the relevant and requisite knowledge and skill—in large part because the teacher has appropriately eased the cognitive burden at the relevant points for students as they learn. Then, the teacher can present subject matter that is more demanding to the student or that allows for greater independence and open inquiry (Kalyuga et al., 2003). In these ways, after adequate explicit and structured instruction (i.e., LRI principles #1–4), students are at a point in the learning process when they benefit from relatively greater independence (i.e., LRI principle #5) (Liem & Martin, 2012; Martin, 2016; Martin & Evans, 2018; Mayer, 2004). This being the case, there is no question as to whether learners benefit more from explicit (and structured) instruction or more from independent learning—they clearly benefit from both; but it is the sequencing of these two that is pivotal to learning, with students benefiting from explicit instruction in the early stages of their academic development before being immersed in the more independent phase of learning as their knowledge and skill develop.

Academic Engagement as a Potential Mediating Mechanism?

As described below, these instructional principles have been connected to enhanced learning and achievement in many research studies. However, an issue that has been somewhat unaddressed relates to the mechanism/s that may be implicated in this connection. Researchers have speculated the role of academic engagement in this process, but relatively little research has attended to this. This chapter, therefore, explores the theory and research that provide some insight into how academic engagement may mediate the link between LRI (and related instructional approaches) and students' learning and achievement—as shown in Fig. 3.

Academic Engagement

In the first edition of this handbook, Martin (2012) contributed a commentary on the chapters elucidating ideas around academic motivation and engagement. In synthesizing the key ideas, Martin drew on the multidimensional Motivation and Engagement Wheel (Martin, 2007, 2009). Building on that line of analysis, the present chapter also draws on the Wheel as one means to consider the relationship between LRI and students' academic engagement and the role of engagement in mediating the association between LRI and academic outcomes such as learning and achievement. In the discussion further below, the chapter also considers the "classic" tripartite engagement framework (behavioral, cognitive, social-emotional;

Fredricks et al., 2004; Martin et al., 2021a) and how its component engagement factors may mediate the link between LRI and academic outcomes. Thus, as relevant to the 4M Academic Engagement Framework (Fig. 1), this chapter focuses on the Wheel and tripartite dimensions (meso-level constructs) of academic engagement (meta-level construct).

Academic Engagement in the Motivation and Engagement Wheel

As Fig. 4 shows, the Motivation and Engagement Wheel is demarcated into positive (adaptive) and negative (maladaptive) motivation and engagement factors. Positive (adaptive) academic engagement comprises planning and monitoring behavior, task management, and persistence. Negative (maladaptive) academic engagement comprises self-handicapping and disengagement. Although not the focus of the present discussion

(see Martin, 2012 in the first edition of this volume), positive motivation comprises self-efficacy, valuing, and mastery orientation and negative motivation comprises anxiety, failure avoidance, and uncertain control.

Following Martin (2012, 2016), the positive and negative academic engagement (meso) factors comprise specific (micro/measured) factors as follows:

Positive (adaptive) academic engagement:

– *Planning (and monitoring)* refers to how much students plan assignments, homework and study and, how much they actively keep track of their progress as they do this work.
– *Task management* refers to how students use their study or homework time, organize a study or homework timetable, choose and arrange where they study or do homework, and increasingly, how they manage their digital world (e.g., self-regulation with regards to mobile technology while doing schoolwork).

Fig. 4 Motivation and Engagement Wheel (Reproduced with Permission from Andrew J. Martin; Download Wheel from www. lifelongachievement. com)

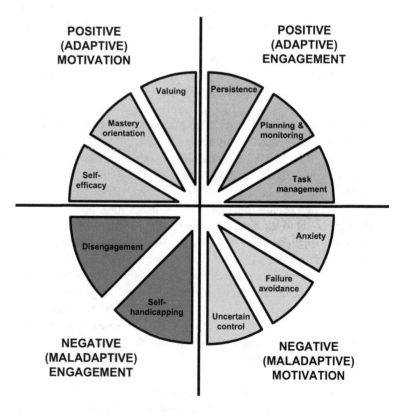

– *Persistence* refers to how much students keep trying to work out an answer or to understand a problem, even if that problem is difficult or challenging.

Negative (maladaptive) academic engagement:

– *Self-handicapping* refers to strategic behaviors that reduce students' prospects of success at school (e.g., waste time, procrastinate, do little or no study, manage time poorly, misbehave in class) to establish an alibi or excuse in case they do not perform well.
– *Disengagement* refers to thoughts and feelings of giving up, trying less each week, detachment from school and schoolwork, feelings of helplessness, and little or no involvement in class or school activities.

Academic Engagement in the Tripartite Framework

The tripartite perspective conceptualizes academic engagement as a meta-construct comprising factors such as behavioral engagement, cognitive engagement, and social-emotional engagement (Fredricks & McColskey, 2012; Martin et al., 2021a). Behavioral engagement draws on ideas around participation and involvement; cognitive engagement draws on ideas around being thoughtful, willing, and strategic as one invests academically and exerts necessary scholarly effort; social-emotional engagement draws on ideas around positive and negative emotional and interpersonal responses relevant to learning and instruction (Fredricks et al., 2004; Martin et al., 2021a). Similar to the Wheel, these constructs might be considered as meso-level constructs, with specific micro/measured constructs as the means by which the meso constructs are assessed and operationalized. In the present chapter three micro/measured engagement constructs will be considered: participation (for behavioral engagement), aspirations and intentions (for cognitive engagement), and enjoyment (for social-emotional engagement).

Multilevel Engagement

Most academic engagement research is conducted at the student level, without accounting appropriately for the classrooms that students belong to. As Fig. 1 shows, the 4M Academic Engagement Framework is clear that engagement resides at multiple levels of an educational structure (e.g., classrooms, schools). The importance of analyzing nested data in appropriate ways is now well known (Marsh et al., 2012), such as when seeking to understand academic engagement in the class or schools as a whole. Single-level research designs can present statistical biases (e.g., within-group dependencies; confounding variables between and within groups) and multilevel analyses seek to address these sorts of biases (see Goldstein, 2003; Marsh et al., 2009; Raudenbush & Bryk, 2002). There are also known reciprocities between individual and group dynamics such that the group may influence individuals and individuals may influence the group (Goldstein, 2003; Marsh et al., 2009; Raudenbush & Bryk, 2002)—thus, classroom- or school-level academic engagement may affect individual students' academic engagement and vice versa. It is therefore important, for example, to ascertain the role of classroom-level academic engagement in mediating the relationship between classroom-level instruction (classroom-level LRI) and classroom-level achievement—beyond the extent to which these relationships occur at the student level. To the extent academic engagement does mediate this link at the classroom level (beyond the student level), there are implications for research and practice in accommodating both students' own engagement and also that of the classrooms to which they belong.

Links Between Instruction and Academic Engagement

In the original development of the LRI framework, Martin (2016) drew several links between LRI and academic engagement. He identified how key LRI factors (e.g., sufficient practice and feedback-feedforward) underpin personal investment in learning. He also pointed to research finding that greater academic engagement occurred when there was an appropriate pedagogical structure in place (i.e., teachers provided explicit plans for the lesson, clear directions, feedback, and guidance; e.g., Jang et al., 2010; Sierens et al., 2009). Martin and Evans (2018) also contended that key LRI factors—such as easing the difficulty of tasks to match learners' level of prior knowledge—may result in lower levels of disengagement (Ashcraft & Kirk, 2001; Martin, 2016). There is thus a basis for considering that LRI and related instructional approaches may lead to academic engagement (see Fig. 3).

Specific and Salient Instructional Factors Under CLT and LRI

CLT researchers have identified many specific instructional factors that are the means by which broader CLT principles are operationalized. Similarly, Martin (2016) identified the specific CLT (and related) instructional factors that are a means to operationalize the LRI principles. These can include the following instructional approaches and techniques: mental practice, worked examples, guided practice, checking for understanding, prompts, templates, reducing split attention, integrating information, using different modalities, reducing redundancy, and increasing coherence. Drawing on Martin (2016), the discussion now turns to each of these specific instructional approaches and techniques and their links to each academic engagement factor in the Wheel and the tripartite framework.

Motivation and Engagement Wheel: Positive Academic Engagement

Planning (and Monitoring) and Task Management Planning, monitoring, and task management are undergirded by skills in self-regulated learning (Zimmerman, 2002). As Martin (2016) explained, self-regulation relies on

students' capacity to organize learning material, pace learning, identify and follow the steps involved in learning, self-monitor, and adjust as required (also see Martin, 2007, 2009, 2010). There are specific elements of CLT, LRI and related instructional approaches that are associated with students' planning, monitoring, and task management, including mental practice, worked examples, and guided practice. In *mental practice* (sometimes referred to as the "imagination effect"; Sweller, 2012) learners are asked to mentally rehearse a procedure or concept. The planning and monitoring part of the Wheel benefits from learners mentally representing their various demands—such as the important parts of a task or schedule of activities (Martin, 2010, 2016). In addition, how well learners can monitor their progress will rely on how well the representation of important parts are stored in long-term memory. *Worked examples* are completed samples of work that show students how a problem can be solved or how a task can be completed. They help learners acquire schemas that they can then apply to solve problems quickly and efficiently (Atkinson et al., 2000; Renkl, 2014; Renkl & Atkinson, 2010; Rosenshine, 1995, 2009; Sweller, 2012). Worked examples identify the parts of a task that the learner needs to plan, emphasize the components important to monitor to stay on task, and taken together optimize processes involved in effectively managing task demands. In *guided practice* (Hunter, 1984) students are linearly guided through the steps of learning. This makes it clear what components of a task are to be performed or what components are to be learned. The teacher may demonstrate these steps first and then guide the students as they practice each step—or, depending on the novice status of the students and/or the nature of the learning task, the teacher may move immediately to guided practice with the students. Knowing these components is essential for planning, knowing what to monitor, how to manage oneself, and one's resources for task completion (Martin, 2016). Taken together, then, there are plausible grounds on which to conject a relationship between specific CLT and LRI factors and students' academic engagement.

Persistence Theory and research also suggest specific CLT and LRI factors that are associated with academic persistence, including checking for understanding, using templates, and using procedural prompts. Rosenshine (1995, 2009; see also Hunter, 1984) identified that effective teachers give sufficient time to *check student understanding*. Others propose frequent intra-lesson assessments to check for student understanding (Black & Wiliam, 2004). For example, "rapid formative assessment" (Wiliam, 2011) three to five times each week has also been proposed (see also Hattie, 2012). Through these, students remain on task and maintain persistence in the task, reducing the inclination to give up or switch off (Martin, 2016). *Templates* can be helpful to enhance persistence where there is a risk that students may get lost or confused midway through a task. Templates tend to be structured and may comprise a checklist that scaffolds a student through a task or could involve "process worksheets" that list the steps involved in completing tasks (Van Merriënboer, 1992). Procedural *prompts* can also assist persistence, particularly through less structured tasks (Rosenshine, 1995; see also Purdie & Ellis, 2005). Procedural prompts reduce distractions from tangential information, help extract central and specific information, and help frame an answer. In summary, theory and research provide a basis for positing a link between specific instructional factors and academic engagement by way of persistence.

et al., 2021b)—thus, LRI can play a part in easing the cognitive burden on students and in turn ease the anxiety that undergirds maladaptive engagement in the form of self-handicapping. In addition to the specific CLT and LRI factors described above (mental practice, worked examples, etc.), two other factors linked with lower instructional cognitive burden are: reducing split attention and integrating information sequencing. Splitting students' attention across two or more aspects of learning content can impose an unnecessary cognitive burden and may elevate anxiety. It occurs when information to learn or solve a problem is presented in different parts of the learning space (Ginns, 2006; Mayer & Moreno, 2010; Sweller, 2012). For example, a diagram or figure may be presented in one part of a screen or page and the associated explanatory material necessary for understanding the diagram is presented somewhere else on the screen or page. CLT researchers have shown that teachers *reduce split attention* by integrating the two informational spaces into one space to reduce the cognitive burden on the learner—for example, the equation for finding an angle might be drawn into the angle itself (Sweller, 2012). Material presented at different points in time can also present a burden on working memory (Mayer & Moreno, 2010), whereas *integrating information sequencing* removes this cognitive load. For example, if teaching students about how lighting works via multi-media, the narration would accompany each part of the animation. By integrating instructional content better, the cognitive load on learners is eased and they are less likely to feel overwhelmed and fearful about the task—this may reduce the potential for maladaptive engagement by way of self-handicapping.

Motivation and Engagement Wheel: Negative Academic Engagement

Self-handicapping The likelihood of self-handicapping is heightened when a student is fearful of failure or anxious (Covington, 2000; Martin & Marsh, 2003). Anxiety may be elevated when the student experiences excessive cognitive burden (Chadwick et al., 2015; Martin, Ginns,

Disengagement Disengagement is a result of poor instructional practices such as inappropriate repetition, uninteresting learning material, and exceeding the capacities of cognitive resources such as visual and auditory processors (Sweller, 2012). CLT, LRI, and related instructional frameworks identify numerous factors that may address disengagement arising from these poor instructional practices, including using different modalities, avoiding redundancy, and increasing coherence. If too much visual information is presented (e.g., via a diagram, text, a table, or call-out boxes), the learner's visual processor reaches capacity and they must dedicate increasing energy to maintain it (Mayer & Moreno, 2010; Sweller, 2012). This imposes an excessive burden on the learner who struggles to keep up and this risks disengagement. In such cases, the teacher may *use different modalities* by offloading some of the information onto the auditory processor as an audible narrative (Mayer & Moreno, 2010; Sweller, 2012). Disengagement can also arise when the same information is presented twice and the learner cannot reconcile the two sources of information, as it exceeds the processing capacity of working memory (Mayer & Moreno, 2010). For example, if a diagram includes the necessary information, it is not necessary to also have the same information placed in a caption below. *Avoiding redundancy* and *increasing coherence* by presenting only the essential information optimize the capacity of working memory to process information (Mayer & Moreno, 2010) and reduce the possibility that students switch off due to being cognitive overwhelmed (Martin, 2016). Again, there is a link between specific instructional factors and students' academic engagement.

Tripartite Academic Engagement

The discussion thus far has identified specific elements of CLT and LRI that are associated with the academic engagement factors in the Motivation and Engagement Wheel. Consideration is also given to how instructional factors under LRI are associated with academic engagement factors in Fredricks et al.'s (2004) tripartite framework. With regard to behavioral engagement (e.g., participation), LRI is aimed at freeing cognitive resources so students are able to keep up with class activities and learning material that is central to the lesson. When students are abreast of subject matter and classroom activities, they are better able to meaningfully partici-

pate in class (Finn & Zimmer, 2012). In terms of social-emotional engagement (e.g., enjoyment), alleviating unnecessary cognitive burdens as students learn may help them better enjoy and immerse in what they are doing. Regarding cognitive engagement (e.g., intentions and aspirations), reducing cognitive burden optimizes understanding and efficacy (Feldon et al., 2018), which are foundations for positive intentions with regard to investing in one's academic future (Burns et al., 2018). Indeed, key principles of LRI seek to make instruction more accessible to students and this may instill in students more positive self-conceptions and more positive orientations to their academic future (Martin, 2016).

Links Between Instruction, Academic Engagement, and Achievement

Most CLT and related research have centered on learning outcomes (typically assessed via achievement and task performance) when testing for effects that are core to their underlying principles (e.g., effects related to worked examples, split attention, expertise reversal, etc.; Sweller et al., 2011). There has been relatively little CLT research exploring the role of academic engagement in the learning process (but for examples, see Lambert et al., 2009; Swann, 2013). Martin et al. (2020b) argue that because much of LRI is related to teachers' instructional practices, it is vital to consider factors known to be implicated in these instructional practices—such as academic engagement. To the extent there is a significant place for academic engagement in mediating the link between LRI and learning, there is a need for theories and research into instruction to accommodate the role of academic engagement in their processes. This notion is not uncommon in major theories of academic engagement. For example, Reschly and Christenson (2012) are clear that instruction and academic engagement are interconnected in how students learn and achieve academically. In addition, as noted earlier, because LRI is a predominantly cognitive model of instruction, there are likely alignments in the processing implicated in how learners acquire their knowledge and skill and how they are psychologically oriented to their academic subject matter, such as by way of their cognitive engagement.

It is therefore notable that many researchers identify academic engagement as a means by which learning and achievement occur. Indeed, the salient role of academic engagement in students' achievement is consistent with major perspectives on engagement and its place in the learning process (Pekrun & Linnenbrink-Garcia, 2012). For example, the agentic elements of academic engagement in which students exert control over their learning are key to understanding how learning and achievement take place (Reeve, 2012; Schunk & Mullen, 2012). Academic engagement also is linked to learning and achievement in the two engagement frameworks under focus in this chapter. In the case of the Motivation and Engagement Wheel factors, significant positive links have been identified between students' planning, task management, and persistence and students' achievement; at the same time, significant inverse links are established between students' self-handicapping and disengagement behaviors and students' achievement (see Liem & Martin, 2012 for review). In the case of the three main factors under the tripartite academic engagement framework, research suggests that behavioral engagement in the form of participation assists students to attain a better understanding of a topic or subject area (Credé et al., 2010; Green et al., 2012; Lysakowski & Walberg, 1982). In terms of cognitive engagement, students' conceptions of their academic futures (e.g., by way of aspirations) impact their present learning (e.g., Burns et al., 2021; de Bilde et al., 2011; Kauffman & Husman, 2004). In relation to social-emotional engagement, factors such as enjoyment encompass affective/social connections and immersion with a topic or learning peers that enhance knowledge and skill acquisition (Burns et al. 2019; Martin & Jackson, 2008; Nakamura & Csikszentmihalyi, 2009).

To summarize, there are links between diverse CLT and LRI instructional factors and students' academic engagement. There is also clear evidence of links between academic engagement and students' learning and achievement. To the extent this is so, we can ascertain a sense of how academic engagement may mediate the link between LRI and achievement—as shown in Fig. 3. However, it is only recently that these links have been formally investigated in a programmatic way. A summary of relevant findings is now presented.

Links Between LRI, Academic Engagement, and Achievement: Empirical Findings

Martin and Evans (2018) developed a survey to assess the five LRI principles. This instrument—the Load Reduction Instruction Scale (LRIS)—comprised five factors, in line with the five principles of LRI. It is a scale that aims to characterize the teacher's instruction on each of the five LRI principles in broad terms (i.e., what a teacher does most of the time)—but, as described by Martin and Evans (2018), has sufficient flexibility to be administered in real-time, or in relation to specific aspects of a lesson to capture any variability relevant to the specific nature of the lesson, its content, and its pace. Martin and Evans (2018) administered the LRIS to 393 students from 40 mathematics classrooms in two comprehensive (mixed ability) high schools. Participants were in year 9, year 10, or year 11. The average age was 15–16 years and slightly over half (57%) of the sample comprised girls. Just under 20% spoke a language other than English at home and, based on their home postcode, their socioeconomic status was slightly above the national average. As well as the LRIS, students were assessed on various academic outcomes, including their positive academic engagement (planning and monitoring, persistence, task management), and negative academic engagement (self-handicapping, disengagement) from the Motivation and Engagement Wheel. Students were also administered items that assessed intrinsic cognitive load and extraneous cognitive load in the mathematics class. Martin and Evans (2018) found that LRI was significantly negatively associated with both intrinsic cognitive load (small effect size) and extraneous cognitive load (large effect size)—hence, significantly more so for extraneous cognitive load than intrinsic cognitive load, in line with theoretical contentions for LRI (Martin, 2016). LRI was also significantly and positively associated with positive academic engagement and significantly inversely associated with negative academic engagement.

In a subsequent study linking the Martin and Evans (2018) data with a previous survey of the same students, analyses revealed that LRI yielded large effect sizes by way of its association with significant gains in academic engagement and achievement at both the student-level and classroom-level (Evans & Martin, 2022). Thus, they provided empirical support for the link between LRI and academic engagement and achievement among students and also demonstrated a link between classroom-level LRI and class-average academic engagement and class-average achievement, beyond links among these factors at the student level. However, this study assessed academic engagement and achievement as outcomes alongside each other—when, as explained above, there is a contended mediating role for academic engagement in linking LRI and achievement.

Accordingly, Martin et al. (2020b) explored the potential of academic engagement as a mediator in the learning process. They employed the LRIS in a multilevel study of more than 180 science classrooms (in 8 comprehensive high schools of mixed ability—though slightly higher in ability than the national average), investigating the extent to which the link between LRI in science and science achievement (at student- and classroom-levels) was mediated by academic engagement, harnessing a tripartite perspective (e.g., Fredricks et al., 2004) via Martin and Liem's (2010) measures of participation, future aspirations, and enjoyment. They operationalized academic engagement as a higher-order factor comprising these three lower-order academic engagement measures (thus, aggregating the micro/measured and meso factors to represent the meta construct). Participants were in years 7–10. The average age was 14–15 years and 60%

of the sample comprised girls. Around one in 10 students spoke a language other than English at home and, based on their home postcode, their socio-economic status was slightly above the national average. Findings revealed that academic engagement mediated the link between LRI and achievement at both student-level and classroom-level: student-level LRI → academic engagement → achievement, $\beta = 0.19$, $p < 0.001$; classroom-level LRI → academic engagement → achievement, $\beta = 0.48$, $p < 0.001$. Interestingly, there was no significant direct effect of LRI on achievement—it was via academic engagement.

All these studies linking LRI to academic engagement and achievement are variable-centered. There is also person-centered work being conducted with these variables. In a recent study Martin et al. (2021b) explored different students' psychological orientations to cognitive load and subsequent links to these students' academic engagement and achievement. They hypothesized that some students would perceive cognitive load in an approach- and challenge-oriented way, while other students would perceive cognitive load in an avoidant- and threat-oriented way. They were also interested to explore how these different orientations would be connected to students' academic engagement and disengagement (via persistence and disengagement in the Wheel), and achievement. They used latent profile analysis to identify the network of instructional-psychological profiles based on students' reports of instructional load (LRI) and their accompanying psychological challenge and threat orientations. They identified five instructional-motivational profiles that represented different presentations of instructional cognitive load, challenge orientation, and threat orientation: Instructionally-Overburdened and Psychologically-Resigned students, Instructionally Burdened and Psychologically Fearful students, Instructionally Supported and Psychologically Composed students, Instructionally Optimized and Psychologically Self-Assured students, and Instructionally Supported and Psychologically Pressured students. They also found that these profiles were significantly different in academic engagement such that the Instructionally Overburdened and Psychologically Resigned profile reflected high disengagement and low engagement and achievement, while the Instructionally Optimized and Psychologically Self-Assured profile reflected low disengagement and high engagement and achievement. Thus, preliminary person-centered research is also suggesting links between LRI and students' academic engagement and achievement outcomes. They are also all amenable to operationalizing at the micro/measured level of the 4M Academic Engagement Framework.

Implications for Academic Engagement Assessment

These findings and the concepts underpinning them suggest that a comprehensive assessment of academic engagement would benefit from also assessing contexts and factors that may shape it. Instructional and cognitive burdens represent a significant source of difficulty for many students and may adversely impact student engagement if not effectively managed. This being the case, it is proposed that to comprehensively assess academic engagement, researchers and practitioners would benefit from also assessing instructional practices that are relevant to easing (or not) the cognitive load on students as they learn. The Load Reduction Instruction Scale (LRIS; Martin & Evans, 2018) was identified as a valid tool to assess LRI. Martin and Evans (2018, 2019; Martin et al., 2020b, 2021b) have suggested numerous ways that the LRIS can be used. It can be readily administered in and across different school subjects, it can be used as an observation checklist for classroom/teacher practice, and it can be used as a tool for teachers' self-reflection.

Of course, there is also the matter of assessing academic engagement itself. There are many validated instruments used to assess tripartite and other engagement frameworks, including the Motivation and Engagement Scale (Martin, 2007, 2009), Patterns of Adaptive Learning Survey (PALS; Midgley et al., 1997), the Motivated Strategies for Learning Questionnaire (MSLQ; Pintrich et al., 1991), the Student Engagement Instrument (SEI; Appleton et al., 2006), and the Inventory of School Motivation (ISM; McInerney et al., 2001). These are forms that are all amenable to inclusion in surveys of instructional and engagement practices—including at student- and classroom levels (see Fredricks, chapter "The Measurement of Student Engagement: Methodological Advances and Comparison of New Self-Report Instruments", this volume).

Implications for Academic Engagement Practice

To the extent that LRI impacts students' academic engagement, the various pedagogical strategies that follow the five principles of LRI are informative for enhancing academic engagement (for detail, see Martin, 2016; Martin & Evans, 2018, 2019). For example, as described in Martin et al. (2020b), to reduce difficulty in the initial stages of learning as appropriate to learners' level of knowledge and skill (principle #1): segmenting (or, "chunking") and pre-training are possible approaches (e.g., Mayer & Moreno, 2010; Pollock et al., 2002). For scaffolding and support (principle #2): worked examples, structured templates, advanced and graphic organizers, and prompting have been suggested (e.g., Berg & Wehby, 2013; Hughes et al., 2019; Renkl, 2014; Renkl & Atkinson, 2010; Sweller, 2012). For ample practice (principle #3): mental rehearsal and deliberate practice have been identified (e.g., Ginns, 2005; Nandagopal & Ericsson, 2012; Purdie & Ellis, 2005; Sweller, 2012). For feedback-feedforward (principle #4): corrective and improvement-oriented information has been proposed, as has personal best goal-setting (e.g., Basso & Belardinelli, 2006; Burns et al., 2019; Hattie, 2009; Martin & Liem, 2010). To promote independence (principle #5): guided discovery learning has been suggested (e.g., Mayer, 2004).

The mediating role of academic engagement suggests it also be a focus for educational practice. Considering academic engagement in terms of the Motivation and Engagement Wheel, Martin (2007, 2009, 2010; Liem & Martin, 2012) has identified numerous strategies at the micro level of the 4M Framework. Students' *planning* can be developed by enhancing their self-regulation skills, e.g., encouraging students to record their homework or assignment in their diary along with the due date and a brief description of what is required. To assist in *monitoring* behavior, the teacher would remind students to check their diaries at appropriate intervals. Teaching students how to use time effectively and how to prioritize can be effective in enhancing their *task management*. Particularly for novices, to reduce the burden on working memory teachers may consider explicitly instructing how to identify the essence of what is required for assignments, how to manage time, and how to check that tasks are being completed in good time—all key aspects of task management. Goal setting can be an effective strategy for enhancing students' *persistence* (Locke & Latham, 2002). Recent research has demonstrated success with personal best goals and the role of these goals in students' engagement, including their persistence (Martin & Elliot, 2016; Martin & Liem, 2010). Reducing *self-handicapping* involves reducing students' fear of failure (that underlies their motive to self-protect; Covington, 2000) and can involve showing students how mistakes are diagnostic feedback and an opportunity for them to improve. Finally, reducing students' *disengagement* can be assisted by empowering students away from helplessness and towards a greater sense of personal control (Covington, 2000). This can be achieved by focusing students' attention on factors that are within their control (e.g., their effort, strategy, attitude; Martin, 2007, 2009). It is also a reality that disengagement may be a result of problems with literacy, numeracy, or a possible disability affecting learning—all requiring intensive and high-quality intervention (Martin et al., 2020a).

There are also practice implications for teachers when seeking to enhance academic engagement at the micro level of the 4M Framework from a tripartite perspective. In terms of *behavioral engagement*, teachers might look to strategies that enhance students' participation in tasks and activities—such as class discussion, small group work, collaboration, help-giving, coopera-

tion, etc. For *cognitive engagement*, teachers might encourage students to develop positive future plans and goals for investing in their schoolwork. In relation to *social-emotional engagement*, teachers might seek to develop tasks and activities that are interesting, fun (where appropriate), pro-social, and arouse curiosity (see also Burns et al., 2019; Martin & Liem, 2010; Martin et al., 2020b; Nagro et al., 2019).

Conclusion

Many students find school difficult, in part because there are instructional burdens that impose a significant cognitive load as they strive to learn. As these burdens escalate, there is the risk of declining academic engagement that in turn adversely impacts learning and achievement. It is important for teachers to deliver instruction in a way that eases the burden on students as they learn and thereby supports students' academic engagement and subsequent academic outcomes. In so doing, educators are in a stronger position to promote young people's positive development, with academic development (at the apex of the 4M Academic Engagement Framework) being one important part of that overall development. LRI (and other instructional perspectives such as CLT) is an instructional approach aimed at managing the cognitive demands experienced by students as they learn. This chapter identified different factors implicated in LRI that are contended to enhance positive academic engagement and reduce negative academic engagement—and in turn, enhance academic outcomes such as achievement. A summary of recent empirical research supported these contentions and the role of academic engagement in mediating the link between instruction and achievement. The chapter also introduced a novel engagement framework—the 4M Academic Engagement Framework—that hierarchically conceptualizes engagement in terms of students' engagement with their broad academic development (the mega level) through to the granular operationalization of specific engagement variables (the micro/measured level). The theoretical and empirical nexus between LRI and the academic engagement dimensions of the 4M Framework was also described. Taken together, it is evident that academic engagement plays an important part in young people's academic development and the instructional factors aimed at supporting that development.

References

Adams, G., & Engelmann, S. (1996). *Research on direct instruction: 25 years beyond DISTAR*. Educational Achievement Systems.

Ainley, M. (2012). Students' interest and engagement in classroom activities. In S. L. Christenson, A. L. Reschly, & C. Wylie (Eds.), *Handbook of research on student engagement* (pp. 283–302). Springer. https://doi.org/10.1007/978-1-4614-2018-7_13

Anderman, E. M. (2013). Middle school transitions. In J. Hattie & E. M. Anderman (Eds.), *International guide to student achievement*. Routledge.

Anderman, E. M., & Mueller, C. E. (2010). Middle school transitions and adolescent development. In J. L. Meece & J. S. Eccles (Eds.), *Handbook of research on schools, schooling, and human development*. Routledge.

Anderman, E. M., & Patrick, H. (2012). Achievement goal theory, conceptualization of ability/intelligence, and classroom climate. In S. L. Christenson, A. L. Reschly, & C. Wylie (Eds.), *Handbook of research on student engagement* (pp. 173–191). Springer. https://doi.org/10.1007/978-1-4614-2018-7_8

Appleton, J. J., Christenson, S. L., Kim, D., & Reschly, A. L. (2006). Measuring cognitive and psychological engagement: Validation of the student engagement instrument. *Journal of School Psychology, 44*, 427–445. https://doi.org/10.1016/j.jsp.2006.04.002

Ashcraft, M. H., & Kirk, E. P. (2001). The relationships among working memory, math anxiety, and performance. *Journal of Experimental Psychology: General, 130*, 224–237. https://doi.org/10.1037/0096-3445.130.2.224

Atkinson, R. K., Derry, S. J., Renkl, A., & Wortham, D. (2000). Learning from examples: Instructional principles from the worked examples research. *Review of Educational Research, 70*, 181–214. https://doi.org/10.3102/00346543070002181

Australian Academy of Science. (2020). *Learning outcomes for online versus in-class education*. Australian Academy of Science. https://www.science.org.au/covid19/learning-outcomes-online-vs-inclass-education

Basso, D., & Belardinelli, M. O. (2006). The role of the feedforward paradigm in cognitive psychology. *Cognitive Processing, 7*, 73–88. https://doi.org/10.1007/s10339-006-0034-1

Berg, J. L., & Wehby, J. (2013). Preteaching strategies to improve student learning in content area classes. *Intervention in School and Clinic, 49*, 14–20. https://doi.org/10.1177/1053451213480029

Bergdahl, N., Nouri, J., & Fors, U. (2020). Disengagement, engagement and digital skills in technology-enhanced learning. *Education and Information Technologies, 25*(2), 957–983.

Bernard, R. M., Borokhovski, E., Schmid, R. F., Tamim, R. M., & Abrami, P. C. (2014). A meta-analysis of blended learning and technology use in higher education: From the general to the applied. *Journal of Computing in Higher Education, 26*(1), 87–122.

Black, P., & Wiliam, D. (2004). The formative purpose: Assessment must first promote learning. *Yearbook of the National Society for the Study of Education, 103*, 20–50. https://doi.org/10.1111/j.1744-7984.2004.tb00047.x

Brophy, J., & Good, T. (1986). Teacher behavior and student achievement. In M. C. Wittrock (Ed.), *Handbook of research on teaching* (3rd ed.). McMillan.

Burns, E. C., Martin, A. J., & Collie, R. J. (2018). Adaptability, personal best (PB) goals setting, and gains in students' academic outcomes: A longitudinal examination from a social cognitive perspective. *Contemporary Educational Psychology, 53*, 57–72. https://doi.org/10.1016/j.cedpsych.2018.02.001

Burns, E. C., Martin, A. J., & Collie, R. J. (2019). Understanding the role of personal best (PB) goal setting in students' declining engagement: A latent growth model. *Journal of Educational Psychology, 111*, 557–572. https://doi.org/10.1037/edu0000291

Burns, E. C., Martin, A. J., & Collie, R. J. (2021). A future time perspective understanding of high school students' engagement and disengagement: A longitudinal investigation. *Journal of School Psychology, 84*, 109–123. https://doi.org/10.1016/j.jsp.2020.12.003

Campbell, D. T., & Fiske, D. W. (1959). Convergent and discriminant validation by the multitrait-multimethod matrix. *Psychological Bulletin, 56*, 81–105.

Chadwick, D., Tindall-Ford, S., Agostinho, S., & Paas, F. (2015). *Using cognitive load compliant instructions to support working memory for anxious students*. 8th Cognitive Load Theory Conference: CO, USA.

Christenson, S., Reschly, A., & Wylie, C. (Eds.). (2012). *Handbook of research on student engagement*. Springer. https://doi.org/10.1007/978-1-4614-2018-7

Christenson, S. L., Reschly, A. L., Appleton, J. J., Berman, S., Spanjers, D., & Varro, P. (2008). Best practices in fostering student engagement. In A. Thomas & J. Grimes (Eds.), *Best practices in school psychology* (5th ed.). National Association of School Psychologists.

Christenson, S. L., Ysseldyke, J. E., & Thurlow, M. L. (1989). Critical instructional factors for students with mild handicaps: An integrative review. *Remedial and Special Education, 10*(5), 21–31.

Cleary, T. J., & Zimmerman, B. J. (2012). A cyclical self-regulatory account of student engagement: Theoretical foundations and applications. In S. L. Christenson,

A. L. Reschly, & C. Wylie (Eds.), *Handbook of research on student engagement* (pp. 237–257). Springer. https://doi.org/10.1007/978-1-4614-2018-7_11

Covington, M. V. (2000). Goal theory, motivation, and school achievement: An integrative review. *Annual Review of Psychology, 51*, 171–200. https://doi.org/10.1146/annurev.psych.51.1.171

Credé, M., Roch, S. G., & Kieszczynka, U. M. (2010). Class attendance in college: A meta-analytic review of the relationship of class attendance with grades and student characteristics. *Review of Educational Research, 80*, 272–295. https://doi.org/10.3102/0034654310362998

Cromley, J. G., & Byrnes, J. P. (2012). Instruction and cognition. *Wiley Interdisciplinary Reviews: Cognitive Science, 3*, 545–553. https://doi.org/10.1002/wcs.1192

de Bilde, J., Vansteenkiste, M., & Lens, W. (2011). Understanding the association between future time perspective and self-regulated learning through the lens of self-determination theory. *Learning and Instruction, 21*, 332–344. https://doi.org/10.1016/j.learninstruc.2010.03.002

Escueta, M., Quan, V., Nickow, A., & Oreopoulos, P. (2017). *Education technology: An evidence-based review (No. w23744)*. National Bureau of Economic Research.

Evans, P., & Martin, A. J. (2022). *Load reduction instruction: Multilevel effects on motivation, engagement, and achievement in mathematics*. Submitted for publication. https://doi.org/10.4324/9780429283895-2

Feldon, D. F., Franco, J., Chao, J., Peugh, J., & Maahs-Fladung, C. (2018). Self-efficacy change associated with a cognitive load-based intervention in an undergraduate biology course. *Learning and Instruction, 56*, 64–72. https://doi.org/10.1016/j.learninstruc.2018.04.007

Finn, J. D., & Zimmer, K. S. (2012). Student engagement: What is it? Why does it matter? In S. L. Christenson, A. L. Reschly, & C. Wylie (Eds.), *Handbook of research on student engagement* (pp. 97–131). Springer. https://doi.org/10.1007/978-1-4614-2018-7_5

Fredricks, J. A., Blumenfeld, P. C., & Paris, A. H. (2004). School engagement: Potential of the concept, state of the evidence. *Review of Educational Research, 74*, 59–109. https://doi.org/10.3102/00346543074001059

Fredricks, J. A., & McColskey, W. (2012). The measurement of student engagement: A comparative analysis of various methods and student self-report instruments. In S. L. Christenson, A. L. Reschly, & C. Wylie (Eds.), *Handbook of research on student engagement* (pp. 763–782). Springer.

Ginns, P. (2005). Meta-analysis of the modality effect. *Learning and Instruction, 15*, 313–331. https://doi.org/10.1016/j.learninstruc.2005.07.001

Ginns, P. (2006). Integrating information: A meta-analysis of the spatial contiguity and temporal contiguity effects. *Learning and Instruction, 16*, 511–525. https://doi.org/10.1016/j.learninstruc.2006.10.001

Goldstein, H. (2003). *Multilevel statistical models* (3rd ed.). Hodder Arnold.

Graham, C., & Hill, M. (2003). *Negotiating the transition to secondary school*. Scottish Council for Research in Education.

Green, J., Liem, G. A. D., Martin, A. J., Colmar, S., Marsh, H. W., & McInerney, D. (2012). Academic motivation, self-concept, engagement, and performance in high school: Key processes from a longitudinal perspective. *Journal of Adolescence, 35*, 1111–1122. https://doi.org/10.1016/j.adolescence.2012.02.016

Hattie, J. (2009). *Visible learning: A synthesis of over 800 meta-analyses relating to achievement*. Routledge.

Hattie, J. (2012). *Visible learning for teachers*. Routledge. https://doi.org/10.4324/9780203181522

Hughes, M. D., Regan, K. S., & Evmenova, A. (2019). A computer-based graphic organizer with embedded self-regulated learning strategies to support student writing. *Intervention in School and Clinic, 55*(1), 13–22. https://doi.org/10.1177/1053451219833026

Hunter, M. (1984). Knowing, teaching and supervising. In P. Hosford (Ed.), *Using what we know about teaching* (pp. 169–192). ASCD.

Jang, H., Reeve, J., & Deci, E. L. (2010). Engaging students in learning activities: It is not autonomy support or structure but autonomy support and structure. *Journal of Educational Psychology, 102*(3), 588–600. https://doi.org/10.1037/a0019682

Kalyuga, S. (2007). Expertise reversal effect and its implications for learner-tailored instruction. *Educational Psychology Review, 19*, 509–539. https://doi.org/10.1007/s10648-007-9054-3

Kalyuga, S., Ayres, P., Chandler, P., & Sweller, J. (2003). The expertise reversal effect. *Educational Psychologist, 38*, 23–31. https://doi.org/10.1207/S15326985EP3801_4

Kalyuga, S., Chandler, P., Tuovinen, J., & Sweller, J. (2001). When problem solving is superior to studying worked examples. *Journal of Educational Psychology, 93*, 579–588. https://doi.org/10.1037/0022-0663.93.3.579

Kalyuga, S., Rikers, R., & Paas, F. (2012). Educational implications of expertise reversal effects in learning and performance of complex cognitive and sensorimotor skills. *Educational Psychology Review, 24*(2), 313–337. https://doi.org/10.1007/s10648-012-9195-x

Kauffman, D. F., & Husman, J. (2004). Effects of time perspective on student motivation: Introduction to a special issue. *Educational Psychology Review, 16*, 1–7. https://doi.org/10.1023/B:EDPR.0000012342.37854.58

Kirschner, P. A., & De Bruyckere, P. (2017). The myths of the digital native and the multitasker. *Teaching and Teacher Education, 67*, 135–142.

Kirschner, P. A., Sweller, J., & Clark, R. E. (2006). Why minimal guidance during instruction does not work: An analysis of the failure of constructivist, discovery, problem-based, experiential, and inquiry-based teaching. *Educational Psychologist, 41*, 75–86. https://doi.org/10.1207/s15326985ep4102_1

Lambert, J., Kalyuga, S., & Capan, L. A. (2009). Student perceptions and cognitive load: What can they tell us about e-learning Web 2.0 course design?

E-Learning and Digital Media, 6, 150–163. https://doi.org/10.2304/elea.2009.6.2.150

Lawson, M. A., & Lawson, H. A. (2013). New conceptual frameworks for student engagement research, policy, and practice. *Review of Educational Research, 83*(3), 432–479.

Lee, H. S., & Anderson, J. R. (2013). Student learning: What has instruction got to do with it? *Annual Review of Psychology, 64*, 445–469. https://doi.org/10.1146/annurev-psych-113011-143833

Liem, G. A., & Martin, A. J. (2012). The motivation and engagement scale: Theoretical framework, psychometric properties, and applied yields. *Australian Psychologist, 47*, 3–13. https://doi.org/10.1111/j.1742-9544.2011.00049.x

Locke, E. A., & Latham, G. P. (2002). Building practically useful theory of goal setting and task motivation. *American Psychologist, 57*, 705–717. https://doi.org/10.1037/0003-066X.57.9.705

Lysakowski, R. S., & Walberg, H. J. (1982). Instructional effects of cues, participation, and corrective feedback: A quantitative synthesis. *American Educational Research Journal, 19*, 559–572. https://doi.org/10.3102/00028312019004559

Marsh, H. W. (2002). A multidimensional physical self-concept: A construct validity approach to theory, measurement, and research. *Psychology: The Journal of the Hellenic Psychological Society, 9*, 459–493.

Marsh, H. W., Lüdtke, O., Nagengast, B., Trautwein, U., Morin, A. J., Abduljabbar, A. S., & Köller, O. (2012). Classroom climate and contextual effects: Conceptual and methodological issues in the evaluation of group-level effects. *Educational Psychologist, 47*, 106–124. https://doi.org/10.1080/00461520.2012.670488

Marsh, H. W., Lüdtke, O., Robitzsch, A., Trautwein, U., Asparouhov, T., Muthén, B., & Nagengast, B. (2009). Doubly-latent models of school contextual effects: Integrating multilevel and structural equation approaches to control measurement and sampling error. *Multivariate Behavioral Research, 44*, 764–802. https://doi.org/10.1080/00273170903333665

Marsh, H. W., Martin, A. J., & Hau, K. T. (2006). A multiple method perspective on self-concept research in educational psychology: A construct validity approach. In M. Eid & E. Diener (Eds.), *Handbook of multimethod measurement in psychology*. American Psychological Association Press.

Martin, A. J. (2007). Examining a multidimensional model of student motivation and engagement using a construct validation approach. *British Journal of Educational Psychology, 77*, 413–440. https://doi.org/10.1348/000709906X118036

Martin, A. J. (2009). Motivation and engagement across the academic lifespan: A developmental construct validity study of elementary school, high school, and university/college students. *Educational and Psychological Measurement, 69*, 794–824. https://doi.org/10.1177/0013164409332214

Martin, A. J. (2010). *Building classroom success: Eliminating academic fear and failure*. Continuum.

Martin, A. J. (2012). Motivation and engagement: Conceptual, operational and empirical clarity. In S. L. Christenson, A. L. Reschly, & C. Wylie (Eds.), *Handbook of research on student engagement*. Springer. https://doi.org/10.1007/978-1-4614-2018-7_14

Martin, A. J. (2015). Teaching academically at-risk students in middle school: The roles of explicit instruction and guided discovery learning. In S. Groundwater-Smith & N. Mockler (Eds.), *Big fish, little fish: Teaching and learning in the middle years*. Cambridge University Press.

Martin, A. J. (2016). *Using load reduction instruction (LRI) to boost motivation and engagement*. British Psychological Society.

Martin, A. J., Burns, E. C., Collie, R. J., Cutmore, M., Macleod, S., & Donlevy, V. (2021a). *The role of engagement in immigrant students' academic resilience*. Submitted for publication.

Martin, A. J., & Elliot, A. J. (2016). The role of personal best (PB) and dichotomous achievement goals in students' academic motivation and engagement: A longitudinal investigation. *Educational Psychology, 36*, 1285–1302. https://doi.org/10.1080/01443410.2015.1093606

Martin, A. J., & Evans, P. (2018). Load Reduction Instruction: Exploring a framework that assesses explicit instruction through to independent learning. *Teaching and Teacher Education, 73*, 203–214. https://doi.org/10.1016/j.tate.2018.03.018

Martin, A. J., & Evans, P. (2019). Load reduction instruction: Sequencing explicit instruction and guided discovery to enhance students' motivation, engagement, learning, and achievement. In S. Tindall-Ford, S. Agostinho, & J. Sweller (Eds.), *Advances in cognitive load theory: Rethinking teaching*. Routledge.

Martin, A. J., & Evans, P. (2021). Load reduction instruction policy. In K.-A. Allen, A. Reupert, & L. Oades (Eds.), *Building better schools with evidence-based policy: Adaptable policy for teachers and school leaders*. Routledge.

Martin, A. J., Ginns, P., Burns, E., Kennett, R., Munro-Smith, V., & Pearson, J. (2021b). *Assessing and validating instructional cognitive load in the context of students' psychological challenge and threat orientations: A multi-level latent profile analysis of students and classrooms*. Submitted for publication.

Martin, A. J., Ginns, P., Burns, E., Kennett, R., & Pearson, J. (2020b). Load reduction instruction in science and students' science engagement and science achievement. *Journal of Educational Psychology, 113*(6), 1126–1142. https://doi.org/10.1037/edu0000552

Martin, A. J., & Jackson, S. A. (2008). Brief approaches to assessing task absorption and enhanced subjective experience: Examining 'Short' and 'Core' flow in diverse performance domains. *Motivation and Emotion, 32*, 141–157. https://doi.org/10.1007/s11031-008-9094-0

Martin, A. J., & Liem, G. A. (2010). Academic Personal Bests (PBs), engagement, and achievement: A cross-lagged panel analysis. *Learning and Individual Differences, 20*, 265–270. https://doi.org/10.1016/j.lindif.2010.01.001

Martin, A. J., & Marsh, H. W. (2003). Fear of failure: Friend or foe? *Australian Psychologist, 38*, 31–38. https://doi.org/10.1080/00050060310001706997

Martin, A. J., Sperling, R., & Newton, K. (Eds.). (2020a). *Handbook of educational psychology and students with special needs*. Routledge. https://doi.org/10.4324/9781315100654

Martin, A. J., Way, J., Bobis, J., & Anderson, J. (2015). Exploring the ups and downs of mathematics engagement in the middle years of school. *Journal of Early Adolescence, 35*, 199–244. https://doi.org/10.1177/0272431614529365

Marzano, R. J. (2003). *What works in schools*. ASCD.

Marzano, R. J. (2011). Art and science of teaching/The perils and promises of discovery learning. *Educational Leadership, 69*, 86–87.

Mayer, R. E. (2004). Should there be a three-strikes rule against pure discovery learning? The case for guided methods of instruction. *American Psychologist, 59*, 14–19. https://doi.org/10.1037/0003-066X.59.1.14

Mayer, R. E., & Moreno, R. (2010). Techniques that reduce extraneous cognitive load and manage intrinsic cognitive load during multimedia learning. In J. L. Plass, R. Moreno, & R. Brunken (Eds.), *Cognitive load theory* (pp. 131–152). Cambridge University Press.

McGuinness, C., & Fulton, C. (2019). Digital literacy in higher education: A case study of student engagement with e-tutorials using blended learning. *Journal of Information Technology Education: Innovations in Practice, 18*, 1–28.

McInerney, D. M., Yeung, A. S., & McInerney, V. (2001). Cross-cultural validation of the Inventory of School Motivation (ISM): Motivation orientations of Navajo and Anglo students. *Journal of Applied Measurement, 2*, 135–153.

Means, B., Toyama, Y., Murphy, R., Bakia, M., & Jones, K. (2009). *Evaluation of evidence-based practices in online learning: A meta-analysis and review of online learning studies*. U.S. Department of Education, Office of Planning, Evaluation, and Policy Development.

Midgley, C., Maehr, M., Hicks, L., Roesser, R., Urdan, T., Anderman, E., Kaplan, A., Arunkumar, R., & Middleton, M. (1997). *Patterns of adaptive learning (PALS)*. University of Michigan. https://doi.org/10.1037/t19870-000

Moreno, R. (2010). Cognitive load theory: More food for thought. *Instructional Science, 38*, 135–141. https://doi.org/10.1007/s11251-009-9122-9

Moreno, R., & Mayer, R. E. (2007). Interactive multimodal learning environments. *Educational Psychology Review, 19*, 309–326. https://doi.org/10.1007/s10648-007-9047-2

Nagro, S. A., Fraser, D. W., & Hooks, S. D. (2019). Lesson planning with engagement in mind: Proactive classroom management strategies for curriculum instruction. *Intervention in School and Clinic, 54*, 131–140. https://doi.org/10.1177/1053451218767905

Nakamura, J., & Csikszentmihalyi, M. (2009). Flow theory and research. In C. R. Snyder & S. J. Lopez (Eds.), *Oxford handbook of positive psychology* (pp. 195–206). Oxford University Press. https://doi.org/10.1093/oxfordhb/9780195187243.013.0018

Nandagopal, K., & Ericsson, K. A. (2012). Enhancing students' performance in traditional education: Implications from the expert performance approach and deliberate practice. In K. R. Harris, S. Graham, & T. Urdan (Eds.), *APA educational psychology handbook* (pp. 257–293). American Psychological Association. https://doi.org/10.1037/13273-010

Nguyen, T. (2015). The effectiveness of online learning: Beyond no significant difference and future horizons. *MERLOT Journal of Online Learning and Teaching, 11*(2), 309–319.

OECD. (2015). *Students, computers and learning: Making the connection*. OECD Publishing.

Paas, F., Renkl, A., & Sweller, J. (2003). Cognitive load theory and instructional design: Recent developments. *Educational Psychologist, 38*, 1–4. https://doi.org/10.1207/S15326985EP3801_1

Patall, E. A., Pituch, K. A., Steingut, R. R., Vasquez, A. C., Yates, N., & Kennedy, A. A. (2019). Agency and high school science students' motivation, engagement, and classroom support experiences. *Journal of Applied Developmental Psychology, 62*, 77–92.

Pekrun, R., & Linnenbrink-Garcia, L. (2012). Academic emotions and student engagement. In S. L. Christenson, A. L. Reschly, & C. Wylie (Eds.), *Handbook of research on student engagement* (pp. 259–282). Springer. https://doi.org/10.1007/978-1-4614-2018-7_12

Pintrich, P. R., Smith, D. A. F., Garcia, T., & McKeachie, W. J. (1991). *A manual for the use of the Motivated Strategies for Learning Questionnaire (MSLQ)*. National Center for Research to Improve Postsecondary Teaching and Learning.

Pollock, E., Chandler, P., & Sweller, J. (2002). Assimilating complex information. *Learning and Instruction, 12*, 61–86. https://doi.org/10.1016/S0959-4752(01)00016-0

Purdie, N., & Ellis, L. (2005). *A review of the empirical evidence identifying effective interventions and teaching practices for students with learning difficulties in Years 4, 5, and 6*. Australian Council for Educational Research.

Raudenbush, S. W., & Bryk, A. S. (2002). *Hierarchical linear models: Applications and data analysis methods* (2nd ed.). Sage.

Reeve, J. (2012). A self-determination theory perspective on student engagement. In S. L. Christenson, A. L. Reschly, & C. Wylie (Eds.), *Handbook of research on student engagement* (pp. 149–172). Springer. https://doi.org/10.1007/978-1-4614-2018-7_7

Reeve, J. (2013). How students create motivationally supportive learning environments for themselves: The concept of agentic engagement. *Journal of Educational Psychology, 105*(3), 579–595.

Reeve, J., & Shin, S. H. (2020). How teachers can support students' agentic engagement. *Theory Into Practice, 59*(2), 150–161.

Renkl, A. (2014). Toward an instructionally oriented theory of example-based learning. *Cognitive Science, 38,* 1–37. https://doi.org/10.1111/cogs.12086

Renkl, A., & Atkinson, R. K. (2010). Learning from worked-out examples and problem solving. In J. L. Plass, R. Moreno, & R. Brunken (Eds.), *Cognitive load theory* (pp. 91–108). Cambridge University Press. https://doi.org/10.1017/CBO9780511844744.007

Reschly, A. L., & Christenson, S. L. (2012). Jingle, jangle, and conceptual haziness: Evolution and future directions of the engagement construct. In S. L. Christenson, A. L. Reschly, & C. Wylie (Eds.), *Handbook of research on student engagement* (pp. 3–19). Springer.

Rosenshine, B. V. (1995). Advances in research on instruction. *The Journal of Educational Research, 88,* 262–268. https://doi.org/10.1080/00220671.1995.9941309

Rosenshine, B. V. (2009). The empirical support for direct instruction. In S. Tobias & T. M. Duffy (Eds.), *Constructivist instruction: Success or failure?* Routledge.

Rosenshine, B. V., & Stevens, R. (1986). Teaching functions. In M. C. Wittrock (Ed.), *Handbook of research on teaching* (3rd ed., pp. 376–391). McMillan.

Schunk, D. H., & Mullen, C. A. (2012). Self-efficacy as an engaged learner. In S. L. Christenson, A. L. Reschly, & C. Wylie (Eds.), *Handbook of research on student engagement* (pp. 219–235). Springer. https://doi.org/10.1007/978-1-4614-2018-7_10

Shute, V. J. (2008). Focus on formative feedback. *Review of Educational Research, 78,* 153–189. https://doi.org/10.3102/0034654307313795

Sierens, E., Vansteenkiste, M., Goossens, L., Soenens, B., & Dochy, F. (2009). The synergistic relationship of perceived autonomy support and structure in the prediction of self-regulated learning. *British Journal of Educational Psychology, 79,* 57–68. https://doi.org/10.1348/000709908X304398

Skinner, E. A., & Pitzer, J. R. (2012). Developmental dynamics of student engagement, coping, and everyday resilience. In S. L. Christenson, A. L. Reschly, & C. Wylie (Eds.), *Handbook of research on student engagement* (pp. 21–44). Springer.

Slavin, R. E. (1995). A model of effective instruction. *The Educational Forum, 59*(2), 166–176.

Swann, W. (2013). The impact of applied cognitive learning theory on engagement with e-learning courseware. *Journal of Learning Design, 6,* 61–74. https://doi.org/10.5204/jld.v6i1.119

Sweller, J. (2004). Instructional design consequences of an analogy between evolution by natural selection and human cognitive architecture. *Instructional Science, 32,* 9–31. https://doi.org/10.1023/B:TRUC.0000021808.72598.4d

Sweller, J. (2012). Human cognitive architecture: Why some instructional procedures work and others do not. In K. R. Harris, S. Graham, & T. Urdan (Eds.), *APA educational psychology handbook* (pp. 295–325). American Psychological Association. https://doi.org/10.1037/13273-011

Sweller, J., Ayres, P., & Kalyuga, S. (2011). *Cognitive load theory.* Springer. https://doi.org/10.1007/978-1-4419-8126-4

Van Merriënboer, J. J. (1992). Training complex cognitive skills: A four-component instructional design model for technical training. *Educational Technology Research and Development, 40,* 23–43. https://doi.org/10.1007/BF02297047

Voelkl, K. E. (2012). School identification. In S. L. Christenson, A. L. Reschly, & C. Wylie (Eds.), *Handbook of research on student engagement* (pp. 193–218). Springer. https://doi.org/10.1007/978-1-4614-2018-7_9

Wiliam, D. (2011). *Embedded formative assessment.* Solution Tree Press.

Winne, P. H., & Nesbit, J. C. (2010). The psychology of academic achievement. *Annual Review of Psychology, 61,* 653–678. https://doi.org/10.1146/annurev.psych.093008.100348

Zimmerman, B. J. (2002). Achieving self-regulation: The trial and triumph of adolescence. In F. Pajares & T. Urdan (Eds.), *Academic motivation of adolescents.* Information Age Publishing.

Achievement Goal Theory and Engagement

Eric M. Anderman, Helen Patrick, and Seung Yon Ha

Abstract

Achievement goal theory (AGT) is a framework for examining student motivation. The theory emphasizes both students' personal goals, as well as their perceptions of the goal structures that are emphasized in classrooms. In this chapter, we examine the relations of AGT constructs to students' cognitive, behavioral, and emotional engagement. We focus in particular on the relations between students' perceptions of classroom goal structures (i.e, mastery, performance, and extrinsic goal structures) and various indicators of engagement. The research, both from an AGT perspective and from an engagement perspective, converges on the importance of students' perceptions of teachers' instructional practices as determinants of a variety of academic outcomes.

E. M. Anderman (✉) · S. Y. Ha
The Ohio State University, Columbus, OH, USA
e-mail: anderman.1@osu.edu

H. Patrick
Purdue University, West Lafayette, IN, USA

Introduction

Achievement goal theory (AGT) is a framework for understanding student motivation. The theory addresses why and how people engage in academic activities (i.e., their goal orientations) and contexts that foster those orientations (i.e., goal structures). The theory has been one of the foremost frameworks for studying achievement motivation since the 1980s, informing both educational research (Elliot & Hulleman, 2017; Maehr & Zusho, 2009) and practice (e.g., Maehr & Midgley, 1996). In this chapter, we examine relationships between constructs central to AGT and engagement. We focus on aspects of the environment that foster different types of motivational orientations (i.e., goal structures), particularly classroom goal structures. We use Fredricks' and her colleagues' (2004) conception of engagement as differentiated into cognitive, emotional, and behavioral dimensions. There have been considerable developments in AGT, in addition to more research relevant to engagement, since our chapter in the previous edition of this handbook. Although the constructs utilized by achievement goal theorists are different from those used by researchers who study engagement, there is much overlap. Indeed, both motivation and engagement researchers are focused on promoting students' learning, and see students as being agentic in their learning (Martin, 2012).

We believe that a more thorough examination and possible integration of research conducted by achievement goal theorists and by engagement researchers will lead to a broader and more conceptually useful understanding of academic motivation.

The Basic Tenets of Achievement Goal Theory

The study of achievement goals began in the late 1970s to explain people's achievement motivation. It incorporated many contemporary motivational constructs (e.g., attributions, perceived competence, conceptions of ability, learned helplessness), in addition to earlier conceptions of achievement motivation (e.g., approach and avoid distinctions). Since its inception, researchers have tended to focus on either personal goal orientations or on classroom goal structures. Therefore, the theoretical and empirical developments over the past four decades have resulted in the two strands moving in somewhat different directions. Accordingly, we review goal orientations and goal structures, and their associations with engagement, separately, although our focus is primarily on goal structures.

Personal Goals or Goal Orientations

Personal goals, or goal orientations, represent "the purposes that individuals have for engaging in specific behaviors" (Anderman & Wolters, 2006, p. 371). Achievement goal theorists originally posited two types of personal goal orientations: *mastery* (i.e., a focus on understanding and personal improvement) and *performance* (i.e., a focus on out-performing others) (e.g., Ames, 1987; Dweck & Leggett, 1988; Maehr, 1984; Nicholls, 1989). When students pursue mastery goals, they are interested in becoming competent at the task. They are concerned with increasing their skills and knowledge and view success in terms of personal improvement or absolute standards. They choose challenging tasks, persist when experiencing difficulty, and are willing to

eager to exert effort to achieve mastery. In contrast, when students pursue performance goals, they view success in normative terms (i.e., compared to others) and are interested in demonstrating their ability relative to others, in outperforming others, in being judged by others as being competent at academic tasks, or in not appearing to have low ability compared to others. In line with these concerns, they also tend to choose tasks they believe they will be successful at, and tend not to persist when faced with difficulty (particularly when they are concerned about not appearing to be less able than others) because they view expending effort as an indicator of insufficient ability (Midgley et al., 2001). Goals are typically independent of each other, or orthogonal (Midgley et al., 1998). Moreover, although these goals are student-specific, they are affected by the larger context of classrooms and schools, which we discuss in the section on goal structures.

Elliot and Harackiewicz (1996) noted that when achievement goal theory was established, two of its founders, Dweck and Nicholls (e.g., Dweck & Elliott, 1983; Jagacinski & Nicholls, 1990; Nicholls et al., 1990), considered performance goals to have two forms—approach (wanting to appear more able than others) and avoid (not wanting to appear less able). Recognizing that this distinction became lost in later definitions, several researchers in the mid-1990s argued that the AGT should differentiate between "approach" and "avoid" types of performance goal orientations, and they provided evidence of this distinction (e.g., Elliot & Harackiewicz, 1996; Middleton & Midgley, 1997). When students are focused on performance-approach goals, they are concerned with demonstrating their ability (i.e., outperforming others). In contrast, when students are focused on performance-avoid goals, they are concerned with not appearing to lack ability (i.e., not looking worse than others) (Elliot, 1999).

The approach-avoid distinction was also applied to mastery goal orientations, resulting in a 2 X 2 framework for achievement goals (Elliot & McGregor, 2001). In this model, mastery goals were divided into two constructs—mastery-approach and mastery-avoid goals—matching the separation of performance-approach and performance-avoid goals. Although mastery goals were already construed in purely approach terms, mastery-avoid was a new addition to the model. Theoretically, students who endorse mastery-avoid goals want to avoid misunderstanding or becoming less competent. The 2 X 2 model has been supported across several international samples. Conroy et al. (2003) tested the model with a sample of 356 recreational university athletes. Participants completed measures of the four achievement goals, as well as a measure of fear of failure, at four-time points. All scales exhibited both structural invariance and stability over 3 weeks. In addition, the goals were related to fear of failure across all time points; for example, the correlations between performance-avoidance goals and fear of failure ranged from 0.28 to 0.34. Bong (2009) provided validity evidence for the 2 X 2 model using a sample of 1196 Korean elementary and middle grades students. She reported that the correlations between all pairs of achievement goals were related inversely to students' age (i.e., correlations were higher for the younger students). For example, the correlation between mastery approach and performance-approach goals was $r = 0.81$ for first and second-grade students, but only $r = 0.45$ for students in grades 7–9.

Despite evidence supporting the 2 X 2 model, some research suggests that some students may have difficulty distinguishing between performance-approach and performance-avoid goals and that the two constructs tend to be highly correlated. For example, Urdan and Mestas (2006) interviewed 53 high school students to examine their reasons for endorsing performance goals. When probed, students provided a range of explanations for their pursuit of performance goals, such as maintaining appearances, being competitive, and pleasing their parents. Bong et al. (2013) examined the structure of performance goals in a sample of 239 Korean middle school students. Although students could distinguish between mastery and performance goals, they were unable to reliably distinguish between different sub-types of performance goals. Other studies have called the validity of mastery-avoid goals into question. Although mastery-avoidance goals have been demonstrated to represent a unique construct (e.g., Baranik et al., 2010), studies to date have not clearly established the face-validity of the construct (i.e., whether students actually actively think about avoiding misunderstanding or becoming less competent). For example, Ciani and Sheldon (2010) interviewed a sample of Division I collegiate baseball players about their understanding of items assessing mastery-avoidance goals. Results suggested that these goals may be somewhat uncommon and may be misunderstood by some respondents.

Another development involved some researchers redefining achievement goals. Specifically, they argued for paring down the definition to include only the person's objective for the task, removing other components such as the reasons for engaging in the task and beliefs about the nature of success and ability (e.g., Elliot & Murayama, 2008). Some researchers adopted this conceptual revision while others did not. Therefore, studies with the new, narrower, definition of achievement goals were published concurrently with other studies that used the traditional conceptualization. Researchers using the original, holistically defined achievement goals sometimes refer to them as goal orientations, to differentiate them from the narrower (i.e., newer) goals, however, this is not always the case. Consequently, there are considerable challenges to consolidating findings across studies.

More recently, researchers have argued that a more comprehensive approach to understanding students' motivation is to consider goal complexes—a combination of students' goals or objectives when pursuing a task with their reasons for completing the task (either autonomous and controlled, from self-determination theory) (Elliot & Thrash, 2001; Vansteenkiste et al., 2014). To illustrate, an autonomous mastery goal complex is represented by the item "My goal is to learn as much as possible because I find this a highly stimulating and challenging goal," whereas "My goal is to perform well relative to other students because I can only be proud of myself if I do so" (Sommet & Elliot, 2017,

p. 1162) represents a controlled performance-approach goal complex.

In addition to differing views about how goals are conceptualized in general, there have been changes with respect to performance goals. Performance goals originally involved normative comparisons (i.e., wanting to do better than, or not worse than, others), although some researchers conceptualize performance goals as involving only a desire to gain rewards (e.g., grades) or avoid punishments, without concern about relative comparisons with others (e.g., Anderman et al., 1998). Performance goals that involve students comparing their achievement with others' have also been termed *normative goals* (Grant & Dweck, 2003), whereas the non-normative goal to gain rewards is also termed *extrinsic goals* (Urdan, 1997) or *outcome goals* (Grant & Dweck, 2003). In summary, the AGT research involving personal achievement goals has become disparate and fragmented, with diverse conceptualizations and measurements. Integrating this research is difficult because researchers conceptualize goals in markedly different ways, leading to the literature becoming significantly less useful. Furthermore, personal goals are affected by the goal structures in one's environment, and the effects do not differ depending on students' personal goals (Linnenbrink, 2005). Therefore, efforts to encourage students' engagement are arguably best achieved through attention to goal structures, which we discuss next.

Goal Structures

Achievement goal theory includes a contextual aspect, premised on the principle that individuals' motivation is influenced not only by their personal dispositions and beliefs but also by aspects of the contexts they experience (Ames, 1992b; Nicholls, 1989). Central to these contexts are *goal structures*, or perceptions of the purposes of schooling and academics, and meanings of success and ability emphasized in the environment (Ames, 1984, 1992b). Goal structures are related to a wide range of constructs; they differentially promote personal goals and encourage some types of engagement while discouraging others.

Researchers consider mastery and performance goal structures most often and conceptualize them to be consistent with the original definitions of mastery and performance goal orientations. That is, a *mastery goal structure* involves a perception that students' real learning and understanding are encouraged, and that success is accompanied by effort and indicated by personal improvement or achieving absolute standards. A *performance goal structure* involves a perception that learning is predominantly a means of achieving recognition of one's ability, worth and extrinsic rewards, and that success is indicated by outperforming others or surpassing normative standards (Ames, 1992b). There has also been recent interest in a purely *extrinsic goal structure*—a perception that grades and rewards are emphasized, with a focus on individuals' accomplishments but not normative comparison. For example, using a sample of over 5000 high school students, Anderman et al. (2011a) adapted a measure of perceived goal structures to assess students' perceptions of an emphasis on extrinsic outcomes in health classrooms. The scale demonstrated good internal consistency ($\alpha = 0.89$). In addition, longitudinal analyses indicated that perceived extrinsic goal structure was related to subsequent outcomes including lower levels of refusal self-efficacy (i.e., feeling confident in one's ability to refuse unwanted sexual overtures) a year after health instruction had ended ($\gamma = -0.24$, $p < 0.001$; see also Won et al., 2020).

Goal structures are not "objective" characteristics but instead depend on how individual students perceive and give meaning to their experiences in that context (Ames, 1992b). Because students' individual past and current experiences and interpretations contribute to their current perceptions, students in the same context do not perceive goal structures in the same way (Ames, 1992b). Goal structures are also independent or unrelated to each other (i.e., orthogonal), in the same way, that personal mastery, performance, and extrinsic goal orientations are. Therefore, a classroom may be viewed as, for example, high in both mastery and performance goal structure, high in just one, low in both, or any other configuration.

Researchers have considered goal structures within schools (e.g., E. Anderman et al., 1998; Cho & Shim, 2013; Gonida et al., 2009; Maehr & Midgley, 1991; Roeser et al., 1996) and families (e.g., Friedel et al., 2010), although the preponderance of research has focused on classrooms. Reflecting on this situation, we focus on classroom goal structures in this chapter.

Students interpret classroom mastery and performance goal structures from their interpretations of teachers' practices and from classroom and school norms, rules, routines, and relationships. These perceptions typically vary among students in the same classroom, although there is usually also some degree of shared agreement. Therefore, classrooms differ in terms of mean goal structures. Because goal structures represent individuals' interpretations, they are usually assessed via self-report surveys (an exception is Boden et al.'s (2020) use of discourse analysis). In some studies, students' perceived goal structures are aggregated at the classroom level, as a measure of the overall environment (e.g., Turner et al., 2002), whereas in others they are treated as individual differences (e.g., Murdock et al., 2001). A few researchers have supplemented surveys with qualitative data, including observations (e.g., Anderman et al., 2002, Anderman et al., 2011b; Patrick et al., 2001; Urdan, 2004) and teacher and student discourse (e.g., Turner et al., 2002).

Mastery Goal Structure

Mastery goal structures are characterized by perceptions that students' learning and understanding, rather than just rote learning and memorization, are valued and that success is accompanied by effort and indicated by personal improvement (Ames, 1992b). Theoretically, it influences students' invoking personal mastery goals for themselves in that context. That is, students are likely to focus on their own improvement and understanding when these aspects of instruction are emphasized. Mastery goals, in turn, influence students' effort, affect use of adaptive learning strategies, and, ultimately, achievement (Ames, 1992b).

A classroom mastery goal structure constitutes a holistic system of instructional practices, and students' perceptions of those practices. Accordingly, it is associated with all aspects of engagement—emotional (e.g., enjoyment, interest, efficacy, commitment), cognitive (e.g., thoughtfulness, use of learning strategies, self-regulation), and behavioral (e.g., persistence, asking for help). From both theoretical and practical standpoints, all aspects of engagement should be high in classrooms that are perceived as emphasizing mastery. Specifically, when the overarching focus in the classroom is perceived as increasing each student's understanding and skill, with success gauged by personal improvement (i.e., classroom mastery structure), it is adaptive and beneficial for students to be fully and thoroughly engaged with those tasks.

Classroom mastery goal structures are created by an array of different types of teacher practices that, working together, communicate the importance of understanding, effort, and improvement (Ames, 1992a). Ames (1992a) identified six practices undergirding classroom mastery goal structure, represented by the acronym TARGET, which was originally developed by Joyce Epstein (Epstein, 1987). These practices include tasks; authority; student recognition; grouping; evaluation; and use of time.

Classroom mastery goal structure is generally measured as a single construct, whereby students report their perceptions of the classroom or the teacher; not all TARGET practices are typically included in these measures, however (e.g., Midgley et al., 1996, 2000). More recently, Lüftenegger and his colleagues created scales for each of the six types of TARGET practices, and scores from samples of Austrian middle and secondary school students provided evidence of validity (Lüftenegger et al., 2014, 2017). Although each scale is empirically distinct, they form a higher-order factor representing a mastery goal structure. Similarly, Tapola and Niemivirta (2008) constructed items corresponding to each TARGET practice and examined the scores' validity with 208 Finnish sixth graders. Interestingly, however, the items did not form six factors as intended, but comprised factors representing five different types of classroom meaning systems. One factor—learning orientation—was analogous to mastery goal structure, based on associations with a range of student-reported beliefs and behavior. The resultant Learning Orientation scale included items about student recognition and evaluation and teacher authority (A. Tapola, personal communication, October 28, 2020).

In another line of scholarship, researchers examined associations between classroom mastery goal structure and social aspects of the classroom and provided support for the argument that perceptions of interpersonal relationships and classroom environments are interconnected (Patrick, 2004). For example, a mastery goal structure is related positively to students' perceptions that their teacher is supportive emotionally and academically; rs range from 0.64 to 0.71 for samples of US middle-grade students (Patrick et al., 2011) and, at the classroom level, $r = 0.77$ with 1171 Norwegian eighth graders (Stornes et al., 2008). Furthermore, factor analysis and multidimensional scaling indicate that US students in the middle grades do not view classroom mastery structure as conceptually distinct from teacher support and respect (Patrick et al., 2011). Interestingly, however, another study with US sixth and seventh graders showed that the conceptual overlap between mastery goal structure and teacher support is evident at the end, but not the beginning, of the year (Turner et al., 2013) Finally, studies of US middle-grade and high-school classrooms using observations (L. Anderman et al., 2011b); Patrick et al., 2001, 2003) and discourse analysis (Turner et al., 2002) indicate that teachers' supportive and respectful practices and interactions vary relative to student-perceived mastery goal structure. Such evidence led to the addition of social interaction to TARGET (i.e., TARGETS; Kaplan & Maehr, 1999; Patrick, 2004).

Researchers in the US have also conducted qualitative studies to understand classroom mastery goal structure. These include observing regular middle grade and high school classrooms and linking observations with student reports of the classroom goal structure (Anderman et al., 2011b; Patrick et al., 2001, 2003), and asking students open-ended questions about the practices that led to their classroom perceptions (Patrick & Ryan, 2008). These studies provide support for the survey measures, and also identify additional dimensions. The broader set of practices and perceptions includes (1) provision of meaningful, challenging, and interesting tasks, (2) feedback and recognition that is constructive, encouraging, and that emphasizes personal improvement and effort, (3) student input and responsibility for rules and decision-making, (4) opportunities for active student participation, (5) flexible use of time, (6) use of effective pedagogical practices, (7) warm, supportive, and respectful teacher-student relationships, (8) respectful interactions among students, and (9) teacher commitment to helping students learn.

Performance Goal Structure

A classroom performance goal structure conveys to students that learning is predominantly a means of achieving recognition and prestige, and is characterized by relative ability comparisons among students. Success is indicated by outperforming others or surpassing normative standards (Ames, 1992b). An integral characteristic of a classroom performance goal structure is that students are compared to each other, with an inherent assumption that this hierarchy is relatively stable and reflects some aspect of students' ability.

A classroom performance goal structure differs from what has been labeled as an *extrinsic goal structure*; the latter conveys that the purpose of engaging in academic tasks is to gain external incentives, although the success of any one student does not affect the success of others (see Urdan, 1997). For example, if students are graded on a curve, with grades indicating relative position, a classroom performance goal structure is invoked, however, if grades (or other incentives) are very salient but do not signify students' relative placement, a classroom extrinsic goal structure is involved.

After the recognition that personal performance goal orientations could be separated, theoretically and empirically, into approach and avoidance dimensions, there have been efforts to make the same distinction with performance goal structure (e.g., Cho et al., 2018; Karabenick, 2004; Peng et al., 2018). That is, these studies suggest that some performance-focused classrooms emphasize approach characteristics, such as scoring better than others, whereas others emphasize avoidance characteristics, such as not doing worse than others. The distinction between performance-approach and performance-avoid goal structures is less compelling than that for personal goals, however. A recent meta-analysis found that a performance-approach goal structure is associated with both performance-approach and performance-avoid goals (Bardach et al., 2020). Furthermore, performance approach and -avoid goal structures are highly correlated. For example, Steuer et al. (2013) reported a correlation of 0.82 with 1116 German middle-grade students, and even when researchers reported distinct approach and avoid goal structures, correlations ranged from 0.43 to 0.53; Cho et al., 2018; Karabenick, 2004; Peng et al., 2018). This pattern of results led researchers to question whether students actually differentiate between the two constructs (e.g., Michou et al., 2013). We also question the ecological validity of this distinction. When observing regular classrooms, we see teachers suggesting, implicitly or explicitly, that students who score the highest are "smarter" or more able than are those with lower scores; however, we have not observed teachers or classrooms promoting either a distinguishably approach or avoidance orientation. We think that students in performance-focused classrooms evaluate, perhaps subconsciously, their likelihood of being ranked highly. If they view outperforming others as realistic they will likely take an approach orientation, and if they are pessimistic about their chances of out-scoring others they will instead likely adopt an avoidance orientation. Therefore, a general classroom performance goal structure may invoke some students taking a performance-approach orientation

and others in the same classroom being performance-avoid oriented.

How Goal Structures Promote Engagement and Research that Supports the Process

In trying to understand how perceived goal structures either promote or hinder student engagement, it is important to recognize that motivation and engagement are extremely similar meta-constructs, with substantial overlap. Eccles and Wang (2012) noted that definitions of both motivation and engagement that are either too broad or too specific can be problematic, but for different reasons. Broad, overly general definitions do little to provide direction to classroom teachers in their daily efforts to support their students' learning, whereas highly specific definitions are not particularly useful to either policymaker or theoreticians. In this chapter, we have conceptualized motivation in terms of achievement goal theory, and we have conceptualized engagement in terms of the trichotomy of cognitive, behavioral, and emotional engagement. We believe that these conceptualizations establish at least some balance between being either too broad or too myopic and allow for an analysis of how aspects of motivation can promote engagement.

Classroom goal structures encompass students' subjective perceptions of the meaning of academic tasks, competence, success, and purposes for students to engage in schoolwork. These integrated meaning systems are communicated, in large part, by teachers' practices, and classroom norms, rules, routines, and relationships. Consequently, classroom goal structures help to create a climate that can either promote or hinder students' behavioral, emotional, and cognitive engagement. For example, students' beliefs about how academic challenges and mistakes are viewed in their classrooms (e.g., indicating deficits in their ability or simply knowledge or skills yet to be learned) influence the amount of effort they expend when experiencing difficulty, how much time they spend at the task, and whether they admit their difficulty to another person and ask for help (i.e., behavioral engagement). The perceived environment also influences students' emotional engagement, including their task-related interest, anxiety, enjoyment, and achievement goals, and the range, quality, and appropriateness of various learning and metacognitive strategies (i.e., cognitive engagement).

In the following sections, we discuss processes whereby three types of classroom goal structures—mastery, performance, and extrinsic—are posited to promote different patterns of behavioral, emotional, and cognitive engagement. We also include results from research studies that support the theoretical premises. From an AGT perspective, instructional practices influence perceptions of mastery, performance, or extrinsic goal structures, which in turn lead to the adoption of various personal goal orientations (e.g., mastery approach goals). Both perceptions of the goal structures and students' personal goals consequently can support or hamper student engagement.

Mastery Goal Structure

Mastery Goal Structures and Cognitive Engagement

Perceptions of a classroom mastery goal structure generally support students' cognitive engagement. Research indicates that perceptions of a mastery goal structure are associated positively with hallmarks of cognitive engagement, including the use of effective metacognitive and self-regulatory strategies. For example, using a sample of 189 fifth and sixth graders in Greece, Michou et al. (2013) found that perceptions of a mastery-approach goal structure were related to the endorsement of personal mastery approach goals ($\beta = 0.17$, $p < 0.05$), as well as to the use of effective learning strategies. Klug et al. (2016) operationalized goal structures in terms of task, autonomy, and evaluation/recognition goal structures. They found that a latent factor combining the three goal structures was related positively to the use of metacognitive strategies ($\beta = 0.43$, $p < 0.001$) in a sample of 5366 children and ado-

lescents (9–21 years old, mean = 15.35). Young (1997) found, in a sample of 316 fifth and sixth graders in the USA, that perceived mastery goal structure (referred to as a "task goal structure" in that study) positively predicted the use of effective cognitive strategies in both English ($\beta = 0.54$, $p < 0.001$) and math ($\beta = 0.34$, $p < 0.001$), after controlling for prior strategy usage (see also Bergsmann et al., 2013; Linnenbrink, 2005).

Mastery Goal Structures and Emotional Engagement

A perceived mastery goal structure also is likely to support students' emotional engagement. Mastery goal structure involves the perceived use of instructional practices that promote academic success as judged by self-improvement, rather than in terms of comparisons with peers. These perceptions are likely to lead to positive emotional responses. Indeed, research indicates that students do tend to experience positive affect and motivational beliefs when they perceive an emphasis on mastery and personal improvement in the classroom (Bardach et al., 2020; Rolland, 2012).

Related research indicates that mastery goal structure is related positively to several emotion-laden outcomes. For example, Diseth and Samdal (2015) examined the relations between perceived classroom goal structures and both motivational engagement (i.e., wanting to do well in school) and affective engagement (i.e., enjoying school). A sample of 1239 Norwegian tenth graders completed surveys assessing perceptions of classroom goal structures and engagement. Using structural equation modeling, they found that perceptions of a mastery goal structure predicted motivational engagement for both males ($\beta = 0.49$, $p < 0.01$) and females ($\beta = 0.26$, $p < 0.01$), and also predicted affective engagement for both males ($\beta = 0.59$, $p < 0.01$) and females ($\beta = 0.62$, $p \leq 0.01$). Anderman (2003) examined the relations between a perceived mastery goal structure and school belonging in a sample of 618 American sixth, seventh, and eighth graders, and reported a positive relationship between perceptions of a mastery goal structure and belonging ($\beta = 0.41$, $p < 0.001$).

Anderman and Anderman (1999) examined changes in perceptions of a mastery (task) goal structure across the transition from elementary to middle school. They found that after transition, perceptions of a mastery goal structure were related positively to school belonging ($r = 0.40$); moreover, both perceptions of a mastery goal structure ($\beta = 0.14$, $p < 0.001$) and school belonging ($\beta = 0.23$, $p < 0.001$) predicted greater personal mastery goals after the transition. They also found that perceptions of a mastery goal structure were related to a desire to follow the school's expectations (i.e., social responsibility goals; $r = 0.46$, $p < 0.001$)) Walker (2012) also found, in a sample of 227 rural high school students, that perceived mastery goal structure was related positively to school belonging ($\beta = 0.51$, $p < 0.001$). Polychroni et al. (2012) examined the relations between perceptions of a mastery goal structure and students' perceptions of a variety of social relationships. Using a sample of 1493 fifth and sixth grade students in Greece, they found that perceived mastery goal structure was related positively to student-student relationships ($b = 0.49$, $p < 0.001$), teacher-student relationships ($b = 0.64$, $p < 0.001$), and home-school relationships ($b = 0.42$, $p < 0.001$). Moreover, mastery goal structure was related positively to perceptions of peer inclusion ($b = 0.13$, $p < 0.05$) and negatively to peer conflict ($b = -0.20$, $p < 0.05$) (see also Madjar, 2017).

Students in mastery-focused classrooms tend to express adaptive motivational beliefs, such as personal mastery goals (e.g., Bardach et al., 2020; Wolters, 2004), self-efficacy (Lüftenegger et al., 2016; Wolters, 2004), positive self-concept (Murayama & Elliot, 2009), and intrinsic or autonomous motivation (Fast et al., 2010; Kim et al., 2010; Murayama & Elliot, 2009; Wolters, 2004). For example, in a sample of 909 Swedish adolescents in grades six through ten, perceptions of a mastery goal structure were related positively to autonomous motivation ($\beta = 0.071$, $p < 0.05$) (Hofverberg & Winberg, 2020). Moreover, students' positive views about their schoolwork, including interest (Khajavy et al., 2018), the usefulness of learning strategies (Nolen & Haladyna, 1990), satisfaction with

their learning (Nolen, 2003), and adaptive coping responses after failure (Kaplan & Midgley, 1999) are related positively to the mastery goal structure perceived in their classrooms. For example, Lazarides et al. (2018) examined the relations between perceptions of a mastery goal structure and students' valuing of mathematics in a sample of 803 German students in grades 9 and 10. They found that students who perceived a mastery goal structure reported greater intrinsic value ($\beta = 0.62$, $p < 0.05$), attainment value ($\beta = 0.81$, $p < 0.05$), and utility value ($\beta = 0.65$, $p < 0.05$) in math. Interestingly, they also found that students were more likely to perceive a mastery goal structure when their teachers reported feeling efficacious at managing classroom behavior ($\beta = 0.48$, $p < 0.05$). In addition, some research also indicates that perceptions of a mastery goal structure are related negatively to unpleasant emotional responses, such as anxiety (Federici et al., 2015).

Mastery Goal Structures and Behavioral Engagement

Underscoring the close connections of emotional and cognitive engagement with behavior, perceiving a classroom mastery goal structure is related positively to many forms of adaptive behavioral engagement. This is because working to learn the material is likely to pay off for students if all students can experience success, rather than just a few. Classroom mastery goal structure is associated positively with students' effort (Lazarides & Rubach, 2017; Peng et al., 2018), persistence (Peng et al., 2018; Wolters, 2004), and use of adaptive help-seeking strategies such as asking for explanations but not answers (Federici et al., 2015; Karabenick, 2004).

A perceived mastery goal structure also is also related negatively to maladaptive student behaviors. Perceptions of an emphasis on mastery are related to fewer reports of students not asking for help when it is needed (Karabenick, 2004; Ryan et al., 1998), self-handicapping behaviors (i.e., purposefully withdrawing effort; Lau & Nie, 2008; Midgley & Urdan, 2001; Urdan & Midgley, 2003), procrastinating (Wolters, 2004), reacting negatively to classmates' errors (Bardach et al., 2019), and cheating (Murdock et al., 2001; Tas & Tekkaya, 2010). Midgley and Urdan (2001) examined the relations between perceptions of a mastery goal structure and self-handicapping in a sample of 484 seventh graders in the United States. They found that after controlling for gender, ethnicity, achievement, and personal goal orientations, perceptions of a mastery goal structure were related to lesser use of self-handicapping strategies ($\beta = -0.09$, $p < 0.05$). Moreover, in addition to adaptive academic behaviors, a perceived mastery goal structure is related inversely to disruptive behavior as well (Kaplan et al., 2002).

Performance Goal Structures

Whereas the relations between perceptions of a mastery goal structure and engagement are generally positive, relations with performance goal structures are less clear. As mentioned earlier, it has been challenging to operationalize performance goal structures. Indeed, performance goal structures may be interpreted somewhat differently by students, depending on the types of instructional practices used, and students' perceived competence (Urdan & Schoenfelder, 2006; Wolters, 2004). Perceiving a classroom performance goal structure is associated with affective, cognitive, and behavioral engagement. In contrast to the mixed findings associated with a personal performance-approach goal orientation, perceiving a classroom performance goal structure is generally associated with students' beliefs and behaviors that are less conducive, and often detrimental, to learning and achievement. We review this research briefly next.

Performance Goal Structures and Cognitive Engagement

There has not been much scholarship that has directly examined the relations between perceptions of a performance goal structure and cognitive engagement. Moreover, classroom performance goal structure is less relevant to cognitive engagement than mastery goal structure is.

For example, a common finding is that performance goal structure is not related to learning or metacognitive strategies. Wolters (2004) examined the relation of students' perception of a performance-approach goal structure to the use of both cognitive and metacognitive strategies and found no significant relations for either ($\beta s = 0.06$ and 0.09, respectively) (see also Michou et al., 2013).

Performance Goal Structures and Emotional Engagement

Students' perceptions that their teacher and classroom emphasize relative ability comparisons (i.e., have a high classroom performance goal structure) are related to the adoption of personal performance approach and/or avoid goals (Wolters, 2004). A pervasive focus on how students 'stack up' against each other can provoke students to focus on the outcomes of their efforts, rather than on the process of learning. This state of affairs is not comfortable for many students, not just those near the bottom of the achievement continuum, and therefore students tend to experience negative affect and motivational beliefs in these types of classrooms.

Classroom performance goal structure is related positively to negative affect on school (Ames & Archer, 1988; Anderman, 1999; Kaplan & Midgley, 1999). In addition, students who perceive a performance classroom goal structure at times feel less of a sense of school belonging (Anderman & Anderman, 1999; Walker, 2012). Moreover, perceptions of a performance goal structure are related to students reporting having less positive relationships at school. For example, Polychroni et al. (2012) found that fifth and sixth graders' perceptions of a performance goal structure related to perceptions of lower peer inclusion ($b = -0.43$, $p < 0.001$) and greater peer conflict ($b = 0.48$, $p < 0.001$). And perceptions of a performance goal structure also are related to affect toward teachers. Murdock and her colleagues found that students view teachers who are perceived as using performance-focused classrooms as less fair (Murdock et al., 2004) and more to blame for student dishonesty (Murdock et al.,

2007), compared to teachers who use mastery-focused practices.

Classroom performance goal structure is related negatively to students' intrinsic and autonomous motivation, and academic self-concepts (Ames & Archer, 1988; Kim et al., 2010; Murayama & Elliot, 2009). Moreover, it is related positively to anxiety (Federici et al., 2015), controlled motivation (i.e., perceiving that one's actions are largely controlled or coerced by others, such as parents) (Kim et al., 2010), and both the adoption of personal performance-approach and -avoid goals (Bardach et al., 2020). There is also greater use of maladaptive coping strategies by students after failure, such as denial or projecting blame onto other people or events (Kaplan & Midgley, 1999), or attributing failures to one's own lack of ability (Ames & Archer, 1988).

Performance Goal Structures and Behavioral Engagement

When classrooms are perceived as emphasizing a hierarchy of ability and students' relative position within that hierarchy, students are likely to report engaging in behaviors that are not condu-cive, and often detrimental, to learning. With an emphasis on outcomes but not process, students may feel encouraged to disregard *how* they come to out-score others and to be concerned only what they *do*. In performance-focused classrooms, students who are not successful at a task immedi-ately may be unlikely to continue trying, given both that a hierarchy of ability tends to invoke an entity view of ability, and high effort without suc-cess is suggestive of low ability.

Accordingly, perceptions of a classroom per-formance goal structure are related inversely to students' task persistence (Wolters, 2004), par-ticipation (Lau & Nie, 2008), and paying atten-tion (Lau & Nie, 2008). Furthermore, in classrooms perceived as emphasizing a perfor-mance goal structure, students who are pessimis-tic about their chances of placing near the top of the hierarchy may find ways to avoid engaging in academic work, and therefore may protect their self-worth by not providing evidence that their ability is lower than their classmates'. Indeed,

classroom performance goal structure is related positively to maladaptive behaviors. Ryan, Gheen, and Midgley et al. (1998) found that, in a sample of 563 US sixth graders, perceptions of a classroom focus on differences in ability among students were predictive of students' avoiding seeking help when needed ($\gamma = 0.245$, $p < 0.05$). Other research indicates that a perceived perfor-mance goal structure is related to procrastinating (Wolters, 2004), self-handicapping (Lau & Nie, 2008; Midgley & Urdan, 2001; Peng et al., 2018; Urdan et al., 1998; Urdan, 2004), cheating (Murdock et al., 2004), and being disruptive (Kaplan et al., 2002; Ryan & Patrick, 2001).

Extrinsic Goal Structure

There has been substantially less research that has examined perceptions of a purely extrinsic goal structure with correlates of engagement. By definition, when students perceive an extrinsic goal structure, they report that the instructional practices being used focus on the value of con-crete outcomes, such as getting the correct answers or obtaining a good grade. The major distinction between an extrinsic goal structure and a performance goal structure is that, whereas performance goal structures are focused on stu-dents' relative ability, extrinsic goal structures are focused on obtaining the desired outcome. The limited research that has been conducted in this area suggests that a perceived extrinsic goal structure is related to maladaptive indicators of engagement.

There is some research examining the rela-tionship between extrinsic goal structures and aspects of cognitive engagement. Vansteenkiste et al. (2006) discuss several studies wherein they found that when students' academic goals are oriented toward extrinsic outcomes, students' conceptual understanding of the content may be diminished. In addition, Fryer and Oga-Baldwin (2019) found that when secondary school stu-dents perceive that their teachers use controlling instructional strategies, they are more likely to adopt an extrinsic orientation toward their aca-demic work; nevertheless, although students tended to adopt this extrinsic orientation, that orientation was not found to be related to achievement.

In terms of behavioral engagement, studies suggest that a perceived extrinsic goal structure is also related to maladaptive outcomes, such as greater involvement in academic cheating (e.g., E. Anderman et al., 1998; Anderman & Won, 2019). The results of Anderman et al.'s study of motivation in health classrooms indicated that, in a sample of over 5000 adolescents, perceptions of an extrinsic goal structure were related to a lower likelihood of waiting to have sex during adolescence (Anderman et al., 2011b). Nevertheless, it is important to note that Murdock et al. (2001) found no relation between an extrinsic goal structure and academic cheating in a sample of 495 seventh and eighth graders. Although research has not examined the relations of a perceived extrinsic goal structure to major indicators of emotion such as depression and optimism, some research has been conducted on variables assessing efficacy beliefs and attitudes. In one study focusing on middle school students' science classes, results indicate that a perception of an extrinsic goal structure is related to students reporting that they are more likely to believe in the acceptability of cheating (Anderman et al., 1998).

Summary

Students' perceptions of classroom goal structures are related to valued outcomes. In terms of the relations between classroom goal structures and a wide range of types of engagement, the goal structures that are perceived in the classroom are related to the quality of engagement experienced by the student. As we have reviewed, perceptions of classroom mastery, performance, and extrinsic goal structures are related to cognitive, emotional, and behavioral engagement in different ways. The fact that classroom goal structures are related to the types of instructional practices used by teachers in classrooms suggests that changes in instructional practices may yield benefits for student engagement (Gresalfi & Barab, 2011). Most of this research has been con-

ducted in the middle grades (i.e., fifth through eighth grades), however, more studies in the earlier grades, in particular, are needed.

Conclusion

In this chapter, we have reviewed the relations between both students' personal achievement goals and their perceptions of their classroom goal structures with a variety of indicators of academic engagement. Specifically, we reviewed both theoretical processes and empirical evidence relevant to behavioral (e.g., time spent, effort expended, avoidance behaviors such as cheating and disruptiveness), emotional (e.g., confidence in learning or self-efficacy, reasons for doing schoolwork [achievement goals], and emotions such as enjoyment, frustration, or anxiety), and cognitive (e.g., use of adaptive or maladaptive learning and metacognitive strategies) engagement. Whereas motivation researchers who study achievement goals and researchers who study academic engagement operationalize and discuss constructs in different ways, there is substantial and important overlap. Future research that draws upon both AGT and research on student engagement will be fruitful, particularly in terms of developing interventions designed to more fully engage students with academic tasks.

We briefly reviewed the history of the development of AGT, and we noted that the measurement of achievement goal constructs has changed in important ways over the past three decades (for more comprehensive reviews, see Elliot, 2005, and Maehr & Zusho, 2009). We noted in particular that although some of the newer developments in AGT have informed scholarship and further development of the theory, some of the newer conceptions may not have sufficient face validity to be useful for practitioners. We then reviewed research on classroom goal structures. We noted in particular that facets of classroom contexts that are focused on extrinsic outcomes or on demonstrations of ability affect students' engagement in generally deleterious ways; in contrast, facets of instruction that are focused on task mastery and individual improvement are associated with more adaptive types of engagement. We also noted that goal orientation theorists are concerned with students' involvement with academic tasks. When students pursue mastery goals or perceive a mastery goal structure, the students' goal is to truly learn or "master" the task. Goals can be adopted by students for many types of learning, including specific activities (e.g., a particular science lab experiment), more general academic tasks (e.g., book reports), or different subject domains (e.g., mathematics) (Anderman, 2021; Anderman & Wolters, 2006).

Our analysis of the relations between perceived goal structures and engagement aligns with the views expressed by several engagement researchers, suggesting that precursors of engagement need to be clearly distinguished from engagement itself (e.g., Reschly & Christenson, 2012; Skinner & Pitzer, 2012). Consequently, we treated the three-goal structures as precursors to engagement. Our discussion of engagement also distinguished between cognitive, behavioral, and emotional engagement; we find this conceptualization of engagement particularly useful, as it strikes a balance between definitions of engagement that are either too general to be useful to classroom teachers, or too specific to be useful to researchers and policymakers (Eccles & Wang, 2012).

From an engagement perspective, students who hold mastery goals or who perceive a mastery goal structure are likely to be more cognitively, emotionally, and behaviorally engaged with tasks, because the overarching "goal" is task mastery. When teachers use instructional practices that are likely to foster perceptions of a mastery goal structure and the adoption of mastery goals, students' cognitive, emotional, and behavioral engagement can benefit (e.g., Zhang, 2014). In contrast, when students pursue various types of performance goals, or when they perceive a performance goal structure in the classroom, students often focus on demonstrating their ability at the task, or, in the case of avoidance goals, to avoid appearing incompetent at the task. When students hold such goals and when teachers utilize instructional practices that emphasize that such goals are valued, engagement is likely not as deep as with mastery goals; rather, students typically engage with less challenging tasks or at

more of a surface-level, to merely demonstrate ability.

Future research examining the relations between teachers' instructional practices and engagement more specifically will be important. In particular, research that examines students' perceptions of goal structures and engagement while students are participating in actual academic tasks may be particularly fruitful. Studies that utilize the experience sampling method (e.g., Shernoff, 2010), where students report on their motivation and engagement during actual task participation, maybe especially worthwhile. Moreover, it will be particularly important to address developmental shifts in academic motivation and engagement. Given that much research indicates that goal orientations and classroom goal structures change as students move from elementary schools into middle schools (e.g., Anderman & Midgley, 1997), it will be important to examine changes in the relations between goals and engagement across developmental shifts. Furthermore, most of the research that has investigated classroom goal structures, and especially teacher practices associated with goal structures, was conducted in middle grade (i.e., fifth through eighth grades) classrooms. Much more research is needed in both earlier and later grades.

In summary, both achievement goal orientation researchers and engagement researchers can benefit greatly from collaborative efforts. Although achievement goal researchers and engagement researchers use different terminologies and constructs, we all are concerned with students' involvement with academic tasks, and with supporting student learning. In classrooms, students' engagement in academic activities can be prompted, guided, and fostered (or diminished) by the perceived goal structures of the classroom. In a classroom with a mastery goal structure, where students perceive the instruction as challenging and believe that asking questions and intellectual risk-taking is welcome, students actively participate in the learning process and are more likely to develop adaptive motivational beliefs and retain new knowledge. Therefore, classroom achievement goals and engagement can positively affect students' academic competence and development. As these two lines of research continue to develop, a convergence and sharing of ideas should lead to richer interventions for students, more effective training for teachers, and the promotion of deeper learning among youth.

References

Ames, C. (1984). Competitive, cooperative, and individualistic goal structures: A cognitive-motivational analysis. In R. Ames & C. Ames (Eds.), *Research on motivation in education, Volume 1: Student motivation* (pp. 177–207). Academic.

Ames, C. (1987). The enhancement of student motivation. In M. Maehr & D. Kleiber (Eds.), *Advances in motivation and achievement, Volume 5: Enhancing motivation* (pp. 123–148). JAI Press.

Ames, C. (1992a). Achievement goals and the classroom motivational climate. In D. H. Schunk & J. L. Meece (Eds.), *Student perception in the classroom* (pp. 327–348). Erlbaum.

Ames, C. (1992b). Classrooms: Goals, structures, and student motivation. *Journal of Educational Psychology, 84*(3), 261–271. https://doi.org/10.1037/0022-0663.84.3.261

Ames, C., & Archer, J. (1988). Achievement goals in the classroom: Students' learning strategies and motivation processes. *Journal of Educational Psychology, 80*, 260–267. https://doi.org/10.1037/0022-0663.80.3.260

Anderman, E. M. (2021). *Sparking student motivation: The power of teachers to rekindle a love of learning*. Corwin.

Anderman, E. M., Griesinger, T., & Westerfield, G. (1998). Motivation and cheating during early adolescence. *Journal of Educational Psychology, 90*(1), 84–93. https://doi.org/10.1037/0022-0663.90.1.84

Anderman, E. M., & Midgley, C. (1997). Changes in achievement goal orientation, perceived academic competence, and grades across the transition to middle-level schools. *Contemporary Educational Psychology, 22*(3), 269–298. https://doi.org/10.1006/ceps.1996.0926

Anderman, E. M., & Wolters, C. (2006). Goals, values, and affect: Influences on student motivation. In P. Alexander & P. Winne (Eds.), *Handbook of educational psychology* (2nd ed., pp. 369–389). Erlbaum.

Anderman, E. M., & Won, S. (2019). Academic cheating in disliked classes. *Ethics & Behavior, 29*(1), 1–22. https://doi.org/10.1080/10508422.2017.1373648

Anderman, E. M., Cupp, P. K., Lane, D. R., Zimmerman, R., Gray, D., & O'Connell, A. (2011a). Classroom goal structures and HIV/pregnancy prevention education in rural high school health classrooms. *Journal of Research on Adolescence, 21*(4), 904–922. https://doi.org/10.1111/j.1532-7795.2011.00751.x

Anderman, L. H., Andrzejewski, C. E., & Allen, J. L. (2011b). How do teachers support students' motivation and learning in their classrooms? *Teachers College Record, 113*(5), 969–1003.

Anderman, L. H. (1999). Classroom goal orientation, school belonging, and social goals as predictors of students' positive and negative affect following the transition to middle school. *Journal of Research and Development in Education, 32*(2), 89–103.

Anderman, L. H. (2003). Academic and social perceptions as predictors of change in middle school students' sense of school belonging. *The Journal of Experimental Education, 72*(1), 5–22. https://doi.org/10.1080/00220970309600877

Anderman, L. H., & Anderman, E. M. (1999). Social predictors of changes in students' achievement goal orientations. *Contemporary Educational Psychology, 25*(1), 21–37. https://doi.org/10.1006/ceps.1998.0978

Anderman, L. H., Patrick, H., Hruda, L. Z., & Linnenbrink, E. A. (2002). Observing classroom goal structures to clarify and expand goal theory. In C. Midgley (Ed.), *Goals, goal structures, and patterns of adaptive learning* (pp. 243–278). Erlbaum.

Baranik, L., Stanley, L., Bynum, B., & Lance, C. (2010). Examining the construct validity of mastery-avoidance achievement goals: A meta-analysis. *Human Performance, 23*(3), 265–282. https://doi.org/10.1080/08959285.2010.488463

Bardach, L., Lüftenegger, M., Yanagida, T., Schober, B., & Spiel, C. (2019). The role of within-class consensus on mastery goal structures in predicting socioemotional outcomes. *British Journal of Educational Psychology, 89*(2), 239–258. https://doi.org/10.1111/bjep.12237

Bardach, L., Oczlon, S., Pietschnig, J., & Lüftenegger, M. (2020). Has achievement goal theory been right? A meta-analysis of the relation between goal structures and personal achievement goals. *Journal of Educational Psychology, 112*(6), 1197–1220. https://doi.org/10.1037/edu0000419

Bergsmann, E. M., Lüftnegger, M., Jöstl, G., Schober, B., & Spiel, C. (2013). The role of classroom structure in fostering students' school functioning: A comprehensive and application-oriented approach. *Learning and Individual Differences, 26*, 131–138. https://doi.org/10.1016/j.lindif.2013.05.005

Boden, K. K., Zepeda, C. D., & Nokes-Malach, T. J. (2020). Achievement goals and conceptual learning: An examination of teacher talk. *Journal of Educational Psychology, 112*(6), 1221–1242. https://doi.org/10.1037/edu0000421

Bong, M. (2009). Age-related differences in achievement goal differentiation. *Journal of Educational Psychology, 101*(4), 879–896. https://doi.org/10.1037/a0015945

Bong, M., Woo, Y., & Shin, J. (2013). Do students distinguish between different types of performance goals? *The Journal of Experimental Education, 81*(4), 464–489. https://doi.org/10.1080/00220973.2012.745464

Cho, Y., & Shim, S. S. (2013). Predicting teachers' achievement goals for teaching: The role of perceived school goal structure and teachers' sense of efficacy. *Teaching and Teacher Education, 32*, 12–21. https://doi.org/10.1016/j.tate.2012.12.003

Cho, E., Lee, M., & Toste, J. R. (2018). Does perceived competence serve as a protective mechanism against performance goals for struggling readers? Path analysis of contextual antecedents and reading outcomes. *Learning and Individual Differences, 65*, 135–147. https://doi.org/10.1016/j.lindif.2018.05.017

Ciani, K. D., & Sheldon, K. M. (2010). Evaluating the mastery-avoidance goal construct: A study of elite college baseball players. *Psychology of Sport and Exercise, 11*(2), 127–132. https://doi.org/10.1016/j.psychsport.2009.04.005

Conroy, D. E., Elliot, A. J., & Hofer, S. M. (2003). A 2 X 2 achievement goals questionnaire for sport: Evidence for factorial invariance, temporal stability, and external validity. *Journal of Sport & Exercise Psychology, 25*(4), 456–476.

Diseth, A., & Samdal, O. (2015). Classroom achievement goal structure, school engagement, and substance use among 10th grade students in Norway. *International Journal of School and Educational Psychology, 3*(4), 267–277. https://doi.org/10.1080/21683603.2015.1084250

Dweck, C. S., & Elliott, E. S. (1983). Achievement motivation. In E. M. Hetherington (Ed.), *Socialization, personality, and social development* (pp. 643–691). Wiley.

Dweck, C. S., & Leggett, E. L. (1988). A social-cognitive approach to motivation and personality. *Psychological Review, 95*(2), 256–273. https://doi.org/10.1037/0033-295X.95.2.256

Eccles, J., & Wang, M.-T. (2012). Part I commentary: So what is student engagement anyway? In S. L. Christenson, A. L. Reschly, & C. Wylie (Eds.), *Handbook of research on student engagement* (pp. 133–145). Springer Science + Business Media. https://doi.org/10.1007/978-1-4614-2018-7_6

Elliot, A. J. (1999). Approach and avoidance motivation and achievement goals. *Educational Psychologist, 34*(3), 169–189. https://doi.org/10.1207/s15326985ep3403_3

Elliot, A. J. (2005). A conceptual history of the achievement goal construct. In A. J. Elliot & C. S. Dweck (Eds.), *Handbook of competence and motivation* (pp. 52–72). Guilford.

Elliot, A. J., & Harackiewicz, J. M. (1996). Approach and avoidance achievement goals and intrinsic motivation: A mediational analysis. *Journal of Personality and Social Psychology, 70*(3), 461–475. https://doi.org/10.1037/0022-3514.70.3.461

Elliot, A. J., & Hulleman, C. S. (2017). Achievement goals. In A. J. Elliot, C. S. Dweck, & D. S. Yeager (Eds.), *Handbook of competence and motivation: Theory and application., 2nd ed.* (pp. 43–60). The Guilford Press

Elliot, A. J., & McGregor, H. A. (2001). A 2 * 2 achievement goal framework. *Journal of Personality and Social Psychology, 80*(3), 501–519. https://doi.org/10.1037/0022-3514.80.3.501

Elliot, A. J., & Murayama, K. (2008). On the measurement of achievement goals: Critique, illustration, and application. *Journal of Educational Psychology, 100*(3), 613–628. https://doi.org/10.1037/0022-0663.100.3.613

Elliot, A. J., & Thrash, T. M. (2001). Achievement goals and the hierarchical model of achievement motivation. *Educational Psychology Review, 13*(2), 139–156.

Epstein, J. L., & Center for Research on Elementary and Middle Schools, B., MD. (1987). *TARGET: An examination of parallel school and family structures that promote student motivation and achievement*. Report No. 6. Center for Research on Elementary and Middle Schools Report.

Fast, L. A., Lewis, J. L., Bryant, M., Bocian, K. A., Cardullo, R. A., Rettig, M., & Hammond, K. A. (2010). Does math self-efficacy mediate the effect of the perceived classroom environment on standardized math test performance? *Journal of Educational Psychology, 102*(3), 729–740. https://doi.org/10.1037/a0018863

Federici, R. A., Skaalvik, E. M., & Tangen, T. N. (2015). Students' perceptions of the goal structure in mathematics classrooms: Relations with goal orientations, mathematics anxiety, and help-seeking behavior. *International Education Studies, 8*(3), 146–158. https://doi.org/10.5539/ies.v8n3p146

Fredricks, J. A., Blumenfeld, P. C., & Paris, A. H. (2004). School engagement: Potential of the concept, state of the evidence. *Review of Educational Research, 74*(1), 59–109. https://doi.org/10.3102/00346543074001059

Friedel, J. M., Cortina, K. S., Turner, J. C., & Midgley, C. (2010). Changes in efficacy beliefs in mathematics across the transition to middle school: Examining the effects of perceived teacher and parent goal emphases. *Journal of Educational Psychology, 102*(1), 102–114. https://doi.org/10.1037/a0017590

Fryer, L. K., & Oga-Baldwin, W. L. Q. (2019). Succeeding at junior high school: Students' reasons, their reach, and the teaching that h(inders)elps their grasp. *Contemporary Educational Psychology, 59*, 201778. https://doi.org/10.1016/j.cedpsych.2019.101778

Gonida, E. N., Voulala, K., & Kiosseoglou, G. (2009). Students' achievement goal orientations and their behavioral and emotional engagement: Co-examining the role of perceived school goal structures and parent goals during adolescence. *Learning and Individual Differences, 19*(1), 53–60. https://doi.org/10.1016/j.lindif.2008.04.002

Grant, H., & Dweck, C. S. (2003). Clarifying achievement goals and their impact. *Journal of Personality and Social Psychology, 85*(3), 541–553. https://doi.org/10.1037/0022-3514.85.3.541

Gresalfi, M., & Barab, S. (2011). Learning for a reason: Supporting forms of engagement by designing tasks and orchestrating environments. *Theory Into Practice, 50*(4), 300–310. https://doi.org/10.1080/00405841.2011.607391

Hofverberg, A., & Winberg, M. (2020). Achievement goals and classroom goal structures: Do they need to match? *The Journal of Experimental Education, 113*(2), 145–162.

Jagacinski, C. M., & Nicholls, J. G. (1990). Reducing effort to protect perceived ability: "They'd do it but I wouldn't.". *Journal of Educational Psychology, 82*(1), 15–21. https://doi.org/10.1037/0022-0663.82.1.15

Kaplan, A., & Maehr, M. L. (1999). Enhancing the motivation of African American students: An achievement goal theory perspective. *Journal of Negro Education, 68*(1), 23–41. https://doi.org/10.2307/2668207

Kaplan, A., & Midgley, C. (1999). The relationship between perceptions of the classroom goal structure and early adolescents' affect in school: The mediating role of coping strategies. *Learning and Individual Differences, 11*(2), 187–212. https://doi.org/10.1016/S1041-6080(00)80005-9

Kaplan, A., Gheen, M., & Midgley, C. (2002). The classroom goal structure and student disruptive behaviour. *British Journal of Educational Psychology, 72*(2), 191–211. https://doi.org/10.1348/000709902158847

Karabenick, S. A. (2004). Perceived achievement goal structure and college student help seeking. *Journal of Educational Psychology, 96*(3), 569–581. https://doi.org/10.1037/0022-0663.96.3.569

Khajavy, G. H., Bardach, L., Hamedi, S. M., & Lüftenegger, M. (2018). Broadening the nomological network of classroom goal structures using doubly latent multilevel modeling. *Contemporary Educational Psychology, 52*, 61–73. https://doi.org/10.1016/j.cedpsych.2017.10.004

Kim, J. I., Schallert, D. L., & Kim, M. (2010). An integrative cultural view of achievement motivation: Parental and classroom predictors of children's goal orientations when learning mathematics in Korea. *Journal of Educational Psychology, 102*(2), 418–437. https://doi.org/10.1037/a0018676

Klug, J., Lüftenegger, M., Bergsmann, E., Spiel, C., & Schober, B. (2016). Secondary school students' LLL competencies, and their relation with classroom structure and achievement. *Frontiers in Psychology, 7*, 680. https://doi.org/10.3389/fpsyg.2016.00680

Lau, S., & Nie, Y. (2008). Interplay between personal goals and classroom goal structures in predicting student outcomes: A multilevel analysis of person-context interactions. *Journal of Educational Psychology, 100*(1), 15–29. https://doi.org/10.1037/0022-0663.100.1.15

Lazarides, R., & Rubach, C. (2017). Instructional characteristics in mathematics classrooms: Relationships to achievement goal orientation and student engagement. *Mathematics Education Research Journal, 29*(2), 201–217. https://doi.org/10.1007/s13394-017-0196-4

Lazarides, R., Buchholz, J., & Rubach, C. (2018). Teacher enthusiasm and self-efficacy, student-perceived mastery goal orientation, and student motivation in mathematics classrooms. *Teaching and Teacher Education, 69*, 1–10. https://doi.org/10.1016/j.tate.2017.08.017

Linnenbrink, E. A. (2005). The dilemma of performance-approach goals: The use of multiple goal contexts to promote student' motivation and learning. *Journal of*

Educational Psychology, 97(2), 197–213. https://doi.org/10.1037/0022-0663.97.2.197

Lüftenegger, M., van de Schoot, R., Schober, B., Finsterwald, M., & Spiel, C. (2014). Promotion of students' mastery goal orientations: Does TARGET work? *Educational Psychology, 34*(4), 451–469. https://doi.org/10.1080/01443410.2013.814189

Lüftenegger, M., Finsterwald, M., Klug, J., Bergsmann, E., van de Schoot, R., Schober, B., & Wagner, P. (2016). Fostering pupils' lifelong learning competencies in the classroom: Evaluation of a training programme using a multivariate multilevel growth curve approach. *European Journal of Developmental Psychology, 13*(6), 719–736. https://doi.org/10.1080/17405629.2015.1077113

Lüftenegger, M., Tran, U. S., Bardach, L., Schober, B., & Spiel, C. (2017). Measuring a mastery goal structure using the TARGET framework: Development and validation of a classroom goal structure questionnaire. *Zeitschrift für Psychologie, 225*(1), 64–75. https://doi.org/10.1027/2151-2604/a000277

Madjar, N. (2017). Stability and change in social goals as related to goal structures and engagement in school. *The Journal of Experimental Education, 85*(2), 259–277. https://doi.org/10.1080/00220973.2016.1148658

Maehr, M. L. (1984). Meaning and motivation: Toward a theory of personal investment. In R. Ames & C. Ames (Eds.), *Research on motivation in education: Student motivation* (Vol. 1, pp. 115–143). Academic.

Maehr, M. L., & Midgley, C. (1991). Enhancing student motivation: A schoolwide approach. *Educational Psychologist, 26*(3–4), 399–427.

Maehr, M. L., & Midgley, C. (1996). *Transforming school cultures.* Westview Press.

Maehr, M. L., & Zusho, A. (2009). Achievement goal theory: The past, present, and future. In K. R. Wentzel & A. Wigfield (Eds.), *Handbook of motivation at school* (pp. 77–104). Routledge.

Martin, A. J. (2012). Part II commentary: Motivation and engagement: Conceptual, operational, and empirical clarity. In S. L. Christenson, A. L. Reschly, & C. Wylie (Eds.), *Handbook of research on student engagement.* (pp. 303–311). Springer Science + Business Media. https://doi.org/10.1007/978-1-4614-2018-7_14

Michou, A., Mouratidis, A., Lens, W., & Vansteenkiste, M. (2013). Personal and contextual antecedents of achievement goals: Their direct and indirect relations to students' learning strategies. *Learning and Individual Differences, 23*, 187–194. https://doi.org/10.1016/j.lindif.2012.09.005

Middleton, M. J., & Midgley, C. (1997). Avoiding the demonstration of lack of ability: An underexplored aspect of goal theory. *Journal of Educational Psychology, 89*(4), 710–718. https://doi.org/10.1037/0022-0663.89.4.710

Midgley, C., & Urdan, T. (2001). Academic self-handicapping and achievement goals: A further examination. *Contemporary Educational Psychology, 26*(1), 61–75. https://doi.org/10.1006/ceps.2000.1041

Midgley, C., Maehr, M. L., Hicks, L., Roeser, R., Urdan, T., Anderman, E. M., & Kaplan, A. (1996). *The patterns of adaptive learning survey (PALS).* University of Michigan.

Midgley, C., Kaplan, A., Middleton, M., Maehr, M. L., Urdan, T., Anderman, L. H., Anderman, E. M., & Roeser, R. (1998). The development and validation of scales assessing students' achievement goal orientations. *Contemporary Educational Psychology, 23*(2), 113–131. https://doi.org/10.1006/ceps.1998.0965

Midgley, C., Maehr, M. L., Hruda, L. A., Anderman, E., Anderman, L., Gheen, M., Kaplan, A., Kumar, R., Middleton, M. J., Nelson, J., & Urdan, T. (2000). *Manual for the patterns of adaptive learning scale.* University of Michigan.

Midgley, C., Kaplan, A., & Middleton, M. J. (2001). Performance-approach goals: Good for what, for whom, under what circumstances, and at what cost? *Journal of Educational Psychology, 93*(1), 77–86. https://doi.org/10.1037/0022-0663.93.1.77

Murayama, K., & Elliot, A. J. (2009). The joint influence of personal achievement goals and classroom goal structures on achievement-relevant outcomes. *Journal of Educational Psychology, 101*(2), 432–447. https://doi.org/10.1037/a0014221

Murdock, T. B., Hale, N. M., & Weber, M. J. (2001). Predictors of cheating among early adolescents: Academic and social motivations. *Contemporary Educational Psychology, 26*(1), 96–115. https://doi.org/10.1006/ceps.2000.1046

Murdock, T. B., Miller, A., & Kohlhardt, J. (2004). Effects of classroom context variables on high school students' judgments of the acceptability and likelihood of cheating. *Journal of Educational Psychology, 96*(4), 765–777. https://doi.org/10.1037/0022-0663.96.4.765

Murdock, T. B., Miller, A., & Goetzinger, J. (2007). Effects of classroom context variables on university students' judgments about cheating: Mediating and moderating processes. *Social Psychology of Education, 106*, 141–169. https://doi.org/10.1007/s11218-007-9015-1

Nicholls, J. G. (1989). *The competitive ethos and democratic education.* Harvard University Press.

Nicholls, J. G., Cobb, P., Wood, T., Yackel, E., & Patashnick, M. (1990). Assessing students' theories of success in mathematics: Individual and classroom differences. *Journal of Research in Mathematics Education, 21*(2), 109–122.

Nolen, S. B. (2003). Learning environment, motivation, and achievement in high school science. *Journal of Research in Science Teaching, 40*(4), 347–368. https://doi.org/10.1002/tea.10080

Nolen, S. B., & Haladyna, T. M. (1990). Motivation and studying in high school science. *Journal of Research in Science Teaching, 27*(2), 115–126. https://doi.org/10.1002/tea.3660270204

Patrick, H. (2004). Re-examining classroom mastery goal structure. In P. R. Pintrich & M. L. Maehr (Eds.), *Advances in motivation: Vol. 13. Motivating students, improving schools: The legacy of Carol Midgley* (pp. 233–263). Elsevier JAI Press.

Patrick, H., & Ryan, A. M. (2008). What do students think about when evaluating their classroom's mastery goal structure? An examination of young adolescents' explanations. *Journal of Experimental Education, 77*(2), 99–123. https://doi.org/10.3200/JEXE.77.2.99-124

Patrick, H., Anderman, L. H., Ryan, A. M., Edelin, K., & Midgley, C. (2001). Teachers' communication of goal orientations in four fifth-grade classrooms. *The Elementary School Journal, 102*(1), 35–58. https://doi.org/10.1086/499692

Patrick, H., Turner, J. C., Meyer, D. K., & Midgley, C. (2003). How teachers establish psychological environments during the first days of school: Associations with avoidance in mathematics. *Teachers College Record, 105*(8), 1521–1558. https://doi.org/10.1111/1467-9620.00299

Patrick, H., Kaplan, A., & Ryan, A. M. (2011). Positive classroom motivational environments: Convergence between mastery goal structure and the classroom social climate. *Journal of Educational Psychology, 103*(2), 367–382. https://doi.org/10.1037/a0023311

Peng, S., Cherng, B., Lin, Y., & Kuo, C. (2018). Four-dimensional classroom goal structure model: Validation and investigation of its effect on student' adoption of personal achievement goals and approach/avoidance behaviors. *Learning and Individual Differences, 61*, 228–238. https://doi.org/10.1016/j.lindif.2017.12.004

Polychroni, F., Hatzichristou, C., & Sideridis, G. (2012). The role of goal orientations and goal structures in explaining classroom social and affective characteristics. *Learning and Individual Differences, 22*(2), 207–217. https://doi.org/10.1016/j.lindif.2011.10.005

Reschly, A. L., & Christenson, S. L. (2012). Jingle, jangle, and conceptual haziness: Evolution and future directions of the engagement construct. In S. L. Christenson, A. L. Reschly, & C. Wylie (Eds.), *Handbook of research on student engagement* (pp. 3–19). Springer Science + Business Media. https://doi.org/10.1007/978-1-4614-2018-7_1

Roeser, R. W., Midgley, C., & Urdan, T. C. (1996). Perceptions of the school psychological environment and early adolescents' psychological and behavioral functioning in school: The mediating role of goals and belonging. *Journal of Educational Psychology, 88*(3), 408–422. https://doi.org/10.1037/0022-0663.88.3.408

Rolland, R. G. (2012). Synthesizing the evidence on classroom goal structures in middle and secondary school: A meta-analysis and narrative review. *Review of Educational Research, 82*(4), 396–435. https://doi.org/10.3102/0034654312464909

Ryan, A. M., & Patrick, H. (2001). The classroom social environment and changes in adolescents' motivation and engagement during middle school. *American Educational Research Journal, 38*(2), 437–460. https://doi.org/10.3102/00028312038002437

Ryan, A. M., Gheen, M., & Midgley, C. (1998). Why do some students avoid asking for help? An examination of the interplay among students' academic efficacy, teacher's social-emotional role and classroom goal structure. *Journal of Educational Psychology, 90*(3), 528–535. https://doi.org/10.1037/0022-0663.90.3.528

Shernoff, D. J. (2010). Engagement in after-school programs as a predictor of social competence and academic performance. *American Journal of Community Psychology, 45*(3), 325–337. https://doi.org/10.1007/s10464-010-9314-0

Skinner, E. A., & Pitzer, J. R. (2012). Developmental dynamics of student engagement, coping, and everyday resilience. In S. L. Christenson, A. L. Reschly, & C. Wylie (Eds.), *Handbook of research on student engagement* (pp. 21–44). Springer Science + Business Media. https://doi.org/10.1007/978-1-4614-2018-7_2

Sommet, N., & Elliot, A. J. (2017). Achievement goals, reasons for goal pursuit, and achievement goal complexes as predictors of beneficial outcomes: Is the influence of goals reducible to reasons? *Journal of Educational Psychology, 109*(8), 1141–1162. https://doi.org/10.1037/edu0000199

Steuer, G., Rosentritt-Brunn, G., & Dresel, M. (2013). Dealing with errors in mathematics classrooms: Structure and relevance of perceived error climate. *Contemporary Educational Psychology, 38*(3), 196–210. https://doi.org/10.1016/j.cedpsych.2013.03.002

Stornes, T., Bru, E., & Idsoe, T. (2008). Classroom social structure and motivational climates: On the influence of teachers' involvement, teachers' autonomy support and regulation in relation to motivational climates in school classrooms. *Scandinavian Journal of Educational Research, 52*(3), 315–329. https://doi.org/10.1080/00313830802025124

Tapola, A., & Niemivirta, M. (2008). The role of achievement goal orientations in students' perceptions of and preferences for classroom environment. *British Journal of Educational Psychology, 78*(2), 291–312. https://doi.org/10.1348/000709907X205272

Tas, Y., & Tekkaya, C. (2010). Personal and contextual factors associated with students' cheating in science. *The Journal of Experimental Education, 78*(4), 440–463. https://doi.org/10.1080/00220970903548046

Turner, J. C., Midgley, C., Meyer, D. K., Gheen, M., Anderman, E., Kang, Y., & Patrick, H. (2002). The classroom environment and students' reports of avoidance behaviors in mathematics: A multi-method study. *Journal of Educational Psychology, 94*(1), 88–106. https://doi.org/10.1037/0022-0663.94.1.88

Turner, J. C., Gray, D. L., Anderman, L. H., Dawson, H. S., & Anderman, E. M. (2013). Getting to know my teacher: Does the relation between perceived mastery goal structures and perceived teacher support change across the school year? *Contemporary Educational Psychology, 38*(4), 316–327. https://doi.org/10.1016/j.cedpsych.2013.06.003

Urdan, T. (1997). Achievement goal theory: Past results, future directions. In M. L. Maehr & P. R. Pintrich (Eds.), *Advances in motivation and achievement* (Vol. 10, pp. 99–141). JAI Press.

Urdan, T. (2004). Predictors of academic self-handicapping and achievement: Examining achievement goals, classroom goal structures, and culture. *Journal of Educational Psychology, 96*(2), 251–264. https://doi.org/10.1037/0022-0663.96.2.251

Urdan, T., & Mestas, M. (2006). The goals behind performance goals. *Journal of Educational Psychology, 98*(2), 354–365. https://doi.org/10.1037/0022-0663.98.2.354

Urdan, T., & Midgley, C. (2003). Changes in the perceived classroom goal structure and pattern of adaptive learning during early adolescence. *Contemporary Educational Psychology, 28*(4), 524–551. https://doi.org/10.1016/S0361-476X(02)00060-7

Urdan, T., & Schoenfelder, E. (2006). Classroom effects on student motivation: Goal structures, social relationships, and competence beliefs. *Journal of School Psychology, 44*(5), 331–349. https://doi.org/10.1016/j.jsp.2006.04.003

Urdan, T., Midgley, C., & Anderman, E. M. (1998). The role of classroom goal structure in students' use of self-handicapping strategies. *American Educational Research Journal, 35*(1), 101–122. https://doi.org/10.3102/00028312035001101

Vansteenkiste, M., Lens, W., & Deci, E. L. (2006). Intrinsic versus extrinsic goal contents in self-determination theory: Another look at the quality of academic motivation. *Educational Psychologist, 41*(1), 19–31. https://doi.org/10.1207/s15326985ep4101_4

Vansteenkiste, M., Lens, W., Elliot, A. J., Soenens, B., & Mouratidis, A. (2014). Moving the achievement goal approach one step forward: Toward a systematic examination of the autonomous and controlled reasons underlying achievement goals. *Educational Psychologist, 49*(3), 153–174. https://doi.org/10.1080/00461520.2014.928598

Walker, C. O. (2012). Student perceptions of classroom achievement goals as predictors of belonging and content instrumentality. *Social Psychology of Education, 15*(1), 97–107. https://doi.org/10.1007/s11218-011-9165-z

Wolters, C. A. (2004). Advancing achievement goal theory: Using goal structures and goal orientations to predict students' motivation, cognition, and achievement. *Journal of Educational Psychology, 96*(2), 236–250. https://doi.org/10.1037/0022-0663.96.2.236

Won, S., Anderman, E. M., & Zimmerman, R. S. (2020). Longitudinal relations of classroom goal structures to students' motivation and learning outcomes in health education. *Journal of Educational Psychology, 112*(5), 1003–1019. https://doi.org/10.1037/edu0000399

Young, A. J. (1997). I think, therefore I'm motivated: The relations among cognitive strategy use, motivational orientation and classroom perceptions over time. *Learning and Individual Differences, 9*(3), 249–283. https://doi.org/10.1016/S1041-6080(97)90009-1

Zhang, Q. (2014). Assessing the effects of instructor enthusiasm on classroom engagement, learning goal orientation, and academic self-efficacy. *Communication Teacher, 28*(1), 44–56. https://doi.org/10.1080/17404622.2013.839047

Student Engagement: The Importance of the Classroom Context

Wendy M. Reinke, Keith C. Herman, and Christa B. Copeland

Abstract

Effective classroom management is associated with positive student outcomes including active student engagement and academic achievement. This chapter reviews the importance of the teachers' use of effective classroom management in creating a positive and culturally inclusive classroom climate that supports positive student engagement. The critical features of effective classroom management are reviewed. In addition, models for supporting teachers in their use of effective practices are discussed. Lessons learned and future direction are provided.

Effective classroom management is associated with positive student outcomes including active student engagement and academic achievement (Herman, Reinke, Dong, & Bradshaw, in press; Kleinert et al., 2017; Reinke et al., 2018). This chapter reviews the importance of the teachers' use of effective classroom management in creating a positive and culturally inclusive classroom climate that supports positive student engage-

W. M. Reinke (✉) · K. C. Herman · C. B. Copeland
University of Missouri, Missouri Prevention Science Institute, Columbia, MO, USA
e-mail: reinkew@missouri.edu;
hermanke@missouri.edu; cbhgg6@missouri.edu

ment. First, we discuss and define student engagement and the connection between classroom management and student engagement. Then, the importance of effective classroom management and the impact of ineffective classroom management on student outcomes and on teachers is reviewed. Next, the connection between effective classroom management and positive and culturally inclusive classroom climates is highlighted. The crucial features of effective classroom management, including proactive preventative classroom management strategies, relationship building, and responding to disruptive or disengaged behavior, are discussed. Next, models for training and supporting teachers in the use of effective classroom management are reviewed. Finally, lessons learned and future directions for supporting teachers in the use of effective classroom management are discussed.

Student Engagement

Theory and research have operationalized student engagement in several ways (see Christenson, Reschly & Wylie, 2012). One prominent theory establishes student engagement along three dimensions: behavioral, affective, and cognitive (Fredericks et al., 2004). Behavioral engagement refers to observable actions students take to participate in learning including participation, task completion, and persistence (Bakker et al., 2015).

Affective engagement refers to the relational aspects and emotional reactions to school, including a sense of bonding with learning, classmates, teachers, and school (Finn, 1989). Finally, cognitive engagement refers to the psychological investment in learning and includes flexibility and openness to challenge and effort (Connell & Wellborn, 1991). Other research has designated a fourth dimension, an academic engagement which is a result of improvements in the other dimension of engagement (Christenson et al., 2012). This chapter draws on these ideas to conceptualize how effective classroom management can increase each dimension of engagement and how increased engagement is linked to positive behavioral and academic outcomes for students.

The connection between effective classroom management and student engagement can be explained by understanding how contextual and psychological variables determine academic performance. Connell and colleagues (1995) outlined a causal model for understanding the contributions of contextual and psychological variables in determining student academic success using an influential theory of motivation (Deci & Ryan, 1985). In this model, student motivation refers to the cognitive, emotional, and behavioral indicators of student investment in and connection to education (Skinner & Belmont, 1993). Only student engagement directly affects academic achievement. All other variables (e.g., teacher behaviors) act through engagement by enhancing or undermining student engagement in learning. Therefore, variables such as effective classroom management indirectly influence student success in school because students become engaged in schoolwork if their basic psychological needs for relatedness, competence, and autonomy are met (Connell et al., 1995). Teachers can fulfill these needs by respectively building positive teacher-student relationships, providing structure (e.g., utilizing proactive management strategies), and supporting student autonomy (i.e., giving choices). For instance, a recent study conducted in secondary schools with a sample of 26,849 students found that observed proactive classroom management by teachers was posi-

tively and significantly associated with student reports of active engagement in that classroom (Larson et al., 2021). Students' higher engagement will, in turn, lead to academic success (Skinner et al., 1990). In this way, teachers' use of effective classroom management practices affects students' achievement through their impact on students' engagement (See Fig. 1).

Importance of Effective Classroom Management

The classroom context plays an important role in the success of students. In particular, a teacher's use of effective classroom management can positively impact the academic, social, emotional, and behavioral outcomes of students in their classroom by increasing student engagement in learning. Whereas, poorly managed classrooms can contribute to negative student outcomes (Reinke & Herman, 2002) by inhibiting student engagement in learning. For instance, students in poorly managed classrooms where little structure or support for consistent behavioral expectations are provided become off task and engage in higher rates of disruptive behaviors, resulting in less time for academic instruction (Jones & Jones, 2004). Negative teacher-student interactions are also more likely to occur in poorly managed classrooms (Conroy et al., 2009), and ineffective classroom environments contribute to students' risk for developing behavior problems (Kellam et al., 1998). Poor classroom management also has been linked to long-term negative academic, behavioral, and social outcomes for students (National Research Council, 2002; Reinke & Herman, 2002).

Furthermore, teachers who struggle with implementing effective classroom management practices exhibit higher levels of stress and burnout, and are more likely to leave the field. When teachers are stressed and do not have good coping strategies, they are less likely to provide engaging instruction. For instance, in a recent study, elementary teachers who reported high levels of stress and low levels of coping were

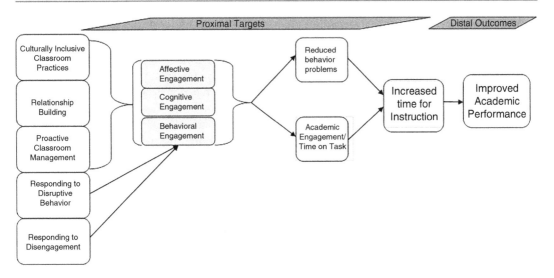

Fig. 1 Conceptual framework for effective classroom management leading to student academic performance

associated with lower student academic achievement and prosocial behavior than teachers who reported lower levels of stress (Herman et al., 2018). A similar study with middle school teachers found that teachers with high levels of stress and low coping reported higher levels of burnout, lower efficacy had higher rates of observed reprimands, and higher levels of student reported depressive symptoms in their classroom in comparison to other teachers. Whereas, teachers with low stress and high coping had lower levels of burnout, more parental involvement, and higher levels of student prosocial behavior in their classrooms in comparison to others (Herman et al., 2020).

Nearly half of teachers leave the field in their first five years of employment. Many of these teachers indicate that challenges in managing student behavior are the main reason for leaving (Ingersoll & Strong, 2011). Teaching is a challenging profession, and the need for qualified, effective teachers is imperative to student success. The cost of teacher turnover in public schools costs billions of dollars a year (Alliance for Excellent Education, 2014). Thus, preparing teachers for the use of effective classroom management is essential. In the next section, we highlight the critical features of effective classroom management.

Critical Features of Effective Classroom Management

Features of effective classroom management practices have long been known. In particular, the use of proactive classroom management practices, such as teaching classroom rules and expectations, providing positive attention to a student displaying these expectations, and providing precorrections—or prompting expected behaviors during times that students struggle—can support a predictable and safe classroom context (Reinke, Herman, & Sprick, 2011). Other important aspects of a positive classroom climate include being culturally inclusive, building positive relationships, and responding to disruptive behavior and disengaged behavior appropriately (Gregory et al., 2016; Reinke et al., 2016; Simonsen et al., 2008).

Being Culturally Inclusive

Youth from minority ethnic backgrounds experience racism that is systemic, meaning that racial bias and discrimination are weaved into all facets of society, including the schooling system (see also Galindo et al., chapter "Expanding an Equity Understanding of Student Engagement: The Macro (Social) and Micro (School) Contexts" this volume). This leads to disproportionately administered harsh discipline (Skiba et al., 2011), negative student-teacher interactions (Reinke et al., 2016), and overrepresentation of students of color in certain special education categories (Skiba et al., 2005), resulting in poorer outcomes for students of color Black students are three times more likely to be suspended than their White peers and are more likely to receive suspension or expulsion for similar behaviors compared to students from other racial groups (Losen & Skiba, 2010). In a sample of over 15,000 students, Morris and Perry (2016) found that even after controlling for socioeconomic status (SES), Black students were three times as likely to be suspended compared to White students. After controlling for school-level differences (e.g., school size, school composition), analyses indicated that both Black and Latinx students had received a disproportionate number of suspensions compared to their White peers. This finding is consistent with several prior studies showing that racial and ethnic disparities in discipline persist even when accounting for SES (Skiba et al., 2011; Wallace et al., 2008).

As such, a critical, yet widely overlooked (and often misinterpreted; see Sleeter, 2012) aspect of effective classroom management, is the adoption and sustained use of culturally relevant pedagogy and practices. When students feel respected, valued, challenged, and supported within a classroom community, they are much more likely to engage in the learning environment (McKinley, 2010). This requires teachers to address the *whole* student, including students' own identities and how they relate to the school and community contexts. Culturally relevant teaching does just that, providing a comprehensive approach to learning through the students' own cultural lenses. These practices are strength-based, facilitating learning through a student's existing knowledge, and function to foster creativity, liberate and empower (Gay, 2010). For consistency, we refer to the practices described above as culturally inclusive practices throughout this section.

Culturally inclusive practices acknowledge and celebrate student differences, encourage and support individualized learning and success,

and challenge existing societal and educational structures and beliefs (Ladson-Billings, 2009). Instead of being a standalone practice, culturally inclusive practices can and should be woven into all aspects of a classroom. To some degree, culturally inclusive practices allow teachers to more appropriately employ common evidence-based classroom practices to meet the cultural needs of their classrooms (Larson et al., 2018). For example, culturally inclusive classroom management can "look" like developing positive student-teacher relationships through affirming and validating cultural backgrounds, emphasizing collectivism and classroom community through reciprocal learning, and extending the learning environment to the home and community settings (e.g., Weinstein et al., 2003). The difference between simply implementing evidence-based practices and using culturally inclusive practices (which are evidence-based practices) is differentiated by the extent that students' "cultural characteristics, experiences and perspectives" are used alongside them as "conduits" to reshape the curriculum and promote meaningful activities and conversations in the classroom (Gay, 2002, p. 106).

Culturally inclusive practice has also been embedded within school-wide approaches to discipline [e.g., Positive Behavior Interventions and Supports (PBIS)] to promote teacher introspection, modify culturally neutral school and classroom practices, and consciously engage with inequitable social issues at the institutional level (e.g., Banks & Obiakor, 2015; Banks & Banks, 2019; Cramer & Bennett, 2015; Diamond & Gomez, 2004; McIntosh et al., 2014; Milner, 2011). For an abundance of rich descriptions of these classroom practices in action, we point our readers to Ladson-Billings (2009). For schools implementing PBIS, see Leverson et al. (2016).

Teacher Bias Several important aspect of culturally inclusive practice are for teachers to reflect on their own culture, the differences between their culture and the culture of the students in their classroom and understanding one's biases. A classroom reflects a teacher's internal values and interests. Therefore, the beliefs, values, and attitudes they bring into their classrooms, directly influence the practices they choose to implement. Culturally inclusive practices begin with changing teacher perspectives through exploration, self-reflection, discovery, and education about how current educational practices can hinder the potential of students with diverse backgrounds. Culturally inclusive practices require personal reflection and a deeper understanding of students, asking the questions: "Who are my students?" and "How do they see themselves at home, in my classroom, and in society?" It also requires teachers to become critically conscious, reflecting on how privilege, values, and culture influence their classrooms (Ladson-Billings, 1995). Practices that support and empower students of diverse backgrounds have repeatedly been shown to be more effective than when these practices are not used, helping to increase student self-identity, autonomy, self-esteem, effective engagement, and academic success (Milner, 2011; Tucker et al., 2002).

Truly effective teachers maintain the belief that students already possess the ability to succeed in a safe and affirming classroom context. By striving to create a culturally inclusive classroom, teachers are acknowledging that embedding individual student experiences and backgrounds into student learning is just as important as the learning process itself. Until culturally inclusive practices are no longer considered to be something "else" we must do, but rather how we should have been doing it all along, we believe that classroom management will continue to be one of the top concerns in education and continue to underserve our diverse students.

Building Positive Relationships

When teachers do not truly know their students, they are much more likely to negatively attribute their classroom behavior as misbehavior (Gay, 2002). Foundational to building a culturally inclusive and positive classroom climate is having positive relationships with students. Classrooms in which students feel supported, respected, and valued are characterized by effective teacher-

student relationships. Teacher-student relationships are most effective when they are warm, engaged, and responsive, and when teachers have high demands and high expectations and provide the class with structure and clear limits (Pianta, 1999; see also Hofkens & Pianta, chapter "Teacher–Student Relationships, Engagement in School, and Student Outcomes", this volume). Theoretically, students who feel respected and who respect their teacher will place greater value on feedback (positive or negative) provided by the teacher and are more likely to be behaviorally and academically engaged in the classroom. When students do not value their relationship with a teacher, praise or positive feedback will be less reinforcing and they will be less likely to comply with directives, even resorting to acting out/misbehavior in the classroom setting (see Simonsen et al., 2008).

Effective teacher-student relationships are associated with increased academic engagement and achievement (Roorda et al., 2017). For instance, a recent meta-analysis investigated whether students' engagement acts as a mediator between teacher-student relationships and achievement (Roorda et al., 2017). They reviewed 189 studies that included students in preschool through high school and found that student engagement partially mediated the associations between positive and negative relationships and student achievement. Some ways that teachers can work to support effective teacher-student relationships is by utilizing the strategies outlined in this chapter for creating effective classrooms, including, creating a classroom structure that is consistent with clear expectations and ongoing reinforcement for appropriate behavior, having more positive than negative interactions with students, providing engaging and meaningful instruction, and providing respectful corrections and constructive feedback (Reinke et al., 2011, Simonsen et al., 2008). Other areas on which teachers can focus their attention when building effective relationships with students include taking a conscious interest in each student, providing noncontingent interactions, and holding appropriately high expectations that they share with their students (Alexander & Rubie-Davies, 2017; Good & Lavigne, 2018).

Researchers recently evaluated a teacher training intervention focused on creating and maintaining positive student-teacher relationships, called *Establish-Maintain-Restore* approach (EMR; see Cook et al., 2018). Teachers attend a 3-h training focused on learning the three components of the intervention. In the first phase, teachers are trained to establish relationships by banking time or having one on one interactions with students that arenondirective and validating. The second phase, maintaining relationships, reinforces that positive relationships with students require ongoing work. The primary practice for maintaining relationships is having teachers deliver a ratio of 5:1 positive to negative interactions with students. Lastly, the restore phase occurs when a relationship has been challenged in some way. Teachers have several strategies that they learn that can help restore positive relationships with students (e.g., acknowledge students feeling; letting go of a previous event, etc.). A randomized control trial with teachers and students in elementary schools found that EMR improved student–teacher relationships, observer-rated disruptive behavior and academically engaged time, with moderate to large effect sizes (Cohen's $d = 0.61$–0.89; Cook et al., 2018). A more recent randomized trial with teachers and students in middle schools found similar results with EMR demonstrating significant improvements in student–teacher relationships (Hedge's $g = 0.61$), academically engaged time ($g = 0.81$), and disruptive behavior ($g = 1.07$; Duong et al., 2019). Results indicate potential promise for EMR as a method for supporting teachers in building positive teacher-student relationships which can then result in improved academic engagement.

Noncontingent Interactions A noncontingent interaction is one in which a teacher spends positive time with students without making that time dependent on the student's behavior. Examples of noncontingent interactions include asking a student about their weekend, greeting students as they enter the door with a "Welcome to class. So glad you are here" and telling a student in the hallway as you pass, "It's great to see you today".

These interactions show the teachers are interested in the student and demonstrate that they are important and valued. In fact, one study evaluated the impact of greeting middle school students as they entered the classroom and found that this simple intervention increased student on task behavior from a mean of 45% to 72% (Allday & Pakurar, 2007). In another study, teachers used noncontingent attention with students with emotional and behavioral disorders and found that classroom observations of disruptive behavior and on-task behavior improved. Additionally, teachers were more likely to provide more praise than reprimands, whereas they used more reprimands before using noncontingent attention (Rubow et al., 2019). This indicates that using noncontingent attention can likely improve teacher-student relationships and support student affective, behavioral, and cognitive engagement. These noncontingent interactions are a vital component of the teacher's effort to build a positive relationship with the student.

Using Proactive Strategies

Proactive classroom management strategies are preventive in nature, meaning that they reduce the likelihood of student disruptive and disengaged behaviors. Examples of proactive strategies include having clear classroom expectations and teaching these expectations to students. When students understand the social and behavioral expectations of the classroom they are more likely to remain engaged in instruction and have a better relationship with their teachers. Another important proactive strategy is the use of praise. Teachers who provide positive and behavior-specific attention to students who are behaviorally and academically engaged and meeting expectations increase the likelihood that students will display these behaviors in the future (see Floress et al., 2018). The recommended ratio of positive to negative attention is 5:1 (Flora, 2000). Classrooms with predictable routines and structures where teachers provide more positive than negative attention to students create a positive and safe climate which is conducive to increasing engagement across all dimensions. See Table 1 for a list of recommended practices for use of praise (see Reinke et al., 2011).

Another important proactive strategy is the use of precorrective statements, or behavioral instructions setting up students for success (see Stormont & Reinke, 2009). For instance, in a classroom where the teacher has noticed that students get distracted and become off-task during group work could set up the activity by noting exactly what they want to see (e.g., "Class, when we move into math group work, everyone should be focused on the activity using a level one voice."). A proactive teacher would also use active supervision to monitor student behavioral and academic engagement by walking around the classroom, redirecting as needed, answering questions, and providing positive attention to students who are on-task.

Responding to Misbehavior and Student Disengagement

While culturally responsive classroom environments that promote positive relationships between teachers and students that utilize proactive classroom management strategies will be

less likely to have students who are disruptive or behaviorally and academically disengaged, teachers also need to have strategies to respond to misbehavior and disengagement when it occurs. For instance, for students who display a behavior seeking attention when they are off task, a teacher can use planned ignoring. Planned ignoring is a strategy where you ignore the attention-seeking behavior and then provide attention when the student is meeting expectations. While this is a great strategy, it is less effective if a student is really just avoiding an activity (e.g., puts head down on desk during instruction). Ignoring a student who is disengaged with instruction will not cause them to suddenly engage. In these instances, a calm redirect that states the expectation to the student (e.g., "Kennedy, please sit with your head up and eyes on me.") can be useful in getting them re-engaged in instruction. Of course, following up with positive attention for being academically engaged and continuation of building a positive relationship with the student will lead to more engagement with learning over time.

Engaging the Disengaged Student Sometimes teachers will find that students are rather difficult to engage in the classroom. It is important to determine the reason for disengagement. Is the student disengaged because they find the academic content difficult and maybe avoiding engaging because of this, or do they just not want to engage? For instance, if a student tends to not engage during math, it could be that they are not understanding or have fallen behind. To determine if this is the cause of disengagement, you would first want to assess the current performance level of the student in that topic (e.g., math) and compare this to the level of performance expected. If there is a mismatch, in that the student has fallen behind or in some instance is too advanced in the topic (i.e., content is boring), then adjustments to the level of instruction would need to occur. So, if a 3rd grader is reading at a 1st grade level, they are likely to be academically disengaged if they are expected to read 3rd grade materials. This student would need extra instruction, tutoring and support to get to a point where they could read 3rd grade materials.

Table 1 Recommended practices for using praise

Praise should be contingent on a behavior and occur after the behavior is observed.	Identify a behavior you want to see more, teach students to use the behavior, and provide praise at a high rate when the behavior occurs.
A 5:1 ratio of positive to negative interaction is the gold standard.	Teachers often use low rates of praise in their classrooms. A ratio of 5:1 positive to negative interaction with students is recommended.
Behavior specific praise is more effective than general praise.	Behavior specific praise describes the behavior of receiving attention, indicating students' clear expectations. This is higher quality praise than general praise.
Praise should be genuine and authentic.	Teachers should only provide praise when they really mean it and the behavior is something that is important and valued.

If the assessment of the student's academic performance level does not find a mismatch, then it may be that the student just does not *want* to do the work. In this case, the teacher would need to find a way to motivate the student to engage in the work. There are several strategies for helping to motivate a student to engage when they do not want to do so. One strategy is the use of a behavioral contract (see Majeika et al., 2020). When using a behavioral contract the teacher and student meet to discuss a goal that if achieved would earn the student something they find reinforcing. As an example, if a student does not engage in the classroom during math or complete any work during math, a reasonable goal may be to answer one question in class and complete the assignments for 3 out of 5 days. For doing so, they might receive computer time (i.e., something that is fun that they are willing to work for). If they do even better than 3 days in one week the student can earn extra computer time or something even more reinforcing. The teacher and student determine how they will decide if the goal was met. Then, the teacher and student review and sign the contract.

Another strategy for working with students who do not want to engage in an activity or topic is to allow them to escape doing some of the work, but with limitations. One intervention called *Take a Break* (see Stormont, Reinke, Herman, & Lembke, 2012; Stormont et al., 2016), involves allowing a student to escape from a task that they are actively avoiding (e.g., academics, social interaction). It seems simple enough. Once you determine that a student is escape maintained, or the disengaged or off-task behavior is because they find it more reinforcing to avoid the task than to complete it, allowing a student to escape some portion of the activity can be helpful. Often students who are trying to escape an activity or task may either sit idly trying to stay off the radar of the teacher or they act out in ways that get them out of completing the task (e.g., display aggressive behavior that gets them sent out of the classroom). Thus, the first step is to identify and teach them a replacement behavior. In this case, it is to ask for a break. Each day they have a certain number of times they can ask for a break without consequence (e.g., 3 times per day for 5 min each time). The student should earn something for only taking the number of breaks allocated per day. The student should also be reinforced for not using all their breaks each day (e.g., get out of a small homework assignment if they only use 2 breaks during the day). A response cost can also be put into place if the student takes more than 3 breaks per day. The goal is to allow the student to get out of some of the tasks they are avoiding while also slowly encouraging the completion of more tasks. The goal is to get students who are very academically disengaged and completing little work to begin completing some work with a goal of getting them to a higher level of engagement. By giving choices and opportunities for success teachers can increase a student's autonomy, which is associated with increased engagement in learning.

It is important that provide positive attention during times when students are behaviorally and academically engaged. One important concept is that students who are escape maintained are less likely to find attention reinforcing, and in fact, may find it aversive. It is important to find ways to let them know, however, that they are valued and appreciated (e.g., quietly whisper to them in their seat, hand them a sticky note with a positive message). It has been our experience in practice that even when it seems like a student doesn't like encouragement and validation (e.g., they shrug off when the teacher privately praises their effort), many times these students are taking this in and do notice teacher efforts to build relationships.

Barriers to Teacher Use of Effective Classroom Management

Although effective classroom practices are known and seem as though they can be easily implemented, many teachers struggle to implement these practices in their classrooms. There are several reasons for the disconnect between what we know is effective and what is actually implemented in the classroom. First, many teachers feel underprepared to use effective classroom management practices in their classroom (Reinke et al., 2011). In particular, teachers who enter the field may have had little to no training in classroom management in their pre-service training. In a recent review of pre-service teacher preparation programs, findings indicated less than half of the reviewed general education programs contained evidence of research-based content in classroom management, demonstrating a significant gap in teacher training program requirements (Freeman et al., 2014). Thus, when new teachers enter the field they are surprised by the complexities of teaching, particularly when they are attempting to provide academic instruction and find students to be disengaged. This lack of knowledge and lack of efficacy in using effective classroom management are barriers.

Another barrier to the use of effective practices is lack of a teacher's knowledge of evidence-based practices (Stormont et al., 2011) or their willingness to use effective classroom management practices. For instance, some teachers may not believe that evidence-based behavior management practices have utility or are appropriate for their classroom. For instance, some teachers are trained to believe that praise is not good for students because it reduces intrinsic motivation or instils a sense of contingent self-worth that leads to helplessness in students (see Kamins & Dweck, 1999). However, for many students, particularly those who are disengaged or displaying challenging behaviors, the use of praise or positive attention can help build positive relationships and reinforce behaviors that you want to see more of in the classroom.

Consultation Models and Strategies to Support Teachers in Using Effective Practices

Research has shown that high-quality induction programs, including mentoring with classroom coaching, are effective support for novice teachers (Ingersoll & Strong, 2011; Smith & Ingersoll, 2004; Stormont et al., 2015). Smith and Ingersoll (2004) showed that early career teachers who were provided with induction programs featuring basic training and the assignment of a mentor were twice as likely to persist as early career teachers who were provided with no induction activities.

Further, any teacher who is struggling with effectively managing student behavior will benefit from coaching. However, despite the need for onsite coaching, few schools have personnel with the behavioral expertise or access to tools that would allow them to effectively support teachers with coaching in classroom management (Stormont et al., 2011). School psychologists can play a key role in this area, either by coaching teachers or providing training to other staff to become coaches.

Coaches need training and information in effective consultation as well as tools for evaluating current practices, providing constructive objective feedback to teachers, developing classroom interventions with teachers, and evaluating the effectiveness of interventions. Without these system-level mechanisms, there is little incentive for teacher change or guidance for teachers (Myers et al., 2011). Utilization of models of support that can be easily accessed would be an essential step in reducing teacher attrition and bridging the gap between the availability of evidence-based practices and their adoption in classrooms.

Classroom Check-up

One such model is the Classroom Check-up (CCU; Reinke et al., 2008; Reinke, Herman, & Sprick, 2011). The CCU is a classroom management intervention that combines data-based decision making and evidence-based classroom management practices with ongoing onsite coaching for teachers. It is an assessment-based consultation intervention that addresses the need for classroom-level support for teachers struggling with classroom management (Reinke et al., 2008; Reinke et al., 2011). The model provides a systematic structure for coaches supporting teachers and is conducted in a series of steps: (1) assessing the classroom, (2) providing the teacher with personalized feedback, (3) developing a menu of options in collaboration with the teacher for intervention, (4) choosing the intervention, (5) planning the intervention and having the teacher self-monitor implementation, and (6) ongoing monitoring which when appropriate includes providing performance feedback. A vital and unique component of the CCU is that it links assessment to intervention by including an assessment of the teachers' current use of critical classroom management variables followed by feedback to the teacher and the collaborative design of classroom intervention. Classroom interventions are tailored to the needs of the classroom and based on objective data. Areas of need are identified (e.g., positive to negative ratio) and a menu of potential interventions are explored by the teacher and coach (e.g., teach expectations and provide behavior-specific praise to students meeting expectations).

Recently, through an Institute of Education Sciences funded Development and Innovation project, a web version of the CCU was developed. The purpose of the CCU website (http://classroomcheckup.org/) is to make the behavioral expertise needed to support teachers in learning new classroom management strategies through coaching and feedback accessible to anyone in a school building. As such, a peer teacher or principal could sit down with a teacher to use the website to readily determine areas of need for support, and learn the needed skill identified through web-based brief intervention descriptions, intervention tools, and exemplary video examples. The website was developed to support anyone in becoming a CCU coach and includes tools for teachers to self-assess and discover new strategies for use in their classroom. Table 2 reiterates the CCU process.

A small pilot study was conducted to evaluate the efficacy of the CCU website. A total of 39 teachers and 617 students were recruited. Teachers completed pre and post-intervention measures on student disruptive behavior, academic competence, and social behaviors. The results indicated, although not statistically significant ($p = 0.18$), teachers in the CCU condition used more behavior-specific praise than control teachers across time points with time point 1

Table 2 CCU coaching framework

Step 1: Interview with teacher	The coach meets with the teacher to conduct a brief interview to build rapport and understand their approach to classroom management
Step 2: Classroom assessment	The coach conducts two or more classroom observations, gathering data on teacher and student behaviors (e.g., use of praise, number of disruptions)
Step 3: Personalized feedback	The coach meets with the teacher to review the data gathered through observations and interview. These data are provided back using a red, yellow, and green feedback form. The meeting is conversational and focuses on both strengths and areas of growth
Step 4: Develop menu of options	The coach and teacher develop a menu of options for strategies or interventions to use in the classroom. The menu is based on the areas the teacher identifies during feedback that they would like to improve
Step 5: Implement intervention	The teacher selects one or more strategies to use from the menu of options. The coach and teacher plan together next steps for implementation
Step 6: Evaluate intervention	The coach visits the classroom when the teacher is using a new strategy. The same data gathered in step 2 occurs. The coach provided feedback to the teacher and supports any changes to the intervention in the classroom

serving as baseline. Within subjects contrasts found that time point one was significantly lower than time point 2 [$F(1, 18) = 5.66$, $p = 0.03$, $\eta^2 = 0.24$], and marginally lower than time point 3 [$F(1, 18) = 3.66$, $p = 0.07$, $\eta^2 = 0.17$], and time point 4 [$F(1, 18) = 3.81$, $p = 0.07$, $\eta^2 = 0.18$], meaning that teacher use of behavior-specific praise improved significantly after receiving the intervention and then maintained over time (see Fig. 2).

Further, a series of two-level hierarchical linear models (HLM), in which students (level 1) are nested within teachers (level 2) were conducted to examine the overall treatment effects on student behavior and academic outcomes. Each student's pretest ($n = 617$) and demographic

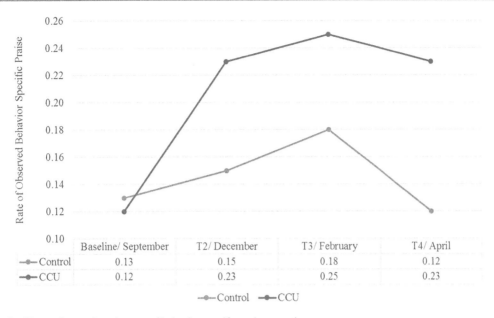

Fig. 2 Observed rate of teacher use of behavior specific praise over time

	Baseline/ September	T2/ December	T3/ February	T4/ April
Control	0.13	0.15	0.18	0.12
CCU	0.12	0.23	0.25	0.23

Table 3 Overview of double check 5 CARES elements

C	Connection to curriculum
A	Authentic relationships
R	Reflective thinking about culture
E	Effective communication
S	Sensitivity to student's culture

information were included at level 1, and the treatment variable was at level 2. The observed effect for each outcome was in the right direction but there were not enough observations to reach significance. The main effect analysis demonstrating marginal significance in the underpowered sample included, teacher-reported disruptive behavior ($b = 0.08$, $p = 0.14$; $d = 0.12$), indicating that CCU teachers increased their use of praise versus reprimands toward individual student in their classroom in comparison to control teachers. This finding was not statistically significant given we only had 30% power to detect an effect. To find a significant improvement in disruptive behavior we will need to find an effect of $d = 0.22$ with 80% power to find an effect. Future studies will target teachers in need of support with classroom management, such as first-year teachers, to increase the likelihood of a larger effect. The cur-

rent study was applied universally to a teacher regardless of risk.

Double Check

Double check is a consultation model that utilizes the CCU coaching model to support teachers in the use of culturally responsive classroom practices (see Pas et al., 2016). As noted earlier, effective classroom management is culturally responsive, but double check is a framework designed to improve teacher culturally responsive behavior management with the goal of decreasing disproportional disciplinary referrals for culturally and linguistically diverse students. Double check utilizes the acronym CARES for the five domains that have been found to successfully engage students from culturally diverse backgrounds at school. See Table 3 for an overview of the CARES elements.

The model includes a series of professional development trainings on each of the CARES elements as well as coaching to support teachers use of the practices learned during the professional development trainings. Double check coaching uses the CCU model described above, incorporating personalized feedback on cultural responsiveness as well as classroom behavior management. Data used to provide feedback are assessed through teacher self-report of culturally responsive behavior management and self-efficacy, classroom observations that gather data on teacher behavior with an eye toward differential rate of praise or reprimands based on student race or gender, and review of office discipline referral data for students from the teachers classroom.

A recent randomized controlled trial evaluating the impact of the double check coaching model with 158 elementary and middle school teachers randomly assigned to either receive coaching or not. All teachers were exposed to the professional development components of the double check model. Findings indicated that there were improvements in self-reported culturally responsive behavior management and self-efficacy for teachers in both conditions following professional development exposure. Teachers who received coaching were observed to be significantly more likely to use proactive behavior management and anticipate student problems, had higher student cooperation, and fewer disruptive behaviors relative to comparison teachers. These findings suggest the promise of coaching combined with school-wide professional development for improving classroom management practices and possibly reducing office discipline referrals among Black students (Bradshaw et al., 2018).

Personalized Performance Feedback

The CCU, double check, and several other consultation models (e.g., My Teaching Partner, see Hofkens & Pianta, chapter "Teacher-Student Relationships, Engagement in School, and Student Outcomes", this volume) utilize personalized performance feedback to support teachers in using new practices in their classrooms. Personalized feedback, or giving back information specific to their classroom, their skills, and their behaviors, has been demonstrated to improve teacher implementation of new practices (Reinke et al., 2007; Reinke et al., 2008;

Reinke, Stormont, Herman, & Newcomer, 2014). A recent meta-analysis of the use of performance feedback with teachers found that performance feedback was effective in increasing the fidelity to a new strategy or intervention and helped to curb the declines in fidelity following skill training (Solomon et al., 2012). Performance feedback was utilized across pre-Kindergarten through high school, with general education and special education teachers, and feedback was provided either immediately, within the day, or weekly among the studies reviewed. Immediate and daily feedback had nearly equal effects, and both outperformed weekly feedback (Solomon et al., 2012). Further, another study found that performance feedback was one of the most effective strategies used by coaches when working with teachers (Stormont et al., 2015). Lastly, a study that looked at teachers who received more performance feedback from a coach in comparison to the teacher who received less performance feedback found that teachers receiving more performance feedback demonstrated a greater increase in their use of proactive classroom management (Reinke et al., 2014). Thus, performance feedback seems like a key ingredient when supporting teachers in using effective classroom management practices.

Pre-implementation Feedback Another method of supporting teacher use of effective classroom practices includes implementation-directed strategies to enhance skill-building before and throughout the use of these practices by teachers (e.g., Hagermoser Sanetti et al., 2018). Performance feedback is an evidence-based strategy regularly used for both student and teacher achievement and development in schools (Stormont et al., 2015; Fallon et al., 2015), yet it is rarely considered viable support during the pre-adoption phase of classroom interventions. Additionally, because of the variability in background, experience and expertise, one-size-fits-all approaches to teacher intervention support are not always effective, as some often need different levels of support to embed these practices in their classroom successfully (Collier-Meek et al., 2019).

The use of personalized, web-based feedback is an emerging tool that offers a sustainable method for enhancing and informing teacher-delivered interventions that address the need for differentiation across teachers, as well as attend to underlying factors associated with low usage of classroom management evidence-based practices (Copeland, 2019). Within this model, teachers are first given a brief measure that assesses research-based variables specific to the implementation process (e.g., behavior attributions, self-efficacy, attitudes toward evidence-based interventions), then provided with a targeted feedback report that includes personalized recommendations with embedded web-based resources, and an action plan template to guide development efforts. This process is completed entirely electronically, making it efficient and flexible for school communities, as well as improving accessibility for schools in more remote areas with less access to expert consultation. By increasing teacher efficacy and attitudes surrounding evidence-based, behavior practices before embedding new strategies in the classroom (see Copeland, 2019), this pre-implementation support can greatly enhance teacher success, especially when used in conjunction with more common consultation methods (Reinke et al., 2011), or a tiered approach to teacher support delivery throughout the implementation process (e.g., Sanetti & Collier-Meek, 2015).

Lessons Learned and Future Directions

The importance of teachers' use of effective classroom management has been highlighted. When teachers struggle with managing their classroom they experience high levels of stress and students experience poorer academic and behavioral outcomes. Thus, supporting teachers in training before entering the field at the pre-service level is needed. The lack of attention to course work and or applied practice using effective classroom management skills will continue to produce in-service teachers who struggle, lack

efficacy, and leave the field early. One idea is to develop pre-service training models that include coaching when pre-service teachers are doing field training. Coaches could observe the pre-service teachers in the field and give performance feedback in a systematic process. These coaches could be graduate students in school psychology programs, giving these students the opportunity to use coaching and learning the use models such as the CCU and learn effective consultation alongside pre-service teachers. The teachers with whom pre-service teachers are placed could be part of the meetings and learn the process as well, providing them with tools for supporting other teachers who may struggle (e.g., mentor/induction programs).

Another area for future and long-term work is the need to support teachers in overcoming biases, understanding culturally inclusive practices, and providing coaching or consultation to teachers to ensure that they are using these practices. Systemic racism is well-embedded in the educational system and teachers will need ongoing support to examine their own biases and enact anti-racist practices in their classrooms. Although excellent books and training materials to promote culturally inclusive teaching practices have been around for decades (see Banks & Banks, 2019; Diamond & Gomez, 2004; Ladson-Billings, 1995; Milner, 2011), professional development materials alone will not move teaching practices. Mentoring and coaching are needed to help teachers improve hidden and sometimes entrenched attitudes, beliefs, and interaction patterns. Coaching models are emerging to fill this void, most notably the previously described double check model which has strong empirical evidence (Bradshaw et al., 2018). However, these models will need continued refinement as they tend to focus on behavioral practices. More work is needed on how best to coach a teacher in examining their biases and reflecting on the structural aspects of racism that disrupt child development, engagement in schooling, and educational success. In addition, often overlooked is the importance of training and supporting coaches and mentors in this process. Obviously, to be effective consultants on this topic, coaches also need to engage in a similar level of self-reflection and discovery to support teacher development in these areas. Lastly, research on the connection between classroom management practices and their association with the dimensions of student engagement is needed. Findings of how specific strategies can lead to improvements across the affective, behavioral, and cognitive engagement can inform teacher training and consultation models.

References

Alexander, P., & Rubie-Davies, C. (2017). *Teacher expectations in education* (1st ed.). Routledge.

Allday, A., & Pakurar, K. (2007). Effects of teacher greeting on students on-task behavior. *Journal of Applied Behavior Analysis, 40*, 317–320.

Alliance for Excellent Education. (2014). *On the path to equity: Improving the effectiveness of beginning teachers.* https://all4ed.org/wp-content/uploads/2014/07/PathToEquity.pdf

Bakker, A. B., Vergel, A. I. S., & Kuntze, J. (2015). Student engagement and performance: A weekly diary study on the role of openness. *Motivation and Emotion, 39*, 49–62.

Banks, J. A., & Banks, C. A. M. (Eds.). (2019). *Multicultural education: Issues and perspectives.* Wiley.

Banks, T., & Obiakor, F. E. (2015). Culturally responsive positive behavior supports: Considerations for practice. *Journal of Education and Training Studies, 3*, 83–90.

Bradshaw, C. P., Pas, E. T., Debnam, K., Bottiani, J., Reinke, W. M., Herman, K. C., & Rosenberg, M. (2018). Promoting cultural responsivity and student engagement through Double Check Coaching of classroom teachers: An efficacy study. *School Psychology Review, 47*, 118–134.

Christenson, S. L., Reschly, A. L., & Wylie, C. (Eds.). (2012). *Handbook of research on student engagement.* Springer Science + Business Media. https://doi.org/10.1007/978-1-4614-2018-7

Collier-Meek, M. A., Sanetti, L. M. H., & Boyle, A. M. (2019). Barriers to implementing classroom management and behavior support plans: An exploratory investigation. *Psychology in the Schools, 56*(1), 5–17. https://doi.org/10.1002/pits.22127

Connell, J. P., Halpern-Felsher, B. L., Clifford, E., Crichlow, W., & Usinger, P. (1995). Hanging in there: Behavioral, psychological, and contextual factors affecting whether African-American adolescents stay in school. *Journal of Adolescent Research, 10*, 41–63.

Connell, J. P., & Wellborn, J. G. (1991). Competence, autonomy, and relatedness: A motivational analysis of self-system processes. In M. R. Gunnar & L. A. Sroufe (Eds.), *Self processes and development* (pp. 43–77).

Conroy, M., Sutherland, K., Haydon, T., Stormont, M., & Harmon, J. (2009). Preventing and ameliorating young children's chronic problem behaviors: An ecological classroom-based approach. *Psychology in the Schools, 46*, 3–17.

Cook, C. R., Coco, S., Zhang, Y., Fiat, A. E., Duong, M. T., Renshaw, T. L., ... Frank, S. (2018). Cultivating positive teacher-student relationships: Preliminary evaluation of the Establish-Maintain-Restore (EMR) method. *School Psychology Review, 47*, 226–243.

Copeland, C. B. (2019). *The use of electronic feedback to strengthen teacher intervention beliefs, knowledge, attitudes and intentions.* (Publication No. 22587293) [Doctoral dissertation, University of Missouri-Columbia]. ProQuest Dissertations Publishing.

Cramer, E. D., & Bennett, K. D. (2015). Implementing culturally responsive positive behavior interventions and supports in middle school classrooms. *Middle School Journal, 46*, 18–24.

Deci, E. L., & Ryan, R. M. (1985). *Intrinsic motivation and self-determination in human behavior.* Plenum Press.

Diamond, J. B., & Gomez, K. (2004). African American parents' educational orientations: The importance of social class and parents' perceptions of schools. *Education and Urban Society, 36*(4), 383–427.

Duong, M. T., Pullmann, M. D., Buntain-Ricklefs, J., Lee, K., Benjamin, K. S., Nguyen, L., & Cook, C. R. (2019). Brief teacher training improves student behavior and student–teacher relationships in middle school. *School Psychology, 34*, 212–221. https://doi.org/10.1037/spq0000296

Fallon, L., Collier-Meek, M., Maggin, D., & Sanetti, L. (2015). Is performance feedback an evidence-based practice? A systematic review and evaluation. *Exceptional Children, 81*, 227–246.

Finn, J. D. (1989). Withdrawing From School. *Review of Educational Research, 59*(2), 117–142. https://doi.org/10.3102/00346543059002117

Flora, S. R. (2000). *Praise's magic reinforcement ratio: Five to one gets the job done. Behavior Analyst Online, gale, cengage learning.* http://www.thefreelibrary.com/Praise's+magic+reinforcement+ratio%3A+five+to+one+gets+the+job+done.-a0170112823

Floress, M., Jenkins, L., Reinke, W. M., & McKown, L. (2018). General education teachers' natural rates of praise: A preliminary investigation. *Behavioral Disorders, 43*, 411–422.

Fredericks, J. A., Blumenfeld, P. C., & Paris, A. H. (2004). School engagement: Potential of the concept, state of the evidence. *Review of Educational Research, 74*, 59–109.

Freeman, J., Simonsen, B., Briere, D., & MacSuga-Gage, A. S. (2014). Pre-service teacher training in classroom management: A review of state accreditation policy and teacher preparation programs. *Teacher Education and Special Education, 37*(2), 106–120. https://doi.org/10.1177/0888406413507002

Gay, G. (2002). Preparing for culturally responsive teaching. *Journal of Teacher Education, 53*, 106–116. https://doi.org/10.1177/0022487102053002003

Gay, G. (2010). *Culturally responsive teaching: Theory, research, and practice* (2nd ed.). Teachers College Press.

Good, T., & Lavigne, A. (2018). *Looking in Classrooms* (11th ed.). Routledge.

Gregory, A., Hafen, C., Ruzek, E., Mikami, A., Allen, J., & Pianta, R. (2016). Closing the racial discipline gap in classrooms by changing teacher practice. *School Psychology Review, 45*, 171–191.

Hagermoser Sanetti, L. M., Williamson, K. M., Long, A. C. J., & Kratochwill, T. R. (2018). Increasing in-service teacher implementation of classroom management practices through consultation, implementation planning, and participant modeling. *Journal of Positive Behavior Interventions, 20*(1), 43–59. https://doi.org/10.1177/1098300717722357

Herman, K. C., Hickmon-Rosa, J., & Reinke, W. M. (2018). Empirically derived profiles of teacher stress, burnout, self-efficacy, and coping and associated student outcomes. *Journal of Positive Behavior Interventions, 20*, 90–100.

Herman, K. C., Prewett, S. L., Eddy, C. L., Savala, A., & Reinke, W. M. (2020). Profiles of middle school teacher stress and coping: Concurrent and prospective correlates. *Journal of School Psychology, 78*, 54–68.

Ingersoll, R. M., & Strong, M. (2011). The impact of induction and mentoring programs for beginning teachers: A critical review of the research. *Review of Educational Research, 81*(2), 201–233. https://doi.org/10.3102/0034654311403323

Jones, V. F., & Jones, L. S. (2004). *Comprehensive classroom management, creating communities of support and solving problems* (7th ed.). Allyn & Bacon.

Kamins, M. L., & Dweck, C. S. (1999). Person versus process praise and criticism: Implications for contingent self-worth and coping. *Developmental Psychology, 35*(3), 835–847. https://doi.org/10.1037/0012-1649.35.3.835

Kellam, S. G., Ling, X., Merisca, R., Brown, C. H., & Ialongo, N. (1998). The effect of the level of aggression in the first grade classroom on the course and malleability of aggressive behavior into middle school. *Development and Psychopathology, 10*, 165–185.

Kleinert, W. L., Silva, M. R., Codding, R. S., Feinberg, A. B., & St. James, P. S. (2017). Enhancing classroom management using the classroom check-up consultation model with in-vivo coaching and goal setting components. *School Psychology Forum, 11*, 5–19.

Ladson-Billings, G. (1995). Toward a Theory of Culturally Relevant Pedagogy. *American Educational Research Journal, 32*(3), 465–491. https://doi.org/10.3102/00028312032003465

Ladson-Billings, G. (2009). *The dreamkeepers: Successful teachers of African American children* (2nd ed.). Jossey-Bass Publishers.

Larson, K., Pas, E., Bottiani, J., Kush, J., & Bradshaw, C. (2021). A multidimensional and multilevel examination of student engagement and secondary school teachers' use of classroom management practices. *Journal of Positive Behavior Intervention, 23*, 149–162.

Larson, K. E., Pas, E. T., Bradshaw, C. P., Rosenberg, M. S., & Day-Vines, N. L. (2018). Examining how proactive management and culturally responsive teaching relate to student behavior: Implications for measurement and practice. *School Psychology Review, 47*(2), 153–166. https://doi.org/10.17105/SPR-2017-0070.V47-2

Leverson, M., Smith, K., McIntosh, K., Rose, J., & Pinkelman, S. (2016). *PBIS culturally responsive field guide: Resources for trainers and coaches.* http://www.pbiscaltac.org/resources/culturally%20responsive/PBIS%20Cultural%20Responsiveness%20Field%20Guide.pdf

Losen, D. J., & Skiba, R. J. (2010). *Suspended education: Urban middle schools in crisis.* Southern Poverty Law Center.

Majeika, C., Wilkinson, S., & Kumm, S. (2020). Supporting student behavior through behavioral contracting. *Teaching Exceptional Children, 53*, 132–139.

McIntosh, K., Moniz, C., Craft, C., Golby, R., & Steinwand-Deschambeault, T. (2014). Implementing school-wide positive behavioural Iinterventions and supports to better meet the needs of indigenous students. *Canadian Journal of School Psychology, 29*, 236–257.

McKinley, J. (2010). *Raising black students' achievement through culturally responsive teaching.* ASCD. http://www.ascd.org/publications/books/110004.aspx

Milner, H. R. (2011). Culturally relevant pedagogy in a diverse urban classroom. *The Urban Review, 43*(1), 66–89. https://doi.org/10.1007/s11256-009-0143-0

Morris, E. W., & Perry, B. L. (2016). The punishment gap: School suspension and racial disparities in achievement. *Social Problems, 63*, 68–86.

Myers, D., Simonsen, B., & Sugai, G. (2011). Increasing teachers' use of praise with a response-to-intervention approach. *Education and Treatment of Children, 34*(1), 35–59.

National Research Council. (2002). Minority students in special and gifted education. Committee on Minority Representation in Special Education. In M. S. Donovan & C. Cross (Eds.), *Division of behavioral and social sciences and education.* National Academy Press.

Pas, E., Larson, K., Reinke, W. M., Herman, K., & Bradshaw, C. P. (2016). Applying the classroom check-up coaching model to promote culturally-responsive classroom management. *Education and Treatment of Children, 39*, 467–492.

Pianta, R. (1999). *Enhancing relationships between children and teachers.* American Psychological Association.

Reinke, W., & Herman, K. (2002). Creating school environments that deter antisocial behaviors in youth. *Psychology in the Schools, 39*, 549–559.

Reinke, W. M., Herman, K. C., & Dong, N. (2018). The incredible years teacher classroom management program: Findings from a group randomized trial. *Prevention Science, 19*, 1043–1054.

Reinke, W. M., Herman, K. C., & Newcomer, L. (2016). The Brief Student-Teacher Interaction Observation: Using dynamic indicators of behaviors in the classroom to predict outcomes and inform practice. *Assessment for Effective Intervention, 42*, 32–42.

Reinke, W. M., Herman, K. C., & Sprick, R. (2011). *Motivational interviewing for effective classroom management: The classroom check-up.* Guilford Press.

Reinke, W. M., Lewis-Palmer, T., & Martin, E. (2007). The effect of visual performance feedback on teacher behavior-specific praise. *Behavior Modification, 31*, 247–263.

Reinke, W. M., Lewis-Palmer, T., & Merrell, K. (2008). The classroom check-up: A classwide consultation model for increasing praise and decreasing disruptive behavior. *School Psychology Review, 37*, 315–332.

Reinke, W. M., Stormont, M., Herman, K. C., & Newcomer, L. (2014). Using coaching to support teacher implementation of classroom-based interventions. *Journal of Behavioral Education, 23*, 150–167.

Reinke, W. M., Stormont, M., Herman, K. C., Puri, R., & Goel, N. (2011). Supporting children's mental health in schools: Teacher perceptions of needs, roles, and barriers. *School Psychology Quarterly, 26*, 1–13.

Reinke, W. M., Stormont, M., Herman, K. C., Wang, Z., Newcomer, L., & King, K. (2014). Use of coaching and behavior support planning for students with disruptive behavior within a universal classroom management program. *Journal of Emotional and Behavioral Disorders, 22*, 74–82.

Roorda, D., Jak, S., Zee, M., Oort, F., & Koomen, H. (2017). Affective teacher–student relationships and students' engagement and achievement: A meta-analytic update and test of the mediating role of engagement. *School Psychology Review, 46*, 239–261.

Rubow, C., Noewl, C., & Wheby, J. (2019). Effects of noncontingent attention on the behavior of students with emotional/ behavioral disorders and staff in alternative settings. *Education and Treatment of Children, 42*, 201–223.

Sanetti, L. M. H., & Collier-Meek, M. A. (2015). Data-driven delivery of implementation supports in a multi-tiered framework: A pilot study. *Psychology in the Schools, 52*(8), 815–828. https://doi.org/10.1002/pits.21861

Simonsen, B., Fairbanks, S., Briesch, A., Myers, D., & Sugai, G. (2008). Evidence-based practices in classroom management: Considerations for research to practice. *Education & Treatment of Children, 31*, 351–380.

Skiba, R. J., Horner, R. H., Chung, C. G., Rausch, M. K., May, S. L., & Tobin, T. (2011). Race is not neutral: A national investigation of African American and Latino disproportionality in school discipline. *School Psychology Review, 40*, 85–107.

Skiba, R. J., Poloni-Staudinger, L., Simmons, A., Feggins-Azziz, R., & Chung, C. (2005). Unproven links: Can poverty explain ethnic disproportionality in special education? *Journal of Special Education, 39*, 130–144.

Skinner, E. A., & Belmont, M. J. (1993). Motivation in the classroom: Reciprocal effects of teacher behavior and student engagement across the school year. *Journal of Educational Psychology, 85*, 571–581.

Skinner, E. A., Wellborn, J. G., & Connell, J. P. (1990). What it takes to do well in school and whether I've got it: A process model of perceived control and children's engagement and achievement in school. *Journal of Educational Psychology, 82*, 22–32.

Sleeter, C. E. (2012). Confronting the marginalization of culturally responsive pedagogy. *Urban Education, 47*(3), 562–584. https://doi.org/10.1080/10665680802400006

Smith, T. M., & Ingersoll, R. M. (2004). What are the effects of induction and mentoring on beginning teacher turnover? *American Educational Research Journal, 41*(3), 681–714. https://doi.org/10.3102/00028312041003681

Solomon, B., Klein, S., & Polityo, B. (2012). Treatment integrity: A meta-analysis of the single-case literature. *School Psychology Review, 41*, 160–175.

Stormont, M., & Reinke, W. M. (2009). The importance of precorrective statements and behavior-specific praise and strategies to increase their use. *Beyond Behavior, 18*, 26–32.

Stormont, M., Reinke, W. M., & Herman, K. C. (2011). Teachers' knowledge of evidence-based interventions and available school resources for children with emotional or behavioral problems. *Journal of Behavioral Education, 20*, 138–147.

Stormont, M., Reinke, W.M., Herman, K.C., & Lemke, E. (2012). *Academic and behavior supports for at-risk students: Tier 2 interventions.* New York: Guilford Press.

Stormont, M., Reinke, W. M., Newcomer, L., Marchese, D., & Lewis, C. (2015). Coaching teachers' use of social behavior interventions to improve Children's outcomes: A review of the literature. *Journal of Positive Behavior Interventions, 17*, 69–82.

Stormont, M., Rodriguez, B., & Reinke, W. M. (2016). Teaching students with behavior problems to take a break. *Intervention in School and Clinic, 5*, 301–306.

Tucker, C. M., Zayco, R. A., Herman, K. C., Reinke, W. M., Trujillo, M., Carraway, K., Wallack, C., & Ivery, P. D. (2002). Teacher and child variables as predictors of academic engagement among low-income African American children. *Psychology in the Schools, 39*(4), 477. https://doi.org/10.1002/pits.10038

Wallace, J. M., Goodkind, S., Wallace, C. M., & Bachman, J. G. (2008). Racial, ethnic, and gender differences in school discipline among US high school students: 1991–2005. *The Negro Educational Review, 59*(1–2), 47.

Weinstein, C., Curran, M., & Tomlinson-Clarke, S. (2003). Culturally responsive classroom management: Awareness into action. *Theory Into Practice, 42*(4), 269–276.

Student Engagement and Learning Climate

Howard Adelman and Linda Taylor

Abstract

Research indicates a strong relationship between student engagement and school climate and this has contributed to making these prominent topics in discussions of school improvement. What often goes unstated, however, is that student engagement is a transactional process, and school climate is an emergent quality. Furthermore, addressing these concerns requires particular attention to how schools deal with barriers to learning and teaching. This chapter starts with a discussion of engagement as a transactional process and the implications with respect to student differences in motivation and ability. We then explore what schools do wrong in addressing these differences and what is involved in creating an engaging and supportive learning climate. We conclude with recommendations for moving forward.

H. Adelman (✉) · L. Taylor
University of California, Los Angeles, Los Angeles, CA, USA
e-mail: adelman@psych.ucla.edu; Ltaylor@ucla.edu

Student Engagement and Learning Climate

Every teacher would like students who are motivationally ready and able to engage in what is being taught. For such students, the teacher's role mainly involves facilitating reasonably good conditions for learning (e.g., in terms of content and instructional processes). However, since students' motivation and ability vary, so does engagement (e.g., the degree to which a student is interested and involved in what is being taught at a given time).

For instance, students differ motivationally based on developed attitudes and current cognitive, emotional, and physiological states of being. A student who has developed a positive attitude toward math will tend to be highly engaged, as contrasted to a student who has come to dislike the subject; a student who is experiencing emotionally upsetting events is unlikely to be motivated to engage in the lessons of the day. As educators long have stressed, such differences among students make teaching a much more complex matter.

Research findings stress that students who are not engaged in their schooling are more likely to misbehave, have poor academic outcomes, and dropout (Chapman et al., 2011; Halverson & Graham, 2019; Rumberger & Rotermun, 2012). Studies also indicate a strong relationship between student engagement and school climate (e.g., Daily et al., 2019; Hopson et al., 2014; Sherblom et al., 2006).

Research findings aside, the desirability of student engagement and a positive school climate are a given and certainly have been prominent topics in discussions of school improvement for some time (Adelman & Taylor, 2005; Fredricks et al., 2004; Zullig et al., 2010). What often goes unstated, however, is that student engagement is a transactional process, and school climate emerges from the complex daily interactions at a school and between a school and its neighborhood. Furthermore, addressing these concerns requires particular attention to how schools deal with barriers to learning and teaching.

In this chapter, we start with a discussion of engagement as a transactional process, and the implications with respect to student differences in motivation and ability. We then explore what schools do wrong in addressing these differences and what is involved in creating an engaging and supportive learning climate. We conclude with recommendations for moving forward.

Student Engagement: A Transactional Process

As the literature on reciprocal determinism stresses, student learning and behavior are a function of the ongoing transactions between an individual and environmental factors (Adelman & Taylor, 1994; Bandura, 1978). From an intervention perspective, good outcomes are a function of an appropriate match between the individual's accumulated capacities and attitudes and current state of being and an intervention's processes, content, context, and expected outcomes. From a psychological perspective, an individual's (e.g., a student's) perception is a critical criterion for evaluating whether an appropriate match exists with any intervention (e.g., teaching).

The commonsense view of good teaching is captured by the old adage: *Good teaching meets learners where they are.* Unfortunately, this adage often is interpreted only as a call for matching a student's current capabilities (e.g., knowl-

edge, skills). The irony in this is that most school staff recognize that motivational factors usually play a key role in accounting for poor instructional outcomes. Indeed, a common lament among teachers is: "That student could do it, if only he wanted to!"

Teachers know that good abilities are more likely to emerge when students are motivated not only to pursue class assignments but also when students are interested in using what they learn in other contexts. So, while matching current knowledge and skills are necessary, it is evident that good teaching and student engagement also involve matching motivation (e.g., attitudes, interests). Moreover, enhancing student engagement and reengaging disconnected students require practices that reflect an appreciation of intrinsic motivation and what must be done to overcome avoidance motivation (Ryan & Deci, 2017; Skinner et al., 2008; Taylor & Adelman, 1999).

Expectancy-times-valuing (E x V) theory is a widely used heuristic paradigm for understanding motivation and engagement (Eccles, 1983; Eccles & Wigfield, 2002). Moving beyond the manipulation of reinforcers (e.g., extrinsic motivators), such theory recognizes that human beings are thinking and feeling organisms and that intrinsic factors can be powerful motivators. Within some limits (which space precludes discussing here), high expectations and high valuing produce high motivation and encourage engagement, while high expectations (E) and low valuing (V) or low expectations and high valuing produce relatively weak motivation (and sometimes avoidance motivation) and work against engagement. Two common reasons people give for not engaging are "I know I won't be able to do it" (E) and "It's not worth it" (V). In general, the amount of time and energy spent on an activity seems dependent on how much the activity is valued by the student and on the student's expectation that what is valued will be attained without too great a cost. Over time, motivation plays a fundamental role in the development not only of knowledge and skills but attitudes about what aspects of schooling are worth investing time and energy in and what are not.

Attending the Range of Engaged and Disengaged Students

As will be remembered during the COVID-19 school closures, the increase in disengaged students was dramatic (National League of Cities, 2020). Some were reacting to the situation; others were repeating behavior tendencies from before. As the circumstances underscored, engaging students is a constant motivational concern; reengaging disconnected students is a major motivational problem.

In our professional development work with teachers and schools, most teachers tell us they usually have received at least a bit of preparation for engaging students, but they indicate having had almost no professional development for reengaging disconnected students. And those trying to help at home often are at a loss when youngsters act disinterested in doing homework.

Motivational differences have profound implications for successful engagement and reengagement in instruction. A youngster may proactively disconnect (e.g., to pursue a desired or preferred activity). Or the disconnection may be reactive – a protective form of coping stemming from motivation to avoid and protest against situations in which s/he feels unable to perform and/or is coerced to participate (e.g., instruction that is too challenging; activities that seriously limit options; activities where those providing instruction are over-controlling).

An intrinsic motivational interpretation of student disengagement stresses that a youngster may perceive school tasks and activities as threats to feelings of competence, autonomy, and/or relatedness to significant others (Ryan & Deci, 2017). Under such circumstances, individuals (especially those with learning, behavior, and emotional problems) can be expected to react by trying to protect themselves from the unpleasant thoughts and feelings associated with activities where they do poorly and experience negative interpersonal interactions, including being controlled by others. It is not surprising when, over time, they tend to develop strong motivational dispositions to avoid such activities.

The transactional nature of learning and instruction must be accounted for in any discussion of student engagement; so must the reality that teachers and student support staff are faced with a continuum of student engagement, including students who are hard to engage and those who have totally disengaged from classroom instruction. A particular concern for many teachers is how to *reengage* a student who has disengaged and is misbehaving. Clearly, greater attention is called for in personnel development on attending to differences in student motivation and capability and understanding the role played by intrinsic motivation, as well as the counterintuitive relationship between intrinsics and extrinsics (Deci et al., 2001).

About Differences in Student Motivation and Capability

Diversity among students and school personnel is a given. Diversity arises from many factors (e.g., gender, ethnicity, race, socioeconomic status, religion, capability, disability, interests). While students differ in many ways, concern for engagement in instruction focuses on how motivationally ready and able a student is with respect to what they are being taught. From this perspective, we think in terms of the following continuum of students:

- Students who are fully engaged – motivationally ready and able
- Students with low engagement – not motivated by what they are asked to do (e.g., having negative attitudes toward school because of past experiences; lacking some prerequisite knowledge and skills for assigned school work; having minor learning vulnerabilities).
- Students who are disengaged – significantly motivated to *avoid* what they are asked to do (e.g., having negative attitudes toward school because of past experiences; having extreme deficits in current performance capabilities; having a learning disability or major health problem).

There are, of course, gradations along the continuum, and the proportion of students in each group differs among schools. And it is widely recognized that too many of those who start out engaged become less engaged over their years of schooling (Hodges, 2018).

Whatever the current numbers and trends, basic concerns in improving schools continue to include dealing effectively with a full continuum of differences in student engagement, countering declines in engagement, and reducing the number who disengage.

What's Wrong with How Schools Address Critical Individual Differences?

In trying to meet learners where they are, teachers strive to differentiate instruction. However, classroom instruction in most schools is not designed to account for a wide range of critical individual differences and circumstances (Czerkawski & Lyman, 2016; Scott et al., 2014; Tomlinson, 2017). Moreover, too little accommodation and specific help are provided to students who manifest learning, behavior, emotional, and physical problems (Ontario Human Rights Commission, n.d.; Wattam et al., 2019).

As a result, soon after a school year begins, schools are inundated with referrals from teachers asking for help with students who are not doing well and who usually are misbehaving. Such referrals include students who may need special education, but most referrals are for students manifesting commonplace learning, behavior, and emotional problems. Unfortunately, the referrals often contribute to the escalating number of youngsters who are misdiagnosed as ADHD, LD, clinically depressed, or some other pathological label (Adelman & Taylor, 2020a; Center for Mental Health in Schools, 2012; Fresson et al., 2019; Hinshaw & Scheffler, 2014).

Commonplace problems can and should be addressed through personalized instruction and special assistance rather than by expensive special education and clinical services that consume

resources needed to help prevent and respond immediately after the onset of problems However, professional preparation generally has not equipped teachers to provide the type of personalized instruction and special assistance necessary to address critical individual differences (Reed, 2019; Schifter, 2016). In too many schools, this state of affairs has contributed to the following:

- Differentiated instruction that does not adequately attend to motivational differences and often assumes that instruction is personalized when differences are addressed through the use of technology.
- Overemphasis on establishing a manageable context for *teaching* and insufficient attention to creating stimulating and caring conditions for *learning*.
- Inadequate understanding of intrinsic motivation contributes to the tendency to over rely on rewards and punishment as primary strategies for teaching and controlling behavior.[1]
- Classrooms organized in ways that presume classroom teachers can do the job alone. For example, too little emphasis on reducing the need for out of the classroom referrals by bringing student/learning support staff into classrooms to collaborate in (a) preventing

---

[1] While student motivation always is a concern of personnel preparation programs, what such programs emphasize often is a narrow focus on using extrinsic motivators. In particular, generations of teachers and student/learning support staff (and parents) have been taught about manipulating and controlling behavior using reinforcers. As a result, control strategies continue to dominate how schools and homes react to engagement problems and misbehavior.

Such strategies can be somewhat effective in the short-run. The price paid, however, is that social control practices often decrease intrinsic motivation for engaging in instruction and generate psychological reactance on the part of students which can lead them to act in undesired ways as they try to restore their feelings of self-determination. Given that such practices can be counterproductive over the long-term, schools and homes are being called upon to move toward more autonomy-supportive approaches to enhance engagement in instruction and reengage disconnected students (Ryan & Deci, 2017).

problems, (b) responding as soon as feasible after problems arise, and (c) providing appropriate special assistance when students display specific problems.

The above matters hinder and undermine efforts to engage students in learning. Moreover, they contribute to the type of psychological reactance among students that generates behavior and emotional problems and works against reengaging disconnected students.

Addressing the above matters is basic to accounting for a wider range of individual differences and preventing and handling problems experienced by many students. Even more is involved in enhancing student engagement and school climate as we discuss now.

What's Involved in Creating an Engaging and Supportive Learning Climate

> Many students say that . . .they feel their classes are irrelevant and boring, that they are just passing time . . . (and) are not able to connect what they are being taught with what they feel they need for success in their later life. This disengagement from the learning process is manifested in many ways, one of which is the lack of student responsibility for learning. In many ways the traditional educational structure, one in which teachers "pour knowledge into the vessel" (the student), has placed all responsibility for learning on the teacher, none on the student. Schools present lessons neatly packaged, without acknowledging or accepting the "messiness" of learning-by-doing and through experience and activity. Schools often do not provide students a chance to accept responsibility for learning, as that might actually empower students. Students in many schools have become accustomed to being spoon-fed the material to master tests, and they have lost their enthusiasm for exploration, dialogue, and reflection – all critical steps in the learning process. American Youth Policy Forum (2000)

As noted, student engagement requires (a) arranging and organizing instruction in ways that establish an appropriate match with a student's motivation and capabilities and (b) providing effective student and learning supports. This involves ensuring that the context and conditions for learning are stimulating, caring, and comfortable. To these ends, priorities for school improvement policy and practice include (1) enhancing personalized instruction and (2) transforming how schools address barriers to learning, development, and teaching.

Personalized Instruction: Building Relationships by Addressing Differences

Definitions and formulations of personalized learning and instruction abound. Missing in most presentations is a psychological perspective. Personalization is a construct. From a psychological perspective, we define personalization as the process of matching learner *motivation and capabilities* and stress that it is the learner's perception that determines whether the match is a good one (Adelman & Taylor, 1994; Adelman & Taylor, 2019; Taylor & Adelman, 1999).

Good working and learning relationships emerge when students perceive instruction as a personal fit. Thus, a basic assessment concern is to elicit student perceptions to determine how well classroom practices and schoolwide experiences match with significant differences in interests and abilities. Such assessments enable appropriate attention to intrinsic motivation and clarify when special assistance is needed and are especially important considerations in reengaging disconnected students.

Personalized classroom instruction is designed to enhance positive attitudes and support learning by ensuring that

- Available options encourage active, engaged learning (e.g., authentic, project- and problem-based discovery learning, blended and flipped learning practices, enrichment opportunities),
- Students are grouped in ways that turn big classes into smaller learning units to enable teacher-student relationship building (Adelman & Taylor, 2006, 2019; Park & Lim, 2019).

We recognize that inappropriately grouping students can be stigmatizing and increase inequities in schooling. We stress diversity in the grouping. For example, a multi-ethnic classroom enables grouping students across ethnic lines to bring different perspectives to a learning activity. This allows students not only to learn about other perspectives but also to enhance critical thinking and other higher-order conceptual abilities. It also can foster the type of intergroup understanding and relationships essential to establishing a school climate of caring and mutual respect.

Teachers Can't Do It Alone

Prevailing policies and practices have tended to leave much of the burden of engaging and reengaging students on teachers. We suggest that it is patently unfair and unreasonable to believe that teachers *alone* can do their job effectively, especially in situations where many youngsters are manifesting learning, behavior, and emotional problems.

While schools have relatively few student/learning support professionals (counselors, psychologists, social workers, nurses, etc.), these personnel have a critical role to play at schools. Given this, it is ironic that school planning so often involves relatively little discussion of the roles and functions of the various district-employed student/learning support professionals (Center for MH in Schools & Student/Learning Supports, 2018).

The reality is that teachers need student/learning support staff, and they need them to do more than consult and be a referral source. Such staff can play an essential collaborative role by teaming with teachers *in classrooms* for part of each day. Moreover, these personnel are key to transforming how schools address barriers to learning into a unified, comprehensive, and equitable system of learning supports at schools throughout a district.

Needed: A Schoolwide System to Address Barriers to Learning and Teaching

Events such as the COVID-19 pandemic underscored what has been evident for some time: continuing with prevailing approaches for addressing barriers to learning and teaching is a recipe for maintaining a terribly unsatisfactory status quo. Equity of opportunity for success at school and beyond is not feasible for many students as long a student/learning supports are fragmented and school improvement policy and practice continue to marginalize the work (Adelman & Taylor, 2018, 2020b; Moore, 2014).

The problems encountered by students and schools are complex and overlapping. The number of students not doing well in some schools is staggering. Student/learning supports as currently provided can't meet the need, especially for schools serving low wealth families. And with tightening school budgets the situation is worse. Rivalry for sparse resources leads to counterproductive competition among school support staff and with community-based professionals who link with schools.

It has become critical to end the system deficiencies that arise from maintaining separate, narrow agenda for student/learning supports.[2] Needed is a system that improves the way schools provide learning supports for all students and especially for those already manifesting learning, behavior, and emotional problems.

Proposed improvements often are referred to as comprehensive and integrated (Hoover et al., 2019; Jacob et al., 2020; Moore, 2014). Our analyses indicate that, while various groups call their approach *comprehensive*, the reality is that the

---

[2]Ultimately, all school interventions to address barriers to learning and teaching are about supporting learning. As defined for policy purposes, *learning supports are the resources, strategies, and practices that support physical, social, emotional and intellectual development and well-being to enable all students to have an equal opportunity for success at school.* Learning Supports are deployed in classrooms and schoolwide.

nature and scope of prevailing proposals are too limited to address the needs of many schools (Center for MH in Schools & Student/Learning Supports, 2018). And references to "integrated" approaches tend to emphasize coordinating services rather than *unifying* student/learning supports in ways that transcend professional affiliations.

Unifying student/learning supports requires braiding together efforts designed to prevent and minimize the impact of factors interfering with learning and teaching. Such efforts include programs, services, initiatives, and projects that provide compensatory and special assistance and promote and maintain safety, physical and mental health, school readiness, early school-adjustment, and social and academic functioning. The need is to transform student/learning supports into a *unified, comprehensive, and equitable system*.

Most school improvement plans do not prioritize efforts to enhance student outcomes by addressing barriers to learning and teaching *directly and comprehensively*. Schools, working with home and community stakeholders, can correct this deficiency by devoting a portion of their limited time and sparse resources to reframing and redeploying how existing resources are used and ending the marginalization of student/learning supports in school improvement policy.

Elevating the Emphasis on Transforming Student and Learning Supports: A Critical Facet of Improving School Climate

Policy makers can end the marginalization of student/learning supports by establishing a component dedicated directly to both (1) addressing barriers to learning and teaching and (2) reengaging disconnected students. An emphasis on both these concerns is essential because interventions that do not ensure students are engaged meaningfully in classroom learning usually are insufficient in sustaining, over time, student engagement, good behavior, and effective learning at school (Adelman, 1995; Adelman & Taylor, 2011, 2017, 2020b).

Our analysis of school improvement policy and planning indicates that districts and schools tend not to directly and comprehensively address barriers to learning and teaching. Policy and practice planning are guided primarily by a two-component framework, namely (1) instruction and (2) governance/management. School improvement plans focus on these two components; interventions for addressing learning barriers and reengaging disconnected students are given secondary consideration at best. The marginalization is a fundamental cause of the widely observed fragmentation and disorganization of student and learning supports. An enhanced policy framework is needed to ensure that efforts to address barriers to learning and teaching are pursued as a primary and essential component of school improvement (see Fig. 1). Early adopters have designated this third facet of school improvement policy and practice as a *learning supports component* (see http://smhp.psych.ucla.edu/summit2002/trailblazing.htm).

About Operationalizing a Learning Supports Component

Besides expanding the policy framework, moving toward a comprehensive and equitable system requires

- Reframing traditional student and learning supports (a) unifying all student/learning supports designed to address barriers to learning and teaching and reengage disconnected students; (b) redeploying resources to enable the development, implementation, and sustainability of the new system),
- Reworking the organizational and operational infrastructure (i.e., institutionalizing a leadership infrastructure for developing a comprehensive and equitable system over several years).

A major emphasis in reframing student and learning supports is placed on developing a system to address a wide range of barriers to learning, development, and teaching. Minimally,

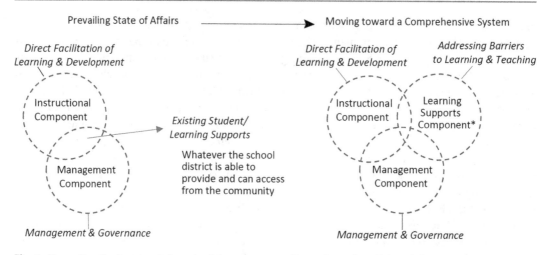

Fig. 1 Expanding the framework for school improvement policy and practice. (Adapted from Adelman and Taylor (2019))

equity of opportunity requires that student/learning supports address barriers interfering with the learning of a majority of students, as well as a potent approach for reengaging students in classroom instruction.

To be effective, the learning supports component requires reworking existing operational infrastructures in ways that fully enmesh the component with instructional efforts and professional development. To be equitable, the component must be established at all schools in a district.

Reframing Student and Learning Supports

Research and development have produced an intervention prototype for a unified, comprehensive, and equitable system to address barriers and reengage students (e.g., see Adelman & Taylor, 2018, 2019, 2020a, 2020b). The prototype has two facets:

- One facet conceives levels of intervention as a full continuum of integrated intervention subsystems that weave together school-community-home resources,
- The other facet organizes programs, services, and specific activities into a circumscribed set of domains of support.

Conceptualizing a Continuum of Intervention as an Integrated System

The Every Student Succeeds Act (ESSA) emphasized a schoolwide tiered model (e.g., a *multitier* system of supports – widely referred to as MTSS) as a framework for preventing and addressing problems. The tiered model is defined as "a comprehensive continuum of evidence-based, systemic practices to support a rapid response to students' needs, with regular observation to facilitate data-based instructional decision-making."[3]

Emphasis on the tiered model is a carryover from previous federal policy guidelines for Response to Intervention and Positive Behavioral

---

[3]The multitier student support (MTSS) model as emphasized in ESSA and as widely portrayed in school improvement plans usually is illustrated simply in terms of levels rather than as a set of intervention subsystems. The simplicity of the tiered presentation is appealing, and the framework does help underscore differences in levels of intervention. However, the simple graphic illustration is not a powerful way to depict the continuum, and it is an insufficient framework for organizing student/learning supports. Specific concerns about the MTSS framework are that (1) it mainly stresses levels of intensity, (2) it does not address the problem of systematically connecting interventions that fall into and across each level, and (3) it does not address the need to connect school and community interventions. As a result, most adoptions of MTSS in school improvement plans do little to guide better directions for addressing barriers to learning and teaching (Center for MH in Schools & Student/Learning Supports, 2020a, 2020b).

Interventions and Supports. The result of these guidelines over the last few years is that schools increasingly are framing student and learning supports in terms of tiers or levels. As currently conceived, however, the multitier model is an insufficient organizing framework for developing a unified, comprehensive, and equitable system for addressing barriers to learning and teaching. As we have stressed, it and other conceptualizations of a continuum of intervention provide a good *starting point* for framing the nature and scope of student and learning supports. Fig. 2 portrays such a continuum in ways that take the multitier system several steps beyond prevailing conceptualizations.

As illustrated, the intervention continuum is presented as an overlapping and intertwined set of *subsystems*. The intent at each subsystem level is to braid together a wide range of school and community (including home) resources. The subsystems focus on:

- Promoting whole child development and preventing problems.
- Addressing problems as soon as they arise.
- Providing for students who have severe and chronic problems.

The subsystems are illustrated as tapering from top to bottom to convey that if the top is well designed and implemented, the numbers needing early intervention are reduced, and then, as more are helped through early-after-onset assistance, fewer students will need "deep-end" interventions.

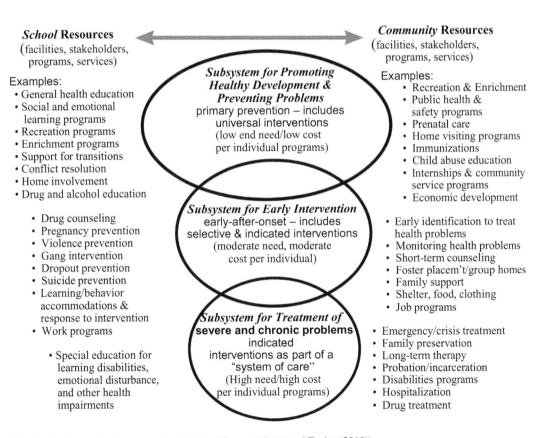

Fig. 2 Framing a school-community. (Adapted from Adelman and Taylor (2018))

Domains of Support

Framing a unified and comprehensive system of student/learning supports requires more than designating a continuum of intervention. It also is necessary to organize interventions cohesively into a circumscribed set of well-designed and delimited domains that reflect the daily efforts at a school to provide student and learning supports in the classroom and schoolwide.

Moving from the typical "laundry list" of programs and services, our Center's research and development efforts have categorized activities aimed at addressing barriers into six domains reflecting basic concerns that schools are confronted with regularly. In organizing the activity, it becomes clearer what supports are needed in and out of the classroom to enable the learning of students who are not doing well.

The six domains are:

- *Embedding student/learning supports into regular classroom strategies to enable learning* and teaching (e.g., working collaboratively with other teachers and student support staff to ensure instruction is personalized with an emphasis on enhancing intrinsic motivation and social-emotional development for all students and especially those experiencing mild-moderate learning and behavior problems; reengaging those who have become disengaged from instruction; providing learning accommodations and supports as necessary; using response to intervention in applying for special assistance; addressing external barriers with a focus on prevention and early intervention).
- *Supporting transitions* (i.e., assisting students and families as they negotiate the many hurdles encountered related to reentry or initial entry into school, school and grade changes, daily transitions, program transitions, accessing special assistance, and so forth).
- *Increasing home and school connections and engagement* (e.g., addressing barriers to home involvement, helping those in the home enhance supports for their children, strengthening home and school communication, increasing home support of the school).
- *Responding to, and where feasible, preventing school and personal crises* (e.g., preparing for emergencies, implementing plans when an event occurs, countering the impact of traumatic events, providing follow-up assistance, implementing prevention strategies; creating a caring and safe learning environment).
- *Increasing community involvement and collaborative engagement* (e.g., outreach to develop greater community connection and support from a wide range of resources -- including enhanced use of volunteers, developing a school-community collaborative infrastructure).
- *Facilitating student and family access to special assistance,* first in the regular program and then, as needed, through referral for specialized services on- and off-campus.[4]

Continuum + Domains = A Comprehensive and Unified System

Combining the continuum and the six domains of supports provide an intervention framework that can guide the development of a system that unifies the resources a school devotes to addressing barriers to learning and teaching (e.g., student/learning supports), as well as braiding in community resources to fill critical gaps and strengthen the system. As illustrated in Fig. 3, operationalizing the third component in this way underscores why the component is an essential facet of a school's accomplishing its instructional mission and doing so with a focus on whole child, whole school, and whole community.

Using the framework to map and analyze resources provides a picture of system strengths and gaps. Strategically, given limited budgets, developing a comprehensive system involves

---

[4]Each of the six domains are discussed in detail in Adelman and Taylor (2019) and have been explored in a variety of venues across the country over the last decade (see http://smhp.psych.ucla.edu/summit2002/nind7.htm)

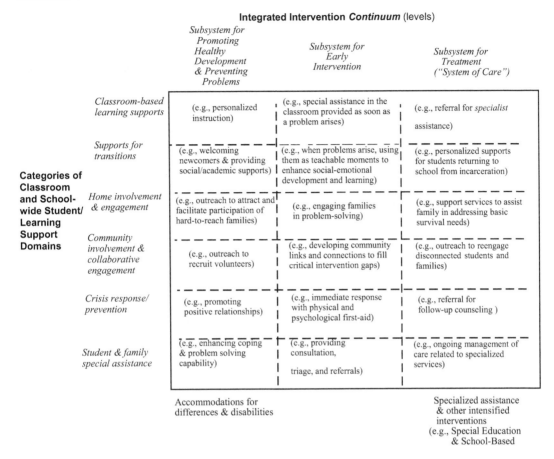

Integrated Intervention *Continuum* (levels)

	Subsystem for Promoting Healthy Development & Preventing Problems	Subsystem for Early Intervention	Subsystem for Treatment ("System of Care")
Classroom-based learning supports	(e.g., personalized instruction)	(e.g., special assistance in the classroom provided as soon as a problem arises)	(e.g., referral for *specialist* assistance)
Supports for transitions	(e.g., welcoming newcomers & providing social/academic supports)	(e.g., when problems arise, using them as teachable moments to enhance social-emotional development and learning)	(e.g., personalized supports for students returning to school from incarceration)
Home involvement & engagement	(e.g., outreach to attract and facilitate participation of hard-to-reach families)	(e.g., engaging families in problem-solving)	(e.g., support services to assist family in addressing basic survival needs)
Community involvement & collaborative engagement	(e.g., outreach to recruit volunteers)	(e.g., developing community links and connections to fill critical intervention gaps)	(e.g., outreach to reengage disconnected students and families)
Crisis response/ prevention	(e.g., promoting positive relationships)	(e.g., immediate response with physical and psychological first-aid)	(e.g., referral for follow-up counseling)
Student & family special assistance	(e.g., enhancing coping & problem solving capability)	(e.g., providing consultation, triage, and referrals)	(e.g., ongoing management of care related to specialized services)

Categories of Classroom and School-wide Student/ Learning Support Domains (left label)

Accommodations for differences & disabilities

Specialized assistance & other intensified interventions (e.g., Special Education & School-Based

Fig. 3 Intervention framework for the third component*. *The above matrix provides a guide for organizing and evaluating a system of student and learning supports and is a tool for mapping existing interventions, clarifying which are evidence-based, identifying critical intervention gaps, and analyzing resource use with a view to redeploying resources to strengthen the system. As the examples illustrate, the framework can guide efforts to embed supports for compensatory and special education, English learners, psychosocial and mental health problems, use of specialized instructional support personnel, adoption of evidence-based interventions, integration of funding sources, and braiding in of community resources. The specific examples inserted in the matrix are just illustrative of those schools already may have in place. For a fuller array of examples of student/learning supports that can be applied in classrooms and schoolwide, see the set of surveys available at http://smhp.psych.ucla.edu/pdf-docs/surveys/set1.pdf. (Adapted from Adelman and Taylor (2018))

deploying, redeploying, and weaving together all existing resources used for student and learning supports. Priorities for filling gaps can then be included in strategic plans for system improvement; outreach to bring in community resources can be keyed to filling critical gaps and strengthening the system.

Developing the system requires an operational infrastructure that is dedicated to enabling the learning supports component. Such an infrastructure calls for administrative and team leadership and workgroups that assume responsibility and accountability for the successful daily operation and continuous development of a unified, comprehensive, and equitable system of learning supports (see Adelman & Taylor, 2018).

Properly implemented, the component increases the likelihood that a school will be experienced as a welcoming, supportive place that accommodates diversity, prevents problems, enhances youngsters' strengths, and is committed to assuring equity of opportunity for all students to succeed at school. This, of course, has relevance to concerns about enhancing a positive school climate (Ryberg et al., 2020).

Appreciating That the Learning Climate at School Is an Emerging Quality

School and classroom climates range from hostile/toxic to welcoming and supportive and can fluctuate daily and over the school year. A variety of studies indicate that a positive climate can have a beneficial impact on students and staff; a negative climate can be another barrier to learning and teaching (Thapa et al., 2013). Such studies suggest significant relationships between classroom climate and matters such as student engagement, behavior, self-efficacy, achievement, social and emotional development, principal leadership style, stages of educational reform, teacher burnout, and overall quality of school life. Research also suggests that the impact of classroom climate may be greater on students from low-income homes and on groups that often are discriminated against (Berkowitz et al., 2017; Bodovski et al., 2013; Bradshaw et al., 2014; Daily et al., 2019; Lombardi et al., 2019; Thapa et al., 2013).

Because of the correlational nature of school climate research, cause and effect interpretations remain speculative. The broader body of organizational research does indicate the profound role accountability pressures play in shaping organizational climate (Laratta, 2011; Schneider et al., 2013). For example, pressing demands for higher achievement test scores and control of student behavior often contribute to a classroom climate that is reactive, over-controlling, and over-reliant on external reinforcement to motivate (McEvoy & Welker, 2000).

A positive school climate is described by the U.S. Department of Education as "essential to providing a safe and supportive learning environment for students" (https://oese.ed.gov/resources/safe-school-environments/school-climate/). A range of concepts have been put forth for consideration in discussing school and classroom climate. These include social system organization; social attitudes; staff and student morale; power, control, guidance, support, and evaluation structures; curricular and instructional practices; communicated expectations; efficacy; accountability demands; cohesion; competition; "fit" between learner and classroom; respectful, trusting, and caring relationships; system maintenance, growth, and change; orderliness; and safety. Insel and Moos (1974) brought order to the work by grouping such concepts into three dimensions: (1) *relationship* (i.e., the nature and intensity of personal relationships within the environment; the extent to which people are involved in the environment and support and help each other); (2) *personal development* (i.e., basic directions along which personal growth and self-enhancement tend to occur); and (3) *system maintenance and change* (i.e., the extent to which the environment is orderly, clear in expectations, maintains control, and is responsive to change).

School and classroom climate reflect the influence of the underlying, institutionalized values and belief systems, norms, ideologies, rituals, traditions, and practices that constitute the school culture. And the climate and culture at a school also are shaped by surrounding political, social, cultural, and economic contexts (e.g., home, neighborhood, city, state, country).

What research and theorizing have not articulated well is that school and classroom climate are *emerging* qualities. That is, climate is a temporal, fluid quality of the immediate setting, and it emerges from the complex *transactions* that characterize daily classroom and schoolwide life (Adelman & Taylor, 2005; Center for Mental Health in Schools, 2011).

The focus on enhancing student engagement, addressing barriers, and reengaging disconnected students are critical facets of improving school climate. Along with the systemic changes discussed above, we also recognize that schools and those at home must take greater advantage of the natural opportunities that occur each day and over the school year for promoting students' personal and social growth and countering daily problems (Center for MH in Schools & Student/Learning Supports, 2019).

In sum, we stress that for a positive school climate to emerge, schools and classrooms must diligently enhance the quality of life for students and staff not only in the classroom but school-wide. This includes supporting whole-child learning and wellness and pursuing a unified, comprehensive, and equitable approach to preventing learning, behavior, emotional, and health problems.

A cautionary note: The Every Student Succeeds Act (ESSA) mandated that school accountability include a measure of school quality or student success. As of 2019, about 20 states were planning to use school climate measures for purposes of public accountability. However, researchers caution that existing measures have insufficient validation data to warrant their use in making comparisons among schools (Ryberg et al., 2020; Wang & Degol, 2016). This caution applies to all school climate surveys in current use, including the U.S. Department of Education's (ED) School Climate Survey (EDSCLS).

Recommendations for Moving Forward

Do not follow where the path may lead.
Go, instead, where there is no path and leave a trail. (Anonymous).

Fundamental and innovative change is essential to enhancing and maintaining student engagement and a positive school climate (Adelman & Taylor, 2020b). The following are some steps recent research and development suggest should be taken.

First and foremost, schools need to expand their policy and practice framework for school improvement. As we have discussed, current policy appropriately improves two components of schooling: (1) instruction and (2) management/governance. In doing so, however, it marginalizes efforts to transform student/learning supports. Ending the marginalization requires elevating such efforts by adopting a third primary and essential component that directly addresses barriers to learning, development, and teaching. While it is desirable that such a three component policy

be adopted at all levels (SEA, LEA, and schools), most schools can move forward once their district enacts such a policy. Given the reality of sparse budgets, the initial emphasis is on mapping and effectively redeploying district funds already allocated for addressing barriers to learning and teaching, braiding in community resources to fill system gaps, and working collaboratively with other local schools to garner economies of scale.[5]

Second, in operationalizing the component, it is essential to develop a design document and a strategic plan. These are critical guides over the several years it takes to fully establish a unified, comprehensive, and equitable system of learning supports in classrooms and schoolwide (in-person and online). Note that the design and strategic plans for the third component must be fully integrated with strategic plans for improving instruction and management at schools.

Third, the existing operational infrastructure needs to be reworked so that mechanisms are in place that are dedicated to the third component's implementation, development, and sustainability.[6] Our prototype calls for assigning administrative and team leadership and workgroups with responsibility and accountability for the successful development and daily operation of a unified, comprehensive, and equitable system of learning supports. Examples of functions include aggregating data across students and from teachers to analyze school needs, mapping school and community resources, analyzing resources, identifying the most pressing program development needs at the school, coordinating and integrating school resources and connecting with community resources, establishing priorities for strengthening programs and developing new ones, planning and facilitating ways to fill intervention gaps, recommending how resources should be deployed and redeployed, developing strategies for enhanc-

---

[5] For examples of policy statements and design and strategic plans, see Sections A and B of our Center's System Change Toolkit at http://smhp.psych.ucla.edu/summit2002/resourceaids.htm

[6] See Adelman and Taylor (2018) for a discussion of the operational infrastructure needed for and the problems associated with making sustainable system changes.

ing resources, social marketing, and helping with enhancing personnel and stakeholder development related to addressing barriers to learning and teaching.

Fourth, capacity building plans and their implementation must include a specific focus on developing a unified, comprehensive, and equitable system. Critical in this respect is personnel development. On the job opportunities and specific times must be allocated to enhance the capability of those directly involved in the learning supports component. More generally, all teachers, administrators, other staff and volunteers, and community stakeholders need more development related to how best to address barriers to learning and teaching.

Fifth, essential facets in the ongoing development of a transformed system of learning supports involve (a) continuous monitoring of all factors that facilitate and hinder transformation progress and then (b) ensuring actions are taken to deal with interfering factors and facilitate system development. As significant progress is made in developing the system, the monitoring expands to evaluate the impact on student outcomes with specific reference to direct indicators of the effectiveness of learning supports (e.g., increased attendance, reduced misbehavior, improved learning).

None of the above recommendations is meant to detract from the fundamentals that permeate all efforts to improve schools and schooling and that should continue to guide policy, practice, research, and training. For example:

- The curriculum in every classroom must include a major emphasis on whole child development. This involves promoting all areas of human development and functioning.
- Every classroom must address student motivation as an antecedent, process, and outcome concern, with an emphasis on intrinsic motivation.
- To enhance the ability of teachers to enable learning, learning supports must be implemented in the classroom, but only after personalized instruction is found insufficient. Such accommodations and special assistance

must be designed to build on strengths and must not supplant the ongoing promotion of healthy development.

- Schools must have policy, leadership, and mechanisms for developing schoolwide enrichment programs before, during, and after school.
- Families of schools (e.g., feeder schools or a neighborhood cluster) need to work together with respect to shared concerns and to effect economies of scale.
- School-community connections are needed to capitalize on the many ways community resources can enhance instruction, enrichment, and learning supports.

Concluding Comments

As Andy Hargreaves and Dean Fink (Hargreaves & Fink, 2000) remind us:

> Ultimately, only three things matter about educational reform. Does it have depth: does it improve important rather than superficial aspects of students' learning and development? Does it have length: can it be sustained over long periods of time instead of fizzling out after the first flush of innovation? Does it have breadth: can the reform be extended beyond a few schools, networks or showcase initiatives to transform education across entire systems or nations?

From this perspective and in keeping with the type of changes we have discussed in this chapter, we conclude by stressing that plans for enhancing student engagement and school climate should begin with a clear vision of what a classroom and school must do to effectively promote whole child development and equity of opportunity. Particular attention must be paid to engaging all students by personalizing instruction and providing a unified and comprehensive system for addressing barriers to learning and teaching. Transformative system changes must be implemented with integrity and commitment to the vision, replicated to scale across districts, and substantively sustained with creative renewal. Doing less contributes to an unsatisfactory status quo.

References

Adelman, H. S. (1995). Education reform: Broadening the focus. *Psychological Science, 6*, 61–62.

Adelman, H. S., & Taylor, L. (1994). *On understanding intervention in psychology and education*. Praeger. http://smhp.psych.ucla.edu/pdfdocs/contedu/understandingintervention.pdf

Adelman, H. S., & Taylor, L. (2005). Classroom climate. In S. W. Lee, P. A. Lowe, & E. Robinson (Eds.), *Encyclopedia of school psychology*. Sage. http://smhp.psych.ucla.edu/publications/46classroomclimate.Pdf

Adelman, H. S., & Taylor, L. (2006). *The implementation guide to student learning supports: New directions for addressing barriers to learning*. Corwin Press.

Adelman, H. S., & Taylor, L. (2011). Expanding school improvement policy to better address barriers to learning and integrate public health concerns. *Policy Futures in Education, 9*, 431–436. https://doi.org/10.2304/pfie.2011.9.3.431

Adelman, H. S. & Taylor, L. (2017). *Addressing barriers to learning: In the classroom and schoolwide*. Los Angeles: Center for MH in Schools & Student/Learning Supports. http://smhp.psych.ucla.edu/pdfdocs/barriersbook.pdf

Adelman, H. S., & Taylor, L. (2018). *Addressing barriers to learning: In the classroom and schoolwide*. Center for MH & Student/Learning Supports at UCLA. https://escholarship.org/uc/item/55w7b8x8

Adelman, H. S., & Taylor, L. (2019). *Improving school improvement*. Center for MH & Student/Learning Supports at UCLA. https://escholarship.org/uc/item/5288v1c1

Adelman, H. S., & Taylor, L. (2020a). *Embedding mental health as schools change*. Center for MH & Student/Learning Supports at UCLA. http://smhp.psych.ucla.edu/pdfdocs/mh20a.pdf

Adelman, H. S., & Taylor, L. (2020b). *Restructuring California schools to address barriers to learning and teaching in the COVID 19 context and beyond*. PACE. https://edpolicyinca.org/publications/restructuring-california-schools-address-barriers-learning-and-teaching-covid-19?utm_source=PACE+All&utm_campaign=61b8aabde4-EMAIL_CAMPAIGN_2020_11_17_07_36_COPY_05&utm_medium=email&utm_term=0_9f1af6b121-61b8aabde4-522725185

American Youth Policy Forum. (2000). High schools of the millenium report. : Author . Retrieved from https://www.aypf.org/resource/high-schools-of-the-millennium-report-of-the-workgroup/

Bandura, A. (1978). The self-system in reciprocal determinism. *American Psychologist, 33*, 344–358.

Berkowitz, R., Moore, H., Astor, R. A., & Benbenishty, R. (2017). Research synthesis of the associations between socioeconomic background, inequality, school climate, and academic achievement. *Review of Educational Research, 87*, 425–469.

Bodovski, K., Nahum-Shani, I., & Walsh, R. (2013). School climate and students' early mathematics learning: Another search for contextual effects. *American Journal of Education, 119*, 209–234.

Bradshaw, C. P., Waasdorp, T. E., Debnam, K. J., & Johnson, S. L. (2014). Measuring school climate in high schools: A focus on safety, engagement, and the environment. *Journal of School Health, 84*, 593–604.

Center for Mental Health in Schools (2011). Designing school improvement to enhance classroom climate for all students. Los Angeles: Center for MH in Schools & Student/Learning Supports. http://smhp.psych.ucla.edu/pdfdocs/schoolclimate.pdf

Center for MH in Schools & Student/Learning Supports at UCLA. (2012). *Schools and the challenge of LD and ADHD misdiagnoses*. Author. http://smhp.psych.ucla.edu/pdfdocs/ldmisdiagnoses.pdf

Center for MH in Schools & Student/Learning Supports at UCLA. (2018). *ESSA and addressing barriers to learning and teaching: Is there movement toward transforming student/learning supports?* Author. http://smhp.psych.ucla.edu/pdfdocs/2018%20report.pdf

Center for MH in Schools & Student/Learning Supports at UCLA. (2019). *About promoting social emotional development at school: "Kernels" and natural Opportunities*. Author. http://smhp.psych.ucla.edu/pdfdocs/socemotdev.pdf

Center for MH in Schools & Student/Learning Supports at UCLA. (2020a). *MTSS: It's just a starting point for transforming student/learning supports*. Author. http://smhp.psych.ucla.edu/pdfdocs/MTSSbuild.pdf

Center for MH in Schools & Student/Learning Supports at UCLA. (2020b). *Much discussion of MTSS, little discussion of student/learning support staff and developing MTSS into a unified, comprehensive, and equitable system*. Author. http://smhp.psych.ucla.edu/pdfdocs/july19init.pdf

Chapman, C., Laird, J., & Kewalramani, A. (2011). *Trends in high school dropout and completion rates in the United States: 1972–2008. Population*. National Center for Educational Statistics.

Czerkawski, B. C., & Lyman, E. W. (2016). An instructional design framework for fostering student engagement in online learning environments. *TechTrends, 60*, 532–539 . Retrieved from https://link.springer.com/article/10.1007/s11528-016-0110-z#citeas

Daily, S. M., Mann, M. J., Kristjansson, A. L., Smith, M. L., & Zullig. K. J. (2019). School climate and academic achievement in middle and high school students. *Journal of School Health, 89*, 173–180 . Retrieved from https://onlinelibrary.wiley.com/doi/full/10.1111/josh.12726

Deci, E. L., Koestner, R., & Ryan, R. M. (2001). Extrinsic rewards and intrinsic motivation in education: Reconsidered once again. *Review of Educational Research, 71*, 1–27. Retrieved from http://www.psych.rochester.edu/SDT/documents/2001_DeciKoestnerRyan.pdf

Eccles, J. (1983). Expectancies, values, and academic behaviors. In J. T. Spence (Ed.), *Achievement and achievement motives: Psychological and sociological approaches* (pp. 75–146). W. H. Freeman.

Eccles, J. S., & Wigfield, A. (2002). Motivational beliefs, values, and goals. *Annual Review of Psychology, 53*, 109–132.

Fredricks, J. A., Blumenfeld, P. C., & Paris, A. H. (2004). School engagement: Potential of the concept, state of the evidence. *Review of Educational Research, 74*, 59–109. Retrieved from http://rer.sagepub.com/content/74/1/59.short

Fresson, M., Meulemans, T., Dardenne, B., & Geurten, M. (2019). Overdiagnosis of ADHD in boys: Stereotype impact on neuropsychological assessment. *Applied Neuropsychology: Child, 8*, 231–245. Retrieved from https://www.tandfonline.com/doi/full/10.1080/21622965.2018.1430576

Halverson, L. R., & Graham, C. R. (2019). Learner engagement in blended learning environments: A conceptual framework. *Online Learning, 23*, 145–178. Retrieved from https://files.eric.ed.gov/fulltext/EJ1218398.pdf

Hargreaves, A., & Fink, D. (2000). The three dimesnions of reform. *Educational Leadership, 57*, 30–34.

Hinshaw, S. P., & Scheffler, R. M. (2014). *The ADHD explosion: Myths, medication, money, and today's push for performance*. Oxford University Press.

Hodges, T. (2018). School engagement is more than just talk. *Education*. Gallop online https://www.gallup.com/education/244022/school-engagement-talk.aspx

Hoover, N., Lever, N., Sachdev, N., Bravo, N., Schlitt, J., Acosta Price, O., Sheriff, L., & Cashman, J. (2019). *Advancing comprehensive school mental health: Guidance from the field*. National Center for School Mental Health. University of Maryland School of Medicine.www.schoolmentalhealth.org/AdvancingCSMHS.

Hopson, L. M., Schiller, K. S., & Lawson, H. A. (2014). Exploring linkages between school climate, behavioral norms, social supports, and academic success. *Social Work Research, 38*, 197–209. Retrieved from https://academic.oup.com/swr/article/38/4/197/1624992

Insel, P. M., & Moos, R. H. (1974). Psychological environments: Expanding the scope of human ecology. *American Psychologist, 29*, 179–188. https://doi.org/10.1037/h0035994

Jacob, I., Temkin, D., Rodriguez, Y., Okogbue, O., Greenfield, S., & Roemerman, R. (2020). *Setting the foundation for safe, supportive, and equitable school climates*. Child Trends. https://www.childtrends.org/publications/setting-the-foundation-for-safe-supportive-and-equitable-school-climates

Laratta, R. (2011). Ethical climate and accountability in nonprofit organizations. *Public Management Review, 13*, 43–63. https://doi.org/10.1080/14719037.2010.501620

Lombardi, E., Traficante, D., Bettoni, R., Offredi, I., Giorgetti, M., & Vernice, M. (2019). The impact of school climate on Well-being experience and school engagement: A study with high-school students. *Frontiers in Psychology, 10*, 2482. https://doi.org/10.3389/fpsyg.2019.02482

McEvoy, A., & Welker, R. (2000). Antisocial behavior, academic failure, and school climate: A critical review. *Journal of Emotional and Behavioral Disorders, 8*, 130–140. https://doi.org/10.1177/106342660000800301

Moore, K. A. (2014). Making the grade: Assessing the evidence for integrated student supports. *Child trends*. Retrieved from https://www.childtrends.org/wp-content/uploads/2014/02/2014-07ISSPaper2.pdf

National League of Cities. (2020). *Addressing student reengagement in the time of COVID-19*. Author. https://www.nlc.org/article/2020/11/04/addressing-student-reengagement-in-the-time-of-covid-19/

Ontario Human Rights Commission. (n.d.). *The opportunity to succeed: Achieving barrier-free education for students with disabilities*. Author. http://www3.ohrc.on.ca/sites/default/files/attachments/The_opportunity_to_succeed%3A_Achieving_barrier-free_education_for_students_with_disabilities.pdf

Park, T., & Lim, C. (2019). Design principles for improving emotional affordances in an online learning environment. *Asia Pacific Educational Review, 20*, 53–67. Retrieved from https://link.springer.com/article/10.1007/s12564-018-9560-7#Sec14

Reed, A.C. (2019). Why we need personalized professional development in our schools.. Teach Plus. Online at https://medium.com/whats-the-plus/why-we-need-personalized-professional-development-in-our-schools-2322c0178982

Rumberger, R. W., & Rotermun, S. (2012). The relationship between engagement and high school dropout. In S. L. Christenson, A. L. Reschly, & C. Wylie (Eds.), *Handbook of research on student engagement* (pp. 491–513). Springer.

Ryan, R., & Deci, E. (2017). *Self-determination theory: Basic psychological needs in motivation, development, and wellness*. Guilford Press.

Ryberg, R., Her, S., Temkin, D., Madill, R., Kelley, C., Thompson, J., & Gabriel, A. (2020). Measuring school climate: Validating the education department school climate survey in a sample of urban middle and high school students. *AERA Open., 6*, 1–2. Retrieved from https://journals.sagepub.com/doi/pdf/10.1177/2332858420948024

Schifter, C. C. (2016). Personalizing professional development for teachers. In M. Murphy, S. Redding, & J. Twyman (Eds.), *Handbook on personalized learning for states, districts, and schools* (pp. 221–235). Temple University, Center on Innovations in Learning. http://www.centeril.org/2016Handbook/resources/Schifter_chapter_web.pdf

Schneider, B., Ehrhart, M. G., & Macey, W. H. (2013). Organizational climate and culture. *Annual Review of Psychology, 64*, 361–388.

Scott, T. M., Hirn, R. G., & Alter, P. J. (2014). Teacher instruction as a predictor for student engagement and disruptive behaviors. *Preventing School Failure, 58*,

193–200. Retrieved from https://www.tandfonline.com/doi/full/10.1080/1045988X.2013.787588

Sherblom, S. A., Marshall, J. C., & Sherblom, J. C. (2006). The relationship between school climate and math and reading achievement. *Journal of Character Education, 4*, 19–31.

Skinner, E., Furrer, C., Marchand, G., & Kindermann, T. (2008). Engagement and disaffection in the classroom: Part of a larger motivational dynamic? *Journal of Educational Psychology, 100*, 765–781. https://doi.org/10.1037/a0012840

Taylor, L., & Adelman, H. S. (1999). Personalizing classroom instruction to account for motivational and developmental differences. *Reading and Writing Quarterly, 15*, 255–276. http://smhp.psych.ucla.edu/publications/19%20PERSONALIZING%20CLASSROOM%20INSTRUCTION.pdf

Thapa, A., Cohen, J., Guffey, S., & Higgins-D'Alessandro, A. (2013). A review of school climate research. *Review of Educational Research, 83*, 357–385.

Retrieved from https://journals.sagepub.com/doi/full/10.3102/0034654313483907

Tomlinson, C. A. (2017). *How to differentiate instruction in academically diverse classrooms* (3rd ed.). ASCD.

Wang, M. T., & Degol, J. L. (2016). School climate: A review of the construct, measurement, and impact on student outcomes. *Educational Psychology Review, 28*, 315–352. Retrieved from https://link.springer.com/article/10.1007/s10648-015-9319-1

Wattam, D. K., Benson, K., & Reyes, K. (2019). K-12 teacher candidates' understanding of ADHD student protections under section 504. *National Social Science Journal, 53*, 67–72. https://nssa.us/journals/pdf/NSS_Journal_53_1.pdf#page=67

Zullig, K. J., Koopman, T. M., Patton, J. M., & Ubbes, V. A. (2010). School climate: Historical review, instrument development, and school assessment. *Journal of Psychoeducational Assessment, 28*, 139–152. Retrieved from https://journals.sagepub.com/doi/10.1177/0734282909344205

Engaging High School Students in Learning

Marcia H. Davis, Crystal L. Spring,
and Robert W. Balfanz

Abstract

Although increasing student engagement may seem to be a daunting task for schools and educators, several strategies have been shown to predict improved engagement and achievement. This chapter provides an overview of strategies that have been studied and supported with research evidence. First, we discuss why it is important for teacher teams to track engagement and implement multi-tiered response systems for students who have disengaged from school. Next, we discuss the importance of increasing students' sense of belonging through building positive adult and peer relationships, implementing nonpunitive behavior systems, connecting with parents and the community, and supporting social–emotional skills. Then, we explore strategies for building student confidence, which should, in turn, lead to increased engagement. Finally, we overview the ways for school teams to support student agency through supporting autonomy in the classroom and making connections between school and students' future postsecondary success. We argue that schools and students will likely see the most benefits if they implement several of these strategies in tandem.

M. H. Davis (✉) · R. W. Balfanz
School of Education, Johns Hopkins University, Baltimore, MD, USA

Center for Social Organization of Schools, School of Education, Johns Hopkins University, Baltimore, MD, USA
e-mail: marcy@jhu.edu

C. L. Spring
School of Education, Johns Hopkins University, Baltimore, MD, USA

Engaging High School Students in Learning

A high school diploma should be seen not as the end of schooling, but as a necessary step toward postsecondary education and training. Securing a well-paying job now requires schooling past the twelfth grade, such as an occupational certificate, industry training, or a college degree. Those who graduate from high school with a high level of success are more likely to succeed in college or trade school. According to the US Bureau of Labor Statistics (2009), the difference between the average weekly earnings of high school dropouts ($595) was somewhat lower than that of high school graduates ($742) but much lower than that of those with a bachelor's or professional degree ($1248 and $1861, respectively). Unemployment among adults with less than a high school degree (5.4%) is also greater than among high school diplomas (3.7%), bachelor's (2.2%), or professional degrees (1.6%).

In the USA, high school success determines students' trajectories toward decent employment. This success is largely dependent upon their level of motivation and engagement in school. We define motivation as the anticipation of potential enjoyment, challenge, or usefulness that causes people to invest effort in a particular experience. Students can be motivated for many different reasons. Some are just motivated to "get through school" as a step toward a future job; others are motivated by high grades and recognition from teachers and parents, and still, others are motivated by learning new topics and ideas. Motivations for school fall on a continuum of extrinsic motivation, based on the pressure from teachers, peers, and family members, to intrinsic motivation, based on the internal drives to learn and do well. Students can experience motivation from multiple sources at once.

Engagement in school, however, is defined as students' behavioral, cognitive, affective, and social involvement in instructional activities (Lutz et al., 2006) and can be considered a visible manifestation of their motivation (Skinner & Pitzer, 2012). We espouse Fredricks et al.'s (2004) definitions of affective or emotional engagement as a physical display of emotion, behavioral engagement as active participation in academic activities, and cognitive engagement as a mental investment in learning. In addition, however, we include social engagement as a core dimension of the construct. As Guthrie and Wigfield (2000) have noted, the exchange of ideas about academic subject matters with peers in "communities of literacy" is an important aspect of school and learning.

Research indicates that both motivation and engagement decline in middle school and continue to decline throughout high school (Gnambs & Hanfstingl, 2016; Guthrie & Davis, 2003; Skinner et al., 2008; Wang & Eccles, 2012; Wigfield, 1994). For example, in an examination of data from 23 Maryland public middle schools over three data collection waves at seventh, ninth, and eleventh grade, Wang and Eccles (2012) found that average growth trajectories of engagement, measured by school participation, perception of school belonging, and self-regulated learning, decreased.

Since motivation and engagement are inextricably linked, strategies to increase motivation should also improve engagement. According to the basic needs theory, which is a micro theory within the larger self-determination theory, students are motivated by activities that support relationships, competence, and autonomy (Deci & Ryan, 2000). We argue that interventions to increase student motivation, and thus engagement, should address one or more of these basic needs. First, schools need to increase students' sense of belonging in their school environments by increasing the relationships between adults and students, students and their peers, school staff and parents, and by reducing harsh and punitive punishments while increasing the use of positive behavior systems. Second, educators need to work together to increase students' feelings of competence in their schoolwork by matching instruction to students' level, providing helpful feedback, and recognizing the progress made. Finally, interventions should focus on supporting students' autonomy by giving them a sense of control in their school and classroom and helping them feel in control of their futures through career exploration. According to self-determination theory, humans need to feel related to others, competent, and autonomous to be fulfilled in their natural psychological needs and flourish. By helping students become more engaged and motivated in school, schools can not only help students become better students and future employees, but also support their development as human beings.

Supporting student engagement at school and with learning is a complicated process, but there are strategies that have been shown, individually, to correlate with improved engagement and achievement. Such strategies may be even more effective when implemented together. In this chapter, we cover the strategies listed in Table 1. First, we discuss why it is important for teacher teams to track engagement and implement multi-tiered response systems for students who have disengaged from school. Next, we discuss the importance of increasing students' sense of

Table 1 Interventions to Increase Engagement of High School Students

1. Tracking engagement	Using predictive indicators of engagement
	Teacher teams focused on improving engagement
	Using multi-tiered response systems
2. Building a sense of belonging	Building positive relationships with adults
	Building connection with peers
	Building communication with parents
3. Building student confidence	Matching the level of instruction to the student
	Checks for understanding and helpful feedback
4. Giving students agency over learning	Student choice
	Building connections to careers

out is something that can be tracked, but that interventions can be put in place to remove the barriers that deter students from graduation and postsecondary success (Allensworth, 2013; Allensworth & Easton, 2005; Davis et al., 2018). The following section summarizes the research on indicators used to track disengagement from school, schools' use of teacher teams to track these indicators and develop student-level interventions, and multi-tiered response systems that provide the magnitude of response necessary for individual students.

Using Predictive Indicators of Engagement

The identification of early warning indicators to predict graduation started with work by Allensworth and Easton (2005). They found that one indicator, sufficient credits to be promoted to 10th grade, predicts high school graduation with 80% accuracy and is thus more predictive than student test scores or background characteristics (Allensworth, 2012; Allensworth & Easton, 2005). However, knowing whether students earned enough credits by the end of ninth grade does not help school staff intervene mid-year. Yet schools already track behavioral manifestations of disengagement, such as absenteeism, lack of attention and assignment completion, and misbehavior. Research on data from Chicago and Philadelphia schools shows that these disengagement indicators (poor attendance, behavior, and course performance) not only predict failure to graduate (Allensworth & Easton, 2005, 2007; Balfanz & Herzog, 2005; Balfanz et al., 2007; Neild & Balfanz, 2006) but can be used to intervene mid-year (Mac Iver et al., 2019). These indicators have been found to be predictive of non-graduation in other districts as well (Balfanz & Boccanfuso, 2007; Balfanz & Byrnes, 2010; Baltimore Education Research Consortium, 2011; Mac Iver et al., 2009; Meyer et al., 2010; Silver et al., 2008).

belonging through building positive adult and peer relationships, implementing nonpunitive behavior systems, connecting with parents and the community, and supporting social–emotional skills. Then, we explore strategies for building student confidence, which should, in turn, lead to increased engagement. Finally, we overview ways for school teams to support student agency through supporting autonomy in the classroom and making connections between school and students' future postsecondary success.

Tracking Engagement

A student's decision to drop out is not often based on an unanticipated life event or a disinterest in graduation but on a gradual process of disengagement that occurs over years prior to and during high school (Anderson et al., 2004; Fine, 1991; Orfield, 2004). Yet the many factors that enter into this decision, such as mobility, safety, peer influence, and family history, could make dropout prevention seem to be an impossible challenge. However, work in Chicago and Philadelphia has shown not only that this supposedly "intractable" problem of high school disengagement and drop-

Recent research has shown that high school graduation predictors, including attendance, behavior, and course performance, are also predictive of college enrollment and persistence when different thresholds are used (Balfanz & Byrnes, 2019). In particular, findings from a study of Boston high school students show that good attendance (94% or above) and a strong GPA (2.7 or above) are very predictive of earning a 4-year college degree (Balfanz & Byrnes, 2019). These findings also suggest that taking challenging courses, such as the sequence of qualifying courses for admission to the state university system or college-level courses offered in high school (e.g., AP, dual enrollment), is also a key metric for being on track to postsecondary success.

In response to the predictive nature of early warning indicators, nationwide attention has focused on developing early warning systems (e.g., Dynarski et al., 2008; Pinkus, 2008; Therriault et al., 2013). A U.S. Department of Education survey indicated that at least half of American high schools use a system that monitors and flags students with early warning indicators (2016). However, there is only minimal evidence that examining alone will have an effect on student outcomes. Of six studies reviewed by Rumberger et al. (Rumberger et al., 2017), only two found that examining data reduced student dropout rates.

Teacher Teams Focused on Improving Engagement

Just tracking students' engagement in school is not enough. Teachers and school staff must reach out to struggling students to focus on getting them engaged in school and on track to graduation. Interventions in the ninth grade are particularly important since there is a documented drop in engagement and grades over the transition from middle to high school (Benner, 2011; Benner & Graham, 2009; Roderick & Camburn, 1999; Seidman et al., 1996; Simmons & Blyth, 1987). Through interviews with teachers and students, and observation of English and mathematics courses in eighth and ninth grade, Allensworth (2013) reported that the decrease in engagement was not aligned with increased academic rigor; many students reported less academic pressure in

their ninth-grade classes. However, the study noted a decline in adult monitoring and support in ninth grade compared to eighth grade. This suggests that monitoring ninth-grade students' engagement and effort and providing support for those falling behind is important to improve their likelihood of graduation from high school.

Grade-level teacher teams, which have long been a staple of successful middle-grade schools, are increasingly being used in ninth grade, especially in high-needs schools (Krone, 2019). The benefits of using teams have been acknowledged in business (e.g., Guttman, 2008) as well as education (e.g., Clark & Clark, 1994). The term "distributed leadership" is used to describe how successful educational leadership can be exercised through the relationships built among faculty and staff rather than a single individual, such as a principal or headmaster (Scribner et al., 2007). Research indicates that shared decision-making is the *impetus* for school change (Preskill & Torres, 1999).

Using Multi-tiered Response Systems to Increase Engagement

In an early warning response system, timely interventions in response to early warning indicator data are the key to getting students back on track. Early warning teams should provide "intensive, individualized support to students who have fallen off track and face significant challenges to success" (Rumberger et al., 2017, p. 20). Further, an adult advocate should lead the support for each student. We suggest that interventions also be tiered so that teams develop interventions that are school or grade wide (Tier 1), targeted interventions for small groups of students with similar indicators (Tier 2), or intensive individual interventions for focus students (Tier 3). Especially in recent years, such a tiered approach has been well documented and supported by research (Fredricks et al., 2019; Reschly, 2020). Even when targeting particular sub-constructs of engagement, such multi-tiered frameworks may be employed (Cook et al., 2020). Of the eight studies that examined the use of individualized supports for students who have fallen off the track to graduation and met the What Works Clearinghouse standards "without reservations," Rumberger et al. (Rumberger et al., 2017) found that four of the studies indicated improvements in either attendance, behavior, or course performance of students. In addition, two of the three of these studies that examined high school graduation found significant improvements in graduation outcomes.

Although many schools have a system of early warning identification (U.S. Department of Education, 2016), many do not have an intervention system in place to help struggling students. A recent randomized control study suggests that data monitoring and team meetings may not be sufficient to effect changes in student outcomes; an organized intervention plan is necessary for an early warning system to be effective (Davis et al., 2018). Implementing and monitoring interventions for struggling students, and using a diversity of interventions, were the factors related to improved outcomes. Recent research using randomized control trials to evaluate two early warning and intervention systems that use teams, the "Early Warning Intervention and Monitoring System" (EWIMS, Faria et al., 2017) and the "Early Warning Intervention (EWI) Team Model" (Mac Iver et al., 2019; Davis et al., 2018), confirm that these systems lead to improvements in student attendance and course performance.

Interventions should re-engage students who have fallen off the path to graduation. However, school teams often reuse the same interventions over and over (e.g., phone calls to parents or individual tracking sheets that students carry to their classes), rather than trying new ideas. Our research shows that teams using a varied approach have better outcomes for attendance and grades than those that used only a few intervention types (Davis et al., 2018). Schools may benefit from taking advantage of the growing literature on effective and promising interventions. For example, the Peer Assisted Learning Strategies (PALS) intervention, designed to enhance academic engagement (Reschly, 2020), could be paired with the Establish-Maintain-Restore approach,

which cultivates affective engagement through teacher–student relationships (Cook et al., 2020).

Increasing Students' Sense of Belonging

According to the basic needs theory (Deci & Ryan, 2000), which is a part of the larger self-determination theory, students' motivation will increase if their basic need for relationships is fulfilled. In the field of education, fulfillment of the need for relationships can be measured by students' sense of connectedness to school. We define school connectedness as believing that one is welcome, wanted, cared about, and needed in school. Research on school belonging shows that students who are connected to their school are less likely to demonstrate negative behaviors such as drug use, violence, absenteeism, and risky activities that could lead to injury, such as drinking and driving (Blum et al., 2002; Resnick et al., 1993); they also have greater school achievement (Booker, 2004; Hughes et al., 2015) than less-connected students. However, a recent national study found that only 39% of high school students reported feeling that they belonged in their school, only 36% reported having supportive relationships with adults in their school, and only 40% reported having supportive relationships with their peers (Margolius et al., 2020). The sense of belonging begins to decrease in middle school (Centre for Education Statistics and Evaluation, 2017).

Building Positive Relationships with Adults

For students to feel that they belong and are welcomed in their school, they need to know that adults in the school not only want them there but also are actively trying to support their success both in school and in life. However, building connections between adults and students takes work. Not only do the adults need to understand the difficulties students face in life and work completion, but they must actively reach out to students in caring and thoughtful ways and be accepting and aware of students' cultures.

Teacher–Student Relationships The strength of relationships built between students and the adults in their school, especially with their teachers, can influence student engagement (Pianta et al., 2012; see also Hoefkens & Pianta, chapter "Teacher-Student Relationships, Engagement in School, and Student Outcomes", this volume; Scales et al., chapter "Developmental Relationships and Student Academic Motivation: Current Research and Future Directions", this volume). For example, Roorda et al. (2011) used a meta-analytic approach to examine correlations between student-teacher relationships and both engagement and achievement. From the 99 studies that matched their criteria, they found correlations between positive teacher–student relationships and both engagement and achievement, as well as negative associations between negative teacher–student relationships and engagement and achievement. The associations for negative associations were stronger than those for the positive associations, showing that it is even more important for teachers to reduce any negative aspects of relationships than it is to increase positive aspects of these relationships. An interesting and unexpected finding was that teacher–student relationships were even more important for older students than younger students. Further, in a more recent meta-analysis, Roorda et al. (2017) examined 189 studies and found that engagement acts as a significant mediator between affective student–teacher relationships and student achievement. This finding held across grade levels, but the direct association between positive relationships and engagement was stronger in middle and high schools than in elementary schools.

Since the quality of teacher–student relationships decreases as students get older (Furrer & Skinner, 2003), and teacher–student relationships are highly related to engagement and achievement for older students, teachers of adolescents and the school structures that support them have to work harder to build these relationships than do their elementary school counterparts. One challenge with teenagers is that getting along well with

one's teacher is not considered as "cool" as it is among younger children. Additionally, the time students have with each of their teachers decreases as they have different teachers for different classes. While some younger students may see one or two teachers during the day, older adolescents can see six to ten teachers who may vary from one semester to the next. In addition to the shorter chunks of the time these teachers have to get to know their students, the sheer quantity of students—sometimes numbering in the hundreds—may be daunting. Teachers of adolescents need to actively get to know their students personally and model caring behavior, and interventions aimed at boosting these relationships must acknowledge and accommodate the significant constraints these teachers face.

Teacher support, demonstrated in a teacher's caring, dependability, and friendliness, has an impact on students' interest in and enjoyment of their schoolwork (Skinner & Belmont, 1993) and may play an even larger role in motivation for adolescents than for elementary school children. For example, Ryan and Patrick (2001) found that during the transition from seventh to eighth grade, students who perceived their teacher was supportive and promoted interactions and mutual respect had greater positive changes in motivation and engagement than students who did not perceive themselves as having a supportive teacher. Interactions between teachers and students in a classroom can also make the difference between a friendly, safe space characterized by encouragement and recognition for trying, and an unpleasant negative space filled with criticism and insults (Anderson et al., 1988). Teachers can build personal relationships with students by sharing information about their hobbies and interests, or by seeing and connecting with students and parents during school functions such as sports, academic competitions, or cultural events.

Positive Behavior Systems Although many secondary schools focus on consequences for poor behavior, excessively harsh and punitive discipline policies decrease students' connectedness to school (Hagan & Foster, 2012; Gregory et al., 2016), which negatively affects their engagement in school and learning. This is especially true for minoritized students who often experience harsher discipline policies than do white students for comparable offenses (Anyon et al., 2014; Ritter & Anderson, 2018; Rocque & Paternoster, 2011).

Positive behavior interventions and supports (PBIS) is a framework to improve school climate through strategies such as setting school-wide expectations for behavior, teaching expectations and rules to the students, acknowledging good behavior, using data for decision-making, and providing administrative and district support (Swain-Bradway et al., 2015). Many districts around the country have adopted this framework in response to increased demand for evidence-based practices (Kittelman et al., 2019). School teams in secondary schools can decrease the use of harsh punishments by using PBIS or other positive behavior systems and improving classroom management. Supporting good classroom management is especially important since students present fewer behavior issues when there are set routines and fair consequences for poor behavior (Blum et al., 2002). When teachers' response to poor behavior is both fair and predictable, students feel they have some control over how they are treated. Further, established school and classroom routines can make students feel secure in knowing what they can expect out of their school day. One important step a school team can take is to institute school-level classroom management guidelines to be implemented across teachers and classrooms so that students do not face different behavior expectations in different classrooms.

While PBIS has been shown to reduce suspensions and promote positive student outcomes (Bradshaw et al., 2010, 2012), many scholars also caution against relying solely on PBIS. Without culturally responsive adaptations and proper teacher training to accompany PBIS, racial disparities may perpetuate themselves (McIntosh et al., 2014), and scholars recommend further research into which specific adaptations best reduce disparities and increase engagement (Gregory & Skiba, 2019).

Restorative Practices Since the development of the Restorative Practices Intervention in 1999, there has also been a push for schools to use more restorative practices that focus less on discipline and more on building relationships and improving school climate. There are 11 "essential Elements" of restorative practices, with one being the use of a restorative "circle." These circles can be large or small and are used to bring individuals (students, teachers, administration) together to set expectations for behavior, resolve conflicts, or respond to inappropriate behavior. Adults are also taught to reduce shaming the students, using questioning to support students thinking about problems rather than reacting to them, and allowing for student input. In a study of 29 high school classrooms, Gregory et al. (2016) found that student-reported implementation of restorative practices related to higher perceived teacher respect and fewer misconduct referrals issued to Latino-African American students. In a review of studies on restorative practices, Velez et al. (2020) stated that although restorative practices offer a lot of potential and have shown to influence improvements in teachers feeling more connected to students and promote a sense of school belonging among students, implementing them can be complex and very dependent on the dynamics and interpersonal relations of particular schools. And as with PBIS, restorative practices without targeted attention to issues of racial inequity may perpetuate disparities and lessen the potential benefits of interventions (Gregory et al., 2018).

Positive Reinforcement Teacher teams should also develop opportunities to positively reinforce good behavior and improvements in attendance, behavior, and grades over a set period. Extrinsic rewards can provide motivation for tasks students do not find motivating for their own sake (Cameron et al., 2001; Deci et al., 1999). In one of our own studies, students who reported liking receiving recognition (I feel proud when I am recognized as a good reader) and good grades for reading (Getting good grades in reading is important to me) also reported more reading behavior and reading engagement (Davis et al., 2020). However, extrinsic rewards could negatively impact motivation in some circumstances, especially if rewards are seen as manipulative rather than informative (Cameron et al., 2005). Further, students who receive rewards or excessive praise for activities they would already do, such as receiving straight As or having perfect attendance, may realize that what they did was extraordinary compared to other students and may try less hard the following semester. Also, if students feel that the rewards are unattainable or given in an unfair way, motivation can decrease. Therefore, teacher teams need to think carefully regarding how and when to give out rewards or praise.

Small Learning Communities Another strategy to connect adults and students is to encourage small learning communities (SLCs). Creating smaller communities makes it easier for teachers who share students to monitor student engagement and create personalized interventions to mitigate disengagement. By sharing their experiences and successes with particular students, they can identify the teacher each student connects with most easily. Also, the teacher with the most connection with each student can share strategies that have worked well for that individual student. Further, after the best team member to be an advocate for each student is identified, that team member can check in regularly with the student to make sure he or she is keeping up with schoolwork. In this way, an SLC becomes a smaller school within a school, encouraging higher quality relationships between adults and students. Since the optimal school size for increasing school connectedness is fewer than 600 students (Blum et al., 2002), creating SLCs and ninth-grade academies can give a large school a small-school feel.

The use of small learning communities can have a positive effect on attendance, behavior, and course performance. Authors of the U.S. Department of Education report on preventing dropout in secondary schools (Rumberger et al., 2017) reviewed eight studies showing moderate evidence for the impact of small learning communities on student outcomes. They found that SLCs decreased student dropout rates and had positive effects on high school graduation.

Report Card Conferences Another strategy school teams can use to increase adult-to-student relationships in their schools, and one encouraged in the Early Warning System literature (Davis et al., 2018; Mac Iver et al., 2019), is the use of report card or progress report conferences. During these conferences, each student in a grade meets with an adult advisor who is not one of his/her current teachers. In some schools, other school personnel volunteer as adult advisors (e.g., teachers from other grades or other school staff), while other schools bring in trusted community members, such as retired teachers, faculty from a nearby college, or adults from a local community center. The adult and student discuss the student's grades to determine the next steps and goals. Ideally, schools try to have these conferences three to four times a year, maintaining the same adult–student pairs each time. This ensures that all students in the target grade receive consistent encouragement. In our recent study of promotion coaches, we found schools that implemented two or more report card conferences with ninth-grade students had significantly higher student attendance than those that implemented one or less conferences (Davis, 2019).

Building Connections with Peers

Not only do connections with adults in the school matter, but secondary students who feel supported by their peers feel more comfortable and connected to their school (Allen et al., 2016; Juvonen et al., 2012), put in more effort (Wentzel et al., 2017), and have a greater academic achievement (Juvonen, 2006). As a part of feeling welcome at school, whether in person or online, students need to know that the students in their classes care whether they show up and encourage them to do well. Students who have many friends usually report feeling connected to their school, while those with few friends in school often feel disconnected (Juvonen et al., 2012). Peers have a strong influence on how students view school and their affiliation with it (Faircloth & Hamm, 2005). Socialization is even more important for adolescents than for younger students (Juvonen et al., 2012). Students, especially shy or less social teenagers, may find it difficult to make these connections in classrooms, especially when they do not see the same peers throughout the day. It is important that students not only make friends in school, but also have positive experiences with peers from other races, genders, and religions. Teams need to brainstorm ways to increase the amount of positive, supportive, and diverse peer relationships among students in their schools. More information on the importance of peer relationships for motivation and engagement with school can be found in this handbook (Knifsend et al., 2021).

Extracurricular Activities One way to build student interactions is through shared interests and affiliations. Teacher teams can support these interactions through group structures such as sports teams, arts activities, student government, robotics clubs, and debate teams. If students are left to organize friendships and organizations without school support, there is a chance that some will be left out. Some educators may see these groups as secondary in importance to instruction or as taking up the energy and time that students should be investing in academic pursuits. However, we believe that as important as it is for students to focus on instruction and complete their schoolwork, they still need to feel a connection to their school and to their peers for instruction to be effective. These activities are particularly helpful to connect students to others with similar interests and life goals. For example, students in an art club for future artists will be able to connect with others who share similar goals. Students can encourage each other and share information, for example, regarding colleges or competitions.

Students who participate in extracurricular activities tend to perform better academically than those who do not. For example, Darling et al. (2005) examined data from six California high schools in a longitudinal analysis and found that students participating in extracurricular activities showed improved grades, attitudes toward school, and academic aspirations. Although extracurricular activities have been shown to improve student outcomes, teachers and administrators may view these activities as a reward for high performance or consider that only students who can handle their schoolwork have time to give to these activities. However, we argue that students who are struggling in school may also be suffering from low levels of belongingness, and therefore may become more motivated in their academics if they are given opportunities to build positive peer connections. In this way, students who teachers may be tempted to "bench" from extracurriculars may actually have more to gain from these activities than those who are doing well.

Many reviews have been written on outcomes of extracurricular activity involvement. Holland and Andre (1987), in a review of studies prior to 1987, found that participation in extracurricular activities was correlated to greater self-esteem, involvement in political activities, academic ability and grades, educational aspirations, feelings of control, and lower delinquency rates. Feldman and Matjasko's (2005) review found that school-based structured activities, in contrast to unstructured activities, were associated with positive outcomes such as better academic performance, lower dropout rates, higher self-esteem, and reduced delinquent and antisocial behavior. However, research at that time also indicated that such participation could be related to poorer outcomes if the number of activities or the amount of time invested exceeded a certain threshold. Farb and Majasko (Farb & Matjasko, 2012) built on the previous review to explore how breadth, intensity, and duration affect the benefit of extracurricular activities, specifically examining an "overscheduling" hypothesis. They found positive outcomes in proportion to the time spent in organized activities, up to a specific point at which there were diminishing returns.

Prosocial Skills Students who are prosocial are more successful in school. In one of our own studies, we found that students in grades 5–8 who were more prosocial in regard to reading (e.g., "I like to help my classmates understand what they have read") were more likely to report higher reading behavior, engagement, and achievement, while those who reported being antisocial ("My friends and I laugh at classmates who do not read well") were likely to report lower levels of reading behavior, engagement, and achievement (Davis et al., 2020). Students, however, may not know how to interact with each other in these healthy ways. School teams need to determine how and when they can teach their student's prosocial skills such as conflict resolution, clear communication, negotiation, appropriate manners, problem-solving in difficult situations, active listening, managing stress, and self-control. Learning social competence can have positive long-term effects on school bonding.

This is important because secondary students' motivation and engagement in school can be influenced, in part, by teachers' and peers' expectations of prosocial behavior. For example, Wentzel et al. (2017) studied teachers' and middle and high school students' expectations for compliant and helping behavior. They found that perceptions of peer expectations for helping behavior and caring were related to effort to learn. If students receive consistent messaging that they should help one another and follow the class rules, they will expend more energy on their schoolwork.

Further, as adolescents near graduation, they start to think about possible future identities and consider how their future work will contribute to the world. Adolescents who understand how their schoolwork may lead to such purposeful work will be motivated to try harder. For example, Yeager and Bundick (2009) interviewed middle and high school students to determine the relationship between future work goals, purpose, and meaning. Work goals were categorized as either purposeful (i.e., students provided a reason for a particular work goal that would benefit the world) or self-oriented (i.e., students provided reasons that pertained to their own benefit from being in a particular career). Only 30% of students in their sample mentioned purposeful work goals during their interviews. Students' responses were also evaluated regarding their sense of purpose in life, sense of meaning in life, and meaningfulness in their schoolwork. Students who stated purposeful work goals in the interviews reported higher scores on the three measures of purpose and meaningfulness than students who did not report purposeful goals, even when controlling for demographics and type of career. The authors' conclusion was that students with purposeful work goals may be more mastery-oriented because they are seeking knowledge to help others, rather than just grades.

Service Learning Another way to foster both prosocial behavior and peer connection is through service-learning opportunities. Service learning is the combination of academic learning and community service (Baker, 2019) that has the dual goal of strengthening student character and increasing student learning (Pak, 2018; Rossi, 2002). Students should not only participate in service-learning opportunities, both in school (peer tutoring, school beautification) and in their communities (environmental projects, assisted living facilities), but should also have time to reflect on what they learned during the experience.

Service learning that follows four recommended practices of "(a) linking programs to academic and program curriculum or objectives, (b) incorporating youth voice, (c) involving community partners, and (d) providing opportunities for reflection" (Celio et al., p. 66) has been shown to relate to student gains in "attitudes toward self, attitudes toward school and learning, civic engagement, social skills, and academic performance" in a review of 62 studies (Celio et al., 2011, p. 164).

Students also benefit from being asked to contribute ideas about what they could do to solve a problem in their community. It is especially helpful for a group of students to be challenged to work together to improve their community; for example, by forming an environmental club. Service learning can teach valuable lessons such as empathy, kindness, and social responsibility. When matched appropriately to students' personal strengths, service-learning opportunities can also help them explore interests and possible careers.

Building Communication with Parents

Parents and the community can influence students' success in ways that teachers and peers cannot. Parents are often the support system students rely on for homework and those who set expectations for their children's school success (Boonk et al., 2018; Shute et al., 2011). Parents can be involved in their child's school experience in many ways including participation in educational activities at home (home-based: such as supporting homework), parents' interactions with their children's school (school-based: such as attending school events and parent-teacher conferences) and supporting their children's academic success by communicating developmental strategies (academic socialization: such as communicating the value of education) (Hill & Tyson, 2009). In addition to traditional conceptualizations of parental involvement, Huguley et al. (2021) found that African American families often engage in racialized parenting strategies such as advocating for systematic change to counteract racial inequalities and poor school quality.

Parents have a significant influence on their child's level of school engagement (Bempechat et al., chapter "Parental Influences on Achievement Motivation and Student Engagement", this volume; Bempechat & Shernoff, 2012; Reschly & Christenson, 2019). However, not all students have strong support at home, depending on family dynamics and circumstances. School teams should discuss how to connect with parents, sharing strategies and information they can use at home to help their children succeed and making them aware of opportunities and resources.

Regular Contact The first step in connecting with parents is to make school feel like a welcoming place for both students and their parents.

This can be challenging as some parents have negative memories of their own high school experiences or school experiences related to discrimination. Also, schools need to remove barriers that prevent minoritized parents from visiting and participating at their children's school (Kim, 2009). To make school a welcoming place, school staff need to make regular contact with parents and respond promptly when parents reach out to them. The first contact from the school to a parent should be positive; teachers should not wait until there is a problem to reach out. Regular contact can be maintained through emails or calls home to report good behavior as well as what students can do to improve (Kraft & Rogers, 2015). Parents should be invited to visit the school, as their schedules permit, e.g., to assist in the classroom or during school events or to attend after-school events or celebrations; schools should encourage an active parent organization. When possible, information should be translated as needed for families that do not speak English. Finally, when parents reach out for help, school staff should try to provide the support the parent requests without making him/her feel like a burden or less knowledgeable regarding his/her child's needs (Smith et al., 2020).

Parental Academic Support Parents' school advice and support to their children is often based on their own school experiences many years earlier. Some of these coping and learning strategies are not well adapted to current schooling (Räty, 2007). Parents' expectations for their children may be too high or too low, which can affect the level and quality of students' engagement in classes. School teams can plan training workshops to provide parents with skills and strategies to create a supportive learning environment, help their children complete homework, develop students' time management skills, communicate with teachers, manage behavior, and support prosocial practices at home (Ferlazzo & Hammond, 2009). To make it easier for parents to attend these events, schools should provide babysitting and transportation. Parents should be invited to share their own viewpoints and cultural norms during these events. Due to the level of coordination required to plan parental support activities and resources, the school may need to assign a staff member to serve as a parent and community liaison (Hill & Tyson, 2009).

Meeting Home Needs Students and parents often need help beyond academic support. Many families need resources for dental health, food access, GED opportunities, childcare options, job placement, or substance abuse support. School teams need to be aware of the resources available in the community so they can provide this information to parents as needed. Providing students with necessities like school breakfast and healthcare will increase their feelings of safety and belonging at school, which will lead to improved attendance (Baumeister & Leary, 1995; Mhurchu et al., 2013; Strolin-Goltzman et al., 2014). School teams can also share information about students to identify reasons why students are struggling. One teacher may perceive a struggling student as lazy and unfocused, while another may know more about what that student is going through at home and be more understanding. Discussing the student's situation in a team meeting can provide an opportunity to meet the family's resource needs and bring all team members to the same understanding of the issues facing the child.

Building Student Confidence

According to basic needs theory, which is a part of the larger self-determination theory, competence is one of three basic needs that must be met for someone to be motivated (Ryan & Deci, 2000). For students to be motivated to complete their schoolwork and engage in their classes, they need to feel like they can succeed if they try. Self-efficacy, defined as a person's perceived capabilities for performing actions (Schunk & Mullen, 2012), has a very strong relationship to both engagement and achievement (Schunk & Mullen, chapter "Self-Efficacy and Engaged Learners", this volume). In one study, we found that students in grades 5–8 who reported higher levels of self-efficacy (e.g., "I am one of the best readers in my class") were likely to report higher reading

behavior, engagement, and achievement, while students who reported that reading is challenging (e.g., "The books that teachers assign are often hard for me to read") were likely to report lower levels of reading behavior, engagement, and achievement (Davis et al., 2020, p. 438).

However, building the confidence of adolescents who may have spent many years in unsuccessful attempts to achieve school success will be difficult. For many, doubts about their ability to succeed in school undermine their effort and engagement in academics (Anderman & Maehr, 1994; Eccles & Midgley, 1989). Such students need a few big wins to believe that they have what it takes to succeed. They need both academic and emotional support. Teachers need to meet them where they currently are by matching instruction to the level of the learner, give them useful feedback they can use to improve, recognize and praise their early wins, and provide supports such as tutoring and extra classes to bring them up to grade level learning.

Matching the Level of Instruction to the Student

Matching the level of the instruction to the level of the student is a key component of Vygotsky's "zone of proximal development" (Vygotsky, 1978). This zone is that space between what students can do on their own and what they can do with full support from another. This sweet spot will be different for different students in each classroom. School teams must decide how to meet students where they are at their varying levels in learning. To meet this need for individualized instruction, teams can establish structures enabling students to receive focused extra help and encourage teachers to reteach topics when necessary and give students opportunities to resubmit work.

Focused Extra Help One way to match students' level of instruction is providing focused extra help outside the classroom. Many teachers provide one-on-one or small group assistance through coach classes during advisory periods or after school. In a meta-analysis study examining the effectiveness of interventions to improve achievement of low SES students, tutoring, defined as intensive academic instruction, had the highest average effect size (0.36), compared to other interventions such as small-group instruction (0.24), computer-assisted instruction (0.11), and incentives (0.01; Dietrichson, 2017).

Second Chances   Another way to provide extra help and decrease the emotional impact of a poor grade is for teachers to allow students to resubmit coursework and quizzes if they fail the first attempt, and to provide an opportunity to submit late work. This aligns to the recent emphasis on standards-based grading, which reflects students' mastery of skills rather than non-academic factors such as behavior and effort (Wisch et al., 2018). Teachers focusing on standards rather than traditional grades allow students to retake, revise, and redo assignments. Although some teachers strongly prefer one or the other extreme (traditional or standards-based grading), many fall somewhere in between. To examine the approaches teachers take and how these relate to their school policies, content area, and personal beliefs, Wisch et al. (2018) surveyed 429 teachers on mastery approaches to grading. They found that more than 90% of teachers implemented some redos or retakes in their classrooms; this occurred more often when teachers believed that a school-wide policy existed allowing late work and revisions.

Checks for Understanding and Helpful Feedback

Students who want to improve cannot do so without helpful feedback and support from their teachers. When students lack agency because they do not know how they can improve their learning and success, motivation and engagement will suffer. Helpful feedback not only tells students what to do, but it also helps students fix errors and provides them with new strategies to accomplish a task. In a meta-analysis of the effectiveness of interventions to improve low SES students' achievement, feedback and prog-

ress monitoring, including any intervention that provided either the teachers or students with information on development, had one of the highest average effect sizes (0.32); only tutoring had a greater effect (0.36; Dietrichson, 2017).

Grades   The most common feedback secondary students receive from their teachers is in the form of grades, which are very important predictors of engagement. In an examination of National Longitudinal Study data from students in the eighth grade, You and Sharkey (2009) found that the previous achievement was the strongest predictor of engagement (effect size = 0.356) compared to other predictors such as gender, race, SES, parental expectations, self-concept, college aspiration, and having a friend drop out. The grades students receive not only trigger emotional reactions but also determine how much time and effort students will continue to invest in school. For instance, Poorthuis et al. (2015) examined secondary school students' reactions to fall report card grades and their engagement the following spring. Lower report card grades predicted lower levels of both emotional and behavioral engagement. The authors concluded that grades were both the outcome of engagement and a motivator for continued engagement. They also found that the relationship between grades and engagement was mediated by positive and negative affective reactions to their first report cards: grades that produced a positive reaction were associated with an increase in emotional and behavioral engagement, but grades that produced a negative reaction were associated with decreased emotional engagement.

Feedback   Students are frustrated when they receive poor grades with little to no feedback from a teacher on what they did wrong or how they can improve. If students receive enough poor grades without feedback, especially if they tried hard to succeed in a particular task, they often conclude that they are just not competent enough to do well in a particular class; over time, they may decide that school is just too difficult. Hattie and Timperley (2007) reviewed 12 meta-analyses examining the influence feedback has on student learning and achievement and found a high average effect size (0.79) of feedback on achievement. However, they noted that studies in which the feedback focused on a specific task, providing information on how to do it more effectively, had larger effect sizes on achievement than feedback that merely praised, rewarded, or censured a student. They concluded that feedback needs to be clear, purposeful, meaningful, and prompt.

One reason that feedback is such a strong predictor of achievement is its impact on engagement. In a large-scale observation of the UK primary classrooms, Apter et al. (2010) found that student on-task behavior during lessons was related to the frequency with which their teachers provided positive feedback. Sutherland et al. (2000) also examined the effect of praise on the engagement of students with emotional and behavioral disorders. Students' on-task behavior increased proportionately to behavior-specific praise.

Teachers can also raise or undermine students' self-efficacy through appraisals of their schoolwork. Usher and Pajares (2006) examined social persuasion, defined as encouragement students receive from significant others, as a means of raising students' self-efficacy in middle school students, finding that social persuasion accounted for 17% of the variance in self-efficacy for girls (though it was not a predictor for boys). This suggests that adolescent girls are more attuned to the messages they receive from teachers and other trusted adults than boys.

Giving Students Agency Over Their Learning

Students, especially adolescents, need to feel that they have some agency over their lives and their education (see also Reeve & Jang, chapter "Agentic Engagement", this volume). In self-determination theory, this feeling of agency is referred to as autonomy, which has been defined as "regulation by the self" and is compared to heteronomy, "regulation that occurs without self-

endorsement" (Ryan & Deci, 2006, p. 1557). According to the basic needs theory, which is a part of the larger self-determination theory, autonomy is one of three basic needs that must be met for someone to be motivated (Ryan & Deci, 2000). In a recent study, we found that a preference for autonomy, as it relates to reading, (e.g., "Choosing what I want to read is important to me") was significantly related to reading behavior, engagement, and achievement in grades 5–8 (Davis et al., 2020). However, adolescents are not often given agency in their education. In a recent study of 3300 high school students in the USA., only 41% reported feeling that they have a voice or power in their schools (Margolius et al., 2020). Further, Guthrie and Davis (2003) found that autonomy support for literacy (e.g., "My teacher lets me decide what science topic I should read and write about") was highest for third-grade students, lower for fifth-grade students, and even lower for eighth-grade students.

Student Choice

One way to increase autonomy is to allow students to make choices related to their learning. When students are given a choice (e.g., which book to read in ELA class), they take ownership in the choice and are more motivated to try hard than students who are not provided a choice (e.g., told which book to read) (Beymer & Thomson, 2015). The provision of choice relates to the outcomes such as effort, task performance, perceived competence, and preference for the challenge (Patall et al., 2008). Schools with a high percentage of low-income students often offer students less choice in learning than schools in wealthier districts (Duke, 2000; Flowerday & Schraw, 2000). Some teachers are reluctant to give their students choices for fear of losing control over the classroom (Flowerday & Schraw, 2000; Netcoh, 2017).

The provision of choice is one of the five components of motivational support in the Concept-Oriented Reading Instruction program (Guthrie et al., 2004). A study of this program found that support for motivation increased reading comprehension, motivation, and strategy use compared to students who received only strategy instruction or traditional instruction. Further, in a study on homework completion, Patall et al. (2010) found that students given a choice of homework options reported higher levels of intrinsic motivation, competency levels, and achievement on the unit test, compared to students who did not have a choice.

The way choice is offered may determine how effective it is. For example, in a review of research on choice, Katz and Assor (2007) found that providing choice is more effective when the choice is relevant to students' interests and goals, is not complex, does not offer too many options, and is congruent with the values of the student's culture. In a meta-analysis of articles related to the provision of choice, Patall et al. (2008) found that the effect of choice on intrinsic motivation was stronger when certain conditions were met: when participants were given two to four options, were children, and were not also offered an extrinsic reward for completing the task.

Merely providing choice to students may not be as effective as using choice along with other strategies to support autonomy. In reviewing articles on support for autonomy, Patall and Zambrano (2019) found that in addition to providing choice, teachers must also give a rationale that helps students understand the value of learning activities and seek out and validate students' perspectives during instruction. All three of these strategies increase students' feelings of autonomy. For example, Patall et al. (2013) asked high school students and their teachers to report on teacher practices and autonomy need satisfaction. Both the provision of choice and teacher attentiveness to students' perspectives were correlated to higher autonomy need satisfaction.

It may also be that some students benefit from the provision of choice more than others. For example, Patall et al. (2014) found that students with high levels of confidence are more motivated by choice than students with lower levels of confidence in a task. It may also be that those with low confidence, when provided a choice, will select the easier task. For example, Parkhurst (2011) examined if college students would select to either complete an assignment that was already started, but had 10 more problems to finish, or start a new assignment that would be slightly less work with only nine more problems to finish. Instead of feeling motivated to finish the original assignment as might have been expected from past research on assignment completion (Hawthorn-Embree et al., 2011), most students in the Parkhurst study (77.6%) elected to do the easier assignment, showing that college students may be more likely to take effort into account over the drive to finish a particular assignment. The selection of completing a task was positively related to students' value of hard work; students who valued hard work were more likely to select to finish the higher effort assignment. Therefore, the provision of choice may benefit those with higher confidence and those who value hard work compared to those with less confidence and hold hard work in less value.

Building Connections to Careers

Another way to build a student's feelings of agency in school is by helping them explore future careers. This enables students to select courses that will help them in their life beyond high school, rather than taking courses just because their parents or counselors suggest them. In addition, when students have a career goal in view, their classwork becomes more meaningful as a steppingstone to their future success. Students become motivated to do well because it matters to their personal goals, rather than to please a teacher, parent, or other external influencer. This can be seen in a study on work-based learning by Kenny et al. (2010), who found that students with "work hope," defined as students with goals for future employment, a plan for obtaining it, and confidence that they will do well in it, had higher levels of academic efficacy, mastery goals, and understanding of the relevance of school for future success.

Career preparation is significantly related to student engagement and grades for secondary students. Using structural equation modeling on survey responses of secondary students, Perry et al. (2010) found that career preparation (a combination of career decision-making self-efficacy and career planning readiness) had a significant direct effect on school engagement (defined in this study as identification with school and behavioral engagement) and a significant indirect positive effect on grades through school engagement. Further, Kenny et al. (2006) examined student engagement over time and found that higher levels of career planning and expectations at the start of ninth grade were associated with increased engagement (defined in this study as belonging and valuing) during the year. In our own study, we found that for ninth-grade students, the amount of career focus in a school (e.g. "This school has really helped me understand the jobs or careers that fit me best.") was related positively and significantly to interest in schoolwork (e.g., "I think that what we are learning in my classes is interesting"), self-efficacy for schoolwork (e.g., "If I try hard, I believe I can do my schoolwork well"), and effort (e.g., "If I don't understand my schoolwork, I keep trying until I do"; Davis et al., 2015). Career focus was negatively correlated to disengagement (e.g., "I cut class or skipped school") and giving up interest (e.g., "I don't really care about school").

Career Explorations and Experiences In the mid-to late 1990s, the School-to-Work Opportunities Act (STWOA) provided funding to states and school districts for programs that would support high school students in job selection and preparation. However, since the act expired in 2002, many high schools have offered less career exploration, instead preferring to focus on academic study and college preparation. Some may have worried that presenting both vocational and college options might confuse students who should be aspiring to attend college. Or perhaps they feel that vocational courses could pull lower performing students into low-paying vocational tracks and away from higher paying career options. In any case, school counselors do not have the time or resources to provide career exploration and experiences for all of their students. However, an examination of STW programs found that students in career explora-

tion programs, including job shadowing, mentoring, and tech prep opportunities, were *more* likely to take college entrance and advanced placement exams than those not participating in these programs (Visher et al., 2004), indicating that these programs did not deflect students from applying to college. In addition, participating students were more likely to graduate from high school, enroll in college, and attend a 2-year rather than a 4-year college; this strongly suggests that these programs encouraged students to attend college who would not have otherwise done so.

Use of Success Mentors Adult and peer role models are necessary to help students develop career goals. In a study of ninth-grade urban students, Kenny and Bledsoe (2005) found that social support from family, teachers, and peers contributed to career outcome expectations. Further, Perry et al. (2010) found that both parental career support and teacher career support had significant direct effects on career preparation and significant indirect effects on engagement, through career preparation.

College-educated adults serving as mentors help increase students' aspirations for postsecondary education and training. One recommendation of the U.S. Department of Education practice guide on helping students navigate the path to college by Tierney et al. (2009) is to "surround students with adults and peers who build and support their college-going aspirations" (p. 26). Studies reviewed found that factors with the highest impact on college enrollment included mentoring services. In these programs, students regularly met one-on-one with college-educated adults who helped them with college guidance and preparation. The guide suggests that schools consider using near-peer mentors: recent high school graduates who were enrolled in college.

Putting It All Together

In this chapter, we reviewed ways in which schools can track student engagement and actions they can take to get secondary students who have become disengaged in school back on track.

Student engagement in middle and high school is important for both their success in school, which leads to graduation, and their postsecondary success. Those who become disengaged during their secondary schooling will limit their options for future careers and earning potential.

The first step in getting students back on track is to track engagement. Although it is very easy for teachers and administrators to focus on the students who are the most disruptive, only through tracking indicators, such as attendance, behavior, and course performance can educators see who needs support before they get too far behind. If data is tracked regularly and interventions are assigned, they may be able to catch a student mid-quarter rather than at the end of the year when little to nothing can be done.

The next step is implementing interventions. We suggest interventions that have been used to successfully increase secondary student school engagement. Each set of recommended interventions is based on one of the three basic needs from the self-determination theory. The first set of interventions are those that increase relationships in their school. These interventions, such as those that strengthen teacher–student, peer–peer, and school–parent connections, have shown to increase student engagement. The second set of interventions are those that increase students' feelings of competence and include matching the level of instruction to the student, afterschool tutoring, and informative adequate feedback. Finally, the last set of interventions are those that support student agency and autonomy over their own learning. These include providing student choice and helping students explore careers.

Interventions should be tiered in that they apply both individual student interventions (Tier 3) such as a phone call home or discipline tracking sheet as well as interventions that apply to groups of students (Tier 2) such as tutoring groups, or interventions for whole-school reforms (Tier 1) such as changing disciplinary practices for the whole school or implementation of job explorations for a grade. Since there is only so much a school can do, they will need to prioritize based on the school's specific population and needs. For example, some schools may select one

Tier 1 goal each month, such as building teacher–student relationships or integrating into job explorations. However, this is a large undertaking for a school, especially those that are under-resourced. Below are strategies we have used to make this work doable within a school.

We began this chapter by considering the importance of using school teams to track engagement and implement interventions. We then explored interventions that school teams can use to increase engagement. However, this is a large undertaking, especially for under-resourced schools. Below are strategies we have seen used to make this work doable in such schools.

Organizing a team The work is too much for one individual. In our research, we have seen Early Warning Indicator teams used to track student data, organize team meetings, and identify, implement, and monitor interventions (Davis et al., 2018; Mac Iver et al., 2019). School teams often consist of core teachers (math, science, English, and history) and an administrator. Some teams have included other school personnel, such as elective and special education teachers, school behavior specialists, guidance counselors, sports coaches, volunteers, and school nurses.

Community partners School teams may need external help to begin or maintain the process. Teams can reach out to community organizations to help with report card conferences or as career mentors. Teams should create a list of partners that can help families with job placement, financial support, and other needs.

Networking As more school teams focus on engagement, it is helpful for teams to meet and share information, strategies, and best practices. From our work with supporting districts and states in implementing early warning systems (Davis, 2012; Mac Iver & Balfanz, 2021; MDRC, 2015), we have seen firsthand the power of connecting adults doing similar work in different schools, or even within schools to share learnings and work collectively to solve common problems of practice. Teachers are more often willing to adopt new practices when they hear from a peer that it works. Participants in the multiple networks in the Everyone Graduates Center have organized a number of networks such as the network of Diplomas Now schools and the ECHO EWS network in New Mexico. These groups report that networking enabled them to see that they were not alone, that they were not the only ones struggling with an issue or a challenge, and that they had good ideas to share with others, which increased their sense of agency in increasing student engagement.

Conclusion

In conclusion, as we have stated, although it takes a great deal of dedication and organization, school teams can both accurately track student engagement and effectively implement interventions to get students back on track to graduation and postsecondary success. Interventions should focus on one or more of the three basic needs from the self-determination theory that are related highly to motivation and engagement: relatedness, competence, and autonomy. Schools and students will likely see the most benefits if they implement several interventions that align with each of these needs in tandem.

References

Allen, K., Kern, M. L., Vella-Brodrick, D., Hattie, J., & Waters, L. (2016). *What schools need to know about fostering school belonging: A meta-analysis.* https://doi.org/10.1007/s10648-016-9389-8

Allensworth, E. (2012). Want to improve teaching? Create collaborative, supportive schools. *American Educator, 36*(3), 30–31. https://eric.ed.gov/?id=EJ986682

Allensworth, E. (2013). The use of ninth grade early warning indicators to improve Chicago schools. *Journal of Education for Students Placed at Risk, 18,* 68–83. https://doi.org/10.1080/10824669.2013.745181

Allensworth, E. M., & Easton, J. Q. (2005). *The on-track indicator as a predictor of high school graduation.* Consortium on Chicago School Research. Retrieved from https://consortium.uchicago.edu/publications/track-indicator-predictor-high-school-graduation

Allensworth, E. M., & Easton, J. Q. (2007). *What matters for staying on-track and graduating in Chicago public high schools.* Consortium on Chicago School Research. https://consortium.uchicago.edu/sites/

default/files/2018-10/07%20What%20Matters%20Final.pdf

Anderman, E. M., & Maehr, M. L. (1994). Motivation and schooling in the middle grades. *Review of Educational Research, 64*(2), 287–309. https://doi.org/10.3102/00346543064002287

Anderson, L. M., Stevens, D. D., Prawat, R. S., & Nickerson, J. (1988). Classroom task environments and students' task-related beliefs. *The Elementary School Journal, 88*(3), 281–295. https://doi.org/10.1086/461539

Anderson, A. R., Christenson, S. L., Sinclair, M. F., & Lehr, C. A. (2004). Check & connect: The importance of relationships for promoting engagement with school. *Journal of School Psychology, 42*(2), 95–113. https://doi.org/10.1016/j.jsp.2004.01.002

Anyon, Y., Jenson, J., Altschul, I., Farrar, J., McQueen, J., Greer, E., … Simmons, J. (2014). The persistent effect of race and the promise of alternatives to suspension in school discipline outcomes. *Children & Youth Services Review, 44,* 379–386. https://doi.org/10.1016/j.childyouth.2014.06.025

Apter, B., Arnold, C., & Swinson, J. (2010). A mass observation study of student and teacher behaviour in British primary classrooms. *Educational Psychology in Practice, 26*(2), 151–171. https://doi.org/10.1080/02667361003768518

Baker, C. (2019). *Experiences of nontraditional high school English language learner students partaking in service learning* (Unpublished doctoral dissertation). Capella University. https://search.proquest.com/docview/2281091874?pq-origsite=gscholar&fromopenview=true

Balfanz, R., & Boccanfuso, C. (2007). *Falling off the path to graduation: Middle grade indicators in [an unidentified northeastern city].* Center for Social Organization of Schools.

Balfanz, R., & Byrnes, V. (2010). *Dropout prevention through early warning indicators: A current distribution in West Virginia schools.* Everyone Graduates Center.

Balfanz, R., & Byrnes, V. (2019). *College, career, and life readiness: A look at high school indicators of post-secondary outcomes in Boston.* Retrieved from the Everyone Graduates Center website: http://new.every1graduates.org/wp-content/uploads/2019/02/BOA_ReadinessReport2019-03_FINAL.pdf.

Balfanz, R., & Herzog, L. (2005). *Keeping middle grades students on-track to graduation: Initial analysis and implications.* Presentation at the second Regional Middle Grades Symposium, .

Balfanz, R., Herzog, L., & Mac Iver, D. J. (2007). Preventing student disengagement and keeping students on the graduation path in urban middle-grades schools: Early identification and effective interventions. *Educational Psychologist, 42*(4), 223–235. https://doi.org/10.1080/00461520701621079

Baltimore Education Research Consortium. (2011). *Destination graduation: Sixth grade early warning indicators for Baltimore City schools—Their preva-*

lence and impact. Author. http://baltimore-berc.org/pdfs/SixthGradeEWIFullReport.pdf

Baumeister, R. F., & Leary, M. R. (1995). The need to belong: Desire for interpersonal attachments as a fundamental human motivation. *Psychological Bulletin, 117*(3), 497.

Bempechat, J., & Shernoff, D. J. (2012). Parental influences on achievement motivation and student engagement. In *Handbook of research on student engagement* (pp. 315–342). Springer. https://link.springer.com/chapter/10.1007/978-1-4614-2018-7_15

Benner, A. D. (2011). The transition to high school: Current knowledge, future directions. *Educational Psychology Review, 23*(3), 299. https://link.springer.com/content/pdf/10.1007/s10648-011-9152-0.pdf

Benner, A. D., & Graham, S. (2009). The transition to high school as a developmental process among multiethnic urban youth. *Child Development, 80*(2), 356–376. https://doi.org/10.1111/j.1467-8624.2009.01265.x

Beymer, P. N., & Thomson, M. M. (2015). The effects of choice in the classroom: Is there too little or too much choice? *Support for Learning, 30*(2), 105–120. https://doi.org/10.1111/1467-9604.12086

Blum, R. W., McNeely, C., & Rinehart, P. M. (2002). *(2002). Improving the odds: The untapped power of schools to improve the health of teens.* Center for Adolescent Health and Development, University of Minnesota. https://www.casciac.org/pdfs/ImprovingtheOdds.pdf

Booker, K. C. (2004). Exploring school belonging and academic achievement in African American adolescents. *Curriculum and Teaching Dialogue, 6*(2), 131. https://search.proquest.com/docview/230426476?accountid=11752

Boonk, L., Gijselaers, H. J., Ritzen, H., & Brand-Gruwel, S. (2018). A review of the relationship between parental involvement indicators and academic achievement. *Educational Research Review, 24*, 10–30. https://doi.org/10.1016/j.edurev.2018.02.001

Bradshaw, C. P., Mitchell, M. M., & Leaf, P. J. (2010). Examining the effects of schoolwide positive behavioral interventions and supports on student outcomes: Results from a randomized controlled effectiveness trial in elementary schools. *Journal of Positive Behavior Interventions, 12*(3), 133–148. https://doi.org/10.1177/1098300709334798

Bradshaw, C. P., Waasdorp, T. E., & Leaf, P. J. (2012). Effects of school-wide positive behavioral interventions and supports on child behavior problems. *Pediatrics, 130*(5), e1136–e1145. https://doi.org/10.1542/peds.2012-0243

Cameron, J., Banko, K. M., & Pierce, W. D. (2001). Pervasive negative effects of rewards on intrinsic motivation: The myth continues. *The Behavior Analyst, 24*(1), 1–44. https://doi.org/10.1007/BF03392017

Cameron, J., Pierce, W. D., Banko, K. M., & Gear, A. (2005). Achievement-based rewards and intrinsic motivation: A test of cognitive mediators. *Journal of educational psychology, 97*(4), 641. https://doi.org/10.1037/0022-0663.97.4.641

Celio, C. I., Durlak, J., & Dymnicki, A. (2011). A meta-analysis of the impact of service-learning on students. *The Journal of Experimental Education, 34*(2), 164–181. https://doi.org/10.1177/105382591103400205

Centre for Education Statistics & Evaluation, NSW Department of Education (2017). *The role of student engagement in the transition from primary to secondary school (Learning Curve 19).* Retrieved from https://www.cese.nsw.gov.au//images/stories/PDF/transition-primary_secondary_AA.pdf

Clark, S. N., & Clark, D. C. (1994). *Restructuring the middle level school: Implications for school leaders.* SUNY Press.

Cook, C. R., Thayer, A. J., Fiat, A., & Sullivan, M. (2020). Interventions to enhance affective engagement. In A. L. Reschly, A. J. Pohl, & S. L. Christenson (Eds.), *Student engagement: Effective academic, behavioral, cognitive, and affective interventions at school* (pp. 203–237). Springer International Publishing. https://doi.org/10.1007/978-3-030-37285-9_12

Darling, N., Caldwell, L. L., & Smith, R. (2005). Participation in school based extracurricular activities and adolescent adjustment. *Journal of Leisure Research, 37*(1), 51–76. https://doi.org/10.1080/00222216.2005.11950040

Davis, M. (2012). *Using data to keep all students on-track for graduation: Team playbook.* Retrieved from the Everyone Graduates Center website: http://new.every1graduates.org/wp-content/uploads/2012/01/Team_Playbook_MarciaDavis.pdf

Davis, M. H. (2019). *Predicting early warning indicators: Attendance and course performance.* Annual Meeting of the American Educational Research Association, Toronto, Canada. https://www.aera.net.

Davis, M. H., Mac Iver, M. A., & Stein, M. L. (2015). *Effects of an early-warning indicator and intervention system on student engagement.* Annual meeting of the American Educational Research Association, Chicago. https://www.aera.net

Davis, M. H., Mac Iver, M., Balfanz, R., Stein, M., & Fox, J. (2018). Implementation of an early warning indicator and intervention system. *Preventing School Failure.* https://doi.org/10.1080/1045988X.2018.1506977

Davis, M. H., Wang, W., Kingston, N., Hock, M., Tonks, S. M., & Tiemann (2020). A computer adaptive measure of reading motivation. Journal of Research in Reading. https://onlinelibrary.wiley.com/doi/full/10.1111/1467-9817.12318

Deci, E. L., Koestner, R., & Ryan, R. M. (1999). The undermining effect is a reality after all—Extrinsic rewards, task interest, and self-determination: Reply to Eisenberger, Pierce, and Cameron (1999) and Lepper, Henderlong, and Gingras (1999). https://doi.org/10.1037/0033-2909.125.6.692

Deci, E. L., & Ryan, R. M. (2000). The "what" and "why" of goal pursuits: Human needs and the self-determination of behavior. *Psychological Inquiry, 11*(4), 227–268. https://doi.org/10.1207/S15327965PLI1104_01

Dietrichson, J., Bøg, M., Filges, T., & Jørgensen, A. M. (2017). Academic interventions for elementary and middle school students with low socioeconomic status: A systematic review and meta-analysis. *Review of Educational Research, 87*(2), 243–282. https://doi.org/10.3102/2F0034654316687036

Duke, N. K. (2000). For the rich it's richer: Print experiences and environments offered to children in very low-and very high-socioeconomic status first-grade classrooms. *American Educational Research Journal, 37*(2), 441–478. https://doi.org/10.3102/00028312037002441

Dynarski, M., Clarke, L., Cobb, B., Finn, J., Rumberger, R., & Smink, J. (2008). *Dropout prevention: A practice guide (NCEE 2008–4025)*. U.S. Department of Education, Institute of Education Sciences, National Center for Education Evaluation and Regional Assistance. http://eric.ed.gov/?id=ED502502

Eccles, J. S., & Midgley, C. (1989). Stage-environment fit: Developmentally appropriate classrooms for young adolescents. *Research on motivation in education, 3*(1), 139–186.

Faircloth, B. S., & Hamm, J. V. (2005). Sense of belonging among high school students representing 4 ethnic groups. *Journal of Youth and Adolescence, 34*(4), 293–309. https://doi.org/10.1007/s10964-005-5752-7

Farb, A. F., & Matjasko, J. L. (2012). Recent advances in research on school-based extracurricular activities and adolescent development. *Developmental Review, 32*(1), 1–48. https://doi.org/10.1016/j.dr.2011.10.001

Faria, A.-M., Sorensen, N., Heppen, J., Bowdon, J., Taylor, S., Eisner, R., & Foster, S. (2017). *Getting students on track for graduation: Impacts of the Early Warning Intervention and Monitoring System after one year (REL 2017–272)*. U.S. Department of Education, Institute of Education Sciences, National Center for Education Evaluation and Regional Assistance, Regional Educational Laboratory Midwest. Retrieved from https://ies.ed.gov/ncee/edlabs/regions/midwest/pdf/REL_2017272.pdf

Feldman, A. F., & Matjasko, J. L. (2005). The role of school-based extracurricular activities in adolescent development: A comprehensive review and future directions. *Review of Educational Research, 75*(2), 159–210. https://doi.org/10.3102/00346543075002159

Ferlazzo, L., & Hammond, L. A. (2009). *Building parent engagement in schools*. ABC-CLIO.

Fine, M. (1991). *Framing dropouts: Notes on the politics of an urban public high school*. State University of New York Press.

Flowerday, T., & Schraw, G. (2000). Teacher beliefs about instructional choice: A phenomenological study. *Journal of Educational Psychology, 92*, 634–645. https://doi.org/10.1037/0022-0663.92.4.634

Fredricks, J. A., Blumenfeld, P. C., & Paris, A. H. (2004). School engagement: Potential of the concept, state of the evidence. *Review of Educational Research, 74*(1), 59–109. https://doi.org/10.3102/00346543074001059

Fredricks, J. A., Reschly, A. L., & Christenson, S. L. (2019). Handbook of student engagement interventions: Working with disengaged students. *Elsevier*. https://doi.org/10.1016/C2016-0-04519-9

Furrer, C., & Skinner, E. (2003). Sense of relatedness as a factor in children's academic engagement and performance. *Journal of Educational Psychology, 95*(1), 148. https://doi.org/10.1037/0022-0663.95.1.148

Gnambs, T., & Hanfstingl, B. (2016). The decline of academic motivation during adolescence: An accelerated longitudinal cohort analysis on the effect of psychological need satisfaction. *Educational Psychology, 36*(9), 1691–1705. https://www.tandfonline.com/doi/full/10.1080/01443410.2015.1113236

Gregory, A., & Skiba, R. J. (2019). Reducing suspension and increasing equity through supportive and engaging schools. In J. A. Fredricks, A. L. Reschly, & S. L. Christenson (Eds.), *Handbook of student engagement interventions* (pp. 121–134). Academic Press. https://doi.org/10.1016/B978-0-12-813413-9.00009-7

Gregory, A., Clawson, K., Davis, A., & Gerewitz, J. (2016). The promise of restorative practices to transform teacher-student relationships and achieve equity in school discipline. *Journal of Educational and Psychological Consultation, 26*(4), 325–353. https://doi.org/10.1080/10474412.2014.929950

Gregory, A., Huang, F. L., Anyon, Y., Greer, E., & Downing, B. (2018). An examination of restorative interventions and racial equity in out-of-school suspensions. *School Psychology Review, 47*(2), 167–182.

Guthrie, J. T., & Davis, M. H. (2003). Motivating struggling readers in middle school through an engagement model of classroom practice. *Reading and Writing Quarterly, 19*, 59–85. https://doi.org/10.1080/10573560308203

Guthrie, J. T., & Wigfield, A. (2000). Engagement and motivation in reading. In M. L. Kamil, P. B. Mosenthal, P. D. Pearson, & R. Barr (Eds.), *Handbook of reading research*. Routledge.

Guthrie, J. T., Wigfield, A., Barbosa, P., Perencevich, K. C., Taboada, A., Davis, M. H., Scafiddi, N. T., & Tonks, S. (2004). Increasing reading comprehension and engagement through concept-oriented reading instruction. *Journal of Educational Psychology, 96*(3), 403–423. https://doi.org/10.1037/0022-0663.96.3.403

Guttman, H. M. (2008). *Great business teams: Cracking the code for standout performance*. Wiley.

Hagan, J., & Foster, H. (2012). Intergenerational educational effects of mass imprisonment in America. *Sociology of Education, 85*(3), 259–286. https://doi.org/10.1177/0038040711431587

Hattie, J., & Timperley, H. (2007). The power of feedback. *Review of Educational Research, 77*(1), 81–112. https://doi.org/10.3102/003465430298487

Hawthorn-Embree, M. L., Skinner, C. H., Parkhurst, J., & Conley, E. (2011). An investigation of the partial-assignment completion effect on students' assignment choice behavior. *Journal of School Psychology, 49*(4), 433–442.

Hill, N. E., & Tyson, D. F. (2009). Parental involvement in middle school: A meta-analytic assessment of the strategies that promote achievement. *Developmental*

Psychology, 45(3), 740–763. https://doi.org/10.1037/a0015362

Hirsch, B. J. (1988). *Moving into adolescence: The impact of pubertal change and school context*, Simmons, R.G., Blyth, D. A. (1987) (Aldine De Gruyter). https://doi.org/10.4324/9781315124841.

Holland, A., & Andre, T. (1987). Participation in extracurricular activities in secondary school: What is known, what needs to be known? *Review of Educational Research, 57*, 437–466. https://doi.org/10.3102/00346543057004437

Hughes, J. N., Im, M. H., & Allee, P. J. (2015). Effect of school belonging trajectories in grades 6–8 on achievement: Gender and ethnic differences. *Journal of School Psychology, 53*(6), 493–507. https://doi.org/10.1016/j.jsp.2015.08.001

Huguley, J. P., Delale-O'Connor, L., Wang, M. T., & Parr, A. K. (2021). African American parents' educational involvement in urban schools: Contextualized strategies for student success in adolescence. *Educational Researcher, 50*(1), 6–16. https://doi.org/10.3102/0013189X20943199

Juvonen, J. (2006). Sense of belonging, social bonds, and school functioning. In P. A. Alexander & P. H. Winne (Eds.), *Handbook of educational psychology* (pp. 655–674). Lawrence Erlbaum Associates Publishers. https://psycnet.apa.org/record/2006-07986-028

Juvonen, J., Espinoza, G., & Knifsend, C. (2012). The role of peer relationships in student academic and extracurricular engagement. In *Handbook of research on student engagement* (pp. 387–401). Springer. https://doi.org/10.1007/978-1-4614-2018-7_18

Katz, I., & Assor, A. (2007). When choice motivates and when it does not. *Educational Psychology Review, 19*(4), 429. https://link.springer.com/content/pdf/10.1007/s10648-006-9027-y.pdf

Kenny, M. E., & Bledsoe, M. (2005). Contributions of the relational context to career adaptability among urban adolescents. *Journal of Vocational Behavior, 66*(2), 257–272. https://doi.org/10.1016/j.jvb.2004.10.002

Kenny, M. E., Blustein, D. L., Haase, R. F., Jackson, J., & Perry, J. C. (2006). Setting the stage: Career development and the student engagement process. *Journal of Counseling Psychology, 53*(2), 272. https://doi.org/10.1037/0022-0167.53.2.272

Kenny, M. E., Walsh-Blair, L. Y., Blustein, D. L., Bempechat, J., & Seltzer, J. (2010). Achievement motivation among urban adolescents: Work hope, autonomy support, and achievement-related beliefs. *Journal of Vocational Behavior, 77*(2), 205–212. https://doi.org/10.1016/j.jvb.2010.02.005

Kim, Y. (2009). Minority parental involvement and school barriers: Moving the focus away from deficiencies of parents. *Educational Research Review, 4*(2), 80–102. https://doi.org/10.1016/j.edurev.2009.02.003

Kittelman, A., McIntosh, K., & Hoselton, R. (2019). Adoption of PBIS within school districts. *Journal of School Psychology, 76*, 159–167. https://doi.org/10.1016/j.jsp.2019.03.007

Knifsend, C., Espinoza, G., & Juvonen, J. (2021). Title here. In *Handbook of research on student engagement* (2nd ed., pp. X–X). Springer.

Kraft, M. A., & Rogers, T. (2015). The underutilized potential of teacher-to-parent communication: Evidence from a field experiment. *Economics of Education Review, 47*, 49–63. https://doi.org/10.1016/j.econedurev.2015.04.001

Krone, E. (2019). *The make-or-break year: Solving the dropout crisis one ninth grader at a time*. The New Press.

Lutz, S. L., Guthrie, J. T., & Davis, M. H. (2006). Scaffolding for engagement in elementary school reading instruction. *Journal of Educational Research, 100*(1), 3–20. https://doi.org/10.3200/JOER.100.1.3-20

Mac Iver, M.A. & Balfanz, R. (In press, forthcoming Fall 2021). *Continuous improvement in high schools: Helping more students succeed* (Harvard Education Press).

Mac Iver, M. A., Balfanz, R., & Byrnes, V. (2009). *Advancing the "Colorado Graduates" agenda: Understanding the dropout problem and mobilizing to meet the graduation challenge*. Colorado Children's Campaign. https://files.eric.ed.gov/fulltext/ED539116.pdf

Mac Iver, M. A., Stein, M., & L., Davis, M. H., Balfanz, R., & Fox, J. (2019). An efficacy study of a ninth grade early warning indicator intervention. *Journal of Research on Educational Effectiveness, 12*, 363–390. https://doi.org/10.1080/19345747.2019.1615156

Margolius M., Lynch, A D., Hynes, M., Glanagan, S., & Jones E. P. (2020). *What drives learning: Young people's perspectives on the importance of relationships, belonging, and agency*. https://www.americaspromise.org/resource/what-drives-learning-young-peoples-perspectives-importance-relationships-belonging-agency

McIntosh, K., Girvan, E. J., Horner, R. H., & Smolkowski, K. (2014). Education not incarceration: A conceptual model for reducing racial and ethnic disproportionality in school discipline. *Journal of Applied Research on Children: Informing Policy for Children at Risk, 5*(2), article 4. https://files.eric.ed.gov/fulltext/EJ1188503.pdf

MDRC. (2015). *Moving down the track*. https://www.mdrc.org/publication/moving-down-track

Meyer, R., Carl, B., & Cheng, H. E. (2010). *Accountability and performance in secondary education in Milwaukee Public Schools*. Council for Great City Schools. https://files.eric.ed.gov/fulltext/ED518089.pdf

Mhurchu, C. N., Gorton, D., Turley, M., Jiang, Y., Michie, J., Maddison, R., & Hattie, J. (2013). Effects of a free school breakfast programme on children's attendance, academic achievement and short-term hunger: Results from a stepped-wedge, cluster randomized controlled trial. *Journal of Epidemiology & Community Health, 67*(3), 257–264. https://doi.org/10.1136/jech-2012-201540

Neild, R. C., & Balfanz, R. (2006). *Unfulfilled promise: The dimensions and characteristics of Philadelphia's dropout crisis, 2002–2005*. Philadelphia Youth Transitions Collaborative. https://files.eric.ed.gov/fulltext/ED538341.pdf

Netcoh, S. (2017). Balancing freedom and limitations: A case study of choice provision in a personalized learning class. *Teaching and Teacher Education, 66*, 383–392. https://doi.org/10.1016/j.tate.2017.05.010

Orfield, G. (2004). *Dropouts in America: Confronting the graduation rate crisis*. Harvard Education Press. https://eric.ed.gov/?id=ed568740

Pak, C. S. (2018). Linking service-learning with sense of belonging: A culturally relevant pedagogy for heritage students of Spanish. *Journal of Hispanic Higher Education, 17*(1), 76–95. https://doi.org/10.1177/1538192716630028

Parkhurst, J. T., Fleisher, M. S., Skinner, C. H., Woehr, D. J., & Hawthorn-Embree, M. L. (2011). Assignment choice, effort, and assignment completion: Does work ethic predict those who choose higher-effort assignments? *Learning and Individual Differences, 21*(5), 575–579. https://doi.org/10.1016/j.lindif.2011.04.003

Patall, E. A., & Zambrano, J. (2019). Facilitating student outcomes by supporting autonomy: Implications for practice and policy. *Policy Insights From the Behavioral and Brain Sciences, 6*(2), 115–122. https://doi.org/10.1177/2372732219862572

Patall, E. A., Cooper, H., & Robinson, J. C. (2008). The effects of choice on intrinsic motivation and related outcomes: A meta-analysis of research findings. *Psychological Bulletin, 134*(2), 270–300. https://doi.org/10.1037/0033-2909.134.2.270

Patall, E. A., Cooper, H., & Wynn, S. R. (2010). The effectiveness and relative importance of providing choices in the classroom. *Journal of Educational Psychology, 102*, 896–915. https://doi.org/10.1037/a0019545

Patall, E. A., Dent, A. L., Oyer, M., & Wynn, S. R. (2013). Student autonomy and course value: The unique and cumulative roles of various teacher practices. *Motivation and Emotion, 37*(1), 14–32. https://doi.org/10.1007/s11031-012-9305-6

Patall, E. A., Sylvester, B. J., & Han, C. (2014). The role of competence in the effects of choice on motivation. *Journal of Experimental Social Psychology, 50*, 27–44. https://doi.org/10.1016/j.jesp.2013.09.002

Perry, J. C., Liu, X., & Pabian, Y. (2010). School engagement as a mediator of academic performance among urban youth: The role of career preparation, parental career support, and teacher support. *The Counseling Psychologist, 38*(2), 269–295. https://doi.org/10.1177/0011000009349272

Pianta, R. C., Hamre, B. K., & Allen, J. P. (2012). Teacher-student relationships and engagement: Conceptualizing, measuring, and improving the capacity of classroom interactions. In *Handbook of research on student engagement* (pp. 365–386). Springer. https://link.springer.com/chapter/10.1007/978-1-4614-2018-7_17

Pinkus, L. (2008). *Using early-warning data to improve graduation rates: Closing cracks in the education system (policy brief)*. Alliance for Excellent Education. http://eric.ed.gov/?id=ED510882

Poorthuis, A. M., Juvonen, J., Thomaes, S., Denissen, J. J., Orobio de Castro, B., & Van Aken, M. A. (2015). Do grades shape students' school engagement? The psychological consequences of report card grades at the beginning of secondary school. *Journal of Educational Psychology, 107*(3), 842. https://doi.org/10.1037/edu0000002

Preskill, H., & Torres, R. T. (1999). *Evaluative inquiry for learning in organizations*. Sage.

Räty, H. (2007). Parents' own school recollections influence their perception of the functioning of their child's school. *European Journal of Psychology of Education, 22*(3), 387–398. https://doi.org/10.1007/BF03173434

Reschly, A. L. (2020). Interventions to enhance academic engagement. In A. L. Reschly, A. J. Pohl, & S. L. Christenson (Eds.), *Student engagement: Effective academic, behavioral, cognitive, and affective interventions at school* (pp. 91–108). Springer International Publishing. https://doi.org/10.1007/978-3-030-37285-9_5

Reschly, A. L., & Christenson, S. L. (2019). The intersection of student engagement and families: A critical connection for achievement and life outcomes. In J. Fredricks, A. L. Reschly, & S. L. Christenson (Eds.), *Handbook of student engagement interventions: Working with disengaged youth*. Elsevier.

Resnick, M. D., Harris, L. J., & Blum, R. W. (1993). The impact of caring and connectedness on adolescent health and well-being. *Journal of Paediatrics and Child Health, 29*, S3–S9. https://doi.org/10.1111/j.1440-1754.1993.tb02257.x

Ritter, G. W., & Anderson, K. P. (2018). Examining disparities in student discipline: Mapping inequities from infractions to consequences. *Peabody Journal of Education, 93*(2), 161–173. https://doi.org/10.1080/0161956X.2018.1435038

Rocque, M., & Paternoster, R. (2011). Understanding the antecedents of the "school to jail" link: The relationship between race and school discipline. *The Journal of Criminal Law and Criminology*, 633–665. https://www.jstor.org/stable/23074048

Roderick, M., & Camburn, E. (1999). Risk and recovery from course failure in the early years of high school. *American Educational Research Journal, 36*(2), 303–343. https://doi.org/10.3102/00028312036002303

Roorda, D. L., Koomen, H. M., Spilt, J. L., & Oort, F. J. (2011). The influence of affective teacher–student relationships on students' school engagement and achievement: A meta-analytic approach. *Review of Educational Research, 81*(4), 493–529. https://doi.org/10.3102/0034654311421793

Roorda, D. L., Jak, S., Zee, M., Oort, F. J., & Koomen, H. M. Y. (2017). Affective teacher–student relationships and students' engagement and achievement: A meta-analytic update and test of the mediating role of engagement. *School Psychology Review, 46*(3), 239–261. https://doi.org/10.17105/SPR-2017-0035.V46-3

Rossi, B. R. (2002). *Impacts and effects of service-learning on high school students*. https://digitalcommons.unomaha.edu/slcedt/45/.

Rumberger, R. W., Addis, H., Allensworth, E., Balfanz, R., Bruch, J., Dillon, E., … Newman-Gonchar, R. (2017). *Preventing dropout in secondary schools. Educator's practice guide. What Works Clearinghouse. NCEE 2017–4028*. What Works Clearinghouse. https://ies.ed.gov/ncee/wwc/Docs/PracticeGuide/wwc_dropout_092617.pdf

Ryan, R. M., & Deci, E. L. (2000). The darker and brighter sides of human existence: Basic psychological needs as a unifying concept. *Psychological Inquiry, 11*(4), 319–338. https://doi.org/10.1207/S15327965PLI1104_03

Ryan, R. M., & Deci, E. L. (2006). Self-regulation and the problem of human autonomy: Does psychology need choice, self-determination, and will? *Journal of Personality, 74*(6), 1557–1586. https://doi.org/10.1111/j.1467-6494.2006.00420.x

Ryan, A. M., & Patrick, H. (2001). The classroom social environment and changes in adolescents' motivation and engagement during middle school. *American Educational Research Journal, 38*(2), 437–460. https://doi.org/10.3102/00028312038002437

Schunk, D. H., & Mullen, C. A. (2012). Self-efficacy as an engaged learner. In *Handbook of research on student engagement* (pp. 219–235). Springer. https://link.springer.com/chapter/10.1007/978-1-4614-2018-7_10

Scribner, J. P., Sawyer, R. K., Watson, S. T., & Myers, V. L. (2007). Teacher teams and distributed leadership: A study of group discourse and collaboration. *Educational Administration Quarterly, 43*(1), 67–100. https://doi.org/10.1177/0013161X06293631

Seidman, E., Aber, J. L., Allen, L., & French, S. E. (1996). The impact of the transition to high school on the self-system and perceived social context of poor urban youth. *American Journal of Community Psychology, 24*(4), 489–515. https://link.springer.com/article/10.1007%2FBF02506794

Shute, V. J., Hansen, E. G., Underwood, J. S., & Razzouk, R. (2011). A review of the relationship between parental involvement and secondary school students' academic achievement. *Education Research International, 2011*. http://downloads.hindawi.com/journals/edu/2011/915326.pdf

Silver, D., Saunders, M., & Zarate, E. (2008). *What factors predict high school graduation in the Los Angeles Unified School District* (California Dropout Research Project Report 14). Retrieved December 2, 2020, from https://www.issuelab.org/resources/11619/11619.pdf .

Skinner, E. A., & Belmont, M. J. (1993). Motivation in the classroom: Reciprocal effects of teacher behavior and student engagement across the school year. *Journal of Educational Psychology, 85*(4), 571. https://doi.org/10.1037/0022-0663.85.4.571

Skinner, E. A., & Pitzer, J. R. (2012). Developmental dynamics of student engagement, coping, and everyday resilience. In *Handbook of research on student engagement* (pp. 21–44). Springer. https://link.springer.com/chapter/10.1007/978-1-4614-2018-7_2

Skinner, E., Furrer, C., Marchand, G., & Kindermann, T. (2008). Engagement and disaffection in the classroom: Part of a larger motivational dynamic? *Journal of Educational Psychology, 100*, 765–781. https://doi.org/10.1037/a0012840

Smith, T. E., Sheridan, S. M., Kim, E. M., Park, S., & Beretvas, S. N. (2020). The effects of family-school partnership interventions on academic and social-emotional functioning: A meta-analysis exploring what works for whom. *Educational Psychology Review, 32*(2), 511–544. https://doi.org/10.1007/s10648-019-09509-w

Strolin-Goltzman, J., Sisselman, A., Melekis, K., & Auerbach, C. (2014). Understanding the relationship between school-based health center use, school connection, and academic performance. *Health & Social Work, 39*(2), 83–91. https://doi.org/10.1093/hsw/hlu018

Sutherland, K. S. (2000). Promoting positive interactions between teachers and students with emotional/behavioral disorders. *Preventing School Failure: Alternative Education for Children and Youth, 44*(3), 110–115. https://doi.org/10.1177/106342660000800101

Swain-Bradway, J., Pinkney, C., & Flannery, K. B. (2015). Implementing schoolwide positive behavior interventions and supports in high schools: Contextual factors and stages of implementation. *Teaching Exceptional Children, 47*(5), 245–255. https://doi.org/10.1177/0040059915580030

Therriault, S.B., O'Cummings, M., Heppen, J., Yerhot, L., & Scala, J. (2013). *High school early warning intervention monitoring system implementation guide*. Retrieved from http://www.earlywarningsystems.org/wp-content/uploads/2013/03/EWSHSImplementationguide2013.pdf.

Tierney, W. G., Bailey, T., Constantine, J., Finkelstein, N., & Hurd, N. F. (2009). *Helping students navigate the path to college: What high schools can do*. National Center for Education Evaluation and Regional Assistance, Institute of Education Sciences, US Department of Education. https://ies.ed.gov/ncee/wwc/Docs/PracticeGuide/higher_ed_pg_091509.pdf

U.S. Bureau of Labor Statistics. (2009). *Unemployment rates and earning by educational attainment*. https://www.bls.gov/emp/chart-unemployment-earnings-education.htm

U.S. Department of Education. (2016). *Issue brief: Early warning systems*. https://files.eric.ed.gov/fulltext/ED571990.pdf

Usher, E. L., & Pajares, F. (2006). Inviting confidence in school: Invitations as a critical source of the academic self-efficacy beliefs of entering middle school students. *Journal of Invitational Theory and Practice, 12*, 7–16. https://eric.ed.gov/?id=EJ766998

Velez, G., Hahn, M., Recchia, H., & Wainryb, C. (2020). Rethinking responses to youth rebellion: Recent growth and development of restorative practices in schools. *Current Opinion in Psychology*. https://doi.org/10.1016/j.copsyc.2020.02.011

Visher, M. G., Bhandari, R., & Medrich, E. (2004). High school career exploration programs: Do they work? *Phi Delta Kappan, 86*(2), 135–138. https://journals.sagepub.com/doi/pdf/10.1177/003172170408600210

Vygotsky, L. S. (1978). *Mind in society: The development of higher psychological processes*. Harvard University Press.

Wang, M. T., & Eccles, J. S. (2012). Adolescent behavioral, emotional, and cognitive engagement trajectories in school and their differential relations to educational success. *Journal of Research on Adolescence, 22*(1), 31–39. https://doi.org/10.1111/j.1532-7795.2011.00753.x

Wentzel, K. R., Muenks, K., McNeish, D., & Russell, S. (2017). Peer and teacher supports in relation to motivation and effort: A multi-level study. *Contemporary Educational Psychology, 49*, 32–45. https://doi.org/10.1016/j.cedpsych.2016.11.002

Wigfield, A. (1994). Expectancy-value theory of achievement motivation: A developmental perspective. *Educational Psychology Review, 6*, 49–78. https://doi.org/10.1007/BF02209024

Wisch, J. K., Ousterhout, B. H., Carter, V., & Orr, B. (2018). The grading gradient: Teacher motivations for varied redo and retake policies. *Studies in Educational Evaluation, 58*, 145–155. https://doi.org/10.1016/j.stueduc.2018.06.005

Yeager, D. S., & Bundick, M. J. (2009). The role of purposeful work goals in promoting meaning in life and in schoolwork during adolescence. *Journal of Adolescent Research, 24*(4), 423–452. https://doi.org/10.1177/0743558409336749

You, S., & Sharkey, J. (2009). Testing a developmental–ecological model of student engagement: a multilevel latent growth curve analysis. *Educational Psychology, 29*(6), 659–684. https://doi.org/10.1080/01443410903206815

The Role of Policy in Supporting Student Engagement

Cathy Wylie

Abstract

Student engagement in schools and learning needs research and evidence-informed policy to support schools and teachers. School leaders and teachers can find their efforts thwarted by system policies such as tracking or punishment-focussed discipline, rigid curriculum, and insufficient roles and time for teachers and others to work together and continually improve. This commentary uses recent policy around engagement in one schooling system, Aotearoa New Zealand, to show how it can affect schools' work to better engage students.

The chapters in this handbook provide rich research testimony to the importance of understanding student engagement in its different dimensions so that it can be nurtured in ways that benefit students, and those who work directly or live with them. Nurturing student engagement however often takes more than the individual knowledge or willingness of teachers and par-

C. Wylie (✉)
New Zealand Council for Educational Research, Wellington, New Zealand
e-mail: cathy.wylie@nzcer.org.nz

ents. The context in which student engagement in school and learning occurs can be traced to wider social structures and forces and to long-standing associated cultural beliefs that enter school and teaching practices, as Galindo, Brown, and Lee, chapter "Expanding an Equity Understanding of Student Engagement: The Macro (Social) and Micro (School) Contexts", this volume. There are encouraging signs that principals and teachers are now aware of unconscious bias and more focussed on using a lens of strengths rather than deficits. At the same time, such efforts can be undercut if the school or school system they work in continues with policies that discourage student belonging and motivation, such as tracking, or punishment-focussed discipline, and policies that tightly structure learning experiences, such as mandated curriculum and pacing calendars. Staffing policies also matter. For example, time for professional learning together, sharing what is working, and continually improving practice is not well-resourced as a regular part of school days. Few schooling systems resource schools sufficiently to provide a web of paraprofessionals or programmes that can make a difference for students starting to disengage or mired in disengagement. Often research-based and well-evaluated programmes that show improvements for such students are only funded for a limited time, or they become dependent on uncertain philanthropic funding.

In this commentary, I hope to underline the importance of intentionally thinking about policies that can enhance individual schools' work to improve student engagement: their attendance, their active emotional and cognitive participation in learning, their positive participation in school activities, seeing themselves as playing their part in a school community they value, and their motivation to learn and achieve. Policy includes mandates and funding related to engagement in the sense of attendance and participation, and sufficient staff in schools to work meaningfully with students. Policy also includes the framing of teaching and learning: qualifications, curriculum, and pedagogy, and how well these are included in teacher and leader preparation and professional development, so that students can be well engaged intellectually and motivated. How well are schools supported to do things differently where there is good reason to do so from research and evidence and changes in the social and cultural contexts? How well are schools supported to make the most of human and other resources for student – and staff – benefit?

What Does Policy Relating to Engagement Look Like with a System Lens? An Illustration

I had the opportunity to think about how policy can support student engagement when I co-edited the first version of this handbook, and again when reading several chapters for this second version. I come from a small country, Aotearoa New Zealand, a schooling system with 826,347 students in mid-2021, in just over 2500 self-managing schools. Our policy settings around curriculum and school management tend to the permissive. The national curriculum provides high-level guidance rather than prescription. By comparison with other systems, schools also have more latitude in how they run and use their resources, within national guidelines. Each school must report each year against their annual plan and goals, which invariably include academic achievement, student wellbeing, and some measure of engagement, usually attendance. But local Ministry of Education offices have not had a clear supportive role with schools, because they are self-managing. So, these annual reports are rarely used as input to ongoing work with a school. Another government agency, the Education Review Office (ERO) has notionally been the policy avenue to hold schools to account. ERO evaluated each school on a regular basis (most recently, on a cycle of every 3 years for most schools; 1–2 years for struggling schools and 4–5 years for schools deemed to be doing well). It has now changed this model of short visits to schools that schools often approached in a spirit of impression management and compliance because it had become clear that periodic evaluation on its own does not contribute to schools' ongoing capability to keep improving.

So much of what students experience depends on the quality of school leadership, teaching practices, and community engagement and resources at their individual schools. The cost of a policy framework centred on self-managing schools has become apparent: too much variability between schools, and insufficient progress in tackling the inequities apparent in lower rates of indigenous Māori and other disadvantaged students' engagement and achievement (Tomorrow's Schools Independent Taskforce, 2018; Wylie, 2012).

A change of government in late 2017 led to a major review of our schooling system (Tomorrow's Schools Independent Taskforce, 2019). The government has largely accepted its recommendations as the basis for significant change (Ministry of Education, 2019). Somewhat disrupted by COVID, work is now underway to develop more of an ecosystem, with closer relations between individual schools and a more supportive and local education government agency, and mutual work together to tackle local issues and share learnings with the central government so that other geographical areas can benefit. The changes will also see more staffing and resources going to schools serving disadvantaged students. As a back-stop to support a fair process, independent local panels will be set up to resolve learner or parent issues with schools relating to enrolment, discipline, and discrimination, including racism.

Policy Relating to Behaviour

Policy interest in student engagement – or rather disengagement – has not been lacking over the years. It has been spurred by schools and others expressing concern about student engagement and behaviour, and it was best-resourced under a Prime Minister's Youth Mental Health package.

Pivotal to a more supportive policy was the 2-day Taumata Whanongo behaviour summit in 2009, hosted by the then Special Education section of the Ministry of Education, with the active involvement of the national teacher unions and other education organisations, keynote speeches from international and local researchers, and discussions. The then Minister for Education from a National government said:

> This summit is about developing an action plan to address the whole range of behaviours that can impede learning, and at their worst, threaten student and teacher safety….
> If a student is going to make the most of their education, they have to be interested in learning, be in a positive learning environment, and, of course they have to attend school.
> Positive environments need the type of leadership that ensures schools are free of student bullying and harassment. They need good relationships between teachers and students. They need informed and involved parents, whānau and communities involved with student learning. (Tolley, 2009).

The Minister for Education also referred to Ka Hikitia, the government's strategy to improve the performance of the education system so that Māori would succeed:

> What works for learners is recognition of their language, culture and identity, personalised teaching and learning, the concept of teacher as learner. When dealing with behaviour issues, similar things make a difference – providing individualised responses, getting alongside the person with the issue to tackle problems together, and working within a person's culture.

But she also pointed to limited resources.

What came out of this summit was a greater sense of shared commitment to improve practice and support, a desire to use research-based practices with good evidence, and to ensure that they worked well for Māori and in Aotearoa New Zealand. That led to a suite of professional learning and development as well as more targeted support for individual students, under the Positive Behaviour for Learning banner (PB4L).

Some whole-school approaches to student engagement within Aotearoa New Zealand, existed, particularly the significant Te Kotahitanga work, which focussed on culturally responsive pedagogy and relationships of trust and respect (Alton Lee, 2015; Bishop et al., 2014; Wearmouth & Berryman, 2012). But these had less evidence of their efficacy at the time than some longer running American approaches that specifically targeted behaviour that impeded learning.

PB4L Schoolwide started in 2010, building on Positive Behavioural Interventions and Supports (PBIS). Incredible Years Teachers (IYT) and Incredible Years Parents (IYP) programmes were trialled and then offered, using the IYT and IYP training and accreditation processes. There was some criticism that the videos and examples used were not reflective of the local context. A Restorative Practices programme was added, and again with some criticism that local work in this area using Māori frameworks was not built on. Check & Connect programmes were added to PB4L in a few locations as a trial through the Youth Mental Health project. Other supports that were funded were a small increase in school health nurses for schools in disadvantaged areas, and a trial of the Friends programme to counter anxiety and depression.

Evaluation ran alongside the PB4L supports for several years, with the intention to identify implementation issues as well as to check that overseas approaches worked well in the local context. The New Zealand Council for Educational Research (NZCER), where I worked, undertook some of these evaluations. There were positive gains from PB4L School-Wide, though it often took some years for the approach to bed in, and it needed ongoing leadership support and focus (Boyd & Felgate, 2015). Taking part in the Incredible Years Teachers' professional development generally had a positive impact on teaching practice, and as a result, on student engagement in classwork, with more focus on their learning work, better self-regulation and problem-solving skills, and less disruptive behaviour (Wylie & Felgate, 2016a). Check & Connect worked well where youth workers were well chosen and supported, and were seen by schools as part of their team (Wylie & Felgate, 2016b).

For a few years, there was a real sense of education sector 'ownership' of PB4L. Annual conferences from 2012 to 2017 were organised by the Ministry and sector groups working together. Evaluation findings were shared and discussed. International and local experts shared their latest research and thinking. Presentations from schools describing their own development changed ways of working, and evidence of improvement in student engagement became more prevalent.

NZCER runs periodic national surveys of principals and teachers to get a picture of what is happening in schools and classrooms. Analysis of the 2016 primary (elementary) school data showed that principals and teachers whose schools had worked with the PB4L School-Wide framework and external advisors reported more systematic support for students' positive behaviour.

However, a policy focus on well-being that produces some gains for student engagement can be undercut by other education policies. Much to the dismay and opposition of the primary teaching profession, National Standards for reading, writing, and mathematics for each primary year of schooling were hastily mandated from 2010 after the government changed in the 2008 national elections. Schools were tasked with measuring student performance against these standards each half-year and giving an annual account. The National-led government set a goal for each school of 85% of students performing 'at or above' the standard: a goal which was not met nationally or by many schools, especially those in disadvantaged areas. Principals were most likely to report that a focus on literacy and mathematics was taking attention away from other curriculum aspects when they had only one or no well-embedded practice to support student well-being. Principals least likely to be distracted by the National Standards were those who had many well-embedded practices to support student well-being (Boyd et al., 2017). The National Standards

came to an end with the change to a Labour-led government in late 2017.

The 2018 secondary school survey data showed that just over half were currently part of PB4L School-Wide, most for more than 3 years, and 42% were part of the Restorative Practices work. At the same time, 40% of the principals also used other restorative practices. PB4L School-Wide practices can also be found in secondary schools whose leaders do not want to be part of the Ministry of Education programme. So national policy to support student engagement can have some influence on school practices beyond those who directly participate in activities that have some additional government resourcing, where school leaders encounter convincing evidence of gains.

In 2018, there were some promising signs that secondary schools were more confident in their work around student behaviour. External expertise to help improve student behaviour was not needed by 38% of the secondary principals in 2018, almost double the 20% who said this in 2015. Fewer saw student behaviour as a major issue for their school (22% compared with 33% in 2009).

But at the same time, responses related to student wellbeing and mental health indicated more concern than previously, with 27% of secondary principals saying they could not readily access external expertise to keep improving student well-being compared with 8% in 2015. Student mental health was much more of a concern: 62% could not readily access external expertise to support students with mental health issues, a marked increase from 36% in 2015. Student mental health as a barrier to engagement in learning is much more to the fore, in both primary and secondary schools. Policy that can make a positive difference here lies at the intersection of social provision more generally, including health, housing, employment, and income sufficiency, as well as education.

A system-level focus on student behaviour and well-being using evidence-based approaches that were centrally funded and which gave a sense of shared ownership of the work and learnings from it, bringing different parties together, did make a positive difference for student engagement and for many schools' and teachers' understanding of what they could change in their practices. But such a system-level focus needs to be sustained if it is to reach all schools.

Policy Encouraging Student Engagement in Learning

School attendance in New Zealand has been slipping in recent years – though it did increase in late 2020 after COVID lockdowns enhanced awareness of the value of schools for wellbeing as well as stimulation (Ministry of Education, 2020). The slip in attendance is noticeable across schools in all socioeconomic areas, though it mostly affects those in the most disadvantaged areas. Despite the system-level attention to inequities for Māori and other students, attendance is lowest for Māori students in schools teaching the English language (the majority of state-funded schools in Aotearoa New Zealand). The overall trend raises questions about possible reasons, including the role of digital experience as it extends further into children's and young people's lives.

Concern about student attendance also contributes to a growing interest among educators in curriculum design to motivate learning and to develop student agency. There is an increased understanding of the linkages between these different facets of student engagement, and the need to tackle attendance in more depth than simply having students physically (or digitally now) in class.

At the policy level, there has been a recognition that the well-received NZ Curriculum, with its vision of *Confident, connected, actively involved, lifelong learners* published in 2007 and made mandatory in 2010, needed refreshing, not least because it was not leading to richer curriculum and more engaging learning opportunities within all schools. A major Curriculum Refresh has now begun. More guidance will be provided about how to weave through capabilities such as agency and critical thinking into different curriculum areas, and pedagogy that engages students well. Key knowledge and understanding will be identified, including Matauranga Māori, and Aotearoa New Zealand Histories, in a long-overdue commitment to a bicultural curriculum that lives up to the commitments made to Māori in the country's founding document, Te Tiriti o Waitangi. If the Curriculum Refresh is done well, schools should be able to focus more on 'rich' and deeper learning that engages more students cognitively and emotionally.

However, this essential work has been complicated and potentially put at risk because curriculum design expertise has been run down in the Ministry of Education. Perhaps this is because the 2007 New Zealand Curriculum was seen as a completed project, rather than an ongoing national responsibility, and there were other pressing calls on education funding. But if individual schools are to fully engage their learners, they need curriculum frameworks, resources, materials, guidance (knowledgeable people, not simply digital postings), and suitable assessments: these are a policy responsibility.

Secondary school qualification and assessment policy also frames students' motivation, as well as their learning opportunities. Aotearoa New Zealand school-leavers do not sit one final examination or leave with a grade point average to signal the level of their school academic achievements to tertiary institutions and employers. The country has an unusual three-level secondary school qualification, the National Certificate of Educational Achievement (NCEA), that frames the final 3 years of schooling. Students can gain credits at each level by meeting teacher-assessed and externally examined standards. Achieving a given number of credits at Level 1 is needed to tackle Level 2, and a Level 2 pass is needed to tackle Level 3. This modular system originally aimed to give parity between 'academic' and 'vocational' subjects and simply signal achievement. But students, teachers, and parents thought that a simple pass/fail for each standard was insufficiently motivating for students to do their best. The policy changed to allow standards, and then courses, to be achieved with merit or excellence from 2007.

The previous National-led government set a goal of 85% of students at a school as well as at the national level achieving a Level 2 NCEA qualification. Schools increasingly focussed on standards that their students did well on, and students focussed their attention on work that would gain them credits. More students gained credits – but teaching and learning both narrowed. Policy that relies on such targets to motivate schools and students comes at a high price. Assessment dominated and intensified the work of students and teachers, resulting in a loss of motivation for deeper learning (and experiences to build strength and confidence for such learning), and increased student and teacher stress. These costs were among the prime reasons for a major review of NCEA in 2018–2019.

Framing the secondary school qualification in terms of credit accumulation also fostered some 'pick and mix' of subject areas, resulting too often in qualifications that were not coherent or sound for employers or tertiary education providers, and often precluded students from pursuing the further education or work that they thought would be open to them (Hipkins & Vaughan, 2019). A school could do this with the best of intentions in terms of wanting to engage students. Schools have also continued to timetable in ways that limit subject choice based on the subject hierarchies, and perceptions of student ability: tracking by another means.

Many schools also continue timetables that curtail more innovative integration of new and traditional curriculum areas and continue to run disciplines in separate streams, such as 'the arts' and 'sciences'. This limits opportunities to engage students living in a much more fluid world with challenges such as climate change that engage them, and that need multidisciplinary understanding.

The NCEA review should provide a clearer framework for schools, by identifying 'big ideas', and fewer standards for each curriculum area, and involving post-school educators and employers in the work. It needs to be coherent with the Curriculum Refresh work to make a tangible difference to student learning opportunities that really will nourish deep engagement. One concern is that the NCEA Review and identification of new standards has started ahead of the Curriculum Refresh, with the potential for the standards to limit the Curriculum Refresh and confuse.

Policy decisions on what is taught, the supports provided for teaching and learning, and the frameworks used for assessment and end-of-school qualifications all have a strong bearing on student engagement. They matter as much as attendance and behaviour policies, and the supports and programmes that are associated with them.

Whose Voices Are Heard to Ensure Policy Supports Student Engagement Equitably?

The change in government in late 2018 led to a new momentum in education, identifying through a wide range of Education Conversations what was most important to students, parents, educators, and the wider community, and where the system had become stuck. Student voices played a powerful role, particularly where they spoke of being ignored, treated as dumb, not recognised for who they were and what they brought to learning, and not being given opportunities to flourish, and confined to 'cabbage' (easy or limited) classes (Office of the Children's Commissioner and New Zealand School Trustees' Association, 2018). Research has shown that teachers' expectations make a difference to how teachers engage the students in their classes, and the opportunities students have for learning (Rubie-Davies, 2015). Currently, there is real momentum around a campaign to stop streaming of students by ability, and grouping students within classes, supported by research that shows the advantages of mixed-ability grouping (Anthony & Hunter, 2017, who note the role played by a government-funded mathematics professional learning programme that suggested benefits from ability grouping; Tokona Te Raki, 2021).

What the Aotearoa New Zealand schooling system is grappling with is distinct in some ways, but far from unique. Every country has some compulsory schooling. Every school system grapples with students who do not want to be in school, who sit in class but with minds and hearts elsewhere, and who do the minimum needed to stay under the radar or act out their frustrations at feeling cut out or unable to achieve.

Student engagement is now better understood in many ways than it was and is increasingly given weight as something that has to be actively nurtured. But individual teachers' and schools' work to nourish engagement can only flourish if it is well-framed and supported in policies by the system responsible for it. The policies that will make a positive difference to student engagement are not just those directly addressed to attendance and behaviour, but just as importantly – sometimes I think more so – what students experience in classes: the curriculum their teachers can share, and how they teach and assess it. The COVID pandemic has highlighted the importance of teaching in ways that build and enhance student well-being, at the same time as their knowledge, skills, and understanding. Researchers of student engagement have much to offer those who work on policies that affect the way schools work, and what students experience.

References

Alton Lee, A. (2015). *Ka Hikitia A demonstration report. Effectiveness of Te Kotahitanga Phase 5 2010-2012.* Ministry of Education. Microsoft Word – BES Ka Hikitia Report 270515 Arial.docx (educationcounts. govt.nz).

Anthony, G., & Hunter, R. (2017). Grouping practices in New Zealand mathematics classrooms: Where are we at and where should we be? *NZ Journal of Educational Studies, 52*(1), 73–92. https://doi.org/10.1007/s40841-016-0054-z

Bishop, R., Berryman, M., & Wearmouth, J. (2014). *Te Kotahitanga: Towards effective education reform for indigenous and other minoritised students.* NZCER Press.

Boyd, S., & Felgate, R. (2015). *A positive culture of support: PB4L school-wide final evaluation report.* A positive culture of support: PB4L school-wide final evaluation report | education counts.

Boyd, S., Bonne, L., & Berg, M. (2017). *Finding a balance—Fostering student wellbeing, positive behaviour, and learning.* NZCER. National Survey_Wellbeing_for publication_0.pdf (nzcer.org.nz).

Hipkins, R., & Vaughan, K. (2019). *Subject choice for the future of work. Insights from research literature.* NZCER & the Productivity Commission. Insights-from-research-literature-NZCER.pdf (productivity.govt.nz).

Ministry of Education. (2019). *Supporting all schools to succeed. Reform of the tomorrow's schools system.* Ministry of Education. https://conversation.education.govt.nz/assets/TSR/November-2019/TSR-Government-Response-WEB.pdf

Ministry of Education. (2020). *Students/ākonga attending school/kura regularly.* Education Indicator. Students/ākonga attending school/kura regularly (education-counts.govt.nz).

Office of the Children's Commissioner and the New Zealand School Trustees' Association. (2018). *Education matters to me: Key insights.* OCC-STA--Education-Matters-to-Me-Key-Insights-24Jan2018.pdf

Rubie-Davies, C. (2015). *Becoming a High Expectation Teacher. Routledge.*

Tokona Te Raki. (2021). *Ending streaming in Aotearoa.* TTR_Streaming_Document.pdf (maorifutures.co.nz)

Tolley, A. (2009). Minister of Education's Speech at Taumata Whanonga. Taumata Whanonga | Beehive.govt.nz

Tomorrow's Schools Independent Taskforce. (2018). *Our schooling futures: Stronger together Whiria Ngā Kura Tūātinitini.* Ministry of Education. Tomorrows-Schools-Review-Report-13Dec2018.PDF (education.govt.nz).

Tomorrow's Schools Independent Taskforce. (2019). *Our schooling futures: Stronger together Whiria Ngā Kura Tūātinitini final report.* Ministry of Education. https://conversation-space.s3-ap-southeast2.amazonaws.com/Tomorrows+Schools+FINAL+Report_WEB.pdf

Wearmouth, J., & Berryman, M. (2012). Viewing restorative approaches to addressing challenging behaviour of minority ethnic students through a community of practice lens. *Cambridge Journal of Education, 42*(2), 253–268.

Wylie, C. (2012). *Vital connections. Why we need more than self-managing schools.* NZCER Press.

Wylie, C. & Felgate, R. (2016a). *"My classroom is a much more positive place".* Incredible years teacher programmes — NZCER evaluation summary report. "My classroom is a much more positive place"Incredible Years—Teacher Evaluation summary (education-counts.govt.nz).

Wylie, C., & Felgate, R. (2016b). *"I enjoy school now": Outcomes from check and connect trials in New Zealand (New Zealand Council for Educational Research).* Ministry of Education. I enjoy school now - Outcomes from the Check and Connect trials in New Zealand | Education Counts.

Part IV

Measurement

The Measurement of Student Engagement: Methodological Advances and Comparison of New Self-report Instruments

Jennifer A. Fredricks

Abstract

The purpose of this chapter is to describe advances in the measurement of student engagement. First, different methods used to assess engagement are outlined including student self-report surveys, teacher ratings, observations, administrative data, experience sampling methods, and real-time measures. Benefits, limitations, and methodological considerations of each of these methods are described. Next, 13 self-report measures that have been developed since 2009 are presented. These measures are compared on a variety of dimensions including what is measured (scale name and items), samples, and the extent of reliability and validity of information. Finally, ongoing challenges with the measurement of engagement and future directions are discussed.

Student Engagement and Positive Youth Development

There has been an explosion of interest in the construct of student engagement by researchers, practitioners, and policymakers. Increasing student engagement is seen as a mechanism to both promote positive developmental outcomes and reduce involvement in negative behaviors. Youth who are engaged in school build a stronger connection to the institution, which helps them to develop the skills, values, and mindsets that are critical to academic achievement and a successful transition to adulthood. Engagement also can serve as a protective factor that helps students cope more effectively with the challenges they face in school, bounce back from setbacks and failures, and constructively re-engage with academic tasks (Skinner et al., 2009). In contrast, youth who are disengaged have fewer opportunities to develop academic and social skills, resulting in them becoming more alienated from their teachers, peers, and academic norms. In turn, this lack of participation and devaluing of school may lead youth to seek solace in problem behaviors.

A growing body of research demonstrates the positive relations between student engagement and indicators of adjustment. Student engagement is associated with higher grades, test scores, and school completion rates (Christenson et al., 2012; Fredricks et al., 2004; Wang & Holcombe, 2010). Student engagement is also correlated with favorable mental health outcomes (Li & Lerner, 2011; Marraccini & Brier, 2017) and is a protective factor that can buffer students from risky behaviors, including substance use, delinquency, and problem behaviors (Henry et al., 2012; Li & Lerner, 2011; Wang & Fredricks, 2014). These relations between engagement and

J. A. Fredricks (✉)
Psychology Department, Union College,
Schenectady, NY, USA
e-mail: fredricj@union.edu

indicators of adjustment are reciprocal, with initial differences in engagement and disengagement being magnified over time (Hughes et al., 2008; Wang & Fredricks, 2014).

The goal of this chapter is to update the original chapter on the measurement of student engagement for the first edition of the *Handbook of Research on Engagement* (Fredricks & McColskey, 2012). First, an overview of definitions of engagement and different reasons for measuring this construct are presented. Second, different methods for assessing engagement are discussed, paying particular attention to methodological advances since the last review. Third, self-report survey measures that have been developed since 2009 are presented and compared on several dimensions. Finally, ongoing limitations with the measurement of student engagement and suggestions for how to address each of these challenges are discussed.

What Is Engagement?

The most prevalent conceptualization of student engagement is that it is a multidimensional construct that includes three distinct, yet interrelated dimensions: behavior, emotion/affective, and cognitive engagement, though there has been variation in how each of these components has been defined and measured. A multidimensional conceptualization of engagement provides a richer picture of how students act, feel, and think in school than research on any single dimension can offer. *Behavioral engagement* focuses on students' involvement in and participation in learning and school contexts; positive conduct; and absence of disruptive behaviors (Fredricks et al., 2004). *Emotional engagement* focuses on positive and negative reactions to teachers, classmates, academics, or school; sense of belonging; and identification with school or subject domains (Finn, 1989; Voelkl, 1997). Finally, *cognitive engagement* is defined in terms of students' cognitive investment in learning and includes being self-regulated and use of deep rather than surface learning strategies (Fredricks et al., 2004). Some scholars have included a fourth component of

engagement including academic (Appleton et al., 2006; Appleton et al., 2008), social engagement (Finn & Zimmer, 2012; Wang et al., 2019), and agentic engagement (Reeve & Tseng, 2011), though more research is necessary to determine whether these are additional unique dimensions of engagement.

Disengagement is also considered to be multidimensional, though there are different perspectives about how engagement relates to disengagement. In most studies, engagement and disengagement are viewed on a single continuum, with lower levels of engagement indicating disengagement. More recently, others have begun to view engagement and disengagement as separate and distinct constructs with different indicators that are associated with different learning outcomes (Skinner et al., 2009; Wang et al., 2015; Wang et al., 2019).

Reasons to Measure Engagement

Scholars are increasingly including engagement as a construct in educational research. This work has emerged out of a variety of theoretical and disciplinary traditions. Motivational scholars have used self-determination, self-regulation, flow, goal theory, and expectancy-value theories to examine the links between contextual factors, patterns of engagement, and academic outcomes. One prominent model is self-determination theory, which links contextual factors (i.e., classroom structure, autonomy support, and involvement) to patterns of engagement (i.e., engagement versus disaffection), through self-system processes, or an individual's appraisals of how well the context meets their needs for competence, autonomy, and relatedness (Skinner et al., 2008).

Other scholars have used sociological theories to examine the role of engagement in the process of dropping out of school. For example, the participation-identification model (Finn, 1989) assumes that early forms of participation (e.g., behavioral engagement) lead students to experience academic success, which in turn leads to increased identification with school (e.g., emotional engagement) and ongoing participation. Conversely, the failure to participate in school and class activities leads students to feel alienated from school, disengaged, and can eventually lead to school withdrawal.

Engagement data also play a key role in the identification, design, and evaluation of interventions (Fredricks et al., 2019b). Many schools collect data on student engagement and disengagement to help identify those students who are in need of additional support, as well as using this data to determine the types of and levels of this support. In multi-tiered systems, increasingly intensive interventions serve a smaller population of disengaged students (MacIver & MacIver, 2010; Reschly & Bergstrom, 2009). Universal interventions (Tier 1) are given to all students to support engagement and performance at school. Engagement can then be monitored among these students to assess if they are in need of more intensive intervention supports (Tier 2 and 3). Engagement data can also be used to differentiate students who have begun to show signs of disengagement and need additional intervention supports to reduce the risk of negative outcomes (Tier 2) from students with chronic and severe disengagement who need immediate and intensive interventions (Tier 3) (Hofkens & Ruzek, 2019).

Increasing student engagement is a key goal of many prevention and intervention efforts (Christenson et al., 2008; Fredricks et al., 2019b). Some examples of interventions to increase engagement include whole-school reforms, project-based learning, social and emotional learning programs, individualized counseling, family support, mentoring, and extracurricular activities (Fredricks et al., 2019b). Collecting data on engagement can help to inform how well an intervention is working, for whom, and whether these effects vary across student and school characteristics. This information can help schools, districts, and communities select the interventions with the strongest evidence base and which aligns with the needs of their particular context.

Engagement is an important construct for practice because it is easily understood by practi-

tioners and describes the conditions that they see in many of their classrooms and schools (Fredricks, 2014). Student disengagement is rated by teachers as one of the biggest stressors they experience in the classroom and one of the factors responsible for high rates of teacher burnout (Chang, 2009; Fredricks, 2014). Teachers can monitor their students' engagement both within and across different instructional contexts (i.e., whole class, small group, seatwork, large discussions) and across different subject areas. Teachers can use data on variations in engagement to make adjustments to their instruction, as well as helping to identify the individual and contextual factors that either help to increase or decrease student engagement.

Methods for Measuring Engagement

In this section, I review methods that have been used to measure engagement, outlining benefits, limitations, and methodological considerations of each method. Particular attention is paid to advances in methodologies over the past decade.

Student Self-report Surveys

The most common method of assessing student engagement is self-report surveys because they are low cost and easy to administer to large and diverse groups of students in classroom settings. Self-report surveys allow researchers to track changes in engagement over time, compare results within and across schools, and test the relations between contextual factors and engagement. Furthermore, this methodology captures students' subjective perceptions and how they make meaning of their classroom experience. As a result, it may be a more valid way of understanding emotional and cognitive engagement than other methods that can be highly inferential (Appleton et al., 2008).

There are methodological considerations when using self-report measures to assess engagement. These measures are more likely to be worded broadly to reflect engagement at either the school or class level as opposed to worded to reflect engagement in a specific subject area or task. Additionally, self-report surveys are based on the assumption that engagement is static and can be measured outside of students' actual involvement in learning tasks (Greene & Azevedo, 2010). When responding to survey questions, students need to reflect on their experiences across multiple tasks to assign an aggregate level of engagement. As a result, self-report methods often do not align with actual or real-time behaviors or strategy use (Greene, 2015; Winne & Perry, 2000). Surveys also are subject to concerns about social desirability, with the potential for students to either over-report or under-report certain behaviors. Finally, self-report surveys do not work well for younger students who have lower reading comprehension levels.

Teacher Ratings

Another way to assess engagement is to have teachers rate students on a variety of indicators. Some of these rating scales include items for behavioral engagement (Rimm-Kaufman et al., 2015; Pagani et al., 2010), and some include items for both behavioral and emotional engagement (Skinner et al., 2009), while still others include items that reflect a multidimensional model of engagement (i.e., behavioral, emotional, and cognitive) (Wang et al., 2016; Wigfield et al., 2008). Teacher surveys are cost-effective and relatively easy to administer. One teacher can report on the engagement of a large number of students either during instruction or outside of instructional time. They also may be more appropriate than self-report survey methods for younger children due to their limited literacy skills. In addition to use in research studies, teacher ratings have been extensively used by practitioners to screen children for social and behavioral problems to help inform intervention-related decisions (Kilgus et al., 2016).

There are also methodological considerations when using teacher ratings of student engage-

ment. Teachers tend to be more accurate reporters of behavior than of emotional and cognitive indicators because behavior is directly observable. Students can hide their emotions and thinking. As a result, teachers need to infer their level of emotional and cognitive engagement based on the behavioral indicators (Skinner et al., 2009). There are also concerns about biases in teacher ratings both as a result of student characteristics (e.g., disability, gender, and socioeconomic status) and teacher characteristics (e.g., knowledge of disability and prior experience) (Mason et al., 2014).

Observational Measures

There are a growing number of observational measures of engagement. Many of these measures use prespecified observational categories and focus on whether behavioral indicators, such as on- and off-task behavior, participation in learning activities, asking and answering questions, listening, and behavioral disruptions, are present or absent during a defined period of time (e.g., Rimm-Kaufman et al., 2015; Volpe et al., 2005). Behavioral engagement can be observed among individual students or groups of students in classrooms. Some studies score the average engagement of students in a class (e.g., Pianta et al., 2007), while others aggregate individual measures of behavioral engagement to form a single global indicator of behavioral engagement at the classroom level (e.g., Briesch et al., 2015). Other studies have used narrative and discourse analysis to assess engagement (Engle & Conant, 2002; Gresalfi, 2009; Ryu & Lombardi, 2015). These studies have observed the quality of instructional discourse between the individual and the group in a specific course and have assessed teacher questioning and the development of student argumentation as evidence of cognitive engagement.

Observational methods can provide a rich description of both engagement and classroom context. These observations can enhance our understanding of how engagement emerges and changes over time, as well as identify individual and contextual triggers of engagement and disengagement (Renninger & Bachrach, 2015). Observations may be more amenable to administrators and teachers because this methodology tends to be less disruptive because it can happen during instructional time. An additional benefit is that observations are grounded in practice. Thus, they are particularly useful to practitioners because they can provide deep insight into a particular case (Renninger & Bachrach, 2015).

Despite these benefits, this technique does have some methodological challenges. First, because of variations in the types of observations and indicators of engagement, scholars who use this technique will need to make decisions about how often to measure, over what periods of time (e.g., continuous, momentary time sampling, partial recordings, or whole-interval recording), with what unit of analysis (individual students, groups, or whole classrooms), and in what settings (e.g., whole class, small group work, seat work). Additionally, we do not know how much the presence of a video camera changes instruction, teacher–student interactions, or students' engagement in class. Furthermore, collecting observational data can require extensive training to support and maintain validity. For example, the Classroom Assessment Scoring System (CLASS) (Pianta et al., 2007), a widely used observational measure that includes a global measure of student engagement, requires a two-day training (Rimm-Kaufman et al., 2015). Finally, since observations can be time-consuming to conduct and analyze, they tend to include a smaller number of students. This raises questions regarding the generalizability of findings to students with different backgrounds or schools in different social and cultural contexts (Waxman et al., 2004).

Administrative Data

Another way to assess student engagement and disengagement is through the use of administrative data, which is already being collected by schools. For example, schools collect data on attendance, truancy, problem behaviors, credit earned, graduation rates, and course enrollment and completion (Appleton et al., 2008; Mandernach, 2015). The majority of these indicators are measures of behavioral engagement and disengagement. A significant advantage of using administrative data to assess engagement is that it is collected regularly on all students across school systems and throughout the academic year allowing school personnel to monitor and track changes over time.

Indicators like attendance, problem behaviors, and course enrollment tend to be meaningful, easily understood, and valued by practitioners and are often aligned with district and school priorities. Furthermore, many school districts collect data on indicators of student disengagement (e.g., problem behaviors, absenteeism, course failure) as part of an early warning system to identify students who are struggling earlier in their school career and to use these data to direct students to appropriate tier of interventions (Balfanz & Brynes, 2019; Balfanz et al., 2007; Heppen & Bowles, 2008). There are several case studies of how schools have used this data to identify students in need of intervention support and facilitate discussions around the district and school-wide responses to disengagement (Appleton, 2012; Appleton & Silberglitt, 2019; Hofkens & Ruzek, 2019).

Despite these benefits, there are a few concerns with using administrative data to assess engagement. One concern is that there is often not a clear demarcation between indicators and outcomes of engagement, such as grades, discipline, and number of credits. This lack of clear demarcation between indicators and outcomes makes it more difficult to explore the consequences of engagement (Lam et al., 2012). Additionally, there are concerns about potential biases in reporting of some indicators of disengagement (e.g., suspensions, problem behavior) by student characteristics (e.g., race, socioeconomic status, special education status) (Skiba et al., 2002). Finally, variations in how schools collect data on indicators like suspension, course marks, and attendance can make it more difficult to compare this data across different school contexts (Balfanz & Brynes, 2019).

Experience Sampling Methods

Experience sampling methods (ESM) is another technique for assessing student engagement. ESM techniques grew out of research on "flow," a high level of engagement where individuals are so deeply absorbed in a task that they lose awareness of time and space (Shernoff & Csikszentmihalyi, 2009). In this methodology, students are randomly contacted throughout the day as they go about their daily lives. In response to ESM signals, they fill out short surveys with a series of questions about their location, activities, behaviors, and cognitive and affective responses.

One benefit of ESM methods is that it offers a time- and context-dependent measure of students' subjective experiences. This allows researchers to collect data on engagement as it is happening, which reduces problems with recall failure and answering in socially desirable ways (Hektner et al., 2007; Zirkel et al., 2015). Additionally, this technique can be used to compare engagement levels within individuals over time and across contexts. There are also statistical advantages to using ESM techniques. The repeated nature of ESM data increases the data reliability, offers greater statistical power, and allows researchers to include participants with variable response rates (Zirkel et al., 2015).

There are several methodological considerations with this methodology. Data collection requires a high level of commitment from participants who are often asked the same questions on multiple occasions. This leads to concerns about participant fatigue, hasty completion, exaggeration, and deliberation falsification (Shernoff et al., 2003; Zirkel et al., 2015). Additionally, it is very labor-intensive for researchers and can be expensive, though new technologies have helped to reduce both the cost and labor. Since the data collected through this technique is relatively limited, it also provides limited insight into individual characteristics and aspects of classroom

context that may help to explain variations in engagement. Furthermore, there are concerns that the multidimensional nature of engagement may not be adequately captured by the small number of items included in ESM studies (Fredricks & McColskey, 2012). For example, in a series of studies, Shernoff and his colleagues (e.g., Shernoff, 2013, 2016; Shernoff et al., 2003) measured engagement with only three items: enjoyment, concentration, and interest.

Real-time Measures

One of the biggest advances in methods to assess engagement since the 2012 review is the increase in the use of real-time measures to capture the dynamics of and fluctuations of engagement. Unlike other measurement techniques, real-time measures collect fine-grained data at time scales ranging from seconds to a few minutes and focus on discrete and objective indicators. For example, some scholars have assessed engagement with log files, or the electronic interactions that occur as students work in online learning environments (Azevedo et al., 2010; D'Mello et al., 2017; Gobert et al., 2015). Some examples of indicators of behavioral and cognitive engagement collected through log files include: (1) number of posts to a discussion board, (2) number of pages viewed in an online resource, (3) number of edits made to a writing task, and (4) number of times reading a text (Fredricks et al., 2019a). Other studies have used log files to measure the amount of time students are off task and the presence of behaviors that indicate a desire to finish quickly instead of doing well on the task (Azevedo et al., 2010; Gobert et al., 2015; Henrie et al., 2015).

Eye-tracking techniques is another method used to collect data on engagement in real-time. In this methodology, an eye-tracking machine records the pattern of eye movements over text and images, including whether a student fixates on a work or object, whether a student looks back and forth over a text, how much time they spend looking at different objects on a page, and how much information they miss (Boucheix et al.,

2013; Duchowski, 2007; Miller, 2015). The assumption is that people look longer at some words or images because they are thinking more deeply about these objects, or are more cognitively engaged (Miller, 2015).

Others have measured facial expressions and body language during online learning as indicators of students' emotional and behavioral engagement (D'Mello & Graesser, 2012; D'Mello et al., 2017). For example, researchers have used the Baker-Rodrigo Observation Monitoring Protocol (BROMP) (Occumpaugh et al., 2015) to make online observations of students' boredom, frustration, engaged concentration, and confusion based on their interactions with peers and teachers, body movements, gestures, and facial expression. These observational data are synchronized to log data files, and then data mining algorithms are used to determine patterns of engagement.

Researchers have also begun measuring engagement with physiological data. Engagement is associated with physiological changes, such as an increase in heart rate, perspiration, muscle tension, or rapid respiration (Kim, 2018). One such technique to measure these physiological changes is a galvanic skin response, a technique in which the conductance of the skin is measured through one or two sensor(s) attached to a part of the hand or foot. Galvanic skill response techniques have been used to assess affective processes and emotional arousal as indicators of emotional engagement (Arroyo et al., 2009; Kim, 2018; McNeal et al., 2014; Poh et al., 2010). Another method to measure engagement is an electroencephalogram (EEG), a neurological technique where electrodes are placed on the scalp during learning tasks to assess cognitive effort (Antonenko et al., 2010). Others have used galvanic skin response techniques in combination with blood pressure and electroencephalography to measure emotional engagement (Shen et al., 2009).

There are several benefits to using real-time measures to assess engagement. First, these measures are more precise and provide rich information on how engagement occurs in real-time in the context of discrete activities. This allows researchers to collect large amounts of data over short periods of time allowing them to model changes in engagement during and across tasks and learning environments. Another benefit of this methodology is that a student does not need to stop the activity to respond to survey questions (Miller, 2015). These measures can also provide insights into aspects of engagement that are difficult to observe or report, are objective, and therefore not suspect to social desirability. There also are potential practical applications to using these techniques. For example, scientists are using facial recognition and physiological data on emotional engagement to build adaptive learning systems that can apply behavioral strategies and emotional supports to support learning (Kapoor et al., 2007; Shen et al., 2009).

Despite these benefits, there are several limitations and many unanswered methodological questions with these new methods. First, data using real-time measures tend to be collected with well-structured laboratory tasks and as part of small studies because of the cost, privacy/ethical considerations, and technical expertise required to use the technology (Antonenko et al., 2010; D'Mello et al., 2017; Miller, 2015). Devices used to collect this data can be expensive, complex, and more difficult to use in the classroom or school settings. Additionally, the physiological phenomena they are measuring are affected by other physiological processes, like sweating or movement (Henrie et al., 2015). Data on nervous system arousal can also be difficult to interpret without supplemental self-report or observational information that indicates whether the physiological arousal detected is indicative of positive or negative emotions (Henrie et al., 2015).

Because these methods are relatively new, there are also questions about the appropriate sampling frequency, time between observations, and the level of granularity. The data collected through these methods can be complex and difficult to analyze, and there are questions about how to ensure accurate data collection, manage the large amount of data that is produced, and interpret the results in a way that is accurate and usable for schools (Henrie et al., 2015). As a result, it is not clear whether, and if so, how this technique can be used to assess engagement in more complex and less structured learning environments and tasks.

Comparison of Self-report Measures

The goal of this chapter is to update the review of self-report measures of engagement described in the first edition of this handbook (Fredricks & McColskey, 2012). This earlier review compared 11 self-report measures that were developed from 1979 to 2009. Table 1 includes the list of measures identified in this review. In addition, several methodological issues were noted in this review. The first was definitional clarity. They noted variation in how defined and measured within and across the different dimensions of engagement. For example, similar items were sometimes used to assess different dimensions of engagement (e.g., class participation as an indicator of both behavioral and cognitive engagement and students' valuing of school was used as an indicator of both emotional and cognitive engagement). Second, the majority of measures assessed general engagement rather than engagement in specific subject areas. These items were rarely worded to reflect specific situations or tasks.

Finally, there was a large variation in the psychometric support for these 11 measures, with only a few examples of the surveys having been validated across different subgroups of students.

As a first step toward identifying self-report surveys published since the 2009 review (See Table 1), a literature search was conducted using terms that were broad enough to capture both subject-specific and general measures of student engagement. PsycARTICLES and ERIC databases were searched for citations between January 2009 and July 2020 using the terms student engagement or school engagement and the terms instrument or survey. First, all citations were screened for entries that included a self-report survey that measured either engagement or a related motivational construct. A large number of the citations were excluded at this stage because either the article did not include any form of data collection or the data was collected using other methods than self-report surveys. The remaining citations were screened for the inclusion of an engagement self-report survey administered to kindergarten to twelfth-grade students. Citations were excluded for the following reasons: (1) developed for college-age samples, (2) measured another construct (e.g., school belonging, school climate, self-concept, parent involvement, goal orientation), (3) developed for a non-academic area (e.g., music, physical education), (4) included in 2012 review (see Table 1),

Table 1 Overview of 11 Instruments from Fredricks and McColskey (2012)

Instrument name	Availability
Attitude Towards Mathematics Survey (ATM)	Miller, Greene, Montalvo, Ravindran, and Nichols (1996)
Engagement versus Disaffection with Learning – Student Report (EvsD)	Skinner et al. (2009) or www. pdx.edu/psy/ellen-skinner-1
High School Survey of Student Engagement (HSSSE)	www.indiana.edu/~ceep/hssse/
Identification with School Questionnaire (ISQ)	(Voelkl, 1997)
Motivated Strategies for Learning Questionnaire (MSLQ)	Pintrich and DeGroot (1990)
Motivation and Engagement Scale (MES)	www.lifelongachievement.com
Research Assessment Packages for Schools (RAPS)	irre.org/sites/default/files/publication_pdfs/RAPS_manual_entire_1998.pdf
School Engagement Measure (SEM) – MacArthur	Fredricks, Blumenfeld, Friedel, and Paris (2005)
School Engagement Scale/Questionnaire (SEQ)	Available by contacting Dr. Steinberg at Temple University
School Success Profile (SSP)	www.schoolsuccessprofile.org
Student Engagement Instrument (SEI)	Appleton et al. (2006)

(5) used measures developed prior to 2009, (6) not available in English, and 7) did not have enough published information.

What Is Measured?

This screening process resulted in 13 new self-report measures. The measures are listed in Table 2 and include a citation where one can access the full scales, the subscales/domains measured, and sample items for each of the subscales.

The surveys were compared in terms of what was measured, samples, and psychometric information. First, the surveys differed in terms of whether they focus on general engagement or subject-specific engagement. Ten of the survey measures include items worded to reflect general engagement in school or in class, while three of the surveys are worded to reflect engagement in a subject-specific area [Math and Science

Table 2 Measures and sample items

Instrument name	Citation	Sample items
Agentic Engagement	Reeve and Tseng (2011)	Agentic Engagement (5 items) *During class, I ask questions* Behavioral Engagement (5 items) *I listen carefully in class* Cognitive Engagement (8 items) *When doing schoolwork, I try to connect what I am learning with my own experiences* Emotional Engagement (4 items) *I enjoy learning new things in class*
Classroom Engagement Inventory	Wang et al. (2014)	Affective Engagement (5 items) *I feel excited* Behavioral Engagement: compliance (3 items) *I complete my assignments* Behavioral Engagement: effortful class participation (5 items) *I work with other students and we learn from each other* Cognitive Engagement (8 items) *I search for information from different places and think about how to put it together* Disengagement (3 items) *I am "zoned out", not really thinking or doing class work*
Delaware School Engagement Survey	Yang et al. (2020)	Cognitive-Behavioral Engagement (5 items) *I follow the rules in school* Emotional Engagement (5 items) *I like most of my teachers*
Math and Science Engagement Scales	Wang et al. (2016)	Behavioral Engagement in Math/Science (8 items) *I put effort into learning science/math* Cognitive Engagement in Math/Science (8 items) *I think about different ways to solve a problem* Emotional Engagement in Math/Science (10 items) *I look forward to science/math class* Social Engagement in Math/Science (7 items) *I try to understand people's ideas in science/math class*
Motivation and Engagement Survey	Lee et al. (2016)	Affective Engagement in Science (5 items) *My science classroom is a fun place to be* Behavioral Engagement in Science (5 items) *I pay attention to all of the learning activities in my science class* Cognitive Engagement in Science (7 items) *I look for extra information (books or internet) to learn more about things we do in science*

(continued)

Table 2 (continued)

Instrument name	Citation	Sample items
School Engagement	Wang et al. (2011)	Behavioral Engagement: attentiveness (3 items) *How often do you get schoolwork done on time?* Behavioral engagement: school compliance (4 items) *How often have you skipped class (reverse coded)?* Cognitive Engagement: Self-regulated learning (4 items) *How often do you try to figure out problems and planning how to solve them?* Cognitive Engagement: Cognitive strategy use (4 items) *How often do you try to plan what you have to do for homework before you get started?* Emotional Engagement: School belonging (3 items) *I feel happy and safe at school* Emotional Engagement: Valuing of school education (5 items) *I have to do well in school if I want to be a success in life*
School Engagement Inventory	Salmela-Aro and Upadyaya (2012)	Energy (Emotional engagement) (3 items) *At school I am bursting with energy* Dedication (Cognitive engagement) (3 items) *I find the schoolwork full of meaning and purpose* Absorption (Behavioral engagement) (3 items) *I feel happy when I am working deeply at school*
School Engagement Scale	Wang et al. (2019)	Behavioral Engagement (4 items) *I always try my best in school* Behavioral Disengagement (8 items) *I don't follow school rules* Cognitive Engagement (5 items) *I plan out how to finish my homework* Emotional Engagement (5 items) *I have fun at school* Emotional Disengagement (4 items) *I feel worried at school* Social Engagement (5 items) *I help my peers when they are struggling* Social Disengagement (4 items) *I don't feel like people notice me at school*
Student Engagement Instrument: Elementary Version	Carter et al. (2012)	Teacher Student Relationships (affective engagement) (9 items) *Teachers at my school care about students* Peer Support for Learning (affective engagement) (6 items) *I have friends at school* Family Support for Learning (affective engagement) (4 items) *My family/guardians are there when I need them* Future Goals and Aspirations (cognitive engagement) (5 items) *I plan to go to college after I graduate from high school*
Student Engagement in Math (SEMS)	Leis et al. (2015)	Cognitive Engagement in Math (5 items) *Today in math class I worked as hard as I could* Emotional Engagement in Math (5 items) *Math class was fun today* Social Engagement in Math (4 items) *Today I talked about math with other kids in the class*
Student Engagement in School	Lam et al. (2014)	Affective Engagement (9 items) *I am very interested in learning* Behavioral Engagement (12 items) *I try to do well in school* Cognitive Engagement (12 items) *When I study, I try to understand the material better by relating it to things I already know*

(continued)

Table 2 (continued)

Instrument name	Citation	Sample items
Student Engagement in School-Four-Dimensional Scale (SES-4DS)	Veiga and Robu (2014)	Agency *I make suggestions to my teachers about how to improve classes* Affective Engagement (5 items) *My school is a place where I make friends easily* Behavioral Engagement (5 items) *I absent from school without a valid reason (reverse coded)* Cognitive Engagement (5 items) *I spend a lot of my free time looking for more information on topics discussed in class*
Student School Engagement Measure (SSEM)	Hazel et al. (2013)	Aspirations (4 items) *Being successful in school will help me in the future* Belonging (6 items) *I am proud to be a student at this school* Productivity (12 items) *I look for more information about things I am learning in school*

Engagement Scales (Wang et al., 2016), Motivation and Engagement Survey (Lee et al., 2016) & Student Engagement in Math (Leis, Schmidt, & Rimm-Kaffman (Leis et al., 2015)].

The self-report measures differed in whether and how they conceptualized disengagement. The majority of the measures assume that a low engagement score indicates disengagement. Many of the scales include reverse coded items that are indicators of disengagement (e.g., get in trouble, doing just enough to get by, do not care about learning, class is boring, give up easily). Two of the measures include separate subscales for disengagement [Classroom Engagement Inventory (Wang et al., 2014); School Engagement Scale (Wang et al., 2019)]. Additionally, the School Engagement Inventory (Salmela-Aro & Upadyaya, 2012) builds on a separate prior measure of student disengagement (School Burnout Inventory; Salmela-Aro et al., 2009).

Finally, a few of the scales blurred the lines between indicators, which describe what engagement looks like in a setting, and facilitators, which are contextual factors that influence engagement (Sinclair et al., 2003: Hofkens & Ruzek, 2019). For example, the Student Engagement Instrument (SEI): Elementary Version (Carter et al., 2012) measures engagement with scales about students' relationships with teachers and peers and support for learning from families. Additionally, the Student School

Engagement Measure includes both indicators (e.g., I am proud to be at school) and facilitators (e.g., teachers help me to be successful at school) in the same scale (Hazel et al., 2013). In contrast, other self-report measures include separate scales for the aspects of classroom or school context that are assumed to influence or be related to engagement.

All of the measures considered engagement as a multidimensional construct, though they differed in both the number and conceptualization of engagement. Two of the measures include two dimensions of engagement [The Delaware School Engagement Survey (Yang et al., 2020) and the Student Engagement Instrument: Elementary Version (Carter et al., 2012)]. Five of the surveys include three dimensions: behavioral, emotional, and cognitive engagement [Classroom Engagement Inventory (Wang et al., 2014); Motivational and Engagement Survey (Lee et al., 2016), School Engagement Inventory (Salmela-Aro & Upadyaya, 2012; School Engagement (Wang et al., 2011), and School Student Engagement in School (Lam et al., 2014)]. Two others include three dimensions: (1) The Student Engagement in Math (cognitive, emotional, and social engagement) (Leis et al., 2015) and (2) The Student School Engagement Measure (SSEM) (aspirations, belonging, and productivity) (Hazel et al., 2013). Finally, four of the measures include four different dimensions of engagement: agentic engagement (Reeve & Tseng, 2011; Veiga & Robu, 2014) and social engagement (Wang et al., 2016; Wang et al., 2019)]. Below we describe the subscales and items found across the 13 instruments by each of the dimensions of engagement.

Behavioral Engagement

Nine of the self-report measures have scales either by the subscale name or sample items that include indicators of behavioral engagement (see Table 2). Across the various behavioral engagement scales/subscales, students are asked to report on their effort, attention, concentration, participation in class, participation in school-based activities, persistence, asking questions, working with peers, attendance, adherence to classroom rules, and absence of risk behaviors. The two behavioral disengagement subscales ask students to report zoning out, lack of effort, not completing work, and problem behaviors.

Emotional/Affective Engagement

All of the self-report measures, either by subscale name or items, have indicators that reflect emotional/affective engagement. Some subscales assess emotional reaction to class or school, while others assess the quality of students' relationships with peers and teachers as an indicator of emotional engagement. Across the various emotional/affective engagement scales/subscales, students are asked about positive emotions such as happiness and pride; liking school and class; enjoying learning new things; experiencing interest and fun; having supportive or positive relations with peers and teachers; making friends; school belonging; feeling safe at school; having family support for learning; and school value. In addition, the emotional disengagement scale includes items about negative emotions including worry, anxiety, and frustration.

Cognitive Engagement

All of the self-report measures either by subscale name or by items have indicators measuring cognitive engagement. Across these various scales, students are asked about their use of deep learning strategies (e.g., connecting material to what already know, planning how to study, making up own examples), going beyond what is required in a class, thinking deeply, searching additional sources for information, persisting when faced with difficulties, asking questions, participating outside of class, effort, paying attention, enthusiasm for learning, school value, and learning from mistakes.

Additional Subscales

In addition to the tripartite conceptualization of engagement, some surveys include additional dimensions of engagement. These include agentic engagement (Reeve & Tseng, 2011; Veiga & Robu, 2014) and social engagement (Leis et al., 2015; Wang et al., 2016, 2019). The agentic engagement scales include items about expressing one's preferences, offering input, asking questions, and communicating what one is thinking and needing from their teacher. The social engagement subscale includes items about enjoying time with peers, working with and learning from peers, sharing with and discussing ideas with peers, helping others who are struggling, and being open to making friends.

As noted above and similar to the earlier review, there is a large variation in how each of the constructs is defined and measured (see Fredricks & McColskey, 2012). Similar items are sometimes used as indicators of different dimensions of engagement. For example, asking questions is included as an indicator of behavioral, cognitive, and agentic engagement. Feeling supported by peers is included as an indicator of both emotional and social engagement. Persistence, effort, attention, and participation are included as indicators in both behavioral and cognitive engagement subscales. Finally, students' valuing of school is included as an indicator in both emotional and cognitive engagement subscales.

Samples

Another way to compare the 13 self-report measures is to examine variations in the samples. The self-report measures have been administered to students in the elementary school years (third through fifth grades) through the high school years, with the majority of the surveys administered to middle and high school students. As seen in Table 3, the majority of measures have been used with ethnically and economically diverse samples.

One of the advances in the last decade is the large involvement of international scholars in the measurement of engagement. A large number of these measures were developed and validated in English and non-English speaking countries throughout the world. The most ambitious of these international efforts is a 12-country collaboration of the International School Psychology Association that included scholars from Austria, Canada, China, Cyprus, Estonia, Greece, Malta, Portugal, Romania, South Korea, the United Kingdom, and the United States. This project was designed to investigate the personal (e.g., demographic factors, emotions, academic performance) and contextual antecedents (i.e., teacher, parents, and peer support; instructional practices) of student engagement. This international collaboration resulted in the development of the Student Engagement in School Survey, a scale that could measure affective, behavioral, and cognitive dimensions of engagement across these countries (Lam et al., 2014).

Psychometric Support

One of the limitations noted with the prior review of self-report measures was variation in the amount and type of psychometric support (Fredricks & McColskey, 2012). One exception is the Student Engagement Instrument (SEI; Appleton et al., 2006). This measure was identified in the first review as one of the earliest measures of student engagement and has strong psychometric support. In a series of studies, researchers have demonstrated the reliability, factor invariance, and convergent, divergent, and predictive validity of the SEI (Appleton et al., 2006; Betts et al., 2010; Fraysier et al., 2020; Lovelace et al., 2014; Reschly et al., 2014).

Table 3 Self-report measures and samples

Measures	Samples
Agentic Engagement	Original sample: 369 high school students from Urban high school in Taiwan Versions used with American high school students with disabilities, Italian high school students, Israel high school students, Korean high school students, Turkish middle school students; college students
Classroom Engagement Inventory	Original sample: 3925 students from fourth to twelfth grades in medium sized city (84.5% white) Version used with Turkish high school students
Delaware School Engagement Survey	Original sample:16,237 students in sixth to twelfth grade from 43 secondary public schools in Delaware Version used with Chinese students in elementary, middle, and high schools; Brazilian public schools
Math and Science Engagement Scales	Original sample 3883 students in sixth through twelfh grades, economically diverse, 38.2% qualify for free or reduced lunch Version used with Chinese middle school students
Motivation and Engagement Survey	Original sample: 2094 middle schools, ethnically and economically diverse sample
School Engagement	Multiple studies using a large longitudinal sample which followed students from seventh grade to 3 years post high school, 56% African American (Wave 1–1452 students) Version used with high school students in Jordan
School Engagement Inventory	Multiple studies using a large longitudinal tracking student of ninth grades students from all comprehensive schools in a city in Finland Version used with Spanish 12–16 years old
School Engagement Scale	Original sample: large racially and ethnically diverse sample of fifth through twelfth grade students ($N = 3632$)

(continued)

One of the advances over the past decade is increased evidence of psychometric support. All of the developers presented technical information

Table 3 (continued)

Measures	Samples
Student Engagement Instrument: Elementary School Version	Original sample: 1493 students in third through fifth grade in a large diverse urban school district
Student Engagement in Math	Original sample: 387 fifth grade students. Version used with Australia sixth to tenth grade students and Turkish secondary school students
Student Engagement in School	Original sample: 3420 in seventh to ninth grades in schools in 12 countries (Austria, Canada, China, Cyprus, Estonia, Greece, Malta, Portugal, Romania, South Korea, the United Kingdom, and United States). Version used among high school students in Italy
SES-4DS	Original sample: 377 Portuguese students between 13 and 17 years of age and 365 ninth and tenth grade Romanian students
Student School Engagement Measure (SSEM)	Original sample: 396 eighth grades in urban district, 80% of students Hispanic

Table 4 Reliability information

Measure	Cronbach's alphas
Agentic Engagement	0.72–0.87
Classroom Engagement Inventory	0.84–0.91
Delaware School Survey	0.84–0.88
Math and Science Engagement Scale	0.73–0.93
Motivation and Engagement Survey	0.76–0.83
School Engagement	0.70–0.78
School Engagement Inventory	0.80–0.87
School Engagement Scale	N/A
Student Engagement Instrument: Elementary Version	0.64–0.82
Student Engagement in Math	0.74–0.91
Student Engagement in School	0.80–0.89
SES-4D	0.69–0.87
Student School Engagement Measure	0.83–0.92

to support both the reliability and validity of these new self-report surveys.

Internal consistency is the extent to which individuals who respond in one way to items tend to respond the same way to other items intended to measure the same construct. A Cronbach's alpha of the engagement scales/subscales was reported for all but one measure. A Cronbach's alpha of 0.70 or higher for a set of items is considered acceptable (Leary, 2004). The reliabilities of these scales range from 0.62 to 0.92, with most scales in the range of 0.70–0.80 (see Table 4).

All of the developers used either exploratory and/or confirmatory factor analyses techniques to examine how the survey items loaded onto the engagement subscales. However, because of the variation in the number of items (ranging from 10 to 42 items), indicators, and subscales (ranging from 2 to 8 subscales) it is difficult to compare the results from these analyses. Two examples

illustrate this variation and challenge with comparisons across different studies where researchers define and name factors differently. For example, Wang and his colleagues (Wang et al., 2016) used confirmatory factor analysis with 33 items on the Math and Science Engagement scale with a sample of 3883 sixth through eighth grade students. These analyses confirmed four subscales: behavioral engagement, cognitive engagement, emotional engagement, and social engagement. Hazel et al. (2013) conducted an exploratory factor analysis with 50 items on a sample of 396 eighth graders. After removing items with low loading, confirmatory factor analyses on the remaining 22 items confirmed three subscales: aspirations, belonging, and productivity.

As noted by Fredricks and McColskey (2012), one limitation with prior self-report measures is we do not know if the engagement can be measured similarly for all groups of students.

To address this concern, five of the developers tested for measurement invariance in the models by race, gender, age, and/or SES. For all five of these measures [Classroom Engagement Inventory (Wang et al., 2014), Delaware School Engagement Survey (Yang et al., 2020), Math and Science Engagement Scale (Wang et al., 2016), School Engagement (Wang et al., 2011), and School Engagement Scale (Wang et al., 2019)], the engagement scales were found to operate similarly across the sub-groups. This finding suggests that most of the engagement items were perceived or interpreted similarly across the different demographic groups.

The majority of the developers provided evidence to support the construct validity of the newly developed measures. For example, the three engagement scales in the Student Engagement in School Survey (Lam et al., 2014) were positively correlated with teacher support, peer support, and family support. Additionally, all four scales of the Classroom Engagement Inventory (Wang et al., 2014) were correlated positively with teacher behavior and motivational constructs (self-efficacy, interest, mastery, performance goals). Evidence of related validity or the extent to which a measure is associated with a key behavior or outcome (Leary, 2004) also was documented on the majority of measures. In 9 out of 13 self-report measures, correlations between engagement and indicators of academic adjustment including GPA, achievement, suspensions, disciplinary referrals, and educational aspirations were documented in the expected direction.

A few of the developers used qualitative methods to further validate their scales (Fredricks et al., 2016; Wang et al., 2019). For example, Wang and his colleagues (Wang et al., 2019) used a mixed-method methodology to both develop and validate their School Engagement Scale. First, they conducted semi-structured interviews with a racially diverse sample of middle and high school students to learn how they thought about engagement and disengagement and what terminology they used in describing these dimensions. Potential indicators of school engagement that emerged from these interviews were then subject to an expert validation process. Finally, they used a cognitive pretesting procedure with students to enhance the cognitive validity of the scales and see if students understood the question in the way that was intended by the researcher.

In sum, the psychometric information on these measures suggests that student engagement can be reliably measured through self-report methods. The results of exploratory and confirmatory factor analyses demonstrate the variability in the different conceptualizations of engagement. Additionally, there is some evidence of the measurement invariance across different demographic groups. This allows researchers to make more appropriate comparisons in engagement between certain groups such as boys and girls and those from different cultural groups (Wang et al., 2011). Furthermore, the measures of engagement relate to both contextual variables in expected directions. Finally, evidence that engagement has been shown to positively relate to indicators of academic adjustment demonstrates that it could serve as a worthwhile intermediate outcome to assess.

Future Research

In sum, this review describes advances in the measurement of engagement since our last review (Fredricks & McColskey, 2012). Highlights which are described in more detail below include (1) the development and validation of 13 new self-report measures, (2) the increase in the use of methods to assess engagement in real-time, and (3) the increase in the use of engagement data to inform policy and practice.

In this chapter, the strengths and limitations of these different approaches to assessing engagement are presented. These measures vary in the extent to which they can accurately capture how students behave, think, and feel in school. The use of multiple methods is recommended to give a fuller picture of engagement and capitalize on the strengths of these different methodologies. Unfortunately, to date, there are few examples of how to triangulate data on engagement collected from different methods, as well as how to reconcile when these methodologies and different reporters provide discrepant and sometimes contradictory information about students' engagement levels (Fredricks et al., 2019a). For example, prior research has shown only moderate correlations between teachers' and students' reports of engagement (Rimm-Kaufman et al., 2015; Skinner et al., 2009). Although students may be more accurate reporters of internal states like emotion and cognition than either outside observers or teachers, students may also not always be aware of them. As a result, combining self-report data with teacher, observer, or physiological data can help obtain a more holistic and accurate assessment of engagement levels (Hofkens & Ruzek, 2019).

One of the biggest advances in the last decade has been the development of new methodologies like log files and physiological data to assess engagement in real-time. These methods have some advantages over traditional methods in that they allow researchers to collect fine-grained data, are more precise, and assess engagement in real-time in the context of real-learning activities. In contrast, traditional methods like student self-reports are much easier to administer but often measure engagement outside of a learning context and fail to capture the dynamic and fluctuating nature of engagement across different contexts (Fredricks et al., 2019b). Despite the benefits of real-time methods, there are significant questions about the practicality of using these methods, as well as unanswered methodological questions about the appropriate time frames and temporal sequences for collecting these types of data.

Definitional clarity is one of the biggest challenges facing research on engagement (Azevedo, 2015; Fredricks & McColskey, 2012). Unfortunately, our review of new self-report measures shows that variation in the operationalization of engagement still remains a concern. There was a large variation in how researchers defined engagement both within and across different dimensions. Although there is a general understanding that engagement is a multidimensional construct, the measures varied in both the number and conceptualization of each dimension. Similar items were often used to assess different indicators of engagement, which makes it difficult to compare and meaningfully interpret findings across different studies. In future research, scholars need to articulate with clarity how they define engagement, describe how their conceptualization is similar or different from other conceptualizations of engagement, and outline similarities and differences with other related

motivational and cognitive constructs. Furthermore, it is critical that both theory and research questions drive the choice of methods, as opposed to the assessment technique determining the theoretical perspective and question (Azevedo, 2015; Sinatra et al., 2015; Fredricks et al., 2019a).

Finally, another advance over the past decade is an increase in the use of engagement data to inform policy and practice. Many schools use engagement data as part of early warning systems to identify students most in need of intervention support (Balfanz & Brynes, 2019). Additionally, schools are collecting data on engagement to help determine the effectiveness of different classroom and school-wide reforms. For example, Hokfens & Rusek (Hofkens & Ruzek, 2019) present three case studies of how school districts, researchers, organizations, and educators have measured engagement including (1) chronic absenteeism in Connecticut, (2) Advancement Via Individual Determination (AVID) intervention, and (3) engagement in Chicago public schools.

Unfortunately, the different surveys and methods for assessing engagement are often not accessible in a way that allows schools to compare these methodologies and decide which can be most easily adopted for use in policy and practice. For example, although there are benefits to developing differentiated sub-scales of engagement for use in research, schools may benefit more from a single global measure of engagement. More research is needed to determine in which situations a global measure or a more differential measure of engagement is more appropriate. Finally, in order for data on engagement to inform practice, educators will need time, opportunities to collaborate with their peers, and professional development related to collecting, analyzing, and using engagement data (Fredricks et al., 2019a).

In sum, this chapter outlines the wide range of options available to scholars, practitioners, and policymakers to assess student engagement. Although significant progress has been made over the past decade in the measurement of this construct, this review also notes ongoing challenges which need to be addressed in future research for the potential of engagement as a construct to be fully realized.

Acknowlegdments I would like to thank Sophia Zacher and Katherine Pink for their help with screening citations.

References

Antonenko, P., Paas, F., Grabner, R., & van Gog, T. (2010). Using electroencephalography to measure cognitive load. *Educational Psychology Review, 22,* 425–438. https://doi.org/10.1007/s10648-010-9130-y

Appleton, J. J. (2012). Systems consultation: Developing the assessment-to-intervention link with the student engagement instrument. In S. Christenson, A. Reschly, & C. Wylie (Eds.), *Handbook of research on student engagement* (pp. 725–742). Springer.

Appleton, J. J., & Silberglitt, B. (2019). Student Engagement Instrument as a tool to support the link between assessment and intervention: A comparison of two districts. In J. Fredricks, A. Reschly, & S. Christenson (Eds.), *Handbook of student engagement interventions: working with disengaged youth* (pp. 225–243). Academic Press.

Appleton, J. J., Christenson, S. L., Kim, D., & Reschly, A. L. (2006). Measuring cognitive and sychological engagement: Validation of the Student Engagement Instrument. *Journal of School Psychology, 44,* 427–445. https://doi.org/10.1002/pits.20303

Appleton, J. J., Christenson, S. L., & Furlong, M. J. (2008). Student engagement with school: Critical conceptual and methodological issues of the construct. *Psychology in the Schools, 45,* 369–386. https://doi.org/10.1002/pits.20303

Arroyo, I., Cooper, D. G., Burleson, W., Woolf, B. P., Muldner, K., & Christopherson, R. (2009). Emotion sensors go to school. *Conference on Artificial Intelligence in Education, 200,* 17–24.

Azevedo, R. (2015). Defining and measuring engagement and learning in science: Conceptual, theoretical, methodological, and analytical issues. *Educational Psychologist, 50,* 84–94. https://doi.org/10.1080/00461520.2015.1004069

Azevedo, R., Moos, D., Johnson, A., & Chauncey, A. (2010). Measuring cognitive and metacognitive regulatory processes used during hypermedia learning: Issues and challenges. *Educational Psychologist, 45,* 210–223. https://doi.org/10.1080/00461520.2010.515934

Balfanz, R., & Brynes, V. (2019). Early warning indicators and intervention systems: state of the field. In J. Fredricks, A. Reschly, & S. Christenon (Eds.), *Handbook of student engagement interventions: working with disengaged youth* (pp. 45–55). Academic Press.

Balfanz, R., Herzog, L., & MacIver, P. J. (2007). Preventing student disengagement and keeping students on graduation path in urban middle grade schools: Early identification and effective interventions. *Educational Psychologist, 42,* 223–235. https://doi.org/10.1080/00461520701621079

Betts, J. E., Appleton, J. J., Reschly, A. L., Christenson, S. L., & Huebner, E. S. (2010). A study of the factorial invariance of the Student Engagement Instrument (SEI): Results from middle and High School students. *School Psychology Quarterly, 25,* 84–93. https://doi.org/10.1037/a0020259

Boucheix, J. M., Lowe, R. K., Putri, D. K., & Groff, J. (2013). Cueing animations: Dynamic signaling aids information extraction and comprehension. *Learning and Instruction, 25,* 71–84. https://doi.org/10.1016/j.learninstruc.2012.11.005

Briesch, A. M., Hemphill, E. M., Volpe, R. J., & Daniels, B. (2015). An evaluation of observational methods for measuring response to class-wide intervention. *School Psychology Quarterly, 30,* 37–49. https://doi.org/10.1037/spq0000065

Carter, C. P., Reschly, A. L., Lovelace, M. D., Appleton, J. J., & Thompson, D. (2012). Measuring student engagement among elementary students: Pilot of the Student Engagement Instrument—Elementary Version. *School Psychology Quarterly, 27*(2), 61–73. https://doi.org/10.1037/a0029229

Chang, M. L. (2009). An appraisal perspective of teacher burnout: Examining the emotional work of teachers. *Educational Psychology Review, 21*(3), 193–218. https://doi.org/10.1007/s10648-009-9106-y

Christenson, S. L., Reschly, A. L., Appleton, J. J., Berman, S., Spanjers, D., & Varro, P. (2008). Best practices in fostering student engagement. In A. Thomas & J. Grimes (Eds.), *Best practices in school psychology* (5th ed., pp. 1099–1199). National Association of School Psychologists.

Christenson, S., Reschly, A., & Wylie, C. (Eds.). (2012). *Handbook of research on student engagement.* Springer.

D'Mello, S., & Graesser, A. (2012). Dynamics of affective states during complex learning. *Learning and Instruction, 22,* 145–157. https://doi.org/10.1016/j.learninstruc.2011.10.001

D'Mello, S., Dieterele, E., & Duckworth, A. (2017). Advanced, analytic, automated (AAA) measurement of engagement during learning. *Educational Psychologist, 52,* 104–123. https://doi.org/10.1080/00461520.2017.1281747

Duchowski, A. (2007). *Eye tracking methodology: Theory and practice* (2nd ed.). Springer.

Engle, R. A., & Conant, F. R. (2002). Guiding principles for fostering productive disciplinary engagement: Explaining an emergent argument in a community of learners' classroom. *Cognition and Instruction, 20,* 399–483. https://doi.org/10.1207/S1532690XCI2004_1

Finn, J. D. (1989). Withdrawing from school. *Review of Educational Research, 59*, 117–142. https://doi.org/10.3102/00346543059002117

Finn, J. D., & Zimmer, K. (2012). Student engagement: What is it? Why does it matter? In S. L. Christenson, A. L. Reschly, & C. Wylie (Eds.), *Handbook of research on student engagement* (pp. 97–131). Springer.

Fraysier, K., Reschly, A. L., & Appleton, J. J. (2020). Predicting postsecondary enrollment and persistence with secondary student engagement data. *Journal of Psychoeducational Assessment, 38*, 882–899. https://doi.org/10.1177/0734282920903168

Fredricks, J. (2014). *Eight myths of student disengagement: Creating classrooms of deep learning*. Sage.

Fredricks, J. A., & McColskey, W. (2012). The measurement of student engagement: A comparative analysis of various methods and student self-report instruments. In S. Christenson, A. L. Reschy, & C. Wylie (Eds.), *Handbook of research on student engagement* (pp. 763–783). Springer.

Fredricks, J. A., Blumenfeld, P. C., & Paris, A. (2004). School engagement: Potential of the concept: State of the evidence. *Review of Educational Research, 74*, 59–119. https://doi.org/10.3102/00346543074001059

Fredricks, J. A., Wang, M.-T., Schall Linn, J., Hofkens, T. L., Sung, H., Parr, A., & Allerton, J. (2016). Using qualitative methods to develop a survey measure of math and science engagement. *Learning and Instruction, 43*, 5–15. https://doi.org/10.1016/j.learninstruc.2016.01.009

Fredricks, J. A., Hofkens, T., & Wang, M. (2019a). Addressing the challenge of measuring student engagement. In A. Renninger & S. Hidi (Eds.), *The Cambridge handbook of motivation and learning* (pp. 689–712). Cambridge University Press.

Fredricks, J., Reschly, A., & Christenson, S. (Eds.). (2019b). *Handbook of student engagement interventions: working with disengaged students*. Academic Press.

Gobert, J. D., Baker, R. S., & Wixon, M. B. (2015). Operationalizing and detecting disengagement within online science microworlds. *Educational Psychologist, 50*, 43–57. https://doi.org/10.1080/00461520.2014.999919

Greene, B. (2015). Measuring cognitive engagement with self-report scales: reflections from over 20 years of research. *Educational Psychologist, 50*, 13–40. https://doi.org/10.1080/00461520.2014.989230

Greene, J. A., & Azevedo, R. (2010). The measurement of learners' self-regulated cognitive and metacognitive processes while using computer-based learning environments. *Educational Psychologist, 45*, 203–209. https://doi.org/10.1080/00461520.2014.989230

Gresalfi, M. S. (2009). Taking up opportunities to learn: Constructing dispositions in mathematics classrooms. *Journal of the Learning Sciences, 18*, 327–369. https://doi.org/10.1080/10508400903013470

Hazel, C. E., Vazirabadi, G. E., & Gallagher, J. (2013). Measuring aspirations, belonging, and in secondary students: Validation of the student school engagement measure. *Psychology in the Schools, 50*, 689–714. https://doi.org/10.1002/pits.21703

Hektner, J. M., Schmidt, J. A., & Csikzentmihalyi, M. (2007). *Experience sampling method: measuring the quality of everyday life*. Sage Publications.

Henrie, C. R., Halverson, L. R., & Graham, C. R. (2015). Measuring student engagement in technology-mediated learning: A review. *Computers and Education, 90*, 36–53. https://doi.org/10.1016/j.compedu.2015.09.005

Henry, K. L., Knight, K. E., & Thornberry, T. P. (2012). School disengagement as a predictor of dropout, delinquency, and problem substance use during adolescence and early adulthood. *Journal of Youth and Adolescence, 41*, 156–166. https://doi.org/10.1007/s10964-011-9665-3

Heppen, J. B., & Bowles, T. S. (2008). *Developing early warning systems*. National High School Center.

Hofkens, T. L., & Ruzek, E. (2019). Measuring student engagement to inform interventions in schools. In J. Fredricks, A. Reschly, & S. Christenon (Eds.), *Handbook of student engagement interventions: working with disengaged youth* (pp. 309–324). Academic Press.

Hughes, J. N., Luo, W., Kwok, O., & Loyd, L. K. (2008). Teacher-student support, effortful engagement, and achievement: A 3-year longitudinal study. *Journal of Educational Psychology, 100*, 1–14. https://doi.org/10.1037/0022-0663.100.1.1

Kapoor, A., Burleson, W., & Picard, R. W. (2007). Automatic prediction of failure. *International Journal of Human Computer Studies, 65*, 724–726. https://doi.org/10.1016/j.ijhcs.2007.02.003

Kilgus, S. P., Eklund, K., & von de Embse, N. P., Taylor, C. N., & Sims, W. S. (2016). Psychometric defensibility of the social, academic, and emotional behavioral risk screener (SAESBRS) teacher rating scale and multiple gating procedures within elementary and middle school samples. *Journal of School Psychology, 58*, 21–39. https://doi.org/10.1016/j.jsp.2016.07.001

Kim, P. W. (2018). Real-time bio-signal-processing of students based on an intelligent algorithm for internet of things to assess engagement levels in a classroom. *Future Generation Computer Systems, 86*, 716–722. https://doi.org/10.1016/j.future.2018.04.093

Lam, S., Wong, B. P. H., Yang, H., & Liu, Y. (2012). Understanding student engagement with a contextual model. In S. Christenson, A. L. Reschy, & C. Wylie (Eds.), *Handbook of research on student engagement* (pp. 403–419). Springer.

Lam, S. F., Jimerson, S., Wong, B. P. H., Kikas, E., Shin, H., Veiga, F. H., Hatzichristou, C., Polychroni, F., Cefai, C., Negovan, V., Stanculescu, E., Yang, H., Liu, Y., Basnett, J., Duck, R., Farrell, P., Nelson, B., & Zollneritsch, J. (2014). Understanding and measuring student engagement in school: the results of an international study from 12 countries. *School Psychology Quarterly, 29*, 213–232. https://doi.org/10.1037/spq0000057

Leary, M. R. (2004). *Introduction to behavioral research methods* (4th ed.). Pearson Education, Inc..

Lee, C. S., Hayes, K. N., Seitz, J., DiStefano, R., & O'Connor, D. (2016). Understanding motivational structures that differentially predict engagement and achievement in middle school science. *International Journal of Science Education, 38*, 2, 192-215/. https://doi.org/10.1080/09500693.2015.1136452

Leis, M., Schmidt, K., & Rimm-Kaufman, S. (2015). Using the partial credit model to evaluate the student engagement mathematics scale. *Journal of Applied Measurement, 16*, 251–267.

Li, Y., & Lerner, R. M. (2011). Trajectories of school engagement during adolescence: Implications for grades, depression, delinquency, and substance use. *Developmental Psychology, 47*, 233–247. https://doi.org/10.1037/a0021307

Lovelace, M. D., Reschly, A. L., Appleton, J. J., & Lutz, M. E. (2014). Concurrent and predictive validity of the student engagement instrument. *Journal of Psychoeducational Assessment, 32*, 509–520. https://doi.org/10.1177/0734282914527548

MacIver, M. A., & MacIver, D. J. (2010). How do we ensure that everyone graduates? An integrated prevention and tiered intervention model for schools and districts. *New Directions for Student Leadership, 2010*(127), 25–35. https://doi.org/10.1002/yd.360

Mandernach, J. (2015). Assessment of student engagement in higher education: a synthesis of literature and assessment tools. *International Journal of Learning, Teaching, and Educational Research, 12*, 1–14.

Marraccini, M. E., & Brier, Z. M. F. (2017). School connectedness and suicidal thoughts and behaviors: A systematic meta-analysis. *School Psychology Quarterly, 32*, 5–21. https://doi.org/10.1037/spq0000192

Mason, B., Gunersel, A. B., & Ney, E. (2014). Cultural and ethnic bias in teacher ratings of behavior: a criterion-focused review. *Psychology in the Schools, 51*, 1017–1030. https://doi.org/10.1002/pits.21800

McNeal, K. S., Spry, J. M., Mitra, R., & Tipton, J. L. (2014). Measuring student engagement, knowledge, and perceptions of climate change in an introductory environment geology course. *Journal of Geoscience Education, 62*, 655–667. https://doi.org/10.5408/13-111.1

Miller, B. W. (2015). Using reading times and eye-movements to measure cognitive engagement. *Educational Psychologist, 50*, 31–42. https://doi.org/10.1080/00461520.2015.1004068

Miller, R. B., Greene, B. A., Montalvo, G. P., Ravindran, B., & Nichols, J. D. (1996). Engagement in academic work:The role of learning goals, future consequences, pleasing others, and perceived ability. *Contemporary Educational Psychology, 21*(4), 388–422. https://doi.org/10.1006/ceps.1996.0028

Occumpaugh, J., Baker, R. S., & Rodrigo, M. M. T. (2015). *Baker Rodriuo Occumpaugh Monitoring Protocol (BROMP) 2.0 Technical and Training Manual.* Teachers College, Columbia University and Ateneo Laboratory for the Learning Sciences.

Pagani, L. S., Fitzpatrick, C., Archambault, I., & Janosz, M. (2010). School readiness and later achievement: A French-Canadian replication and extension. *Developmental Psychology, 46*(5), 984–994. https://doi.org/10.1037/a0018881

Pianta, R. C., Hamre, B. K., Haynes, N. J., Mintz, S. L., & La Paro, K. M. (2007). *Classroom Assessment Scoring System manual, middle/secondary version.* University of Virginia Press.

Poh, M., Swenson, N. C., & Picard, R. W. (2010). A wearable sensor for unobtrusive, long-term assessment of electrodermal activity. *IEE Transactions on Biomedical Engineering, 57*, 1243–1257.

Pintrich, P. R., & DeGroot, E. (1990). Motivational and self-regulated learning components of classroom academic performance. *Journal of Educational Psychology, 82*, 33–40. https://doi.org/10.1037/0022-0663.82.1.33

Reeve, J., & Tseng, C.-M. (2011). Agency as a fourth aspect of students' engagement during learning activities. *Contemporary Educational Psychology, 36*(4), 257–267. https://doi.org/10.1016/j.cedpsych.2011.05.002

Renninger, K. A., & Bachrach, J. E. (2015). Studying triggers for interest and engagement using observational methods. *Educational Psychologist, 50*, 58–69. https://doi.org/10.1080/00461520.2014.999920

Reschly, D. J., & Bergstrom, M. K. (2009). Response to intervention. In T. B. Gutkin & C. R. Reynolds (Eds.), *The handbook of school psychology* (4th ed., pp. 434–460). Wiley.

Reschly, A. L., Betts, J., & Appleton, J. J. (2014). An examination of the validity of two measures of student engagement. *International Journal of School & Educational Psychology, 2*, 106–114. https://doi.org/10.1080/21683603.2013.876950

Rimm-Kaufman, S. E., Baroody, A. E., Larsen, R. A., Curby, T. W., & Abruy, T. (2015). To what extent do teacher-student interaction quality and student gender contribution to fifth graders' engagement in mathematics learning? *Journal of Educational Psychology, 107*, 17–185. https://doi.org/10.1037/a0037252

Ryu, S., & Lombardi, D. (2015). Coding classroom interactions for collective and individual engagement. *Educational Psychologist, 50*, 70–83. https://doi.org/10.1080/00461520.2014.1001891

Salmela-Aro, K., & Upadyaya, K. (2012). The schoolwork Engagement Inventory: Energy, dedication, and absorption (EDA). *European Journal of Psychological Assessment, 28*, 60–67. https://doi.org/10.1027/1015-5759/a000091

Salmela-Aro, K., Kiuru, N., Leskinen, E., & Nurmi, J. E. (2009). School burnout inventory: Reliability and validity. *European Journal of Psychological Assessment, 25*, 48–57. https://doi.org/10.1027/1015-5759/a000091

Shen, L., Wang, M., & Shen, R. (2009). Affective e-Learning: Using "emotional" data to improve learning in pervasive learning environment. *Educational Technology & Society, 12*(2), 176–189.

Shernoff, D. J. (2013). *Advancing responsible adolescent development*. Springer Science + Business Media. https://doi.org/10.1007/978-1-4614-7089-2

Shernoff, D. J., & Csikszentmihalyi, M. (2009). Flow in schools: Cultivating engaged learners and optimal learning environments. In R. Gilman, E. S. Huebner, & M. Furlong (Eds.), *Handbook of Positive Psychology in Schools* (pp. 131–145). Routledge.

Shernoff, D. J., Csikzentmihalyi, M., Schneider, B., & Shernoff, E. S. (2003). Student engagement in high schools from the perspective of flow theory. *School Psychology Quarterly, 18*, 158–176. https://doi.org/10.1521/scpq.18.2.158.21860

Shernoff, D. J., Kelly, S., Tonks, S. M., Anderson, B., Canvanagh, R. F., Sinha, S., & Abdi, B. (2016). Student engagement as a function of environmental complexity in high school classrooms. *Learning and Instruction, 43*, 52–60. https://doi.org/10.1016/j.learninstruc.2015.12.003

Sinatra, G., Heddy, B. C., & Lombard, D. (2015). The challenge of defining and measuring student engagement in science. *Educational Psychologist, 1*, 1–13. https://doi.org/10.1080/00461520.2014.1002924

Sinclair, M. F., Christenson, S. L., Lehr, C. A., & Anderson, A. R. (2003). Facilitating student engagement: Lessons learned from Check & Connect Longitudinal studies. *The California School Psychologist, 8*(1), 29–42.

Skiba, R. J., Michael, R. S., Nardo, A. C., & Peterson, R. L. (2002). The color of discipline: Sources of racial and gender disproportionality in school punishment. *The Urban Review, 34*, 317–342. https://doi.org/10.1023/A:1021320817372

Skinner, E. A., Furrer, C., Marchand, G., & Kindermann, T. (2008). Engagement and disaffection in the classroom: Part of a larger motivational dynamic? *Journal of Educational Psychology, 100*, 765–781. https://doi.org/10.1037/a0012840

Skinner, E. A., Kindermann, T. A., & Furrer, C. J. (2009). A motivational perspective on engagement and disaffection. Conceptualization and assessment of children's behavioral and emotional participation in academic activities in the classroom. *Educational and Psychological Measurement, 69*, 493–525. https://doi.org/10.1177/0013164408323233

Veiga, F. H., & Robu, V. (2014). Measuring student engagement with school across cultures: Psychometric findings from Portugal and Romania. *Romanian Journal of School Psychology, 7*.

Voelkl, K. E. (1997). Identification with school. *American Journal of Education, 105*, 204–319. https://doi.org/10.1086/444158

Volpe, R. J., DiPerna, J. C., Hintze, J. M., & Shapiro, E. S. (2005). Observing students in classroom settings: A review of seven coding schemes. *School Psychology Review, 34*(4), 454–474. https://doi.org/10.1080/02796015.2005.12088009

Wang, M. T., & Fredricks, J. A. (2014). The reciprocal links between school engagement and youth problem behavior during adolescence. *Child Development, 85*, 722–737. https://doi.org/10.1111/cdev.12138

Wang, M.-T., & Holcombe, R. (2010). Adolescents' perceptions of school environment, engagement and academic achievement in middle school. *American Educational Research Journal, 47*, 633–662. https://doi.org/10.3102/000281209361209

Wang, M. T., Willett, J. B., & Eccles, J. S. (2011). The assessment of school engagement: Examining dimensionality and measurement invariable by gender and race/ethnicity. *Journal of School Psychology, 49*, 465–480. https://doi.org/10.1016/j.jsp.2011.04.001

Wang, Z., Bergin, C., & Bergin, D. A. (2014). Measuring engagement in fourth to twelfth grade classrooms: The classroom engagement inventory. *School Psychology Quarterly, 4*, 527–535. https://doi.org/10.1037/spq0000050

Wang, M. T., Chow, A., Hofkens, T., & Salmela-Aro, K. (2015). The trajectories of student emotional engagement and school burnout with academic and psychological development: Findings from Finish adolescents. *Learning and Instruction, 36*, 57–65. https://doi.org/10.1016/j.learninstruc.2014.11.004

Wang, M. T., Fredricks, J. A., Ye, F., Hofkens, T., & Schall, J. (2016). The math science engagement scale: development, validation, and psychometric properties. *Learning and Instruction, 43*, 16–26. https://doi.org/10.1016/j.learninstruc.2016.01.008

Wang, M. T., Fredricks, J. A., Ye, F., Hofkens, T., & Schall, J. (2019). Conceptualization and assessment of adolescents' engagement and disengagement in school: A multidimensional school engagement scale. *European Journal of Psychological Assessment, 35*(4), 592–606. https://doi.org/10.1027/1015-5759/a000431

Waxman, H. C., Tharp, R. G., & Hilberg, R. S. (2004). Future directions for classroom observation research. In H. C. Waxman, R. S. Hilberg, & R. G. Tharp (Eds.), *Observational research in U.S. classrooms: New approaches for understanding cultural and linguistic diversity* (pp. 266–277). Cambridge University Press.

Wigfield, A., Guthrie, J. T., Perencevich, K. C., Taboada, A., Klauda, S. L., McRae, A., & Barbosa, P. (2008). Role of reading engagement in mediating the effects of reading comprehension instruction on reading outcomes. *Psychology in the Schools, 45*, 432–445. https://doi.org/10.1002/pits.20307

Winne, P. H., & Perry, N. E. (2000). Measuring self-regulated learning. In M. Boekaerts, P. Pintrich, & M. Zeidner (Eds.), *Handbook of self-regulation* (pp. 531–566). Academic Press.

Yang, C., Sharkey, J. D., Reed, L. A., & Dowdy, E. (2020). Cyberbullying victimization and student engagement among adolescents: Does school climate matter? *School Psychology, 35*, 158–169. https://doi.org/10.1037/spq0000353

Zirkel, S., Garcia, J. A., & Murphy, M. C. (2015). Experience-sampling research methods and their potential for education research. *Educational Researcher, 44*(1), 7–16. https://doi.org/10.3102/0013189X14566879

Measuring Student Engagement with Observational Techniques

Jennifer A. Fredricks

Abstract

The purpose of this chapter is to describe the use of observational methods to assess student engagement. These observational measures range from standardized rating scales of behavior to qualitative studies of classroom context and student engagement. Benefits, limitations, and methodological considerations with observational methods are described. Next, nine observational instruments with indicators of student engagement are presented. These instruments are compared on a variety of dimensions including what is measured, uses, samples, and the extent of reliability and validity of information. Finally, ongoing challenges with the use of observational methods of student engagement are discussed.

Engagement is a multidimensional construct that describes the quality of involvement in an activity or learning context. The most prevalent conceptualization of student engagement is that it consists of three distinct, yet interrelated dimensions: behavioral, emotional, and cognitive engagement (Fredricks et al., 2004). *Behavioral engagement* includes indicators of involvement in classroom and school contexts such as attention, participation, and effort; positive conduct; and the absence of disruptive behaviors (Fredricks et al., 2004). *Emotional engagement* focuses on positive and negative reactions to teachers, peers, academics, and school; a sense of belonging; and identification with school or subject domains (Finn, 1989; Voelkl, 1997). Finally, *cognitive engagement* is defined in terms of students' cognitive investment in learning and includes indicators such as being self-regulated and using deep learning strategies (Fredricks et al., 2004). Additionally, some scholars have added a fourth component of engagement including academic (Appleton et al., 2006, 2008), social (Finn & Zimmer, 2012; Wang et al., 2019), and agentic engagement (Reeve & Tseng, 2011).

Scholars, practitioners, and policymakers have used a variety of methods to assess these different dimensions of student engagement. These methods include self-report surveys, teacher rating scales, observations, administrator data (e.g., attendance, suspensions), experience sampling methods, and a new group of real-time measures that collect fine-grained data at time scales ranging from seconds to a few minutes (e.g., computer log files, galvanic skin responses). A detailed description of these different methodologies, including information on the benefits and limitations of these methods, is outlined in

J. A. Fredricks (✉)
Union College, Schenectady, NY, USA
e-mail: fredricj@union.edu

other sources (See Fredricks, 2021; Fredricks, Hofkens, & Wang, 2019a, for more details).

In this chapter, I focus specifically on measuring engagement using observational techniques. First, I review the different reasons to use observational techniques to assess engagement, outline the benefits and limitations of this methodology, provide an overview of different types of observational measures, and describe questions to consider when using observational methods to assess engagement. Next, nine observational instruments that have been used to assess engagement are presented and compared on several dimensions. These observations range from tools with standardized rating scales to studies that use qualitative techniques to describe the classroom context and level of student engagement. On one end of the continuum are systematic direct observation techniques which measure a specific target behavior(s) using standardized coding schemes (Hintze et al., 2002; Volpe et al., 2005). On the other end of the continuum are studies that have assessed engagement using narrative discourse analysis to examine how students engage in and experience classrooms over time (Engle & Conant, 2002; Gresalfi, 2009; Ryu & Lombardi, 2015). This chapter concludes with a discussion of unanswered questions with observational methods.

Why Use Observational Techniques

There are a variety of reasons to use observational methods to assess engagement. Educational psychologists have developed observational instruments to assess variations in teacher effectiveness and the quality of the classroom environment (Pianta & Hamre, 2009). For example, the Classroom Assessment Scoring System for Secondary School Students (CLASS-S) is an observational tool that includes student engagement as an indicator of teaching effectiveness (Pianta et al., 2007). Data collected on engagement using classroom observational measures

can be used to identify a teacher's strengths and weaknesses and inform professional development efforts (Stulman et al., 2021). Observational techniques also have been used to capture the dynamic interactions by which students come to engage in groups, activities, and communities. This research is grounded in sociocultural theory and focuses on how engagement evolves in a dialectical relationship between the individual and the social context over time (Corno & Mandinach, 2004; Ryu & Lombardi, 2015). For example, Ryu and Lombardi (2015) used both critical discourse analysis and social network analysis to describe the process by which elementary students both individually and collectively engage in scientific argumentation.

Other studies have used observational tools to monitor the effectiveness of educational interventions (Volpe et al., 2005). For example, researchers have used observation techniques to examine the impact of instructional reforms, disciplinary interventions, peer modeling, and socioemotional interventions on changes in student engagement (Fredricks, Reschly, & Christenson, 2019b). It is common in these studies to restrict observations to those students with the highest levels of problem behavior to increase the likelihood of documenting change (Briesch et al., 2015).

Finally, observational measures play a key role in practice. School psychologists have used direct observations of student behavior to screen students for academic, emotional, and behavioral problems and determine appropriate interventions (Volpe & McConaughy, 2005). Direct observational techniques allow practitioners to quantify behavior with standardized procedures at the time and place the behavior occurs (Christ et al., 2009; Hintze et al., 2002). For example, the Behavioral Assessment for Children: Student Observation System (Reynolds & Kampaus, 2015) is used in conjunction with rating scales to identify behavioral problems, eligibility for special education, and aid in the development of intervention plans.

Benefits and Limitations of Observational Methods

There are several benefits to using observational methods to assess behavioral, emotional, and cognitive engagement. First, observers are able to collect information on all three types of engagement in real-time as opposed to asking students to report retroactively on classroom context and their engagement levels (Fredricks & McColskey, 2012). As a result, this methodology has the potential to overcome bias or inaccurate assessments that are a concern with self-report methodologies. Moreover, observational methods may be more amenable to administrators and teachers than using surveys to assess engagement because it does not result in loss of instructional time. Another benefit of observational methods is that they can provide a rich description of variations in engagement and classroom context. Studies using observational methods can enhance our understanding of the factors that explain both the antecedents of and variations in engagement over time. Because observations are grounded in practice and provide detailed information on a specific case, they also can be very useful to practitioners (Renninger & Bachrach, 2015).

Systematic direct observational techniques also have several benefits. These techniques are low inference, objective, and can be used to conduct sequential analyses and test for quantitative differences in behavioral engagement across individuals, time periods, and settings (Hamre et al., 2009; Hintze et al., 2002). There is also a large degree of flexibility in these observational instruments in terms of observable behaviors, sampling period, and the duration of ratings (Ferguson et al., 2018; Hintze et al., 2002). A further benefit of data collected from these measures is that they can be used to inform placement decisions and progress monitoring.

Despite these benefits, there are several limitations to observational methods. First, most observational measures focus on a limited number of behavioral indicators of engagement and fail to capture the multidimensionality of the engagement construct. As a result, these tools can provide valuable information on the frequency of

and variations in student behaviors, but limited information on emotional or cognitive engagement and the quality of this behavioral engagement (Fredricks et al., 2004). Self-report survey methods may be a more valid way to assess emotional and cognitive engagement than observations, which require an observer to infer what students are thinking and feeling from their observed behaviors (Appleton et al., 2008). The large variability in observational tools in terms of the number of behavioral targets (one student versus a larger number of students), time sampling (15 seconds versus 1 minute), behavioral indicators, observational length, and the number of observations makes it difficult to compare findings using different tools (Ferguson et al., 2018). Furthermore, there is limited information on the predictive validity of these observational techniques, and the relation between these indicators and achievement-related outcomes (Fredricks & McColskey, 2012).

Another limitation is the large number of resources that are necessary to train observers, collect, and analyze interview data. Because of the costs and time investments, studies usually include only a small number of participants, which raises concerns about the generalizability of the findings to other settings. Furthermore, collecting observational data can require extensive training to support and maintain validity. Finally, indicators of engagement are culturally determined, as differences in rules around speaking, listening, and taking can impact engagement ratings and may result in some ethnic groups being mislabeled as disengaged (Bingham & Okagaki, 2012).

Methodological Considerations

In this section, I describe the different methodological decisions related to the use of observations. First, there are several decisions related to the timing of observations including how often to observe, in what contexts (e.g., whole group, small group, and individual subject areas), and over what periods of time (e.g., continuous, momentary time sampling, partial recordings, or whole-interval recording) (Waxman et al., 2004). The frequency of observations will also vary depending on whether it is a higher frequency (e.g., on-task behavior) versus a low-frequency behavior (e.g., aggression) (Kamphaus & Dever, 2016).

Another consideration is whether to use a measure that collects data on the frequency of discrete behaviors or includes more holistic and global measures of behavioral engagement (Hamre et al., 2009; Stulman et al., 2021). One advantage of global measures of student engagement is that the data collected can be more meaningful than discrete behaviors measured in isolation and may be more appropriate for examining differences between classrooms and teachers. On the other hand, observational instruments with more global indicators require an observer to make more inferences, which can reduce the reliability of these methods. Additionally, an instrument that measures the frequencies of certain behaviors may be more appropriate for measuring the effectiveness of an intervention (Stulman et al., 2021). For example, researchers used the Behavioral Observational System (Shapiro, 2011) to compare participants in a class-wide peer tutoring program to students in a control group on indicators of behavioral engagement (e.g., active and passive engaged time) (Volpe et al., 2012).

Another important factor in deciding on an observation tool is information on the psychometric properties of the instrument (Stulman et al., 2021). One important question is whether the measure has information on the reliability of the instruments in terms of the consistency in ratings across observers, or interrater reliability, and the stability of observations across different children and time periods. Another important criterion to consider is whether the instrument has information on validity or the extent to which the observational measures are related to teacher and student outcomes in the expected direction (Stulman et al., 2021). To date, there is limited published information on the psychometric properties of these measures.

Finally, one needs to decide who will conduct the observations. Teachers' expertise and knowl-

edge of their students can help them to notice and interpret student behavior, but these experiences may also color their perceptions and can lead to biased observations. Furthermore, it may be difficult for teachers to observe at the same time they are delivering instruction and managing classroom dynamics. On the other hand, outside observers have less knowledge of the students but may have broader and less biased perspectives (Hofkens & Ruzek, 2019).

Review of Measures

In this section, nine observational instruments of student engagement are presented. These instruments were chosen because they have been used extensively in either research or practice, include indicators of more than just on-task behavior, and include at least some information on the psychometric properties of the instrument. The list of instruments is presented in Table 1. These instruments were compared in terms of what is measured, uses, samples, psychometric properties, and uses.

What Is Measured? All nine instruments included indicators of behavioral engagement. Additionally, three of the instruments [BROMP (Ocumpaugh et al., 2015); Collective Engagement (Reeve et al., 2004); and Observed Child Engagement Scale (Rimm-Kaufman, 2005)] also included indicators of emotional/affective engagement. Two of the instruments [(BOSS (Shapiro, 2011) and (CLOCK) (Volpe & Diperna, 2010)] differentiate between active (e.g., reading aloud) and passive behavioral engagement (e.g., silently reading). Eight instruments [BROMP (Ocumpaugh et al., 2015); BASC-3 SOS (Reynolds & Kampaus, 2015); BOSS (Shapiro, 2011); CISSAR-MS (Greenwood et al., 1991); CLOCK (Volpe & Diperna, 2010); COS (Waxman & Padron, 2004); Collective Engagement (Reeve et al., 2004); and Observed Child Engagement Scale (Rimm-Kaufman, 2005)] include indicators of behavioral disengagement.

Table 1 List of observational measures

Instrument name	Citations	Sample indicators
Baker Rodrigo Ocumpaugh Monitoring Protocol (BROMP)	Ocumpaugh et al. (2015)	On-task behavior (e.g., on-task conversation, on-task help seeking, on-task giving/receiving answers) Off-task behavior (e.g., aggression, off-task social, off-task supplies) Gaming the system Affective categories (e.g., boredom, confusion, delight, engaged conversation, frustration, surprise)
Behavior Assessment System for Children–Third Edition: Student Observation System (BASC-3 SOS)	Reynolds and Kampaus (2015)	Adaptive behavior (e.g., responds to teacher/lesson, works on school subjects, transition movements) Inappropriate behavior (e.g., inappropriate interaction, inappropriate movement, inattention)
Behavioral Observation in Schools (BOSS)	Fredricks et al. (2011), Shapiro (2011)	Active engaged time (e.g., writing, reading aloud) Passive engaged time (e.g., listening to a lecture, silently reading) Off-task motor Off-task verbal Off-task passive

(continued)

Table 1 (continued)

Instrument name	Citations	Sample indicators
Code for Instrumental Structure and Student Academic Response-Mainstream Version (CISSAR-MS)	Fredricks et al. (2011), Greenwood et al. (1991)	Academic responding (positive engagement behaviors) (e.g., engaged in writing, playing an academic game, asking or answering an academic question, reading aloud or silently) Task management (neutral engagement behaviors) (e.g., raising a hand to ask for help, looking for materials) Inappropriate behaviors/competing behaviors (being disruptive, talking inappropriately, not paying attention)
Classroom Assessment Scoring System-Secondary Schools (CLASS-S)	Pianta et al. (2012)	Behavioral indicators of engagement (i.e., responding, asking questions, volunteering, active listening, and lack of off-task behavior)
Cooperative Learning Observation Code for Kids (CLOCK)	Volpe and DiPerna (2010)	Active engagement Passive engagement Positive social interaction Nonphysical aggression Interference

(continued)

Table 1 (continued)

Instrument name	Citations	Sample indicators
Collective Engagement	Reeve et al. (2004)	Attention (dispersed vs. focused attention) Effort (passive, slow, minimal effort vs. active, quick, intense effort) Verbal participation (verbally silent vs. verbally participating) Persistence (students give up easily vs. persist) Positive emotion (flat vs. positive emotion tone) Voice
Classroom Observation Schedule (COS)	Waxman and Padron (2004)	On-task Waiting for teacher Disruptive Distracted
Observed Child Engagement Scale	Rimm-Kaufman (2005)	Participation in learning opportunities (involvement in activities, duration, interest) Disruptive behavior (learning disruptions) Positive affect (happiness, verbal expression) Self-reliance (self-management, response to intrusions, initiative)

Behavioral Engagement All nine observational instruments include indicators of behavioral engagement (see Table 1). Examples of behavioral indicators include being on-task, responding to teacher/lessons, giving and receiving answers, writing, volunteering, reading aloud, listening to a lecture, talking to a teacher, playing an academic game, asking for help, positive social interaction, effort, attention, persistence, self-reliance, initiative, and verbal participation. Examples of indicators of behavioral disengagement include aggression, distracted, off-task

behavior, being disruptive, talking inappropriately, inattention, inappropriate interactions, and interference.

Affective/Emotional Engagement Three of the observational instruments include indicators of affective/emotional engagement and disengagement [BROMP (Ocumpaugh et al., 2015); Collective Engagement (Reeve et al., 2004); & Observed Child Engagement Scale (Rimm-Kaufman, 2005)]. Indicators of affective/emotional engagement include happiness, delight, surprise, engaged conversation, verbal expression, and positive emotion, and indicators of affective/emotional disengagement include boredom, confusion, frustration, and flat emotional tone.

Uses Another way to compare the nine observational measures is to examine variations in the purposes and uses (See Table 2). Six of the measures [(BOSS) (Shapiro, 2011); CLASS-S (Pianta et al., 2012); CISSAR-MS (Greenwood et al., 1991); CLOCK (Volpe & Diperna, 2010); COS (Waxman & Padron, 2004) & Collective Engagement (Reeve et al., 2004)] have been used in evaluations of the effectiveness of a variety of disciplinary, social, and instructional interventions. For example, the CLOCK was used in an evaluation of the effectiveness of a positive behavioral program on student engagement and learning (Diperna et al., 2016) and the Collective Engagement Scale (Reeve et al., 2004) was used to evaluate the effectiveness of an intervention aimed to increase teachers' autonomy support. The CLASS-S (Pianta et al., 2012) has been used both to monitor engagement at the teacher, district, and school level, and with professional development for teachers.

Six of the observational measures [(BROMP (Ocumpaugh et al., 2015); CLASS-S (Pianta et al., 2012); CLOCK (Volpe & Diperna, 2010); COS (Waxman & Padron, 2004): Collective Engagement (Reeve et al., 2004); & Observed Child Engagement Scale (Rimm-Kaufman,

Table 2 Observational uses, samples, and psychometric information

Instrument name	Uses	Samples	Psychometric information
Baker Rodrigo Ocumpaugh Monitoring Protocol (BROMP)	Research on engagement of students in range of classroom activities (both with technology and more traditional activities) Educational data mining to develop and refine automated models of student engagement for commercial systems	Wide range of samples in United States, India, Philippines, United Kingdom, United Arab Emirates and Mexico Kindergarten to undergraduate to populations	Observers are trained and certified; to be certified, observed must achieve a Kappa of 0.6 Predictive validity-relationship between engagement and disengagement and achievement in expected direction
Behavior Assessment System for Children–Third Edition: Student Observation System (BASC-3 SOS)	Individual clinical assessment by school psychologists Identification of behavioral problems and development of individualized education plans Autism related research	Ages 2–21	Published reliability and validity information for teacher and parent ratings scales; no published psychometric specific to the observation
Behavioral Observation in Schools (BOSS)	Individual clinical assessment by school psychologists Research on the effectiveness of educational interventions	Developed for use with pre-kindergarten to grade 12 students Ethnically diverse groups of both typically developing and special needs Most published studies have used with elementary school students	High interrater reliability after training (90–100%) Discriminant validity: Evidence that measure can differentiate between children with ADHD and typically developing students
Code for Instrumental Structure and Student Academic Response-Mainstream Version (CISSAR-MS)	Individual clinical assessment by school psychologists Research on effectiveness of educational interventions	Developed and validated for both elementary and middle school students in both regular and special educational classes	Interrater reliability at 80% of higher after training Construct validity: academic responding is correlated with academic achievement
Classroom Assessment Scoring System-Secondary Schools (CLASS-S)	Data on teacher effectiveness at school and district level Professional development with teachers Research on teacher student interactions and engagement Research on the effectiveness of educational interventions	Secondary classrooms in United States, Norway, Sweden	With training, fair interrater reliability [Exact or adjacent agreement (76.6%)] Predictive validity: engagement related to achievement outcomes Concurrent validity: evidence of association between CLASS and teacher self-ratings
Cooperative Learning Observation Code for Kids (CLOCK)	Research on the effectiveness of educational interventions Research on classroom context, motivation, and engagement	Elementary school students	Concurrent validity: moderate correlation between engagement and teacher ratings
Collective Engagement	Research on effectiveness of educational intervention	High school	Interrater reliability ranged from 0.63 to 0.92

(continued)

Table 2 (continued)

Instrument name	Uses	Samples	Psychometric information
Classroom Observation Schedule (COS)	Research on effectiveness of educational interventions Research on classroom instruction and student behavior Professional development with teachers	Diverse samples of elementary and middle school students	High interrater reliability (over 0.95) Discriminant validity evidence that can differentiate between resilient and non-resilient students
Observed Child Engagement Scale	Research on classroom quality, teacher-student interactions and engagement	Kindergarten and first grade classrooms	Concurrent validity: correlation between behavioral engagement and duration of time engaged Behavioral engagement associated with indicators of classroom quality and achievement in expected direction High interrater reliability

2005) have been in used in research on classroom context, motivation, and engagement. Another common usage of observational measures by school psychologists is in the diagnosis and monitoring of behavioral, social, and emotional problems (Shapiro & Heick, 2004). Three of the observational measures included in this review [BASC-3 (Reynolds & Kampaus, 2015; BOSS (Shapiro, 2011); CISSAR-MS (Greenwood et al., 1991)] were used primarily for child and adolescent individual assessments. Finally, the BROMP has been used to develop and refine automated models of student engagement for commercial systems such as the Cognitive Tutor and the Reasoning Mind (Baker et al., 2018; Mulqueeny et al., 2015).

Samples The observational instruments were used with a range of populations from early childhood samples to undergraduate student populations, with the majority administered to elementary school students. As seen in Table 2, these observations have been used with both typically developing and special needs students. Two of the observation instruments have been used in international studies [BROMP (Ocumpaugh et al., 2015) & CLASS-S (Pianta et al., 2012)]. For example, the BROMP has been used in samples in India, Philippines, the

United Kingdom, United Arab Emirates, and Mexico (Baker et al., 2018).

Psychometric Support The final way to compare these nine observational instruments is the extent of psychometric support. Information on both reliability and validity is presented in Table 2. Eight of the instruments included some published information on interrater reliability or the degree to which two or more raters assign consistent ratings for the same behavior [BROMP (Ocumpaugh et al., 2015); BOSS (Shapiro, 2011); CLASS-S (Pianta et al., 2012); (CISSAR-MS (Greenwood et al., 1991); COS (Waxman & Padron, 2004); Collective Engagement (Reeve et al., 2004); & Observed Child Engagement Scale (Rimm-Kaufman, 2005)]. All report at least moderate agreement between raters, with an increase in interrater reliability with training.

In contrast, there is much less detailed information on the validity of these measures. Four of the instruments include some published evidence that engagement is associated with indicators of achievement either concurrently or over time [BROMP (Ocumpaugh et al., 2015; CLASS-S (Pianta et al., 2012), CISSAR-MS (Greenwood et al., 1991) & Observer Child Engagement Scale (Rimm-Kaufman, 2005)]. Additionally, three of the developers provide evidence of concurrent validity or the extent to which the instrument correlates with previously validated measures [CLASS-S (Pianta et al., 2012), CLOCK (Volpe & Diperna, 2010), and Observed Child Engagement Scale (Rimm-Kaufman, 2005)]. Finally, two of the instruments [BOSS (Shapiro, 2011) and COS (Waxman & Padron, 2004)] included published information on discriminant validity or the extent to which the measure can differentiate between the type of students. For example, BOSS (Shapiro, 2011) has been shown to differentiate the behavioral engagement of students with ADHD from their typically developing peers.

Unanswered Questions

Despite the increased use of observational techniques to assess student engagement, several unanswered questions remain. One question concerns the number of observations that need to be completed to adequately sample classroom-level processes. We know from prior research that there is both stability and variability in engagement across time and different contexts (Azevedo, 2015; Fredricks et al., 2004; Lawson & Lawson, 2013). This is an important question because classroom observations are expensive and time-consuming to conduct. Furthermore, there are questions about the scalability of these measures for research due to the necessary investments in training and coding classroom videos. Advances in the automated coding of videos may help to reduce these costs. For example, a few scholars have captured observational behavior data using computer system such as intelligent tutoring and learning management systems (Baker et al., 2012; Henrie et al., 2015; Morris et al., 2005).

As noted in this review, the extent of information on the reliability and validity of these measures is limited. This makes it more challenging for both researchers and practitioners to choose an appropriate instrument for their population and target use (Stulman et al., 2021). Furthermore,

it is important to validate these observational measures across culturally and linguistically diverse samples of students because variations in the type of and frequency of behaviors may lead to differences in the interpretation of student engagement (Bingham & Okagaki, 2012; Kamphaus & Dever, 2016). Moreover, there are tensions between the feasibility of collecting data, the ability to establish reliability and validity, and the degree of information obtained from these measures. On one hand, standardized and defined observational rating scales require less training to obtain a high degree of reliability but provide much more limited information on engagement. On the other hand, more holistic and qualitative measures provide a more comprehensive picture of engagement and disengagement but require more training and are more difficult to establish the reliability and compare across contexts.

Finally, as noted in this chapter, observational measures have both strengths and limitations in the amount and types of data collected. One of the biggest challenges with this methodology is the cost in terms of time and labor. The cost is even greater if numerous observations are required to establish reliability and validity (Kamphaus & Dever, 2016). As a result, observations are rarely used in used isolation for research, diagnosis, or outcome assessment. In sum, observations that are paired with other techniques to assess student engagement (e.g., surveys, real-time measures, interviews) will provide the most comprehensive and complete picture of student engagement.

References

Appleton, J. J., Christenson, S. L., Kim, D., & Reschly, A. L. (2006). Measuring cognitive and psychological engagement: Validation of the Student Engagement Instrument. *Journal of School Psychology, 44*, 427–445. https://doi.org/10.1002/pits.20303

Appleton, J. J., Christenson, S. L., & Furlong, M. J. (2008). Student engagement with school: Critical conceptual and methodological issues of the construct. *Psychology in the Schools, 45*, 369–386. https://doi.org/10.1002/pits.20303

Azevedo, R. (2015). Defining and measuring engagement and learning in science: Conceptual, theoretical, methodological, and analytical issues. *Educational Psychologist, 50*, 84–94. https://doi.org/10.1080/0046 1520.2015.1004069

Baker, R. S. J., Gowda, S. M., Wixon, M., Kalka, J., Wagner, A. Z., Aleven, V., et al. (2012). Towards sensor-free affect detection in cognitive tutor algebra. In K. Yacef, O. Zaïane, H. Hershkovitz, M. Yudelson, & J. Stamper (Eds.), *Proceedings of the 5th International Conference on Educational Data Mining* (pp. 126–133). International Educational Data Mining Society.

Baker, R. S., Ocumpaugh, J. L., & Andres, J. M. A. L. (2018). BROMP quantitative field observations: A review. In R. Feldman (Ed.), *Learning science: Theory, research, and practice*. McGraw-Hill.

Bingham, G. E., & Okagaki, L. (2012). Ethnicity and student engagement. In S. L. Christenson, A. L. Reschly, & C. Wylie (Eds.), *Handbook of research on student engagement* (pp. 65–95). Springer Science + Business Media.

Briesch, A. M., Hemphill, E. M., Volpe, R. J., & Daniels, B. (2015). An evaluation of observational methods for measuring response to class-wide intervention. *School Psychology Quarterly, 30*, 37–49. https://doi.org/10.1037/spq0000065

Christ, T. J., Riley-Tillman, T. C., & Chafouleas, S. M. (2009). Foundation for the development and use of Direct Behavior Rating (DBR) to assess and evaluate student behavior. *Assessment for Effective Intervention, 34*, 201–213. https://doi.org/10.1177/1534508409340390

Corno, L., & Mandinach, E. B. (2004). What have we learned about student engagement in the past twenty years. In D. M. McInerney & S. Van Etten (Eds.), *Big theories revisited: Vol 4. Research on sociocultural influences on motivation and learning* (pp. 299–328). Information Age Publishing.

Diperna, J. C., Lei, P., Bellinger, J., & Cheng, W. (2016). Effects of a positive behavioral program on student learning. *Psychology in the Schools, 53*, 189–205. https://doi.org/10.1002/pits.21891

Engle, R. A., & Conant, F. R. (2002). Guiding principles for fostering productive disciplinary engagement: Explaining an emergent argument in a community of learners' classroom. *Cognition and Instruction, 20*, 399–483. https://doi.org/10.1207/S1532690XCI2004_1

Ferguson, T. D., Briesch, A. M., Volpe, R. J., Donaldson, A. R., & Feinberg, A. B. (2018). Psychometric considerations for conducting observations using time-sampling procedures. *Assessment for Effective Intervention, 44*(1), 45–57. https://doi.org/10.1177/1534508417747389

Finn, J. D. (1989). Withdrawing from school. *Review of Educational Research, 59*, 117–142. https://doi.org/10.3102/00346543059002117

Finn, J. D., & Zimmer, K. (2012). Student engagement: What is it? Why does it matter? In S. L. Christenson, A. L. Reschly, & C. Wylie (Eds.), *Handbook of research on student engagement* (pp. 97–131). Springer.

Fredricks, J. (2021). The measurement of student engagement: Methodological advances and comparisons of new self-report measures. In S. Christenson, A. L. Reschy, & C. Wylie (Eds, 2nd edition.), *Handbook of research on student engagement* (2nd ed). Springer.

Fredricks, J. A., & McColskey, W. (2012). The measurement of student engagement: A comparative analysis of various methods and student self-report instruments. In S. Christenson, A. L. Reschly, & C. Wylie (Eds.), *Handbook of research on student engagement* (pp. 763–783). Springer.

Fredricks, J. A., Blumenfeld, P. C., & Paris, A. (2004). School engagement: Potential of the concept: State of the evidence. *Review of Educational Research, 74*, 59–119. https://doi.org/10.3102/00346543074001059

Fredricks, J., & McColskey, W., with Meli, J., Mordica, J., Montrosse, B., & Mooney, K. (2011). *Measuring student engagement in upper elementary through high school: a description of 21 instruments*. (Issues & Answers Report, REL 2010–No. 098). Washington, DC: U.S. Department of Education, Institute of Education Sciences, National Center for Education. Available at http://ies.ed.gov/ncee/edlabs/projects/project.asp?projectID=268

Fredricks, J. A., Hofkens, T., & Wang, M. (2019a). Measuring student engagement: An overview of methods, challenges, and new directions. In A. Renninger & S. Hidi (Eds.), *The Cambridge handbook of motivation and learning* (pp. 689–712). Cambridge University Press. https://doi.org/10.1017/9781316823279

Fredricks, J., Reschly, A., & Christenson, S. (Eds.). (2019b). *Handbook of student engagement interventions: Working with disengaged students*. Academic.

Greenwood, C. R., Carta, J., & Atwater, J. (1991). Ecobehavioral analysis in the classroom: Review and implications. *Journal of Behavioral Education, 1*, 59–77. https://doi.org/10.1007/BF00956754

Gresalfi, M. S. (2009). Taking up opportunities to learn: Constructing dispositions in mathematics classrooms. *Journal of the Learning Sciences, 18*, 327–369. https://doi.org/10.1080/10508400903013470

Hamre, B. K., Pianta, R. C., & Chomat-Mooney, L. (2009). Conducting classroom observations in school-based research. In L. M. Dinella (Ed.), *Conducting science-based psychology research in schools* (pp. 79–105). American Psychological Association. https://doi.org/10.1037/11881-004

Henrie, C. R., Halverson, L. R., & Graham, C. R. (2015). Measuring student engagement in technology-mediated learning: A review. *Computers and Education, 90*, 36–53. https://doi.org/10.1016/j.compedu.2015.09.005

Hintze, J. M., Volpe, R. J., & Shapiro, E. S. (2002). Best practices in the systematic direct observation of student behavior. In A. Thomas & J. Grimes (Eds.), *Best practices in school psychology IV* (pp. 993–1006). National Association of School Psychologists.

Hofkens, T. L., & Ruzek, E. (2019). Measuring student engagement to inform interventions in schools. In J. Fredricks, A. Reschly, & S. Christenon (Eds.), *Handbook of student engagement interventions: Working with disengaged youth* (pp. 309–324). Academic.

Kamphaus, R. W., & Dever, B. V. (2016). Behavioral observation and assessment. In J. C. Norcross, G. R. VadenBos, & D. K. Freedheim (Eds.), *APA handbook of clinical psychology: Vol. 3* (pp. 17–29). Applications and Methods.

Lawson, M. A., & Lawson, H. A. (2013). New conceptual frameworks for student engagement research, policy, and practice. *Review of Educational Research, 83*(3), 432–479. https://doi.org/10.3102/0034654313480891

Morris, L. V., Finnegan, C., & Wu, S.-S. (2005). Tracking student behavior, persistence, and achievement in online courses. *The Internet and Higher Education, 8,* 221–231. https://doi.org/10.1016/j.iheduc.2005.06.009

Mulqueeny, K., Kostyuk, V., Baker, R. S., & Ocumpaugh, J. (2015). Incorporating effective e-learning principles to improve student engagement in middle-school mathematics. *International Journal of STEM Education, 2.* https://doi.org/10.1186/s40594-015-0028-6

Ocumpaugh, J., Baker, R. S., & Rodrigo, M. M. T. (2015). *Baker Rodriguo Occumpaugh monitoring protocol (BROMP) 2.0 technical and training manual.* Teachers College, Columbia University and Ateneo Laboratory for the Learning Sciences.

Pianta, R. C., & Hamre, B. K. (2009). Conceptualization, measurement, and improvement of classroom processes: Standardized observation can leverage capacity. *Educational Researcher, 38*(2), 109–119. https://doi.org/10.3102/0013189X09332374

Pianta, R. C., Hamre, B. K., Haynes, N. J., Mintz, S. L., & La Paro, K. M. (2007). *Classroom Assessment Scoring System manual, middle/secondary version.* University of Virginia Press.

Pianta, R. C., Hamre, B. K., & Mintz, S. L. (2012). *Classroom assessment scoring system (CLASS): Secondary class manual.* Teachstone.

Reeve, J., & Tseng, C. M. (2011). Agency as a fourth aspect of students' engagement during learning activities. *Contemporary Educational Psychology, 36*(4), 257–267. https://doi.org/10.1016/j.cedpsych.2011.05.002

Reeve, J., Jang, H., Carrell, D., Jeon, S., & Barch, J. (2004). Enhancing students' engagement by increasing teachers' autonomy support. *Motivation and Emotion, 28,* 147–169. https://doi.org/10.1023/B:MOEM.0000032312.95499.6f

Renninger, K. A., & Bachrach, J. E. (2015). Studying triggers for interest and engagement using observational methods. *Educational Psychologist, 50,* 58–69. https://doi.org/10.1080/00461520.2014.999920

Reynolds, C. Z., & Kampaus, R. W. (2015). *Reynolds, intellectual assessment scales* (2nd ed.). Psychological Assessment Resources.

Rimm-Kaufman, S. E. (2005). *Classroom observation protocol for Early Learning Study* (Unpublished protocol). University of Virginia.

Ryu, S., & Lombardi, D. (2015). Coding classroom interactions for collective and individual engagement. *Educational Psychologist, 50,* 70–83. https://doi.org/10.1080/00461520.2014.1001891

Shapiro, E. S. (2011). Behavioral observation of students in schools. In E. S. Shapiro (Ed.), *Academic skills problems fourth edition workbook* (pp. 35–56). The Guilford Press.

Shapiro, E. S., & Heick, P. (2004). School psychologist assessment practices in the evaluation of students referred for social/behavioral/emotional problems. *Psychology in the Schools, 41,* 551–561. https://doi.org/10.1002/pits.10176

Stulman, M. W., Hamre, B. K., Downer, J. T., & Pianta, R. C. (2021). *How to select the right observation tool.* CASTL, University of Virginia.

Voelkl, K. E. (1997). Identification with school. *American Journal of Education, 105,* 204–319. https://doi.org/10.1086/444158

Volpe, R. J., & DiPerna, J. C. (2010). *Cooperative learning observation code for kids.* Unpublished observation code.

Volpe, R. J., & McConaughy, S. H. (2005). Systematic direct observational assessment of student behavior: Its use and interpretation in multiple settings: An introduction to the miniseries. *School Psychology Review, 34*(4), 451–453. https://doi.org/10.1080/02796015.2005.12088008

Volpe, R. J., DiPerna, J. C., Hintze, J. M., & Shapiro, E. S. (2005). Observing students in classroom settings: A review of seven coding schemes. *School Psychology Review, 34*(4), 454–474.

Volpe, R., Young, G., Piana, M., & Zaslofsky, A. (2012). Integrating classwide early literacy intervention and behavioral supports: A pilot investigation. *Journal of Positive Behavior Interventions, 14,* 56–64. https://doi.org/10.1177/1098300711402591

Wang, M. T., Fredricks, J. A., Ye, F., Hofkens, T., & Schall, J. (2019). Conceptualization and assessment of adolescents' engagement and disengagement in school: A multidimensional school engagement scale. *European Journal of Psychological Assessment, 35*(4), 592–606. https://doi.org/10.1027/1015-5759/a000431

Waxman, H. S., & Padron, Y. N. (2004). The use of classroom observation to improve student instruction. In H. W. Waxman & R. J. Tharp (Eds.), *Observational research in U.S. classrooms: New approaches for understanding cultural and linguistic diversity* (pp. 72–96). Cambridge University Press.

Waxman, H. C., Tharp, R. G., & Hilberg, R. S. (2004). Future directions for classroom observation research. In H. C. Waxman, R. S. Hilberg, & R. G. Tharp (Eds.), *Observational research in U.S. classrooms: New approaches for understanding cultural and linguistic diversity* (pp. 266–277). Cambridge University Press.

Multicultural and Cross-Cultural Considerations in Understanding Student Engagement in Schools: Promoting the Development of Diverse Students Around the World

Shane R. Jimerson and Chun Chen

Abstract

In the last decades, student engagement has captured the attention and curiosity of researchers across the world, because of its importance in promoting positive development outcomes. This chapter highlights the role of culture in student engagement at school. The first section of this chapter offers definitions of culture, multiculturalism, multicultural psychology, cross-cultural research, and student engagement at school to establish a shared understanding of these constructs. The second section of the chapter describes the similarities and differences regarding the conceptualization of student engagement across races and ethnicities in the United States and internationally across countries around the world. Next, the chapter contributes a review of current student engagement measures that have been validated for use with diverse cultural populations around the world. The fourth section summarizes relevant research about how student engagement pro-

motes positive outcomes for students across cultures. This chapter concludes with the implications for future empirical research incorporating cross-cultural considerations in understanding student engagement in schools.

Introduction

Amidst the increasingly diverse populations of children and families in many communities throughout the United States and around the world, it is imperative that scholars and professionals focused on understanding and advancing student engagement at school are knowledgeable of multicultural and cross-cultural considerations. The American Psychological Association emphasizes the importance of diversity and multicultural considerations in the *Multicultural Guidelines: An Ecological Approach to Context, Identity, and Intersectionality* (APA, 2017; i.e., APA Multicultural Guidelines). The APA Multicultural Guidelines (APA, 2017) highlights the importance of, and encourage professionals to consider, how knowledge and understanding of cultural identities develops and the implications for scholarship and professional practice. Central to this understanding is an approach that incorporates developmental and contextual antecedents of cultural identity and how these ante-

S. R. Jimerson (✉)
University of California, Santa Barbara, CA, USA
e-mail: Jimerson@ucsb.edu

C. Chen
Chinese University of Hong Kong, Shenzhen, China
e-mail: chenchun@cuhk.edu.cn

© The Author(s), under exclusive license to Springer Nature Switzerland AG 2022
A. L. Reschly, S. L. Christenson (eds.), *Handbook of Research on Student Engagement*,
https://doi.org/10.1007/978-3-031-07853-8_31

cedents can be acknowledged, addressed, and embraced to engender more effective models of scholarship and professional engagement (APA Multicultural Guidelines, 2017). Furthermore, it is important to incorporate broad reference group identities (e.g., Black/African American/Black American, White/White American, and Asian/ Asian American/Pacific Islander) to acknowledge within-group differences and the role of self-definition in identity, as well as intersectional considerations (APA Multicultural Guidelines, 2017). The APA Multicultural Guidelines (APA, 2017) provide a valuable framework from which to consider the understanding of diversity and its considerations within the practice, research, consultation, and education to directly address how development unfolds across time and intersectional experiences and identities and to recognize the highly diverse nature of individuals and communities in their defining characteristics. Table 1 provides a summary of considering the multicultural guidelines relevant to understanding and advancing student engagement in school scholarship and practice. Considering the importance of these topics in our scholarship and practice, this chapter begins with a brief definition of key terms invoked throughout this chapter.

> For purposes of this module we are going to define **culture** as patterns of learned and shared behavior that are cumulative and transmitted across generations. … Patterns emerge from adapting, sharing, and storing cultural information. Patterns can be both similar and different across cultures. … Behaviors, values, norms are acquired through a process known as enculturation that begins with parents and caregivers, because they are the primary influence on young children. … Humans cooperate and share knowledge and skills with other members of their networks. The ways they share, and the content of what they share, helps make up culture. … Cultural knowledge is information that is "stored" and then the learning grows across generations. … Passing of new knowledge and traditions of culture from one generation to the next, as well as across other cultures is cultural transmission. In everyday life, the most common way cultural norms are transmitted is within each individuals' home life. (Worthy et al., 2021, pp. 10–11)

Table 1 Multicultural Guidelines Relevant to Understanding and Advancing Student Engagement in Schools Scholarship and Practice

Guideline 1. Recognize and understand that identity and self-definition are fluid and complex and that the interaction between the two is dynamic. Thus, scholars and practitioners working to understand and advance student engagement at school need to appreciate that intersectionality is shaped by the multiplicity of the individual's social contexts.

Guideline 2. Recognize and understand that as cultural beings, scholars and practitioners hold attitudes and beliefs that can influence their perceptions of and interactions with others as well as their clinical and empirical conceptualizations. As such, in our efforts to understand and advance student engagement at school, we must strive to move beyond conceptualizations rooted in categorical assumptions, biases, and/or formulations based on the limited knowledge about individuals and communities.

Guideline 3. Recognize and understand the role of language and communication through engagement that is sensitive to the lived experience of the individual, family, group, community, and/or organizations with whom they interact. Scholars and practitioners must seek to understand how they bring their own language, communication, and conceptualizations to these interactions and implications for understanding and advancing student engagement at school.

Guideline 4. Be aware of the role of the social and physical environment in the lives of students and families, as the implications for student engagement at school.

Guideline 5. Recognize and understand historical and contemporary experiences with power, privilege, and oppression that influence student engagement at school. As such, in understanding and advancing student engagement at school, scholars and practitioners must address institutional barriers and related inequities, disproportionalities, and disparities of law enforcement, administration of criminal justice, educational, mental health, and other systems as they seek to promote justice, human rights, and access to quality and equitable mental and behavioral health services.

Guideline 6. Develop and promote culturally adaptive supports, interventions and advocacy within and across systems, including prevention and early intervention in order to promote understanding and advance student engagement at school.

Guideline 7. Examine the profession's assumptions and practices within an international context, whether domestically or internationally based, and consider how this globalization has an impact on the definition, purpose, role, and function of student engagement at school.

(continued)

Table 1 (continued)

Guideline 8. Develop awareness and understanding of how developmental stages and life transitions intersect with the larger sociocultural contextual influences, how identity evolves as a function of such intersections, and how these different socialization and maturation experiences influence worldview and identity to further understand and promote student engagement at school.

Guideline 9. Conduct culturally appropriate and informed research, consultation, assessment, interpretation, diagnosis, dissemination, and evaluation of efficacy in understanding and advancing student engagement at school, addressing the first four levels of the Layered Ecological Model of the Multicultural Guidelines.

Guideline 10. Take a strength-based approach when working with individuals, families, groups, communities, and organizations that seeks to build resilience, decrease trauma within the sociocultural context, and promote student engagement at school.

Note: Adapted from the APA Multicultural Guidelines (2017)

Multiculturalism is the quality or condition of a society in which different ethnic and cultural groups have equal status and access to power but each maintains its own identity, characteristics, and mores. Multiculturalism also refers to the promotion or celebration of cultural diversity within a society. Also called cultural pluralism. (American Psychological Association, 2021a)

Multicultural education is a progressive approach to education that emphasizes social justice, equality in education, and understanding and awareness of the traditions and language of other cultures and nationalities. Multicultural programs involve two or more ethnic or cultural groups and are designed to help participants define their own ethnic or cultural identity and to appreciate that of others. The purpose is to promote inclusiveness and cultural pluralism in society. (American Psychological Association, 2021b)

Multicultural psychology is an extension of general psychology that recognizes that multiple aspects of identity influence a person's worldview, including race, ethnicity, language, sexual orientation, gender, age, disability, class status, education, religious or spiritual orientation, and other cultural dimensions, and that both universal- and culture-specific phenomena should be taken into consideration when psychologists are helping clients, training students, advocating for social change and justice, and conducting research. (American Psychological Association, 2021b)

Cross-cultural research is the systematic study of human psychological processes and behavior across multiple cultures, involving the observation of similarities and differences in values, practices, and so forth between different societies. Cross-cultural research offers many potential advantages, informing theories that accommodate both individual and social sources of variation, but also involves numerous risks, notable among them the production of cultural knowledge that is incorrect because of flawed methodology. Indeed, there are a host of methodological concerns that go beyond monocultural studies, including issues concerning translation, measurement, equivalence, sampling, data analytic techniques, and data reporting. (American Psychological Association, 2021c)

As educational professionals aim to promote "school engagement" in an effort to enhance student outcomes, it is important that a shared definition is established and appropriate measures are clarified. Thus, based on this review of the literature, it is suggested that **school engagement** is a multifaceted construct that includes affective, behavioral, and cognitive dimensions. Furthermore, in measuring this multifaceted construct the primary contexts include: a) academic performance, b) classroom behavior, c) extracurricular involvement, d) interpersonal relationships and e) school community. (Jimerson et al., 2003, pp. 11–12)

The extant research has consistently shown that student engagement plays an important role in the development of positive student outcomes, including academic achievement (e.g., Christenson et al., 2012; Lee, 2014) and social–emotional and behavioral wellbeing (e.g., Bond et al., 2007; Christenson et al., 2012; Li & Lerner, 2011). The significance of student engagement has attracted researchers in the past decades to develop measures that quantify the construct, and use the findings to inform interventions. It is important that we consider cultural and contextual factors relevant to measuring, understanding, and promoting student engagement at school (Gordon et al., 2017). In this chapter, we describe cultural and contextual considerations salient to measuring student engagement and discuss the construct in a culturally responsive context. The chapter explores the question of "does student engagement look the same in students across different cultural backgrounds?" A review of cross-cultural measures of student engagement that have been validated among different races/

ethnicities and among different countries informs this discussion. The chapter also explores the question "does student engagement have the same impact on student outcomes across different cultures?" by reviewing cross-cultural research on student engagement and student outcomes. Overall, this chapter aims to guide and challenge the readers to explore some of the foundational questions of student engagement considering broader cultural and contextual factors.

Student Engagement Theory and Conceptualization

Student engagement is generally used to describe the quality of meaningful relationships between students and school (Christenson et al., 2012; Lam et al., 2014; Skinner et al., 2009). The concept of student engagement first emerged in the late 1980s. It was initially viewed as the degree of students' active involvement in their academic tasks to understand school dropout and completion (Finn, 1989; Jimerson et al., 2003; Christenson et al., 2012). However, academic engagement is not enough to fully conceptualize the purpose of students' goals of schooling, which goes beyond academic engagement and also includes social–emotional and behavioral engagement. Thus, recent researchers have argued that student engagement shall not be conceptualized solely as students' academic attributes but rather a multidimensional construct including affective, behavioral, and cognitive aspects (Christenson et al., 2012; Jimerson et al., 2003).

Early research conceptualized student engagement as a two-dimensional construct comprised of behavioral and affective/emotional dimensions (Finn, 1989; Finn & Voelkl, 1993; Jimerson et al., 2003; Ryan, Stiller, & Lynch, 1994). The behavioral dimension includes students' observable actions or performance, such as participation in extracurricular activities (e.g., sports, clubs), completion of homework, as well as grades, grade point averages, and scores on achievement tests (Jimerson et al., 2003). The affective dimen-

sion includes students' feelings about the school, teachers, and/or peers (e.g., positive feelings toward teachers and other students (Jimerson et al., 2003). In recent decades, researchers have incorporated a third dimension, namely, cognitive dimension. The cognitive dimension includes students' perceptions and beliefs related to self, school, teachers, and other students (e.g., self-efficacy, motivation, perceiving that teachers or peers care, aspirations, and expectations) (Jimerson et al., 2003). A considerable amount of literature in recent years describes student engagement as a construct that includes these three interrelated dimensions, namely, cognitive, emotional, and behavioral engagement (e.g., Christenson et al., 2012; Fredricks et al., 2004; Jimerson et al., 2003; Lam et al., 2014; Wang et al., 2011). It is also worth noticing that some researchers have attempted to develop a fourth dimension, which is academic engagement, into the student engagement construct (Appleton, Christenson, Kim, & Reschly, 2006). Although the consensus among the authors in defining the concept of student engagement has long been elusive, the nonuniformity of the definition reflects the multidimensional nature of the construct (Ciric & Jovanovic, 2016; Jimerson et al., 2003). During the past decade, increasing yet limited research has started to pay more attention to quantifying student engagement in a cross-cultural context.

For those who are not familiar with the literature in this area, it is also important to note that there are other terms that have been used across the decades related to the discussion of student engagement including school bonding, belonging, school community, affiliation, school membership, motivation, and school attachment (see Jimerson et al., 2003 for a full discussion). Each of these terms is used to describe various aspects of what is delineated in this chapter as student engagement. For instance, a popular notion regarding school bonding is that it reflects the degree of closeness or attachment to teachers and commitment to conventional school goals, although the measurement of school bonding varies considerably in the literature (Jimerson et al., 2003). Commitment is another aspect that is frequently invoked in articles addressing school bonding and appears to reflect both behavioral and cognitive dimensions. Relatedly, belonging, affiliation, and school membership are frequently characterized by feelings of connectedness to school or community, or feelings of inclusion and support in the school social environment. Similar to school bonding, these terms include affective and cognitive dimensions in their definitions. School community involves a more reciprocal relationship between student and community in which the needs of both are satisfied.

Herein, we explore whether it is practical and/or beneficial for student engagement to be represented as the same construct for students across different countries and diverse cultural backgrounds. If yes, what are the similarities and differences of student engagement cross-culturally and/or cross-nationally? This chapter addresses these two questions by discussing some recent cross-cultural and/or cross-national measurement studies conducted. Although most researchers have reached an agreement upon student engagement being considered as a multidimensional construct with different facets interrelated with each other, differences in the multidimensionality and the types of student engagement dimensions included in the definition of student engagement vary across research. Therefore, the descriptions of the scholarship herein use the definitions of student engagement based on the individual cited research. The following section provides a general framework for cross-cultural research in understanding the role of race and ethnicity on student engagement locally in the United States and the role of cultural values on student engagement internationally across countries.

Berry (2013) described three putative stages of the development of cross-cultural psychology. The first stage involves an initial use of the imposed etic approach (i.e., research that studies cross-cultural differences) that aims to transport findings obtained in Western cultures to other cultures. The second stage involves an emic search (i.e., research that studies solely one culture with no cross-cultural focus) for local phenomena. In the third stage, the approaches in the previous two stages are synthesized to create a global psychology. This chapter highlights the importance of the third stage, advocating the advantages of a more comprehensive perspective by looking for both cultural differences and similarities.

Contextual Considerations and Student Engagement in Schools

Researchers and educators are eager to learn more about contextual factors influencing student engagement in schools. The understanding of these contextual factors is essential for developing suitable interventions to promote student engagement. Consistent with Bronfenbrenner's (1977) ecological systems theory, human development occurs within a set of nested systems. Thus, with the interplay of families, peers, and schools, in communities around the world, student engagement develops in an intricate web of reciprocal, dynamic, and mutually influencing systems. Among the most immediate and salient systems in which student engagement develops are the family and the school. Within these microsystems, important agents of socialization (e.g., teachers, peers, and parents) exert a direct impact on student engagement. For instance, research reveals that the quality of instruction and teacher–student relationship are positively associated with student engagement (Dotterer & Lowe, 2011, Hofkens & Pianta, chapter "Teacher-Student Relationships, Engagement in School, and Student Outcomes", this volume). Reinke et al., chapter "Student Engagement: The Importance of the Classroom Context", this volume). Furthermore, peer support in school has also been documented as a strong predictor of student achievement (Cowie & Fernandez, 2006). As for family context, research indicates that parental support contributes to student academic performance (Waanders et al., 2007, Bempechat et al., chapter "Parental Influences on Achievement Motivation and Student Engagement", this volume).

The extant literature reveals that support from teachers, peers, and parents facilitates student engagement in school. Nevertheless, with a few exceptions (e.g., McInerney, 2008; McInerney et al., 1998), most of the studies about these agents of socialization have been conducted in the West. Thus, it is uncertain to what extent the results of these studies can be applied to non-Western contexts. Although some studies about the effects of contextual factors on student engagement have been conducted in Eastern countries, it is common for such studies to be published in their vernacular languages and in local journals (e.g., Kim & Lee, 2012). Thus, whether the impact of contextual factors on student engagement is culturally universal or not is largely unknown.

The broader culture and economy in which an individual is situated are macrosystems that have undeniable influences on human development (Bronfenbrenner, 1977). However, they are often neglected in the scientific research regarding human development, and as Henrich, Heine, and Norenzayan (Henrich et al., 2010) previously noted, most of the psychological literature is built on studies from Western, Educated, Industrialized, Rich, and Democratic (WEIRD) societies. Thus, to have a comprehensive understanding of the contextual antecedents of student engagement, there is a pressing need to investigate how support from teachers, parents, and peers in the microsystems functions in macrosystems with different cultures.

There are contextual considerations related to individualistic versus collectivist societies. For instance, Markus and Kitayama (1991) described that many Asian countries endorse collectivism and insist on the fundamental relatedness of individuals to each other. In contrast, many Western countries advocate individualism and autonomy. Markus and Kitayama argued that this contrast has important consequences for cognition, emotion, and motivation. However, little research has been conducted to examine directly how the pursuit of collectivism or individualism moderates the association between support in the microsystems and student engagement (Castella et al., 2013). Socioeconomic development is another prominent factor within the macrosys-

tem. There has been a paucity of scholarship examining student engagement in schools across developed and developing countries (Lam et al., 2016; Salili et al., 2007). It is important to investigate whether the associations between support in the microsystems and student engagement are the same, stronger, or weaker in developed countries than in developing countries. Further cross-cultural studies are warranted to examine the moderating effects of culture and socioeconomic development on the associations between student engagement and support from important agents of socialization (e.g., teachers, peers, and parents).

Cross-Cultural Measurement of Student Engagement in Schools

Cross-Racial/Ethnic Comparisons of Student Engagement in Schools

While the content of academic achievement differences among racial and ethnic groups have been examined in numerous studies, the similarities and differences of student engagement among different groups and the underlying mechanisms of how student engagement functions across different racial and ethnic groups warrant further emphasis. In the context of cross-racial/ethnic research, various researchers have categorized races and ethnicities differently. Thus, race and ethnicity defined in one study might be very different from how it was represented in another study. It is also important to acknowledge that there is great diversity within each ethnic group label. For example, the label of "Asian" is usually comprised of people from Asian countries who have huge differences in their cultural values (Truong et al., 2021). Therefore, in this chapter, we intend to use the definitions of ethnicities, according to the individual cited research. However, we also aim to use the most inclusive language. For example, in this chapter, we use "Latinx" instead of "Latino" or "Latina" and use "Black" instead of "African American."

Cultural Context Sociocultural differences between racial/ethnic groups and within each group are important to consider (Lam, Wong, et al., 2012). One study conducted by Uekawa et al. (2007) used a student engagement measure in National Science Foundation's Urban Systemic Initiative (USI) to compare student engagement levels in math and science class across high school students from four different ethnic groups (i.e., White, Black, Asian, and Latinx). Student engagement in this study was measured using self-report from students (e.g., attention, listening, motivation level, boredom, enjoyment, focused, and interest). Uekawa and colleagues found that Black, White, and Asian students reported relatively higher levels of student engagement on average, while Latinx students reported the lowest level of engagement. When examining engagement in different settings, they found Asian students were the only group who reported to be significantly more engaged in individual work than lecture, whereas White students favored lecture to individual work, which was also unique to this group. Importantly, Uekawa and colleagues also considered the location of the cities when interpreting the within-group differences in Latinx students' engagement. They revealed significant differences in engagement level between Latinx students in El Paso and those in Chicago, with students in El Paso endorsing higher engagement levels on average. One explanation proposed is the wide differences in the percentage constitution of Latinx students in each city, with El Paso having a large percentage of Latinx students in the school (69%) vs. the schools in Chicago that constitute only 13% of Latinx students. At the same time, their engagement level in different classroom activities (i.e., group, lecture, and individual) varies significantly across Latinx students in three different cities (i.e., Chicago, El Paso, and Miami). These data further reflect the importance of considering racial/ethnic, as well as cultural and contextual considerations when investigating and interpreting studies of student engagement.

However, when reviewing cross-racial/ethnic studies on student engagement, it became evident that very few studies [e.g., Delaware Student Engagement Scale- Student (DSES-S; Bear et al., 2014) and Student Engagement Scale in the National Education Longitudinal Study of 1988 (NELS:88; Glanville & Wildhagen, 2007)] have conducted invariance testing of the student engagement measure that they used before they compared the means of diverse racial/ethnic groups (see summary in Table 2). In detail, DSES-S has been validated across White, Black, Asian, and multiracial/multiethnic student groups from elementary to high school (Bear et al., 2014). Furthermore, the Student Engagement Scale in NELS:88 has been proven to be culturally valid to use across White, Black, Latinx, and Asian eighth-grade students (Glanville & Wildhagen, 2007). One potential problem underlying the lack of measurement invariance is that it is not possible to know whether the dimensions of engagement operate similarly across races/ethnicities. Without such invariance testing, the interpretation of some measures of student engagement is not clear. Therefore, it is important that future research examining race/ethnicity should consider conducting measurement invariance of the measures used since rigorous comparisons of student engagement cannot be achieved without establishing measurement invariance. For further discussion, see Lam et al. (2014).

Social Justice Lens Besides factoring in cultural factors to explain statistical differences in student engagement across students of diverse races/ethnicities, it is also important to consider potential underlying reasons for differences through a social justice lens (García-Vázquez et al., 2020). Previous race and ethnicity researchers have argued that "race and ethnicity research must be contextualized within the milieu of histories of oppression, power, and resistance" (Omi & Winant, 2014). For example, student engagement among Asian American populations, which is comprised of several diverse cultures, still remains as one of the most under-researched

Table 2 Summary of cross-cultural research related to student engagement measures

Measure	Item Domains	Cross-Cultural Groups	Measurement Invariance Validation	Citation
Across Races and Ethnicities				
Student Engagement Scale in the National Science Foundation's Urban Systemic Initiative (USI): *(a) I was paying attention, (b) I did not feel like listening, (c) My motivation level was high, (d) I was bored, (e) I was enjoying class, (f) I was focused more on class than anything else, (g) I wished the class would end soon, and (h) I was completely into class.*	Engagement in Math and Science Classroom	White, Black, Latinx, and Asian	No	Uekawa et al. (2007)
Delaware Student Engagement Scale- Student (DSES-S)	Cognitive-Behavioral Engagement; Emotional Engagement	White, Black, Hispanic/ Latinx, Asian, and other race/ethnicity including multirace/ multiethnicity	Yes	Bear et al. (2014)
Questionnaire not indicated; Data from the Educational Longitudinal Study (ELS) – Student and Teacher Report	Cognitive Engagement; Behavioral Engagement; Emotional Engagement	Native American, Black, White, Asian, and Latinx	No	Sciarra and Seirup (2008)
Engagement Scale (Shernoff et al., 2003)	Engagement (i.e., concentration, interest, and enjoyment)	White, Black, Asian, and Latinx	No	Shernoff and Schmidt (2008)
Student Engagement Scale in the National Education Longitudinal Study of 1988 (NELS:88)	Behavioral Engagement; Psychological Engagement; Time Spent of Homework	White, Black, Latinx, and Asian	Yes	Glanville and Wildhagen (2007)
Across Countries				
Student Engagement in Schools Questionnaire (SESQ; Lam et al., 2014)	Affective Engagement; Behavioral Engagement; Cognitive Engagement	Austria, Canada, China, Cyprus, Estonia, Greece, Malta, Portugal, Romania, South Korea, the United Kingdom, and the USA	Yes	Hart et al. (2011), Lam and Jimerson, (2009), Lam et al. (2012a, b, 2014, 2016), Nelson et al. (2020)
Delaware Student Engagement Scale- Student (DSES-S)	Cognitive-Behavioral Engagement; Emotional Engagement	China, the USA	Yes	Bear et al. (2018)

(continued)

Table 2 (continued)

Measure	Item Domains	Cross-Cultural Groups	Measurement Invariance Validation	Citation
Student Engagement Instrument Brief Version (SEI; Appleton et al., 2006)	Affective Engagement: Teacher-Student Relationships, Peer Support at School, and Family Support for Learning; Cognitive Engagement: Control and Relevance of School Work, and Future Aspirations and Goals	Denmark, Finland, Portugal	Yes	Virtanen et al. (2018)
Three-item scale for Observing Student academic engagement in a lesson	Academic Engagement	South Korea, the Netherlands	Yes	Van de Grift et al. (2017)
Goal Orientation and Learning Strategies Survey (Dowson and McInerney, 2004)	Cognitive Engagement	The USA, China	Yes	Qu and Pomerantz (2015)
Student Engagement in School – Four-Dimensions Scale (SES-4DS; Veiga, 2012, 2008)	Cognitive Engagement; Affective Engagement; Behavioral Engagement; Agentic Engagement	Portugal, Romania	Yes	Veiga and Robu (2014)

racial groups in the United States(Corley & Young, 2018; Truong et al., 2021). When considering recent research comparing Asian American students' engagement levels to students of other racial/ethnic groups, there is a consistent pattern of Asian American students having greater engagement in both cognitive-behavioral (e.g., engagement on homework completion) and emotional domains (e.g., peer relationship) (Bingham G.E. & Okagaki L., 2012; Yang et al., 2018). For example, Yang et al. (2018) found that Asian American students reported higher engagement levels on average using the Delaware Student Engagement Scale-Student (DSES-S), which has been statistically validated across different racial/ethnic groups. Moreover, Sciarra and Seirup (2008) reported student engagement in terms of cognitive (i.e., eight student items and two teacher items [one from the math teacher and the other from the English teacher]) concerning the student's commitment to learning, importance of good grades, perseverance in the face of difficulty, homework completion, and amount of hours per week spent on homework), behavioral

(i.e., 14 items divided into eight responses from students, three from the math teacher, and three from the English teacher, items dealt with frequency of lateness, cutting, absences, disruptive versus attentive behaviors, disciplinary actions, and time dedicated to extracurricular activities and emotional (i.e., student responses to 24 items dealing with the quality of student–teacher relationships, school safety, relationships with peers, and harmony among different racial groups) engagement across five racial/ethnic groups (i.e., White, Black, Latinx, Asian, and American Indian) in the US high schools.

Although there was not a statistical comparison of student engagement across these groups, from their reported descriptive table in the paper, Asian students clearly reported the highest behavioral and cognitive engagement compared to the other groups. However, what are the underlying reasons behind the Asian American students' report of higher student engagement? Some researchers have provided some justification in the context of model minority stereotype for Asian students' having higher student engagement. The model minority stereotype refers to a concept used to portray Asian American people as minorities who are hard-working and problem-free (Kiang et al., 2017). They explained that teachers are more likely to perceive Chinese and other Asian students as exemplifying the model minority stereotype, defined by high academic achievement, effort, self-regulation, reliability, and compliance with classroom norms, according to studies in the US schools (Yang et al., 2018). Then, how might the model minority stereotype help to explain the self-report of student engagement in Asian American students? Under the model minority stereotype, this might resemble the self-fulfilling prophecy (Jussim et al., 1996). Thompson and Kiang (2010) found that adolescents who perceived more stereotyping tended to report more positive academic and psychological outcomes. Despite the positive expectations, it is also important for scholars and practitioners to reflect on the potential challenges that Asian American students may face, and implications on their identity development.

Multiple studies report that student engagement levels for many other minority groups were consistently being reported lower than for White students. For example, in Sciara and Seirup's study (Sciarra & Seirup, 2008), White students reported the highest level of emotional engagement across the board. In their definition, emotional engagement includes feelings of belongingness (Osterman, 2000), safety, comfort, pride in the institution (Maddox & Prinz, 2003), and relationships with teachers and peers (Jimerson et al., 2003). Several studies have found that Black students to be less engaged in terms of engagement with instructions than White students (Yair, 2000), particularly when their engagement level was rated by teachers (Downey & Pribesh, 2004). Binghan and Okagaki have also pointed out that the academic underachievement of minority students, particularly Black, Latinx, and American Indian students in the United States, has been partially explained by the reported lower engagement in school (2012). The engagement discrepancies across ethnic groups should raise our awareness

to think deeply about the daily experience of being a minority student in a classroom. Previous sociolinguistic studies have claimed that racial/ethnic minority students are sometimes alienated in class due to differences between patterns of home and school interactions (Mehan, 1992). Thus, the education experience might become hostile to historically underprivileged and/or minoritized students, because most mainstream classrooms still struggle with multicultural education that purposefully and intentionally considers the importance of cultural diversity (Galindo et al., chapter "Expanding an Equity Understanding of Student Engagement: The Macro (Social) and Micro (School) Contexts", this volume).

Cross-Country Comparisons of Student Engagement

Despite a significant increase in research on student engagement in recent years, evidence-based student engagement measurements that have been statistically validated across different cultures are still in an early phase of development (Samuelsen, 2012). Among these previous cross-country measurement studies, an underlying pattern of findings is that there are more cultural similarities than differences when it comes to how student engagement is related to its contexts, antecedents, and outcomes, although different countries have very different economic development and cultures (e.g., Lam & Jimerson, 2009; Lam et al., 2012a, b, 2014, 2016). One potential reason behind finding cultural similarities in cross-country research on student engagement is that it is possible that the underlying mechanism of how to promote student engagement is universal (Liem & Chong, 2017). For example, a healthy and positive school climate is believed to be beneficial to increase student engagement across different cultures and diverse contexts. However, we also cannot overlook the fact that the concept and measurement of student engagement are developed in a Eurocentric context (e.g., Western, educated, industrialized, rich, and democratic WEIRD societies). Additional studies outside of WEIRD societies are needed to understand and define student engagement from a bottom-up approach (e.g., conducting qualitative to understand the constitution of student engagement in a specific culture).

Within the few cross-country measurement studies of student engagement, the Student Engagement in School Questionnaire (SESQ) (Lam & Jimerson, 2009; Lam et al., 2012a, b, 2014, 2016) is the measure that has been validated across the largest number of countries. Beginning in 2010, within the context of the research committee of the International School Psychology Association (Lam & Jimerson, 2009; Lam et al., 2012a, b, 2014, 2016), colleagues from more than 20 countries contributed to the development of the SESQ that is consistent with the definition of student engagement being a multidimensional construct comprised of behavioral, cognitive, and emotional domains (Jimerson et al., 2003). The impetus to develop a conceptually and psychometrically sound measure of student engagement that could be used internationally was described by Lam et al. (2014, p. 214), *"Despite increasing interest in student engagement in countries around the world, there is no clear understanding of the construct. Indeed, there has been much confusion regarding its definition and measurement. In an effort to overcome these problems and to also advance knowledge and understanding related to student engagement in school around the world, an international project was initiated to clarify the concept of student engagement and to develop a measurement tool appropriate for use in countries around the world."*

The SESQ (Lam et al., 2012a, b, 2014, 2016) has already been validated across 12 countries (i.e., Austria, Canada, China, Cyprus, Estonia, Greece, Malta, Portugal, Romania, South Korea, the United Kingdom, and the USA;). Lam, Jimerson, et al. (2012) reported that the intraclass correlation of the SESQ full-scale scores of student engagement between countries revealed that it was appropriate to aggregate the data from the 12 countries for further analyses. Furthermore, the SESQ coefficient alphas revealed good internal consistency (α ranged from 0.78 to 0.89), and the test–retest reliability coefficients were also acceptable (coefficient ranged from 0.60 to 0.74). In addition, confirmatory factor analyses of the SESQ indicated that the data fit well to a second-order model with affective, behavioral, and cognitive engagement as the first-order factors and student engagement as the second-order factor. Lam, Jimerson, et al. (2012a) highlight that the results support the use of the SESQ to measure student engagement as a meta-construct. Additionally, the significant correlations of the scale with instructional practices, teacher support, peer support, parent support, emotions, academic performance, and school conduct indicated good concurrent validity of the scale. The results from Lam et al. (2014 & 2016) using the SESQ further extend the cross-country analyses by further comparing male and female students, as well as cultural universality and specificity in student engagement at school. In addition, additional development and analyses related to the SESQ have revealed a teacher engagement report form that also yielded strong psychometric data (Hart et al., 2011; e.g., α ranged from 0.78 to 0.95, except 0.65 in Attributions domain), thus providing another perspective to measure student engagement in schools.

Another study examined a cross-cultural measurement among high school students in Portugal and Romania (Veiga & Robu, 2014). Their results indicate that the School Engagement in School-Four-Dimensions Scale (SES-4DS) is a measure that captures the same underlying dimensions of engagement in schools across two countries (see Table 2 for more details). The exploratory factor analysis revealed a four-factor measurement model in both samples. The correlations coefficients across the affective, behavioral, cognitive, and agentic engagement dimensions were each good, as well as the internal consistency.

In addition, Virtanen and colleagues (2018) examined a modified version of the SEI (Appleton et al., 2006) across seventh-grade students in three countries (i.e., Demark, Finland, and Portugal). Divergent from the original five (Betts et al., 2010) or six (Appleton et al., 2006) interrelated first-order factors, the brief version in their study revealed a second-order five-factor model on two second-order factors as affective and cognitive engagement and five first-order factors as teacher–student relationships, peer support at school, family support for learning, control and relevance of school work, and future aspirations and goals. Virtanen and colleagues report that among the total 33 original instrument items, 15 items indicated acceptable psychometric properties of the Brief-SEI. Using these 15 items, analyses revealed cross-national factorial validity and invariances across genders and students with different levels of academic performance (samples from Finland and Portugal). Virtanen and colleagues revealed the highest overall engagement among Portuguese students followed by Danish and Finnish students.

Recent cross-country research focused on student engagement in school has focused on comparing and contrasting engagement between students in East Asia and students in the United States or European countries. Different from cross-racial/ethnic research in the United States, that Asian American students tended to have higher engagement than students of other racial/ethnic backgrounds, mixed findings have been reported on cross-country research about student engagement between East Asian and the US students. For example, the differences in student engagement between the US students and Chinese students vary over time. Bear et al. (2018) reported that during elementary school, the US students reported greater cognitive-behavioral (e.g., engagement on homework completion) and emotional engagement (e.g., peer relationships) than Chinese students. However, in middle and high school students, Chinese students started to report higher emotional engagement than the US students, whereas no significant differences in cognitive-behavioral engagement were found between the US and Chinese students. Besides higher emotional engagement in Chinese middle and high school students, Van de Grift et al. (2017) reported higher levels of academic engagement, with an emphasis on psychological and behavioral engagement (e.g., students show that they are interested in learning) in South Korean students compared to students from the Netherlands in the secondary educational context. However, this study focused on measuring only academic engagement. Instead of students' self-report, academic engagement was measured through observation (i.e., observers used a Likert-type rating for the level of student engagement by watching a class videotape, and rating engagement in learning, demonstrating that they are interested in learning, and other dimensions), which could provide us with a diverse perspective in understanding cross-cultural engagement. Van de Grift and colleagues attributed some of the differences to South Korean students' having access to teachers with more advanced teaching skills regarding how students should learn. They also proposed some other explanatory factors for future cross-cultural research to examine, which include demographic homogeneity, cultural settings, student motivation, private tutoring, and amount of illiteracy.

To explain higher academic engagement in East Asian students, some researchers have argued that historically East Asian students (e.g., Chinese students) scored relatively higher in standardized universal academic achievement (Bear et al., 2018), such as the Program for International Student Assessment (Hsin & Xie, 2014; Kastberg et al., 2016). The heavy emphasis on academic learning in East Asian schools may cultivate the level of academic engagement (i.e., students' active involvement in their academic tasks) to be higher in this population. Some other speculations include unique cultural values to be a major factor to explain the differences, such as Chinese students' higher value of authority (i.e., teachers in the context of schooling especially beyond elementary school), social harmony (i.e., how Chinese students view and regulate peers and their own behaviors), and Chinese teachers' classroom management skills. Particularly for Chinese students who are in middle and high schools, these cultural values tend to become more consolidated, which might impact their attitude toward schools. Thus, in Bear and colleagues' study (Bear et al., 2018), they found that when going beyond elementary school, Chinese students tended to report more positive perceptions of school climate than the US students, which was likely to be the reason to explain the stronger emotional engagement in Chinese middle and high school students. Considering the relative paucity of cross-country investigations of student engagement in school, further research is warranted to advance our collective understanding.

Relevant Research on Student Engagement and Outcomes

Student engagement has been considered among the primary conceptual foundations for understanding school outcomes of students both short-term and long-term (Archambault et al., 2009; Christenson et al., 2008). However, in a recent meta-analysis focused on school belongingness, Korpershoek et al. (2020) argue that the concept of student engagement is used to place the school belongingness construct in a broader theoretical framework. School belongingness is conceptually similar to emotional engagement (i.e., positive and negative reactions to teachers, classmates, academics, and school) (Allen & Boyle, chapter "School Belonging and Student Engagement: The Critical Overlaps, Similarities, and Implications for Student Outcomes", this volume). Korpershoek and colleagues found that samples of studies conducted on student engagement outside the USA and Canada are relatively few. Moreover, little is known about the potential moderating role of country and culture on the relationship between student engagement and student outcomes. The next section of this chapter highlights some empirical studies conducted in the recent decades to exemplify the importance of considering cultural differences in student engagement and directions for future research.

Cross-Racial/Ethnic Comparisons of Student Engagement and Outcomes

Several previous studies have shown that the impact of student engagement on academic achievement differs substantially due to an individual's social–cultural background in the USA. For example, Sciarra and Seirup (2008) examined the role of race and ethnicity in the relationship between student engagement and math achievement among high school students. Overall, student engagement was found to significantly predict math achievement for all five racial groups included in the study (i.e., Native American, Asian, Black, Latinx, and White adolescents); the effect size was the smallest in Latinx and Black students. When broken into each dimension of student engagement (i.e., behavioral [e.g., learning, compliance of school norms, and participation in extracurricular activities], emotional [e.g., feelings of belongingness, safety, comfort, pride in the institution, and relationships with teachers and peers], and cognitive engagement [e.g., investment in learning, beliefs about the importance of academics and good grades, degree of studying and homework completion, capacity to confront the challenge, and willingness to go beyond the minimum requirements]), cognitive and behavioral engagement were stronger indicators of math achievement relative to emotional engagement in all racial groups, with the exception that emotional engagement was found to be a significant factor in predicting achievement in Latinx students. This was explained by the cultural differences that Latinx culture might place more emphasis on the tendency of people defining themselves through relationships, which may explain why emotional engagement emerged as a significant predictor within this group of students.

Cross-Country Comparisons of Student Engagement and Outcomes

An analysis of 20 recent research studies of "school belonging" found significant differences in the correlation between behavioral engagement and school belongingness between the USA/Canada and Asia, with the correlation higher in Asian countries, and nonsignificant in Europe (see, Korpershoek et al., 2020 for further details). However, the results need to be interpreted with caution, given the small samples of studies in Asian countries (Korpershoek et al., 2020).

Lam et al. (2014) examined gender differences in student engagement and academic performance in school with a sample of 3420 students (seventh, eighth, and ninth graders) from Austria, Canada, China, Cyprus, Estonia, Greece, Malta, Portugal, Romania, South Korea, the United Kingdom, and the USA. The results indicated that, compared to boys, girls reported higher levels of engagement in school and were rated higher by their teachers in academic performance. Student engagement accounted for gender differences in academic performance, but gender did not moderate the associations among student engagement, academic performance, or contextual supports. Analysis of multiple-group structural equation modeling revealed that perceptions of teacher support and parent support, but not peer support, were related indirectly to academic performance through student engagement. This partial mediation model was invariant across gender. The findings from this study advance the understanding about the contextual and personal factors associated with girls' and boys' academic performance around the world.

Lam et al. (2016) investigated how student engagement in school is associated with grade, gender, and contextual factors across 12 countries using the SESQ (Lam & Jimerson, 2009), as well as whether these associations vary across countries with different levels of individualism and socioeconomic development. Hierarchical linear modeling was used to examine the effects at both student and country levels. Overall, the results across countries revealed a decline in student engagement from Grade 7 to Grade 9, with girls reporting higher engagement than boys. Notably, these trends did not vary across the 12 countries according to the Human Development Index and Hofstede's Individualism Index. Most of the contextual factors (instructional practices, teacher support, and parent support) were positively associated with student engagement. With the exception that parent support had a stronger association with student engagement in countries with higher collectivism, most of the associations between the contextual factors and student engagement did not vary across countries. The results of Lam et al.' (2016) study revealed both cultural universality and specificity regarding contextual factors associated with student engagement in school. They illustrate the advantages of integrating etic and emic approaches in cross-cultural investigations.

Directions for Future Research

Considering the results of research from the past decade revealing that the Student Engagement in Schools Questionnaire (SESQ) is reliable and valid across at least 12 diverse countries, there is a tremendous opportunity for further investigations to advance our understanding of student engagement in schools around the world. The following are a few reflections on future research that would be valuable to further advance our understanding of multicultural, cross-cultural, cross-country, and contextual considerations related to student engagement in schools.

Further research is required to understand the interplay of socioeconomic status, race/ethnicity, the composition of the student population, and school climate in facilitating student engagement in schools, both within and across countries. Students who differ in social class, race and ethnicity, and schooling experiences may interpret questionnaire items about their engagement differentially, which could further limit our understanding. Therefore, more bottom-up research (i.e., a research methodology that aims to piece micro-information to answer a complex macro question) would be helpful to understand student engagement experiences of students with a diverse background, such as using qualitative data to inform measurement designs. Furthermore, comparisons of student engagement would not be considered rigorous without establishing measurement invariance of the measures. We urge future researchers to either select student engagement measures that have been found to be culturally representative in diverse racial/ethnic groups or conduct measurement invariance before cross-cultural comparisons.

When examining cross-cultural differences on student engagement, besides solely looking at between cultural differences, we also need to examine within cultural differences, such as the experiences of racial/ethnic minority students when they reside in a cultural enclave compared to those when they constitute only a small percentage of the population in the community. Besides, it would be informative for researchers to further examine the settings of engagement across different cultures, as informed by Uekawa et al.'s research (Uekawa et al., 2007).

Student engagement is a potentially malleable target for intervention (Korpershoek et al., 2020; Lazowski & Hulleman, 2016). Thus, it would be valuable for further research to examine the effectiveness of specific intervention programs focusing on promoting student engagement in schools around the world. The research regarding systems-level interventions to transform the school climate is a related area of scholarship that would benefit from including established measures of student engagement in schools, to further examine the association between these constructs and student outcomes.

The emergence of student engagement has also become a significant line of research in higher education contexts across the world, due to its being a core element of institutional learning and teaching strategies (Coates & McCormick, 2014, Tinto, chapter "Exploring the Character of Student Persistence in Higher Education: The Impact of Perception, Motivation, and Engagement", this volume). Given the scope of the present chapter (i.e., student engagement in grades K–12), we look forward to future scholarship that provides a more thorough understanding of student engagement in higher education (Tinto, chapter "Exploring the Character of Student Persistence in Higher Education: The Impact of Perception, Motivation, and Engagement", this volume).

Further efforts are warranted in the development of a more comprehensive perspective of assessing student engagement, for example, using self-, teacher-, and parent reports. Information from multiple sources may provide a better understanding of students. Additionally, multi-informant student engagement data collected at the school level can provide administrators with additional school climate information, and may direct interventions at the universal, school-wide level. Ongoing efforts related to the conceptualization and measurement of student engagement also need to seek out helpful information about how the construct relates directly to positive student outcomes.

It is important for school personnel to be aware of the literature and the ongoing research efforts in the area of student engagement in the schools. School psychologists can provide a context that is consultation- and collaboration friendly; they can advocate with teachers about the importance of engagement in the classroom, in addition to strategies to enhance student engagement in school. Through further scholarship focused on informing multicultural and cross-cultural considerations related to student engagement in schools, it is anticipated that further work in this area will increase attention to conducting culturally sensitive and responsive research with the aim of increasing positive outcomes for students from culturally and linguistically diverse backgrounds.

References

American Psychological Association. (2017). *Multicultural guidelines: An ecological approach to context, identity, and intersectionality.* Available online http://www.apa.org/about/policy/multicultural-guidelines.pdf

American Psychological Association. (2021a). Multiculturalism. *APA Dictionary of Psychology.* Available online https://dictionary.apa.org/multiculturalism

American Psychological Association. (2021b). Multicultural education. *APA Dictionary of Psychology.* Available online https://dictionary.apa.org/multicultural-education

American Psychological Association. (2021c). Cross-cultural research. *APA Dictionary of Psychology.* Available online https://dictionary.apa.org/cross-cultural-research

Appleton, J. J., Christenson, S. L., Kim, D., & Reschly, A. L. (2006). Measuring cognitive and psychological engagement: Validation of the student engagement instrument. *Journal of School Psychology, 44,* 427–445. https://doi.org/10.1016/j.jsp.2006.04.002

Archambault, I., Janosz, M., Fallu, J., & Pagani, L. S. (2009). Student engagement and its relationship with early high school dropout. *Journal of Adolescence, 32,* 651–670. https://doi.org/10.1016/j.adolescence.2008.06.007

Bear, G. G., Yang, C., Chen, D., He, X., Xie, J.-S., & Huang, X. (2018). Differences in school climate and student engagement in China and the United States.

School Psychology Quarterly, 33(2), 323–335. https://doi.org/10.1037/spq0000247

Bear, G. G., Yang, C., Mantz, L., Pasipanodya, E., Boyer, D. & Hearn, S. (2014). Technical manual for Delaware surveys of school climate, bullying victimization, student engagement, and positive, punitive, and social emotional learning techniques University of Delaware, Center for Disabilities Studies, Positive Behavioral Supports and School Climate Project. Retrieved from: http://wordpress.oet.udel.edu/pbs/technical-manual-for-school-climate-surveys

Berry, J. W. (2013). Achieving a global psychology. *Canadian Psychology/Psychologie Canadienne, 54*, 55–61. https://doi.org/10.1037/a0031246

Bingham G.E. & Okagaki L. (2012). Ethnicity and Student Engagement. In S. Christenson, A. Reschly, & C. Wylie (Eds.), *Handbook of research on student engagement*. Springer. https://doi.org/10.1007/978-1-4614-2018-7_4

Betts, J. E., Appleton, J. J., Reschly, A. L., Christenson, S. L., & Huebner, E. S. (2010). A study of the factorial invariance of the Student Engagement Instrument (SEI): Results from middle and high school students. *School Psychology Quarterly, 25(2)*, 84–93. https://doi.org/10.1037/a0020259

Bond, L., Butler, H., Thomas, L., Carlin, J., Glover, J., Bowes, G., et al. (2007). Social andStudent Engagement 28 school connectedness in early secondary school as predictors of late teenage substance use, mental health, and academic outcomes. *Journal of Adolescent Health, 40*(4), 9–18.

Bronfenbrenner, U. (1977). Toward an experimental ecology of human development. *American Psychologist, 32*, 513–531. https://doi.org/10.1037/0003-066X.32.7.513

Castella, D., Krista, D. B., & Covington, M. (2013). Unmotivated or motivated to fail? A cross-cultural study of achievement motivation, fear of failure, and student disengagement. *Journal of Educational Psychology, 105*(3), 861–880.

Christenson, S. L., Reschly, A. L., Appleton, J. J., Berman, S., Spanjers, D., & Varro, P. (2008). Best practices in fostering student engagement. In A. Thomas & J. Grimes (Eds.), *Best practices in school psychology* (5th ed.). National Association of School Psychologists.

Christenson, S. L., Reschly, A. L., & Wylie, C. (2012). *Handbook of Research on Student Engagement* (1st ed.). Springer Science.

Ciric, M., & Jovanovic, D. (2016). Student engagement as a multidimensional concept. In *Multidimensional concept. WLC 2016: World LUMEN Congress. Logos Universality Mentality Education Novelty 2016. LUMEN 15th Anniversary Edition* (pp. 187–194). https://doi.org/10.15405/epsbs.2016.09.24

Coates, H., & McCormick, A. C. (Eds.). (2014). *Engaging university students: International insights from system-wide studies*. Springer.

Corley, N. A., & Young, S. M. (2018). Is social work still racist? A content analysis of recent literature. *Social Work, 63(4), 317–326.* https://doi.org/10.1093/sw/swy042

Cowie, H., & Fernandez, F. J. (2006). Peer support in school, implementation and challenges. *Electronic Journal of Research in Educational Psychology, 4*, 291–310. Retrieved from http://www.investigacion-psicopedagogica.org/revista/new/english/LeerArticulo.php

Dotterer, A. M., & Lowe, K. (2011). Classroom context, school engagement, and academic achievement in early adolescence. *Journal of Youth and Adolescence, 40*, 1649–1660. https://doi.org/10.1007/s10964-011-9647-5

Downey, D. B., & Pribesh, S. (2004). When race matters: Teachers' evaluations of students' classroom behavior. *Sociology of Education, 77*, 267.

Dowson, M., & McInerney, D. M. (2004). The development and validation of the goal orientation and learning strategies survey (GOALS-S). *Educational and Psychological Measurement, 64(2), 290–310.* https://doi.org/10.1177/0013164403251335

Finn, J. D. (1989). Withdrawing from school. *Review of Educational Research, 59, 117–142.* https://doi.org/10.2307/1170412

Finn, J. D., & Voelkl, K. E. (1993). School characteristics related to student engagement. *Journal of Negro Education, 62, 249–268.* https://doi.org/10.2307/2295464

Fredricks, J. A., Blumenfeld, P. C., & Paris, A. H. (2004). School engagement: Potential of the concept, state of the evidence. *Review of Educational Research, 74*(1), 59–109.

García-Vázquez, E., Reddy, L., Arora, P., Crepeau-Hobson, F., Fenning, P., Hatt, C., Hughes, T. L., Jimerson, S., Malone, C., Minke, K., Radliff, K., Raines, T., Song, S., & Vaillancourt Strobach, K. (2020). School psychology unified anti-racism statement and call to action. *School Psychology Review, 49*(3), 209–211. https://doi.org/10.1080/2372966X.2020.1809941

Glanville, J. L., & Wildhagen, T. (2007). The measurement of school engagement: Assessing dimensionality and measurement invariance across race and ethnicity. *Educational and Psychological Measurement, 67*(6), 1019–1041.

Gordon, R. K., Taichi, A., Cynthia McDermott, J., & Lalas, J. W. (2017). *Challenges associated with cross-cultural and at-risk student engagement.* IGI Global. Advances in Early Childhood and K-12 Education (AECKE) Book Ser. Web.

Hart, S. R., Stewart, K., & Jimerson, S. R. (2011). The Student Engagement in Schools Questionnaire (SESQ) and the Teacher Engagement Report Form-New (TERF-N): Examining the Preliminary Evidence. *The Contemporary School Psychologist, 15*, 67–79.

Henrich, J., Heine, S. J., & Norenzayan, A. (2010). Most people are not WEIRD. *Nature, 466*, 29. https://doi.org/10.1038/466029a

Hsin, A., & Xie, Y. (2014). Explaining Asian Americans' academic advantage over whites. *PNAS Proceedings of the National Academy of Sciences of the United States of America, 111*, 8416–8421. https://doi.org/10.1073/pnas.1406402111

Jimerson, S., Campos, E., & Greif, J. (2003). Towards an understanding of definitions and measures of school engagement and related terms. *The California School Psychologist, 8*, 7–28.

Jussim, L., Eccles, J., & Madon, S. (1996). Social perception, social stereotypes, and teacher expectations: Accuracy and the quest for the powerful self-fulfilling prophecy. In M. P. Zanna (Ed.), *Advances in experimental social psychology* (Vol. 28, pp. 281–388). Academic Press. https://doi.org/10.1016/S0065-2601(08)60240-3

Kastberg, D., Chan, J. Y., & Murray, G. (2016). *Performance of U.S. 15-year-old students in science, reading, and mathematics literacy in an international context: First look at PISA 2015 (NCES 2017–048).* National Center for Education Statistics. Retrieved from https://nces.ed.gov/pubs2017/2017048.pdf

Kiang, L., Huynh, V. W., Cheah, C. S., Wang, Y., & Yoshikawa, H. (2017). Moving beyond the model minority. *Asian American Journal of Psychology, 8*(1), 1.

Kim, J. R., & Lee, E. J. (2012). The structural relationship among classroom goal structures, basic psychological needs, and academic engagement of elementary and middle school students. *The Korean Journal of Educational Psychology, 26*, 817–835.

Korpershoek, H., Canrinus, E. T., Fokkens-Bruinsma, M., & de Boer, H. (2020). The relationships between school belonging and students' motivational, social-emotional, behavioural, and academic outcomes in secondary education: A meta-analytic review. *Research Papers in Education, 35*(6), 641–680.

Lam, S.-F., & Jimerson, S. R. (2009). Advancing International Knowledge of Student Engagement. *International School Psychology Association – World Go Round, 36*(4), 9–12.

Lam, S.-F., Jimerson, S. R., Kikas, E., Cefai, C., Veiga, F. H., Nelson, B., Hatzichristou, C., Polychroni, F., Basnett, J., Duck, R., Farrell, P., Liu, Y., Negovan, V., Shin, H., Stanculescu, E., Wong, B., Yang, H., & Zollneritsch, J. (2012a). Do girls and boys perceive themselves as equally engaged in school? The results of an international study from 12 countries. *Journal of School Psychology, 50*, 77–94. https://doi.org/10.1016/j.jsp.2011.07.004

Lam, S.-F., Wong, B. P. H., Yang, H., & Liu, Y. (2012b). Understanding student engagement with a contextual model. In S. L. Christenson, A. L. Reschly, & C. Wylie (Eds.), *Handbook of research on student engagement* (pp. 403–420). Springer.

Lam, S.-F., Jimerson, S., Wong, B. P. H., Kikas, E., Shin, H., Veiga, F. H., Hatzichristou, C., Polychroni, F., Cefai, C., Negovan, V., Stanculescu, E., Yang, H., Liu, Y., Basnett, J., Duck, R., Farrell, P., Nelson, B., & Zollneritsch, J. (2014). Understanding and measuring student engagement in school: The results of an international study from 12 countries. *School Psychology Quarterly, 29*, 213–232. https://doi.org/10.1037/spq0000057

Lam, S.-F., Jimerson, S. R., Shin, H., Cefai, C., Veiga, F. H., Nelson, B., Hatzichristou, C., Polychroni, F., Kikas, E., Wong, B., Stanculescu, E., Basnett, J., Duck, R., Farrell, P., Liu, Y., Negovan, V., Yang, H., Shin, H., & Zollneritsch, J. (2016). Cultural universality and specificity of student engagement in school: The results of an international study from 12 countries. *British Journal of Educational Psychology, 86*(1), 137–153. https://doi.org/10.1111/bjep.12079

Lazowski, R. A., & Hulleman, C. S. (2016). Motivation interventions in education: A meta-analytic review. *Review of Educational Research, 86*(2), 602–640. https://doi.org/10.3102/0034654315617832

Lee, J. S. (2014). The relationship between student engagement and academic performance: Is it a myth or reality? *The Journal of Educational Research, 107*(3), 177–185.

Li, Y., & Lerner, R. M. (2011). Trajectories of school engagement during adolescence: Implications for grades, depression, deliquency, and substance use. *Developmental Psychology, 47*(1), 233–247.

Liem, G. A. D., & Chong, W. H. (2017). Fostering student engagement in schools: International best practices. *School Psychology International, 38*(2), 121–130. Web.

Maddox, S. J., & Prinz, R. J. (2003). School bonding in children and adolescents: Conceptualization, assessment, and associated variables. *Clinical Child and Family Psychology Review, 6, 31–49.* https://doi.org/10.1023/A:1022214022478

Markus, H., & Kitayama, S. (1991). Culture and the self: Implications for cognition, emotion and involvement. *Psychological Review, 98*, 224–253. https://doi.org/10.1037/0033-295X.98.2.224

McInerney, D. M. (2008). Personal investment, culture and learning: Insights into school achievement across Anglo, Aboriginal, Asian and Lebanese students in Australia. *International Journal of Psychology, 43*, 870–879. https://doi.org/10.1080/00207590701836364

McInerney, D. M., Hinkley, J., Dowson, M., & Van Etten, S. (1998). Aboriginal, Anglo, and immigrant Australian students' motivational beliefs about personal academic success: Are there cultural differences? *Journal of Educational Psychology, 90*, 621–629. https://doi.org/10.1037/0022-0663.90.4.621

Mehan, H. (1992). Understanding inequality in schools: The contribution of interpretive studies. *Sociology of Education, 65(1), 1–20.* https://doi.org/10.2307/2112689

Nelson, R. B., Asamsama, O. H., Jimerson, S. R., & Lam, S.-F. (2020). The association between student wellness and student engagement in school. *Journal of Educational Research and Innovation, 8*(1), 2–26. Available at: https://digscholarship.unco.edu/jeri/vol8/iss1/5

Omi, M., & Winant, H. (2014). *Racial formation in the United States* (3rd ed.). Routledge.

Osterman, K. E. (2000). Students' Need for Belonging in the School Community. *Review of Educational Research, 70,* 323–367.

Qu, Y., & Pomerantz, E. M. (2015). Divergent school trajectories in early adolescence in the United States and China: An examination of underlying mechanisms. *Journal of Youth and Adolescence, 44*(11), 2095–2109.

Ryan, R. M., Stiller, J. D., & Lynch, J. H. (1994). Representations of relationships to teachers, parents, and friends as predictors of academic motivation and self-esteem. *The Journal of Early Adolescence, 14,* 226–249. https://doi.org/10.1177/027243169401400207

Salili, H., Salili, F., & Hoosain, R. (2007). *Culture, motivation, and learning : A multicultural perspective.* IAP. Print. Research in Multicultural Education and International Perspectives.

Samuelsen, K. M. (2012). Part V Commentary: Possible New Directions in the Measurement of Student Engagement. In: Christenson, S., Reschly, A., Wylie, C. (eds) *Handbook of research on student engagement. Springer, Boston, MA.* https://doi.org/10.1007/978-1-4614-2018-7_39

Sciarra, D., & Seirup, H. (2008). The multidimensionality of school engagement and math achievement among racial groups. *Professional School Counseling, 11,* 218–228. https://doi.org/bzv6ft

Shernoff, D. J., & Schmidt, J. A. (2008). Further evidence of an engagement–achievement paradox among US high school students. *Journal of Youth and Adolescence, 37*(5), 564–580.

Shernoff, D. J., Csikszentmihalyi, M., Schneider, B., & Shernoff, E. S. (2003). Student engagement in high school classrooms from the perspective of flow theory. *School Psychology Quarterly, 18,* 158–176.

Skinner, E. A., Kindermann, T. A., & Furrer, C. J. (2009). A motivational perspective on engagement and disaffection conceptualization and assessment of children's behavioral and emotional participation in academic activities in the classroom. *Educational and Psychological Measurement, 69,* 493–525. https://doi.org/10.1177/0013164408323233

Thompson, T. L., & Kiang, L. (2010). The model minority stereotype: Adolescent experiences and links with adjustment. *Asian American Journal of Psychology, 1*(2), 119.

Truong, D. M., Tanaka, M. L., Cooper, J. M., Song, S., Talapatra, D., Arora, P., Fenning, P., McKenney, E., Williams, S., Stratton-Gadke, K., Jimerson, S. R., Pandes-Carter, L., Hulac, D., & García-Vázquez, E. (2021). School psychology unified call for deeper understanding, solidarity, and action to eradicate anti-AAAPI racism and violence. *School Psychology Review, 50*(2–3), 469–483. https://doi.org/10.1080/2372966X.2021.1949932

Uekawa, K., Borman, K., & Lee, R. (2007). Student engagement in US urban high school mathematics and science classrooms: Findings on social organization, race, and ethnicity. *The Urban Review, 39*(1), 1–43. https://doi.org/10.1007/s11256-006-0039-1

Van de Grift, W. J., Chun, S., Maulana, R., Lee, O., & Helms-Lorenz, M. (2017). Measuring teaching quality and student engagement in South Korea and The Netherlands. *School Effectiveness and School Improvement, 28*(3), 337–349.

Veiga, F. H. (2008). Disruptive behavior scale professed by students (DBS-PS): Development and validation. *International Journal of Psychology and Psychological Therapy, 8*(2), 203–216.

Veiga, F. H. (2012). Proposal to the PISA of a new scale of students' engagement in school. *Procedia-Social and Behavioral Sciences, 46,* 1224–1231.

Veiga, F. H., & Robu, V. (2014). Measuring student engagement with school across cultures: Psychometric findings from Portugal and Romania. *Romanian Journal of School Psychology, 7*(14), 57–72.

Virtanen, T., Moreira, P., Ulvseth, H., Andersson, H., Tetler, S., & Kuorelahti, M. (2018). Analyzing measurement invariance of the Students' Engagement Instrument brief version: The cases of Denmark, Finland, and Portugal. *Canadian Journal of School Psychology, 33*(4), 297–313. https://doi.org/10.1177/0829573517699333

Waanders, C., Mendez, J., & Downer, J. (2007). Parent characteristics, economic stress and neighborhood context as predictors of parent involvement in preschool children's education. *Journal of School Psychology, 45,* 619–636. https://doi.org/10.1016/j.jsp.2007.07.003

Wang, M. T., Willet, J. B., & Eccles, J. S. (2011). The assessment of school engagement: Examining dimensionality and measurement invariance by gender and race/ethnicity. *Journal of School Psychology, 49,* 465–480. https://doi.org/10.1016/j.jsp.2011.04.001

Worthy, L. D., Lavigne, T., & Romero, F. (2021). *Culture and psychology: How people shape and are shaped by culture.* Creative Commons Available online https://open.maricopa.edu/culturepsychology

Yair, G. (2000). Educational battlefields in America: The tug-of-war over students' engagement with instruction. *Sociology of Education, 73,* 247–269.

Yang, C., Bear, G. G., & May, H. (2018). Multilevel associations between school-wide social–emotional learning approach and student engagement across elementary, middle, and high schools. *School Psychology Review, 47*(1), 45–61. https://doi.org/10.17105/SPR-2017-0003.V47-1

Measuring Student Engagement: New Approaches and Issues

Joe Betts

Abstract

This commentary reflects upon issues and developments found in chapters on the measurement of student engagement. A variety of issues are discussed and one of the interesting aspects of these chapters is to see the major changes that have taken place since the original publication of this handbook a decade ago. A discussion of some of the specific issues raised is provided along with broader areas that apply across the chapters. Observational methods, self-report measures, real-time measurements, and cross-cultural uses of measures are discussed. Within the discussion, there are interjections of possible fecund areas of research related to these new developments. Overall, the advances in the measurement of student engagement have been broad and have led to increased use and recognition of the importance of student engagement across the world for positive student outcomes.

The study of student engagement has made a lot of advances since the original publication of this handbook (Christenson et al., 2012) as can be seen in the current volume. However, one thing remains consistent: the need to apply the best methods for measuring the construct. Measuring the construct of student engagement in a consistent and meaningful manner is the basis for evaluating research claims and providing evidence of individual differentiation for predictive models in practice. Without strong measurement of the construct, all results-based and data-driven methods for research and practice are moot. All measurement instruments should provide strong, psychometrically sound, and defensible results (American Educational Research Association, American Psychological Association, & National Council on Measurement in Education [AERA, APA, & NCME], 2014; Betts, 2012; Samuelsen, 2012).

One of the consistent issues related to the measurement of student engagement is the definition itself, as can be seen from the variety of insights and positions in the current research. While there are numerous conceptualizations of engagement and unique representations across the varied assessment instruments, one thing that the study of engagement, along with all scientific studies, embodies is the importance of developing and validating those instruments to provide meaningful data (Betts, 2012). One helpful aspect of this endeavor to develop and measure engagement is that there are several well-validated approaches to test development for psychological assessments that can be applied (AERA, APA, &

J. Betts (✉)
National Council of State Boards of Nursing, Chicago, IL, USA
e-mail: jbetts@ncsbn.org

© The Author(s), under exclusive license to Springer Nature Switzerland AG 2022
A. L. Reschly, S. L. Christenson (eds.), *Handbook of Research on Student Engagement*,
https://doi.org/10.1007/978-3-031-07853-8_32

NCME, 2014; Irwing et al., 2018; Lane et al., 2016; Nering & Ostini, 2010; Rao & Sinharay, 2006; Wilson, 2005; van der Linden, 2016).

In the current volume, there are a set of papers that evaluate some specific aspects of measuring student engagement, which will be the focus of this commentary. These three papers highlight some unique and important issues (Fredricks, 2022a; Jimerson & Chen, 2022) along with providing some information about the advances since the first volume (Fredricks, 2022b). The current commentary will provide an extension of the ideas and results developed in these chapters and some general thoughts for researchers as they continue to move the measurement of student engagement forward.

Some Important Developments

Fredricks (2022b) describes some developments over the past decade in student engagement. An exciting finding is that there are now many new measures of engagement. These assessments represent attempts to develop instruments that measure the different characterizations and theories of student engagement. They all were developed and validated using sound test development and psychometric principles. Jimerson and Chen (2022) also show how these assessments are being used across the world in multiple countries.

This expanse of assessments and use across the world highlights the importance of engagement in education. While there are many competing definitions of engagement that can make defining the construct difficult, this plethora of assessments approaching the construct from many different perspectives is quite useful. For instance, this provides numerous opportunities to test out different theories and validate complementary aspects of the construct. Likewise, from a practical perspective, this also provides a large set of tools for practitioners to choose for their specific needs. Having many high-quality assessments in the engagement toolbox can provide significant value to both researchers and practitioners.

Another exciting development is the increased use of these measures to inform policy. This is another welcome finding. Utilizing the results of these measures to help inform systems and intervene more directly in the ecology of the educational environment is needed. Many times, the focus of assessment is on the individual with the unstated assumption that the environment is not an issue and not a force impeding or enhancing problematic behavior. Recognizing that environments can and do affect engagement along with the courage to address interventions at those levels is essential. Having measures to assess the environment either directly or by utilizing aggregated data from individual assessments is an important use case for improving educational delivery and outcomes. However, this brings the issue of measurement to the fore; with these uses comes the imperative to develop and use only high-quality measures that can be justified for use at both the individual and the aggregate level for making decisions.

Observational Methods

Fredricks (2022a) outlines a number of important issues and some notable assessments using observational ratings to evaluate student engagement. These findings show how far the observational methods (see, for example, Bakeman & Gottman, 1997) have come with student engagement. Rosenbaum (2002, 2020) also provides some more introductory material with the benefit of introducing some freely available statistical packages in the R programming language (R Core Team, 2021) to support research and development. Stulman et al. (n.d.) also provide some important practical factors to consider when selecting observation methods and tools.

There are several benefits and limitations noted by Fredricks (2022a) to utilizing this approach. The importance of strong psychometric properties of scores, generally reliability and validity, is well known and highly important and will be discussed below. However, with observational methods and approaches, an equally important consideration is how representative are the specific observations with respect to the totality of the object of measurement. One of the broad issues underlying much of the discussion revolves around the statistical concept of sampling (Casella & Berger, 2006; Thompson, 2012). Whether it be an individual student, a teacher, a classroom, or a school in practice or a research study investing important outcomes of an intervention study, the nature of the sample of observations is important.

One of the first and most important issues relates to how well results are believed to generalize. This can be generalizing from controlled environments, such as those carried out in more homogeneous laboratory conditions, to more naturalistic environments, such as in the classroom or at home. Controlled environments are necessary for replication and making judgments about the variables understudy, for instance, an intervention focused on changing the behavioral engagement of students with high levels of behavioral issues. The controls are necessary to improve the potential for replication of findings.

The naturalistic methods have some positive aspects as it can be completed and carried out in the natural environment. Fredricks (2022a) notes some strengths and limitations of this approach, too. A positive is that it allows for authentic observations of the lived actions and behaviors as they are happening in real-time in the natural environment. This also helps to negate the potential issue of the Hawthorne effect (McCambridge et al., 2014; McCarney et al., 2007) that can be found in the controlled studies when the object of study realizes they are being watched and will potentially act differently than normal to comport with expectations. Natural environmental observations can reduce this when the observer is themselves a participant in that environment, e.g., school psychologists, counselors, or anyone that students see throughout the day in the school.

When it comes to observational methods, sampling becomes quite complex. All humans vary in their comportment from hour to hour and day-to-day. Therefore, obtaining observational measurements needs to be planned to ensure adequate sampling from times of the day, different days, different environments (e.g., teachers,

classrooms, subjects), etc. The importance of this is to ensure adequate representation for generalization. For instance, some basic questions that might be asked if one is sampling appropriately for making inferences about classroom effects might be as follows: are a variety of observations being taken across the day, across the week, during diverse activities, across the various subjects, etc.

Another important aspect of observational methods is the extent to which different raters rate behavior consistently. This is generally not much of an issue with the administration of self-report or class-wide rating scales where a proctor oversees individual completion of the forms. However, with observational methods, the observer becomes part of the measurement process by translating observations into ratings within the measure. It is important in practical use or clinical settings where the focus is on making real-life decisions about students, teachers, or schools to use observational methods that can be used reliably by various observers to consistently rate behavior. Methods that improve consistency across raters are vital for making valid generalizations of results.

One of the most direct ways to address this is by ensuring that the structured or semi-structured rating scales used are specific and easily understood by raters. This means that definitions of how and what behaviors need to be coded should be comprehensive. With sufficient training, the raters should be able to understand and identify the correct behaviors and the appropriate method for scoring them. The more specific and definable, the more consistent the ratings will be. However, as Fredricks (2022a) notes, this can also be a detriment as overly specific measures can have lower levels of predictive validity and make inferences to a broader understanding of student engagement problematic.

Psychometric integrity is a very important goal of all observational approaches. Of which, inter-rater reliability (Gwet, 2014) is a significant component needed to validate claims of consistency of ratings across multiple raters (AERA, APA, & NCME, 2014). In general, the analysis is done by having two or more independent raters rate the same person at the same time using the same instrument, and then compare the ratings between the raters. In essence, it is desirable that two independent raters observe the same individual at that same time and have perfectly consistent ratings. However, in practice, this is not always the case, but for observational methods, controlling the variation between raters is vitally important in making sure that a high level of replication of scores/ratings is produced between independent raters.

One thing that test developers can do to support high levels of inter-rater reliability is to provide exemplars for individuals being trained to benchmark their ratings against the expected standard. This can be accomplished with the use of recorded audio/visual of situations for trainees to rate that come along with standardized scoring for comparison and discussion of the rationale behind the scoring. Users of these methods should also take care to consistently provide dual ratings on all raters during the normal course of practice. This is necessary to make sure raters are maintaining consistency across time and following the prescribed procedures.

There are a number of standard approaches to evaluating inter-rater reliability (Gwet, 2014). Fredricks (2022a) provides evidence that the observational systems reviewed have adequate inter-rater reliability. This should be encouraging for users of the assessment systems that given adequate training, consistency between raters can be accomplished. It is important to note that with inter-rater reliability, both developers of systems must show adequate levels of reliability with some level of training, those practitioners in the field should also provide evidence that the measures are being implemented reliably in practice.

Much of the evidence provided (Fredricks, 2022a) used standard methods, however, there are some more advanced methods that could be used. These advanced methods can be useful for both test development validation and researchers. One possible approach is generalizability theory (Brennan, 2001). The method isolates a number of facets of measurement using analysis of variance (ANOVA) statistical methods for partitioning the variance associated with each facet. A full

explication of this method is not possible in this commentary, but the basic of the approach is to identify those aspects of the measurement process and instrument that can introduce inconsistencies into the observed scores for analysis. Using this theory, variables, such as rater, classroom, time of day, can be introduced into the statistical model and parsed out to evaluate the variance components (Brennan, 2001; Searle et al., 2009). A complementary approach uses explanatory item response models (De Boeck & Wilson, 2004).

Another advanced methodology is the Many-Facet Rasch model (Linacre, 1994). This is a model that allows for the evaluation of numerous facets of measurement. For instance, a common use is to evaluate both raters and the rating scale in a similar way as generalizability theory but uses the Rasch measurement model to ensure that all raters and scores are on the same scale. An aspect of this model can also be used to evaluate specific rater bias as to their leniency or strictness in rating. Another useful outcome of this method is the potential to measure raters over time and provide corrective feedback as necessary over time directed at the specific areas they appear to be deviating from the standard. This can be powerful feedback for raters in the field to help ensure they maintain consistency and if they get off track, they can get remediation. This method like the others above has the potential for adding additional facets of measurement for analysis which makes the potential use for researchers suggestive.

As Fredricks (2022a) notes, a significant limitation is the lack of predictive validity between observational measures and later outcomes. While this is an issue that needs to be addressed by observational systems, there is another way to think about the importance of this issue. Given that observational approaches provide unique information that cannot be gathered in other ways and can be resource-intensive to acquire, is this information needed as a predictive measure? If concurrent evidence can be found to validate the scores on observational systems for identifying normative, at-risk, and problematic levels of behavior, then the observations can be used to validate results from much more efficiently administered measures, such as rating scales like the Student Engagement Instrument (SEI; Appleton et al., 2006). Moreover, the use of the observational methods should provide data from the actual environment that helps to support the selection and implementation of interventions when needed. This data might not be as effective with making future predictions, but expending time and effort to gather this type of data with a validated observational system could be thought of as more informative for making change rather than evaluated as a long-term predictive measure.

A common approach for concurrent validity is to use convergent and divergent methods (see, for example, Reschly et al., 2014). This approach identifies variables that are believed to be related to the construct. Measures of these variables with the construct of interest should show reasonable positive correlations providing convergent evidence in support of the construct representation. Additionally, it is possible to identify variables that should have little to do with the construct. In these instances, one is looking for practically small effect sizes in the relationship between the variables providing divergent evidence.

One research option that could help to shed light across the diverse methods of measuring engagement is to evaluate the multi-trait multi-method (MTMM; Campbell & Fiske, 1959) framework. This approach allows for the investigation of different methods of measuring a student engagement using observational and self-report across the various conceptualizations of divergent aspects like behavioral and cognitive. MTMM can be evaluated by confirmatory factor analytic (CFA) methods (Kenny & Kashy, 1992; Marsh & Bailey, 1991) which are already used to investigate validity research to parse out how different methods of measurement interact with different traits. In a basic case, the MTMM matrix could have a 3x3 design with {observation, self-report, teacher report} as methods and {behavioral, cognitive, emotional} as the traits. Utilization of approaches to analysis such as the MTMM could help to provide comprehensive evidence for the use of common assessment para-

digms in education such as the use of screeners for early identification, rating scales for further follow-up on students identified at risk, and then observational approaches for evaluation of effective interventions.

Additionally, it is important to think about the goal to which the measurements will be used. Care needs to be taken as methods used in research studies could be tailored for specific needs of the study but use in practice stipulates a different degree of psychometric validation and justification may be needed (AERA, APA, & NCME, 2014). For the overall screening of a student population, then more efficient rating scale measures could be used. Once a student is identified as at-risk, then observational methods could be used to provide more specific information on the student in their environment. This can be used to set a baseline for behavior and allow for repeated measures over time if interventions are introduced. Additionally, if the classroom is the level of observation, then again repeated observations, given a well-thought-out sampling plan, could provide more useful specific information for providing feedback to improve performance. With the goal in mind, pick the appropriate methods for gathering evidence and if the goal is to evaluate change over time, then ensure that the measure has enough precision to make decisions about the trends.

Real-Time Measurements

Fredricks (2022b) provides a valuable overview of the status of self-report measures over the past decade. Additionally, Fredricks provides a view into what is suggested to be the biggest change in the measurement of engagement over this decade. This development has been the result of 'real-time' measurements. These methods have the common element of providing measurements on students as they are engaging in activities in real-time. One thing that is clear from the review is that real-time methods need much more research before they could be used in practice. Fredricks (2022b) identifies a number of issues. A few more will be provided here for future researchers and theoreticians to consider.

One of the strengths of these methods is that they could provide additional information that augments the static picture of the student at any single time that common assessments of student engagement provide. These real-time measurements could help to increase information from self-report measures that give only information based on the students reflecting on experiences and responding (Fredricks, 2022b). They also hold out the potential for repeated measurements to help provide information over time that many rating scales are not psychometrically capable of providing. Given the intended use of measuring over time, it would be important to make sure that these measures are sensitive to changes over the time span of intended use to ensure that a reliable level of change can be evaluated.

The potential for repeated, daily assessments on a few key variables using a simple sampling plan across the school or district could provide a great amount of data with minimal disruption of student and teacher time during the day. This potential to gather longitudinal, time-series data allows for within-person, repeated measures analytic methods to be applied when engaging in research (Crowder & Hand, 1990; Diggle et al., 2002; Koepsell & Weiss, 2003; Verbeke & Molenberghs, 2000). In the case of monitoring for intervention effectiveness of a single subject, be it a student in an intervention or a single classroom undergoing an intervention, there are single-subject designs (Kratochwill, 1978; Tate & Perdices, 2018) available to aid in the design and analysis of data.

Likewise, with the potential for rich daily data feeds, the potential for an early warning metric would be in place for more specific usage as indicators can be updated daily as new responses are registered and aggregated. While there are a number of methods for evaluating change (see, references above), one interesting approach researchers might want to investigate is the use of the reliable change index (RCI; Jacobson & Truax, 1991). The index computes the significance of the difference between scores taking into account scale reliability. One of the nice things about this type of index is that, unlike large sample statistical tests, this index can be used in small, local samples.

A review of some case studies utilizing a number of these real-time methods has recently been completed (DiMello et al., 2017). Many of the case studies in this review provide enticing results. However, one issue appears to predominate when thinking about their utility for measuring the more global construct of engagement. This has to do with the validity of the generalization of engagement in a specific task to the more global person-centered construct of engagement usually associated with student engagement. Student engagement tends to be understood as a more global aspect of individuals with individual differences appearing across the main domains (see most chapters in the current volume of this handbook).

For instance, eye-tracking, physical measures, and log files represent specific levels of engagement with specific instruction, reading, games, etc. While this can provide diagnostic information about reading behavior with respect to eye-tracking or decision-making/problem-solving for game logs, the extent to which this particular level of engagement generalizes to a student's overall level of engagement indicative of personal- and school-related problems needs significant work. A simple example of the potential counter-example would be a student that has completely tuned out of school but finds enjoyment in reading (and does not have any eye-tracking issues related to reading problems) and engagement in particular games as the student can do these specific tasks without any proximity or integration with others or the educational environment. Overall, the student could be thought of as 'disengaged' in general but the specific engagement with tasks would be high.

Another counterexample of this could be found in the interpretation of facial or body expressions while engaging in a reading task. A basic question would be, does a series of emotional states reflective of facial comportment elicited during a specific task tell us about the student's overall sense of engagement at school? Beyond the simple issue of generalizing from the specific, imagine a legitimate facial recognition of sadness during the task that is not related to global engagement comportment but to environmental stimuli at the same time. Negative emotions in some situations could suggest high engagement, for instance when it is an appropriate emotional response to environmental triggers. For instance, it could be difficult and frustrating for a student attempting to do their work at a computer when others around them are acting or behaving in inappropriate ways. The frustration would not be an indication of disengagement but a signal of attempted engagement being thwarted by the environmental mischief of others.

The use of facial recognition also brings up a more subtle issue: the use of machine learning or artificial intelligence algorithms (Goodfellow et al., 2016; Hastie et al., 2017; Witten et al., 2011). These approaches utilize training datasets to build models for making predictions and can be developed to continually update with new information. One nice thing about the continual updating is that training can take place on samples from a specific individual, thus individualizing the predictions over time. It is recommended that before engaging in these types of products, one should consult standards developed by experts in the field (IEEE Standards Association, n.d.; National Institute of Standards and Technology, 2019) and also issues that have become a focus in the testing industry (International Privacy Subcommittee of the ATP Security Committee, 2021).

The concern with training data is that the data could have been collected without being representative of the population of interest. Just like observational methods that utilize only the most at-risk students, results from training models on biased data will result in biased predictions. Generalizability, again, is the issue. As all statistical models use training data to help the machine learn and build the predictive algorithm, the representativeness of the data in the training data set needs to be evaluated. This also dovetails with Jimerson and Chen's (2022) concerns with making inferences across different cultures (Jimerson & Chen, 2022).

Take for example, the automated analysis of human faces and facial expressions has become much more commonplace in the past decade with a number of methods and algorithms (Dubey & Singh, 2016; Sariyanidi et al., 2015). It has likewise come a long way from original implementations (Belhumeur et al., 1997). However, even with this technology, there are subtle concerns for use in education. A number of the issues that have been identified with reduced utility and increased error rates would be found quite frequently when working within schools and with children, e.g., illumination issues, head pose changes, etc. (Dubey & Singh, 2016; Grother et al., 2019; Sariyanidi et al., 2015). Additionally, it has also been found that even the recognition algorithms for faces have potentially significant racial/ethnic biases that would call into question their uses in diverse populations (Grother et al., 2019).

Another aspect of real-time measures and those outlined in the case studies (DiMello et al., 2017) is that they generally take place while interacting with technology. However, much of a student's school day takes place away from technology. This could limit the generalizability of the results for making inferences about a general sense of a student's overall engagement. The issue of technology and data capture also brings to the forefront issues related to security and privacy. This is related not only to the actual, physical security of the data but also highlights other privacy concerns; for example, digital/video recording of classrooms could pose some additional legal issues schools would need to contend with. Engaging in this type of data collection for research study purposes or practical/clinical situations in the school imposes responsibilities on school representatives to consider.

One of the interesting opportunities identified by Fredricks (2022b) related to the use of experience sampling methods (ESM; Larson & Csikszentmihalyi, 1983). With the rapid dispersion of personal electronic devices and the potential to distribute these devices throughout the school day to students is a compelling idea. These could be relatively unobtrusive methods for gathering in vivo information about both endogenous variables like student cognitive or emotional status and exogenous variables such as those related to understanding or engagement with the current activity. It is also feasible to think that subsets of the items presented on global screening assessments (Koepsell & Weiss, 2003) could also be used as a small set of indicators for these real-time sampling methods.

Cultural Considerations

Jimerson and Chen (2022) reflect on the importance of cultural considerations in the measurement of constructs. They also provide a though examination of these issues and some important findings. Care should be taken when using measures developed within one cultural framework being applied to different cultural environments (Abedi, 2016; AERA, APA, & NCME, 2014; International Testing Commission, 2017).

One of the most important measurement issues in need of validation before making comparisons between groups is measurement invariance (Meredith, 1964, 1993). Ensuring that measures of any construct by any specific instrument can be used to compare different groups is founded on the assumption that the scales of measurement are the same between the two groups. Measurement invariance is the broad psychometric and statistical conceptualization of this foundational issue. The methods of evaluating invariance focus on ensuring measurements are similar across different groups. This fundamental principle of measurement should not be taken for granted but rather actively analyzed for evidence of its validity before accepting any claims of group differences.

This is not just relevant to the situation where different languages and countries are using measures developed elsewhere. It is also relevant to assure that there is no bias in the measurement of important subgroups of a single population. For instance, evaluating the extent to which items measure individuals from different ethnic groups within the United States in a consistent manner is an important aspect of validity evidence (AERA, APA, & NCME, 2014). If psychological assessments measure groups differently, then this bias could result in making incorrect decisions. This can affect the individual that is being measured in a manner inconsistent with the expected inferences of the scores but also poses a danger to aggregated results comparing those groups.

There are a number of methods for evaluating the possibility of differences in construct representation for measurement instruments (Brown, 2015; Millsap, 2011; Raju et al., 2002; Reise et al., 1993; Wells, 2021). One direct method studies the measurement invariance of an instrument across different subpopulation groups using a confirmatory factor analytic approach (see, for example, Betts et al., 2010). This approach is based on identifying the groups of interest in the population and then structuring a series of confirmatory models of increasing constraints to address the level of equivalence in measurement between the groups. The goal is to find strict equivalence between the groups such that all inferences from scores can be applied equally to each group.

The use of the CFA models for measuring invariance assumes that the items and forms are well structured for analysis. However, there are other methods that utilize item response theory (IRT; Hambleton et al., 1991; van der Linden, 2016) to evaluate these same issues using the methods of differential item functioning (DIF; Holland & Wainer, 1993). While these methods can be applied using well-structured forms, they also can be used for the analysis of independent items with the results being very similar to the CFA methods (Raju et al., 2002; Reise et al., 1993; Stark et al., 2006). The methods of DIF can be used and the logic of testing is the same as above with the use of increasingly constrained models being compared across the groups to ensure items are measuring individuals of the same latent ability similarly.

Another important area of cross-cultural testing is a translation from the base language of the instrument to the language of the new cultural group. Whenever developing translated texts, it is vital to outline a defensible method for validating the translation (Abedi, 2016). Without valid translations, interpretation of responses and scores on those instruments are uninterpretable. The International Test Commission (2017) provides a set of guidelines that research and test developers can use to evaluate the translation process for their work. Providing solid evidence to support the validity of translated text is just as vital as evidence to support comparisons of scores across cultures (AERA, APA, & NCME, 2014).

An important aspect of Jimerson and Chen's (2022) call for care in validating measures across cultures is that when this can be accomplished, the foundation for true cross-cultural research on student engagement can begin. An exciting opportunity is highlighted with respect to the potential to replicate and validate intervention effectiveness across different cultures. With strong evidence of valid translations and measurement invariance, research studies of theoretical interest and practical effects can be studied using a common set of measures. This would allow for important opportunities to directly compare the outcomes across cultures and allow for important replication analyses to be undertaken with the safety and belief that the measures and scores obtained are truly comparable. This comparability of scores across all possible sets of subgroups is the basis for the scientific measurement needed for solid research to be undertaken.

Conclusion

The measurement of student engagement has come a long way over the past decade. Several new measures of engagement have been developed. Additionally, there is also a growing recognition of the importance of positive engagement to strong educational outcomes that have guided use at the systems level. With the expansion of high-quality psychometric measures and the recognition of the importance, the options for schools to choose those measures that fit their system-level needs have increased. This also provides a fertile ground for researching the diversity of characterizations of engagement found in the literature.

Another interesting development has been the expanse of quality observational methods. These provide options for engaging in both individual and system-level evaluations that are sometimes difficult to evaluate with the usual rating scales and individual assessments. More work is needed to help support the use of these measures, but the ability to use them in conjunction with individual measures and large-scale screening measures is intriguing. One of the key aspects of the use of these methods will continue to be an assurance that inter-rater reliability is strong both for the research grounding the measures but also by those using them in practice. Research into the use of these measures using approaches like multi-trait multi-method or generalizability theory is ripe for picking.

A very interesting and fecund area of research is one of the other major developments over the past decade: the use of real-time measures. One of the key areas of interest will be to evaluate the extent to which these measures of specific aspects of engagement with specific tasks can generalize to the broader picture of student engagement as a psychological construct. However, the importance and utility of these measures for advancing educational goals and positive outcomes are not dependent upon this type of correspondence, but the intersection of specific engagement and broader engagement is an interesting and open area of study.

One important aspect of some of the real-time measures which are also found in the area of observational measurement has to do with basic sampling methodologies. Like with observational methods, real-time measures could give misleading results if an understanding of the contexts within which the measurements were taken or judgments about scores on the measures was obtained. One very important aspect of some real-time measures that rely on predictive models developed from machine learning techniques is the evaluation and validation of the sample used to build those models. For instance, facial recognition models have been shown to have biases with respect to specific groups of individuals. Using these approaches in educational settings will need to ensure biases in the predictive algorithms are negated.

On the subject of bias, another vast area for the investigation of student engagement has been the worldwide recognition of its importance. This positive recognition has also spawned the need to adapt measures from culture to culture. The adaptation must be done with care to ensure that both the language components related to the translation of content along with the psychometric properties like measurement invariance are sound. The importance of ensuring similar measurement of the same psychological construct is a foundational axiom of any research exploring cross-cultural comparisons. Without evidence of strict correspondence between the construct and the measurements between groups, no valuable comparisons can be made. This would be a shame if the opportunity was missed with poorly validated measures because the potential for cross-cultural studies of a psychological construct like engagement and the evaluation of intervention outcomes is enormous.

Future research should evaluate the extent to which all of the types of measurement approaches discussed in these chapters are amenable and adaptable to repeated measures. From observational studies to self-report measures to real-time measures, a valuable aspect of all of these is to map trends and changes at the individual and systems levels. One of the future aspects of student engagement appears to revolve around gathering data over time to identify trends and changes to trends given interventions.

Continued evaluation of the validity of the scores from the new measures will be important. These types of studies should continue to look at the measurement properties of the scales or observational systems in unique situations with a diversity of student populations. Replication of results is one of the best ways to continue to grow the research base for both the measures and findings especially when they are done in a variety of settings with a variety of students.

Methods such as ESM have an interesting potential. With the widespread distribution of electronic devices, the potential for providing students with personal devices to provide mea-

surements throughout the day could be a reality. Utilizing the widespread availability of personal electronic devices across schools and districts could allow for the development of an early warning model that keeps school and district officials continually informed. Using a simple sampling method along with an efficient and informative interrogative questioning modality, the potential for gathering significant data is present. Additionally, the simple use of subsets of items from district-wide screening measures could be continually evaluated over time to gauge the 'temperature' of the environments on a daily basis and intervene as needed before issues arise.

Most of the real-time methods are predicated on the use of technology not normally used in educational settings. Therefore, these types of approaches need experts in those areas to coordinate and carry out the evaluations. For instance, with the physiological methods, there is a need for trained experts to operate unique medical equipment that could be difficult to implement within a school environment, let alone the issues related to 'wiring' the students up for evaluation. Even with the ESM system, the expert issue could manifest as a strong technology team that would need to be available to ensure the network is secure and connected, along with ensuring the privacy and safety of all data being acquired. These are issues future researchers and practitioners will have to deal with as the measurement of engagement evolves over the next decade.

Overall, the past decade has seen some interesting advances in the measurement of student engagement. As expounded upon in the chapters in this volume of the handbook, there will be a plethora of research opportunities in the next decade. Likewise, the use of these measures to help prepare and educate students for the future suggests great potential.

References

Abedi, J. (2016). Language issues in item development. In S. Lane, M. R. Raymond, & T. Haladyna (Eds.), *Handbook of test development* (2nd ed., pp. 355–373). Routledge.

American Educational Research Association, American Psychological Association, & National Council on Measurement in Education [AERA, APA, & NCME]. (2014). *The standards for educational psychological testing*. American Educational Research Association.

Appleton, J. J., Christenson, S. L., Kim, D., & Reschly, A. L. (2006). Measuring cognitive and psychological engagement: Validation of the Student Engagement Instrument. *Journal of School Psychology, 44*, 427–445.

Bakeman, R., & Gottman, J. M. (1997). *Observing interaction: An introduction to sequential analysis* (2nd ed.). Cambridge University Press.

Belhumeur, P. N., Hespanha, J. P., & Kriegman, D. J. (1997). Eigenfaces vs. Fisherfaces: Recognition using class specific linear projection. *IEEE Transactions on Pattern Analysis and Machine Intelligence, 19*(7), 711–720. https://doi.org/10.1109/34.598228

Betts, J. (2012). Issues and methods in the measurement of student engagement: Advancing the construct through statistical modeling. In S. L. Christenson, A. L. Reschly, & C. Wylie (Eds.), *Handbook of research on student engagement* (pp. 783–804). Springer.

Betts, J., Appleton, J. J., Reschly, A. L., Christenson, S. L., & Huebner, E. S. (2010). A study of the factorial invariance of the Student Engagement Instrument (SEI): Results from middle and high school students. *School Psychology Quarterly, 25*, 84–93.

Brennan, R. L. (2001). *Generalizability theory*. Springer.

Brown, T. (2015). *Confirmatory factor analysis for applied research* (2nd ed.). The Guilford Press.

Campbell, D., & Fiske, D. (1959). Convergent and discriminant validation by the multitrait-multimethod matrix. *Psychological Bulletin, 56*, 81–105.

Casella, G., & Berger, R. L. (2006). *Statistical inference* (2nd ed.). Thompson Press.

Christenson, S. L., Reschly, A. L., & Wylie, C. (Eds.). (2012). *Handbook of research on student engagement*. Springer.

Crowder, M. J., & Hand, D. J. (1990). *Analysis of repeated measures*. Chapman and Hall.

De Boeck, P., & Wilson, M. (Eds.). (2004). *Explanatory item response models: A generalized linear and nonlinear approach*. Springer-Verlag.

Diggle, P. J., Heagerty, P. J., Liang, K.-Y., & Zeger, S. L. (2002). *Analysis of longitudinal data*. Oxford University Press.

DiMello, S., Dieterle, E., & Duckworth, A. (2017). Advanced, analytic, automated (AAA) measurement of engagement during learning. *Educational Psychologist, 52*(2), 104–123.

Dubey, M., & Singh, L. (2016). Automatic emotion recognition using facial expression: A review. *International Research Journal of Engineering and Technology, 3*(2), 488–492.

Fredricks, J. A. (2022a). Measuring student engagement with observational techniques. In A. L. Reschly & S. L. Christenson (Eds.), *Handbook of research on student engagement* (2nd ed.,). Springer.

Fredricks, J. A. (2022b). The measurement of student engagement: Methodological advances and comparisons of new self-report instruments. In A. L. Reschly & S. L. Christenson (Eds.), *Handbook of research on student engagement* (2nd ed.,). Springer.

Goodfellow, I., Bengio, Y., & Courville, A. (2016). *Deep learning*. The MIT Press.

Grother, P., Ngan, M., & Hanaoka, K. (2019). *Face recognition vendor test (FRVT) Part 3: Demographic effects*. U.S. Department of Commerce: National Institute of Standards and Technology. https://doi.org/10.6028/NIST.IR.8280

Gwet, K. L. (2014). *Handbook of inter-rater reliability* (4th ed.). Advanced Analytics, LLC.

Hambleton, R., Swaminathan, H., & Rogers, H. (1991). *Fundamentals of item response theory*. Sage.

Hastie, T., Tibshirani, R., & Friedman, J. (2017). *The elements of statistical learning: Data mining, inference, and prediction* (2nd ed.). Springer.

Holland, P. W., & Wainer, H. (1993). *Differential item functioning*. Erlbaum.

IEEE Standards Association. (n.d.). *Raising the standards in artificial intelligence systems (AIS)*. Retrieved 12/2/2021. https://standards.ieee.org/initiatives/artificial-intelligence-systems/index.html

International Privacy Subcommittee of the ATP Security Committee. (2021). *Artificial intelligence and the testing industry: A primer*. Association of Test Publishers. https://www.testpublishers.org/assets/ATP%20White%20Paper_AI%20and%20Testing_A%20Primer_6July2021_Final%20R1%20.pdf

International Test Commission [ITC]. (2017). *The ITC guidelines for translating and adapting tests* (2nd ed.). www.intestcom.org

Irwing, P., Booth, T., & Hughes, D. J. (Eds.). (2018). *The Wiley handbook of psychometric testing: A multidisciplinary reference on survey, scale and test development*. Wiley Blackwell.

Jacobson, N. S., & Truax, P. (1991). Clinical significance: A statistical approach to defining meaningful change in psychotherapy research. *Journal of Consulting and Clinical Psychology, 59*, 12–19.

Jimerson, S. R., & Chen, C. (2022). Multicultural and cross-cultural considerations in understanding student engagement in schools: Promoting the development of diverse students around the world. In A. L. Reschly & S. L. Christenson (Eds.), *Handbook of research on student engagement* (2nd ed.,). Springer.

Kenny, D., & Kashy, D. (1992). Analysis of the multitrait-multimethod matrix by confirmatory factor analysis. *Psychological Bulletin, 112*, 165–172.

Koepsell, T. D., & Weiss, N. S. (2003). *Epidemiological methods: Studying the occurrence of illness*. Oxford University Press.

Kratochwill, T. R. (Ed.). (1978). *Single subject research: Strategies for evaluating change*. Academic.

Lane, S., Raymond, M. R., & Haladyna, T. M. (Eds.). (2016). *Handbook of test development* (2nd ed.). Routledge.

Larson, R., & Csikszentmihalyi, M. (1983). The experience sampling method. *New Directions for Methodology of Social and Behavioral Science., 15,* 41–56.

Linacre, J. M. (1994). *Many-facet Rasch measurement.* MESA Press.

Marsh, H., & Bailey, M. (1991). Confirmatory factor analysis of multitrait-multimethod data: A comparison of alternative models. *Applied Psychological Measurement, 15,* 47–70.

McCambridge, J., Witton, J., & Elbourne, D. R. (2014). Systematic review of the Hawthorne effect: New concepts are needed to study research participation effects. *Journal of Clinical Epidemiology, 67*(3), 267–277.

McCarney, R., Warner, J., Iliffe, S., Van Haselen, R., Griffin, M., & Fisher, P. (2007). The Hawthorne Effect: A randomised, controlled trial. *BMC Medical Research Methodology, 7*(1), 1–8.

Meredith, W. (1964). Notes on factorial invariance. *Psychometrika, 29,* 177–185.

Meredith, W. (1993). Measurement invariance, factor analysis and factorial invariance. *Psychometrika, 58,* 525–543.

Millsap, R. E. (2011). *Statistical approaches to measurement invariance.* Routledge.

National Institute of Standards and Technology. (2019). *U.S. leadership in AI: A plan for federal engagement in developing technical standards and related tools.* U.S. Department of Commerce: National Institute of Standards and Technology. https://www.nist.gov/system/files/documents/2019/08/10/ai_standards_fedengagement_plan_9aug2019.pdf

Nering, M. L., & Ostini, R. (Eds.). (2010). *Handbook of polytomous item response models.* Routledge.

R Core Team. (2021). *R: A language and environment for statistical computing.* R Foundation for Statistical Computing. https://www.R-project.org/

Raju, N. S., Laffitte, L. J., & Byrne, B. M. (2002). Measurement equivalence: A comparison of methods based on confirmatory factor analysis and item response theory. *Journal of Applied Psychology, 87,* 517–529.

Rao, S. R., & Sinharay, S. (Eds.). (2006). *Handbook of statistics 26: Psychometrics.* Elsevier.

Reise, S. P., Widaman, K. F., & Pugh, R. H. (1993). Confirmatory factor analysis and item response theory: Two approaches for exploring measurement invariance. *Psychological Bulletin, 114,* 552–566.

Reschly, A. L., Betts, J., & Appleton, J. J. (2014). An examination of the validity of two measures of student engagement. *International Journal of School & Educational Psychology, 2*(2), 106–114. https://doi.org/10.1080/21683603.2013.876950

Rosenbaum, P. R. (2002). *Observational studies* (2nd ed.). Springer.

Rosenbaum, P. R. (2020). *Design of observational studies* (2nd ed.). Springer.

Samuelsen, K. M. (2012). Possible new directions in the measurement of student engagement. In S. L. Christenson, A. L. Reschly, & C. Wylie (Eds.), *Handbook of research on student engagement* (pp. 805–811). Springer.

Sariyanidi, E., Gunes, H., & Cavallaro, A. (2015). Automatic analysis of facial affect: A survey of registration, representation, and recognition. *IEEE Transactions on Pattern Analysis and Machine Intelligence, 37*(6), 1113–1133. https://doi.org/10.1109/TPAMI.2014.2366127

Searle, S. R., Casella, G., & McCulloch, C. E. (2009). *Variance components.* Wiley.

Stark, S., Chernyshenko, O. S., & Drasgow, F. (2006). Detecting differential item functioning with confirmatory factor analysis and item response theory: Toward a unified strategy. *Journal of Applied Psychology., 91,* 1292–1306.

Stulman, M. W., Hamre, B. K., Downer, J. T., & Pianta, R. C. (n.d.). *How to select the right classroom observation tool.* University of Virginia Center for Advanced Study of Teaching and Learning (CASTL). https://curry.virginia.edu/sites/default/files/uploads/resourceLibrary/CASTL_practioner_Part3_single.pdf

Tate, R. L., & Perdices, M. (2018). *Single-case experimental designs for clinical research and neurorehabilitation settings: Planning, conduct, analysis and reporting.* Routledge.

Thompson, S. K. (2012). *Sampling* (3rd ed.). Wiley.

van der Linden, W. (Ed.). (2016). *Handbook of item response theory* (Vol. 1–3). CRC Press.

Verbeke, G., & Molenberghs, G. (2000). *Linear mixed models for longitudinal data.* Springer.

Wells, C. S. (2021). *Assessing measurement invariance for applied research.* Cambridge University Press.

Wilson, M. (2005). *Constructing measures: An item response modeling approach.* Lawrence Erlbaum Associates.

Witten, I. H., Frank, E., & Hall, M. A. (2011). *Data mining: Practical machine learning tools and techniques* (3rd ed.). Morgan Kaufman.

Epilogue

Amy L. Reschly and Sandra L. Christenson

Abstract

Based on the content of 32 chapters across four sections (Defining Student Engagement, Positive Development and Outcomes, Contexts for Engagement, and Measurement), the co-editors summarize the big ideas in the study of student engagement and call on researchers to consider specific conceptual, empirical, and practical aspects of the construct to advance the knowledge base for promoting youth development.

Ten years has passed since the publication of the first edition of the *Handbook of Research on Student Engagement* (Christenson, Reschly, & Wylie, 2012). In the first edition, our goal was to advance research and practice in the field, with contributions from renowned international scholars in student engagement, motivation, and related areas. We gathered their perspectives on the definition of student engagement, differentiation of the construct from motivation, and future directions. The volume also allowed for an exten- sive accounting of the evidence linking student engagement to an array of student outcomes.

The second edition of this *Handbook* high- lights the remarkable growth and advancement in the conceptualization and study of student engagement. We again invited renowned interna- tional scholars to contribute to the volume. Working with the authors has been a wonderful professional and learning experience. Each coed- itor believes that her understanding and knowl- edge of student engagement have been embellished as a result of coediting this *Handbook*. In particular, we noted that many authors raised conceptual, empirical, and applied considerations with respect to advancing the research on student engagement. As a result of such scholarship, we contend the purpose of a focus on student engagement is ultimately to pro- mote youth development–to achieve optimal social, emotional, academic, and behavioral learning outcomes for children, adolescents, and young adults. This purpose demands or requires psychometrically sound assessment and feasible universal and individual interventions. Hence, the bookends are assessment and intervention or the assessment-to-intervention link.

Although there are still questions regarding the differentiation between motivation and stu- dent engagement, we agree that this difference may be thought of as one of focus (Finn & Zimmer, 2012). The broad differentiation of a motivational vs. developmental view on student

A. L. Reschly (✉)
University of Georgia, Athens, GA, USA
e-mail: reschly@uga.edu

S. L. Christenson
University of Minnesota, Minneapolis, MN, USA
e-mail: chris002@umn.edu

engagement may also be helpful, as is the distinction between framework and theory (Tinto, chapter "Exploring the Character of Student Persistence in Higher Education: The Impact of Perception, Motivation, and Engagement", this volume). Student engagement is best characterized as a broad framework or model, albeit one that is influenced by motivational theories in general, and self-determination theory in particular (e.g., Connell & Wellborn, 1991; Fredricks et al., 2019; National Research Council & Institute of Medicine [NRC], 2004; Reeve, 2012). The student engagement framework is useful for conceptualizing contextual influences, interactions between students and their environments, and linking contexts and students to outcomes across development. It would be difficult or even impossible to design a longitudinal study that accounts for all the possible contextual influences, student characteristics, subtypes of engagement, interactions, and possible outcomes of integrated developmental engagement models (Reschly & Christenson, chapter "Jingle-Jangle Revisited: History and Further Evolution of the Student Engagement Construct", this volume); however, a portion of the model or framework can be specified and tested. For example, examining the effects of changes in instruction on students' cognitive and behavioral engagement and subsequent achievement, an investigation of a relationship intervention such as Banking Time (Williford & Pianta, 2020) or Establish-Maintain-Restore (Cook et al., 2020) on students' affective (e.g., belonging) and behavioral engagement (academic engaged time, class behavior), an examination of parenting practices and students' affective, cognitive, and/or behavioral engagement, and subsequent achievement, etc. is feasible. Motivational theories tend to view student engagement more narrowly as the observable manifestation of students' motivation and are more amenable to studies focused on theory testing. Skinner and Raine (chapter "Relationships Between Student Engagement and Mental Health as Conceptualized from a Dual-Factor Model", this volume) provided several suggestions for integrating and strengthening both areas of study.

In this final chapter of the second edition of the *Handbook of Research on Student Engagement*, we offer a summary of what we believe are the big ideas in student engagement and of the conceptual, empirical, and applied considerations that will, in our minds, advance the research on student engagement, enabling efficacious assessment-to-intervention practices for all students.

Big Ideas in Student Engagement

We think it worthwhile to summarize what were, and still are, the big ideas in the study of student engagement.

Student Engagement:

- It is a broad, integrative construct that draws from diverse theoretical perspectives and lines of research.
- It includes aspects of emotion, cognition, and behavior. Regardless of the subtypes and indicators selected, student engagement involves how students think and feel about learning, their classroom and school, the relevance of education, and their relationships with others, as well as how they attend, participate, and behave in class and school.
- It is alterable, directly tied to proximal and distal outcomes of interest across domains of achievement, social–emotional wellbeing, and behavior.
- It is influenced by contexts–families, schools and classrooms, peers, and communities. It may be viewed as a product of interactions between students and contexts over time. Contexts may enhance or hinder students' engagement at school and with learning; however, there is agency or responsibility on the part of students as well. It cannot be ignored.
- There are thought to be Matthew effects, or spirals, in interactions between contexts and students such that as students become engaged, contexts support and further enhance their engagements. Thus, engagement begets engagement. Processes and interactions between disengagement/disaffection and contexts function similarly but in the opposite direction. The notion of developmental cascades, risk/resilience, and student engagement (see Masten et al., chap-

ter "Resilience and Student Engagement: Promotive and Protective Processes in Schools", this volume) and boosting (Salmela-Aro et al., chapter "Study Demands-Resources Model of Student Engagement and Burnout", this volume) are similar in this regard.

- It may be an input, mediator, and outcome, depending on the purpose and time frame of the study.
- It serves as a protective factor among those placed at higher risk for poor educational outcomes.
- It may be differentiated from disengagement/ disaffection/burnout.
- It can be influenced or impacted at several points of intervention (e.g., instruction, classroom management, school climate and discipline, family support for learning) all of which can be studied at different levels.
- It is relevant for all students, from diverse backgrounds and cultures, preschool-age through college.

Themes: The Conceptual, Empirical, and Applied

A major purpose of this volume was to describe scholars' understanding and research regarding how student engagement fosters positive development. Fostering positive youth development is not "owned" by one academic discipline, setting, or point in time. Our beliefs were reinforced in the descriptions in the many outstanding chapters and points raised within. Although a number of themes and directions may be identified in the second Edition, we particularly want to highlight the following:

- There is a far greater emphasis on seeing the child/student/adolescent/young adult as a whole, aligning with Bronfenbrenner's (1979) conceptualization of youth development. We improve the development and learning of youth when they are engaged academically, behaviorally, cognitively, and affectively.
- Student engagement is conceptualized by many authors as a relational process and we concur, having said during the development of

Check & Connect that the quality of the relationship was more important than the specific engagement-focused intervention per se (Christenson & Pohl, 2020). We improve the development and learning when we promote relationship-building in varied forms – student–student, teacher–student or student–teacher, parent–child, and family–school. It is glaringly clear that working at the mesosystemic level is essential to engage disengaged students and to foster optimal engagement for all youth, even those who "appear engaged."

- There is a growing commitment to recognizing the value of student's voice. Listening to the experience of students in specific contexts provides the opportunity to build on or promote "I value," "I can," and "I want to" into "I act," and "I do." Student's voice is particularly important for understanding the experiences of students from different racial, ethnic, and socioeconomic backgrounds and to inform retention efforts (Tinto, chapter "Exploring the Character of Student Persistence in Higher Education: The Impact of Perception, Motivation, and Engagement", this volume). Engaging a student is a process. Behavior does not change quickly or with one or two interventions. For many students the trust building in the relationships is necessary to see an improved trajectory in student behavior and that takes quality time.
- The study and prevention of high school dropouts is one enduring line of research related to current models of student engagement (Archambault et al., chapter "Student Engagement and School Dropout: Theories, Evidence, and Future Directions", this volume; Reschly & Christenson, chapter "Jingle-Jangle Revisited: History and Further Evolution of the Student Engagement Construct", this volume). A consensus among dropout scholars (e.g., Mosher & McGowan, 1985; Natriello, 1982), and the later National Academy Panel (NRC, 2004) on engaging high school students and school reform, is that school-level policies and practices affect students' engagement at school and with learning. As evidenced by authors in this *Handbook*, there is an increasing recognition of the ways

that broader systemic forces, particularly with respect to inequality and racism, at the societal, district-, or school levels, may affect students' engagement at school and with learning as well as their developmental outcomes. Although student engagement is thought to be a protective factor for students placed at risk for poor outcomes, as noted by several authors and addressed eloquently by Galindo et al. (chapter "Expanding an Equity Understanding of Student Engagement: The Macro (Social) and Micro (School) Contexts", this volume), the question of how much students' engagement can buffer the effects of macro-systemic inequalities and racism remains. Students have different opportunities to be engaged at school and with learning. Macro-level conditions are an important consideration in future research and as a target of policy and intervention efforts.

At this juncture, we offer a summary of the conceptual, empirical, and applied considerations that will, in our minds, continue to advance the research on student engagement, enabling efficacious assessment-to-intervention links and practices for all students.

Conceptual Considerations

- The definition of student engagement must be specified. One could ask: How many new subtypes are necessary to intervene and promote youth development? We are advocates of the tripartite model (emotion, cognition, and behavior; see also Fredricks et al., 2019), but respect the conceptualization of other researchers to add the adjective (agentic, social) to engagement. As part of clarity for the construct to be meaningfully understood by others, researchers must clearly specify their definition and indicators within subtypes.
- The overlap with engagement and motivation-to-learn persists, and in our reading, was first used interchangeably by the NRC (2004). Admittedly, in our investigations of the Student Engagement Instrument, we believe

one could describe cognitive engagement as the student perception of motivation-to-learn variables and affective engagement as the student perception of relationships with others in the context of learning (e.g., Appleton et al., 2006). We view motivation and student engagement as overlapping constructs (see also, Skinner and Raine, chapter "Unlocking the Positive Synergy Between Engagement and Motivation", this volume). Again, researchers assist our collective understanding by providing clear definitions as well as noting theoretical frames.

- School engagement or student engagement? These terms seem most confusing when describing school connection or belonging. We are advocates of the use of student engagement. The school context must have "holding power" to promote the development of youth. Hence, what school professionals do to specifically connect with students or to build trusting relationships and provide instrumental support is a necessary variable for promoting school completion – defined as graduating with sufficient academic and social skills to achieve at the next level (e.g., college, work, military, technical school). We advocate for eliminating the use of the term school engagement and use school in conjunction with disengagement, which seems to be similar to school connection and school disengagement. Referring to school disengagement, resulting in student engagement as meaning engagement at school and with learning would, in our minds, foster clarity.
- In reading the many chapters in this *Handbook*, we asked ourselves: Can there be too many subtypes (e.g., study engagement, agentic engagement)? Is there a proliferation of terms? Is there any danger in the proliferation of terms, whether for subtypes or indicators? Although we believe the tripartite model (Fredricks et al., 2004; Fredricks et al., 2019) of cognition, emotion, and behavior represents consensus in the research field, we do not intend to argue against the use of other terms. Rather, we call for clear explanations including examples of relevance. This applies to other related terms as well, such as motiva-

tional resilience and motivational vulnerability.

- We are intrigued by the notion of psychological capital raised by Suldo and Parker (chapter "Relationships Between Student Engagement and Mental Health as Conceptualized from a Dual-Factor Model", this volume). We see this as an opportunity to explore and explicitly include the concepts of psychological capital, hope, and well-being with the student engagement framework and as part of interventions to promote positive outcomes among youth. We suggest that psychological capital is not student engagement, but rather a resource for students (e.g., agency, volition) that protects, supports, and promotes their engagement and further facilitates positive outcomes.

Empirical Considerations

- Construct validity for student engagement has been established. Equally encouraging for researchers is the number of psychometrically sound or reliable and valid measures and approaches for examining student engagement. The significant progress in this area has enabled measures to be more context-specific and to address different purposes (e.g., classification decisions). This progress is needed to refine the assessment-to-intervention link, especially for various student groups (minoritized youth, cultural differences).

- Limitations in measurement hampered efforts to advance the study of student engagement; however, research in the last 10 years has grown increasingly sophisticated, not only with an expansion of measures (Fredricks, chapters "The Measurement of Student Engagement: Methodological Advances and Comparison of New Self-Report Instruments" and "Measuring Student Engagement with Observational Techniques", this volume), but also with longitudinal studies, sophisticated statistical methodologies (Betts, chapter "Measuring Student Engagement: New Approaches and Issues", this volume), and a growing number of person-centered studies of students' engagement and disengagement, with the intention that such studies will inform and enable research-to-practice. Research is needed to address how engagement data may be aggregated and used in combination with other sources. In addition, scale validation is an ongoing endeavor.

- The empirical base for associations between student engagement subtypes and positive learning outcomes has strengthened and cannot be ignored as an avenue for intervention. There is consistent, converging evidence that student engagement is influential in promoting desired learning outcomes in academic as well as social–emotional areas. This reinforces the notion of student engagement as a meta-construct. Most recently, the focus on contextual variables as well as mental health has reinforced our commitment to researching student engagement.

- Engagement versus Disengagement/ Disaffection? Although there is consensus that disaffection/disengagement is separate from engagement (Reschly & Christenson, chapter "Jingle-Jangle Revisited: History and Further Evolution of the Student Engagement Construct", this volume; Wang et al., 2019), the development, process, and interaction of engagement and disaffection processes over time is not yet clear and will be an important direction for basic and intervention research. Archambault et al. (chapter "Student Engagement and School Dropout: Theories, Evidence, and Future Directions", this volume) elaborated on this point, discussing the identification of short- and long-term processes of disengagement related to drop out and the role of protective factors in the multifinality of disengagement trajectories and academic outcomes.

- For this *Handbook* and in other recent work (Fredricks et al., 2019; Reschly, Pohl, & Christenson, 2020), we note that there was an increased interest in intervention programs – those that may be described as student engagement interventions. The focus of the programs included students, teachers, and parents. As researchers interested in data-driven practices to promote positive learning outcomes, we welcome ongoing intervention or applied research in the next decade. The possibility of such research is propelled to the forefront as goals for graduation and the use of progress monitoring procedures become more frequent by school and college professionals.

- As ever, engagement scholars must work to facilitate the research-to-practice link. As our colleague Fredricks (chapter "The Measurement of Student Engagement: Methodological Advances and Comparison of New Self-report Instruments", this volume) notes, accessibility to educators is an important consideration.

- The seminal role of relationships was underscored consistently in ways to facilitate engagement, learning, and positive youth development. In his discussion of microengagements (e.g., peers, faculty), Tinto (chapter "Exploring the Character of Student Persistence in Higher Education: The Impact of Perception, Motivation, and Engagement", this volume) raised a salient question: Do effects depend on with whom one engages? His proposal to conduct a social network analysis offers promise for enhanced discernment or interpretation of the strength and range of a student's affiliations.

- Although there is broad consensus in subtypes and in many indicators of students' engagement, as well as agreement regarding the importance of relationships, less is known about other critical contextual influences and supports. What are the essential characteristics of various contexts that promote and support students' engagement?

Applied Considerations

- There is a growing evidence base for interventions that address specific subtypes and indicators of student engagement (Fredricks et al., 2019; Reschly et al., 2020). Fewer interventions, however, address students' engagement comprehensively (see also Fredricks et al., 2019); an important direction for the next 10 years. There are also questions regarding the timing and length of interventions to re-engage and sustain the engagement of those at greatest risk for poor educational outcomes.

- Although there are several instruments and other sources of data (e.g., attendance, participation) that are useful for assessing the outcomes of interventions at the universal and individual levels, the identification and refinement of data that are sensitive to small changes and that may be used for progress monitoring purposes is needed to complement the growing menu of student engagement interventions.

- As we have noted on several occasions: Context matters (e.g., Christenson & Thurlow, 2004; Fredricks et al., 2019; Reschly, 2020). Therefore, school professionals will access the student engagement research base – assessment and intervention strategies – and apply these to fit their context. Resource availability must also be considered by the educators; however, we argue that there is always something that can be done to improve student engagement. An important question is: *What are the critical contextual variables to enhance student engagement and for whom*? We speculate that the role of successful learning experiences, instructional match, climate, and appropriate cognitive load may be examples of essential components in instructional practices. Further, educators must note collective disengagement among students (see Hoefkens and Pianta, chapter "Teacher–Student Relationships, Engagement in School, and Student Outcomes", this volume) as they seek to target conditions that inhibit students' engagement at school and with learning.

- The student engagement framework is applied in nature. We are advocates of keeping the assessment-to-intervention practical, and appreciate Anderman et al.'s remarks (chapter "Achievement Goal Theory and Engagement", this volume) cautioning of too much fragmentation and proliferation in descriptions of students' engagement. This is another reason we are advocates of the three subtypes as representing a good categorization for the field. We recognize that too many terms create difficulty for the implementers in that there is a practical limit to how much educators can keep track of while still providing instruction for all the students in their classes. As an implementation vs. policy issue, we are reminded of the point about the luxury of theory in contrast to the limits or constraints of practice.

- Successful intervention practices – whether for individual students or at a classroom and school level – are those that develop competence and allow students to demonstrate competence (see Pekrun & Linnenbrink-Garcia, chapter "Academic Emotions and Student Engagement", this volume). Such practices account for and foster students' behavioral, cognitive, and emotional/affective engagement. Most students and situations will require more than attending to attendance, behavior, or work completion to foster significant learning gains.

Conclusion

The first edition of the *Handbook* began a dialogue between motivation and engagement researchers and promoted much interest in research on student engagement. This edition has embellished and expanded our understanding of the construct; therefore, we offer this modified definition for student engagement:

> Student engagement refers to the student's active participation in academic and co-curricular or school-related activities and commitment to educational goals and learning. Engaged students find learning meaningful, are invested in their learning and future, and are more likely to experience well-being and positive developmental outcomes. It is a multidimensional construct that consists of behavioral (including academic), cognitive, and affective subtypes. Student engagement drives learning; requires energy and effort; is affected by multiple contextual influences; and can be achieved for all learners. It is studied at different levels and structures and does represent energy in action.

Across the chapters in this *Handbook*, we suggest two variables explicitly "fit in, but stand out" for improving the quality and utility of research on student engagement and promoting students' academic, behavioral, social, and emotional development: the seminal role of relationships and the value and power of viewing students' presenting behavior holistically. Engagement is a relational process; learning occurs in interaction with others.

Student engagement is a highly relevant, useful construct to school professionals and parents who desire positive, optimal learning outcomes and development for all students. Paired with this goal is the understanding that there are individual differences, hence there is no expectation that all students will attain a similar level of engagement. Rather, there is, and appropriately should be, an expectation that all students can be engaged behaviorally, cognitively, and affectively. In part, the usefulness of the construct is that it provides an integrative framework to understand student performance at school and with learning. The student is viewed as a system or whole, not in a piecemeal fashion (e.g., academic performance separates from motivation, goals, or connections with others about schooling). We add to this point that explicit attention must be paid to contextual influences and supports of students' engagement.

Conceptualizing students' experiences comprehensively is remindful of the book, *Seven Blind Mice*, by Ed Young. In this story, seven blind mice found a strange "something" in their pond. Each mouse visited the pond on subsequent days and offered a suggestion as to what the "something" – the elephant – was. Touching only a part led to suggestions of a pillar, a snake, a spear, a great cliff, a fan, and a rope. Of course, the mice with different information and experiences did not agree. They argued until the last mouse ran up one side, ran down the other, ran across the top and from end to end. Researchers would be wise to heed advice from the mouse moral: "Knowing in part may make a fine tale, but wisdom comes from seeing the whole" (Young, 1992, p. 35).

The purpose of this volume was to address how student engagement can promote positive development and outcomes among youth. We were also able to revisit some past issues (see Reschly & Christenson, chapter "Jingle-Jangle Revisited: History and Further Evolution of the Student Engagement Construct", this volume) and update the state of theory and research in the field. This volume includes 33 chapters across four sections: Defining Student Engagement: Models and Related Constructs, Student Engagement: Positive Development and Outcomes, Contexts for Engagement, and Measurement.

We extend our appreciation to the authors. Our interest in engagement is because it may be the most promising means for understanding students' school experiences and outcomes and, most importantly, that by understanding engagement, we can improve educational and life outcomes for youth. It is our hope that across the next decade this *Handbook* inspires researchers, educators, and other professionals to advance the field so that we may someday accomplish this goal.

References

Appleton, J. J., Christenson, S. L., Kim, D., & Reschly, A. L. (2006). Measuring cognitive and psychological engagement: Validation of the Student Engagement Instrument. *Journal of School Psychology, 44*(5), 427–445.

Bronfenbrenner, U. (1979). *The ecology of human development*. Harvard University Press.

Christenson, S. L., & Pohl, A. J. (2020). The relevance of student engagement: The impact of and lessons learned implementing Check & Connect. In A. L. Reschly, A. J. Pohl, & S. L. Christenson (Eds.), *Student engagement: Effective academic, behavioral, cognitive, and affective interventions at school* (pp. 3–30). Springer Nature.

Christenson, S. L., Reschly, A. L., & Wylie, C. (2012). Handbook of research on student engagement. New York: Springer. https://doi.org/10.1007/978-1-4614-2018-7

Christenson, S. L., & Thurlow, M. L. (2004). School dropouts: Prevention considerations, interventions, and challenges. *Current Directions in Psychological Science, 13*(1), 36–39.

Connell, J. P., & Wellborn, J. G. (1991). Competence, autonomy, and relatedness: A motivational analysis of self-system processes. In M. R. Gunnar & L. A. Sroufe (Eds.), Self processes and development (pp. 43–77). Lawrence Erlbaum Associates, Inc.

Cook, C. R., Thayer, A. J., Fiat, A., & Sullivan, M. (2020). Interventions to enhance affective engagement. In A. L. Reschly, A. J. Pohl, & S. L. Christenson (Eds.), *Student engagement: Effective academic, behavioral, cognitive, and affective interventions at school* (pp. 203–237). Springer Nature.

Finn, J. D., & Zimmer, K. S. (2012). Student engagement: What is it? Why does it matter?. In S. L. Christenson, A. L. Reschly, & C. Wylie (Eds.), Handbook of research on student engagement (pp. 97–131). Springer. https://doi.org/10.1007/978-1-4614-2018-7_5

Fredricks, J. A., Blumenfeld, P. C., & Paris, A. H. (2004). School engagement: Potential of the concept, state of the evidence. *Review of Educational Research, 74,* 59–109.

Fredricks, J. A., Reschly, A. L., & Christenson, S. L. (Eds.). (2019). *Handbook of student engagement interventions: Working with disengaged students*. Elsevier.

Mosher, R., & McGowan, B. (1985). *Assessing student engagement in secondary schools: Alternative conceptions, strategies of assessing, and instruments*. University of Wisconsin, Research and Development Center. (ERIC Document Reproduction Service No. ED 272812).

National Research Council and the Institute of Medicine. (2004). *Engaging schools: Fostering high schools students' motivation to learn*. The National Academy Press.

Natriello, G. (1982). *Organizational evaluation systems and student disengagement in secondary schools*. Final Report.

Reeve, J. (2012). A self-determination theory perspective on student engagement. In S. L. Christenson, A. L. Reschly, & C. Wylie (Eds.), *The handbook of research on student engagement* (pp. 149–172). Springer.

Reschly, A. L. (2020). Dropout prevention and student engagement. In A. L. Reschly, A. Pohl, & S. L. Christenson (Eds.). Student Engagement: Effective Academic, Behavioral, Cognitive, and Affective Interventions at School. (pp. 31–54). New York: Springer. https://doi.org/10.1007/978-3-030-37285-9_2

Reschly, A. L., Pohl, A., & Christenson, S. L. (2020) Student Engagement: Effective Academic, Behavioral, Cognitive, and Affective Interventions at School. New York: Springer. https://doi.org/10.1007/978-3-030-37285-9

Wang, M-T., Degol, J. L., & Henry, D. A. (2019). An integrative development-in-sociocultural-context model for children's engagement in learning. *American Psychologist, 74, 1086–1102*. https://doi.org/10.1037/amp0000522

Williford, A. P., & Pianta, R. C. (2020). Banking time: A dyadic intervention to improve teacher-student relationships. In A. L. Reschly, A. J. Pohl, & S. L. Christenson (Eds.), *Student engagement: Effective academic, behavioral, cognitive, and affective interventions at school* (pp. 239–250). Springer Nature.

Young, E. (1992). *Seven blind mice*. Phimolel Books.

Index

© The Author(s), under exclusive license to Springer Nature Switzerland AG 2022
A. L. Reschly, S. L. Christenson (eds.), *Handbook of Research on Student Engagement*,
https://doi.org/10.1007/978-3-031-07853-8